7.⁰⁰

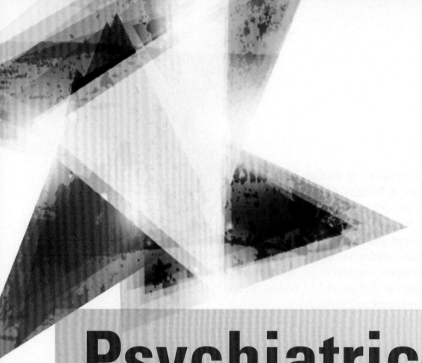

Psychiatric–Mental Health Nursing

EVIDENCE-BASED CONCEPTS, SKILLS, AND PRACTICES

WANDA K. MOHR, PhD, RN, FAAN

University of Medicine and Dentistry of New Jersey
School of Nursing
Newark, New Jersey

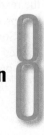

edition 8

. Wolters Kluwer | Lippincott Williams & Wilkins
Health

Philadelphia · Baltimore · New York · London
Buenos Aires · Hong Kong · Sydney · Tokyo

Acquisitions Editor: Patrick Barbera
Product Manager: Mary Kinsella
Design Coordinator: Joan Wendt
Art Director, Illustration: Brett MacNaughton
Manufacturing Coordinator: Karin Duffield

Eighth Edition

9 8 7 6 5 4 3 2 1

Printed in China

Library of Congress Cataloging-in-Publication Data

Psychiatric-mental health nursing : evidence-based concepts, skills, and practices / editor, Wanda K. Mohr.—8th ed.
  p. ; cm.
Includes bibliographical references and index.
ISBN 978-1-60913-708-3 (alk. paper)
I. Mohr, Wanda K.
[DNLM: 1. Mental Disorders–nursing. 2. Evidence-Based Nursing. 3. Psychiatric Nursing–methods. WY 160]
616.89′0231—dc23

2012020808

Care has been taken to confirm the accuracy of the information presented and to describe generally accepted practices. However, the authors, editors, and publisher are not responsible for errors or omissions or for any consequences from application of the information in this book and make no warranty, expressed or implied, with respect to the currency, completeness, or accuracy of the contents of the publication. Application of this information in a particular situation remains the professional responsibility of the practitioner; the clinical treatments described and recommended may not be considered absolute and universal recommendations.

The authors, editors, and publisher have exerted every effort to ensure that drug selection and dosage set forth in this text are in accordance with the current recommendations and practice at the time of publication. However, in view of ongoing research, changes in government regulations, and the constant flow of information relating to drug therapy and drug reactions, the reader is urged to check the package insert for each drug for any change in indications and dosage and for added warnings and precautions. This is particularly important when the recommended agent is a new or infrequently employed drug.

Some drugs and medical devices presented in this publication have Food and Drug Administration (FDA) clearance for limited use in restricted research settings. It is the responsibility of the health care provider to ascertain the FDA status of each drug or device planned for use in his or her clinical practice.

LWW.COM

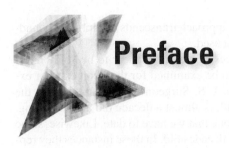

Preface

From the Author: I would like the Preface of this edition to speak to instructors and students alike because the book was written for them. Hence the familiarity of my tone. This preface is written so that you can understand what I have tried to achieve.

While the history of mental health research is at least 200 years old, the heavy work commenced during the 21st century. The biochemical, physiologic, pharmacologic, and structural features of the brain have been described and in many instances defined. So, too, have the basic perceptual, emotional, attention, and cognitive functions. The past few decades have seen an explosion of knowledge of the kind that pioneers such as Hildegard Peplau and Sigmund Freud never dreamed. For those of us who struggle to keep up with this new knowledge, every day brings new and exciting discoveries and challenges. Much more remains for us to learn.

In addition to this explosion of knowledge, the economics of health care have changed dramatically, and not always for the best. The interaction of new science and new economic pressures has contributed to an urgent need for psychiatric–mental health nurses to articulate a new paradigm for conceptualizing, teaching, and practicing this discipline. Over 10 years ago, the late Susan McCabe (2000) argued that psychiatric nursing was in danger of extinction unless the specialty let go of what may be historically interesting but no longer clinically relevant. She also emphasized the need to incorporate the new.

To some extent managed care and the marketplace have forced such change upon us. At the same time, we may have taken a step or two backward. In some ways, things have remained the same. By this, I mean that along with the biologic focus on mental health and mental illnesses, we may be in danger of sacrificing the psychosocial component of care. The rush for efficiency in care provision may contribute to clients and families feeling like they are receiving "short shrift." State and local budgets are strained, leading to cuts in programs already historically underfunded. In addition, the ugliness of stigma continues to undermine efforts toward parity of care for people with mental illnesses. Unwitting "help" from the media continues to poison perceptions of the public regarding people who suffer from these devastating illnesses.

My ongoing vision for the eighth edition included the ongoing quest to let go of the old and articulate the new. I also wanted to begin sensitizing students to themselves, their attitudes, and the experience of mental illness, beyond the confines of the *DSM* and other guideposts for understanding illnesses and their treatments. Certainly the book acknowledges historical figures who made immeasurable additions to the specialty, but it is important for students and instructors to understand that the text minimizes such information, and makes clear what practices are current and, more importantly, which are based in empirical research. We can learn enduring lessons from the past, but there are also concepts that are simply not able to be verified or researched and translated into an evidence base for practice. My aims for the eighth edition of *Psychiatric–Mental Health Nursing* are to focus on the evidence base for our specialty and to discuss rational practice. Rational practice may not always have much supporting research, because such studies may not be feasible or even ethical. An example might be the immorality of examining the noxious effect of physical restraint on clients; but we know from case reports that they are aversive and that they have resulted in injury and death. Other research may be possible, but also unethical, so the studies that we have may not meet the "gold standard" of Type I research. For example, we cannot withhold psychoactive medications from a client with psychosis to measure the effects of new drugs against no medication at all. Nevertheless, we can practice in a way that is targeted to the symptoms and needs of all clients.

In this edition, we made a deliberate decision to reference the DSM that was operational at the time of the textbook's updating process. It may well be that the DSM V is the manual that supercedes the DSM IV-TR at the time of publication. We made this decision for a number of reasons. First, there was no guarantee that the DSM V would be published in 2012. Indeed the publication date had been moved forward several times. Secondly, and most important, the DSM is a psychiatric classification system that is a consensus document describing psychiatric conditions. The DSM categories are descriptions and not explanations. With the exception of assessment, they do not inform nursing care, or for that matter psychiatric care, and there are cultural limitations to the DSM categories. Seeing a need to move forward on updating research that was relevant to actual nursing care, the decision was made to retain the DSM IV-TR classification system. Most textbook authors in the field of nursing, psychiatric medicine, social work, and psychology were faced with this same decision, and no doubt it will be several years before the DSM V informs all current textbooks.

Clearly, the major conceptual approach to psychiatry in the 21st century is grounded in molecular biology. Thus, Chapter 2 explains concepts such as neuroplasticity and genetic expression. Because evidence is increasing that "mental states" have their representation in brain neuronal anatomy and functioning, the text focuses on those psychotherapeutics with a solid grounding in the research literature.

In addition to focusing on the latest research in neurobiology, physiology, and psychopharmacotherapeutics, the textbook articulates service provision changes that have taken place, emphasizing the shift toward care of clients in their community settings and with their families. Discussions throughout give special consideration to portraying people suffering from mental illnesses and their families as human beings who are reacting normally to very stressful and overwhelming experiences. I have devoted much of an entire chapter to sensitize students to this kind of stress and suffering, as told by patients in their own words.

Knowing from experience how frightening and frankly "off-putting" the word "theory" can be, I hope that students will be empowered by the down-to-earth discussion of theory and theoretical frameworks in Chapter 3. Ever mindful of the strong role of the therapeutic alliance, the text conceptualizes psychotherapy as a process of learning new thinking and new behaviors, rather than as a "talking cure," thereby taking the mystery out of it and placing it in understandable terms for students who can in turn de-mystify it to clients. We are past the point in our specialty in which simply "talking" in the absence of hard work on the part of clinician and client can be seen as moving forward the healing and recovery enterprise.

For every silver lining there seems to be a dark side. The exciting new knowledge presented in this book represents a revolution in the arena of the behavioral sciences, one that is analogous to the revolution that came about in orthopedics with the development of radiology. But we live in an era in which scientific advances frequently make even the most recent scientific books and journals dated soon after their publication. Our team recognizes that what was written may have been timely when we wrote it but may be out of date in a decade, given the explosion of knowledge in the field. This underscores the importance and indispensability of reading and keeping abreast of new publications and new editions of texts as they are published.

This brings up another important point. Our team listened carefully to what our readers said about references. At the end of each chapter there are references; all of which are as up to date as we could possibly make them. Sadly, in many areas of research, the nursing voice has been absent and the production of knowledge is dominated by other professions. This is a problem that should be rectified but one that must also be acknowledged. As a result, the research presented in this text has been taken from the medical, psychology, sociology, or social work literature. As many scholarly nursing writings as possible have been included. My intent is to refer to the actual primary source study itself. By primary source I mean the research itself, and not a textbook that interprets the original study. Moreover, the references include the most relevant studies available regardless of what discipline conducted the research. I firmly believe in a journey that includes all disciplines collaboratively moving forward

to help clients. This approach transcends disciplinary boundaries and is client focused.

In other instances, there may appear to be "old" references, which need to be examined for their context. For example, the landmark U.S. Surgeon General's report on the nation's mental health is almost a decade old at this writing. Sadly, it is the only one that we have to date. Likewise, some references are many decades old. In these instances they represent seminal works that may stand as classics in the field, or simply reflect that no further work has been done in the field, because the research community may feel no need to replicate that which has been repeatedly replicated. Or, such as in the case of the Zimbardo and Rosenhan landmark studies discussed in Chapter 8, they simply could not be replicated in the present research environment.

I also wanted to underscore that in writing this book, our team has made every effort to make it readable and user friendly. Keeping in mind that we have an ever growing immigrant population (Dr. Mohr among them), we avoided inaccessibility and the use of idioms to the extent possible, without sacrificing necessary disciplinary terminology. In addition, each chapter is infused with cultural content that reflects the rich diversity of the United States in the third millennium.

Researching and writing this textbook was both tedious and exhilarating. I was struck by the complexity of the emergent knowledge but at the same time excited by its possibilities. My reading highlighted the intricacies of the human condition and made me very aware of how specialized psychiatric–mental health nursing can be. This awareness gave rise to the urgency for providing these vulnerable clients with competent caregivers. It also underscored the importance for this nursing specialty to survive and thrive.

Organization of the Eighth Edition

The Table of Contents emphasizes key foci of the curriculum and logically integrates chapters focused on essential aspects of core nursing care. The current edition contains eight units:

- Unit I, *Foundational Concepts in Psychiatric–Mental Health Nursing,* contains material basic to the study of psychiatric–mental health nursing. Topics include the introduction to the field, neurobiology, conceptual frameworks, evidence-based practice, and legal and ethical issues.
- Unit II, *Client Care Considerations,* presents content on culture and spirituality—core elements of each person that nurses must consider during all interactions and care delivery.
- Unit III, *The Nurse–Client Relationship,* emphasizes the heart of psychiatric–mental health nursing—the therapeutic relationship between the giver and the recipient of care. Topics include values, attitudes, self-awareness, the nursing process, interviewing, mental health assessment, mental status examination, therapeutic communications

and relationships, and working within multidisciplinary teams.

- Unit IV, *Conceptual Bases of Treatment,* explores current methodologies of care and treatment. Chapters focus on therapies and nursing interventions for individuals, groups, and families; psychopharmacology; integrative (complementary and alternative) modalities; and somatic therapies.
- Unit V, *Settings for Care,* addresses similarities and differences across settings for psychiatric–mental health nursing. Individual chapters focus on inpatient settings, community/home environments, and forensic psychiatric nursing.
- Unit VI, *Psychiatric Disorders,* outlines the core features of the most common psychiatric disorders within the following groups: sleep, anxiety, somatoform, dissociative, sexual, personality, eating, depressive, bipolar, thought, substance use, and cognitive. In addition to reviewing aspects of these disorders, including their prevalence, origins, signs and symptoms, and evidence-based treatment approaches, each chapter also contains detailed sections focusing on nursing care and interventions, using a nursing process framework.
- Unit VII, *Psychiatric Emergencies,* includes those situations that require directed, acute interventions from nurses and other health care providers: anger, aggression, violence, abuse, and suicide. The unit also contains a chapter on crisis intervention as a methodology for emergencies, including the burgeoning threats of terrorism and campus violence.
- Unit VIII, *Special Populations,* focuses on key mental health concerns and variations in psychiatric nursing care associated with targeted groups: children and adolescents, older adults, those who are homeless, and clients with medical illnesses.

Changes to the Eighth Edition

Given the importance of research and its everchanging impact on practice, this edition has been thoroughly updated with the most current research available. As already mentioned, that material is presented from primary as opposed to secondary sources. Several chapters that try to convey elements that I believe to be germane to all nurses, and that instructors and students indicated would be significant inclusions.

- Chapter 8, "Nursing Values, Attitudes, and Self-Awareness," presents content that I particularly enjoyed writing for this edition. My aim was to help students reduce the uncertainty of entering a psychiatric–mental health setting and to present them with some interesting influential classic studies from the social psychology literature that might help them understand what they may encounter. Unfortunately, with the amount of nursing knowledge that students must absorb in school, they may not be exposed to some literature that is useful in understanding phenomena encountered in mental health settings. Also unfortunately, disciplines do not often communicate to each other their important and landmark studies. Nor are nursing students often exposed to seminal studies of other disciplines. Space precluded me from discussing more than two, but I hope that it whets the students' appetites to dig deeper into the literature of other fields as their work may generate many insights for the field of nursing.
- Chapter 10, "The Interview and Assessment Process," reviews key elements of the mental health/mental status examination, which provides the foundation of all subsequent interactions with and care for clients.
- Chapter 18, "Somatic Therapies," is concerned with the existing and emerging field of body-based, nonpharmacologic treatments, such as electroconvulsive therapy, phototherapy, and transcranial magnetic stimulation.
- Chapter 19, "Inpatient Care Settings," explores key considerations and variations for care during psychiatric hospitalization at a time when hospitalization lengths have been severely truncated.
- Chapter 34, We included a separate chapter on suicide to address its association with several psychiatric disorders, such as depression, bipolar illness, personality disorders, and substance abuse. The chapter specifically addresses dangerous myths, such as those associated with suicide contracts that have been perpetuated by practice convention.
- Chapter 39, "Clients With Medical Illnesses," speaks to the ubiquity of mental health issues throughout the spectrum of life and within the context of medical disorders. I recognize that not all students of this text will go on to be psychiatric–mental health nurses, which is why I conceived of this chapter. I hope that students will find the discussion useful, because whatever their ultimate specialty, they will generalize some of the material to other numerous disorders to which it applies.

The team decided early that we wanted to produce a textbook that was concise, current, and readable. We carefully edited for redundant material as well as for material that constituted a "nice to know" versus a "need to know." I like to read books that I believe speak to me as an individual. This kind of writing is engaging and makes learning fun, so we strived for readability and student "friendly" writing. I would like each student to come away from each chapter with a feeling of comfort.

Features

In response to opinions from instructors and students about what would make for the most appealing and useful text, this edition has retained the following enhancements:

- **Evidence-Based Practice Spotlights.** More than 25 of these features throughout the book summarize validated studies and findings on topics of relevance. They also supply implications for nursing practice to communicate to students "take-away" points for client care.

- **Evidence-Based Practice Summaries.** These tables compare and contrast levels of evidence for various interventions used to treat different disorders under discussion.
- **Case in Point.** These case studies present detailed client/family scenarios with integrated nursing care plans. Organized according to the steps of the nursing process, these cases include assessment findings; integrated NANDA, NIC, and NOC; examples of documentation; and follow-up to reflect a systematic approach to treatment. Many include photos to help students connect with the clients and families under discussion.
- **Case Vignettes:** More than 30 throughout the book with accompanying Reflection and Critical Thinking Questions pose realistic client scenarios and thought-provoking topics for exploration and discussion.
- **Understanding Biologic Foundations:** These features in selected chapters mix narrative and art to explain core biologic processes, neuroanatomy, neurotransmission, and pathophysiology. They help students better understand the connections between mind and body, cellular and organ functioning, and normal versus abnormal processes.
- **Cultural Spotlight:** These boxes in several chapters cover pertinent points relevant to understanding the cultural context of clients.

Additionally, several well-received and dynamic features from the previous edition have been retained, with revisions as appropriate:

- **Learning Objectives.** This bulleted list highlights the main ideas for students to know or accomplish after reading the chapter.
- **Key Terms.** Each chapter begins with a list of key terms. The terms are bolded in a special color upon first appearance in the chapter with accompanying definitions. The Glossary also provides definitions.
- **Checkpoint Questions.** Found at key points for review within each chapter, these questions ask students to provide quick answers to ensure rapid recall and understanding of essential content.
- **Think About It.** Each chapter contains one or more of these exercises that encourage application and interpretation of client scenarios based on core content explored in the text.
- **Challenging Behaviors.** This feature presents scenarios that many in mental health find challenging and troublesome and details how expert psychiatric nurses can meet those challenges.
- **Therapeutic Communication.** This feature provides sample dialogues to assist nurses in understanding effective versus ineffective communication. Reflection and Critical Thinking at the end help students make choices and interpret why certain communication styles succeed or fail for clients with psychiatric problems.

- **Client-Centered Education.** These boxes contain client- and family-focused teaching points and related resources (Web, organizations, books, etc.) for the condition under discussion.
- **Nursing Spotlight.** These boxes describe important guidelines, approved practice standards, and other key nursing-focused components relevant to care.
- **Assessment Tools.** This designation has been given to relevant boxes and tables that present commonly used checklists, mechanisms for testing, and other documents for evaluating aspects of clients.
- **Reviewing and Applying Your Knowledge.** Each chapter ends with a section for students to process their knowledge and to apply what they have learned.
- **Chapter Summary.** Bulleted lists of key points correspond with the chapter's learning objectives to ensure full understanding and continuity.
- **Study Questions.** These practice tests with questions in NCLEX-style formats test students' comprehension of the chapter's content.
- **Critical Thinking Questions.** These exercises challenge students to expand their thinking about issues discussed within each chapter.

Photography and Art

Recognizing the power of visual appeal, we have included illustrations and graphics that we hope will please. We have woven art and photography throughout the book to illustrate crucial points and assist visual learners to understand symptoms, interventions, biologic mechanisms, and differences and similarities in clients. The visual emphasis is in line with the needs and characteristics of today's student population. It also is a key element of new features, such as the aforementioned "Understanding Biologic Foundations" and the case studies.

Teaching Learning Package

thePoint (http://thepoint.lww.com), a trademark of Wolters Kluwer Health, is a Web-based course and content management system providing every resource that instructors and students need in one easy-to-use site. Advanced technology and superior content combine at thePoint to allow instructors to design and deliver on- and off-line courses, maintain grades and class rosters, and communicate with students. Students can visit thePoint to access supplemental multimedia resources to enhance their learning experience. They can also check the course syllabus, download content, upload assignments, and join an online study group.

For instructors, a wealth of information can be found at thePoint, all designed to make teaching easier:

- Pre-Lecture Quizzes, made up of five True/False and five Fill-in-the-Blank questions, are meant to be given at the beginning of class and help evaluate whether students are keeping up with the reading and the material it covers.

- Assignments, broken into four types—written, group, clinical, and Web—and organized by learning objective, provide opportunities for in- or after-class activities.
- Discussion Topics, also organized by learning objective, allow students to critically think through scenarios and discuss their ideas with other students.
- Guided Lecture Notes organize the chapter objective-by-objective and provide references to appropriate Power-Point slides and figures from the text.

In addition, thePoint package includes an online eBook so students and instructors can search their text electronically.

Student Resources

The accompanying free student resources on thePoint include exciting and instructive learning tools, including such assets as our popular Clinical Simulations and Movie Viewing Guides:

- Clinical Simulations: These interactive case studies, focusing on the acutely manic phrase, major depressive disorder, and paranoid schizophrenia in the acutely psychotic phase, help students gradually take theory and apply it

through practice—without the fear and intimidation that can accompany students fresh from the classroom.
- Movie Viewing Guides: Helping students recognize disorders in "everyday" life, Movie Viewing Guides ask students to view characters in movies as psychiatric clients, and, again, take some of the fear and intimidation out of client contact, all while becoming more and more familiar with such interactions as well as possible diagnoses.
- Psychotropic Drug Monographs: Often a difficult portion of any mental health–psychiatric student's workload, psychotropic drug monographs provide students with information on drugs specific to their area of study.

Also included are a Spanish-English audio glossary, an interactive tutorial that walks students through the alternate-format questions on the NCLEX, and journal articles that offer the most recent research organized by chapter.

Wanda K. Mohr, PhD, RN, FAAN

McCabe, S. (2000). Bringing psychiatric nursing into the 21st century. *Archives of Psychiatric Nursing, 14*(3), 109–116.

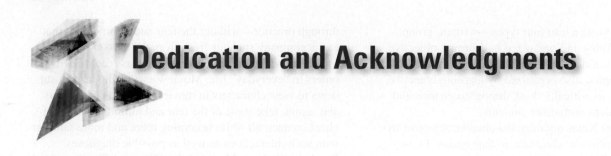

Dedication and Acknowledgments

I would like to acknowledge and dedicate this book to my family. I could not have achieved what I have without my husband, Brian, whose confidence in me and ceaseless cheer-leading gave me the energy and self-assurance to reach even higher than the last time. My children and their spouses are a continuing source of joy and add to the fullness of my life.

I also dedicate this book to the National Alliance for the Mentally Ill (NAMI) who work tirelessly against stigma and on behalf of research and education. As mental health consumers and family members, they have taught me valuable lessons about the devastation of mental illness and the courage of those who suffer from it.

An effort such as this book is made possible by the hard work of dozens of people, the chapter authors, as well as the Editorial, Production, and Marketing teams at Wolters Kluwer.

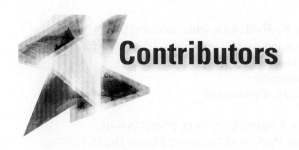
Contributors

Jeffrey A. Anderson, PhD
Associate Professor and Research Faculty
School of Education
Indiana University
Bloomington, Indiana

Kerry Brown, BA, BS, CTRS
Associate Director of Clinical Services
Acadia University & Dalhousie University
Philadelphia, Pennsylvania

Barbara A. Caldwell, PhD, APN-BC
Professor
School of Nursing
University of Medicine & Dentistry of New Jersey
Newark, New Jersey

Phyllis M. Connolly, PhD, PMHCNS-BC
Professor
The Valley Foundation School of Nursing
San Jose, California

Jan Dalsheimer, MS, RN, CNE
Associate Clinical Professor
Texas Woman's University
Dallas, Texas

Susan D. Decker, PhD, RN
Associate Professor of Nursing
University of Portland
Portland, Oregon

Catherine Gray Deering, PhD, APRN-BC
Professor
Clayton State University
Morrow, Georgia

Melissa Garno, EdD, RN
Associate Professor, BSN Program Director
Georgia Southern University
Statesboro, Georgia

Connie S. Heflin, MSN, RN, CNE
Director of Online Learning
West Kentucky Community and Technical College
Paducah, Kentucky

Kevin Ann Huckshorn,
RN, MSN, CADC
State Director of Delaware Division
   of Substance Abuse/Mental Health
New Castle, Delaware

JoAnne DeSanto Iennaco, PhD,
PMHCNS-BC, APRN
Assistant Professor
School of Nursing
Yale University

Barbara Kearney, PhD, RN
Assistant Professor
School of Nursing
Murray State University
Murray, Kentucky

Pamela E. Marcus, RN,
APRN/PMH-BC
Associate Professor of Nursing
Prince George's Community College
Upper Marlboro, Maryland

Sherri Melrose, PhD, RN
Assistant Professor
Athabasca University
Athabasca, Alberta

Mary D. Moller, DNP, PhD(h), MSN,
APRN-PMH-CS, CPRP, FAAN
Associate Professor
School of Nursing
Yale University
New Haven, Connecticut

Sharon L. Moore, PhD, Med. RN
Associate Professor
Faculty of Health Disciplines
Athabasca University
Athabasca, Alberta

Karyn Morgan, RN, MSN, CNS
Senior Instructor
The University of Akron
Akron, Ohio

Geraldine S. Pearson, PhD, PMH-CNS, FAAN
Associate Professor
School of Medicine
University of Connecticut
Farmington, Connecticut

Suzanne Perraud, PMHCNS-BC, PhD
Associate Dean for Academic Affairs
College of Nursing
Rush University
Chicago, Illinois

JoAnn Pietro, RN, JD
Partner
Wahrenberger & Pietro, LLP
Springfield, New Jersey

Nancy S. Redeker, PhD, RN, FAHA, FAAN
Professor and Associate Dean of Scholarly Affairs
School of Nursing
Yale University
New Haven, Connecticut

Wendy Umberger, PhD, PMHCNS-BC
Associate Professor/Director of Mental Health Nursing
College of Nursing
Kent State University
Kent, Ohio

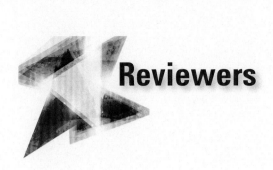 # Reviewers

Cynthia Bostick, MSN, PhD
Lecturer
California State University Dominguez Hills
Carson, California

Carolyn Cleiland, RN
Assistant Professor of Nursing
Virginia Western Community College
Roanoke, Virginia

Jennifer Clymer-Graber, EdDc, APRN, CS, BC
Nursing Instructor
Delaware Technical and Community College

Frances Davis, RN, MSN
Associate Degree Nursing Instructor
Mississippi Gulf Coast Community College

Bonnie Gnadt, PhD, RN
Professor of Nursing
Southwestern Adventist University
Keene, Texas

Marilyn K. Miller, MSN, RN
Professor of Nursing
St. Charles Community College
Cottleville, Missouri

Donna Rye, MSN, RN
Assistant Professor
Cox College
Springfield, Missouri

Koreen W. Smiley, RN, MSN, MSEd
Professor/Dept. Chair, Associate Degree
  Nursing Program
St. Charles Community College
Cottleville, Missouri

Judy G. Walker, MSN
Assistant Professor, Associate Degree
  Nursing Program
Bowling Green Community College
Western Kentucky University

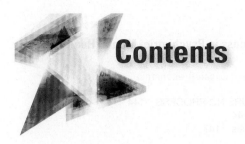

Contents

FOUR Conceptual Bases of Treatment 223

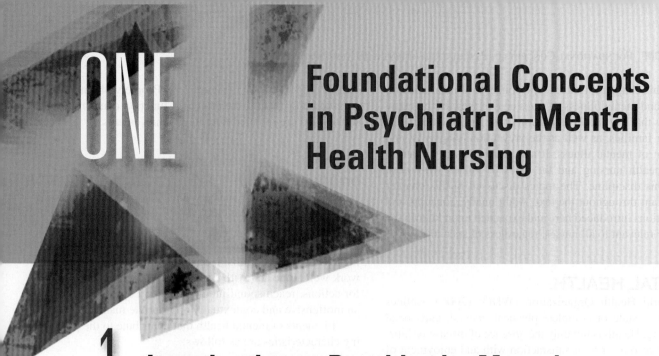

ONE

Foundational Concepts in Psychiatric–Mental Health Nursing

1

Introduction to Psychiatric–Mental Health Nursing

Wanda K. Mohr

KEY TERMS

culturally competent care
dual diagnosis
medication adherence
mental disorders
mental health
mental health nursing
mental illness
psychiatric–mental health nursing
psychiatric nursing
tautology

LEARNING OBJECTIVES

On completion of this chapter, you should be able to accomplish the following:

- Explain elements that contribute to mental health.
- Discuss the significance of *Mental Health: A Report of the Surgeon General.*
- Describe the purposes of the multiaxial diagnostic system used in the *Diagnostic and Statistical Manual of Mental Disorders,* 4th edition, text revision (*DSM-IV-TR*).
- Review trends, problems, and goals related to the delivery of mental health care and treatment of mental illness.
- Identify the contributions of self-help organizations and advocacy movements to understanding client and family adaptation to mental illness.
- Outline the functions and levels of practice of psychiatric–mental health nurses.

This chapter introduces the concepts of mental health and mental illness. It gives an overview of the many problems that psychiatric conditions pose for affected clients and their families, as well as the prevention, diagnosis, and treatment of mental illness. It also introduces psychiatric–mental health nursing and the roles of nurses who work within this discipline. The topics discussed in this chapter are relevant throughout the text. Additionally, concepts and interventions introduced here and expanded upon later in the book are relevant to all nurses, regardless of specialty.

MENTAL HEALTH

The World Health Organization (WHO) (2006a) defines *health* as a state of complete physical, mental, and social well-being. Health is not only the absence of disease or infirmity, but also a sense of satisfaction with and enjoyment of self and the environment.

Mental health means the successful performance of mental function, resulting in productive activities, fulfilling relationships, and the ability to adapt to change and cope with adversity. Mental health provides the capacity for rational thinking, communication, learning, emotional growth, resilience, and self-esteem (National Institute of Mental Health [NIMH], 2006) (Figure 1.1). People with emotional well-being or mental "healthiness" function comfortably in society and are satisfied with their achievements.

Elements of and Influences on Mental Health

Mental health implies mastery and relative contentment in love, work, play, spirituality, and relationships. Mentally healthy people perform meaningful tasks, enjoy life, have a sense of humor, and are satisfied in their interpersonal dealings. They show optimism, benefit from rest and sleep, and work well alone and with others. They accept responsibility for actions, reach sound judgments, and express feelings in an inoffensive and contextually appropriate manner.

Elements of mental health that contribute to the preceding characteristics are as follows:

- *Self-governance:* acting independently, dependently, or interdependently as the need arises without permanently losing autonomy
- *Progress toward growth or self-realization:* being willing to move forward to maximize capabilities
- *Tolerance of the unknown:* facing the uncertainty of life and the certainty of death with faith and hope

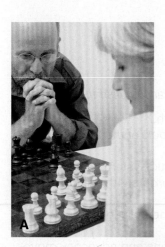

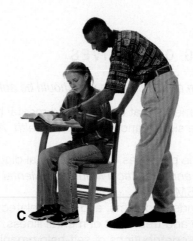

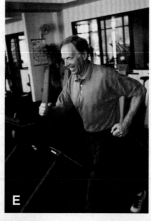

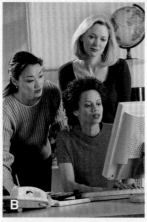

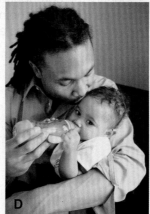

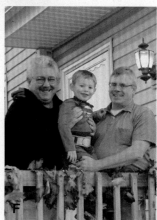

FIGURE 1.1 A state of mental health enables people of all backgrounds to (**A**) think rationally, (**B**) communicate with others, (**C**) learn, (**D**) grow emotionally, (**E**) show resilience, and (**F**) feel a sense of self-esteem.

- *Self-esteem:* being aware of and accepting of personal abilities and limitations through lifelong self-reflection and feedback from others
- *Reality orientation:* distinguishing fact from fantasy and behaving accordingly
- *Mastery of environment:* interacting competently, effectively, and creatively with and influencing environmental contexts
- *Stress management:* experiencing congruent emotions in daily life and tolerating stress-provoking situations in an adaptive, creative, and flexible way, knowing that any negative feelings are time limited

Biologic, psychological, and sociocultural factors influence mental health (Figure 1.2). In addition, society and culture greatly influence views of mental health and mental illness because society largely determines which behaviors are considered acceptable.

Mental Health as a National Priority

In *Mental Health: A Report of the Surgeon General* (U.S. Department of Health and Human Services [USDHHS], 1999), Dr. David Satcher made mental health a national priority. Not only was this the first such report issued by a U.S. Surgeon General, but also, sadly, to date it was the last. Although its information at this writing is 13 years old, it remains relevant. The 1999 report addressed the need to eradicate the stigma attached to mental illness and emphasized the hope that treatment can offer. In fact, the strong message is "There are effective treatments for mental illness" (USD-HHS, 1999). This historic document focused national attention on the following messages:

- Mental health is fundamental to and necessary for a healthy life.

- Mental disorders are real health conditions with enormous consequences for individuals, families, communities, and the nation.
- Effective treatments for mental disorders are available; most combine psychosocial interventions (eg, behavior therapy, counseling) and psychopharmacotherapy.
- A range of treatment options is available for most mental disorders.
- Those with mental disorders or symptoms should seek treatment because it can help.

> **Checkpoint Questions**
> **1.** What three things result from mental health?
> **2.** Which element of mental health reflects a person's ability to take independent, interdependent, or dependent action based on need while maintaining autonomy?

MENTAL ILLNESS

The American Psychiatric Association's *Diagnostic and Statistical Manual of Mental Disorders (DSM)* definition of **mental disorder** or **mental illness** is the one most widely accepted by the clinical community. The *DSM* is a multiaxial classification system that defines a mental disorder as "a clinically significant behavioral or psychological syndrome or pattern that occurs in an individual and that is associated with present distress or disability or with a significantly increased risk of suffering death, pain, disability, or an important loss of freedom." (American Psychiatric Association [APA], 2000, p. 12). Problems result from brain functioning or dysfunctioning, and they cause the person distress, impairment, or both. Related symptoms must be above and beyond expected reactions to everyday events, such as a death in the family.

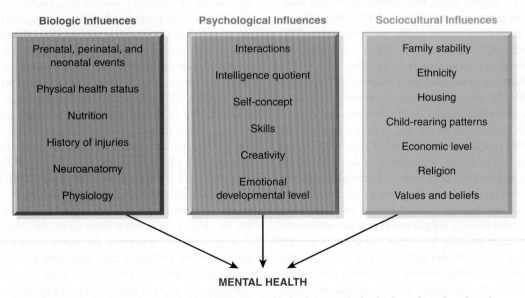

FIGURE 1.2 Influences on mental health include biologic, psychological, and sociocultural factors.

Additionally, the syndrome is not merely a cultural expectation. In other words, practices to which the majority culture in a society objects or that might cause nonmembers of the cultural group distress are *not* mental disorders. For example, some cultures believe that women should be subservient to men and expect the behavior of both sexes to reflect this idea. Western cultures might view such women as dependent or codependent, yet the behavior of these women is normal within their own cultural parameters.

Precise definitions of mental disorders and mental illness are elusive and impractical, and mental health professionals consider the idea of distinguishing physical illness from mental illness a quaint vestige of the past. The term *mental disorder*, although it is convenient, is unfortunate because it implies that a mental disorder is separate from a physical illness, when actually, researchers and scientists have known for some time that this distinction is a fallacy. There is much interaction between brain processes and processes in the rest of the body, and the environment to which humans are exposed affects the whole person. We continue to use the term "mental disorders" because a better term has not yet been found (Keyes, 2005).

Physical, genetic, and physiologic findings related to mental illness are discovered daily. Additionally, the experience and consequences of mental illness are much more complicated than a list of symptoms. Although a person may have a diagnosis of schizophrenia or depression, the person should *not* be labeled a "schizophrenic" or "depressive." He or she is a person with schizophrenia or depression. That is, the person is separate and different from his or her diagnosis (see Chap. 8).

The Mental Health–Illness Continuum

Because mental illnesses are brain illnesses (see Chap. 2), one might think of mental health as complete structural and functional brain integrity. But mental health encompasses much more. Individuals are either mentally ill or presumed mentally healthy; however, experts agree that mental health and mental illness are *not* polar opposites (Keyes, 2005). Nevertheless, many models posit them as end points on a continuum. This approach is oversimplistic, but it is useful in communicating that neither state exists in isolation from the other.

Mental illness is associated with distress and impaired functioning. Mental disorders can be extremely disabling, generating an enormous public health burden. The associated alterations in thought, mood, and behavior can contribute to many other problems, such as loss of personal freedom and heightened risk of death. A limitation of the "continuum model" is that it presumes pure states of mental health and mental illness that serve as bases for comparison. Somewhere between optimal functioning (mental health) and functional impairment (mental illness), people can experience distressful states of insufficient intensity to qualify clinically as mental illness. However, just as health and illness in their broadest sense are not opposite poles, neither is a person completely well or completely ill. Seemingly healthy people still have conditions such as acne and problems with siblings and

friends. Likewise, a person with a diagnosed illness (eg, controlled chronic schizophrenia) may function most optimally in terms of his or her well-being. To summarize, nurses must remember that mental health and mental illness are not defined completely in terms of one or the other.

Overt and covert values, which are built into any definitions of mental health and mental illness, can be powerful determinants of behavior (see Chap. 8). Additionally, concepts of mental illness or mental health in the continuum model have meaning only within the context of certain cultures (Institute of Medicine, 2002, 2004a, 2004b). Chapter 6 explores the complexities of culture; additionally, "Cultural Spotlight" boxes throughout this text emphasize how culture can influence the assessment, diagnosis, and treatment of mental illness.

Incidence and Prevalence

The discipline of epidemiology is at its most basic level in the study of patterns of mental illnesses, including how frequently the disorders occur, their risk factors, and how they are distributed across populations. The current picture that emerges from various agencies, such as the Centers for Disease Control and Prevention and NIMH, suggests that mental disorders occur across the lifespan, affecting people of all ethnicities, genders, and socioeconomic status. In any year, more than 57.7 million Americans have a diagnosable mental disorder (Table 1.1). When applied to the 2004 U.S. census, this number translates to 26.2% of people 18 years or older—about one in four adults (NIMH, 2006; Pan American Health Organization, 2009). Half of all citizens in the United States have a mental illness at some time in their lives; however, most never seek treatment (NIMH, 2006).

Mental illness is the second leading cause of U.S. disability (heart disease is first) and is the leading cause for people 15 to 44 years old. The WHO (2006b) has listed depression, alcohol use, bipolar disorder, schizophrenia, and obsessive-compulsive disorder (OCD) among the 10 leading causes of disability worldwide. Approximately 15% of adults with mental illness also have a co-occurring substance abuse problem (a condition termed **dual diagnosis**), which complicates treatment. Nearly 50% of people with any mental disorder meet the criteria for two or more disorders, with severity strongly related to the comorbidity (NIMH, 2006).

At least 20% of U.S. children have a diagnosable mental disorder, 5% of whom experience severely impaired functioning. More than 5 million U.S. adults experience serious and persistent mental illness in any year. In adults 18 to 54 years old, 18.1% have anxiety disorders, 9.5% have mood disorders, and 1.1% have schizophrenia (NIMH, 2006).

Depression, a serious mental health problem for all age groups, is particularly challenging for older adults. Although 8% to 15% of them have depression, the condition often is undiagnosed and untreated for older clients because they, their families, or health care providers mistakenly confuse signs and symptoms with "normal aging." People 65 years or older have the highest suicide rates. Alzheimer's disease (AD) occurs in 4.5 million Americans, a number that has doubled

TABLE 1.1 **Mental Disorders in the United States**

Type	Prevalence	Median Age of Onset	Points of Interest
Eating disorders	Females are at much greater risk than males. In their lifetimes, an estimated 0.5–3.7% of females experience anorexia; an estimated 1.1–4.2% experience bulimia. An estimated 2–5% of Americans experience binge-eating disorder in any 6-month period.	Teens and 20s	The estimated mortality rate for anorexia in females 15–24 years is 0.56% per year, or approximately 5.6% per decade. This rate is approximately 12 times the annual death rate from all causes for this group. See Chapter 26 for more information.
Attention deficit hyperactivity disorder (ADHD)	One of the most common mental disorders in children and adolescents, it also affects approximately 4.1% of people 18–44 years in any given year.	7 years	It can persist into adolescence and occasionally into adulthood. See Chapter 36 for more information.
Autism	There are approximately 3.4 cases per 1,000 children 3–10 years old; estimating prevalence is difficult and controversial because of differences in how cases are identified and defined, variances in study methods, and changes in diagnostic criteria.	Generally diagnosed by 3 years	Autism is the most debilitating disorder in a group called *autism spectrum disorders* (ASDs) or *pervasive developmental disorders.* Autism is approximately four times more common in boys than girls; however, affected girls tend to have more severe symptoms and greater cognitive impairment. See Chapter 36 for more information.
AD	AD affects approximately 4.5 million Americans.	Increasing age is the greatest risk factor; symptoms usually first appear after 65 years, with rare, inherited forms striking as early as the 30s–40s.	The most common cause of dementia among people 65 years and older, the number of Americans with AD has more than doubled since 1980. From time of diagnosis, people with AD survive about half as long as those of similar age without dementia. See Chapter 31 for more information.
Schizophrenia	Approximately 2.4 million people 18 years and older (1.1%) have schizophrenia in any given year.	Men: late teens or early 20s Women: 20s or early 30s	It affects men and women with equal frequency. See Chapter 29 for more information.
Mood Disorders			
Major depressive disorder	Depression affects approximately 14.8 million people 18 years and older (6.7%) in any given year.	32 years	More prevalent in women than in men, depression is the leading cause of U.S. disability for people 15–44 years. See Chapter 27 for more information.

(continues on page 6)

TABLE 1.1 **Mental Disorders in the United States** (continued)

Type	Prevalence	Median Age of Onset	Points of Interest
Dysthymic disorder	Approximately 3.3 million people 18 years and older (1.5%) in any given year have dysthymia.	31 years	See Chapter 27 for more information.
Bipolar disorder	This disorder affects approximately 5.7 million people 18 years and older (2.6%) in any given year.	25 years	See Chapter 28 for more information.
Anxiety Disorders			
OCD	Approximately 2.2 million people 18 years and older (1%) in any given year have OCD.	19 years	First symptoms tend to emerge during childhood or adolescence. See Chapters 23 and 36 for more information.
Post-traumatic stress disorder (PTSD)	Approximately 7.7 million people 18 years and older (3.5%) have PTSD in any given year.	23 years	It can develop at any age, including childhood. Approximately 30% of Vietnam veterans at some point after the war have experienced PTSD. It frequently follows a violent personal assault, such as rape, mugging, or domestic violence; terrorism; natural or human-caused disasters; and accidents. See Chapters 23, 34, and 35 for more information.
Generalized anxiety disorder (GAD)	Approximately 6.8 million people 18 years and older (3.1%) in any given year have GAD.	31 years	It can begin at any point in the life cycle. See Chapter 23 for more information.
Panic disorder	Approximately 6 million people 18 years and older (2.7%) in any given year have panic disorder.	24 years	Approximately one third of people with panic disorder experience *agoraphobia,* a condition in which the person is afraid of being in any place or situation where escape might be difficult or help unavailable in the event of a panic attack. See Chapter 23 for more information.
Social phobia	Approximately 19.2 million people 18 years and older (8.7%) in any given year have social phobia.	13 years	See Chapter 36 for more information.
Specific phobia	This condition affects approximately 15 million people 18 years and older (6.8%) in any given year.	7 years	See Chapter 36 for more information.
Agoraphobia without panic disorder	This affects approximately 1.8 million people 18 years and older (0.8%) in any given year.	20 years	See Chapter 23 for more information.

Adapted from National Institute of Mental Health. (2006). The numbers count: Mental disorders in America. A fact sheet describing the prevalence of mental disorders in America. Retrieved from http://www.nimh.nih.gov/healthinformation/statisticsmenu.cfm.

since 1980. It affects 10% of those older than 65 years and nearly 50% of those older than 85 years (NIMH, 2006).

Roughly 25% of homeless people have schizophrenia or bipolar disorder. This number equals the populations of such cities as Dayton, Ohio; Des Moines, Iowa; Fort Lauderdale, Florida; Grand Rapids, Michigan; Providence, Rhode Island; Richmond, Virginia; and Salt Lake City, Utah. At any given time, more people with untreated severe psychiatric illnesses are living on U.S. streets than are receiving care in hospitals. Approximately 900,000 people with schizophrenia or bipolar disorder are in hospitals receiving treatment for their disease (Texas Advocacy Center, 2007).

Etiology

The specific causes of mental illnesses are largely unidentified but generally seem to involve enormously complex interactions among genetic predispositions and environmental influences (see Chap. 2). *Mental Health: A Report of the Surgeon General* identifies the roots of mental illness as a combination of biologic and environmental factors; however, the document cautions against thinking that any one gene is responsible for any mental disorder. In all likelihood, small variations in many genes disrupt healthy brain functioning, and under certain environmental conditions, this disruption can result in mental illness (National Alliance for the Mentally Ill [NAMI], 2007). This point cannot be stressed enough. Although some disorders have high heritability (eg, bipolar disorder), genetic transmission is complex and multidimensional. The genes involved are not of the Mendelian variety commonly learned about in elementary science.

What also cannot be emphasized enough is that stress in and of itself is not sufficient to produce a mental illness. The idea that stress can cause a psychiatric disorder is simply a myth. While stress can often be a risk factor in the genesis of mental illness, it does not cause mental illness. For example, people in New York City were exposed to an enormous stressor on September 11, 2001, when the World Trade Center was destroyed by terrorists, but not all of them developed PTSD (see Chap. 23). The causes of mental illness are far more complex, and making simple causal statements diminishes this complexity.

> ### Checkpoint Questions
> 3. How do culture and society influence views of mental health and mental illness?
> 4. What is meant by the term *dual diagnosis*?

Diagnosis

The clinical literature and mental health professionals use two main classification systems to diagnose mental illness. The international classification system, the ICD, refers to the WHO's *Classification of Mental and Behavioural Disorders.* The ICD-10 is the latest in a series that originated in the 1850s. It has become the international diagnostic standard for general epidemiologic and many health management

purposes. Examples include the analysis of the general health of populations and the monitoring of the incidence and prevalence of diseases and other health problems in relation to the characteristics and circumstances of the people affected. The ICD also is used to classify diseases and health problems on many types of records, including death certificates and hospital charts. In addition to enabling the storage and retrieval of diagnostic information for clinical and epidemiologic purposes, these records also provide the basis for the compilation of national mortality and morbidity statistics by WHO member states (WHO, 2006b).

The APA developed the second system, which is currently in its sixth revision, more than five decades ago. The *Diagnostic and Statistical Manual of Mental Disorders,* 4th edition, text revision (*DSM-IV-TR*) (APA, 2000) is most commonly accepted in the U.S. and Canadian clinical community. The *DSM* groups disorders by symptom clusters and differentiates between normality and psychopathology based on the duration and severity of symptoms.

Five Axes of the DSM

The *DSM* categorical classification lists diagnostic criteria for each mental disorder. Its five-axis system gives a comprehensive picture of the client's functioning as follows:

- *Axis I:* clinical disorders
- *Axis II:* personality disorders and mental retardation
- *Axis III:* general medical conditions
- *Axis IV:* psychosocial and environmental problems (*DSM-IV-TR* Box 1.1)

DSM-IV-TR BOX 1.1

Examples of Axis IV (Psychosocial and Environmental) Problems

- **Problems with primary support group:** eg, death of a family member; health problems in family; disruption of family by separation, divorce, or estrangement; removal from the home; remarriage of parent; sexual or physical abuse; parental overprotection; neglect of child; inadequate discipline; discord with siblings; birth of a sibling
- **Problems related to the social environment:** eg, death or loss of friend; inadequate social support; living alone; difficulty with acculturation; discrimination; adjustment to life-cycle transition (such as retirement)
- **Educational problems:** eg, illiteracy; academic problems; discord with teachers or classmates; inadequate school environment
- **Occupational problems:** eg, unemployment; threat of job loss; stressful work schedule; difficult work conditions; job dissatisfaction; job change; discord with boss or coworkers
- **Housing problems:** eg, homelessness; inadequate housing; unsafe neighborhood; discord with neighbors or landlord

(continues on page 8)

DSM-IV-TR BOX 1.1 (continued)

- **Economic problems:** eg, extreme poverty; inadequate finances; insufficient welfare support
- **Problems with access to health care services:** eg, inadequate health care services; lack of transport to health care facilities; inadequate health insurance
- **Problems related to interaction with the legal system/crime:** eg, arrest; incarceration; litigation ; victim of crime
- **Other psychosocial and environmental problems:** eg, exposure to disasters, war, other hostilities; discord with nonfamily caregivers such as counselor, social worker, or physician; unavailability of social service agencies

Reprinted with permission from the *Diagnostic and Statistical Manual of Mental Disorders,* 4th ed., text revision (Copyright © 2000 American Psychiatric Association.)

- *Axis V:* global assessment of functioning (GAF), written as numbers (0 to 100), meaning "current functioning"/"highest level of functioning in past year" (APA, 2000). (The GAF is reproduced in its entirety in Appendix A.)

See Case Vignette 1.1 for an example of the application of the *DSM* axes.

Each disorder's criteria describe its behaviors, symptoms, or signs; duration; and sometimes other qualifiers (eg, severe, recurrent). However, the criteria do not determine the diagnosis. Clinicians who use the criteria as guidelines decide on the diagnosis. Many clients have more than one diagnosis on the first three axes.

Limitations and Criticisms of the DSM

Although the *DSM* is used universally as a classification system, it has serious limitations. The categories are descriptions, not explanations. Nurses must guard against the

Case Vignette 1.1

Judith, 20 years old, lives at college. Three months ago, she broke up with her boyfriend of 2 years. When she calls home, Judith tells her parents that she "feels bad" and cries all the time. Some days, she cannot force herself out of bed to attend class.

Judith's parents decide to visit her. When they arrive, they are troubled by her slovenly, unkempt appearance. Upon questioning, Judith says that she has no energy to shower, wash her hair, or do laundry. Although she tries to study, she cannot concentrate or sleep at night. Her social interactions have dwindled; she usually feels "too tired" to see friends. She has lost 10 pounds in the past month. Her meals consist of food from a vending machine because she's too tired to walk to the dining hall.

The parents persuade Judith to begin visiting a mental health practitioner at the university. In addition to the above findings, Judith's health history reveals episodes of depression in her mother and grandmother. During the initial interview, Judith reports feelings of worthlessness, helplessness, and self-disgust but denies thoughts of self-harm. After follow-up questions, physical examination, and diagnostic tests, the practitioner makes the following diagnoses according to the *DSM-IV-TR* axes:

- **Axis I: Major Depressive Disorder, single episode, moderate 296.22.** Judith reports pervasive sadness; diminished interest in school, friends, and hygiene; fatigue and insomnia; lack of appetite and weight loss; inability to concentrate; and worthlessness. Symptoms have existed for more than 2 weeks; she has a family history of depression. Based on *DSM-IV-TR* criteria, major depression is the likely diagnosis (see Chap. 27).
- **Axis II: Deferred.** Axis II is reserved for mental retardation and personality disorders. Judith does not have mental retardation. Diagnosis of a personality disorder requires extensive history taking and long-term professional evaluation. Judith may have one, but current information is

insufficient for diagnosis. "Deferred" simply means a practitioner is reserving judgment pending more information.
- **Axis III: No diagnosis.** Axis III is reserved for medical conditions (eg, diabetes, asthma). If findings from the history and physical examination are normal, no diagnosis is given.
- **Axis IV: Recent loss of significant other; problems with social interaction; educational problems.** Axis IV is reserved for psychosocial problems or life stressors that might affect diagnosis, treatment, or prognosis of a mental illness (see *DSM-IV-TR* Box 1.1). Judith's recent stressor is breaking up with her boyfriend. Subsequent social isolation and school difficulties further complicate the overall diagnostic picture.
- **Axis V: Current GAF—55/Highest GAF in past year—95.** This axis is a judgment about the client's overall functioning based on the GAF. The GAF's hypothetical continuum of mental health–illness ranges from 100 (superior functioning) to 1 (persistent danger of hurting self or others) (see Appendix A). Based on Judith's present social and school functioning, the diagnostician gives a score of 55.

The practitioner prescribes 20 mg of citalopram (Celexa) each morning. Judith follows the drug regimen and starts attending regular counseling sessions. Eventually, symptoms subside and functioning increases. By semester's end, she feels "like herself" and earns good grades.

Reflection and Critical Thinking

- How do the *DSM-IV-TR* axes reflect different areas of the client's life and functioning?
- What possible risk factors did Judith have for a psychiatric disorder? Could anything have been done to help prevent the episode?
- What factors might contribute to a recurrence of depression? Is Judith at risk for any other current or future problems?

tendency to think that something has been explained when, in fact, it has only been named. In other words, giving a condition a label does not explain or confer any reality on it other than the name itself and the cluster of behaviors subsumed under it. Thus, nurses must avoid explicating a person's behavior based on a diagnostic label. (He acts like a schizophrenic because he has schizophrenia.) This logical error in reasoning is known as a **tautology**.

In addition, as convenient as the *DSM* system is, its categories imply sharp dividing lines between "normal" and "abnormal" behaviors and among different disorders. The reality is that such categories are not so neat; some scholars argue that they are artificial (Mallett, 2006; Widiger & Trull, 2007). For example, three clients may suffer from the same disorder; however, manifestations and the personal experience will differ for each client. As another example, although the *DSM* has criteria that might specify that a person must have six of eight symptoms for 1 month, these criteria are not flexible enough to account for the person who has five of eight symptoms for 3 weeks and is in distress. Moreover, the *DSM* diagnostic categories differ somewhat from the taxonomies of other illnesses (eg, hypertension, diabetes mellitus) in that many psychiatric categories lack an empirical foundation (although research is available to support most major psychiatric illnesses). Many scholars believe that, in particular, the dimension-weighted *DSM-IV-TR* model for classifying the depressive disorders lacks utility and does not inform individual treatment (Parker, 2006).

The *DSM* diagnostic labels for children were derived from adult categories. The most problematic related issue is that the diagnoses are not based on a body of research on children—similar disorders may have different signs and symptoms for each age group. For example, depression in children has different clinical manifestations than it does in adults. Moreover, making categories for children mere downward extensions of adult categories assumes that children are little adults who can have adult illnesses. The reality is that some diagnoses are specific to children and some are specific to adults (Mallett, 2006).

The *DSM* criteria may not apply uniformly to all cultures. Most studies upon which *DSM* criteria are based were conducted in the United States or Canada. Clinicians should take care to avoid diagnosing pathology in people who express unusual beliefs (Morrison, 2006). The *DSM* lists several specific cultural syndromes but is not comprehensive.

The GAF scale used for Axis V has generated criticism and controversy. Its areas of concern overlap considerably with Axes I and II, which may limit the usefulness of Axis V as an assessment of functioning. In addition, the GAF scale does not differentiate physical impairments from behavioral symptoms, but medical conditions may be responsible for behavioral symptoms (see Chap. 39). It does not reflect potentially influential environmental problems. Lack of specificity on how to use the GAF scale has led to its misapplication. One source of confusion is how to operationalize the GAF's "current" time frame. Another involves how to integrate the potentially distinct contributions of a client's psychiatric symptoms and functioning to the final score. The inherent subjectivity of the scale interferes with its usefulness in tracking changes in a client's functioning over time (Morrison, 2006). Finally, some GAF criteria have culture-related problems. An example involves the subject's job and occupational environment. In many countries, young adults remain under both the emotional and the financial protection of the parent or family until 25 to 30 years of age. Using this area of the GAF is challenging because this period is a culturally accepted "prolonged adolescence," but in other cultures it is viewed as "delayed."

Finally, the *DSM* system is not fixed. It is always a "work in progress" and should be thought of as such. As knowledge expands, new categories appear and old ones are revised, refined, or eliminated. However, if the manual omits a disorder, it does not mean that the disorder does not exist. Likewise, a disorder that appears in a manual today may eventually no longer be considered a mental disease. For example, homosexuality was declassified as a disorder in 1973. At this writing, the *Diagnostic and Statistical Manual of Mental Disorders* is in its sixth iteration. It is presently being revised, but because the process involves polling numerous clinicians and collating their feedback and responses, it is a daunting undertaking. Estimates are that the original 2012 deadline for a *DSM V* may not be met.

Prevention and Treatment

National health care priorities focus on the following areas:

- Health promotion and illness prevention
- Attention to medically underserved populations
- Involvement of managed care in behavioral health
- Quality management, including client outcomes
- Expanded practice of advanced clinical health care providers, including nurse practitioners
- Community-based primary care
- Influence of consumer and family advocacy groups
- Decreased benefits through Medicare, Medicaid, and disability programs

As the aging population continues to increase, the incidence of chronic illnesses and disabilities requiring mental health care (eg, AD) also will rise (Figure 1.3). By 2020, violence and self-injury are predicted to be major worldwide disabilities (Rosenbaum & Langhinrichsen-Rohling, 2006). Violence, a public health problem, requires integrated attention from families, schools, neighborhoods, communities, and governments. Within this context, the burden of psychiatric illness is immense and expected to grow, necessitating more mental health services provided by more mental health care professionals.

The importance of preventing and treating mental illness cannot be overestimated. The following sections discuss problems and goals in doing so, as well as the significant contributions of self-help organizations and advocacy groups for clients and their families.

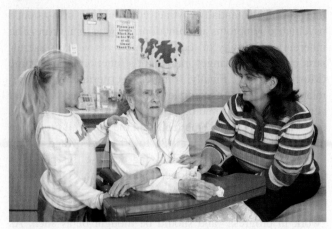

FIGURE 1.3 An increasing aging population means similarly increasing rates of chronic illnesses (including AD). The need for mental health services also will grow.

Problems in Treating Mental Illness

Given the significant numbers of people with mental illness, why do nearly two thirds of them fail to seek treatment? Several factors contribute to this problem.

COST-RELATED ISSUES. The financial cost of mental illness is high and undoubtedly increases annually. Inpatient care is expensive, partly because of the number of skilled professionals required to provide it. Other forms of treatment are also costly. However, untreated mental illness is prohibitively expensive in terms of lost productivity and money spent to maintain criminal justice systems and social service agencies.

As it has become increasingly important to provide and improve access to quality care, mental health administrators have turned to behavioral health managed care. A goal has been to reduce hospital admissions, which are the most expensive form of treatment. Unfortunately, some managed care "gatekeepers" in the past denied or restricted access to needed services and therefore have added to the discouragement, distress, and even despair of clients and their families (Cohn, 2007; Sharfstein et al., 2002). The recent parity legislation described later in this section was designed to improve coverage for mental health care and close the gap between physical and mental health care benefits.

Another reason people do not seek appropriate treatment can be traced to the Internet. Although the Web provides easy access to vast resources, some material is distorted. The Web can also serve as an outlet for unscrupulous people to swindle desperate clients and families seeking help (Friedman et al., 2006; Kennedy et al., 2002). Students can explore government websites and Quackwatch (http://www.quackwatch.org) for more information on medical "quackery" and deceitful practices. See also Chapter 4.

STIGMA. Strong stigma still attaches to people with mental illness, largely related to public misunderstandings, misconceptions, and associated fears. Stigma can greatly exacerbate the experience of mental illness. Diagnostic classifications may intensify this stigma by enhancing the public's sense of "groupness" and "differentness" when perceiving people with mental illness. The objectification of people with mental illness sometimes leads both the professionals and the public to consider such individuals solely within the parameters of their condition. Some people may avoid anyone with a psychiatric label or even treat him or her unkindly or maliciously (Centers for Disease Control and Prevention, 2010; Corrigan, 2007; Sartorius, 2002). See Chapter 8.

Misconceptions have ranged from attributing mental illness to demonic possession to blaming people for their problems. This stigmatization has led to discrimination and intolerance. Perceived stigma is associated with a considerable decrease in quality of life and role functioning (Alonso et al., 2009). Over time, such stereotyping has effectively discouraged public sympathy for the traumatic life dislocation of people with brain disorders and has prevented public policy from allocating resources (eg, medication parity) that would meet their needs. For example, many health plans cover the costs of psychotropic drugs at far lower rates than they do for other medications. Government-sponsored research funds for the treatment of mental illness are often far lower than monies allocated for other diseases. At a personal level, people with mental illness must deal with painful rejection, isolation, and discrimination that erode self-assurance and can systematically undermine self-confidence. Stigma creates or reinforces interpersonal, financial, employment, and social barriers to accessing care and places obstacles to obtaining newer pharmacotherapies.

REVOLVING DOOR TREATMENT. The community mental health movement of the 1960s led many state hospitals and other long-term care facilities to discharge clients with mental illness. The effectiveness of newer psychotropic medications has reduced the need for hospitalization. Even when hospitalization is necessary, lengths of stay have decreased. Managed care companies often mandate certain kinds of treatments. Insurers favor short-term, time-limited, and cognitive–behavioral approaches, even when a client's needs are for longer, more intensive treatment. For these and other reasons, many clients are being discharged from mental health care facilities without the skills to survive in the community. This "deinstitutionalization" has contributed to people living with inadequate or no programs to serve them. Some deinstitutionalized clients have severe and persistent mental illnesses that require many specialized interventions. The term "revolving door" describes the plight of those who enter and leave psychiatric hospitals repeatedly because they cannot effectively manage their care independently or within the community (Figure 1.4).

Psychotropic medications often are not enough to produce positive outcomes for those with mental illness. To recover and become completely well, clients must be reintegrated into their communities and social groups. Money to be used for appropriate and accessible treatment must follow

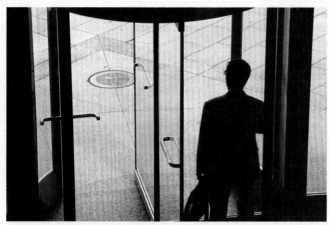

FIGURE 1.4 The metaphor of the "revolving door" reflects the experience of clients who continually enter, leave, and reenter psychiatric hospitals because they cannot independently manage care for their illness or locate sufficient community supports.

clients into their communities. Coordination and collaboration among agencies providing services are needed. Many state mental hospitals have closed, increasing the responsibility of local agencies to provide community-based care.

An attempt to tailor services to those with severe and persistent mental illness led to the development of Assertive Community Treatment (ACT) programs. Such programs serve those in greatest need, such as the homeless, incarcerated clients, clients with dual diagnoses, and clients resistant to usual treatment (see Chap. 20).

> **Checkpoint Questions**
> **5.** Why is use of the *DSM* with children problematic?
> **6.** What term describes the problem of deinstitutionalized clients undergoing repeated entry and discharge from psychiatric hospitals because they cannot manage independently or within the community?

Challenges Remaining

Despite the good news about the increasingly effective treatments becoming available for mental illnesses in the 1999 Surgeon General's report mentioned earlier, the report also stressed that formidable financial and systemic barriers have prevented many people from seeking help for their conditions. The situation involving barriers is not new. It appeared in articles in psychiatric medicine several decades ago (Reiger et al., 1978) and has not changed over time. The situation is as formidable is it was over a decade ago.

THE NEW FREEDOM COMMISSION REPORT. In 2002, the New Freedom Commission (NFC) on Mental Health in America became the first such endeavor since the Carter administration. The NFC was given the task of studying the mental health delivery system, identifying problems and gaps, and recommending change that would facilitate

better outcomes for adults and children with serious mental and emotional conditions. Its work spanned 12 months and in its final report, the NFC described America's mental health system as "fragmented and in disarray . . . leading to unnecessary and costly disability, homelessness, school failure and incarceration" (2003, p.3). It further stated that the mental health services system defies easy description and looks like a maze, and posited that the maze was more complex and more inadequate for children than for adults.

LIMITED ACCESS TO SERVICES. The fragmented U.S. mental health care system often provides inadequate, inappropriate, or no care (Cohn, 2007). It is difficult for clients and families to determine what services are needed and where to find them. Health care providers often lag behind what researchers know about the effectiveness of various treatments. For example, professionals have known for many years that giving a child a "dummy" or punching bag to hit for anger expression actually increases aggressive behavior. Yet some professionals still engage in this practice so that children can achieve catharsis (relief).

Goals of Care and Methods of Achievement

Past health care practitioners generally attributed mental illness to a single pathogen: a toxin, germ, genetic defect, metabolic imbalance, or nutritional deficiency. They geared treatment to "getting to the root" of the problem in search of a cure. However, this approach failed to recognize the reciprocity between humans and their environments. It ignored that people cannot possibly remain uninfluenced by their contexts. Gradually, the mental health profession realized that even if a causative pathogenic agent could be identified, the reactions of clients to it and the resulting life changes were vitally important to gathering a complete clinical picture.

Scholars in mental health have integrated findings from diverse disciplines, such as medicine, sociology, psychology, neurophysiology, biochemistry, genetics, anthropology, and nursing, to better understand mental illness. Their work has been incorporated in the service community, where it has become increasingly apparent that a broader understanding, which includes biologic, psychosocial, and sociocultural factors see (Figure 1.2), offers a more comprehensive approach to mental illness. Today, clinicians integrate these factors into an overall picture that describes clients' problems, the behavioral context for them, the conditions that might add stress, and the conditions that might help or buffer the effects of stress. They synthesize this information to create a unique assessment on which they base individual treatment.

Long-term goals of care in treating mental illness include the following:

- Increase the number of mental health professionals caring for children and adolescents (Figure 1.5).
- Expand mental health services.

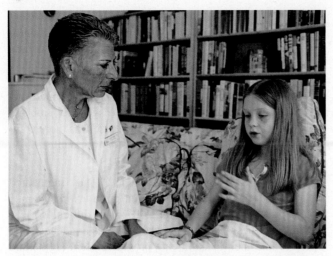

FIGURE 1.5 A long-term goal for mental health treatment services is for more mental health professionals to provide care for children and adolescents.

- Understand mental illness through a cultural lens and deliver services to minority groups in a culturally congruent and sensitive manner.
- Improve public understanding of mental illness.
- Redesign rehabilitation services to meet clients' physical, mental, cultural, and social needs.
- Ensure that interagency coordination and collaboration become the norm.

BEYOND RESPONSE TO RECOVERY. Recovery and quality of life are important treatment goals. Past treatment efforts aimed at reducing distressing symptoms and teaching clients skills to deal with or diminish them. However, clients who are not fully recovered and rehabilitated (as in a partial response to treatment for depression) are more likely to experience relapse or chronic problems (McReynolds, 2002). The aim now is for clients to recover or to experience a remission and be restored to pre-illness functioning in various domains, such as occupationally, socially, and educationally. A true rehabilitation approach employs modes of intervention that include strengthening the client's skills and his or her environmental supports. Client skill-strengthening approaches that have been recognized for their strong positive effects include social and independent living skills training, symptom management, and job-finding clubs. Critical environment-support-strengthening approaches include family behavior management and the use of peer groups in the transition to community living. Supported employment has been cited as a crucial service component that equally emphasizes enhanced client skills and environmental supports.

> Think About It 1.1
> Consider Judith from Case Vignette 1.1. How could health professionals foster recovery and quality of life for her?

REINTEGRATION INTO SOCIETY. The newer psychotropic medications have contributed to clients being able to reclaim aspects of their lives, such as family involvement, employment, continued education, social and recreational activities, and community participation. However, drugs alone cannot treat severe and persistent mental illnesses. The concept of reintegration means coordinating social programs with the goal of assisting people with serious mental illness to lead meaningful and more self-sufficient lives. Examples include finding ways to help clients locate safe housing, achieve gainful employment, experience satisfying family and social relationships, and develop a sense of belonging to the community.

MENTAL HEALTH PARITY. Parity legislation is designed to improve coverage for mental health care and close the gap between physical and mental health care benefits. The federal act requiring such parity is the Paul Wellstone and Peter Domenici Mental Health Parity and Addiction Equity Act of 2008 (MHPAEA). Beginning in 2010, the MHPAEA aligned mental health/substance abuse (MHSA) benefits and medical/surgical benefits for group health plans with more than 50 employees. The new law requires that any group health plan that includes MHSA disorder benefits along with standard medical and surgical coverage must treat them equally in terms of out-of-pocket costs, benefit limits, and practices such as prior authorization and utilization review. These practices must be based on the same level of scientific evidence used by the insurer for medical and surgical benefits. The MHPAEA greatly expands on an earlier law, the Mental Health Parity Act of 1996, which required parity only in aggregate lifetime and annual dollar limits between the categories of benefits and did not extend to substance use disorder benefits (Centers for Medicare and Medicaid Services, 2010).

CULTURALLY COMPETENT CARE. The majority of the U.S. population will have shifted to people of color by the middle of the 21st century. As the population needing services changes, so must the delivery of care. A mental health system should value diversity and make the provision of culturally competent care part of its mission. **Culturally competent care** means care that is acceptable to the client's cultural background, regardless of whether it is given by someone from the same or from a different ethnic or minority group as the client (Figure 1.6). Health care professionals must be able to incorporate cultural factors, including language, customs, beliefs, and traditions, into plans of care. See Chapter 6.

MEDICATION ADHERENCE. Also called *medication compliance*, **medication adherence** means that clients actually take their drugs as prescribed. To do so, they need information about the medications and the opportunity to discuss issues important to them. Teaching about psychotropic medications should include the following information:

- The medication's generic and brand names
- Dosage, route, frequency, and times to be taken

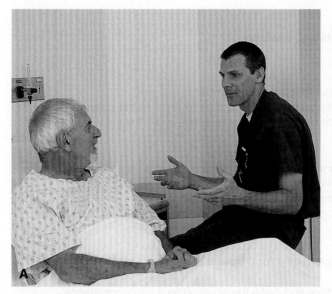
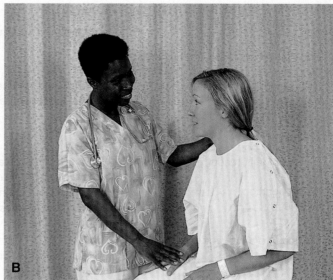

FIGURE 1.6 Culturally competent care is necessary whether clients (**A**) share the same cultural background or (**B**) are of different ages, races, genders, or other parameters. (Copyright © B. Proud.)

- Expected common side effects
- Possible toxic or dangerous effects
- How to treat minor and common side effects

See Client-Centered Education 1.1 for an example of medication teaching.

Self-Help Movements and Advocacy

The consumer movement has changed the role of family involvement and brought attention to the needs of those with mental illness and their loved ones. The influence of mutual support groups, consumer and family education programs, and advocacy services has effected change in treatment services and mental health policy.

NATIONAL ALLIANCE FOR THE MENTALLY ILL

The NAMI is an important self-help group for consumers of mental health services and their social supports. The major thrusts of NAMI are as follows:

- Communicating that mental illnesses are brain disorders
- Advocating for people with mental illness
- Eliminating stigma and discrimination against people with mental illness
- Improving access to treatment services for people with mental illness
- Facilitating accountability to mental health consumers and their families for service delivery
- Integrating mental illness into general health and community life

Client-Centered Education 1.1

Managing Drug Therapy

Psychiatric–mental health nurses need to explain fully the possible toxic or serious side effects of or allergic responses to psychotropic medications. Following is a sample of information that a nurse must provide to clients who are prescribed Haldol (haloperidol) and to their families.

Haldol (haloperidol) is a high-potency neuroleptic that powerfully blocks dopamine to control psychosis. It also blocks dopamine receptors in the "motor strip" of the brain, which controls finely coordinated body movements. This secondary blockade contributes to a group of neurologic movement disorders known as extrapyramidal

symptoms (EPSs). EPSs resemble the symptoms of Parkinson's disease. Akathisia, the most troublesome of these side effects, ranges from an inner feeling of muscular discomfort and restlessness to agitated, desperate, involuntary pacing, "hand-wringing," and weeping. This effect occurs early in treatment, and studies show that it is the one side effect that accounts for most cases of nonadherence to neuroleptic medications. Should EPS occur, notify your health care provider immediately because other medications (atypical antipsychotics) are available.

TABLE 1.2 Family Adaptation Model

Stage	Family's Thoughts and Feelings
1. Dealing with the catastrophic event	
a. Crisis, chaos, shock	Family is overwhelmed, confused, and lost.
b. Denial	This protective response gives family time to process the catastrophe.
c. Hoping against hope	Family members think, "I hope that this is not what I think it is. Maybe it will go away."
2. Learning to cope	
a. Anger, guilt, resentment	Family initially blames the client, wants him or her to "snap out of it," and feels guilty for having such thoughts.
b. Recognition	The illness becomes a reality.
c. Grief	Family expresses grief, fear, and sorrow over lost possibilities and the uncertain future.
3. Moving into advocacy	
a. Understanding	Members develop empathy for the client (other family member) and leave fear behind.
b. Acceptance	Family acknowledges and owns the situation as a life circumstance.
c. Advocacy and action	Family focuses anger and grief on empowerment and involvement with support groups. Members confront systems that fail the family and client.

Adapted from the Provider Education Program with permission from NAMI.

FAMILY ADVOCACY MOVEMENT. Clients with mental illness and their families bear most of the burden of their condition. The family advocacy movement has made enormous contributions to communicating how families and clients experience mental illness. The health care industry once viewed families and clients with mental illness as dysfunctional and their behaviors as pathologic. In fact, it often regarded relatives as contributors to the illness. In reaction to this "blaming" approach, family advocates conducted research that "normalizes" much of the behavior that families and clients display, explaining it as an adaptive process (Mohr et al., 2000; NAMI, 2010a, 2010b). The Family and Client Adaptation Models in Tables 1.2 and 1.3, based on NAMI research, represent chronic mental illness as a catastrophic and challenging life event. To adapt to this intense trauma, the client and family progress through a series of stages that health care providers must understand.

PSYCHIATRIC ADVANCED DIRECTIVES. Many states currently are enacting psychiatric advanced directives, in which clients formally declare their treatment wishes should they become ill. Such directives may include whether the client wishes the use of psychotropic medication, seclusion and restraint, and electroconvulsive treatment. Advanced directives are not meant to supersede care necessary to protect client safety (Schouten, 2006).

TABLE 1.3 Client Adaptation Model

Event	Stage	Emotions	Needs
1. Crisis (episode of serious mental illness)	1. Recuperation (period of exhaustion and dependence)	Denial, depression, humiliation, resentment, anger	Rest, sleep, someone to take care of client, probably medications
2. Decision (time to begin to heal and move forward)	2. Rebuilding (learning to do things for oneself)	Hope, grief, self-doubt, trust, fear, excitement, frustration, pride	Telling one's story, learning about the illness, having someone believe in the client, learning or relearning skills
3. Awakening (realization that the client is a person of worth with dreams)	3. Recovery/discovery (healthy interdependence)	Self-acceptance, appreciation of others, confidence, anger at injustice, assertiveness, helpfulness	A personal vision, social acceptance, meaningful work, someone to love, someone to advocate for self and others

Adapted from the Provider Education Program with permission from NAMI.

PSYCHIATRIC–MENTAL HEALTH NURSING

The term *psychiatric–mental health nursing* refers to two aspects of nursing that interact and overlap. **Psychiatric nursing** focuses on the care and rehabilitation of people with identifiable mental illnesses or disorders. **Mental health nursing** focuses on well and at-risk populations to prevent mental illness or provide immediate treatment for those with early signs of a disorder. Thus, *Psychiatric–Mental Health Nursing: Scope and Standards of Practice* describes **psychiatric–mental health nursing** as committed to promoting mental health through the assessment, diagnosis, and treatment of human responses to mental health problems and psychiatric disorders (American Nurses Association [ANA], American Psychiatric Nurses Association [APNA], and International Society of Psychiatric–Mental Health Nurses [ISPN], 2007).

Psychiatric–mental health nursing uses the study of human behavior as its science and purposeful use of self as its art. It views people holistically, considering their strengths, needs, and problems. In most ways, psychiatric–mental health nursing is similar to other types of nursing. It is based on the physical and social sciences. It is designed to meet the needs of people with health problems. It is provided by caring and knowledgeable professionals. It relies on a problem-solving approach to plan, deliver, and evaluate care. People with mental health or psychiatric problems need services

to recover and return to or improve their previous level of functioning. As with other nursing disciplines, services are tailored for primary, secondary, or tertiary care needs.

In addition to the qualities it shares with other nursing specialties, psychiatric–mental health nursing also has evolved into a unique discipline combining the knowledge, experience, and skills of nursing and the biologic and behavioral sciences. It offers a wide range of preventive strategies and interventions to promote optimal functioning and health (Nursing Spotlight 1.1).

Nursing Process and Standards of Care

The nursing process is the foundation of all clinical nursing decision making (ANA, APNA, & ISPN, 2007). Through this systematic problem-solving approach, nurses provide comprehensive care to individuals, families, groups, and communities. Both U.S. and Canadian standards of care describe activities that nurses demonstrate through assessment, diagnosis, planning, outcome identification, implementation of interventions, and evaluation. The nursing process and standards of care for psychiatric–mental health nursing are discussed extensively in Chapter 9.

Levels of Practice

Psychiatric–mental health nurses are educated and prepared to practice at both the basic and advanced levels. Nurses who have completed a nursing program and passed their state's licensing examination practice at the basic level. Those who have received at least a master's degree in nursing practice at the advanced level as clinical nurse specialists or nurse practitioners.

Basic psychiatric–mental health nurses promote and encourage the maintenance of health and prevention of

---

▲ NURSING SPOTLIGHT 1.1 ▲

Psychiatric–Mental Health Nursing's Phenomena of Concern

Phenomena of concern for psychiatric–mental health nurses include:

- Promotion of optimal mental and physical health and well-being and prevention of mental illness
- Impaired ability to function related to psychiatric, emotional, and physiologic distress
- Alterations in thinking, perceiving, and communicating due to psychiatric disorders or mental health problems
- Behaviors and mental states that indicate potential danger to self or others
- Emotional stress related to illness, pain, disability, and loss
- Symptom management, side effects, or toxicities associated with self-administered drugs, psychopharmacologic intervention, and other treatment modalities
- The barriers to treatment efficacy and recovery posed by alcohol and substance abuse and dependence

- Self-concept and body image changes, developmental issues, life process changes, and end-of-life issues
- Physical symptoms that occur along with altered psychological status
- Psychological symptoms that occur along with altered physiologic status
- Interpersonal, organizational, sociocultural, spiritual, or environmental circumstances or events that have an effect on the mental and emotional well-being of the individual and family or community
- Elements of recovery, including the ability to maintain housing, employment, and social support, that help individuals reengage in seeking meaningful lives
- Societal factors such as violence, poverty, and substance abuse

From American Nurses Association (ANA), American Psychiatric Nurses Association (APNA), & International Society of Psychiatric–Mental Health Nurses (ISPN). (2007). Silver Spring, MD: American Nurses Publishing.

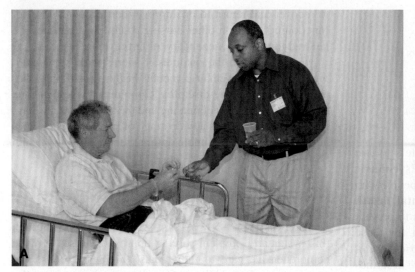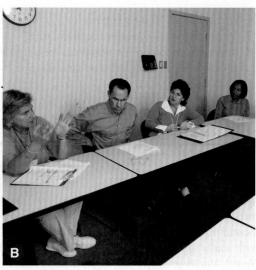

FIGURE 1.7 **(A)** Basic psychiatric–mental health nursing involves activities such as medication management. (Copyright © B. Proud.) **(B)** Advanced psychiatric–mental health nursing may include conducting group therapy.

disorders, assess biopsychosocial functioning, serve as case managers, design therapeutic environments, and promote self-care activities, including medication and symptom management. They also use psychobiologic interventions such as administering drugs (Figure 1.7A) and complementary interventions such as teaching relaxation techniques. They educate clients and families about health, illness, and treatment; provide supportive counseling; intervene in crises; and promote psychiatric rehabilitation (ANA, APNA, & ISPN, 2007).

At the advanced level, psychiatric–mental health nurses deliver comprehensive primary mental health services. Functions include teaching and screening, performing preventive interventions, and evaluating and managing care for people with mental illness. Health teaching is important in that many clients have poor and neglectful health habits. Nurses can play a role in teaching the importance of such things as abstaining from tobacco and alcohol. Teaching is also related to prevention. Preventive strategies might include teaching family and clients about the signs and symptoms of relapse so that treatment can be instituted early and aggressively. Management of mental illnesses includes formulating diagnoses; ordering and interpreting laboratory tests; prescribing and managing psychopharmacologic medications; conducting individual, family, and group therapies (Figure 1.7B); and facilitating psychiatric rehabilitation (ANA, APNA, & ISPN, 2007).

Think About It 1.2

A psychiatric–mental health nurse is to talk to a group of senior-level nursing students about the discipline, focusing on the roles and functions of basic and advanced levels of practice. What information would the nurse incorporate into the presentation?

Guiding Principles

Psychiatric–mental health nursing is built on certain principles or beliefs about people and the care they deserve:

- Every person is worthy of dignity and respect.
- Every person has the potential to change and grow.
- All people share basic human needs.
- All behavior is meaningful and can be understood from the person's perspective.
- People have the right to participate in decisions affecting their health and treatment.
- Through the therapeutic use of self, via therapeutic relationships and communication (see Chap. 11), nurses help people adapt, change, and grow.

The Role of the Psychiatric Nurse as a Team Member

In most psychiatric care settings, an interdisciplinary team functions collaboratively to provide comprehensive care for clients. Such care may include general medical treatment, substance abuse services, psychotherapy, medication management, access to entitlements, and other needed therapies or assistance. Each member brings specialized knowledge to the treatment process, thereby enhancing assessment and management. Teams might include psychologists, nurses, psychiatrists, social workers, and paraprofessionals such as lay volunteers and former clients. The team also includes the client and his or her family. Collaboration implies that members work toward a common goal and share responsibility for outcomes. In Chapter 12, several professionals explain their unique roles within the multidisciplinary team and how they collaborate given their various skill sets.

Development of Appropriate Client Care Skills

There is no one "right" way to intervene therapeutically for clients exhibiting disturbed behavior. Mental health care providers must explore their own thoughts and feelings, follow guidelines and standards of care, search for effective interventions, measure client outcomes, and, if needed, redesign interventions. Nurses new to psychiatric–mental health nursing are likely to discover certain feelings, fears, and impressions that, if left unexamined, may hamper their effectiveness with clients and families. Commonly, students facing their first psychiatric nursing clinical experience feel anxious, fearful of clients' actions and possible rejections, fearful of damaging clients through nontherapeutic interventions, or concerned about their own mental health or mental symptoms. More discussion of these issues is found in Chapter 8.

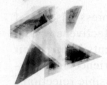

Reviewing and Applying Your Knowledge

Chapter Summary

- Elements that contribute to mental health include self-governance, progress toward growth or self-realization, tolerance of the unknown, self-esteem, reality orientation, mastery of the environment, and stress management.

- *Mental Health: A Report of the Surgeon General* was the first and, to date, last national analysis of the state of mental health in the United States. It analyzed the causes of and treatments for mental illness. Its overriding message was: "There are effective treatments for mental illness. If you have symptoms, seek help."

- The *DSM-IV-TR* represents an ever-evolving, multiaxial classification system with diagnostic criteria for various mental illnesses.

- Stigma, costs, changing needs of the population, denial of illness, limited access to services, and lack of parity are some of the reasons two thirds of people with psychiatric symptoms do not seek treatment. Scientific and technologic advances and improvements in some of the systems of mental health care offer promising options for treatment and recovery.

- Self-help groups and advocacy movements have enhanced the understanding of the public and health care providers about the experience of clients with mental illness and their families. Research of such experience has led to the development of a model that describes these clients and families as adapting to a pathologic catastrophe.

- Psychiatric–mental health nursing is a unique discipline that contributes to the care of people with mental illness and to the promotion of mental health in the general population. Basic and advanced functions and roles of psychiatric–mental health nurses include advocacy, health promotion and maintenance, case management, screening, milieu therapy, health teaching, psychobiologic interventions, and participation in the interdisciplinary mental health team.

Study Questions

1. A client's medical record contains a diagnosis of schizophrenia. Using the *DSM-IV-TR* classification, the nurse would identify this disorder as belonging to which axis?

   a. Axis I

   b. Axis II

   c. Axis III

   d. Axis IV

2. When reviewing a client's history for possible influences on mental health, which of the following would the nurse identify as sociocultural?

   a. History of injuries

   b. Intelligence quotient

   c. Interactions with others

   d. Family stability

3. Which activities would be appropriate for a psychiatric–mental health nurse practicing at the basic level? Select all that apply.

   a. Prescribing psychopharmacologic medications

   b. Conducting individual therapy sessions

   c. Assessing biopsychosocial functioning

   d. Interpreting laboratory test results

References

Alonso, J., Buron, A., Rohas-Farreras, S., de Graaf, R., Haro, J., de Girolamo, G., ... Vilagut, G. (2009). Perceived stigma among individuals with common mental disorders. *Journal of Affective Disorders, 118*(1–3), 180–186.

American Nurses Association (ANA), American Psychiatric Nurses Association (APNA), & International Society of Psychiatric–Mental Health Nurses (ISPN). (2007). *Psychiatric–mental health nursing: Scope and standards of practice.* Silver Spring, MD: American Nurses Publishing.

American Psychiatric Association (APA). (2000). *Diagnostic and statistical manual of mental disorders* (4th ed., text rev.). Washington, DC: Author.

Centers for Disease Control and Prevention. (2010). Attitudes toward mental illness—35 states, District of Columbia, and Puerto Rico, 2007. *Morbidity & Mortality Weekly Report, 59*(20), 619–625.

Centers for Medicare and Medicaid Services. (2010). Mental Health Parity and Addictions Act of 2008. Retrieved from http://cciio .cms.gov/programs/protections/mhpaea/mhpaea_factsheet.html

Cohn, J. (2007). *Sick: The untold story of America's health care crisis and the people who pay the price.* New York, NJ: HarperCollins.

Corrigan, P. W. (2007). How clinical diagnosis might exacerbate the stigma of mental illness. *Social Work, 52*(1), 31–39.

Friedman, R. M., Pinto, A., Behar, L., Bush, N., Chirolla, A., Epstein, M., ... Klokeret, A. (2006). Unlicensed residential programs: The next challenge in protecting youth. *American Journal of Orthopsychiatry, 76*(3), 295–303.

Institute of Medicine. (2002). *Speaking of health: Assessing health communication strategies for diverse populations.* Washington, DC: National Academies Press.

Institute of Medicine. (2004a). *Health literacy: A prescription to end confusion.* Washington, DC: National Academies Press.

Institute of Medicine. (2004b). *In the nation's compelling interest: Ensuring diversity in the health-care workforce.* Washington, DC: National Academies Press.

Kennedy, S. S., Mercer, J., Mohr, W. K., & Huffine, C. (2002). Snake oil, ethics and the first amendment. What's a profession to do? *American Journal of Orthopsychiatry, 72*(1), 5–15.

Keyes, C. L. M. (2005). Mental illness and/or mental health? Investigating axioms of the complete state model of health. *Journal of Consulting and Clinical Psychology, 73*(3), 539–548.

Mallett, C. A. (2006). Behaviorally based disorders: The historical social construction of youths' most prevalent psychiatric diagnoses. *History of Psychiatry, 17,* 437–460.

McReynolds, C. J. (2002). Psychiatric rehabilitation: The need for a specialized approach. *International Journal of Psychosocial Rehabilitation, 7,* 61–69.

Mohr, W. K., Lafuze, J. E., & Mohr, B. D. (2000). Opening caregiver minds: NAMI's Provider Education Program. *Archives of Psychiatric Nursing, 14*(6), 285–295.

Morrison, J. (2006). *Diagnosis made easier: Principles and techniques for mental health clinicians.* New York, NY: Guilford Press.

National Alliance for the Mentally Ill (NAMI). (2007). *Inform yourself about mental illness.* Retrieved from http://www.nami.org/Content/Navigation/Menu/Inform_Yourself/About_Mental_Illness/About_Mental_Illness.htm

National Alliance for the Mentally Ill (NAMI). (2010a). Family to Family Program. Retrieved from http://www.nami.org/Template.cfm?Section=Family-to-Family

National Alliance for the Mentally Ill (NAMI). (2010b). Provider Education Program. Retrieved from http://www.nami.org/template.cfm?section=Provider_Education

National Institute of Mental Health (NIMH). (2006). *Mental health statistics.* Rockville, MD: Office of Consumer, Family and Public Information, Center for Mental Health Services. Retrieved from http://www.nimh.nih.gov/health/publications/the-numbers-count-mental-disorders-in-america/index.shtml

New Freedom Commission on Mental Health. (2003). *Achieving the promise: Transforming mental health care in America* (DHHS Pub. No. SMA-03-3832). Washington, DC: U.S. Department of Health and Human Services.

Pan American Health Organization. (2009). *Mental health in the U.S. and Latin America.* Retrieved from: http://new.paho.org/hq/index.php?option=com_content&task=view&id=1884&Itemid=259

Parker, G. (2006). Through a glass darkly: The disutility of the *DSM* nosology of depressive disorders. *Canadian Journal of Psychiatry, 51*(14), 879–886.

Reiger, D. A., Goldberg, I. D., & Taub, C. A. (1978). The de facto U.S. mental health services system: A public health perspective. *Archives of General Psychiatry, 35*(6), 685–693.

Rosenbaum, A., & Langhinrichsen-Rohling, J. (2006). Meta-research on violence and victims: The impact of data collection methods on findings and participants. *Violence & Victims, 21*(4), 404–409.

Sartorius, N. (2002). Iatrogenic stigma of mental illness. *British Medical Journal, 24,* 1470–1471.

Schouten, R. (2006). Commentary: Psychiatric advance directives as tools for enhancing treatment of the mentally ill. *Journal of the American Academy of Psychiatry & the Law, 34*(1), 58–60.

Sharfstein, S. M., Stoline, A. M., & Koran, L. M. (2002). Mental health services. In A. R. Kovner & S. Jonas (Eds.), *Health care delivery in the United States* (7th ed., pp. 246–247). New York, NY: Springer.

Texas Advocacy Center. (2007). Fact sheet on homelessness and the tragic effects of nontreatment. Retrieved from http://www.treatment.advocacycenter.org

U.S. Department of Health and Human Services (USDHHS). (1999). *Mental health: A report of the Surgeon General.* Rockville, MD: USDHHS, Substance Abuse and Mental Health Services Administration, Center for Mental Health Services, National Institutes of Health, National Institute of Mental Health.

Widiger, T. A., & Trull, T. J. (2007). Plate tectonics in the classification of personality disorder: Shifting to a dimensional model. *American Psychologist, 62*(2), 71–83.

World Health Organization (WHO). (2006a). *Frequently asked questions.* Retrieved from http://www.who.int/suggestions/faq/en

World Health Organization (WHO). (2006b). *The ICD-10 classification of mental and behavioural disorders—Diagnostic criteria for research.* Geneva, Switzerland: Author.

Web Resources

National Alliance for the Mentally Ill: http://www.nami.org/Content/NavigationMenu/Inform_Yourself/About_Mental_Illness/About_Mental_Illness.htm

National Institutes of Mental Health: http://www.nimh.nih.gov/health-information/index.cfm

Quackwatch: http://www.quackwatch.org

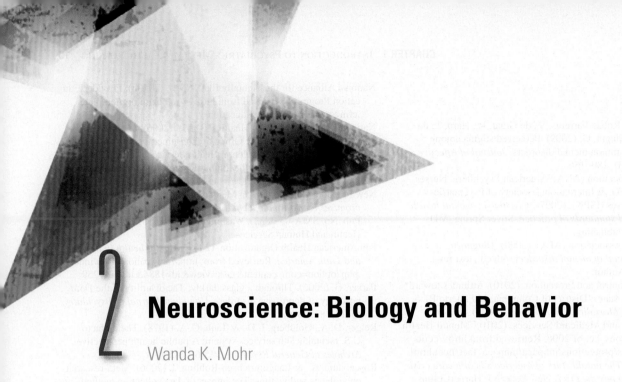

2

Neuroscience: Biology and Behavior

Wanda K. Mohr

KEY TERMS

action potential
adaptive plasticity
apoptosis
axon
blood–brain barrier
cell body
circadian rhythm
concordance rate
critical periods
dendrites
endophenotypes
first messengers
glial cells
learning
memory
neurogenesis
neurons
neuropeptides
neuroplasticity
neurotransmitters
psychoneuroimmunology
reactive plasticity
receptor
second hit
second messengers
stress–diathesis model
synapse
synaptic cleft

LEARNING OBJECTIVES

On completion of this chapter, you should be able to accomplish the following:

- Identify the basic structures of a neuron.
- Describe the process of neurotransmission.
- Discuss the relationship between neurotransmitters and mental illness.
- Describe how major structures of the brain are related to behavior.
- Discuss *neuroplasticity* and how this concept relates to mental health and mental illness.
- Briefly explain the importance of interaction between genes and environment, the role of endophenotypes, and the stress–diathesis model of psychiatric illness.
- Identify the different kinds of memory.
- Describe neuroimaging techniques and their relative advantages and disadvantages.

Research findings during the past few decades have made it abundantly clear that the brain is the organ of the mind. As the major organ of the nervous system, the brain governs *all* behavior of the body, including respiration, locomotion, and sensory activity, as well as cognition, thought, and the actions that constitute our conduct and performance as humans.

Although these statements are not late-breaking news, they are important to internalize completely and make part of a template through which nurses see and understand everything else in psychiatric–mental health nursing. Too often, chapters such as this are "tacked on" to the rest of the textbook, more or less gratuitously, so that authors and instructors can proceed with the "important" work of describing disorders and interventions. This failure to fully integrate the neurosciences into psychiatric–mental health nursing, however, impedes students from connecting nervous system functioning (biology) with behavior.

This problem may be related to difficulty in presenting material about the brain in a meaningful, understandable, and relevant way. Doing so is not easy, but the goals of this chapter are to briefly review the nervous system, neurotransmission, and brain structure and function; introduce the relationships among the brain, neurotransmission, and psychiatric illness; and summarize theories of higher brain functions as they relate to psychiatric–mental health nursing. One operative word is "brief," meaning that the neuroanatomical content is *not* comprehensive. Such vast information expands so rapidly that doing it justice in a single chapter is impossible. Every week, scientific journals publish new insights into the neural sciences, many of which conflict with or at least modify previous observations, hypotheses, or theoretical models. Genetics, neurophysiology, and brain function are so complex that they require their own courses. Detailed information on gray and white matter, membranes, myelin sheaths, and so forth can be found in specialty neuroanatomy texts. This chapter, limited to "need-to-know" material, conveys few minute details and instead focuses on overarching concepts. However, this chapter goes beyond other texts and tries to convey the dynamic nature of nervous system functioning and development by describing anatomical changes in the brain throughout the lifespan and the vital role of and interaction between genetics and environment.

Comprehensiveness in this chapter is impossible. There is simply too much material to convey. The intention is to relate certain aspects of nervous system functioning to what students might see in cases and clients whom they encounter in clinical settings. This chapter can help to inform future clinical experiences and to spur student and practicing nurses to think about interventions creatively, rather than generically. Such an approach may whet students' appetites for further study and "jog" their memories about relevant material learned in anatomy and physiology classes. For those wanting more in-depth information, the chapter's references contain useful current texts and articles.

NEUROANATOMY AND NEUROPHYSIOLOGY

The nervous system (including the brain) contains two broad classes of cells. The first, **glial cells**, provide mechanical and metabolic support for the second, known as neurons. **Neurons**, or nerve cells, are the basic units of structure and function in the nervous system.

Neurons

Approximately 100 billion neurons are in the brain alone. Any single neuron can release multiple types of molecular signals. It also can have receptors and receptor subtypes for multiple different molecular signals. Thus, each individual neuron is capable of exquisite integration and modulation of incoming and outgoing signals.

Each neuron consists of a **cell body** with a nucleus, other organelles, and snakelike extensions called **dendrites** and **axons** that both perform the vital function of transporting information (Figure 2.1). Neurons also synthesize proteins, which are produced as the result of gene activation. Most of the structural and regulatory molecules of a neuron consist of proteins, which means they also carry out orders from the genome.

Between each neuron are spaces called **synapses**, which serve as points of cellular contact. The estimated number of synapses in the human nervous system is staggering—from 10 to 100 trillion.

Neurotransmitters

Every neuron receives information encoded as electrical potentials at its dendritic processes. To transmit the information along the axon, the message must cross the synapse (gap) between adjacent neurons. An axon can make contact anywhere along the second neuron: on the dendrites (*axodendritic synapse*), the cell body (*axosomatic synapse*), or the axons (*axo-axonal synapse*). This complex crossing involves tiny explosive depolarizations and a release of chemical-transmitting substances called *neurotransmitters* (LeDoux, 2002; Porth, 2009). Thus, communication involves both electrical

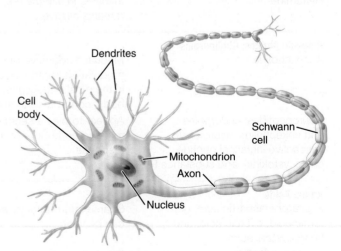

FIGURE 2.1 **Structure of a typical neuron.** Dendrites relay messages to the cell body, which then sends impulses along the axon.

and chemical activity. As a nerve impulse, or action potential, reaches the end of a presynaptic axon, molecules of neurotransmitter are released into the synaptic space.

Neurotransmitters are a diverse group of chemical compounds. Originally, approximately six neurotransmitters were known; current research has revealed several dozen, and several hundred to thousand may remain undiscovered (Stahl, 2008; Stein et al., 2006).

Checkpoint Questions
1. What are the basic units of structure and function in the nervous system?
2. How is information in the nervous system funneled in and out of individual cell bodies?

TYPES OF NEUROTRANSMITTERS. In addition to *acetylcholine*, the three major categories of neurotransmitters are as follows:

- *Amino acids* include glutamic acid, gamma-aminobutyric acid (GABA), aspartic acid, and glycine. They serve as the brain's major "workhorse" neurotransmitters.
- *Peptides* include vasopressin, somatostatin, and neurotensin. They perform specialized functions in the hypothalamus or act as cofactors elsewhere in the brain.
- *Monoamines* include norepinephrine, dopamine, and serotonin. Along with acetylcholine, they perform specialized modulating functions, often confined to specific structures.

More information about neurotransmitters is presented in (Table 2.1) and (Box 2.1).

TABLE 2.1 Some Neurotransmitters and Their Functions

Neurotransmitter	Presumed Function	Possible Implications for Mental Illness
Biogenic Amines: Catecholamines		
Dopamine	Involved in pleasurable feelings and complex motor activities	Schizophrenia
Norepinephrine	Regulates awareness of environment, attention, learning, memory, and arousal	Mood disorders
Epinephrine	Has limited presence in the brain; contributes to the "fight-or-flight" response	
Biogenic Amines: Indolamines		
Serotonin	Contributes to temperature regulation	*Low levels:* depression, aggression, suicidality, and impulsivity *High levels:* anxiety disorders (fearfulness, avoidance)
Histamine	Involved in allergic responses; role in CNS remains elusive	Weight gain associated with psychotropic medications
Biogenic Amines: Cholinergics		
Acetylcholine	Mediates cognitive functioning directly or by modulating another neurotransmitter indirectly; is the most widely used neurotransmitter in the body; contributes to sleep–wake cycles	Sleep disorders
Neuropeptides: endorphins and enkephalins, neurotensin, vasoactive intestinal peptide, cholecystokinin, and substance P	Appear to play a secondary messenger role and contribute to modulating the pain response	Alzheimer's disease, movement disorders
Amino Acids		
Excitatory: aspartic acid, glutamic acid, cysteic acid, and homocysteic acid	Sparse information available; high levels can be toxic	
Inhibitory: GABA	Slows down body activity	Dementia, schizophrenia, and anxiety disorders

BOX 2.1 Neurotransmitters in the Brain

Amines

- Serotonin
- Dopamine
- Norepinephrine
- Epinephrine
- Acetylcholine
- Tyramine
- Octopamine
- Phenylethylamine
- Tryptamine
- Melatonin

Pituitary Peptides

- Corticotropin
- Growth hormone
- Lipotropin
- Alpha-melanocyte-stimulating hormone
- Oxytocin
- Vasopressin
- Thyroid-stimulating hormone
- Prolactin

Circulating Hormones

- Angiotensin
- Calcitonin
- Glucagon
- Insulin
- Leptin
- Atrial natriuretic factor
- Estrogens
- Androgens
- Progestins
- Thyroid hormones

Hypothalamic-Releasing Hormones

- Corticotropin-releasing factor
- Gonadotropin-releasing hormone
- Somatostatin
- Thyrotropin-releasing hormone

Amino Acids

- GABA

- Glycine
- Glutamic acid
- Aspartic acid
- Gamma-hydroxybutyrate

Gut Hormones

- Cholecystokinin
- Gastrin
- Motilin
- Pancreatic polypeptide
- Secretin
- Vasoactive intestinal peptide

Opioid Peptides

- Dynorphin
- Beta-endorphin
- Met-enkephalin
- Leu-enkephalin
- Kyotorphin

Miscellaneous Peptides

- Bombesin
- Bradykinin
- Carnosine
- Neuropeptide Y
- Neurotensin
- Delta sleep factor
- Galanin
- Oxerin

Gases

- Nitric oxide
- Carbon monoxide

Lipid Neurotransmitter

- Anandamide

Neurokinins/Tachykinins

- Substance P
- Neurokinin A
- Neurokinin B

Nurses need a basic working knowledge of the major neurotransmitters because many psychiatric medications work to increase or decrease neurotransmitter levels in the brain (see Chap. 16). Moreover, too much neurotransmitter activity can lead to symptoms. For example, when too much excitatory neurotransmission occurs, it is hypothesized that this overproduction may mediate symptoms such as those associated with panic attacks (Stahl, 2008). However, this way of viewing neurotransmitter action can be an oversimplification and lead to cause-and-effect thinking. Neurotransmitters

can affect each other's levels and functioning, as well as regions and systems *beyond the brain*. For example, serotonin has been implicated as influencing sexual functioning; norepinephrine acts on both alpha-1 and alpha-2 adrenergic receptors to cause vasoconstriction and increase blood pressure.

Although the CNS has many neurotransmitters, the peripheral nervous system has only two: acetylcholine and norepinephrine. Why does the brain have so many neurotransmitters? Because the functions performed by brain neurotransmitters are not as uniform or straightforward as they might appear. Some neurotransmitters (like glutamate) are excitatory; others (like GABA) are primarily inhibitory. In many cases (as with dopamine) the receptor determines whether the neurotransmitter is excitatory or inhibitory. Receptors also can determine whether a neurotransmitter acts rapidly, by direct effect on an ion channel (eg, nicotinic acetylcholine receptors), or slowly, by a second messenger system that enables synaptic plasticity (eg, muscarinic acetylcholine receptors). Speed and mechanism of neurotransmitter inactivation after the signal has been sent are additional variations.

PROCESS OF NEUROTRANSMISSION. Most neurotransmitters are synthesized and stored in the terminal region of the neuron, where they are released after electrical stimulation (an **action potential**) causes the neuron to fire (ie, become depolarized). Depolarization causes changes in the fluxes of particular ions across a cell membrane. The neurotransmitters then diffuse across the **synaptic cleft** to act on and attach to receptors in the membrane of the postsynaptic cell. This postsynaptic cell may be another neuron, a muscle cell, or a specialized gland cell.

Neurotransmitters can either inhibit or excite the receptor cell, making an axon discharge more or less likely. The nerve cell "decides" whether to send output as a result of the number of inhibitory or excitatory inputs it receives. Cells are more likely to become depolarized if the neurotransmitter is excitatory, or less likely if it is inhibitory.

Receptors themselves are proteins and are unique to specific neurotransmitters. They can be located either postsynaptically, on the next neuron that the neuron releasing the transmitter excites or inhibits, or presynaptically, on the neuron that has released the transmitter. See Understanding Biologic Foundations 2.1 for an illustrated guide to neurotransmission.

Neurotransmitters are deactivated in one of two ways. They can be broken down by multiple subtypes of enzymes (eg, monoamine oxidase, peptidases), or they can be broken down by multiple subtypes of transporter proteins (eg, reuptake pumps).

FIRST AND SECOND MESSENGERS. Neurotransmitters are referred to as **first messengers**, which means molecules that communicate information or change *from one cell or cell group to another* cause an immediate effect and are typically found in circuitry that produces behavior (Kandel et al., 2000; Porth, 2009). They fit specific receptors on neurons. The presence of first messengers in varying quantities at the synaptic site is implicated in many conditions, such as schizophrenia, major depression, and bipolar disorder.

Neurotransmitters also can produce their effects by modulating the production of other signal-transducing molecules, called **second messengers**. A second messenger is a substance manufactured from the coupling of a first messenger to a receptor. Second messenger systems are complex and cause delayed effects. In second messenger systems, the activation of a receptor by a neurotransmitter initiates a cascade of intracellular events with the potential to change long-term neurotransmission.

Second messenger systems orchestrate highly elegant activity with many intracellular possibilities (Waxman, 2003). For example, one such system may infuse the nucleus of a neuron and directly affect genes that ultimately fuel the expression of protein and enzymes. Thus, the system may refine genetic expression, leading to genotypic alterations. Again, this complex neuronal behavior represents far more than cellular depolarization. The potential is for lasting changes in the postsynaptic neuron and in the system within which the neuron functions. Because effects on nucleus activity via chromosomal and genetic modifications are complicated, these second messenger systems operate slowly. It can take hours for genetic changes to begin and days for them to be fully operationalized. The actual duration of effect can last weeks.

Research has revealed that there are third and fourth messengers that initiate an entire cascade of signal transduction. Signal transduction at the cellular level refers to the movement of signals from outside the cell to inside. This shower of signal transduction allows for neurons to respond in a wide array of ways to chemical messaging systems.

PSYCHIATRIC NURSING IMPLICATIONS. At one time, students were taught mantras such as "schizophrenia—too much dopamine; depression—too little serotonin." Although the specific contributions of neurotransmitters to mental illness are not known, recent evidence suggests that no single neurotransmitter is responsible for any one disorder. Current findings indicate that psychiatric illnesses are associated with alterations in several neurotransmitters. Moreover, the alterations may result not from a simple abundance or overabundance of neurotransmitters, but from ratios of various neurotransmitters or any number of complex permutations. Later chapters that focus on major psychiatric disorders discuss the latest hypotheses about the role of neurotransmission in specific mental illnesses.

Psychopharmacotherapy involves blocking or enhancing certain neurotransmitters (see Chap. 16). Although neurotransmitters are numerous (see Box 2.1), three major neurotransmitter pathways in the brain are essential to understanding certain psychiatric conditions and the actions of medications used to treat them. These are the dopamine, norepinephrine, and serotonin pathways. See Understanding Biologic Foundations 2.2.

The first and second messenger modulation systems, and the complex cascade of responses from third and fourth messaging systems, account for how long it takes some drugs to exert their therapeutic actions against mental illness. Unlike many medications used for medical–surgical conditions, blood levels of psychotropic medications do not necessarily correlate with clinical response. This outcome can be frustrating for clients who are seeking immediate relief and is an important teaching point for nurses to review with clients and families.

UNDERSTANDING BIOLOGIC FOUNDATIONS 2.1

Neurotransmission

Synthesis and Release. Neurotransmitters are synthesized in the presynaptic neuron, where they are stored in the terminal region. When a nerve impulse stimulates the presynaptic neuron, the neurotransmitters are released into the synaptic cleft.

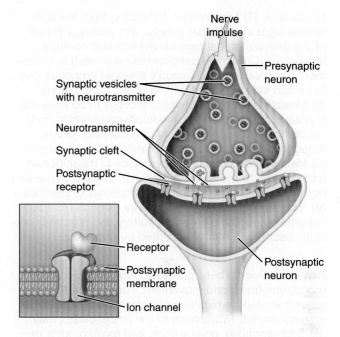

Binding. The neurotransmitters then move across the synaptic cleft to bind to receptors on the postsynaptic neuron. The type of receptor (inhibitory or excitatory) determines the specific action of the neurotransmitter.

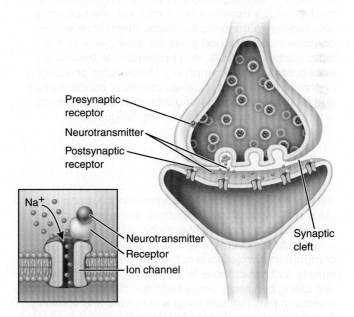

Think About It 2.1

How would you expect imbalances in neurotransmitters to affect mental health? Why does it take some psychotropic medications that affect major neurotransmission systems from 3 weeks to up to 1 year to achieve stabilization of certain psychiatric conditions?

Plasticity

In addition to its transmitting properties, the most significant property of nervous tissue is plasticity. Neuroplasticity is the brain's ability to reorganize itself by forming new neuronal connections throughout life. Neuroplasticity allows neurons to compensate for injury and disease and adjust their activities in response to new situations or to changes in their environment. Neuroplasticity is presented in more detail later in this chapter.

UNDERSTANDING BIOLOGIC FOUNDATIONS 2.2

Major Neurotransmitter Pathways in Mental Health

Dopamine. **(1)** *Nigrostriatal.* Extending from the substantia nigra to the basal ganglia, this pathway is part of the extrapyramidal nervous system and controls movement. Dopamine deficiencies here result in movement disorders (eg, Parkinson's disease) and contribute to certain side effects of antipsychotic medications. **(2)** *Mesolimbic.* This pathway is thought to be involved in pleasurable sensations and euphoria resulting from substance abuse. Overactivity of dopamine here is thought to contribute to hallucinations and delusions. **(3)** *Mesocortical.* This pathway begins in the midbrain and projects to the limbic cortex. It is thought to mediate both the negative and cognitive symptoms of psychosis. **(4)** *Tuberoinfundibular.* This pathway extends from the hypothalamus to the anterior pituitary and regulates prolactin secretion, which is inhibited by dopamine.

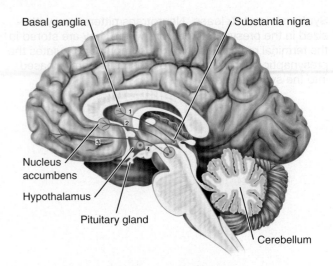

Norepinephrine. These pathways regulate cognitive mood, emotions, and movement. They originate in the locus coeruleus, which focuses attention on internal or external stimuli. Projections to the limbic cortex may mediate emotions, energy level, and psychomotor retardation, whereas projections to the cerebellum may mediate motor movements. Norepinephrine pathways also regulate autonomic functions. Projections to the brainstem control blood pressure, projections to the heart control heart rate, and projections to the urinary tract control bladder emptying. Deficiencies of norepinephrine may lead to impaired attention, concentration, and memory; delayed information processing; depression; psychomotor retardation; and fatigue.

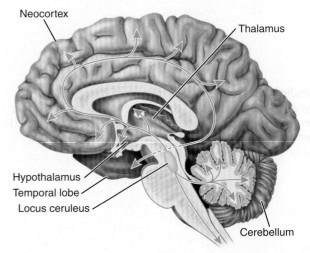

Serotonin. These pathways originate in the raphe nucleus of the brainstem. Projections to the frontal cortex may regulate mood, whereas those to the basal ganglia may regulate movement as well as obsessions and compulsions. Projections to the limbic areas may control anxiety and panic; those to the hypothalamus may regulate eating behaviors. Projections to different areas of the brainstem may regulate sleep and nausea and vomiting. Serotonin neurons that project down the spinal cord may control sexual responses such as orgasm and ejaculation. Last, receptors in the gut may regulate both appetite and gastrointestinal functioning. Deficiencies in serotonin may lead to depressed mood, anxiety, panic, phobia, obsessions, compulsions, food cravings, and bulimia.

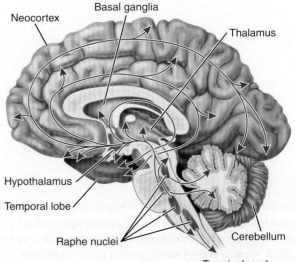

Neurogenesis

Neurogenesis is the process by which neurons are born, and the brain is endowed with the ability to restore itself through the production, differentiation, and migration of precursor or blast cells into new functioning neurons. It was once thought that this process was limited to developing organisms, but we now know that neurogenesis occurs throughout a person's lifespan. Neurogenesis can be stimulated through such activities as learning, psychotherapy, endogenous growth factors, and certain medications.

Apoptosis

In addition to neurogenesis, another important activity of neurons is known as **apoptosis**. Apoptosis, the process of cell death, can be thought of as the opposite of neurogenesis. Under certain conditions throughout the life cycle, cells kill themselves in a kind of suicidal process of fading away. This happens extensively before birth, during fetal development, throughout which billions of redundant neurons undergo apoptosis between conception and birth. Apoptosis is programmed into the human genome of various cells and, when the process is activated, the cell self-destructs. Apoptosis should not be confused with cell necrosis, which occurs as a result of sudden injury or inflammatory response.

Central Nervous System

The neurons enclosed in the bony coverings of the skull and vertebral column make up the CNS, which consists of the spinal cord and brain. Neurons outside the CNS make up the *peripheral nervous system,* which carries information into the CNS. The peripheral nervous system also carries motor impulses outward to muscles and glands.

Spinal Cord

The spinal cord provides a channel through which sensory information from the body reaches the brain. The cord also contains pathways for voluntary control of skeletal muscles and the neural systems that regulate functioning of the internal organs. The neural systems of the spinal cord also are the bases for integrated and coordinated limb movement.

Brain

For years, the remarkable human brain was viewed as relatively static, determined by the interaction of genetic programming and early childhood experiences. Recent contrasting theoretical perspectives, as well as technologic advances in brain imaging, have revealed that the brain is continually built and rebuilt based on experiences (Cozolino, 2002, 2007).

The brain is an exceedingly vital and complex organ relative to its small size (Figure 2.2). It is encapsulated and protected by three lining membranes (*meninges, pia mater,* and *dura mater*) and the bony enclosure of the skull. The inner lining of the cerebral blood vessels provides additional protection, forming tight connections that limit the entry of blood elements (Bear et al., 2006; Beatty, 2001). This protective connection is known as the **blood–brain barrier**.

ORGANIZATION AND STRUCTURE. The brain has a hierarchical organization. "Lower" parts mediate simple regulatory functions, such as respiration, heartbeat, and body

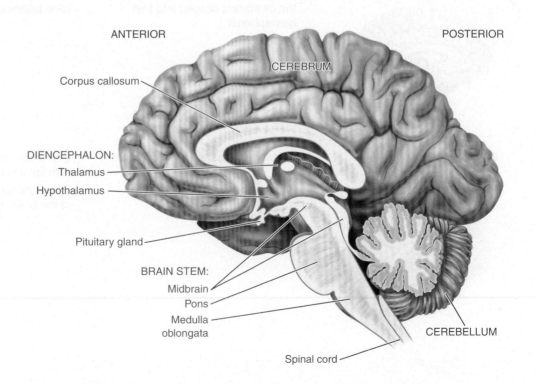

FIGURE 2.2 Sagittal section of the brain, showing major divisions.

temperature. "Higher" cortical structures mediate complex functions, such as language and abstract thought.

Damage to any part of the brain results in functional deficits. For example, damage to two parts of the occipital lobe (Broca's and Wernicke's areas) results is language deficits specific to the section affected. Chronic alcoholism can damage the hippocampus, leading to *Korsakoff's syndrome*, in which a person cannot form new memories despite intact intelligence. Destruction of the amygdala causes a decreased aggressive response in animals (Bear et al., 2006).

Major structures of the brain include the cerebrum, diencephalon, cerebellum, and brainstem (Table 2.2). Additional important structures are the limbic system and basal ganglia. Although the sections below describe the roles and functions

TABLE 2.2 **Organization of the Brain**

Division	Description	Functions
Cerebrum	Largest and uppermost portion of the brain; divided into two hemispheres, each subdivided into lobes	Cortex (outer layer) is site for conscious thought, memory, reasoning, and abstract mental functions, all localized within specific lobes
Diencephalon	Between the cerebrum and the brainstem; contains the thalamus, hypothalamus, and pineal gland	Thalamus sorts and redirects sensory input; hypothalamus maintains homeostasis, controls autonomic nervous system and pituitary gland
Cerebellum	Below the posterior portion of the cerebrum; divided into two hemispheres	Coordinates voluntary muscles; maintains balance and muscle tone
Brainstem	Anterior region below the cerebrum	Connects cerebrum and diencephalon with spinal cord
Pons	Anterior to the cerebellum	Connects cerebellum with other parts of the brain; helps regulate respiration

(continues on page 29)

TABLE 2.2 **Organization of the Brain** (continued)

Division	Description	Functions
Medulla oblongata	Between pons and spinal cord	Links brain with spinal cord; has centers for control of vital functions (eg, respiration, heartbeat)
Midbrain	Below the center of the cerebrum	Has reflex centers concerned with vision and hearing; connects cerebrum with lower brain portions

of various parts of the brain, nurses should keep in mind that the systems of the brain interact and do not operate in isolation. Current evidence shows that correlating one area with one function is an oversimplification. Networks and systems within the brain interact to produce what a person eventually experiences or observes as thoughts, feelings, or behaviors.

Cerebrum. The *cerebrum,* composed of the frontal, parietal, occipital, and temporal regions, contributes to intellectual function, including learning, judgment, reasoning, and memory (Figure 2.3). It also plays a primary role in processing emotions and sensory input from voluntary muscles. The *cerebral cortex* (cortex of the cerebrum) forms the outer layer of the cerebral lobes and plays an important role in processing sensory information from the environment. It can be thought of as a map formation engine, organizing incoming signals and creating dynamic representations of this input. Depending on the frequency and intensity of such input, these representations change through a complex rewiring of cortical connections. These input-driven changes are a function of *neuroplasticity.* Lack of sensory input or severe trauma during crucial periods of a person's life can affect the cerebral cortex negatively and result in future adaptive difficulties.

Diencephalon. The *diencephalon* consists of the thalamus, hypothalamus, and pineal gland. The thalamus acts as a large relay station through which sensory information passes on its way to other cortical regions. Beneath the thalamus is

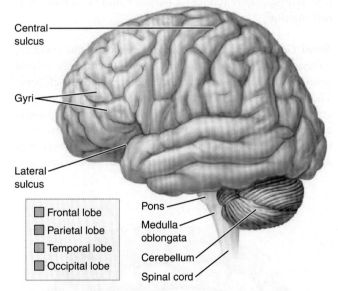

Central sulcus

Gyri

Lateral sulcus

☐ Frontal lobe
☐ Parietal lobe
☐ Temporal lobe
☐ Occipital lobe

Pons
Medulla oblongata
Cerebellum
Spinal cord

FIGURE 2.3 Lobes of the cerebral cortex and relationships of various areas to human function.

the hypothalamus, which is the control center for endocrine, somatic, and autonomic functioning. Hormones from the hypothalamus are released into the bloodstream and modulate many body functions, including drinking, salt balance, sexual activity, feeding, body temperature, and feelings of rage. The pineal gland secretes melatonin, a hormone that affects the sleep–wake cycle.

Cerebellum. The complex *cerebellum* controls and guides movements and maintains muscle tone. Damage to the cerebellum results in characteristic movement disorders. For example, the person may execute normally delicate movements quite violently or show errors in the strength and direction of movements. Impaired gait is an example of alcohol's toxic effects on cerebellar functioning.

Brainstem. The *brainstem* includes the pons, medulla oblongata, reticular formation, and midbrain. The nerve-fiber pathways of the *pons* send information to other areas of the CNS. The *medulla oblongata* controls respiration, gastrointestinal motility, and circulation. The *reticular formation* controls sleep and wakefulness and directs visual and auditory reflexes. The *midbrain* is vital to life. In some tragic circumstances, it is the only brain area maintaining heart and lung function in an otherwise comatose person with no higher-level capacities.

Limbic System. The *limbic system,* located beneath the cerebral cortex, contains the *hippocampus, amygdala,* and *fornix* (Figure 2.4). The limbic system is involved with emotions, memory, and learning. It is also thought to mediate aggressive feelings, sexual impulses, and submissive behaviors. Damage to the limbic system has been implicated in several conditions. For example, because the hippocampus consolidates new information into memories, damage there reduces a person's ability to learn new information.

Basal Ganglia. The *basal ganglia* consist of the *caudate, putamen,* and *globus pallidus.* These functionally related neuron groups initiate and control activities and muscle tone. They elaborate and integrate complex voluntary motor processes to allow smooth actions. In addition, the basal ganglia assume motor skills that have become automatic. Lesions in the basal ganglia cause involuntary or delayed movements and loss of automatic movement and facial expression.

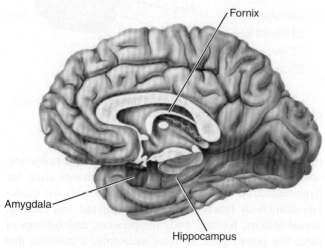

FIGURE 2.4 The limbic system.

Checkpoint Questions
3. What structures are part of the diencephalon?
4. What is the role of the limbic system?

BRAIN DEVELOPMENT. During the intrauterine period, a great excess of neurons is produced—perhaps twice as many as necessary. The fetal brain grows at an amazing rate; at times, 250,000 neurons are added every minute. Excess neurons are eliminated in the final months of pregnancy and in the months just after birth. The brain has all the neurons that it will ever have at birth; however, the brain continues to grow in size for a few years. By age 2 years, the brain is approximately 80% of adult size.

Genetic influences are of primary significance in intrauterine brain development. Nevertheless, the complexity of organization and connections of the nervous system far exceed the capacity of the genome to specify each cell location and axon trajectory. The local chemical milieu of the developing fetus and the maternal uterus collaborate with genetic plans to specify CNS organization. Broad exogenous factors also are involved, including maternal health, nutrition, and contact with potential toxins (eg, tobacco, alcohol and other drugs, certain viruses). The local dynamic intrauterine mechanisms also may be significant, a fact especially pertinent for multiple fetuses, in which intrauterine position may markedly affect the size and vigor of each. Even maternal state of mind may be significant. Some cultures believe that an infant will bear the visible imprint of an object that frightens its mother during her pregnancy. More positively, Japanese women think happy thoughts (taikyo) during pregnancy to ensure the health and well-being of their babies. Recent data suggest that newborns are more likely to respond to sound combinations (words) characteristic of the mother's language than to those of a foreign tongue. By implication, the fetus, especially in the third trimester, may already be sensitive to stimuli in the maternal external environment (Afifi & Bergman, 2005; Snell, 2009).

During infancy and childhood, the human brain develops rapidly, acquiring an entire set of capabilities. Experiences guide the sequential process of development, from less to more complex. The brain modifies and changes itself in response to new events, with neurons and neuronal connections evolving in an "activity-dependent" manner (Bear et al., 2006; National Academy of Sciences [NAS], 2000). In other words, the activity to which neurons are exposed drives their response. For example, visual learning in children causes neurons to develop and neuronal connections to form in the visual pathways. However, without such stimuli, visual development may cease. Scientists demonstrated this phenomenon during a study in which they deprived a sample of kittens of light and visual stimuli for several weeks, both before and after the kittens' eyes opened. Despite no gross anatomical differences between the visually deprived kittens and their littermates, the visually deprived kittens were rendered blind. Their visual neurons were never activated for sight through exposure to the stimuli needed for them to grow and network.

Thus, development of the brain is use dependent. As certain neural systems are activated repeatedly, the brain creates a corresponding internal representation of the experience. This use-dependent capacity to make such representations provides the basis for learning and memory (NAS, 2000).

The capacity and desire for emotional relationships is related to the organization and functioning of specific systems of the human brain, which develop during the first years of life. This capacity peaks during childhood, making children far more malleable and receptive to environmental stimuli than adults. Experiences during this vulnerable period can have critical influences on abilities for intimate and healthy relationships (Figure 2.5). By age 3 years, the brain is 90% of its adult size, and the emotional, behavioral, cognitive, and social foundation is in place for the rest of life. A child's earlier repertoire of experiences provides an organizing framework or template through which he or she filters subsequent experiences.

Children's use-dependent brains mirror the pattern, timing, nature, frequency, and quality of their experiences. For optimal brain development, children must be exposed to appropriate sensory information. The consequences of sequential development are that as different

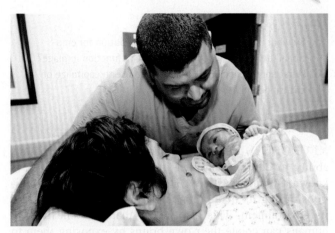

FIGURE 2.5 It is during the human's earliest years that the capacity for developing relationships forms. This begins in the earliest days of life. (Photo courtesy of Joe Mitchell.)

regions organize, they require specific data to develop properly. For example, a child must be exposed to visual input while the visual system is organizing. These developmental times are called **critical periods**. Without a sufficient number and duration of experiences during critical periods, children lose some of their genetic potential to develop commensurate skills. Moreover, a disruption in the timing, intensity, quality, or quantity of normal developmental experiences may have devastating consequences. See Client-Centered Education 2.1.

Client-Centered Education 2.1

Encouraging Optimal Learning in Children

In their teaching role, nurses can educate families about the importance of exposing children to optimal learning experiences. Tips to give parents and adult caregivers include the following:

- Because very young brains are more plastic than older ones, interventions are more likely to succeed with younger children than older children. It will take older children longer to develop new behaviors that will override existing ones.
- Although optimal and critical periods exist during which children should be exposed to certain activities, parents should not make life stressful for their children by enrolling them in every enrichment program available. Activities as simple as play and reading to children positively influence both future prosocial behaviors and language acquisition.
- The interaction of life events and developmental variables, such as genetic characteristics, is important to understanding children's behavior. Behavior comes from somewhere, and it is always meaningful. The meaning of a child's behavior, however, may differ from what parents may think. For example, toddlers may act fussy and difficult during a long religious service. Such behavior is entirely normal; small children are not "wired" to sit

for long periods exposed to things that they perceive as tedium. Exposing children to experiences for which they are not developmentally ready can lead to unintended consequences. In this case, the child may develop an aversion to church. Or a child who normally behaves well during church may simply be hungry or tired. Parents should always look for more than one meaning.

- Children's responses are not "psychological" or "mental" patterns. They are physiologic patterns expressed cognitively and, thereby, behaviorally. The potency of children's behavioral and cognitive responses to like stimuli will correlate strongly with the strength of prior experiences. This is why children like to play the same activity or have the same book read to them over and over. Although adults may find such repetition boring, it is essential and comforting to children.
- Children exposed to rich sensory experiences and many protective factors, as opposed to risk factors, will experience fewer maladaptive responses than their counterparts. Parents should try to decrease risk factors (eg, exposure to violence) and increase protective factors (eg, stable home life) as much as possible for children to become resilient.

Checkpoint Questions

5. By what age is most of a person's foundation for emotional, behavioral, cognitive, and social function in place?

6. What approach is best for parents to use to capitalize on critical periods?

Think About It 2.2

How can neuroplasticity influence psychotherapy? What techniques can health care professionals use to help clients perform new, more adaptive behaviors?

NEUROPLASTICITY. As described previously, the brain's ability to develop and alter in response to experience is known as **neuroplasticity**. The brain adapts to new conditions during its maturation and constant interaction with its environment. This also means that, to some degree, humans can create their own brains by exposing them to certain experiences. Stimuli in the internal or external environment trigger neuroplastic mechanisms. Thus, as mentioned in the preceding section, brain development depends on exposure to certain environmental stimuli and subsequent activation of developing pathways (Bear et al., 2006).

Neuroplasticity not only is responsible for how brains develop, but also enables people to avoid being completely at the mercy of early learning environments. The brain continues to form new connections, and exposure to new learning results in brain changes, even into advanced old age.

Two basic phenomena are involved in neuroplasticity, both of which depend on a structural change in neurons. The first type, **reactive plasticity**, is comparatively simple and brings about functional changes, which usually are reversible. The second type, **adaptive plasticity**, affects the expression of genotype into phenotype. Adaptive plasticity is not reversible.

PSYCHIATRIC NURSING IMPLICATIONS. The concept of neuroplasticity provides the foundation for learning, memory, and other complex mental processes. It is important to remember that all learning is brain based. Learning is a form of adaptation in response to specific life experiences. Psychotherapy is nothing more than assisting people to acquire knowledge or develop the ability to perform new behaviors. It is a form of education. Thus, education in the form of psychotherapy is literally an attempt to change the brain's structure so changes in behavior will follow. This would not be possible without neuroplasticity and its role in new learning.

Neuroscientific findings and brain imaging techniques are providing support for many forms of psychotherapy. For example, research has been conducted on the outcomes of psychotherapy as opposed to psychopharmacotherapy. Studies with positron emission tomography (PET) found that both behavior therapy and fluoxetine (Prozac) produced similar decreases in cerebral metabolic rates in the head of the right caudate nucleus (Cozolino, 2002). This result suggests that behavior psychotherapy and fluoxetine have similar physiologic effects on the brain.

The Role of Genetics

The role of genes on human development and behavior cannot be underestimated. *Genes* are segments of DNA. Their organization may be thought of as templates within chromosomes. *Chromosomes* contain the DNA, which in turn contains the instructions for the development and maintenance of the entire human body. Genes are like bytes of information for the production of proteins. Their enormous amounts of coding information serve as a blueprint for biologic processes. Genes are responsible for transmitting hereditary characteristics (Ridley, 2003).

Cells read genes in two steps: transcription and translation. *Transcription* is the process by which DNA sequences are copied into RNA. *Translation* is the process by which information in RNA produces strings of amino acids, which in turn make up proteins (life's building blocks).

Genetic templates coordinate and maintain all cellular activity. Each person inherits two complements of chromosomes, one from each parent. Parents and their biologic children, full siblings, and nonidentical twins share 50% of their genes. Grandchildren share approximately 25% of their grandparents' genes.

Each gene has a specific location on the chromosome called an *allele*. Variations and combinations in inherited allele patterns determine various traits. Each parent transmits one allele for each gene. When parents transmit the same allele for a given gene, the child is considered *homozygous* for that gene. When they transmit dissimilar alleles, the child is considered *heterozygous*.

Genes are related to the expression of certain traits. Genetic variations are hypothesized to result in individual differences in behavior and emotional responsiveness to environmental stimuli. The combinations of these genetic parameters, altered by environmental influences over time, are referred to as the *phenotype*. For example, if a person is homozygous for a gene that contributes to heightened physiologic arousal, he or she may have an increased inclination to overreact to stressful life events (Ridley, 2003).

Genetics and Psychiatric Disorders

In the 19th century, Gregor Mendel demonstrated certain regularities of trait expression. While conducting research, Mendel deduced that traits were inherited in certain numerical ratios. He derived certain basic laws of heredity:

• Hereditary factors do not combine but are passed intact from one generation to the next.

• Each parent transmits only half of his or her hereditary factors to each offspring.
• Certain hereditary factors are dominant over others.
• Different offspring of the same parents receive different sets of hereditary factors.

Mendel's classic theory of genetics accurately explains the likelihood of certain traits when one hereditary factor is dominant over another. However, his simple model does not explain the heritability of psychiatric illnesses or subtle traits such as temperament. Human genome research has revealed that each chromosome is studded with variations unique to it, and that these variations (called *restriction fragment length polymorphisms* [RFLPs]) may contribute to the expression of certain disorders. The identification of actual RFLPs and their potential role in heredity may soon reveal many mendelian inheritance assumptions to be oversimplifications.

An example of the failure of mendelian inheritance assumptions involves the transmission of schizophrenia. Monozygotic (identical) twins share the same in utero environment and, in most cases, other environments after birth. Studies have shown that their **concordance rate**—that is, the rate at which the second twin will have a disorder if the first one has it—for schizophrenia is approximately 50%. In dizygotic (nonidentical) twins, the concordance rate is considerably lower. Likewise, prevalence studies of dyslexia have shown that if one twin has the disorder, the other twin has a 90% chance of also having dyslexia. In the case of nonidentical twins, the concordance rate for dyslexia falls to 30%.

Such gene studies challenge simplistic ideas about inheritance and suggest that interaction between the genes and the circumstances under which genes are expressed is complex. If identical twins share the same genes, and those genes are programmed toward the development of an illness, then why wouldn't the concordance rate be 100% for schizophrenia? The section that follows may help explain this puzzle.

Interaction Between Genes and Environment

Previous sections explained that how humans develop, adapt, and behave depends on the interaction of physiology and environment. But the picture is not so simple. Genes play an enormous role in the expression of certain talents, conditions, and pathologies. Psychiatric disorders, like all disorders, depend on a complex interaction of genetic and environmental factors, which in turn also affect brain development and subsequent function.

Variable disease patterns in identical twins suggest that factors beyond genes are involved. One might hypothesize that because monozygotic twins have exactly identical genetic material, their development would be exactly identical as well, but this is not so, as evidenced by their concordance rate for schizophrenia (Figure 2.6). Thus, some other factor or factors must contribute to schizophrenia in one twin but not the other.

These other factors, found in the environment, are called **second hits**. Examples might include intense experiential toxins, such as physical abuse or neglect, infections, or prenatal exposure to alcohol (Ridley, 2003). These second hits may also include stress, but mental illness is

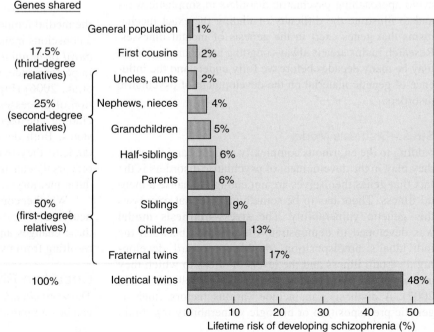

FIGURE 2.6 **The complex etiology of mental disorders involves both biologic elements (eg, genetics) and environmental influences. The chart reflects the familial nature of schizophrenia. Risk increases with the number of genes family members share. However, if genes alone were responsible identical twins (who have the exact same genes) would have a 100% lifetime risk. Thus, other factors also must be involved.** (From: Bear, M. F., Connors, B., & Paradiso, M. [2006]. *Neuroscience: Exploring the human brain* [3rd ed.]. Philadelphia, PA: Lippincott Williams & Wilkins.)

not caused by stress or any other second hit. The limitless expression of second hits, their quality, and whether they are cumulative or one-time occurrences can be seen in the wide range of characteristic illness patterns in different people. To give a simple example, John and Bill have the exact same genes for a certain condition. John lives a benign middle-class existence with occasional minor troubles. Bill, however, spends 5 years in a war zone (eg, Iraq). The second hit in Bill might be devastating and contribute to the expression of illness, whereas John may never manifest that same disorder because his environment has been continuously more stable.

Recent genetic research introduces even greater complexity. In addition to the variability of gene expression and environmental experiences, multiple genes make partial contributions to the picture. Researchers believe that multiple genetic pathways may lead to vulnerability, with no one disorder specifically correlated with any one particular mutation. Thus, multiple changes in gene expression must occur for certain disorders to develop, and these unfold sequentially. The changes are based on the effects of stresses and life experiences, as well as the illness itself.

Further, a relatively new paradigm has emerged in psychiatry that conceptualizes genes not as direct causes of mental illness, but as causes of subtle molecular abnormalities that create the risk for mental illness. The concept applied to this notion is that of an **endophenotype**, which is a kind of biomarker that predisposes a person for a certain illness. Endophenotypes may be neurophysiologic, biochemical, endocrinologic, neuroanatomical, cognitive, or neuropsychological in nature. An endophenotype-based approach has the potential to assist in the genetic dissection of complex psychiatric diseases (Gottesman & Gould, 2003). It is beyond the scope of this text to discuss this approach in depth, but it is mentioned here to emphasize the need to avoid approaching psychiatric disorders in simplistic ways and to illustrate the difficulty of finding the exact mechanisms that genes exert in the genesis of mental illnesses. Research in this area is always ongoing and changing, but it may be many decades before we fully understand the influence of genetic material on the development of psychiatric disorders.

Stress–Diathesis Model

Adding to the enormous complexity of genes and the roles they play in the development of psychiatric disorders is the fact that genes themselves are not enough to cause a mental illness. There has to be something else that expresses this genetic vulnerability. The **stress–diathesis model** was developed to demonstrate the dynamic between the individual's predisposition (diathesis) toward developing a certain illness and the levels of stress to which they are subjected (Grunebaum et al., 2006; Ruelbach et al., 2007). A diathesis can include various factors, such as genetic predisposition or biologic vulnerability (eg, brain

abnormalities). Stress is the response that an individual experiences when presented with life events and experiences that they perceive as exceeding their coping abilities. Examples of some of the causes of stress are abuse, neglect, and exposure to traumatic events, such as war or natural disasters. In an individual with a genetic profile that puts him at risk for mental illness, the experience of trauma notably increases the likelihood of psychiatric symptoms. An individual with a protective gene may be resilient against stress and exhibit a normal phenotype even following a severe trauma.

Checkpoint Questions

7. What is meant by *concordance rate*?
8. What role do *second hits* play in the development of psychiatric disorders?

OTHER TOPICS IN NEUROSCIENCE

Memory, Repetition, and Learning

Because of neuroplasticity, living organisms can change their behavior in response to environmental events (stimuli). This capacity underpins the ability of every organism with a nervous system to learn and remember. **Learning** occurs when organisms take in and store information as a function of experience. **Memory** is the information stored as a result of learning. Learning results in neuronal changes at existing synapses. It also helps new synapses to develop, thereby causing behavioral change (Bear et al., 2006). Structural alterations at the cellular level are thought to result through changes in the effectiveness of existing synapses between cortical cells, the formation of new synapses among existing cortical neurons, and the creation of new neurons to support new memory (Kandel, 2007).

Declarative or *explicit memory storage*, mediated by the medial temporal lobe and the hippocampus, constitutes a conscious memory for people, places, and things. *Procedural* or *implicit memory* is unconscious and evident only in performance, rather than through conscious recall (Bear et al., 2006) (Figure 2.7). Procedural memory is a collection of processes involving several interrelated events, including cue recognition and various associated affective states. Both declarative and procedural memory work in tandem; they overlap. Constant repetition (eg, behavioral rehearsal) can transform declarative memory into procedural memory.

Whether conscious or not, memory is reflected in diffuse neuroanatomical changes. Neuroplasticity is responsible for these changes and may be the key to long-term alterations resulting from psychotherapeutic interventions.

Circadian Rhythm

The word *circadian* means "about a day." **Circadian rhythm** can be compared with a big internal clock that coordinates

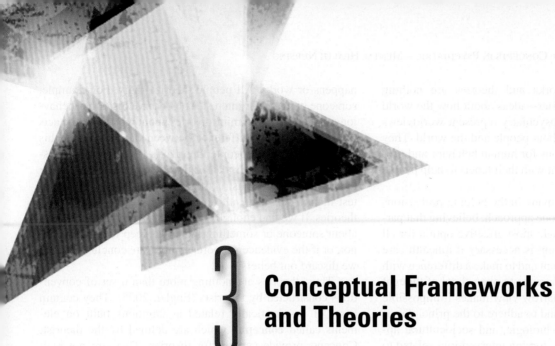

3

Conceptual Frameworks and Theories

Wanda K. Mohr

Conceptual frameworks and theories are nothing more than conjectures—ideas about how the world works. Various theories in psychology inform a would-be clinician's way of thinking. How people and the world think differently about these for human behavior, each may help the clinician with different kinds of psychiatric disorders.

A continuum interested in or dealing with such clients are conversations.

A nurse needs to be able to give attention to all aspects. Scientific examination is necessary for one to understand a why a nurse might make a difference with human behavior and which their client's care. A nurse understands how people behave and contribute to the principles of treatment psychoanalytic therapy, and so particular approach to care. In short, a nurse understands related to approaches may make a transaction to reach and help a person with a problem better in other actions, behaviors and functions.

No one theory can explain and answer a particular behavior or explain and some perspectives have more supporting research than others. Some are completely useless and lack an evidence base. Theodore care and theories have dominated mental health care and society. The assumptions that underlie them may dominate popular beliefs, even though many theories resist these beliefs. Consequently, many of these beliefs are popular and sophisticated as clients or clients' families who may offer behavior as certain complex symptoms (Wylton 1997). Today, clinicians often find that their ideas and beliefs have reached the public, who express and interpret them at the popular press and even in academic texts. This backlash speaks to its importance, and the endurance of popular ideas regarding certain human behaviors; some of these ideas have been discredited through scientific inquiry, and a mental health care provider and clinician change rapidly.

This chapter reviews several theories with which a nurse in psychiatric nursing or other mental health work must be familiar; however, not all theories is not encompassed by one chapter. It deals with only those that have achieved prominence based on their importance. Several theories and provides certain important concepts that the psychiatric nurse uses.

THEORIES: WHO CARES AND SO WHAT?

When we understand why the world seems more caring of human experience. The world seems healthier and dynamics and spatial quality. Use a theory is nothing more than a conjecture, a hunch, a supposition, a

KEY TERMS

- applied behavior analysis
- cognitions
- concepts
- conditioning
- countertransference
- defense mechanisms
- dialectic behavior therapy (DBT)
- discrimination
- generalization
- hypothesis
- modeling
- operant conditioning
- punishment
- reinforcement
- repressed
- respondent conditioning
- shaping
- theory
- transference
- unconscious
- utility

LEARNING OBJECTIVES

On completion of this chapter, you should be able to accomplish the following:

- Describe what is meant by *theory* and why theories are important to nursing practice.
- Differentiate the psychoanalytic, behavioral, cognitive, cognitive–behavioral, humanistic, interpersonal, biophysiologic, and sociocultural theories.
- Give examples of behavioral and cognitive–behavioral interventions.
- Describe a conceptual framework that incorporates several theories and its importance to understanding clients in development and context.

Conceptual frameworks and theories are nothing more than *worldviews*—ideas about how the world works. Various theories in psychiatry represent worldviews and are a way of thinking about people and the world. They all offer different explanations for human behavior and promote interventions consistent with their tenets to help people with psychiatric disorders.

A common mistake of many in the helping professions is overzealously embracing one approach, believing that particular method to be the single most effective option for all people. Although commitment is necessary if a health care professional is to be competent and to make a difference with clients, a single-minded adherence to one school of thought is not helpful. A rigid and narrow view makes it impossible to treat people holistically and to adhere to the principles of an integrated psychosocial, biologic, and sociocultural approach to care. Furthermore, forcing interventions related to one approach may make it impossible to reach and help people who would respond better to other options (Norcross & Goldfried, 2005).

No one theory adequately accounts for human behavior or mental illness, although some perspectives have more supporting research than others, and some are completely unsupported from an evidence-based standpoint. Competing theories have dominated mental health care at one time or another, sometimes to the detriment of both the field and clients. For example, as late as the 1970s, U.S. conventional wisdom posited that psychoanalysis was superior to biologic interventions. Consequently, many clinicians stopped prescribing neuroleptics or antidepressants in an effort to make clients "get to the root of their problems" rather than "covering up their symptoms" (Wyden, 1997). Today, the psychoanalytic movement is less influential, and many of its concepts have been debunked (Esterson, 1999; Kandel, 1998, 1999; Tallis, 1996). However, its vestiges remain in the popular press and even in academic texts. This finding speaks to its enormous past influence and the reluctance of professionals to give up cherished notions. It also underscores that, despite rapid and enormous expansion of knowledge, professional and clinical change happens slowly.

This chapter discusses several theories with which nurses working in psychiatric–mental health should be familiar. It includes historically important theories as well as those supported by solid research. It concludes with a holistic worldview or conceptual frame that incorporates several theories and provides enormous explanatory power for many psychiatric conditions.

THEORIES: WHO CARES AND SO WHAT?

When some students see the word *theory*, they either panic or their eyes glaze over. The word seems instilled with a mysterious or off-putting quality. Yet, a **theory** is nothing more than a person's or group's beliefs about how something

happens or works. All people theorize daily. For example, someone piques your interest. You observe his or her behavior and then construct mini-theories about why he or she acts that way. The only difference between the theories in this chapter and how all people theorize is that "theorists" systematically record their ideas. They then proceed to see if the theory "works" by constructing research studies designed to test it. In a sense, we all do the same with our own mini-theories. If we find enough "evidence" to support our beliefs about someone or something, then we keep them. If we do not, or if the evidence supports an opposite conclusion, then we discard our beliefs.

Thus, theories are nothing more than a set of conventions constructed by theorists (Engler, 2005). They contain a set of systematically related assumptions built on elements called **concepts**, which are defined by the theorist. Concepts provide support for theories. They are not real; they are merely representations. An example of a concept is "self-esteem." Self-esteem is not tangible. You cannot go to the self-esteem store to buy some if you need more! It is a label used to represent a set of cognitions (thoughts) and corresponding behaviors related to the regard with which people hold themselves. A theory related to the concept of self-esteem is that if their self-esteem is high, clients will think and feel well about themselves and behave adaptively.

A **hypothesis** is a prediction about two or more concepts within a certain theoretical perspective. For example, one might hypothesize that certain tragic and unfortunate circumstances might affect self-esteem adversely. If one wanted to test that prediction, one could construct a study that examines many people with unfortunate life circumstances to see if their self-esteem was significantly lower than that of an equal and matched number of people who had not experienced the same circumstances. This simplistic example basically illustrates how theories, hypotheses, and research work.

The next questions readers might ask are "So what?" "Who cares?" and "Why do I need to know this?" Theories are important for many reasons—two stand out as key for nurses. First, because theories lead to the collection of relevant empirical (factual) data or relations not yet observed, they help to expand knowledge in a field. Such knowledge provides the *evidence base* upon which nurses and members of other professions practice. This is crucial because it streamlines what nurses know "works" in the vast array of interventions. For example, if scientists had not discovered bacteria and other pathogens, which led to a theory of infection, people might still be subjected to such "treatments" as purging and bleeding.

Second, theories serve as a way to incorporate known empirical findings within a logically consistent and reasonably simple framework. An adequate theory of psychotherapy should organize all that is known about a certain modality in an understandable and logical system that provides a rationale for practice and choice of intervention, one based on solid research and not on intuition. A logical extension of theoretically validated practice is the movement toward

evidence-based practice. Evidence-based nursing practice is "the process by which nurses make clinical decisions using the best available research evidence, their clinical expertise and patient preferences" (University of Minnesota, 2001). The goal is to apply valid and reliable nursing research to clinical practice and to bring the most current knowledge to clinicians. This is particularly important as a result of the knowledge explosion in nursing and health care. The methodology of evidence-based nursing practice includes identifying a clinical problem, searching for related research, evaluating the research, and identifying the most useful related interventions (Beautler & Levant, 2006; Nathan & Gorman, 2007) (Figure 3.1) (see Chap. 4).

It is crucial for nurses to ground their practice in empirical evidence to ensure that clients not only receive interventions with proven effectiveness, but also are protected from harm. For example, in the weeks after the terrorist attacks of September 11, 2001, well-meaning counselors flocked to New York City to conduct critical incident debriefings of victims and bystanders. Intuitively, one might expect such intervention to be helpful. However, randomized clinical trials 3 and 12 months later showed no significant difference in the incidence of post-traumatic stress disorder (PTSD) in those who had undergone a single debriefing session and those who had experienced none. One trial found that debriefing within 10 hours reduced PTSD, compared with debriefing after 48 hours. Moreover, a systematic review showed an increased risk of subsequent psychological problems in people experiencing intense traumatic exposure who also received critical incident debriefing (see Chap. 35) (Rose et al., 2006).

Among other characteristics, theories are judged on the basis of their **utility** (capacity to generate predictions that are confirmed upon collection of relevant empirical data). Utility involves the scope or completeness of derivations.

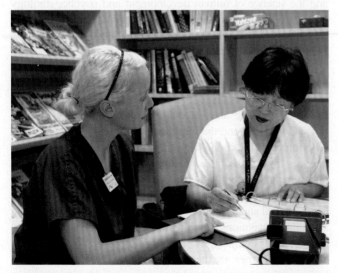

FIGURE 3.1 Evidence-based nursing practice necessitates careful review of current research findings and recommendations and implementation of interventions based on such support.

One theory may generate confirmed consequences but deal with only a few aspects of a phenomenon of interest. For example, a theory of personality that held up only partly under scientific conditions would not be very useful. Ideally, a theory should lead to accurate predictions that deal very generally or inclusively with the empirical events that the theory purports to include. Adequate theories enable their users to predict what will happen and are capable of being tested.

> **Checkpoint Questions**
> 1. What are concepts?
> 2. What is the goal of evidence-based nursing practice?

THEORIES OF HUMAN BEHAVIOR

Many theories purport to explain human behavior, some of which are more useful and verifiable than others. Theories fall into several categories that represent differing viewpoints, including psychoanalytic, behavioral, cognitive, cognitive–behavioral, humanistic, interpersonal, biophysiologic, and sociocultural (Butcher et al., 2006; Engler, 2005).

Psychoanalytic or Psychodynamic Theory

Psychoanalytic/psychodynamic theory derives from the ideas of Sigmund Freud, whom many believe to have been the most overrated figure in the history of science and medicine because his theory led to harm through false etiologies, mistaken diagnoses, and fruitless lines of inquiry (Erwin, 1995; Webster, 1996). However, Freud is important historically because his was the first major attempt to bring order out of the chaos that constituted ideas about human personality and behavior (Butcher et al., 2006). Freud's disciples who revised and modified psychoanalytic theory include Karen Horney, Melanie Klein, Alfred Adler, Ernest Jones, Erik Erikson, Carl Jung, Erich Fromm, and Harry Stack Sullivan. Psychoanalytic practitioners range from orthodox Freudians, who adhere strictly to the original theory, to those who combine psychoanalytic theory with other perspectives.

Psychoanalysis typically involves two to three visits per week and is quite lengthy, with most clients' treatment lasting for years. Today, a relatively small number of psychiatrists practice Freudian psychoanalysis. Not only is it unrealistic in today's cost-conscious health care environment to treat people with this kind of insight-based therapy, but also third-party payers are demanding that treatment approaches be backed by solid supporting research (see Chaps. 4 and 13). Criticism that psychoanalysis is expensive and inefficacious has given way to the graver charge that it may be dangerous and destructive. Psychoanalysts have frequently attributed serious illnesses with organic

origins to psychological causes, sometimes with fatal re-sults (Erwin, 1995).

General Principles

Psychoanalytic thought has been very influential, especially in the United States. The following discussion is not exhaus-tive; interested readers can consult appropriate references at the end of this chapter for a more complete treatment.

Central to psychoanalytic theory is the idea of the **unconscious**. Freud thought that the conscious part of the mind represents a very small area, whereas the unconscious part, like the submerged part of an iceberg, is much larger. The unconscious contains hurtful memories, forbidden de-sires, and other experiences that a person has **repressed**, or pushed from consciousness. Although the person is unaware of such unconscious material, repressed thoughts seek ex-pression, which may be reflected in dreams and fantasies or may lead to irrational and maladaptive behavior. A goal of psychodynamic counseling is to expand awareness of un-conscious functioning and its relation to daily living.

One enduring set of constructs is Freud's notions of what constitutes human personality, which is assumed to result from the interplay of three subsystems: id, ego, and superego.

1. The *id,* the original system of the personality, consists of everything psychological a person inherits at birth, including the instincts.
2. The second subsystem, the *ego,* mediates between the id and the external world. The ego's function is to meet the needs of the id, but in a way that ensures the per-son's well-being.
3. The third subsystem, the *superego,* is essentially what Freud thought of as conscience.

Another of Freud's contributions was his concept of **defense mechanisms**, or unconscious measures that people use to protect their personal stability against anxiety and threat resulting from conflicts among the id, ego, and super-ego. Defense mechanisms are not *real* and cannot be empiri-cally observed, nor can they be "proven." They are inferred from observed bits of behavior. The therapist infers their use based on what a client does or says, and this inference may or may not be correct. Freud thought that defense mecha-nisms resulted from repressed sexuality. One goal of psycho-dynamic counseling is to uncover and understand the nature of a client's defense mechanisms (Butcher et al., 2006).

Defense mechanisms proliferated throughout psychiatric history like the "tribbles" in the classic *Star Trek* episode. Since Anna Freud's (1936/1966) articulation of the initial 12 defense mechanisms, the number of defense mechanisms proposed by psychodynamic scholars has increased dramatically. Symonds (1946) described 25 defense mechanisms. Bibring and col-leagues (1961) listed 39 defense mechanisms, and Kernberg (1994) identified 31 defense mechanisms. The *Diagnostic and Statistical Manual of Mental Disorders,* 4th edition, text revi-sion (*DSM-IV-TR*) (American Psychiatric Association [APA], 2000) lists 31 defense mechanisms and defines 27 of them. Blackman (2004), in the longest compilation to date, lists and defines 101 defense mechanisms, and claims that there is po-tentially an infinite number. Readers are directed to Table 3.1 for a partial list of these defense mechanisms. This is not an exhaustive list of all the defense mechanisms that have been proposed. For a more comprehensive list, readers are referred to the *DSM IV-TR* (APA, 2000), pages 811 through 813.

Historically, Freud was one of the first theorists to view personality development as a succession of stages, as out-lined in Table 3.2. Essentially, he believed that appropriate gratification during each stage is important if the person is not to become *fixated* (stuck) at that stage.

No exploration of psychoanalytic thought would be complete without a discussion of the two fixed constructs and enduring contributions known as transference and coun-tertransference. **Transference** refers to feelings and thoughts that clients have toward the nurse, psychiatrist, or other ser-vice provider. In transference, the client is thought to project an imagined image about the provider, which may be posi-tive or negative and may hamper or move forward the pro-cess of therapy (Evans, 2007). **Countertransference** refers to feelings and thoughts that service providers have toward the client. In countertransference, the provider may harbor certain images of the client that result in "blind spots," which can be destructive or disruptive to therapy. Transference and countertransference are useful conceptualizations and pro-vide a shortcut for exploring what might happen between providers and clients to influence the relationship.

Critiques

Freud's speculations about mental systems, human personality, instincts, and life itself went far beyond any data that he could legitimately claim to have unearthed. As more findings are re-vealed about neurobiology and physiology, the human genome, and the science of human development and psychopathology (see Chap. 2), the verdict on Freud has been uniformly negative: as a scientist, metapsychologist, and diagnostician of society, Freud emerges as a fraud (Erwin, 1995; Webster, 1996).

The major criticism of psychodynamic theory from within and outside the profession is that it is simply "bad" theory (Es-terson, 1999; Tallis, 1996). As previously discussed, a theory must be verifiable and capable of generating logical predic-tions. Critics contend that psychoanalytic theory meets neither criterion. First, deriving any empirical predictions or conse-quences from many of its tenets is impossible. Psychoanalytic phenomena are often "after the fact" explanations. Second, no scientific or respectable procedures have ever substantiated this theory. Freud and his adherents have been disinclined to follow scientific conventions, resulting in the criticism that psychoana-lytic thought is philosophy, not science.

Dead theories are theories that, regardless of merit, have little empirical support and that no one seriously considers true. Several psychoanalytic theories are now considered dead. For example, Freud hypothesized that mental instabil-ity resulted from deliberate interruption of sexual intercourse

TABLE 3.1 Defense Mechanisms

Defense Mechanism	Description	Example from Popular Culture
Acting out	Expressing thoughts and feelings in actions rather than words	*Say Anything* (1989): Lloyd Dobler blasts a love song from a boom box outside his girlfriend's window to communicate his feelings for her.
Compensation	Emphasizing positive traits to make up for real or perceived weaknesses	*The Office* (2005): Michael Scott repeatedly calls attention to his humor and friendliness to distract people from his questionable management skills.
Denial	Refusing to recognize a reality that might be troublesome or traumatic	*The Sopranos* (1998): The family goes along with the idea that Tony, the husband and father, is in "waste management," instead of organized crime.
Devaluation	Maintaining an entirely negative view of another person by ignoring his or her virtues (the opposite is idealization)	*Eternal Sunshine of the Spotless Mind* (2004): Following a nasty breakup, Clementine refuses to acknowledge that her boyfriend had good traits or that they once were happy together.
Identification	Acting and behaving like someone else; taking on another's personality characteristics	*Seinfeld* (1990): George Costanza starts to imitate a new friend he wants to go into business with, constantly referring to himself in the third person.
Intellectualization	Using the powers of the intellect, thinking, and reasoning to blunt reality	*House* (2004): Dr. Gregory House argues, wisecracks, and logically tears apart his colleagues when they confront him about behavior or try to analyze his emotions.
Projection	Refusing to recognize behavior in oneself and instead "projecting" it or seeing it in someone else	*Friends* (1994): Ross insists that his ex-girlfriend Rachel (whom he still loves) is flirting with him and trying to reconcile.
Reaction formation	Doing the opposite of one's unconscious wishes	*It's a Wonderful Life* (1946): George Bailey becomes increasingly mired in the everyday affairs of his small town, despite desperately wanting to leave home to travel the world.
Regression	Going back to an earlier and happier time of development	*American Beauty* (1998): During a midlife crisis, Lester Burnham quits his job at an agency, starts working at a fast-food restaurant, and begins behaving like a teenager.
Repression	Involuntarily placing material of life experience out of the conscious	*The Bourne Identity* (2002): Jason Bourne cannot remember troubling episodes from his career as a spy.
Sublimation	Taking repressed feelings and transforming them into positive and constructive pursuits	*The Pursuit of Happyness* (2006): Chris Gardner represses his anger about separating from his wife and frustration over money troubles into overachieving at his internship.
Suppression	Wishing to put something unpleasant out of awareness and voluntarily doing so	*Lost* (2004): Hugo, a survivor of a plane crash, organizes a makeshift golf game to provide distraction from the harsh challenges of surviving on a deserted island.

TABLE 3.2 Freud's Model of Psychosexual Development

Stage	Characteristics
Oral stage	During the first 2 years of life, the mouth is the principal erogenous zone and the child's primary means of gratification.
Anal stage	From ages 2 to 3 years, the membranes of the anal region provide the greatest source of pleasurable stimulation.
Phallic stage	From ages 3 to 5 or 6 years, self-manipulation of the genitals is the major source of pleasurable stimulation.
Latency stage	From ages 6 to 12 years, sexual motivations recede as children become preoccupied with developing skills and other activities.
Genital stage	After puberty, the deepest feelings of pleasure come from heterosexual relations.

by withdrawal of the penis from the vagina prior to ejaculation (coitus interruptus). No one believes this today, and the theory is dead.

Nursing Applications

Nursing students should be acquainted with some of the major constructs of psychodynamic theory, not necessarily because they are scientifically sound, but simply because the terms are still used in psychiatric settings. From a historical perspective, the psychodynamic school should be given credit for the first systematic approach that showed how human psychological processes result in mental disorders. Although use of psychodynamic theories in psychiatric–mental health nursing is limited and of little treatment value, Freud did demonstrate that certain mental phenomena result from attempts to cope with difficult problems. His perspective and the development of the "talking cure" laid the foundation for modern counseling, as well as the need for therapeutic interpersonal relationships. Perhaps his greatest contribution was to help dispel much of the mystery and fear surrounding people with psychiatric problems.

Behavioral Theory

The behaviorist approach has been praised for its precision and objectivity. The enormous amount of empirical research that this approach has generated has demonstrated the effectiveness of its interventions (Hersen, 2002). However, it also has been criticized for being "mindless," focusing strictly on behavior and ignoring the workings of the brain.

> **Checkpoint Questions**
> 3. According to psychoanalytic theory, what is the underlying basis for maladaptive behavior?
> 4. Which of Freud's constructs refers to the feelings and thoughts that clients have toward the nurse, psychiatrist, or other service provider?

The behaviorist movement emerged in the early 20th century as a direct challenge to psychoanalytic thought (Butcher et al., 2006). Behavioral psychologists believed that the study of subjective experience did not provide acceptable scientific data because psychoanalytic observations and interpretations were not open to verification by others. In the behaviorist view, only the study of directly observable behavior and the stimuli and reinforcing conditions that control it could serve as a basis for formulating scientific principles of human behavior. Moreover, they argued that achieving insight through psychoanalysis did not equate with changing behavior.

Although many schools of thought fall within the behaviorist perspective, they are all organized around a single central theme: the role of learning. They also all operate on the assumption that behavior is lawful (Butcher et al., 2006; Hersen, 2002).

General Principles

Because behavioral theory maintains that all human behavior is learned, its major scholars have concerned themselves with explaining and researching learning. They have focused on how environmental conditions result in the acquisition, modification, maintenance, and elimination of adaptive and maladaptive behaviors.

CONDITIONING. **Conditioning** is a basic type of learning with two forms: respondent (classical) and operant. **Respondent conditioning** happens when a response and a stimulus become connected. Unconditioned responses develop before learning and may be innate to all humans. For example, Ivan Pavlov showed that food, an unconditioned stimulus (US), elicited salivation in dogs, an unconditioned response. One could postulate that similar responses in humans are part of their biologic and physiologic wiring. Conditioned responses develop through the repeated pairing of stimuli and responses. Pavlov demonstrated this by pairing the sound of a bell with food. Eventually he removed the food, and his dogs salivated to the sound of the bell alone. This was a conditioned response to a conditioned stimulus (CS) (Figure 3.2).

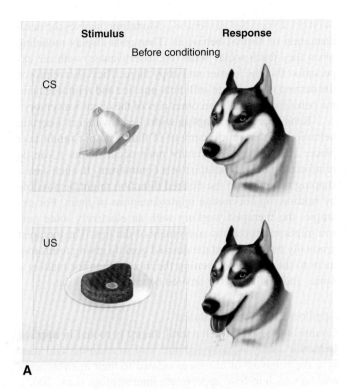

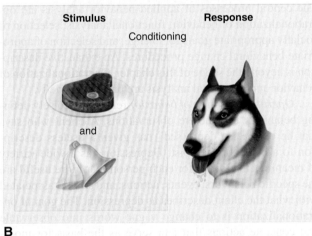

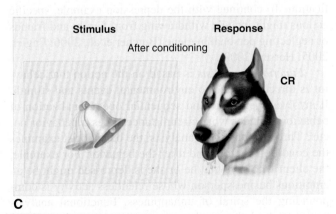

FIGURE 3.2 (**A**) Before conditioning, the sound of a bell elicits no salivary response in the dog, which is opposite to the effect generated by the sight of meat. (**B**) During conditioning, the sound of a bell and the meat are paired. (**C**) After conditioning, the sound of a bell alone elicits the salivary response in the dog.

In **operant conditioning**, people respond to achieve a certain goal. They "operate" on their environment to achieve something rewarding or to avoid something aversive. The response precedes the stimulus. For example, clients in inpatient settings learn that certain behaviors lead to positive events, such as praise from staff or family, more freedom, and better privileges. Thus, they increase that behavior to subsequently increase those positive events. Likewise, they may learn that other behaviors may lead to negative events and thus avoid such actions to prevent the negative circumstances.

REINFORCEMENT. A second important but frequently misunderstood behavioral concept is **reinforcement**. Contrary to popular wisdom, a reinforcer is not a reward. A reinforcer is a stimulus that strengthens a new response by its repeated association with that response. That stimulus may be either pleasant (positive) or aversive (negative). Thus, a person may learn a certain response (behavior) either to receive a reward or to avoid a punishment. In both positive and negative reinforcement, the person is rewarded for an appropriate response. With positive reinforcement, the response happens by *adding* something to increase probability. The nature of the positive reinforcer can differ for different people. One example of a positive reinforcer is a reward for a job well done. This is fairly intuitive, but sometimes human behavior is not so simple. For example, losing one's temper with a nagging spouse might serve as a positive reinforcer if the spouse feels neglected and nags to get any kind of attention. Nagging, unpleasant though it might seem, will likely result in more nagging if it achieves the objective of gaining a response. The nagging has been reinforced.

Negative reinforcement involves the *termination* or *removal* of a consequence after a desired response to increase the probability of a behavior. Negative reinforcers are usually aversive so that the person is motivated to exhibit a desired target behavior to escape from the unpleasant condition. For example, a coach might bench a player for unsportsmanlike behavior. Sitting on the bench is an aversive condition (Figure 3.3). When the benching is over, the player will exhibit better behavior.

High rates of reinforcement are necessary in early learning, with gradual tapering to maintain the response. Responses are particularly persistent when reinforcement is intermittent. The person continually responds based on past reinforcement, hoping for future reinforcement. This is why such activities as habitual gambling, in which winnings are intermittent and unpredictable, may be so difficult to overcome. The person keeps gambling, hoping for elusive reinforcement. Should reinforcement completely stop, the response gradually extinguishes itself or ends, but not before an initial rise in the response rate (Butcher et al., 2006; Hersen, 2002).

PUNISHMENT. **Punishment**, a special stimulus, operates in an opposite way from reinforcement. A punishment is any aversive stimulus introduced after a response to decrease the

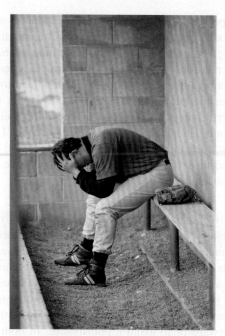

FIGURE 3.3 Benching a player for poor behavior can serve as a negative reinforcer to encourage better actions and performance once the benching is removed.

future likelihood of that response. Negative reinforcers, although aversive, are *removed* and result in certain behaviors. Punishing stimuli are *introduced* to stop certain behaviors. Punishment sometimes results in short-term compliance; however, it does not have long-term effectiveness. Moreover, punishment can be unpredictable and self-defeating. Most people tend to react to punishment by fighting back, withdrawing passively, or avoiding the person with whom the punishment is associated. Despite society's near-universal use of punishment (eg, in child rearing), it has been shown to be less effective than reinforcement in modifying behaviors.

GENERALIZATION AND DISCRIMINATION. Generalization happens when a person associates a conditioned response with similar stimuli. For example, children who engage in polite behavior (eg, saying "please" and "thank you") at home repeatedly are likely to display that behavior in circumstances outside the home given similar conditions. Closely allied with generalization is **discrimination** (distinguishing among and responding differently to similar stimuli). For example, children learn that they should act a certain way within the family but that their peers have different expectations.

Behaviorists believe that generalization and discrimination have important implications for maladaptive behaviors (Hersen, 2002). For example, some people who become frightened in specific social situations may begin to avoid similar situations and gradually develop social phobia, in which they avoid all social situations. Eventually social phobia might expand to full-blown *agoraphobia* (refusal to leave the home or other "safe" environment) (see Chap. 23).

MODELING AND SHAPING. Modeling involves the demonstration of desired behaviors. Therapists display modeling when they teach social skills (eg, assertiveness) with the expectation that the learner will copy them. They also reinforce the desired skills. Given sufficient practice and reinforcement, the behavior gradually becomes part of the client's inventory.

Behaviorists use **shaping** with clients who lack a certain behavior, so that reinforcement of that behavior might take place. The fact that a behavior must occur before it can be reinforced places a therapist in a conundrum. In such cases, shaping behaviors in the desired direction might be possible by reinforcing successive approximations of them. For example, the therapist working with an electively mute person might reinforce any movement of the lips. The therapist gradually builds toward the desired goal by giving reinforcement to the client for opening the mouth, then for making a noise, and finally for the desired behavior—speaking.

Applied Behavior Analysis

Counseling based on behavioral theory is rooted in **applied behavior analysis**, a systematic way to examine and analyze the behavior of clients as related to their environments and on which to base appropriate interventions (Lax, 2002). The central processes of applied behavior analysis are operationalization of behavior, functional analysis, selection of socially appropriate goals for change, and selection of appropriate behavioral change procedures. An exhaustive description is beyond the scope of this chapter. Operationalization of behavior and functional analysis are presented briefly.

Operationalization of behavior refers to precisely defining behaviors in concrete observations. A client who says that he or she is "depressed" has given a useless description to a behavior therapist. Depression has a wide variety of meanings that differ for each person. Far more useful are the specific behaviors, events, actions, and stimuli associated with what the client describes as depression. The goal of operationalization is to change vague words into observable and concrete actions that can serve as the basis for modification. To continue with the depression example, specific actions might include withdrawing from family and friends or neglecting personal hygiene (Butcher et al., 2006; Engler, 2005; Hersen, 2002).

Functional analysis is based on the notion that behavior is directly related to environmental events and stimuli. It involves systematic and sequential operationalization of behaviors—under what circumstances does a behavior occur? Through functional analysis, the behaviorist examines the conditions before and after the behavior. For example, the client who says that he or she is depressed might be an ambitious businessperson whose relentless activity is compounding the spiral of unhappiness. Functional analysis would lead a behavior therapist to discover such a pattern and work with the client to change work habits and introduce more pleasurable activities. This is known as the ABC model, in which *A* is the antecedent preceding *B*, the behavior, which leads to *C*, the consequence. This ABC model is

TABLE 3.3 Behavior Modification Techniques

Learning Principle	Behavior Modification Technique	Example of Treatment
When an established behavior pattern is no longer reinforced, it tends to extinguish itself.	Withdrawal of reinforcement for undesirable behavior	Parents begin to show less concern for their child's temper tantrums or ignore them altogether.
A specified behavior can gradually be established if successive approximations of that behavior are reinforced.	Shaping of desired behavior	Social reinforcement is provided to develop sustained eye contact in clients with schizophrenia who have social-skills deficits.
Behavior patterns are developed and established through repeated associations with positive reinforcers.	Use of positive reinforcers to establish desired behavior	Token economy is used, in which children exchange tokens, earned for desired behaviors, for toys.

an effective, although underused, way of assessing client behaviors (Lax, 2002).

Table 3.3 describes some other techniques that behavior therapists use in their treatment of clients and the learning principles underlying those techniques.

Nursing Applications

Many psychiatric treatment settings and schools use behavioral principles. Such interventions as token economies and privilege systems are rooted in behaviorism; similar interventions are commonly used with children and adolescents. Behavioral modification and management programs are used for eating disorders, anxiety, anger management, substance abuse, and other problems. Many principles of client and family education derive from behavioral approaches.

> **Think About It 3.1**
> A 32-year-old woman is receiving treatment for agoraphobia (fear of open spaces). She tells the nurse that she was able to stand near her open front door for 3 minutes. The nurse praises her for this behavior. How is the nurse applying the concepts of behavioral therapy? Which concept(s) of behavioral therapy is the nurse using?

Cognitive Theory

Cognitive theory guides two major schools of thought (Dobson, 2002; O'Donohue et al., 2005). The first is Albert Ellis's rational emotive theory. The second is Aaron Beck's cognitive theory. Both emphasize the central role of cognitions (thoughts) in how people feel and act.

Rational Emotive Theory

The essence of Ellis's (1962) theory of psychopathology is that activating events do not cause emotional or behavioral consequences directly. Rather, beliefs about these activating events are the most direct and important causes of how people feel and act. Rational emotive therapy (RET) emphasizes the disputation of *irrational beliefs,* or those unlikely to have empirical support in the environment and that do not promote survival and enjoyment.

Cognitions, then, help to determine a person's response to stimuli. The idea behind RET is that clients engage in certain self-statements based on distorted cognitions. These self-statements contribute to maladaptation and related behaviors. See Box 3.1 for examples of such distorted cognitions or beliefs.

RET therapists teach clients to do a kind of functional analysis of their own behaviors in which they examine the *antecedent condition,* or the cognition that precedes behaviors and results in self-statements. Clients then examine the associated consequences. In RET this is known as the "ABCD" approach:

- *A* is the antecedent behavior.
- *B* is the belief.
- *C* is the consequence (of the belief).
- *D* is the disputation of maladaptive beliefs (Ellis, 1962).

BOX 3.1 Examples of Distorted Beliefs

- I must do well at everything that I do. Otherwise, I have no worth as a human being.
- People should act better than they do; if they do not, then they should be punished.
- Avoiding life's difficulties is easier than facing them.
- Because I was hurt or traumatized in the past, that past will forever haunt me, and I must be continuously preoccupied with that event.
- If I do not find an instant and perfect solution to my problems, it is a catastrophe.
- I can't stand feeling anxious, frustrated, uncomfortable, guilty, or otherwise emotionally upset.

The goals of therapy are for clients to monitor their maladaptive thoughts and beliefs, look for evidence supporting their beliefs, dispute their maladaptive self-statements, substitute adaptive thoughts, and thus change their patterns of distorted thinking and, consequently, behavior. This is part of a technique known as *cognitive restructuring* (Corsini, 2000).

Let us consider an example. A woman who has been unemployed for several months is devastated after an unsuccessful job interview. Using cognitive restructuring, a self-help homework exercise might be as follows:

- A *(Antecedent behavior): I went for a job interview and didn't get the job.*
- B *(Beliefs):* How terrible to get rejected! I'm worthless! I'll never get a job.
- C *(Consequences):* I feel blue and hopeless. I am making myself so anxious that I will do poorly on other job interviews.
- D *(Disputation):* I'll do better next time. Perhaps I can practice with my husband before the next interview.

The client describes his or her thoughts systematically, links self-defeating thoughts to present discomfort, and then disputes them.

Beck's Cognitive Theory

Aaron Beck's model (1976; Beck & Beck, 1995; Beck & Rush, 1987) holds that conditions such as depression result primarily from pervasive, negative misinterpretations (Table 3.4). Beck postulates that psychological problems stem from faulty learning and incorrect inferences based on inadequate or wrong information. Cognitive therapy uses an information-processing model directed toward identifying and modifying incorrect cognitions. In collaboration with the therapist, clients address their biased selection of information and distorted beliefs and learn to invalidate them. Cognitive therapy and RET have much in common.

Cognitive–Behavioral Theory

Learning theorists, such as Donald Meichenbaum (1977), enhanced behavioral theory by introducing the role of **cognitions**, or mediating processes between a stimulus and a response. This led to cognitive–behavioral therapy or cognitive–behavioral modification (CBM). Subsumed under CBM are different techniques that incorporate concepts from RET, cognitive therapy, problem-solving training, behavioral therapy, skills training, and self-instructional training.

CBM is implemented in various ways, but generally this therapy is active, directive, highly structured, and time limited. Therapists are seen as teachers or coaches and expect clients to be engaged actively in their treatment, practicing new thoughts and behaviors through homework exercises developed by the therapist. Some techniques in the cognitive–behavioral therapeutic tool kit are described briefly in Table 3.5. The field of CBM has grown immensely in the past several decades, and studies demonstrate empirical support for the techniques in the treatment of several conditions.

A Brief Note on Dialectic Behavior Therapy

Dialectic behavior therapy (DBT), developed by clinician Marsha Linehan (Dimeff, Koerner, & Linehan, 2007), builds on the foundation of cognitive theory. DBT was developed to treat persons with borderline personality disorder. The major premise of this approach is that some people react abnormally to emotional stimulation with extremes of mood. These persons seem to lack adaptive coping mechanisms for dealing with their sudden, intense surges of emotion and this poor coping can be destructive. DBT's goal is to reduce parasuicidal (self-injuring) and life-threatening behaviors. When clients achieve stability they work on reducing behaviors that interfere with the therapy/treatment process and reducing behaviors that impede their quality of life. These goals are accomplished by teaching clients skills that will help in centering them in the moment (mindfulness), making them aware of their dichotomous (black and white) extreme thinking, and modulating their intense responses to distress.

DBT seems to reduce severe dysfunctional behaviors that are targeted for intervention (eg, parasuicide, substance abuse, and binge eating), enhance treatment retention, and reduce psychiatric hospitalization. Additional research is

TABLE 3.4 Types of Cognitions in Cognitive Therapy

Cognition	Type	Example
Cognitive event	Automatic thought	"I'm a lousy parent. How terrible."
Cognitive process	Distorted information processing	"I love my kids very much, but yesterday I lost my temper and yelled at them. On the basis of this one incident, I conclude that I am no longer any good as a parent." (selective abstraction)
Cognitive structure	Irrational belief*	"I must always be competent in every area of life."

*Irrational beliefs lead to dysfunctional schemata upon which the client operates and behaves.

TABLE 3.5 **Cognitive–Behavioral Techniques**

Technique	Description
Cognitive relabeling	The way a person labels something will strongly determine his or her emotional response and behavior. A person who labels things incorrectly will have a maladaptive emotional response and ineffective behavior. This technique involves teaching the client to perceive environmental cues more accurately so that he or she clearly differentiates between realistically dangerous situations and those in which the source of harm is purely imaginary.
Systematic rational restructuring	This technique involves constructing a hierarchy of increasingly difficult situations, with successful coping by the client determining progression to the next, more difficult situation. It is similar to systematic desensitization, except that rational reevaluation replaces relaxation as a coping skill.
Rational problem solving	This technique involves systematic problem-solving training. It consists of five stages: (1) Orientation to the problem (2) Precisely defining the problem (3) Generating alternatives to the problem (4) Making a decision among the alternatives (5) Verifying whether the alternative chosen was useful

warranted to examine which components of DBT contribute to its efficacy.

Nursing Applications

Although actual CBM should be practiced by appropriately trained professionals with advanced degrees, generalist psychiatric nurses can play a supportive role and apply principles of CBM to assessment, planning, and interventions. For example, nurses can teach clients to identify negative cognitions and implement interventions to change them. Nurses can monitor and record improvements in mood and behavior. Furthermore, crucial to the success of CBM is the client's engagement in homework prescribed by therapists. Often a lack of follow-up with homework can sabotage therapeutic efforts. Generalist nurses can support clients' completion of homework in the same way that they encourage medication adherence.

Humanistic Theory

Humanistic theory recognizes the importance of learning and other psychological processes that traditionally have been the focus of research. Such processes include creativity, hope, love, self-fulfillment, personal growth, values, and meaning. Humanists are concerned with the personal growth and potentialities of people. With their positive view of human nature, humanists believe that psychopathology results from the blocking or distortion of personal growth, excessive stress, and unfavorable social conditions.

The humanist perspective has been criticized for its lack of scientific grounding. Indeed, the view is less a theory and more a system of values. Its main importance for psychiatric–mental health nurses lies in its optimistic view of people and their capacity to become fully functional. Some well-known humanists are Carl Rogers, Abraham Maslow, Thomas Szasz, and Fritz Perls (Butcher et al., 2006; Engler, 2005).

> **Checkpoint Questions**
> **5.** What is the emphasis of cognitive theory?
> **6.** How do humanists view psychopathology?

Interpersonal Theory

Adherents to the interpersonal perspective believe that unsatisfactory interpersonal relations are the primary cause of maladaptive behaviors. At present, no systematic view of human nature and behavior is based entirely on interpersonal theory or the social context in which people live and function. The closest approximation may be the viewpoint developed by the neo-Freudian psychologist Harry Stack Sullivan (Butcher et al., 2006; Engler, 2005). Sullivan believed that poor relationships cause anxiety, which serves as the basis for all emotional problems. Others in the psychiatric field elaborated on Sullivan's viewpoint, including his student Hildegard Peplau, the renowned pioneer in psychiatric nursing.

General Principles

Interpersonal theorists emphasize the socialization of humans throughout their developmental stages. Failure to proceed through these stages satisfactorily lays the foundation for later maladaptive behavior. Within this developmental context, the interpersonal perspective emphasizes the role of early childhood in shaping self-concept. Distorted self-concepts can be traced to the person's family. Two results of distorted self-concepts are poor interpersonal functioning and self-defeating "games" people learn to play (Berne, 1964). The interpersonal perspective also is concerned with the anxiety-arousing aspects of interpersonal relationships.

Interpersonal therapy is concerned with alleviating anxiety and pathogenic or problem-causing relationships. It also focuses on helping clients achieve more satisfactory relationships. Such therapy is concerned with verbal and nonverbal communication, social roles, attributions people make about themselves and others, and the general interpersonal context of behavior. It emphasizes remediating the client's interpersonal skills within the therapeutic relationship.

Despite its intuitive appeal and similar to the psychoanalytic and humanistic approaches, incomplete information concerning many aspects of interpersonal functioning handicaps it. As a result, many of its concepts lack adequate scientific grounding.

Hildegard Peplau

Hildegard Peplau (1909–1999) is considered the "mother of psychiatric nursing." Changes in mental health care and advances in biologic psychiatry have necessitated reevaluation of Peplau's nursing theory, which considers nursing to be an interpersonal process between nurse and client. The theory lacks empirical investigation and has not yet been tested regarding the multidisciplinary approach. Moreover, the interpersonal process is not limited to nursing (see Chap. 12). For the theory to gain credibility within the dynamics of the multidisciplinary team, it must be differentially tested within a framework of robust research design involving various diagnostic groups and practice settings. Until such time, the theory's utility remains questionable.

Biophysiologic Theory

The biophysiologic perspective has gained influence slowly as efforts to find the causes and treatments of psychiatric illness have resulted in promising new findings. Enormous strides have been made toward understanding the probable biophysiologic components of many disorders (see Chap. 2). The biophysiologic perspective sometimes is called the "medical model," which is misleading. Although psychiatrists, who are physicians, direct much of the care of clients with psychiatric disorders, nothing is inherently "medical" about this model. Basically, all models seek to explain psychopathology, its cause (pathogenesis), and its cure or treatment, regardless of whether that treatment is purely psychotherapy or purely somatic therapy.

General Principles

The biophysiologic perspective proposes that psychopathology results from a physiologic condition, primarily a deviation within the central nervous system (Leckman et al., 2007). The reasons for these deviations are multifaceted, involving a complex interplay of genetics, temperament, development, brain circuitry, molecular biology, and environment (see Chap. 2). Although much study remains needed, international biologists are making new discoveries about mental illnesses daily.

Until recently, the therapeutic processes associated with the biophysiologic perspective focused on somatic treatments such as medications, sleep deprivation, photo (light) therapies, and electroconvulsive therapy (see Chaps. 16 and 18). As research expands to include the effects of the environment and psychotherapy on brain circuitry, this perspective also will expand its range of options to include more psychosocial modalities.

The Stress–Diathesis Model

The *stress–diathesis model,* a popular variation of the biophysiologic model, assumes that a disposition (or vulnerability) toward a certain disorder may result from a combination of genetics and early learning (Figure 3.4). In this model, the effects of life events cannot be understood without considering innate diatheses, and the effects of constitutional vulnerabilities cannot be understood without considering stressors. However, having a disposition for a disorder does not mean that a person necessarily will develop it. The model posits that the predisposition or constitutional vulnerability is necessary for developing a disorder and that disorders do not occur in its absence (Paris, 1999). For example, some people experience chronic physical abuse yet never show signs of PTSD. Conversely, some people experience less intense or chronic stressors but develop PTSD. The stress–diathesis model may help explain such disparities. No specific therapeutic techniques derive from or are associated with it, but this model has great explanatory power.

> **Checkpoint Questions**
> **7.** According to the interpersonal perspective, what causes maladaptive behavior?
> **8.** What is the major assumption of the stress–diathesis model?

Sociocultural Theory

Early psychology primarily was concerned with the person. Gradually, however, sociocultural influences, such as family, community, and environmental factors, have become recognized for their enormous effects on individuals. Many approaches fall within the sociocultural perspective, and they all focus on the role of social and cultural influences on the person.

Culture can be thought of as the "glue" that holds certain groups together (see Chap. 6). It consists of socially acquired and transmitted symbols, beliefs, techniques, institutions, customs, and norms. Culture has been found to exert a great influence on the birth, development, and death

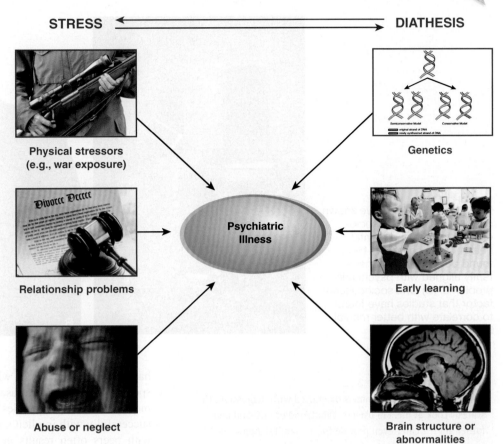

FIGURE 3.4 **In the stress–diathesis model, conditions of vulnerability and environmental stressors combine to produce psychiatric disorders.**

of humans. Culture also affects how the body is treated (Gallagher, 2002; Horowitz, 2002).

A rapidly growing discipline known as *medical anthropology* deals with the cross-cultural study of medical systems and the influence of ecological, biologic, and sociocultural factors on health and disease. Some related areas of interest for health care professionals include the dynamics of health-seeking behaviors, models of mental illness, systems of healing, alcohol-drinking patterns, and special mental states, such as trance and spirit possession. Another is psychiatric syndromes seen in and influenced by the values of non-Western cultures (Cultural Spotlight 3.1).

In terms of social influences, a strong association has been shown between social class or socioeconomic position

Cultural *Spotlight* 3.1

Koro

An example of a culture-bound syndrome is *koro*, an affliction seen in men of Southeast Asian origin. Koro is characterized by intense anxiety and fear that the penis is shrinking and receding (Gallagher, 2002; Mintzer et al., 2005). Koro can and has reached epidemic proportions in some countries and is thought to be influenced by the importance and fragility of male sexuality in specific cultures.

and psychiatric disorders. A classic study by Hollingshead and Redlich (1958) found that the lower the social class, the greater the prevalence of psychotic problems. Since then, findings in dozens of studies have shown that noxious social conditions (eg, poverty) affect humans adversely. Several explanations have been advanced. One is that the complex social stressors associated with poverty and few resources inhibit the abilities of poor people to cope as effectively as their more affluent counterparts. Ineffective coping leads to a constant cycle of extreme stress, subsequent maladaptation, and potential illness. In this view, poverty is a social toxin (Figure 3.5A).

Another sociodemographic factor of interest is marital status. Married people have been found consistently to have better mental health than unmarried people (Figure 3.5B). Race and ethnicity also have been studied in relation to mental health and illness, but race per se has not been found to account for any significant differences in social patterns of mental health. However, clients belonging to racial minorities have been found to experience disproportionate stress resulting from prejudice and because they are more likely to be poor than whites.

Scholars have recognized the importance of cultural and ethnic factors as they relate to mental health and mental illness. How the client with a psychiatric disorder is received, understood, and treated has been found to affect the course of treatment greatly. Moreover, solid empirical data support the sociocultural perspective (Gallagher, 2002; Mintzer et al., 2005). However, it is only one perspective and does not fully explain all facets of mental illness.

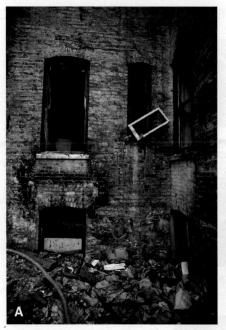
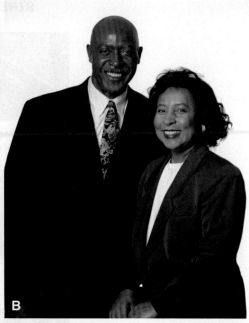

FIGURE 3.5 Studies have shown correlations between sociocultural factors and mental health. (**A**) Researchers have found poverty to be consistently aligned with psychiatric problems. (**B**) One sociocultural factor that studies have found to correlate with better mental health is being married.

Think About It 3.2

A 40-year-old Hispanic man is diagnosed with depression. He states, "Look at me. I'm useless. What kind of husband and father am I? I can't even provide for my family." Applying the sociocultural viewpoint, what areas would be the focus during assessment?

TOWARD A COMPREHENSIVE, MULTIDISCIPLINARY UNDERSTANDING OF PSYCHOPATHOLOGY

With ongoing research, psychiatric–mental health professionals continue to expand their understanding of the roles of biologic, psychosocial, and sociocultural factors in the development of mental illness. Explanations based on only one of these factors are likely to be incomplete. Today, the dominant belief in the field is that an interaction of several factors produces disorders.

Dante Cicchetti and his colleagues developed a useful, all-inclusive conceptual framework incorporating several different theories and perspectives (Cicchetti & Cohen, 2006). It originally was created to explain maladaptation in children, but its application to adults is equally valid. Cicchetti's perspective evolved from the work of ecology theorist Uri Bronfenbrenner (1979, 1989), who asserted that people's contexts are crucial to understanding their development and behavior. Cicchetti also incorporated ideas from various developmental theorists who wrote that humans, during their development, must achieve *critical competencies* (eg, prosocial behaviors) to meet the challenges of later stages successfully. Research

has shown that children who do not master competency-specific tasks are at increased risk for later social maladjustment. For example, studies show that an inability to cope successfully with implicit social rules and exchanges in play with peers often results in peer rejection and detrimental consequences later in development (Kaufman, 2007).

Cicchetti's framework addresses both individual and environmental characteristics, simultaneously emphasizing the interactive and reciprocal influences of the person, his or her family, the community, and the greater sociocultural arena in which the person develops and lives. It includes the broad contexts of development and functioning, and it is solidly informed by the genetic and neurophysiologic variables inherent within each unique human being (see Chap. 2). In addition, this perspective hypothesizes that certain contextual characteristics and events (risk or protective factors) may enhance or hinder a person's development and adaptation (Aber & Cicchetti, 1984). *Risk factors* are variables that impede development and cause hardship (eg, extreme poverty). *Protective factors* are variables that serve as buffers and have a helpful influence (eg, supportive family). See Table 3.6 for examples of risk and protective factors at different levels.

In addition to their unique ontogenic characteristics (eg, genetic endowment, temperament), humans continuously are exposed to many risk and protective factors across proximal and distal systems. *Proximal systems* are those variables with the strongest influence and to which people are exposed most immediately (eg, parents for children). *Distal systems* are less adjacent and exert less powerful effects (eg, school systems). Much of how a child responds and develops depends on this complex web of experiences, risk and protective factors, and proximal and distal systems.

The ecological, developmental view is based on theories with empirical validation. Scholars are testing this model,

TABLE 3.6 **Examples of Risk and Protective Factors**

Type of System	Risk Factors	Protective Factors
Macrosystem	Violent culture Lack of access to health care War	Restricted sales of firearms Governmental support programs (eg, Women, Infants and Children Program, Medicare coverage) Universal lead screening
Exosystem	Violent neighborhood Impoverished neighborhood Paucity of health care providers Substandard housing	Strong alliance with community police officers Supportive and strong family and social networks Neighborhood "free" clinics
Microsystem	Domestic violence No affordable child care Chronic illness of a family member	Extended family support Consistent employment Respite care
Ontogenic	Genetic loading for major psychotic illness Low intelligence	High educational attainment Physical health

which has been advanced as a valuable way in which to frame problems of childhood psychopathology and maladaptation. The National Academy of Sciences endorsed this model in the early 1990s as the paradigm within which child development and psychopathology should be studied (National Research Council, 1993). Moreover, it represents the true complexity of people in their contexts. It also serves as a foundation for the kind of interagency collaboration and integration that has been promoted as a holistic and cost-effective way to deliver comprehensive care to clients with serious and persistent mental illness and their families (Anderson & Mohr, 2003; Walter & Petr, 2000). A schematic of the model is presented in Figure 3.6.

The Emergence of Mental Illness

Cicchetti's model posits that mental illness disrupts the resolution of developmental tasks. This consideration is important because many serious psychiatric disorders begin to manifest in childhood or adolescence. The person's developmental stage and tasks determine the effects of the illness. Thus, to understand the potential effects of any intervention, it is critical to assess and to understand the effects of proximal and distal systems and how those effects might be reflected in the person's behavior. In this view, behavior is developmentally based, with biophysiologic and environmental characteristics interacting and transacting.

Nursing Applications: Assessing Multiple Systems

The developmental–ecological perspective draws attention to the importance of identifying and attending to the multiple systems that affect development. It emphasizes

the need for the nurse and multidisciplinary team to collect information across multiple contexts. Most nurses have extensive preparation in accurate client assessment. However, sometimes time, awareness, or other factors lead nurses to overlook investigations of the client's context or environment and what role it might play in diagnosis and treatment. The next two subsections explain how to incorporate assessment of the microsystem and exosystem into client care (see Figure 3.6).

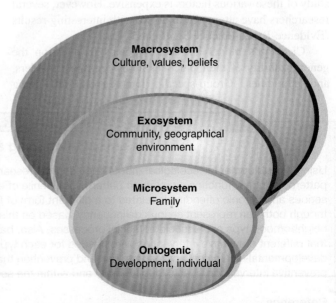

FIGURE 3.6 In the developmental–ecological model, layers of overlapping systems combine to create a specific context within which a person should be considered, assessed, diagnosed, and treated.

Family Characteristics (Microsystem)

Multiple risk factors can increase a child's risk for maladjustment. This finding suggests that children experiencing serious mental illness and environmental risk factors are at increased risk for poor outcomes (Pruett, 2007). Important components to assess when evaluating the client's microsystem include family characteristics and development because they constitute essential elements of the child's ecology. The structure of the parental unit can be an important indicator of support or stress in a family; for example, the presence or absence of marital conflict can affect development. Other microsystem contextual risk factors to consider include poverty; family, employment, or residential instability; child care burden; parental stress; and social isolation.

Community Characteristics (Exosystem)

A second level of salient ecological characteristics is the community. Cohesive neighborhoods with strong support services (eg, churches, community policing partnerships) can help mitigate the effects of community violence (Limbos et al., 2007; Mytton et al., 2006) (Figure 3.7). Conversely, studies have shown chronic community violence to be stressful for those exposed to it (Scarpa et al., 2006). Such violence can tax family resources and generally impede the performance of daily activities. Thus, assessing for community-level variables and factors that might mitigate related challenges is crucial for developing well-informed interventions.

Implications and Criticisms

Ecological theory is not a theory in the formal sense. Rather, it is a structured framework for identifying influences at numerous levels. Thus, it is not falsifiable. Its value is in alerting clinicians to factors that they otherwise might neglect. Research guided by this model is difficult to execute because study of these various factors is expensive. However, several researchers have attempted to do so, with interesting results (Evidence-Based Practice Spotlight 3.1).

Cicchetti's model has led clinicians to question the generalizability of their practices across cultures, genders, and ethnicities. Group-specific interventions are being

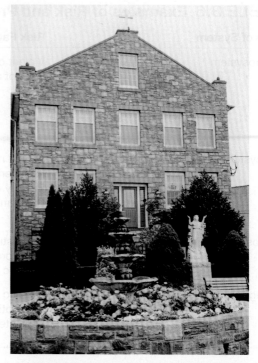

FIGURE 3.7 **Strong sources of community support, such as churches and neighborhood groups, can help to mitigate effects of community violence.**

developed. Ecological theory has led to policy changes in the federal funding of research, in that large studies now must address questions of generalizability across groups. Finally, ecological theorists have pressed clinicians to consider the possibility that interventions at a broader level might exert a powerful effect at the microsystem level.

Checkpoint Questions

9. What type of factors exert the strongest influence on children?

10. How would someone explain mental illness using the developmental–ecological framework?

◭ EVIDENCE-BASED PRACTICE SPOTLIGHT 3.1 ◭

Family Functioning and Juvenile Violence

Using a developmental–ecological model to guide their research, Gorman-Smith and colleagues (2000) examined how patterns of family functioning relate to patterns of juvenile offending. They found that risk for involvement in a pattern of serious and chronic offending is related to a different form of family configuration than a pattern of rapid escalation. Although both can represent serious delinquency, based on this study, the disparities seem to be differentially sensitive to neighborhood type and associated social processes. Also, based on the family configuration differences, they speculate that different preventive interventions are needed for each type of pathway. The patterns they found seem to support the developmental–ecological approach to risk and prevention that emphasizes understanding of predictor-risk relations and preventive intervention effects longitudinally and within the social context.

Reference

Gorman-Smith, D., Tolan, P. H., & Henry, D. B. (2000). Developmental–ecological model of the relation of family functioning to patterns of delinquency. *Journal of Quantitative Criminology, 16,* 169–198.

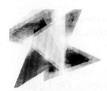

Reviewing and Applying Your Knowledge

Chapter Summary

- Theories and conceptual frameworks are worldviews that provide ways to understand human behavior and systematically frame research studies.

- Several theories have informed psychiatric nursing practice. They include the psychoanalytic, behavioral, cognitive, cognitive–behavioral, humanistic, interpersonal, biophysiologic, and sociocultural theories.

- Although no one theory has been adequate to explain mental health and mental illness, some are more useful than others. Some also have actual empirical evidence to support them.

- Research indicates that biologic, psychological, interpersonal, and sociocultural factors contribute to mental illnesses. However, the same circumstance may affect different people in very different ways.

- Researchers have constructed models that go beyond past reductionistic ones to view the person as a complex organism living, interacting, and transacting with others and negotiating risk and protective factors in ecologies. This dynamic view of humans holds great promise for research and for more precise assessment and interventions in the future.

Study Questions

1. When preparing a teaching plan about psychoanalytic theory for a group of nursing students, which concepts would the instructor expect to include? Select all that apply.
   a. The unconscious represents a small portion of the mind.
   b. People use defense mechanisms to protect against anxiety and threats.
   c. Personality develops through a succession of stages.
   d. Freud's ego represents a person's instinctual drives.
   e. Feelings of a service provider about a client are reflected in transference.
   f. The superego acts as the person's conscience.

2. Parents bring an adolescent female into counseling because she has been skipping school. The client states, "My parents are irresponsible and don't care about my feelings." The nurse interprets this statement as the client using which defense mechanism?
   a. Regression
   b. Reaction formation
   c. Projection
   d. Identification

3. During counseling, a client tells the therapist, "You remind me so much of my mother." The therapist interprets this statement as indicating the client's use of which of the following?
   a. Projection
   b. Transference
   c. Identification
   d. Countertransference

4. When a client is undergoing cognitive restructuring during RET therapy, which of the following would be essential for the client to identify first?
   a. Behavior or event based on the distorted belief
   b. Distorted belief about the behavior or event
   c. End result or consequence of the distorted belief
   d. Correction or debate about the distorted belief

5. When using the developmental–ecological framework, the nurse would assess which factors as important in the client's microsystem? Select all that apply.
   a. Violence in the neighborhood
   b. Family economic level
   c. Structure of the parental unit
   d. Lead screening activities
   e. Intelligence
   f. Stability of the home residence

References

Aber, J. L., & Cicchetti, D. (1984). The social-emotional development of maltreated children: An empirical and theoretical analysis. In H. Fitzgerald, B. Lester, & M. Yogman (Eds.), *Theory and research in behavioral pediatrics* (pp. 123–145). New York, NY: Plenum.

American Psychiatric Association. (2000). *Diagnostic and statistical manual of mental disorders* (4th ed., text rev.). Washington, DC: Author.

Anderson, J. A., & Mohr, W. K. (2003). A developmental ecological perspective in systems of care for children with serious emotional disturbances and their families. *Education and Treatment of Children, 26*(1), 52–74.

Beautler, L. E., & Levant, R. F. (2006). *Evidence-based practices in mental health: Debate and dialogue on the fundamental questions.* Washington, DC: American Psychological Association.

Beck, A. T. (1976). *Cognitive therapy and the emotional disorders.* New York, NY: International Universities Press.

Beck, A. T., & Rush, J. (1987). *Cognitive therapy of depression.* New York, NY: Guilford Press.

Beck, J., & Beck, A. T. (1995). *Cognitive therapy and beyond.* New York, NY: Guilford Press.

Berne, E. (1964). *Games people play.* New York, NY: Grove Press.

Bibring, G. L., Dwyer, T. F., Huntington, D. S., & Valenstein, A. F. (1961). A study of the psychological processes in pregnancy and of the earliest mother–child relationship. *Psychoanalytic Study of the Child, 16*, 9–72.

Blackman, J. S. (2004). *101 defenses: How the mind shields itself.* New York, NY: Brunner-Routledge

Bronfenbrenner, U. (1979). *The ecology of human development: Experiments by nature and design.* Cambridge, MA: Harvard University Press.

Bronfenbrenner, U. (1989). Foreword. In A. R. Pence (Ed.), *Ecological research with children and families: From concepts to methodology* (pp. 1–20). New York, NY: Teachers College Press.

Butcher, J. N., Mineka, S., & Hooley, J. M. (2006). *Abnormal psychology* (13th ed.). Reading, MA: Allyn & Bacon.

Cicchetti, D., & Cohen, J. D. (Eds.). (2006). *Developmental psychopathology, Volume 2: Risk, disorder and adaptation.* New York, NY: Wiley.

Corsini, R. J. (2000). *Current psychotherapies.* Itasca, IL: F. E. Peacock.

Dimeff, L. A., Koerner, K., & Linehan, M. M. (2007). *Dialectical behavior therapy in clinical practice: Applications across disorders and settings.* New York, NY: Guilford Press.

Dobson, K. S. (2002). *Handbook of cognitive behavior therapy* (2nd ed.). New York, NY: Guildford Press.

Ellis, A. (1962). *Reason and emotion in psychotherapy.* New York, NY: Lyle Stuart & Citadel Press.

Engler, B. (2005). *Personality theories: An introduction* (7th ed.). New York, NY: Houghton Mifflin.

Erwin, E. (1995). *A final accounting: Philosophical and empirical issues in Freudian psychology.* Cambridge, MA: MIT Press.

Esterson, A. (1999). *Seductive mirage: An exploration of the work of Sigmund Freud.* Chicago, IL: Open Court Books.

Evans, A. M. (2007). Transference in the nurse–patient relationship. *Journal of Psychiatric Mental Health Nursing, 14*(2), 189–195.

Freud, A. (1966). *The ego and the mechanisms of defense.* New York, NY: International Universities Press. (Original work published 1936)

Gallagher, B. J. (2002). *The sociology of mental illness.* Upper Saddle River, NJ: Prentice Hall.

Hersen, M. (2002). *Clinical behavior therapy: Adolescent and child.* New York, NY: John Wiley & Sons.

Hollingshead, A. M., & Redlich, F. C. (1958). *Social class and mental illness.* New York, NY: John Wiley & Sons.

Horowitz, A. V. (2002). *The social control of mental illness.* Clinton Corners, NY: Eliot Werner Publications.

Kandel, E. R. (1998). A new intellectual framework for psychiatry. *American Journal of Psychiatry, 155*(4), 457–469.

Kandel, E. R. (1999). Biology and the future of psychoanalysis: A new intellectual framework for psychiatry revisited. *American Journal of Psychiatry, 156*(4), 505–524.

Kaufman, J. (2007). Child abuse and neglect. In A. Martin & F. R. Volmar (Eds.), *Lewis's child and adolescent psychiatry: A comprehensive textbook* (4th ed., pp. 692–701). Philadelphia, PA: Lippincott Williams & Wilkins.

Kernberg, O. F. (1994). The psychotherapeutic management of psychopathic, narcissistic, and paranoid transferences. In T. Millon, E. Simonsen, M. Birket-Smith, & R. D. Davis (Eds.), *Psychopathy: Antisocial, Criminal and Violent Behavior* (pp. 372–460). New York, NY: The Guilford Press.

Lax, P. D. (2002). *Functional analysis.* New York, NY: Wiley Interscience.

Leckman, J. F., Vaccarino, F. M., & Lombroso, P. J. (2007). From genes to brain: Developmental neurobiology. In A. Martin & F. R. Volmar (Eds.), *Lewis's child and adolescent psychiatry: A comprehensive textbook* (4th ed., pp. 177–189). Philadelphia, PA: Lippincott Williams & Wilkins.

Limbos, M. A., Chan, L. S., Warf, C., Schneir, A., Iverson, E., Shekelle, P., & Kipke, M. D. (2007). Effectiveness of interventions to prevent youth violence: A systematic review. *American Journal of Preventive Medicine, 33*(1), 65–74.

Meichenbaum, D. H. (1977). *Cognitive behavior modification: An integrative approach.* New York, NY: Plenum.

Mintzer, J. E., Hendrie, H. C., Warachal, C. B., & Faison, E. (2005). Minority and sociocultural issues. In B. J. Sadock & V. A. Sadock (Eds.), *Kaplan and Sadock's comprehensive textbook of psychiatry* (8th ed., pp. 3813–3822). Philadelphia, PA: Lippincott Williams & Wilkins.

Mytton, J., DiGuiseppi, C., Gough, D., Taylor, R., & Logan, S. (2006). School-based secondary prevention programmes for preventing violence. *Cochrane Database of Systematic Reviews, 2006*(3). CD004606.

Nathan, P. E., & Gorman, J. M. (2007). *A guide to treatments that work* (3rd ed.). New York, NY: Oxford University Press.

National Research Council. (1993). *Understanding child abuse and neglect.* Washington, DC: National Academy Press.

Norcross, J. C., & Goldfried, M. R. (2005). *Handbook of psychotherapy integration.* New York, NY: Oxford University Press.

O'Donohue, W. T., Hayes, S. C., & Fisher, J. E. (2005). *Cognitive behavior therapy: Applying empirically supported techniques in your practice.* New York, NY: John Wiley & Sons.

Paris, J. (1999). *Nature and nurture in psychiatry: A predisposition-stress model of mental disorders.* Washington, DC: American Psychiatric Press.

Pruett, K. D. (2007). The art of the science: A child, family, and systems-centered approach. In A. Martin & F. R. Volmar (Eds.), *Lewis's child and adolescent psychiatry: A comprehensive textbook* (4th ed., pp. 2–11). Philadelphia, PA: Lippincott Williams & Wilkins.

Rose, S., Bisson, J., Churchill, R., & Wessely, S. (2006). Psychological debriefing for preventing post traumatic stress disorder. *Cochrane Database of Systematic Reviews, 2006*(4). doi:10.1002/14651858/CD001087.pub3

Scarpa, A., Hurley, J. D., Shumate, H. W., & Haden, S. C. (2006). Lifetime prevalence and socioemotional effects of hearing about community violence. *Journal of Interpersonal Violence, 21*(1), 5–23.

Symonds, P. (1946). *The dynamics of human adjustment.* New York, NY: Appleton-Century- Crofts.

Tallis, R. C. (1996). Burying Freud. *Lancet, 347*(9002), 669–671.

University of Minnesota. (2001). *Evidence-based nursing.* Retrieved from http://evidence.ahc.umn.edu/ebn.htm

Walter, U., & Petr, C. (2000). A template for family-centered interagency collaboration. *Families in Society, 81*(5), 494–503.

Webster, R. (1996). *Why Freud was wrong: Sin, science and psychoanalysis.* London, UK: HarperCollins.

Wyden, P. (1997). *Conquering schizophrenia.* New York, NY: Alfred A. Knopf.

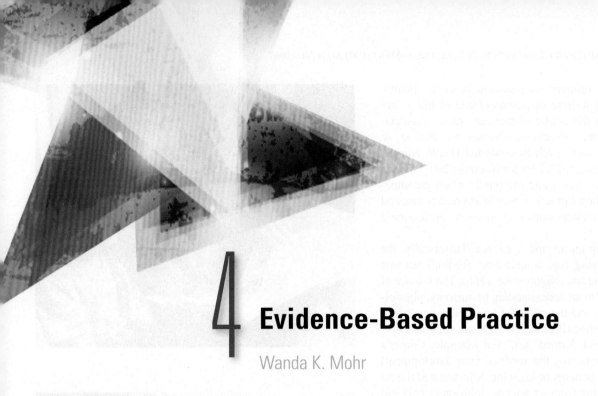

4

Evidence-Based Practice

Wanda K. Mohr

LEARNING OBJECTIVES

On completion of this chapter, you should be able to accomplish the following:

- Define *science*.
- Identify principles of the scientific method.
- Define *evidence-based care*.
- Identify the types of scientific evidence that constitute support for treatments and interventions.
- Differentiate pseudoscience, junk science, and quackery from science.
- Give examples of pseudoscience, junk science, and quackery and how they can have detrimental effects on the public.
- Explain the importance of evidence-based practice to nursing.

The nurse's primary commitment is to the health, safety, and welfare of people placed in his or her care, as well as to the public (American Nurses Association [ANA], American Psychiatric Nurses Association, & International Society of Psychiatric–Mental Health Nurses, 2007). The ANA's Code of Ethics for Nursing (2001) directs nurses to safeguard clients and the public when incompetent, unethical, or illegal practices may affect health care and safety. It further instructs nurses to maintain professional competence.

Nursing is both an art and a science. Historically, the simple acts of nursing (eg, wound care, feeding) became known as the nursing arts (Nightingale, 1860). The science of nursing was rooted in an understanding of anatomy, physiology, and chemistry, and the quest for knowledge was based on the scientific method (Peplau, 1988). Many nursing scholars have debated and defined "art." For example, Carper's (1978) seminal (containing the seeds of later development) article on nursing's patterns of knowing differentiated the art or esthetics of nursing from its science. Johnson (1994) and Wainwright (1999) conceptualized the art of nursing as a craft and an ability to grasp meaning, establish a connection with clients, determine a course of action, and skillfully perform nursing activities. Given this way of thinking, the art of nursing is not a phenomenon or aspect separated from science, but more the means of carrying out the science of nursing in a skillful, knowledgeable, intelligent, and ethical manner.

As competent and moral practitioners, nurses are obligated to provide evidence-based treatment for those in their care. Although similar, **evidence-based practice (EBP)** and **empirically supported treatments (ESTs)** are different. EBP is the integration of research with clinical expertise in the context of the client's characteristics, culture, and preferences. EBP also includes a weighing of benefits against the risks and costs of treatment as well. ESTs are treatments with at least two randomized controlled clinical trials that demonstrate their efficacy. This is a very rigorous standard. Because EBP allows for various kinds of evidence besides randomized, controlled trials to be taken into consideration, it is usually considered less stringent and less controversial than the use of ESTs (Chorpita, 2003).

The scientific and ethical foundations of nursing imply that the profession's interventions and services have validated support. Competent nurses are expected to make decisions based on research findings, to monitor and document the effects of interventions, and to use concrete, observable, and measurable terms and instruments to demonstrate outcomes.

The history of mental health has been distinguished by extraordinary gains in the understanding of human behavior and neurophysiology. Unfortunately, excess, scandal, pseudoscience, and quackery also have proliferated. Extraordinary claims bombard the public through multiple means daily (Figure 4.1). Evaluation of these numerous claims requires sophisticated knowledge and understanding of research methods, professional practice, and the principles and limitations of the scientific method.

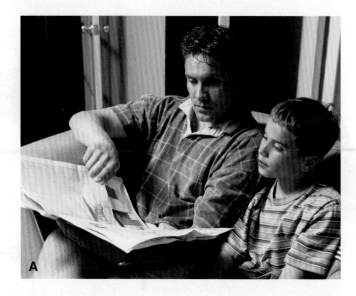

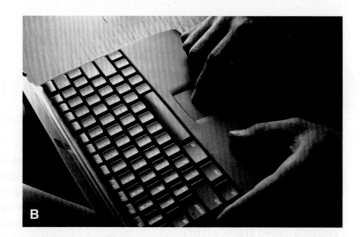

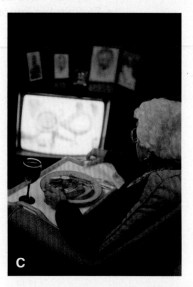

FIGURE 4.1 **People are exposed to multiple outlets that communicate extraordinary claims relative to all sorts of treatments and problems. Examples include (A)** newspapers, **(B)** the Internet, and **(C)** television.

The purpose of this chapter is to differentiate evidence-based from non–EBPs. To help students evaluate and distinguish the mythical and fraudulent from genuine science, this chapter reviews what constitutes science and the scientific method. Using concrete examples, it provides an overview of the potentially harmful effects of practices not grounded in scientifically validated principles. It also describes some pseudoscientific practices that have had negative emotional and financial outcomes for clients with psychiatric problems and their families.

SCIENCE

The words *science* and *research* sometimes intimidate or frighten readers, perhaps because students have not been encouraged earlier in school to develop a passion for science. A less intimidating way of approaching science is to understand it primarily as an attitude toward problem solving. **Science** attempts to explain natural phenomena by creating a relatively simple conceptual framework to account for observed facts. Scientists apply formal and informal reasoning methods to comprehend and predict the world. A fundamental principle is that the natural world is ordered, understandable, and explainable through natural processes. Scientists greatly emphasize what can be observed, measured, and publicly verified. Scientific processes include controlled observation, experimentation, analysis, synthesis, prediction, and confirmation (Table 4.1).

Principles of the Scientific Method

The **scientific method** is a self-correcting system that relies on logic and empirical processes to test theories against observable data. As such, it is the best method humans have of gaining objective knowledge because empirical facts ultimately support this system. The scientific method is not a strict set of rules; however, it has some important principles:

1. Science uses methods of systematic empiricism.
2. Science aims for publicly verifiable knowledge.
3. Science seeks empirically solvable problems that yield testable theories (Stanovich, 2007).

Systematic Empiricism

Empiricism is a philosophical position that all knowledge and all ideas derive from experience. Scientists learn about the world by observing and examining it (Figure 4.2). They do so systematically, not randomly. Systematic empiricism means that scientific observations are structured so that results of those observations reveal something about the world. However, knowledge derived from observations can be no more than generalizations and can never reach more than a very high degree of probability (Stanovich, 2007).

Publicly Verifiable Knowledge

The second principle of the scientific method involves the public nature of scientific knowledge. Knowledge gathered

TABLE 4.1 **Scientific Processes**

Controlled observations	*Observation* basically means watching phenomena and taking note of changes (if any) through some means of measurement. Researchers make observations using direct and indirect methods. The controlled element involves conducting observation under specifically defined protocols.
Experimentation	Experimentation is the process of testing a hypothesis or prediction by carrying out data-gathering procedures under controlled conditions. Such conditions eliminate extraneous influences and facilitate close observations.
Analysis	Analysis of data is the process of determining whether data are reliable and whether they support a given prediction or hypothesis. Scientists analyze data in many ways, including using statistics, interpreting graphs, determining relationships between variables, comparing data with those obtained from other studies, and determining possible sources of experimental error.
Synthesis	Synthesis is the ability to put parts together to form a new whole.
Prediction	To test a hypothesis, a scientist usually makes a prediction that follows from the hypothesis. Predicting is stating in advance the results that one will obtain from testing a hypothesis. A prediction can take the form of an "if–then" statement. If the data collected show a prediction to be false, then they refute the hypothesis. If the data show a prediction to be true, then they support the hypothesis.
Confirmation	Once a researcher collects data through repeated observation and experimentation and reaches conclusions, he or she must publish these results for review by other scientists around the world. Then, other scientists must confirm or replicate the results of the experiment or study and reach similar findings before giving the results validity.

Adapted from Dobson & Fitzgerald (2005).

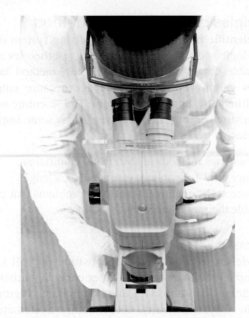

FIGURE 4.2 Science is rooted in the objective study of phenomena.

empirically does not exist solely in the mind of the scientist. In fact, it does not exist at all until he or she disseminates results to the scientific community for critique, testing, and replication. Unverified findings limited to one person or group never attain the status of scientific knowledge. The person or group must present evidence to the scientific community so that others can achieve the same outcomes. This process protects against bias or error in achieving results.

Empirically Solvable Problems and Testable Theories

The third principle is that science limits itself to empirically solvable, specified problems. Scientists deal with questions potentially answerable only through empirical techniques (Stanovich, 2007). Questions such as "Is the death penalty immoral?" "Does God exist?" "What does this dream mean?" and "What is evil?" do not lend themselves to scientific study. They involve matters unanswerable through current scientific techniques.

Many aspects of mental health, psychiatric illness, and related care are unobservable. Some of the previously mentioned questions are typical issues troubling clients with various disorders (eg, depression). Pinpointing what can be studied related to such questions is important. For example, although scientific methodology cannot prove the existence of God, researchers can study the effects of spiritual beliefs on recovery from mental illness (see Chap. 7). Although empirical methods cannot establish the meaning of a dream, studies may be designed to report the physical and mental effects of discussing dreams with a therapist. Again, empirical techniques can be used to examine such questions, and researchers can disseminate their results to others for retesting.

Types of Scientific Evidence

Experimental investigations provide the highest level of scientific support for treatments. In such studies, researchers construct a design in which they assign subjects randomly to various groups. One group receives the treatment under investigation; one group remains untreated for comparison. Other possible groups include those who receive a sham treatment and those who receive a placebo. **Sham treatments** refer to counterfeit forms of therapy. **Placebos** are inert substances, such as sugar pills, given to determine the efficacy of a medication. Both sham treatments and placebos are used in clinical trials that compare their effects against those of a legitimate therapy or active medication. By the rules of research design, a clinical trial is the only approach that enables the interpretation of significant differences between or among groups as indicating that the treatment itself has caused change.

Ideally, investigation of a treatment uses a **double-blind approach**, in which neither clients and their families nor the researchers recording results know what treatment a subject is receiving. Nathan and Gorman (2007) designate these studies as type I. Their typology is elaborated on more fully in Evidence-Based Practice Spotlight 4.1.

Type II studies involve clinical trials, but some component of a type I study is missing. An example is a trial in which researchers cannot maintain a double-blind approach. Type II studies are methodologically flawed, but flaws are not fatal. They provide valuable contributions to scientific knowledge, despite being less rigorous than type I studies.

Type III studies have clear limitations, involve heavy bias, and generally are conducted as pilot research. Scientists do them to determine whether a treatment is worth pursuing with a more extensive or rigorous design. An example is a **case–control study**, in which researchers use specific criteria to identify participants and then interview them retrospectively. Case–control studies provide extensive naturalistic data, but findings are clearly exploratory and not definitive.

Type IV studies involve secondary data analysis, which can be quite helpful, particularly when sophisticated. In a **secondary data analysis**, the analyst is not the person who collected the data or the data were collected for a reason different than that for which they are currently being used. This method can be a creative way to reuse existing information. Conversely, it can be handled irresponsibly (eg, an analyst might manipulate and transform data to lessen the validity of the original research).

Type V studies entail reviews of literature without secondary data analysis. They help consolidate findings on a certain subject but are subject to the biases and opinions of the writer.

Type VI studies involve **uncontrolled case reports** and are of questionable value. They may be of interest in terms of discussing unusual or extreme situations; however,

◣ **EVIDENCE-BASED PRACTICE SPOTLIGHT 4.1** ◢

Typology of Studies

Type I	• Most rigorous
	• Prospective in nature
	• Involve comparison groups with random assignment of subjects, blinded assessments, clear presentation of inclusion and exclusion criteria, state-of-the-art diagnostic methods, adequate sample size for statistical power, and clearly described statistical methods
Type II	• Clinical trial of an intervention or treatment
	• Less rigorous than type I, in that some aspect of a type I study is missing (eg, treatment is not randomized, double blinding is impossible)
	• Important but not definitive
Type III	• Methodologically limited
	• Include open treatment studies aimed at collecting pilot data and subject to observer bias, as well as retrospective studies because they are subject to recall error
Type IV	• Reviews of the literature with secondary data analysis of original studies
	• Although useful, tend to include only positive data and are thus flawed by the omission of negative outcome data
Type V	• Reviews of the literature without secondary data analysis
	• Helpful because they give an overview of literature, but are subject to the writers' opinions and sometimes highly biased
Type VI	• Various reports with marginal value (eg, case studies, essays, opinion papers)

Adapted from Nathan & Gorman (2007).

they are not an appropriate basis for interventions. Moreover, they are subject to the bias of the person reporting them and are often simply "hearsay."

Evidence-Based Practice Spotlight 4.2 provides exemplars of each of the six types of studies. The writers of this text have attempted as much as possible to refer to type I or type II studies when referencing interventions. In psychiatric–mental health nursing, not all interventions have an empirical basis. Some are recommended based on expert consensus by scholars from various professional organizations. Others are based on tradition. The evidence-based movement represents an attempt to apply more rigor and science to interventions for clients and their families.

Checkpoint Questions

1. What three principles are most important to the scientific method?
2. What is meant by a double-blind approach?
3. Which type of scientific study typically is used as pilot research?

PSEUDOSCIENCE

Pseudoscience is the term used for therapies and treatments that have no empirical or theoretical support. Such practices frequently are based on assumptions at odds with paradigms generally accepted by professionals in related areas. They may lead to myths and distortions that influence mainstream practices. Frequently, practitioners of pseudoscience describe their methods as "unconventional" or "unorthodox." Some sincerely believe in the appropriateness and efficacy of their therapies. Others are concerned with enriching themselves at the expense of trusting clients (Wynn & Wiggins, 2001).

Some clients or families become disenchanted with professionally approved treatments and voluntarily seek pseudoscientific therapies. Others habitually reject "establishment" views and readily accept theories that contrast with common professional practices. Pseudoscience may involve underground or unlicensed activities; however, many practitioners function openly and market themselves as mainstream "therapists." Some problematic people come to professional and public awareness only after excesses and abuses result in legal or criminal proceedings. An example is the death of Candace Newmaker, discussed later in this chapter.

By virtue of their sheer numbers alone, nurses are highly visible professionals with daily public contact. As such, they have many excellent opportunities to protect clients and families from pseudoscientific therapies (Figure 4.3). Such faulty practices share several common characteristics that distinguish them from scientifically approved health care interventions.

Pseudoscience Versus Science

Perhaps the most important characteristic that separates pseudoscience from genuine science is the lack of concern

EVIDENCE-BASED PRACTICE SPOTLIGHT 4.2

Exemplars of Levels of Study

Level	Study	Method	Results and Conclusions
Type I	Jensen, H. V., Davidsen, K., Toftegaard, L., Mellerup, E. T., Plenge, P., Aggernaes, H., & Bjorum, N. (1996). Double-blind comparison of the side-effect profiles of daily versus alternate-day dosing schedules in lithium maintenance treatment of manic-depressive disorder. *Journal of Affective Disorders, 36*(3–4), 89–93.	**Double-blind randomized trial.** Researchers compared side-effect profiles with daily versus alternate-day dosing of lithium carbonate for 50 clients with bipolar disorder. After 3 months of daily lithium maintenance treatment, they randomly allocated clients to daily or alternate-day dosing, aiming at maintaining the same 12-h serum concentration as before allocation (median 0.7 mmol/L). Median daily and alternate-day doses were 700 mg and 1200 mg, respectively.	No significant correlation appeared between changes in side-effect scores on the side-effect and lithium dosing schedule (ordinal logistic regression), although analysis revealed a trend in favor of alternate-day dosing in terms of polyuria, polydipsia, and diarrhea. Thus, the study findings lend no support to the hypothesis that extending the interval between lithium doses from 1 to 2 days can diminish side effects.
Type II	Sensky, T., Turkington, D., Kingdon, D., Scott, J., Siddle, R., O'Carroll, M., & Barnes, T. (2000). A randomized controlled trial of cognitive–behavioral therapy for persistent symptoms in schizophrenia resistant to medication. *Archives of General Psychiatry, 57*(2), 165–172.	**Randomized controlled trial non–double blind.** Researchers compared the efficacy of manualized cognitive–behavioral therapy developed particularly for schizophrenia with that of a nonspecific befriending control intervention. Two experienced nurses under regular supervision delivered both interventions. Blind raters assessed clients at baseline, after treatment (up to 9 months), and at a 9-month follow-up visit. Clients continued to receive routine care throughout the study. An assessor blind to the clients' treatment groups rated the technical quality of random audiotaped sessions. Analysis was by intention to treat.	Ninety clients received a mean of 19 individual treatment sessions over 9 months, with no significant between-group differences in treatment duration. Both interventions resulted in significant reductions in positive and negative symptoms and depression. At the 9-month follow-up evaluation, clients who had received cognitive therapy continued to improve, whereas those in the befriending group did not. These results were not attributable to changes in prescribed medication. Cognitive–behavioral therapy is effective in treating negative as well as positive symptoms in schizophrenia resistant to standard antipsychotic drugs, with its efficacy sustained over 9 months of follow-up.
Type III	Jensen, H. V., & Andersen, J. (1989). An open noncomparative study of amoxapine in borderline disorders. *Acta Psychiatrica Scandinavica, 79*(1), 89–93.	**Comparative pilot study with N of 10.** Five clients with borderline personality disorder (BPD) and five with schizotypal personality disorder (SPD) completed at least 3 weeks of treatment with amoxapine. They met *DSM-III* criteria for BPD and scored 7 points or more in Gunderson's Diagnostic Interview for Borderlines (DIB). The final median medication in clients with BPD was 200 mg/day of amoxapine and 42 mg/day of oxazepam. Treatment averaged 28 days. In clients with SPD, corresponding figures were 250 mg/day amoxapine, 36 mg/day oxazepam, and 39 days.	Findings suggest that amoxapine improves schizophrenic-like and depressive symptoms in clients with SPD. No effect could be substantiated in clients with BPD.

EVIDENCE-BASED PRACTICE SPOTLIGHT 4.2

Exemplars of Levels of Study (continued)

Level	Study	Method	Results and Conclusions
Type IV	deLiz, T. M., & Straus, B. (2005). Differential efficacy of group and individual/couple psychotherapy with infertile patients. *Human Reproduction, 20*(5), 1324–1332.	***Meta-analyses*** were conducted to evaluate the efficacy of group and individual/couple therapies on the reduction of negative emotional symptoms and the possible promotion of pregnancy.	Group and individual/couple psychotherapy led to decreased anxiety. Upon termination of therapy, clients had fewer depressive symptoms after 6 months. Psychotherapy accompanying IVF treatment yielded similar conception success rates to psychological interventions administered to clients not in specific medical care. Results suggest positive effects of psychotherapy for clients with infertility; however, these results must be viewed with caution because of methodological and informational bias within the studies analyzed.
Type V	Mohr, W. K. (2006). Spiritual issues in psychiatric care. *Perspectives in Psychiatric Care, 42*(3), 174–183.	***Review of literature with no meta-analysis.*** This article differentiates between spirituality and religion and analyzes the strengths and weaknesses of research findings related to spirituality, religion, and mental health. It discusses the importance of clarifying values and becoming self-aware relative to spiritual and religious interventions. It explains the components of spiritual assessment and spiritual coping practices and interventions that may help when working with clients. Review of literature was obtained from MEDLINE, CINAHL, PSYCHINFO, and current texts.	
Type VI	Amardeep, K., & Balan, S. (2007). Fluoxetine for persistent developmental stuttering. *Clinical Neuropharmacology, 30*(1), 58–59.	***Case Report.*** Stuttering is a disturbance in the normal fluency and time patterning of speech. Developmental stuttering (DS), with or without associated psychiatric illness, is the most common form and includes all cases with gradual onset in childhood that are not the result of acquired brain damage. Persistent developmental stuttering (PDS) is DS that has not undergone spontaneous or speech therapy–induced remission. Adults in speech therapy behavioral programs often show regression and even total relapse if they stop practicing. This case report deals with a client with PDS who responded significantly to treatment with fluoxetine.	

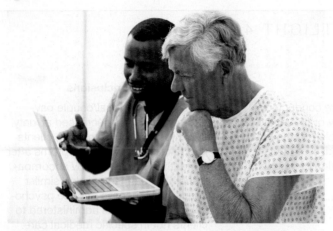

FIGURE 4.3 Nurses can teach clients and families about genuine, scientifically sound treatments and alternatives. They also can work with them to differentiate fraudulent pseudoscientific therapies from legitimate modalities.

with valid evidence (Lilienfeld et al., 2004). Practitioners of pseudoscience rely on eyewitness testimonies and personal anecdotes, rather than well-controlled, publicly verifiable studies. Conversely, the foundations of science are evidence and logical argumentation.

Pseudoscientists operate from **assumptions,** or assertions taken for granted or supposed that may be either explicit or hidden (Mohr & Anderson, 2001). Assumptions are beliefs accepted as true and viewed as representative of reality. They also can misrepresent reality and perpetuate the status quo. For example, an erroneous assumption is that physical restraint of clients is a therapeutic tool in milieu management. In reality, researchers have found that restraint yields no demonstrable therapeutic effects on aggressive clients and indeed is associated with decreased positive behaviors (Delaney, 2006; Mohr & Anderson, 2001).

Scientists make underlying assumptions explicit before presenting evidence for their claims. Pseudoscientists do not do so, nor do they encourage examination of their assumptions by supporters, outside experts, or detractors for soundness or logic (Lilienfeld et al., 2004).

Myths

Within this context, **myths** are complete inventions, often deeply rooted in cultural beliefs, and difficult to dispel. Rather than measuring actual outcomes, practitioners of myths assess performance in terms of behaviors prescribed by the myths themselves. They usually do not question the myths unless they have new myths to replace them. Without myths to embrace, they would have little basis for believing in their own efficacy.

An example involves the concept of *self-esteem.* For nearly two generations, self-esteem has been the foundation of personal growth in the United States. So many societal problems—smoking, drinking, drug use, stealing, lying, cheating, overeating, and underachieving—have been linked to problems with self-esteem. Proponents of

high self-esteem encourage the idea that "we are who we think we are." According to this viewpoint, improvements in individual self-esteem will lead to improved individual outcomes.

However, scientific research on self-esteem challenges these beliefs. Roy Baumeister, professor of psychology at Florida State University, and his colleagues have conducted extensive reviews of research on self-esteem during the past 20 years. Describing society's belief that self-esteem rises with success and declines with corresponding failure, they noted, "This pervasive correlation may well strengthen the impression that one's level of self-esteem is not just the outcome, but indeed the cause, of life's major successes and failures" (Baumeister et al., 1993, p. 150). Baumeister's research has shown that pervasive efforts to boost student self-esteem did not improve, and sometimes hurt, academic performance. Their findings indicate that high self-esteem does not prevent children from smoking, drinking, taking drugs, or engaging in early sex. Indeed, their study supports that high self-esteem fosters experimentation, which may increase early sex or drinking. According to their research, effects of self-esteem, in general, are negligible. An important exception is that high self-esteem reduces the chances of bulimia in girls and women (Presnell et al., 2004).

Nursing texts often promote building self-esteem as an intervention for children with conduct disorder (Stanovich, 2007). A common assumption is that low self-esteem underlies aggressive behavior or violence. Actually, evidence negates this idea. Some studies have shown an association between violent aggression and inflated, not low, self-esteem (Baumeister, 2001; Baumeister et al., 1993; Cale & Lilienfeld, 2006; Stanovich, 2007). This finding has held true across a broad spectrum of behaviors, from bullying to domestic abuse and rape. Violent perpetrators typically have exaggerated self-esteem and are more aggressive than others (Baumeister et al., 1996).

Such findings do not mean that health care providers should engage in interventions that diminish self-esteem or positive self-regard for all clients. They do question ideas and beliefs that have resulted more from conventional wisdom than from collected scientific evidence. They also identify the inherent difficulties in dealing with abstractions such as "self-esteem." What exactly is self-esteem? Does it mean something different to each person? How have various studies measured it? What findings are reliable if operational definitions for self-esteem differ according to study, research team, or both?

Quackery

The definition of a **quack** is "a charlatan; a pretender to medical skill" (*Merriam-Webster's On-line Dictionary*, 2007). Quackery entails methods not scientifically accepted and involves fraudulent medical practices, usually for money, ego gratification, and power. Those who practice quackery give false hope to genuinely suffering people (Dawes, 2001). Sometimes quacks engage in deliberate fraud and deception.

However, often they sincerely believe in what they are doing and may be unwitting victims who share misinformation and personal anecdotes with others (Barrett, 2001).

Quackery and misleading advertising are frequent companions. For example, some quacks attribute nonscientific therapeutic effects and outcomes to herbs, vitamins, minerals, and other food supplements. Quackery also may involve labeling something as harmful (eg, food additives or preservatives) without scientific evidence (Barrett & Jarvis, 2005). Practitioners actually may harm vulnerable clients by causing them to postpone legitimate care, or they may not cause direct harm but lead clients and families to spend financial resources needlessly. Some treatments may involve legitimate therapies or medications. For example, vitamin B_{12} has been shown to be useful in the treatment of pernicious anemia. However, it has not been shown to be effective in the treatment of fatigue (Barrett & Jarvis, 1993). Regardless of the particular circumstances, quackery causes suffering, provides false hope, and misleads people into spending money and time on ineffective, and possibly dangerous, "treatments."

Distinguishing unproven interventions from quackery is important. Unproven treatments consistent with established scientific concepts are considered *experimental;* researchers studying them are engaged in properly designed studies. Treatments promoted without established scientific methodology, replication, and peer review are not experimental (Whitlock, 2001). They are either unvalidated or unproven. In other words, "the jury is still out." They may actually become legitimized through empirical means.

Quacks engage in struggles with legitimate health care providers, mainstream scientists, government regulatory agencies, and consumer protection groups. Despite the strength of scientific opposition, quackery persists. Unfortunately, quacks often target illnesses that are poorly understood by the medical community, difficult to treat, terminal, or characterized by fluctuations. They prey on the frustration of clients who have failed to achieve relief through the services of the legitimate medical community (Whitlock, 2001).

Quacks and pseudoscientists use several strategies to defend themselves against the medical establishment. They may point to instances of persecution of pioneers such as Pasteur or Galileo. They may accuse such authorities as the American Medical Association or U.S. Food and Drug Administration (FDA) of engaging in a conspiracy to suppress their treatment (Barrett & Jarvis, 2005). They also may accuse these organizations and agencies of being "bought off" by insurers or drug companies. They may point out that medical science does not have all the answers. However, medical science does not make such a claim. Rather, its claim is that empirically supported interventions have been subject to rigorous study, peer review, and public scrutiny.

Most recently, several quacks have defended themselves using concepts from postmodernism. The movement is influenced by the writings of philosophers (eg, Jean Baudrillard, Jacques Lacan) who use (and sometimes misuse) terminology and concepts from mathematics and physics (Sokal & Bricmont, 1999). Postmodernists have applied such ideas as Gödel's theorems, relativity, quantum mechanics (particularly the uncertainty principle), chaos theory, and catastrophe theory to literature and psychoanalysis. The postmodern movement also has infiltrated medicine and nursing. It encourages people to believe that health care advice based on scientific research is of no more value than any other health care advice. It is not uncommon to read in some nursing journals discussions of the existence of energy fields or applications of Einstein's equations to ethical relativity. Some authors borrow terms from theoretical physics without regard for what those terms actually mean (Sokal & Bricmont, 1999). For example, the terms *energy* and *field* both have precise (not metaphorical) meanings in physics, but *energy field* is meaningless in physics (Raskin, 2000). Many readers have little understanding of the scientific theory or the philosophical implications of what is being invoked. They may assume that if an author has a doctorate, he or she should be believed without question.

Patterning

Families usually are motivated to obtain the best and most effective services available for relatives with severe disabilities. Staff members usually want to provide their best training and methods. Both recipients and providers are vulnerable to promises offered by unconventional therapeutic techniques, especially when respected authorities misrepresent or misinterpret effects. Probably the best-known quackery treatment precipitously and broadly adopted within the field of developmental disabilities was "patterning," also referred to as the Doman-Delacato technique (Delacato, 1963; Doman et al., 1960). Doman and Delacato asserted that mental retardation represents a person's failure to develop through proper "phylogenetic" (evolutionary) stages. Their modality of patterning is a time-consuming treatment involving passive physical manipulation of the limbs and body to stimulate proper phylogenetic development. According to patterning, the person must master each stage before progressing to the next. The exercises intend to impose the proper "pattern" on the central nervous system. When first used, the intensity of the procedures requires several volunteers to work daily or weekly conducting physical manipulations on each subject.

The American Academy of Pediatrics (AAP) has issued and reaffirmed its position statement (1999, 2006) that patterning has no special merit, that its proponents' claims are unproven, and that the demands on families are so great that in some cases their financial resources become severely depleted, leading to compromised parental and sibling relationships. Nevertheless, patterning services are still available in some areas, despite the lack of credible supporting scientific research. Indeed, ample basic science supports the contrary position that the person's interactive participation and contact with contingencies of reinforcement are essential to establish the neural substrate of organized behavior during development.

Facilitated Communication

Another example of quackery is *facilitated communication* (FC), methods that assist nonverbal people to type letters, words, phrases, or sentences with a typewriter, computer keyboard, or alphabet facsimile. Developed by a special education teacher in Australia during the 1970s, FC was introduced in the United States in 1990. It involves a graduated manual prompting procedure, with the intent of supporting a person's hand sufficiently to make it more feasible to strike the desired keys, without influencing selection (Mulick et al., 1993). Proponents have claimed that FC produces unexpected literacy (Biklen, 1990, 1992a, 1992b) in nonverbal people with a lifelong and unambiguous history of autism, moderate to profound mental retardation, or both. Without scientific evidence of its validity and effectiveness (Federal Trade Commission [FTC], 1995a, 1995b), and despite objective research findings identifying widespread, systematic facilitator control of typed content, FC became pervasive in special education and adult services for people with developmental disabilities.

FC continues to be practiced, with many supporting websites available. However, according to the American Psychological Association, peer-reviewed, scientifically based studies found that therapists who provided FC directed or systematically determined the typed language output (represented through computers, letter boards, and so forth) attributed to clients. As a result, the American Psychological Association adopted a resolution in 1994 (Resolution on Facilitated Communication by the American Psychological Association) stating that FC "is a controversial and unproved communicative procedure with no scientifically demonstrated support for its efficacy" (Jacobson et al., 1995, p. 760). The AAP (1998, 2006) also has reaffirmed its position that FC lacks empirical support.

Although FC is not physically damaging, it causes harm by fostering hope in already stressed families. It also diverts funds that could be better spent for treatments with actual supporting evidence.

The Dangers of "Junk Science"

Junk science means faulty data collection and analysis used to further a special agenda. The media may use junk science for sensational headlines and programming to attract viewers and advertisers. Some members of the media use junk science to advance their or their employers' social and political agendas. In some cases, problems with junk science have wreaked havoc in health care. Two examples involve multiple personality disorder (MPD) and aspartame.

Multiple Personality Disorder

MPD, known in the *Diagnostic and Statistical Manual of Mental Disorders*, 4th edition, text revision (*DSM-IV-TR*; American Psychiatric Association [APA], 2000) as dissociative identity disorder (DID), is a legitimate, albeit rare, diagnostic category that has prompted much controversy (see Chap. 24). During the 1980s and 1990s, thousands of people received this diagnosis indiscriminately. Programs specializing in treatment of DID proliferated across the United States.

This diagnosis arose from relative obscurity with the publication of the 1954 case study and subsequent film *The Three Faces of Eve* (Thigpen & Cleckley, 1957). A second book, *Sybil* (Schrieber, 1973), presented as a semidocumentary, described a woman believed to have 16 separate personalities. The book became a best seller and television movie. These and other books and movies made major contributions to the public's perception and acceptance of MPD. Despite little evidence that abuse is a necessary or sufficient contributor to MPD, conventional wisdom is that early childhood abuse can lead to multiple personalities. This perception has persisted despite evidence that the therapist in the *Sybil* case induced the personalities (Acocella, 1999). After publication of *Sybil*, reports of MPD rose from 50 to more than 20,000 (Piper, 1997).

Several social forces during the 1980s contributed to a proliferation of interest in and publicity for MPD, including the rise of a huge for-profit psychiatric hospital industry, talk shows featuring victims of sexual abuse, the emergence of the child advocacy movement, and widespread allegations of satanic ritual abuse (SRA) of children. SRA is the name given to the allegedly systematic sexual molestation, torture, and murder of U.S. children by well-organized intergenerational satanic cults across the country. In the 1980s panic ensued regarding SRA, with allegations publicized widely on radio and television talk shows.

Many therapists began to uncover in clients "repressed memories" of murderous satanic cults that subjected people to unspeakable horrors. Some therapists claimed to uncover dozens and even hundreds of "alters" (personalities) in clients. One physician uncovered 4,500 alters and described them as flying over the client's hospital by means of astral projection (Acocella, 1999). Families were torn apart by claims of unsubstantiated abuse. Clients were rendered financially bankrupt by "treatment" that included sessions lasting as long as 8 hours and costing as much as $1,560 per day (McDonald, 1994).

A study funded by the National Center on Child Abuse and Neglect and conducted by researchers at the University of California at Davis and University of Illinois at Chicago found allegations of SRA to be without merit. Investigating more than 12,000 accusations and surveying more than 11,000 psychiatric, social service, and law enforcement personnel, researchers found no unequivocal evidence of a single case of SRA (Goodman et al., 1994). An independent study conducted by Kenneth Lanning (1992), a supervisory special agent at the FBI Academy who has been studying SRA since 1981, came to the same conclusion.

It is difficult to say when or why reason reasserted itself. In addition to outlandish claims, allegations of abuse by therapists, and several high-profile scandals exposed by courageous nurses (McDonald, 1994), empirical studies on the nature of memory were published and disseminated in the professional literature (Loftus, 1992; Loftus & Loftus, 1994; Schacter, 1996). In the wake of these revelations and criticism, former clients and families began to file huge malpractice suits, with some settlements running into millions of dollars (Pendergast, 1996). Clients began to recant allegations. Articles in major publications were critical of the recovered memory movement, and talk show hosts apologized for their contributions to the hysteria (Rivera, 1995).

Aspartame

Another case involves critics of the nonnutritive sweetener aspartame, which is found in many soft drinks, yogurts, and dietetic foods. Many websites allege that aspartame causes various illnesses, including multiple sclerosis, systemic lupus erythematosus, Gulf War syndrome, chronic fatigue syndrome, brain tumors, Alzheimer's disease, and diabetes mellitus. Virtually all the information offered is anecdotal, from anonymous sources, and scientifically implausible. The anti-aspartame campaign purports to explain illnesses that are either prominent in the public eye or for which causes remain elusive.

More than 800 citations are found in the Medline data from 1966 to 2007 under the subject heading "aspartame." No citation purports to have evidence that aspartame causes, worsens, or contributes to multiple sclerosis, systemic lupus erythematosus, or fibromyalgia. Repeated studies (rats, children, adults) in peer-reviewed journals show no adverse effects of aspartame on weight; body temperature; cognitive, behavioral, neuropsychiatric, or neurophysiologic function; or hormones or enzymes. They also have not identified aspartame as a cause of brain tumors or other forms of cancer and birth defects. No evidence shows that aspartame worsens diabetes or causes depression. Several small reports have shown that some clients with migraines may have worsened headaches with the use of aspartame. Other studies show no connection in clients who have claimed to have aspartame-related headaches (Park, 2002).

Checkpoint Questions
4. On what do practitioners of pseudoscience rely?
5. What is the American Psychological Association's viewpoint on facilitated communication?
6. What term denotes faulty data collection and analysis used to further a special agenda?

The Dangers of Pseudoscience: Attachment Therapy

Both the *DSM-IV-TR* (APA, 2000) and the *International Classification of Diseases* (ICD-10) from the World Health Organization (1992) describe reactive attachment disorder (RAD) as comprising two clinical patterns: (1) an emotionally withdrawn, unresponsive pattern in which absence of attachment behaviors predominates (*inhibited subtype*), and (2) a pattern in which attachment behaviors are evident but directed nonselectively or indiscriminately, even at relative or complete strangers (*disinhibited subtype*). Each pattern has been described in institutionalized children (Tizard & Hodges, 1978; Tizard & Rees, 1975; Zeanah et al., 2005) and maltreated children (Albus & Dozier, 1999; Boris et al., 2000; Zeanah et al., 2004). Recent diagnoses of RAD have increased. Disagreement on this subject is considerable, particularly in terms of assessments and interventions.

Children with a history of abuse or severe neglect are particularly likely to be diagnosed with RAD because associated behavior problems often are presumed to stem from their maladaptive relationships with abusive caregivers. However, many children diagnosed with RAD have behavior problems that clearly extend beyond *DSM-IV-TR* criteria. Perhaps the most worrisome consequence of the RAD diagnosis is the emergence of "treatments" that lack a sound theoretical basis or empirical support, and may potentially be traumatizing and dangerous (Barlow et al., 2006; Hanson & Spratt, 2000).

One example is attachment therapy, a fringe psychotherapy that the scientific community has neither validated nor accepted (Kennedy et al., 2002). Attachment therapy has many variations, but most involve subjecting the client to physical confrontation and restraint to release repressed anger over abandonment. The process is repeated until the child is exhausted and emotionally reduced to an "infantile" state. Then, parents cradle, rock, and bottle-feed the child, implementing an "attachment" (Mercer, 2001; Mercer et al., 2003).

Despite the lack of validity for attachment therapy in peer-reviewed journals, Internet searches yield thousands of sites promoting attachment therapy and claims by practitioners to have research data showing its efficacy. Although data on attachment theory abound, attachment and holding therapies emanate in no logical way from attachment theory or research (Dozier, 2003).

The potential for tragedy is illustrated dramatically by the case of Candace Newmaker in 2000. Candace's adoptive mother felt that Candace suffered from an emotional disorder that prevented loving attachment and decided to seek attachment therapy. While the mother watched from another room, several "therapists" forcibly held Candace beneath a blanket for 11 hours, suffocating her to death. Despite its dangers, legislators have been unsuccessful in banning attachment therapy (Kennedy et al., 2002).

Think About It 4.1
The parents of a young child report that their child seems distant and withdrawn and is experiencing behavior problems. They state, "When we try to hug or comfort him, he just stares at the walls. We read something on the Internet about attachment therapy. Maybe we should try it?" How would the nurse respond?

IMPLICATIONS FOR PROFESSIONAL NURSES

The vulnerability of consumers invokes questions about the nursing profession's ethical obligation to them. Because of their specialized knowledge, professional nurses presumably should be able to discriminate fact from fiction, science from pseudoscience, and fraudulent health care claims from legitimate ones. Indeed, schools of nursing require students to take a course in research for this very reason.

Advocating for and educating clients and families require nurses to be able to discern "claims" from valid information in professional sources (Client-Centered Education 4.1). To appropriately use their education, nurses must be aware of existing controversies over treatments. They also should be familiar with professional sources (books and journals) and maintain a thorough knowledge of the research standards in their particular field. Professional nurses have numerous ways to advocate and educate themselves and the public.

The Internet is one method for distributing quality information to many people. Unfortunately, it also has been used to post false claims, to mislead, and to steer people away from legitimate information. Many people get health care information from the Internet. When websites are deceptive and untruthful, consumers are at risk. The number of sites touting unproven remedies for serious diseases such as cancer, mental illnesses, heart disease, HIV/AIDS, and arthritis continues to increase.

The FDA, FTC, and Health Canada have joined together to prosecute unscrupulous marketers who use the Internet to prey on the sickest and most vulnerable consumers. The FTC is targeting false and unsubstantiated Internet health claims through Operation Cure All, a law enforcement and consumer education campaign. The FTC's website (http://www.ftc.gov) offers information on how to recognize health fraud and on buying health care products on the Internet. Both the FDA and FTC encourage people to report suspicious health claims at their websites: http://www.fda.gov/oc/buyonline/buyonlineform.htm and http://www.ftc.gov.

In addition, some websites are devoted to exposing quackery and pseudoscience. The most extensive is http://www.quackwatch.com. Quackwatch's mission includes investigating questionable claims, distributing reliable publications, reporting illegal marketing, generating consumer protection lawsuits, improving the quality of health information on the Internet, and attacking misleading advertising on the Internet. On Quackwatch, Dr. Stephen Barrett and volunteer experts from medicine, nursing, psychology, and other fields investigate and publish the latest research on various worthless or actually harmful treatments. The National Council Against Health Fraud (NCAHF) (http://www.ncahf.org) is a nonprofit agency that focuses on health misinformation, fraud, and quackery as public health problems. Both Quackwatch and NCAHF have multiple links to other websites and contain up-to-date information that discusses and distinguishes between legitimate and nonlegitimate health claims.

Client-Centered Education 4.1

Combating Quackery and Fraudulent Claims

The nurse teaches and assists client and family as follows:

- Be suspicious of products that claim to cure a wide range of unrelated diseases, particularly serious diseases, such as cancer and diabetes. No product can treat every disease and condition. For many serious diseases, there are no cures, only therapies to help manage them.
- Personal testimonies can be fraudulent and difficult to prove. Testimonials are personal case histories that have been passed on from person to person. Testimonials are the weakest form of scientific validity, often amounting to compounded hearsay.
- Be wary of talk that suggests a product can bring quick relief or provide a quick cure, especially if the disease or condition is serious.
- Do not be fooled by the term *natural*. It is often used in health fraud as an attention-grabber; it suggests a product is safer than conventional treatments.
- Beware of remedies from companies or practitioners that make paranoid claims suggesting that legitimate health care providers and manufacturers are in cahoots to suppress unorthodox products because they threaten their financial standing.

- Beware of health practitioners who suggest a nonscientific or little-known therapy and then attempt to dissuade you from getting a second opinion.
- Check with the Better Business Bureau or local attorneys general' offices to see whether other consumers have lodged complaints about a product or a product's marketer.
- Check with the appropriate health professional group—for example, the APA, the American Psychiatric Nurses Association, the National Alliance for the Mentally Ill, and government websites (eg, http://www.nimh.gov). Many of these groups have local chapters that can provide various resource materials about diseases. Government websites have information on the latest research available about treatments.
- Contact a nearby FDA office. Look for the number and address in the blue pages of the phone book under U.S. Government, Health and Human Services, or go to http://www.fda.gov/ora/fed_state/dfsr_activities/dfsr_pas.html. The FDA records whether it has taken action against a product or its marketer.

THE FUTURE OF MENTAL HEALTH AND PSYCHIATRIC NURSING

During the past couple of decades, much effort has been put into conducting research on the effectiveness of interventions in mental health, resulting in a number of evidence-based and ESTs. This can be seen as a great advance since the days when few approaches to psychiatric care could boast empirical support. Pharmacologic agents are subjected to type I and type II study, and even psychotherapy has been manualized and subjected to rigorous scrutiny. While psychotherapy may fundamentally be seen as therapeutic conversation, which is by its nature difficult to subject to empirical analysis, financial interests are driving each of the helping professions in mental health to define specific treatments that are effective for treating specific disorders. The time has come when third-party payers are more willing to fund therapy for disabling disorders than they are to pay for talk therapy for vague existential concerns or problems of living. As

EBP becomes more recognized, third-party payers are more likely to require mental health practitioners of all disciplines to use EBP treatments in order to receive payment (Cummings, 2006).

Nursing leaders have recommended that psychiatric nurses begin to examine theory, research, and curriculum in their specialty. They have pointed out the need to examine sacred cows, tradition, and dogma that may be historically valuable but unrepresentative of an evidence base from which practice concepts and research ideas can emerge. One example of such a concept is milieu therapy, something that we teach in psychiatric nursing, but which has not been subjected to systematic study. There are many others. Unfortunately, as a whole, nurses are not contributing to evidence-based care as actively as they should, and, unlike other professions, they have little by way of interventions that meets that gold standard (Stuart, 2001). This must change in order for the profession to remain relevant and competitive in the knowledge enterprise.

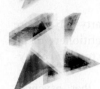

Reviewing and Applying Your Knowledge

Chapter Summary

- Despite the advanced state of mental health services, clients and their families continue to turn to dubious practices.

- The history of mental health services is full of excess and scandal, but it is also one of extraordinary gains in understanding the human brain and behavior.

- Nurses have individual and collective ethical obligations to protect the public from such excesses and educate themselves and others about the differences between legitimate treatments and interventions grounded in research and treatments and interventions grounded in flummery.

Study Questions

1. When explaining evidence-based care to a group of nursing students, which of the following concepts would the instructor address?

   a. Increased emphasis on intuition

   b. Integration of research findings with clinical expertise

   c. Use of pseudoscientific practices and therapies

   d. Increased reliance on assumptions

2. After teaching a group of students about the scientific process, the instructor determines that the teaching has been successful when the students describe synthesis as which of the following?

   a. Watching something carefully and noting events

   b. Testing a hypothesis or prediction

   c. Determining whether data are reliable and supportive

   d. Putting the information together to form a new whole

3. A nurse is participating in a research study that involves a review of the literature and analysis of the data to be used in a new form. The nurse is involved in which type of study?

   a. Type I

   b. Type II

   c. Type III

   d. Type IV

4. When conducting an experimental research study investigating the effects of a medication, one group receives the medication, a second group receives no medication, and a third group receives a capsule containing a sugar solution. The nurse identifies the sugar solution capsule as:

   a. a sham treatment.

   b. a placebo.

   c. empirics.

   d. junk science.

5. Which of the following statements would be appropriate to include in a teaching plan for clients and their families about quackery? Select all that apply.

   a. Fraudulent medicine is typically involved.

   b. Most practitioners sincerely believe in what they are doing.

   c. Advertising is frequently accurate in its description of the practice.

   d. Treatment may involve legitimate therapies or techniques.

   e. Difficult-to-treat illnesses are rarely addressed or involved.

Critical Thinking Questions

1. Quack therapies cost the U.S. public millions of dollars each year, in addition to bringing stress to people hoping for miracle cures. What are your thoughts as to what nurses individually and collectively can do to prevent quackery?

2. Many people depend on unsubstantiated therapies. Why do you think these therapies sometimes seem to "work"?

3. In the past 10 years, the U.S. public has embraced complementary and alternative medicines (CAM; see Chap. 17). What can nurses do to help distinguish legitimate CAM interventions from fraudulent or unsubstantiated ones?

References

Acocella, J. (1999). *Creating hysteria: Women and multiple personality disorder.* San Francisco, CA: Jossey-Bass.

Albus, K. E., & Dozier, M. (1999). Indiscriminate friendliness and terror of strangers in infancy. *Infant Mental Health Journal, 20,* 30–41.

American Academy of Pediatrics (AAP). (1998). Policy statement: Auditory integration training and facilitated communication for autism. *Pediatrics, 102,* 431–433.

American Academy of Pediatrics (AAP). (1999). Policy statement: The treatment of neurologically impaired children using patterning. *Pediatrics, 104,* 1149–1151.

American Academy of Pediatrics (AAP). (2006). AAP publications retired and reaffirmed. *Pediatrics, 117,* 1846–1847.

American Nurses Association (ANA). (2001). *Code of ethics for nurses with interpretive statements.* Washington, DC: American Nurses Publishing.

American Nurses Association, American Psychiatric Nurses Association, & International Society of Psychiatric–Mental Health Nurses. (2007). *Psychiatric–mental health nursing: Scope and standards of practice.* Silver Spring, MD: American Nurses Publishing.

American Psychiatric Association (APA). (2000). *Diagnostic and statistical manual of mental disorders* (4th ed., text rev.). Washington, DC: Author.

Barlow, J., Johnston, I., Kendrick, D., Polnay, L., & Stewart-Brown, S. (2006). Individual and group-based parenting programmes for the treatment of physical child abuse and neglect. *Cochrane Database of Systematic Reviews, 19*;3:CD005463.

Barrett, S. J. (2001). *Quackery: How should it be defined?* Retrieved from http://www.quackwatch.org/01QuackeryRelatedTopics/quackdef.html

Barrett, S. J., & Jarvis, W. (1993). *Health robbers: A close look at quackery in America.* Amherst, NY: Prometheus.

Barrett, S. J., & Jarvis, W. T. (2005). *How quackery sells.* Retrieved from http://www.quackwatch.org/01QuackeryRelatedTopics/quacksell.html

Baumeister, R. F. (2001). Violent pride: Do people turn violent because of self-hate, or self-love? *Scientific American, 284*(4), 96–101.

Baumeister, R. F., Heatherton, T. F., & Tice, D. M. (1993). When ego threats lead to self-regulation failure: Negative consequences of high self-esteem. *Journal of Personality and Social Psychology, 64,* 141–156.

Baumeister, R. F., Smart, L., & Boden, J. M. (1996). Relation of threatened egoism to violence and aggression: The dark side of high self-esteem. *Psychological Review, 103,* 5–35.

Biklen, D. (1990). Communication unbound: Autism and praxis. *Harvard Educational Review, 60,* 291–314.

Biklen, D. (1992a). Autism orthodoxy versus free speech: A reply to Cummins and Prior. *Harvard Educational Review, 62,* 242–256.

Biklen, D. (1992b). Facilitated communication: Biklen responds. *American Journal of Speech and Language Pathology, 1*(2), 21–22.

Boris, N. W., Hinshaw-Fuselier, S., Heller, S. S., Smyke A. T., Scheeringa, M. S., & Zeanah, C. H. (2000, July). *New approaches to assessing reactive attachment disorder.* Presented at the Biennial Meeting of the World Association for Infant Mental Health, Montreal, Canada.

Cale, E. M., & Lilienfeld, S. O. (2006). Psychopathy factors and risk for aggressive behavior: A test of the "threatened egotism" hypothesis. *Law and Human Behavior, 30*(1), 51–74.

Carper, B. A. (1978). Fundamental patterns of knowing. *Advances in Nursing Science, 1,* 13–23.

Chorpita, B. G. (2003). The frontier of evidence based practice. In A. Kazdin & J. Weisz (Eds.), *Evidence based psychotherapies for children and adolescents* (pp. 42–59). New York, NY: Guilford Press.

Cummings, N. A. (2006). Psychology, the stalwart profession, faces new challenges and opportunities. *Professional Psychology: Research and Practice, 37*(6), 598–605.

Dawes, R. M. (2001). *Everyday irrationality: How pseudo-scientists, lunatics, and the rest of us systematically fail to think rationally.* Boulder, CO: Westview Press.

Delacato, C. H. (1963). *The diagnosis and treatment of speech and reading problems.* Springfield, IL: Charles C. Thomas.

Delaney, K. R. (2006). Evidence base for practice: Reduction of restraint and seclusion use during child and adolescent psychiatric inpatient treatment. *Worldviews in Evidence Based Nursing, 3*(1), 19–30.

Dobson, S., & Fitzgerald, L. (2005). *Knowledge to action? Evidence-based health care in context.* Oxford, UK: Oxford University Press.

Doman, R. J., Spitz, E. B., Zucman, E., Delacato, C. H., & Doman, G. (1960). Children with severe brain injuries: Neurologic organization in terms of mobility. *Journal of the American Medical Association, 174,* 257.

Dozier, M. (2003). Attachment-based treatment for vulnerable children. *Attachment & Human Development, 5*(3), 253–257.

Federal Trade Commission. (1995a, January 4). Abovo, Inc., et al.; Proposed consent agreement with analysis to aid public comment. *Federal Register, 60*(2), 464.

Federal Trade Commission. (1995b, January 4). LouisBass, Inc.; Proposed consent agreement with analysis to aid public comment. *Federal Register, 60*(2), 467.

Goodman, G. S., Qin, J., Bottoms, B. L., & Shaver, P. R. (1994). *Characteristics and sources of ritual child abuse. Executive summary of the final report to the National Center for Child Abuse and Neglect Grant #90CA1405.* Washington, DC: National Center for Child Abuse and Neglect.

Guyatt, G. H., & Rennie, D. (2002). *Users' guides to the medical literature: A manual for evidence-based clinical practice.* Chicago, IL: AMA Press.

Hanson, R. F., & Spratt, E. G. (2000). Reactive attachment disorder: What we know about the disorder and implications for treatment. *Child Maltreatment, 5*(2), 137–145.

Jacobson, J. W., Mulick, J. A., & Schwartz, A. A. (1995). A history of facilitated communication: Science, pseudoscience, and antiscience. Science Working Group on Facilitated Communication. *American Psychologist, 50,* 750–765.

Johnson, J. (1994). A dialectical examination of nursing art. *Advances in Nursing Science, 17,* 1–13.

Kennedy, S. S., Mercer, J., Mohr, W. K., & Huffine, C. W. (2002). Snake oil, ethics, and the First Amendment: What's a profession to do? *American Journal of Orthopsychiatry, 72*(1), 5–15.

Lanning, K. V. (1992). *Investigator's guide to allegations of "ritual" child abuse.* Quantico, VA: Behavioral Science Unit, National Center for the Analysis of Violent Crime, FBI Academy.

Lilienfeld, S. O., Lynn, S. J., & Lohr, J. M. (2004). *Science and pseudoscience in clinical psychology.* New York, NY: Guilford Press.

Loftus, E. F. (1992). When a lie becomes memory's truth: Memory distortion after exposure to misinformation. *Current Directions in Psychological Science, 1,* 120–123.

Loftus, E. F., & Loftus, G. R. (1994). The repressed memory controversy. *American Psychologist, 49,* 443–445.

McDonald, S. (1994). An ethical dilemma: Risk vs. responsibility. *Journal of Psychosocial Nursing and Mental Health Services, 32*(1), 19–25.

Mercer, J. (2001). Attachment therapy using deliberate restraint: An object lesson on the identification of unvalidated treatments. *Journal of Child & Adolescent Psychiatric Nursing, 14,* 105–115.

Mercer, J., Sarner, L., & Rosa, L. (2003). *Attachment therapy on trial: The torture and death of Candace Newmaker.* Westport, CT: Praeger.

Merriam-Webster's On-Line Dictionary. (2007). Retrieved from http://www.m-w.com/dictionary/quack.

Mohr, W. K. (2006). Spiritual issues in psychiatric care. *Perspectives in Psychiatric Care, 42*(3), 174–183.

Mohr, W. K., & Anderson, J. A. (2001). Faulty assumptions associated with the use of restraints with children. *Journal of Child and Adolescent Psychiatric Nursing, 14*(3), 141–151.

Mulick, J. A., Jacobson, J. W., & Kobe, F. (1993). Anguished silence and helping hands: Autism and facilitated communication. *Skeptical Inquirer, 17,* 270–280.

Nathan, P. E., & Gorman, J. M. (2007). *A guide to treatments that work* (3rd ed.). New York, NY: Oxford University Press.

Nightingale, F. (Original work published in 1860). *Notes on nursing: What it is, and what it is not.* Philadelphia, PA: Lippincott.

Park, R. (2002). *Voodoo science: The road from foolishness to fraud.* Oxford, UK: Oxford University Press.

Pendergast, M. (1996). *Victims of memory: Sex abuse accusations and shattered lives* (2nd ed.). Hinesburg, VT: Upper Access.

Peplau, H. (1988). The art and science of nursing: Similarities, differences, and relations. *Nursing Science Quarterly, 1,* 8–15.

Piper, A. (1997). *Hoax and reality: The bizarre world of multiple personality disorder.* Northvale, NJ: Jason Aronson.

Presnell, K., Bearman, S. K., & Stice, E. (2004). Risk factors for body dissatisfaction in adolescent boys and girls: A prospective study. *International Journal of Eating Disorders, 36,* 389–401.

Raskin, J. (2000). Rogerian nursing theory: A humbug in the halls of higher learning. *Skeptical Inquirer, 24*(5), 30–36.

Rivera, G. (1995, December 12). *Wrongly accused and convicted of child molestation* [Television broadcast]. New York, NY: Cable National Broadcasting Corporation.

Schacter, D. L. (1996). *The brain, the mind, and the past.* New York, NY: Basic Books.

Schrieber, F. R. (1973). *Sybil.* New York, NY: Warner Bros.

Sokal, A. D., & Bricmont, J. (1999). *Fashionable nonsense: Postmodern intellectuals' abuse of science.* New York, NY: Picador Press.

Stanovich, K. E. (2007). *How to think straight about psychology* (8th ed.). Boston, MA: Allyn & Bacon.

Stuart, G. W. (2001). Evidence based psychiatric nursing practice: Rhetoric or reality? *Journal of the American Psychiatric Nurses Association, 7,* 103–111.

Thigpen, C. H., & Cleckley, H. M. (1957). *Three faces of Eve.* New York, NY: McGraw-Hill.

Tizard, B., & Hodges, J. (1978). The effect of institutional rearing on the development of 8-year-old children. *Journal of Child Psychology and Psychiatry, 19,* 99–118.

Tizard, B., & Rees, J. (1975). The effect of early institutional rearing on the behavior problems and affectional relationships of four-year-old children. *Journal of Child Psychology and Psychiatry, 27,* 61–73.

Wainwright, P. (1999). The art of nursing. *International Journal of Nursing Studies, 356,* 378–385.

Whitlock, C. R. (2001). *Mediscams: How to spot and avoid healthcare scams, medical frauds and quackery, from the local physician to the major healthcare providers and drug manufacturers.* New York, NY: St. Martin's Press.

World Health Organization (WHO). (1992). *The ICD-10 classification of mental and behavioral disorders: Clinical descriptions and diagnostic guidelines.* Geneva, Switzerland: Author.

Wynn, C. M., & Wiggins, A. W. (2001). *Quantum leaps in the wrong direction: Where real science ends and pseudoscience begins.* Washington, DC: Joseph Henry Press.

Zeanah, C. H., Scheeringa, M., Boris, N. W., Heller, S. S., Smyke, A. T., & Trapani, J. (2004). Reactive attachment disorder in maltreated toddlers. *Child Abuse & Neglect, 28,* 877–888.

Zeanah, C. H., Smyke A. T., Koga, S. F., Carlson, E., & Bucharest Early Intervention Project Core Group. (2005). Attachment in institutionalized and community children in Romania. *Child Development, 76*(5), 1015–1028.

Web Resources

Federal Trade Commission: http://www.ftc.gov/bcp/conline/edcams/cureall/index.html

Food and Drug Administration: http://www.fda.gov/oc/buyonline/buyonlineform.htm

Quackwatch: http://www.quackwatch.com.

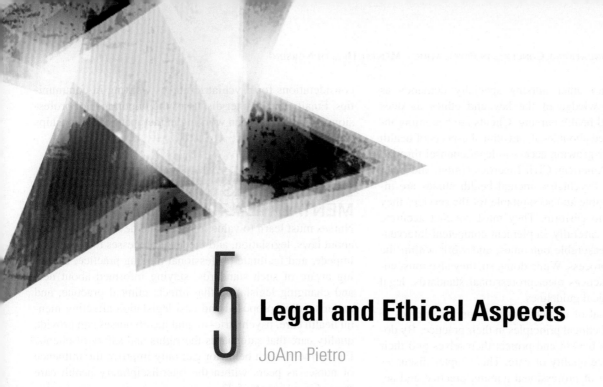

5

Legal and Ethical Aspects

JoAnn Pietro

KEY TERMS

autonomy
battery
beneficence
emergency admission
ethical dilemma
ethics
fidelity
informed consent
involuntary admission
Justice
malpractice
paternalism
respondeat superior
substituted consent
veracity
voluntary admission

LEARNING OBJECTIVES

On completion of this chapter, you should be able to accomplish the following:

- Identify basic legal issues relevant to psychiatric–mental health nursing care.
- Explain the legal function of nursing practice acts.
- Discuss malpractice and measures that health care professionals can take to protect themselves from litigation.
- Identify the basic rights of people with mental illness.
- Describe different types of commitments and states of competency.
- Explain the term *standard of care* as a concept in practice.
- Discuss the importance of ethics in psychiatric–mental health nursing practice.
- Summarize the American Nurses Association's *Code of Ethics for Nurses.*
- Analyze the ethical principles of autonomy, beneficence, paternalism, veracity, fidelity, and justice in relation to care of clients with psychiatric disorders.
- Describe unique aspects of ethics as related to community-based psychiatric nursing.
- Outline steps for resolving conflicts between or among two or more ethical principles.

Probably no other nursing specialty demands as much knowledge of the law and ethics as does psychiatric–mental health nursing. Clients are becoming increasingly informed about legal and ethical aspects of health care and have ever-growing access to legal counsel through legal clinics, the American Civil Liberties Union, and other advocacy groups. Psychiatric–mental health nurses are increasingly responsible and accountable for the services they perform and fail to perform. They must conduct accurate assessments, plan carefully, implement competent interventions, evaluate measurable outcomes, and work within the interdisciplinary process. While doing so, they also must ensure that their practices meet professional standards, legal mandates, and ethical guidelines.

The major goal of this chapter is to prepare nurses to abide by legal and ethical principles in their practice. By doing so, nurses can benefit and protect themselves and their clients and enhance quality of care. This chapter discusses the legal authority of professional nursing practice and acknowledges the expansion of nursing's scope of practice. It addresses basic and evolving client rights and the importance of acknowledging and protecting them. It clarifies differences related to important legal and ethical concepts that may seem similar superficially. It explores the various types of commitment, as well as significant legal issues that apply to special client populations.

The chapter also introduces ethics as basic and obvious moral truths that guide deliberation and action when providing care to those with psychiatric disorders. It reviews the familiar bioethical principles of autonomy, beneficence, nonmaleficence, veracity, and fidelity and discusses ethical considerations for psychiatric nurses working in communities. Finally, the chapter discusses the importance of professional boundaries when working in therapeutic relationships with clients.

LEGAL ISSUES IN PSYCHIATRIC–MENTAL HEALTH NURSING

Nurses must learn to value, respect, and develop knowledge about laws, legislation, and the legal processes that regulate, impede, and facilitate professional nursing practice. By being aware of such standards, staying informed about new and changing legislation that affects clinical practice, and understanding proposed and past legislation affecting mental health care, psychiatric–mental health nurses can provide quality care that safeguards the rights and safety of clients. Furthermore, such behavior can only improve the influence of nurses as peers within the interdisciplinary health care team (Case Vignette 5.1).

Nurse Practice Acts and the Expanding Role of Nursing

Standards of nursing practice are written documents that outline minimum expectations for safe nursing care. They guide nursing care and its evaluation, and the judicial system looks to them during cases of malpractice litigation. Each state's nurse practice act defines nursing, describes its scope, and identifies its limits. Although nurse practice acts vary for each state, the definition of professional nursing in the Texas Code is similar to that in most states:

Case Vignette 5.1

Lillian, an 82-year-old client with schizophrenia, lives alone. Her psychiatric condition is stable and controlled with medications. A psychiatric nurse from the Visiting Nurse Association (VNA) sees Lillian once a week to assess her health and refill her prescriptions. A home health aide assists with ADLs three times a week; during visits, the aide usually cleans. Lillian receives Meals on Wheels; she has no other support.

In the past month, Lillian's physical health has deteriorated. She has fallen several times; twice the aide arrived to find Lillian on the floor. The nurse has attempted to discuss other living arrangements with Lillian, to no avail. Lillian seems not to appreciate the seriousness of her situation. She states that the VNA should provide daily visits so she can remain at home.

The VNA is not sanctioned to provide continuous care. The nurse contacts Adult Protective Services (APS) twice to discuss the circumstances. APS assigns a case manager to investigate; however, it does not rate the case as a high priority.

Thus, the case manager cannot visit immediately or confirm when he will do so.

The nurse feels obligated to continue to see Lillian. She even tries to increase her visits, although she realizes that doing so violates agency procedure. The nurse and aide believe that abandoning Lillian would be unethical. They are torn: Should they follow procedures outlined by the VNA and client's insurance, which would mean discontinuing visits and forcing APS to take action? Would doing so further compromise Lillian's health? Should the nurse keep visiting, citing the need to fill the prescriptions as the rationale, even though doing so would mean using government funding in an unauthorized way?

Reflection and Critical Thinking

- What are possible legal and employment concerns if the nurse continues to make extra visits to Lillian? What if the nurse stops visiting? Can the nurse use any alternative strategies?
- What are the responsibilities of and risks to the VNA? APS?
- What would you do if you were the nurse? Defend your actions.

Professional nursing involves: (A) the observation, assessment, intervention, evaluation, rehabilitation, care and counsel, or health teachings of a person who is ill, injured, infirm, or experiencing changes in normal health processes; (B) the maintenance of health or prevention of illness; (C) the administration of a medication or treatment as ordered by a physician, podiatrist, or dentist; (D) the supervision or teaching of nursing; (E) the administration, supervision, and evaluation of nursing practices, policies, and procedures; (F) the requesting, receiving, signing for, and distribution of prescription drug samples to patients at sites in which a registered nurse is authorized to sign prescription drug orders...; and (G) the performance of an act delegated by a physician.... (*Vernon's Texas Code Annotated*, 2003)

Nursing is expanding its scope and roles as a result of increasing education, health access needs in communities, and the strong political activities of nursing organizations. New challenges, responsibilities, and opportunities accompany this broadened scope. Advanced nurse practitioners have prescriptive authority in every state and receive third-party reimbursement from private insurers and Medicaid in many states. Nurses are making it increasingly possible for consumers to access high-quality and cost-effective care.

Malpractice

Professional negligence, commonly referred to as **malpractice**, is a particular tort action that a consumer *plaintiff* brings against a professional *defendant* when the plaintiff believes that the professional injured him or her within the consumer–professional relationship (Box 5.1). For a plaintiff to successfully be awarded monetary damages in a malpractice suit against a professional nurse, he or she must prove each of the following elements of nursing negligence:

1. That the nurse professional owed a duty of due care toward the plaintiff
2. That the nurse professional's performance breached the duty owed to the plaintiff by falling below or deviating from the accepted standard of care
3. That the nurse professional's act was the proximate cause of the plaintiff's injury, and that it was foreseeable that it would cause an injury; and
4. That the plaintiff consumer sustained injury or harm.

To decrease their chances of liability for malpractice, psychiatric nurses must ensure that their professional behavior always reflects statutory and professional standards. In malpractice actions against nurses, proof of the "standard of care" becomes essential. Both sides usually present expert witness testimony to give the jury perspectives about accepted professional practices and standards. The appropriate expert witness for psychiatric–mental health nursing practice is another psychiatric nurse (or, in some states, a physician) with the requisite knowledge or experience to advise on the standard of care in the same or similar circumstances. Both plaintiffs and defendants include and submit such expert testimony with all other testimony and evidence to the jury for a decision. The defendant nurse is held to providing the level of conduct that an average nurse would exercise using the skill ordinarily possessed by the nurse acting in the same or similar circumstances. It is not a standard for excellence. Rather, the nurse must act as any reasonable nurse would in the particular psychiatric–mental health situation. Thus, when determining a *verdict* (the outcome in a malpractice case), the court instructs the jury to determine from expert testimony what the given standard of care is and determine if the nurse adhered to that standard.

When nurses are found liable in malpractice cases, their employers also are usually found liable under the legal theory of **respondeat superior**. This Latin term means that acts of employees are attributable to the employer, whom the court also will find responsible for damages to injured third parties (Prosser et al., 2005). However, if a nurse acts outside the scope of nursing practice or her actions are intentional, *respondeat superior* may not apply. In such a case, the nurse's employer also may withdraw legal assistance it otherwise would have provided. If the jury finds the nurse liable, the health care facility could file an indemnity action against the nurse.

BOX 5.1 Malpractice Suits Against Nurses

Historically, nurses were largely protected from direct malpractice suits. One contributing factor was a public perception that nurses were dependent on either physicians or hospital authorities for orders. Attorneys tended to sue well-insured physicians or the employer–health care facility, rather than nurses, because doing so generally improved their chances of achieving big monetary victories for their clients. However, in recent years consumer knowledge has grown, and professional nursing is increasingly recognized as an independent discipline. Consequently, the trend to sue individual nurses as codefendants with physicians and health care facilities is becoming more common.

This trend has many implications for the nursing profession. As nurses are held increasingly responsible and monetarily liable for practice and malpractice, the nursing profession must strive to control such issues as staffing, productivity, educational qualifications and competencies, and the nurse's role within the interdisciplinary team. Nurses should purchase independent medical malpractice insurance.

Think About It 5.1

A client who is violent and psychotic is admitted to a psychiatric unit. He is placed in four-point leather restraints and sedated. Hospital policy states that nurses must assess his extremities every 15 minutes. The nurse checks on the client in 15 minutes and notes that his hand is dusky, but his pulses are strong and he can move his fingers. She does not remove his restraint because he is being verbally threatening. When the nurse checks him again in 15 minutes, he cannot raise his wrist. The nurse removes the restraint. It is later determined that the client has a nerve injury. Can the nurse be found guilty of malpractice?

Legal Counsel

Psychiatric–mental health professionals must know how and when to obtain ongoing and appropriate legal consultation. First, consulted attorneys must be aware of issues in mental health law to evaluate the institution's policies and procedures and to provide a review for staff in a problem-solving manner. Second, health care facilities and programs should arrange for an attorney to offer continuing and regular education programs that review with the staff recent court decisions, legislation, and updates that affect care in psychiatric settings. Also, having legal consultation readily available when the staff is endeavoring to ensure legal accountability is extremely valuable. Many institutions provide such legal consultation, if requested, for the benefit of their clients and to protect the institution from potential liability.

Moreover, individual malpractice insurance carriers provide legal representation in the event that a nurse is or may be sued. Attorney representation would be available under a nurse's malpractice insurance even if the nurse is not a party to a lawsuit but has been called to testify as a witness. Nurses should contact their own carriers for advice, representation, or both when asked to give statements or depositions. They also should contact carriers if asked to testify as a nonparty to a lawsuit, in a potential lawsuit, or if named as a party to a lawsuit. Insurance carriers are also available to handle any questions that nurses might have regarding potential or pending lawsuits. Nurses are sued less frequently than are other health care professionals, but it is prudent for nurses to carry individual malpractice policy as the litigation climate changes.

Checkpoint Questions

1. What are standards of practice, and why are they important?
2. When nurses are found liable in malpractice cases, what legal theory is applied when their employers are also found liable to the plaintiff?

Basic Rights of Clients Receiving Psychiatric Nursing Care

Clients receiving psychiatric–mental health care have basic rights (Box 5.2). This issue calls for special attention because the admission and treatment of clients with mental illness tends to be more coercive, less voluntary, and less open to public awareness and scrutiny than are the admission and treatment of clients with other needs or disorders.

Some clients with psychiatric disorders who enter treatment facilities lose normal freedoms to come and go, schedule their time, and choose and control activities of daily living (ADLs). If also adjudicated incompetent, clients lose the freedom to manage financial and legal affairs and make important, usually personal, decisions. Because of the loss of these important freedoms, the courts and advocates for clients with psychiatric disorders closely guard and value

the rights that these clients retain. Some such rights include communicating with an attorney, sending and receiving mail without censorship, having visitors, receiving basic necessities of life, and being protected from harm.

Certainly, some disorders or forms of treatment necessitate limitations on visitors. Behavior modification treatment programs may require that participants earn tokens that they can use to secure certain privileges or articles. Nevertheless, clients retain the right to challenge such restrictions, and treatment facilities may have to prove the value or necessity of associated abridgments to rights.

Application of restraints and use of seclusion are considered high-risk, dangerous modalities that can result in injury or even death (Mohr & Mohr, 2000). Legally, they are high risk because they greatly inhibit the right to freedom, which clients may perceive as a form of punishment. Therefore, accrediting agencies and governmental entities require institutions to have in place policies and procedures to govern the use of restraint and seclusion. Many states have statutes that define the use of restraints and seclusion within psychiatric facilities. The Centers for Medicare and Medicaid Services has issued strict governmental guidelines for the use of restraints and seclusion in facilities that receive federal funds as third-party reimbursement. The Joint Commission continually revises its standards guiding the use of restraints and seclusion. The Joint Commission (2008) standards outline how such methods must be implemented, ongoing client monitoring requirements during their use, and assessment provisions for continuing need of restraint or seclusion. They also specifically require leaders of health care organizations to limit use of restraints and seclusion to clinically justified situations.

Clients have limited rights to be paid for work within long-term residential institutions. Forced or even voluntary labor by clients without payment violates U.S. legal principles.

The nursing profession has long espoused advocacy for clients as one of its most important roles. Discussing rights within treatment teams, including these rights in nursing care plans, and ensuring that facility and unit policies and procedures include methodologies for protecting client rights are examples of advocacy-oriented nursing interventions (Nursing Spotlight 5.1). An important resource that health care facilities and agencies should make available to nurses is ongoing legal advice and consultation about client rights.

Informed Consent

Informed consent means the consent that a recipient of health care gives to treating providers after he or she receives sufficient information that enables the recipient to understand a proposed treatment or procedure. Sufficient information includes the following components:

- The way the treatment or procedure will be administered
- The prognosis if the treatment or procedure is given
- Side effects

BOX 5.2 Federal Bill of Rights for Mental Health Clients

1. The right to appropriate treatment and related services in a setting and under conditions that are the most supportive of such person's personal liberty, and restrict such liberty only to the extent necessary consistent with such person's treatment needs, applicable requirements of law, and applicable judicial orders.
2. The right to an individualized, written, treatment or service plan (such plan to be developed promptly after admission of such person), the right to treatment based on such plan, the right to periodic review and reassessment of treatment and related service needs, and the right to appropriate revision of such plan, including any revision necessary to provide a description of mental health services that may be needed after such person is discharged from such program or facility.
3. The right to ongoing participation, in a manner appropriate to a person's capabilities, in the planning of mental health services to be provided (including the right to participate in the development and periodic revision of the plan).
4. The right to be provided with a reasonable explanation, in terms and language appropriate to a person's condition and ability to understand the person's general mental and physical (if appropriate) condition, the objectives of treatment, the nature and significant possible adverse effects of recommended treatment, the reasons why a particular treatment is considered appropriate, the reasons why access to certain visitors may not be appropriate, and any appropriate and available alternative treatments, services, and types of providers of mental health services.
5. The right not to receive a mode or course of treatment in the absence of informed, voluntary, written consent to treatment except during an emergency situation or as permitted by law when the person is being treated as a result of a court order.
6. The right not to participate in experimentation in the absence of informed, voluntary, written consent (includes human subject protection).
7. The right to freedom from restraint or seclusion, other than as a mode or course of treatment or restraint or seclusion during an emergency situation with a written order by a responsible mental health professional.
8. The right to a humane treatment environment that affords reasonable protection from harm and appropriate privacy with regard to personal needs.
9. The right to access, on request, to such person's mental health care records.
10. The right, in the case of a person admitted on a residential or inpatient care basis, to converse with others privately, to have convenient and reasonable access to the telephone and mails, and to see visitors during regularly scheduled hours. (For treatment purposes, specific individuals may be excluded.)
11. The right to be informed promptly and in writing at the time of admission of these rights.
12. The right to assert grievances with respect to infringement of these rights.
13. The right to exercise these rights without reprisal.
14. The right of referral to other providers upon discharge.

42 U.S.C.A. § 10841.

- Risks
- Possible consequences of refusing the treatment or procedure
- Other alternatives

All clients have the right to give informed consent before health care professionals perform interventions. Administration of treatments or procedures without a client's informed consent can result in legal action against the primary provider and the health care agency. In such lawsuits, clients will prevail, alleging **battery** (touching another without permission), if they can prove that they did not consent to the procedure, that providers did not give adequate information for a decision, or that the treatment exceeded the scope of the consent (Prosser et al., 2005).

In the landmark case of *Canterbury v. Spence* (1972), the court established that clients could truly be informed only if primary providers shared all the things that a prudent client "would find material" in deciding whether to permit or participate in a particular treatment regimen. As well, many legal cases subsequent to *Canterbury v. Spence* address the standards for an informed consent. Informed consent requires that health care professionals give clients adequate and accurate knowledge and information. Of course, subsumed in the equation to secure consent is that providers obtain it from competent adults who are giving it voluntarily. As a broad mandate for informed consent, the U.S. Congress passed the Patient Self-Determination Act (PSDA) in the early 1990s. The PSDA requires health care facilities to provide clear written information to every client concerning his or her legal rights to make health care decisions, including the right to accept or refuse treatment.

Informed consent also protects clients from being subjected to experimental treatments and research projects without their knowledge and agreement. Because issues related to informed consent become even more complex when clients have psychiatric disorders, institutions with programs that involve research or experimental treatments must have review boards that evaluate such projects and programs and approve or reject them based on strict client protection criteria. Human subjects committees usually view favorably research projects that entail no undue risks to clients, have strong expectations of benefit, and allow clients to withdraw at any time, provided that clients give voluntary consent to participate.

NURSING SPOTLIGHT 5.1

Nursing Care Guidelines to Maintain Legal Rights of Clients

Expected Outcome: *Client feedback will reflect satisfaction with nursing care.*

Interventions	Rationales
Provide at least a "reasonable person" standard of care when using the nursing process to deliver client care.	Breach of guidelines for safe practice and standards of care can provide the basis for negligence and malpractice suits.
Attend periodic workshops that review standards and legal and ethical issues.	The responsibility to update one's knowledge base continually is essential to the practice of safe nursing care.

Expected Outcome: *The client's right to informed consent will be maintained.*

Interventions	Rationales
Apply the elements of informed consent, including the following: • The person must be competent. • The person must have the ability to refuse consent. • The person must have adequate information to give consent, including information about risks, benefits, and alternatives. • The person must give consent voluntarily.	A basic client right is control over his or her body. The physician has the legal obligation to ensure that clients are giving informed consent, considering the nurse's observation and assessment of the client.
Observe and document client behavior indicating consent is valid.	The client record must reflect specific nursing assessment of current behaviors, and the nurse needs to take appropriate action if consent is questioned or invalidated.
Record and report any discrepancies in consent or behavior, revocation of consent, or other issues to the client's physician.	The nurse acts as a client advocate and has the interdependent role of assessment of consent, compliance, and consent revocation with the physician.

Expected Outcome: *The client's right to confidentiality of health data will be protected.*

Interventions	Rationales
Protect the client's record and chart and share data only with client authorization.	The client's written authorization is necessary before the nurse can share information in records or charts.
Maintain communication about the client and client care among treatment team members.	The nurse can share information about client care with treatment team members to provide continuity.
Use policies and procedures that reflect the nurse's duty to protect himself or herself or others in cases of threats to harm the nurse or other people.	The nurse has a responsibility to breach confidentiality to protect the client and others from harm.

Expected Outcome: *The client's rights will be protected.*

Interventions	Rationales
Review the policies and procedures of the unit to ensure they are in accordance with client rights.	Policies and procedures need to be in place to support protection of clients' rights.
Attend training on legal issues, such as voluntary or involuntary commitment and treatment consequences.	As a member of the psychiatric treatment team, the nurse has a responsibility to ensure that client care is compliant with laws dealing with commitment and treatment issues.
Suggest that legal consultation be obtained for legal updates, review of policies and procedures, and case consultation.	A legal consultant should be available to staff.
Participate in ongoing performance monitoring.	The nurse must develop or participate in performance improvement strategies to ensure quality care.

SPECIAL CONSIDERATIONS IN PSYCHIATRIC SETTINGS. A major problem with consent and clients who have psychiatric disorders involves their competence to agree to procedures. Many clients with mental illness certainly can give informed consent. These clients are aware of their surroundings, understand others, make decisions based on what they think is best, and agree to treatments or procedures without coercion. However, other clients with psychiatric disorders are not able to give informed consent. It may be questionable whether clients whom the court has already determined to be incompetent for handling civil and business affairs possess the ability to make treatment decisions. Likewise, some clients who have not been so adjudicated are so clearly impaired by their psychiatric illnesses that they cannot truly understand what health care professionals are communicating. They therefore cannot give valid consent.

Because of this unreliability, major considerations for informed consent in psychiatric–mental health nursing involve ongoing monitoring and observing of clients for the following:

• A state of legal capacity or competence when they are asked to give informed consent
• Continuing understanding of the information they have been given
• Power and opportunities to revoke consent at any time during treatment

Ensuring legally adequate informed consent before treatment is an important part of the psychiatric nursing care plan. Nurses serve as the client's advocate, the team's colleague, and the facility's watchful employee by continually evaluating the client's ability to give informed consent and his or her willingness to participate and continue with treatment. Unless serving as the primary provider, nurses are not responsible for obtaining informed consent—that is the role of the primary provider. However, it is the nurse's prerogative actively to pursue the observations previously outlined to protect the client's rights during treatment.

Every agency should clearly define the nurse's role in assisting with obtaining a client's signature on a consent form. A joint signing between the primary provider and the client at the time of the decision is a preferred method of documenting consent; many agency policies and consent forms reflect this preference (Figure 5.1).

SUBSTITUTED CONSENT. When a client cannot give informed consent independently for a necessary procedure or treatment, health care providers must obtain **substituted consent** from another person on the client's behalf. The appointment of a health care proxy is one example of the concept of substituted consent. Substituted consent can come from a court-appointed guardian or, in some instances, from the client's next of kin. If the client has not been adjudicated incompetent previously, no next of kin are available, and the law so permits, the health care agency may initiate a court proceeding to appoint a guardian so that professionals can carry out their interventions. In emergencies, clients in

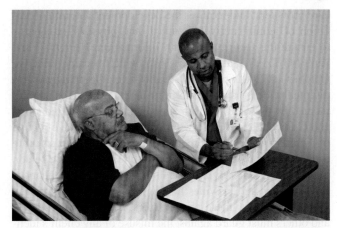

FIGURE 5.1 Many health care agencies have informed consent forms that document the signatures of both the client and the primary health care provider at the time of the decision for a treatment or procedure.

danger of harming themselves or others can be given medication, restrained, or secluded without consent.

Nurses and other health care providers must know the statutory requirements for obtaining substituted consent. In their role as client advocates, nurses also must know whether a client has been adjudicated incompetent and whether consent from a next of kin or guardian is a legally acceptable substitution.

Confidentiality

Nurses have a professional and an ethical duty to use knowledge gained about clients only to enhance their care and not for other purposes, such as gossip, personal gain, or curiosity. Accordingly, nurses must strive to maintain the confidentiality of verbal and written information.

Preserving confidentiality is especially important for clients with mental illness. Despite some advances, society still attaches tremendous stigma to those with psychiatric diagnoses (see Chaps. 1 and 8). Breaches of confidentiality about clients' diagnoses, symptoms, behaviors, and outcomes of treatment can have negative consequences for clients' employment, promotions, marriage, insurance benefits, and so forth. However, health care practitioners must maintain a delicate balance. With managed care companies frequently paying for behavioral health services, providers and institutions must share clinical information with case managers to justify admission and continued treatment. Thus, health care providers must obtain "fiscal informed consent" from clients or their family (Dasco & Dasco, 2001). Providers are responsible for knowing the legal requirements associated with clinical confidentiality and the requirements of managed care companies to be informed of the client's clinical condition for reimbursement.

HEALTH INSURANCE PORTABILITY AND ACCOUNTABILITY ACT. The Health Insurance Portability and Accountability Act (HIPAA) of 1996 outlines appropriate use and disclosure of the health information of clients, identifies privacy rights, requires certain privacy practices of health care providers, and requires the development and implementation of administrative, technical, and physical safeguards to ensure the security of health information. HIPAA's Final Rule (45 C.F.R. Parts 160 & 164), which became effective October 15, 2002, provides standards for the privacy of individually identifiable health information. HIPAA is supplemented by the Health Information Technology for Economic and Clinical Health (HITECH) Act, which became effective on February 17, 2009. Although the main goal of this statute is the utilization of an electronic health record for each person in the United States by 2014, it also strengthens and enhances privacy rules and provides for harsher penalties for privacy violations. Under these privacy rules, health care providers and others must guard against the misuse of any client's identifiable health information. The rules also limit sharing such information and afford significant rights to enable clients to understand and to control the use and disclosure of their health information. Protected health information is defined broadly as any individually identifiable health information and includes demographic data that either identifies or could reasonably be used to identify the person.

The privacy rules govern health care providers who transmit health information electronically. Providers may use and disclose protected health information without consent, authorization, or both when they are conducting treatment, payment, and health care operations. They may disclose information without consent or authorization if so mandated by state or federal reporting requirements, such as those related to public health, abuse, neglect, and domestic violence. Providers may disclose protected information to law enforcement officials under specific circumstances. They also may disclose protected information without authorization to comply with laws related to workers' compensation, to a party responsible for paying the benefits, and to any agency responsible for handling the workers' compensation claim. Special provisions for authorization apply to psychotherapy notes.

Providers need to follow carefully their institution's policies and procedures for HIPAA compliance. Civil penalties for violating the rules are $100 per occurrence, not to exceed $25,000 per year; criminal penalties range from a $50,000 fine and 12 months in prison for a simple knowing violation to a $250,000 fine and 10 years in prison for an intentional disclosure for financial gain or malicious harm. Under HITECH, civil penalties for violating the rules are $100 per occurrence, not to exceed $25,000 per year, if the party did not know of the violation; $1,000 per occurrence, not to exceed $100,000 per year, if the party had reasonable cause to know of the violation; and $10, 000 per occurrence, not to exceed $250,000 per year, if there is willful neglect allowing a breach of confidential information. Additionally, if the violations are not corrected properly, penalties range from $50,000 to $1.5 million.

RESPONSIBLE RECORD KEEPING. Each client has a right to a written record that enhances care (American Hospital Association, 2003). Accrediting agencies such as the

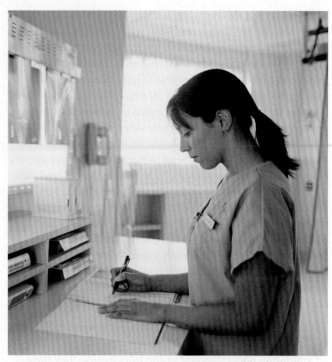

FIGURE 5.2 When documenting care, nurses must take the utmost measures to record information in descriptive, nonjudgmental, and objective terms. They also must do everything possible to safeguard and protect this information.

Joint Commission (2008) also require each client to have a medical record. Examples of forms of documentation include narrative notes, SOAP notes (recording information by subjective data, objective data, assessment, and plan), and clinical pathways. Records, kept manually or electronically, are legal documents that can be used in court; therefore, all nursing notes and progress records should reflect descriptive, nonjudgmental, and objective statements (Figure 5.2). Examples of significant data to include are here-and-now observations of clients through the nurse's critical assessments, accurate reports of verbal exchanges with clients, and descriptions of client outcomes after provided care. The medical record can be the best source of legal protection in malpractice suits.

Verbal communication should be straightforward, forthright, descriptive, unbiased, and limited to those involved in the client's care and treatment. Health care facilities and agencies should have established methodologies for reminding staff members about their professional and legal responsibilities related to confidentiality. Examples include annual requirements for all nurses to sign a form certifying their understanding of and commitment to maintaining confidentiality.

PRIVILEGED COMMUNICATION. Each state has statutes regarding *privileged communication* that delineate which professionals have the legal privilege to withhold conversations and communications. Although statutes vary, they customarily provide this privilege to physicians, attorneys, and clergy. Some states also extend privileged communication to psychologists, nurses, and other health care providers. Psychiatric nurses should be aware of their state's statutorily privileged communication rules. If the privilege for nurses is limited or nonexistent, the nurse should know what specific boundaries to set in therapeutic interviews. Nurses who work in states with no or limited statutory privileges may be required to repeat communications with clients in court through the subpoena process. Therefore, nurses should not encourage clients to share sensitive or incriminating data—they should limit therapeutic communication to the requirements of the treatment plan.

Some cases have involved appropriate circumstances that warrant breach of privileged communication. A leading example is *Tarasoff v. Board of Regents of University of California* (1974), which held that therapists might have a duty to protect a person who is threatened by a client. Subsequent decisions discuss the issues of foreseeable violence and the amount of control that the therapist could reasonably use to prevent the harm (Beck, 1987). In such cases, courts have ruled that mandates to protect client confidentiality end for therapists when confidences include threats against others.

Although courts recognize the duty to maintain confidentiality between client and therapist, they have established that it is superseded by the duty to protect the public safety. There are no nursing cases per se on this point, but nurses must be aware that they cannot ignore or fail to attend to clients' threats against others, especially when the opportunity for clients to act on these threats is reasonable. Other legal situations that may demand breaches of confidentiality include allegations of child abuse, threats of suicide, and allegations of sexual misconduct against a therapist or other health care professional.

Think About It 5.2

A client tells a nurse that she is ashamed about something illegal that she did, even though no one was hurt. The nurse encourages her to discuss it, and the client reveals that she set fire to her neighbor's garage. The conversation is not protected as privileged information in this state, and the nurse later is subpoenaed and testifies in court that the client admitted to setting the fire. Did the nurse violate the client's rights? Explain your answer.

Evolving Legal Rights

U.S. laws constitute the system of binding rules of action or conduct that governs citizens' behavior with one another, as well as with the government itself. Generally, laws are meant to reflect the population's moral values and opinions about the "rightness" or "wrongness" of particular acts. Although guided by foundational ethical principles, laws evolve to reflect changing societal beliefs. Examples of areas affected by recent legal changes include fetal tissue use, abortion, confidentiality for clients with AIDS, and expanded prescriptive privileges for nurses. Nurses need to familiarize themselves with current laws to make informed choices and to ensure that their practices are consistent with established provisions.

Right to Treatment

The idea that clients with psychiatric illnesses have a legally actionable right to treatment emerged in the late 1960s and culminated in the early 1970s in the federal circuit court of appeals case of *Wyatt v. Stickney* (1971). The *Wyatt* case provided innovative statements about the rights of civilly committed clients with mental illnesses in state hospitals. The court stated that such clients have certain treatment rights, which include the following:

- Treatment must give some realistic opportunity for improvement or cure.
- Custodial care is insufficient to meet treatment requirements.
- A lack of funding does not excuse the state from treatment responsibilities.
- Commitment without treatment violates the due process rights of clients.

Perhaps the most important pronouncement in this case concerns the three determinants for adequacy of treatment: (1) a humane environment, (2) adequate numbers of qualified staff, and (3) individualized treatment plans. This case gave the nation guidance about treatment rights; however, the Supreme Court did not review it. The Supreme Court decision on *O'Connor v. Donaldson* (1975) commonly is considered the leading case for the right to treatment. Albeit, that decision sets forth that no state can confine a person with mental illness in a state hospital who is not a threat to self or others if he or she can survive safely in the community alone or with the help of willing, responsible family members or friends.

Right to Treatment in the Least Restrictive Environment

Courts have given guidance to the mental health system on many matters, including standards for treatment settings. As early as 1969, in *Covington v. Harris*, the court held that a person treated involuntarily should receive care in a setting least restrictive to liberty that still meets treatment needs. Least restrictive environments can be community resources instead of hospitalization, open units instead of locked units, or outpatient or home care instead of inpatient care (*Covington v. Harris*, 1969). For this reason, nurses continually assess the condition and status of clients to ensure that more or less restrictive alternatives are consistent with the client's evolving needs.

Right to Refuse Treatment

The doctrine of informed consent implies that clients have the right to choose or refuse medical and health treatment. Certainly, health care providers, through interpersonal relationships and client education, may try to convince clients about the

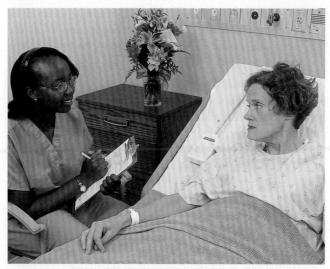

FIGURE 5.3 Nurses may use their roles as educators and advocates for clients to explain to them the importance of agreeing to certain treatments or approaches to care. However, ultimate decisions rest with clients or with those designated as having such authority in extenuating circumstances. (Photo © B. Proud.)

need for certain treatments (Figure 5.3). However, only in rare or life-threatening instances do courts intervene in decisions.

Right to Aftercare

Clients with psychiatric problems who have been hospitalized or admitted to other inpatient facilities need follow-up care in the community after discharge to prevent readmission and to ensure rehabilitation. Nevertheless, no absolute federal legal right currently establishes aftercare programs. Some state statutes may provide such a right. It is conceivable that case law may evolve to mandate aftercare services as a right of clients with mental disorders.

In conjunction with other members of the interdisciplinary team, nurses plan for aftercare treatment. As knowledgeable and responsible citizens, they can voice their concerns at all levels of the political system to ensure that clients with psychiatric illnesses have access to adequate aftercare services. Examples include outpatient counseling, home care, medication follow-up, vocational placement, and sheltered living environments.

Checkpoint Questions

3. What is the best source of legal protection in a malpractice suit?

4. What are the three determinants for adequacy of treatment?

Client Status and Specific Legal Issues

When clients with psychiatric disorders are hospitalized, the type of admission determines the treatment plan. Civil commitment admissions include the following:

- Voluntary admissions
- Emergency admissions
- Involuntary commitments (indefinite duration)

Each state has specific statutory regulations pertaining to each status that mandate procedures for admission, discharge, and commitment for treatment.

Voluntary Admissions

Clients who present themselves at psychiatric facilities and request hospitalization are considered **voluntary admissions** (Figure 5.4). Likewise, clients evaluated as being a danger to themselves or others or who are so seriously mentally ill that they cannot adequately meet their own needs in the community but are willing to submit to treatment and competent to do so have voluntary admission status.

Voluntary clients have certain rights that differ from those of other hospitalized clients. Specifically, they are considered competent (unless otherwise adjudicated) and therefore have the absolute right to refuse treatment, including psychotropic medications, unless they are dangerous to themselves or others. An example of such a danger is a client who has a violent destructive episode while in the treatment unit (*Rennie v. Klein,* 1981).

Voluntary clients do not have an absolute right to discharge at any time, but may be allowed to request discharge. The time delay that this provision affords gives health care personnel an opportunity to initiate a procedure to change a client's admission status to involuntary if he or she meets the necessary statutory requirements. Many people with mental illness can be treated voluntarily; however, the state cannot

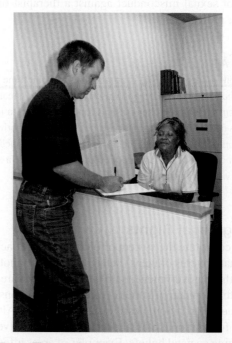

FIGURE 5.4 This man is filling out paperwork for his wife, who has presented to the health care facility for voluntary admission to help manage her substance use problems.

require that a client receive treatment in any setting if he or she refuses. Therefore, many people with psychiatric disorders whose behavior causes family, community, and social problems do not and cannot receive psychiatric care if they are unwilling to be voluntary clients.

Emergency Admissions

Emergency admission status is appropriate when a client's behavior indicates that he or she is mentally ill and, consequently, likely to harm self or others. State statutes will define the exact procedure for the initial evaluation, possible length of detainment, and attendant treatment available (Case Vignette 5.2).

All clients with emergency admission status enter health care facilities for diagnosis, evaluation, and emergency treatment. At the end of the statutorily limited admission period, the facility must discharge the client, change his or her status to voluntary admission, or send representatives to a civil hearing to determine the need for continuing involuntary treatment.

During an emergency admission, the client's right to come and go is restricted. The right to consult with an attorney to prepare for a hearing remains and must be protected. Clients may be forced to take psychotropic medications, especially if they continue to be dangerous to themselves or others. Invasive procedures, such as electroconvulsive therapy (ECT) or psychosurgery, are not permitted unless they are ordered by the court or consented to by the client or his or her legal guardian. No treatment should impair the client's ability to consult with an attorney at the time of a hearing.

Involuntary Admissions

People who refuse psychiatric hospitalization or treatment but pose a danger to themselves or others, are mentally ill, and are not judged suitable for less drastic options may be adjudicated to **involuntary admission** status for an indefinite period. Although the exact legal procedure may differ in each state, the standards for commitment are similar throughout the United States.

To deprive a person of liberty by involuntary commitment is a serious matter, and the legal protections are strict. *Addington v. Texas* (1979) requires that before involuntary commitment, clear and convincing evidence must be used as the standard of proof in a civil hearing to determine if a person is "mentally ill and dangerous to self or others." This high standard differs from a "preponderance of the evidence" (the prior civil commitment standard). The statutes of each state concerning commitment procedures must reflect the Supreme Court's standard of the protection of the right to liberty.

Legal Issues and Special Client Populations

Forensic Clients

Mental health professionals become involved with clients who are charged with criminal acts in two major circumstances:

1. For the evaluation of a defendant's competency to stand trial and administration of concomitant pretrial treatment, if needed
2. For the evaluation of a defendant's mental condition at the time of an alleged crime and administration of concomitant treatment if the defendant pleads and is acquitted on an insanity defense

Case Vignette 5.2

Jim, 20 years old, lives at home with his parents. He is enrolled in classes at the community college. For the past 2 months, Jim's behavior has been increasingly problematic. Currently, he does not attend school. He leaves his house several times day and night, disrupting the neighbors. When Jim's dad tries to discuss these matters, Jim becomes agitated and storms from the room. Jim's parents do not know of any drug use by their son; however, they have seen Jim drinking beer. He has lost 30 pounds and neglects his personal hygiene.

Despite his agitation and erratic behavior, Jim has never threatened nor been aggressive to anyone. Although he has never been especially religious, he has become preoccupied with the Bible. When his parents question this sudden interest, Jim responds that he is an apostle doing what God has told him. One month ago, Jim's parents persuaded him to visit the local mental health center. However, when the therapist suggested inpatient treatment at a psychiatric hospital, Jim angrily left the office.

One night, Jim is standing on the patio. He begins "preaching the gospel." His shouting disturbs the entire neighborhood. His parents, feeling helpless and frightened, call the local police, who transport Jim to the state psychiatric facility. He stays there for 5 days as an emergency admission, after which he attends a hearing.

During the hearing, Jim cannot sit still. Based on the testimony of health care providers about Jim's mental state and behavior, the court finds that Jim meets the standards for civil judicial commitment on two grounds. First, his hyperactivity secondary to his mental illness is resulting in loss of appetite, weight, and sleep, which are compromising his physical health. Second, his increasing agitation and religious preoccupation, also secondary to his mental illness, are potential antecedents to loss of control and harm of self or others. The court returns Jim to the psychiatric hospital for continued treatment on an involuntary committed basis with no judicial pronouncements about his competency status.

Reflection and Critical Thinking

• Could this situation have been averted? How?
• Based on the evidence, do you agree with the court's decision? Why or why not?

This specialized area of mental health care is called *forensic psychiatry* (see Chap. 21). Ideally, the team responsible for forensic evaluations and services is composed of a psychiatrist; clinical psychologist; social worker; psychiatric–mental health nurse, clinical specialist, or nurse practitioner; and other nursing personnel who are actively involved in the client's treatment. Advanced practice nurses are valuable members of such teams (Heitkemper & Bond, 2004; Laurant et al., 2005; Reasor & Farrell, 2005). They are specially trained to perform mental status examinations and to function as individual and group therapists. In some states, they are qualified to be trained in competency evaluations and to testify in court as expert forensic witnesses.

COMPETENCY TO STAND TRIAL. Competency to stand trial refers to a defendant's mental condition at the time of the trial. Mental health professionals determine competence by assessing the following:

- Ability to assist the attorney with defense
- Understanding of the nature and consequences of the charge against him or her
- Understanding of courtroom procedures

The U.S. Supreme Court decision in *Jackson v. Indiana* (1972) resulted in state statutes designed to protect the rights of criminal defendants who continue to be incompetent to stand trial because of mental illness. These defendants cannot be detained indefinitely without the same type of commitment hearing to which all civilly committed clients have a right. In other words, these pretrial defendants should be returned to court as soon as they are competent to stand trial, which should be the primary goal of pretrial treatment.

PLEAS OF INSANITY OR MENTAL ILLNESS. If the defendant chooses to plead insanity, mental health professionals evaluate his or her mental condition at the time of the alleged crime. A person found not guilty by reason of insanity is admitted involuntarily to a psychiatric facility for a statutorily defined evaluation period. During this time, mental health professionals evaluate the need for hospitalization and any other appropriate disposition. On completion of the evaluation, the professionals notify the court of their recommendations, at which time a hearing may be scheduled to determine the court's order for release or for continuation of mandatory commitment for treatment. As soon as clients are considered not committable, they must be released into the community, possibly with some mandatory requirements for aftercare.

Much controversy involves the verdict of not guilty by reason of insanity. A famous example of this outcome is the acquittal of John Hinckley after his assassination attempt against President Ronald Reagan in 1981. Some states have established a plea of "guilty but mentally ill," meant to mandate psychiatric treatment in correctional facilities of criminals with mental illness.

Minors

Minors or juveniles (those younger than 18 years) represent a special population of psychiatric clients. Until recently, parents or guardians had an almost absolute privilege to admit their children younger than 18 years for mental health treatment. However, state recognition of the rights of children 12 to 18 years old to protest such treatment has eroded this absolute right.

In 1979, the U.S. Supreme Court, in *Parham v. J.R.,* gave a more definite standard for juvenile admissions, to which state statutes and hospital policy should conform. The Supreme Court held that parents can authorize the admission of juveniles, but accompanying the admission, some neutral fact-finder should determine whether statutory requirements for admission are satisfied. Nevertheless, an adversarial hearing for admission is not required, nor does due process require that the fact-finder be legally trained or be a hearing officer. By ruling in this way, the Court balanced the competing interests of the rights of parents and guardians to control the lives of their children with the right of children to due process before their liberty is limited.

Psychiatric–mental health nurses must be mindful of these procedural protections for the benefit of their juvenile clients. Limiting hospitalization to statutory requirements is an important advocacy activity on behalf of pediatric clients with mental illness.

Checkpoint Questions

5. How do the rights of clients voluntarily committed differ from those of other hospitalized clients?

6. What factors are assessed to determine if a defendant is competent to stand trial?

ETHICAL ISSUES IN PSYCHIATRIC–MENTAL HEALTH NURSING

Ethics are principles that serve as codes of conduct about right and wrong behaviors to guide actions. Although there are universal ethics, such as respect for others, ethics often are tailored for a specific professional culture, such as business, law, and medicine.

Psychiatric–mental health nurses must understand ethical theories and use ethical principles to guide decisions about client care. They must clarify their own ethical beliefs and then combine them with professional ethical principles to make sound decisions. *Psychiatric–Mental Health Nursing Practice: Scope and Standards* (American Nurses Association [ANA], American Psychiatric Nurses Association, & International Society of Psychiatric–Mental Health Nurses, 2007) outlines expectations for ethical clinical practice in professional standard V.

"Everyday ethics" act as the center of nursing practice and give meaning and purpose to nursing care (Austin, 2007; Erlen, 1997; Roberts, 2004). They focus on interpersonal relationships, demand the confirmation of positive regard, and respect the search for human dignity. They involve not only caring "for" but caring "about" the client.

Nurses display ethical behavior when they listen to and develop trusting and respectful relationships with clients. Other ethical behaviors include maintaining the dignity of clients while guiding and coaching them through the maze of mental illness. A respectful attitude communicates the value of each person's uniqueness and self-determination. Respect and caring together promote ethical nursing.

Responsibility and accountability are additional ethical foundations. As nurses interact with clients, they make many ethical decisions. For example, nurses employ ethics when they request that a client sign a consent form permitting ECT. Does the nurse carefully assess the client's desire or willingness to have the procedure and cognitive ability to understand its full effects? Does the nurse attempt to influence the client into signing because the nurse believes the treatment is in the client's best interest? Whatever a nurse decides, he or she must take full responsibility and accountability for his or her ethical decision making. Such responsibility requires a code of ethics, such as the ANA's *Code of Ethics for Nurses,* to guide decision making (Nursing Spotlight 5.2).

Nurses do not make most ethical decisions about client care in isolation. Rather, they usually collaborate with other health care providers, including physicians, psychologists, social workers, nurses, and perhaps ethicists. Nurses are often in positions to gather and disseminate information about the provision of care to clients. This position is valuable for participating in institutional debates regarding ethical client care decisions. Although all psychiatric–mental

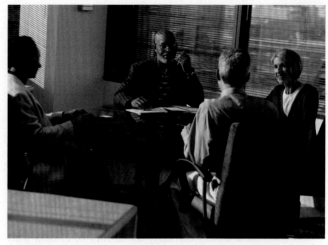

FIGURE 5.5 Many health care facilities have ethics committees that discuss challenges that staff members are encountering. Nurses may benefit from participating in such committees.

health nurses are responsible for acting as advocates for ethical care, some nurses choose to become first-line activists by becoming members of the ethics committees of their health care facilities. Ethics committees discuss and debate ethical dilemmas during meetings (Figure 5.5). Health care professionals develop an ethical climate according to their relationships with one another, managers, and clients. An ethical climate supports organizational practices that foster the discussion of challenging client care issues and the ethical implications (Hart, 2005; Ulrich et al., 2007).

NURSING SPOTLIGHT 5.2

American Nurses Association Code of Ethics for Nurses

1. The nurse, in all professional relationships, practices with compassion and respect for the inherent dignity, worth, and uniqueness of every individual, unrestricted by considerations of social or economic status, personal attributes, or the nature of health problems.
2. The nurse's primary commitment is to the patient, whether an individual, family, group, or community.
3. The nurse promotes, advocates for, and strives to protect the health, safety, and rights of the patient.
4. The nurse is responsible and accountable for individual nursing practice and determines the appropriate delegation of tasks consistent with the nurse's obligation to provide optimum patient care.
5. The nurse owes the same duties to self as to others, including the responsibility to preserve integrity and safety, to maintain competence, and to continue personal and professional growth.
6. The nurse participates in establishing, maintaining, and improving health care environments and conditions of employment conducive to the provision of quality health care and consistent with the values of the profession through individual and collective action.
7. The nurse participates in the advancement of the profession through contributions to practice, education, administration, and knowledge development.
8. The nurse collaborates with other health professionals and the public in promoting community, national, and international efforts to meet health needs.
9. The profession of nursing, as represented by associations and their members, is responsible for articulating nursing values, for maintaining the integrity of the profession and its practice, and for shaping social policy.

From American Nurses Association. (2001). Code of ethics for nurses with interpretive statements. *Washington, DC: American Nurses Publishing.*

Bioethical Principles in Psychiatric Nursing Practice

In addition to the universal principles of respect and responsibility, several other principles guide nurses and other health care professionals in ethical decision-making. They include autonomy, beneficence, paternalism, veracity, fidelity, and justice.

Autonomy

Autonomy is the right to make decisions for oneself. It implies that a person not only chooses to make his or her own decisions but freely accepts their consequences. Health care issues that repeatedly involve debates over the right of absolute autonomy include assisted suicide, abortion, and refusal of treatment (eg, hospitalization, medication).

Nurses must assess carefully the ability of clients with psychiatric disorders to process information, solve problems, and make autonomous decisions. This assessment is critical when nurses are seeking informed consent. For example, when the client gives consent to treatment, does he or she freely decide to sign the consent form? Does the client understand the import of his or her decision?

Voluntary consent implies that the client has freedom of choice. Therefore, nurses must refrain from coercion whenever possible (Husted & Husted, 2008). Coercion can be blatant intimidation such as "Do this or else we cannot help you" or, more likely, subtle with clients sensing a nurse's approval or disapproval for the way a decision should be made.

Certainly, acute mental illness with accompanying unclear or delusional thought processes or suicidal ideation compromises a client's autonomy. However, issues of autonomy can pose an **ethical dilemma** (a situation in which moral and ethical principles conflict with one another) for health care providers. Consider the client with grandiose mania who is roaming the streets and demanding that people stop and listen to his revelations. He refuses to take his medications and chooses not to be hospitalized. His ability to be autonomous is questionable, and health care providers, along with the courts, must balance the client's desire for autonomy against what is in his, and in society's, best interests.

Beneficence and Paternalism

Beneficence is the principle of doing good, not harm. **Paternalism** is similar to beneficence in that the intent is to do good; however, professionals define how to do good, which may override the wishes and self-determination of clients.

Staff members may act benevolently toward clients by providing a safe environment and being available. However, sometimes they also may need to act paternalistically. For example, some clients must be put on suicide alert, even though it is against their wishes. Practicing beneficence and evaluating a need for paternalism require that caregivers carefully analyze interventions, considering their possible good effects versus their possible harmful effects. A similar issue is the possible good versus possible harm of psychotropic medications and physical restraints.

Veracity and Fidelity

The ethical principles of **veracity** and fidelity are related closely. **Veracity** is a systematic behavior of honesty and truthfulness in speech. **Fidelity** is faithfulness to duties, obligations, and promises. Both are basic to establishing therapeutic relationships. It is not unusual for clients to test nursing students or novice psychiatric nurses regarding veracity early in the relationship (see Chap. 11). A client in an inpatient setting might ask the student, "Why do you want to spend time with me?" or "Are you afraid to come here?" Clients need to trust their nurses, and they will test them for honesty.

In a therapeutic relationship, fidelity involves faithfulness to follow through with the client's plan of care and promises made. For example, when a nurse agrees to meet with a client at a certain time, the nurse must follow through on that commitment. If the nurse cannot meet with the client, the client deserves an explanation and perhaps an apology. Even with an explanation and an apology, clients may still question the nurse's commitment to fidelity. The nurse who practices both fidelity and veracity can develop trusting nurse–client relationships (Case Vignette 5.3).

Case Vignette 5.3

Sydney, an adolescent client, is admitted to an inpatient psychiatric unit that follows a behavior modification plan to decrease aggression toward self and others. Sydney knows that if he verbally attacks anyone on the unit, he must take a 15-minute time-out in the side room. During that 15 minutes, if the other clients can leave the unit and go to the recreation room, Sydney will lose his opportunity to join them.

One evening, this scenario happens. As the nurse directs Sydney to go to the side room, he begs and pleads to join the others in the recreation room. He promises to control himself and states he will not be aggressive for the rest of the evening. The nurse wants to do what is best for the client (beneficence) and

appreciates that Sydney is willing to try to control his behavior (autonomy). Nevertheless, Sydney knew what would happen if he became aggressive. If the nurse allows Sydney to go to the recreation room, she endangers her credibility with everyone, which is essential to maintaining veracity and fidelity (Parker, 1995).

Reflection and Critical Thinking

- Would the nurse's failure to exert the imposed behavioral consequences be ethically wrong? Can a child or adolescent who avoids consequences learn veracity and fidelity?
- What obligation does the nurse have in terms of acting as a role model for Sydney and the other teens on the unit?
- What decision would you make?

Justice

The ethical principle of **justice** in health care commonly is seen as the equitableness of benefits, including the right to access care. As health care reform continues, justice as an ethical consideration becomes even more critical. Currently, clients with mental illnesses do not receive the same health care benefits as clients with other illnesses. Managed care providers and insurance companies often severely limit coverage for psychiatric care. Nurses must become advocates for mental health care at both the state and national levels of government.

Nurses also must consider the principle of justice as they provide care to clients. For several reasons, nurses may find that they are spending more time with a select few clients and limiting their time with others. Occasionally, reasons for such inequality are legitimate. However, it is just as likely that a nurse has formed a particular bond with a client or the personalities of some clients motivate the nurse's behavior. When nurses allow this situation, they are not meeting the ethical principle of justice.

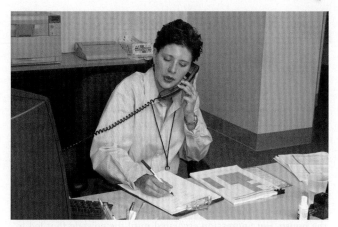

FIGURE 5.6 Community mental health nurses frequently face legal and ethical challenges related to the follow-up care and management of clients with chronic, long-term psychiatric disorders. They may spend much time negotiating with agencies, other health care providers, family, and services to advocate for clients and assist them to obtain needed attention and materials.

Checkpoint Questions

7. Which bioethical principle is a critical aspect of informed consent?

8. The right to access care reflects which ethical principle?

Nursing Ethics in Community Mental Health

Working with clients in community mental health affords nurses an opportunity to practice with greater autonomy than nurses who work in mental health facilities. However, as autonomy increases, so do responsibility and accountability. Community mental health nurses not only are responsible for working with clients, families, and multidisciplinary treatment teams, but also for working with public and private agencies and the community at large (Figure 5.6).

Community mental health nurses must comprehend how, out of necessity, legislation and policies establish boundaries for ethical decision making. In the community, nurses frequently encounter ambiguous situations for client care. For example, what are the nurse's responsibilities if a client with schizophrenia living in the community chooses to stop taking medication? A nurse who believes that a client's autonomy outweighs all other ethical principles may think the client has a right to make that choice and decide not to intervene. This decision may mean that the nurse is placing both the client's life at risk and the community's safety in jeopardy. In general, the interest of the community overrides the interest of the client.

Boundaries in Ethical Nursing Care

As discussed in Chapter 11, nurses must maintain boundaries in therapeutic relationships with clients. Interpersonal boundaries protect clients from emotional harm that would impede their recovery. Boundaries must be initiated when clients begin treatment, continue throughout, and, for the most part, persist even after the therapeutic relationship has ended. During treatment, providers must conduct interactions with clients within appropriate guidelines and focus on the client's growth and movement toward wellness. Members of the health care team must recognize that stepping outside their professional boundaries can compromise a client's movement toward recovery (Case Vignette 5.4).

Boundary violations usually develop insidiously. At first, a health care provider may be unaware that the relationship is drifting from therapeutic interactions into a friendship or social relationship. As this relationship changes, the judgment of the provider becomes clouded, and the client's therapeutic needs become compromised. For example, during a psychiatric–mental health rotation of several weeks, a student nurse was assigned to work with an inpatient sex offender. Toward the end of the rotation, the student shared with the instructor that the client had asked the student to write to him after she completed the rotation. The student explained that she had developed a feeling of friendship toward and felt sorry for the client. The instructor reminded the student of the state policy that students could have no contact with clients after completion of the rotation. The instructor counseled the student about why continued contact would be detrimental to the client's recovery. However, 3 months later, the agency informed the instructor that the student was both calling and writing to the client. In another example, a nurse maintained a therapeutic relationship with a client during a lengthy hospitalization. Once the client was discharged, the nurse entered into an intimate relationship with the client. The relationship ended 6 months later, at which point the client became extremely depressed and suicidal and needed to be readmitted to the hospital.

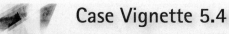

Case Vignette 5.4

A juvenile court judge commits 16-year-old Mary Ann to an adolescent residential treatment facility for attempted suicide and homicide against her brother. Mary Ann's parents have a history of substance use and child neglect and physical abuse. When Mary Ann was 6 years old, a neighbor sexually molested her. In the past 2 years, Mary Ann was suspended twice for bringing marijuana to school. After she joined a gang, Mary Ann began verbally and physically abusing her siblings; she also ran away three times. However, 4 months before her admission, she stopped seeing the gang, dropped out of school, and seldom left the house. Her aggression escalated until the episode that led to her admission. Mary Ann describes obsessive suicidal thoughts and negative feelings, including self-hatred. Her mood is labile. The psychiatrist diagnoses her with major depression, substance use disorder, and post-traumatic stress disorder.

Tom, a 25-year-old psychiatric nurse specialist, is assigned as Mary Ann's primary nurse. He is to meet with Mary Ann for 30 minutes, three times a week, to evaluate her plan of care. Almost immediately Mary Ann responds to Tom's caring and sincerity. Although she shares little with other team members, Mary Ann expresses herself to him. Initially, Tom is careful to let others know what happens in his meetings with Mary Ann. However, over time he becomes more secretive. He does not share his growing fondness for Mary Ann. Sometimes during team meetings Tom states, "I know what is best for her." Without consulting with the team, he increases his meetings with Mary Ann to five times per week.

After several months, Mary Ann is discharged to a group home in the city. Two weeks after her discharge, Tom calls to check on Mary Ann. Phone calls become increasingly frequent. Tom and Mary Ann begin to meet over coffee to "discuss her feelings and concerns."

Soon, Tom and Mary Ann become sexually involved. Tom learns of drug dealing and robberies involving Mary Ann and her friends, but he cannot bring himself to go to the police. After all, he would lose his job. He tells himself that he needs to "protect" Mary Ann. Not until the police come to his place of employment does Tom realize how much trouble he is in.

Reflection and Critical Thinking

- Were Tom's supervisor or team members legally, ethically, or institutionally obligated to insist that Tom report what occurred during his sessions in the mental health unit with Mary Ann?
- What are the nurse's legal and ethical obligations related to contacting a client after discharge from a facility in which the nurse is practicing?
- What are the nurse's legal or ethical obligations when a client reveals that he or she has committed or is going to commit a crime?

Clients with psychiatric disorders are highly vulnerable. Nurses must take responsibility for evaluating and maintaining the boundaries in a nurse–client relationship. Nurses should be alert to the need to reevaluate boundary lines when:

- They provide extraordinary care to one or more particular clients, such as spending an unusual amount of time with them, giving care to them at unusual places or hours, and doing things for clients that are outside of the ordinary nursing role.
- Clients seem more like friends, at times, than clients.
- Limit-setting with clients is difficult, and nurses find themselves "protecting" clients from the natural consequences of their behavior.
- They strongly identify with clients.
- They want or feel compelled to rescue clients.
- They are at odds with the rest of the team as to a client's needs.
- They believe that they understand clients better than other team members do.
- They have recurring sexual thoughts about clients.

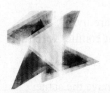

Reviewing and Applying Your Knowledge

Chapter Summary

- A failure to meet the standard of care that results in an injury to a client or consumer makes the nurse liable for nursing negligence or malpractice.

- To provide legally acceptable nursing care in psychiatric–mental health settings, nurses must be informed about various legal issues, including client rights. Nurses must take responsibility, along with other health team members, to see that client rights are protected.

- Nurses must request and secure ongoing continuing education and consultation with attorneys knowledgeable in mental health law.

- Nurses have the responsibility to understand ethical theories and to follow ethical principles in providing care to psychiatric clients.

- Psychiatric–mental health nurses put ethics into practice when they demonstrate respect within the therapeutic relationship and when they protect and build the client's dignity.

- Autonomy, beneficence, paternalism, veracity, fidelity, and justice are ethical principles used by psychiatric nurses in ethical decision making.

- Boundaries are essential in therapeutic relationships, and nurses must evaluate and maintain the boundaries in the nurse–client relationship.

Study Questions

1. When caring for psychiatric–mental health clients whose ability to give informed consent depends on their degree of psychiatric impairment, the nurse's priority obligation is to

   a. assess the client's mental capacity when that client is asked to give consent.

   b. prevent the client from revoking consent.

   c. obtain informed consent when the primary provider cannot be present.

   d. persuade the client to consent.

2. A client with a history of depression is admitted voluntarily to the psychiatric hospital, having been transferred from a medical hospital where he was treated for a self-inflicted gunshot wound to the chest. After a few days of treatment, the client decides he would like to leave the hospital. The treatment team, believing he is still a danger to himself, discusses initiating legal proceedings

to have the client's admission status changed to involuntary. Which ethical concepts are in conflict? Select all that apply.

   a. Beneficence

   b. Fidelity

   c. Paternalism

   d. Autonomy

   e. Veracity

3. A client has developed a therapeutic relationship with the nurse. Upon discharge, she asks for the nurse's home phone number so she can "keep in touch." The nurse likes the client very much but tells her that a friendship would violate the boundaries of the therapeutic relationship. The nurse's response best reflects which ethical concept?

   a. Veracity

   b. Beneficence

   c. Autonomy

   d. Fidelity

4. A 35-year-old man was hospitalized 2 weeks ago for acute mania. Upon admission, he made many lewd and offensive comments to the nurse. The nurse finds it hard to have a conversation with the client now, even though his offensive remarks have ceased. The nurse's ethical dilemma involves which principle?

   a. Justice

   b. Veracity

   c. Beneficence

   d. Paternalism

5. After discussing "everyday ethics" with a group of nursing students, which description would lead the nursing instructor to determine that the students have understood the concept?

   a. The focus is interpersonal relationships, respect, caring with unconditional positive regard, and fostering of human dignity.

   b. The primary focus of everyday ethics is promoting and maintaining the client's autonomy.

   c. It reflects the practice of the principles of beneficence and paternalism in all nurse–client interactions.

   d. The ultimate outcome is the assurance that health care is provided justly.

(continues on page 92)

Critical Thinking Questions

1. How has managed care altered the responsibility of health care providers to release information?

2. Why does the "reasonable person test" seek a peer standard, not a performance standard, of excellence?

3. Consider the community in which you are living. How might the rights of the psychiatric client conflict with the rights of your community?

4. Should a civilly committed adolescent have the same rights as a civilly committed adult? Defend your answer.

References

Addington v. Texas, 99 S. Ct. 1813, 441 U.S. 418 (1979).

American Hospital Association. (2003). *The patient care partnership: Understanding expectations, rights, and responsibilities.* Chicago, IL: Author.

American Nurses Association, American Psychiatric Nurses Association, & International Society of Psychiatric-Mental Health Nurses. (2007). *Psychiatric–mental health nursing: Scope and standards of practice.* Silver Spring, MD: American Nurses Publishing.

Austin, W. (2007). The ethics of everyday practice: Healthcare environments as moral communities. *Advances in Nursing Science, 30*(1), 81–88.

Beck, J. C. (1987, March–April). The psychotherapist's duty to protect third parties from harm. *Mental and Physical Disability Law Reporter, 2.*AU: Page numbers?

Canterbury v. Spence, 464 F.2d 772 (1972).

Covington v. Harris, 419 F.2d 617 (1969).

Dasco, S., & Dasco, C. (2001). *Managed care answer book.* New York, NY: Aspen Publishers.

Erlen, J. A. (1997). Everyday ethics. *Orthopaedic Nursing, 16*(4), 60–63.

Hart, S. E. (2005). Hospital ethical climates and registered nurses' turnover intentions. *Journal of Nursing Scholarship, 37*(2), 173–177.

Health Information Technology for Economic and Clinical Health Act, Title XIII of Division A and Title IV of Division B of the American Recovery and Reinvestment Act of 2009.

Health Insurance Portability and Accountability Act (HIPAA) of 1996, Final Rule, 45 C.F.R. Parts 160 and164 (2002).

Heitkemper, M. M., & Bond, E. F. (2004). Clinical nurse specialists: State of the profession and challenges ahead. *Clinical Nurse Specialist, 18*(3), 135–140.

Husted, G. L., & Husted, J. H. (2008). *Ethical decision making in nursing and healthcare: The symphonological approach* (4th ed.). New York, NY: Springer.

Jackson v. Indiana, 46 U.S. 715 (1972).

Joint Commission. (2008). *2008 Comprehensive accreditation manual for hospitals.* Oakbrook Terrace, IL: Author.

Laurant, M., Reeves, D., Hermens, R., Braspenning, J., Grol, R., & Sibbald, B. (2005). Substitution of doctors by nurses in primary care. *Cochrane Database of Systematic Reviews,2005*(2). CD001271.

Mohr, W. K., & Mohr, B. D. (2000). Mechanisms of injury and death proximal to restraint use. *Archives of Psychiatric Nursing, 14*(6), 285–295.

O'Connor v. Donaldson, 422 U.S. 563 (1975).

Parham, Commissioner, Department of Human Resources of Georgia et al. v. J.R. et al., 442 U.S. 584 (1979).

Parker, J. (1995). Chemical restraints and children: Autonomy or veracity. *Perspectives in Psychiatric Care, 31*(2), 25–29.

Patient Self-Determination Act, Omnibus Budget Reconciliation Act of 1990, Pub. L. No. 101–508, § 4206, 104 Stat. 1388–115 (codified at 42 U.S.C.A. § 1395cc[f]).

Prosser, W. L., Wade, J. W., Schwartz, V. E., Kelly, K., & Partlett, D. F. (2005). *Prosser, Wade, Schwartz, Kelly and Partlett's cases and materials on torts* (11th ed.). New York, NY: Foundation Press.

Reasor, J. E., & Farrell, S. P. (2005). The effectiveness of advanced practice registered nurses as psychotherapists. *Archives of Psychiatric Nursing, 19*(2), 81–92.

Rennie v. Klein, 653 F.2d 836 (1981).

Roberts, M. (2004). Psychiatric ethics: A critical introduction for mental health nurses. *Journal of Psychiatric Mental Health Nursing, 11*(5), 583–588.

Tarasoff v. Board of Regents of University of California, 592 P.S. 553 (1974).

Ulrich, C., O'Donnell, P., Taylor, C., Farrar, A., Danis, M., & Grandy, C. (2007). Ethical climate, ethics stress, and the job satisfaction of nurses and social workers in the United States. *Social Science Medicine, 65*(8), 1708–1719.

Vernon's Texas Code Annotated, Occupations Code, Section 301.002, 2003.

Wyatt v. Stickney, 325 F. Supp. 781 (1971).

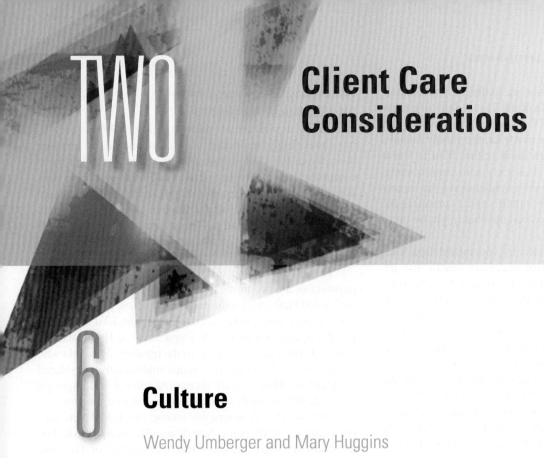

TWO

Client Care Considerations

6

Culture

Wendy Umberger and Mary Huggins

LEARNING OBJECTIVES

On completion of this chapter, you should be able to accomplish the following:

- Describe the importance of culture to human behavior and its influence over the provision of effective mental health services.
- Explain how demographic changes in North America are contributing to the importance of cultural awareness.
- Describe the elements of a culturally congruent service system.
- Identify disparities in mental health for clients from minority cultures.
- Explore barriers that have led to mental health issues for clients from minority cultures.
- Discuss biologic variations and various social, psychological, and spiritual perspectives within ethnic groups and across cultures.
- Identify aspects of transcultural assessment.
- Describe skills essential to the implementation of culturally competent care.
- Explain nurses' unique position in providing culturally competent care.
- Assess one's own heritage, reference group, and personal and cultural biases.

North American societies are undergoing a transformation. By the middle of the 21st century, the average U.S. citizen (as defined by Census Bureau statistics) will likely trace his or her ancestry to Africa, the Pacific Islands, or Hispanic or Middle Eastern lands, rather than to European countries. Nursing reflects society and, consequently, cultural changes. Growing diversity underscores the importance of learning about various cultures and recognizing the needs of people who come from groups that might be unfamiliar to nurses.

This chapter assists nurses to understand how culture influences the behavior of clients in health and illness. When nurses view clients through a cultural lens, they can both expand cultural awareness and provide culturally congruent services for those with psychiatric or emotional stress. Nurses also become better equipped to promote positive mental health within specific cultural environments. This chapter explores the meaning of culture, the relationship between changing demographics and the need for cultural awareness, and the components of a culturally congruent health care system. It discusses disparities found in mental health among minority, refugee, and white populations and explores related barriers to effective health care. It examines various beliefs about health and illness common to different cultural groups. Finally, the chapter focuses on the nurse's role in providing culturally congruent care.

CULTURE

Culture is the integration of human behaviors (which include thoughts, communications, actions, customs, beliefs, values, and institutions) particular to a racial, ethnic, religious, or social group. It represents the vast structure of ideas, attitudes, habits, languages, rituals, ceremonies, and practices found among a specific group of people. Members of such groups share an accepted way of life that provides a general structure for living, as well as patterns by which they interpret reality. Thus, culture provides a collective programming that distinguishes one group from another (Hofstede & Hofstede, 2004).

Culture can influence perceptions of health and illness greatly, as well as how, when, and why people seek treatment for health problems. This factor becomes especially important in mental health. Many aspects of psychiatric care involve self-perception, roles and relationships, family dynamics and interactions, attitudes toward medications, values, and community supports. Before mental health care providers can administer appropriate and effective treatment, they must understand a client's cultural context and how it might influence his or her attitudes toward a particular health concern and its causes and treatment. Culturally relevant care is as diverse as the cultures represented. An understanding of the client's cultural context also is necessary to appreciate the client's attitude toward the provider.

Changing Demographics and Cultural Awareness

The ability to view clients through a cultural lens is becoming increasingly important as a consequence of growing diversity in the United States and Canada. Although these countries always have been composed of people from various ethnic groups, races, and religions, the majority culture has traditionally been white, English-speaking, Christian, and middle class. Members (mostly men) of this majority culture have held power, and traditions and attitudes have supported and reinforced their ideals.

However, dramatic shifts in demographics indicate that populations are becoming incredibly diverse. New arrivals to the United States during the past 50 years have predominantly come from Latin America, Asia, the Middle East, and other non-European locations (U.S. Department of Homeland Security, 2007). They are adding to the numbers of people who belong to racial and ethnic groups traditionally considered "minorities." They also are increasing cultural and linguistic diversity, with English no longer dominant in some areas.

Another U.S. demographic change involves the increasing influence of Hispanic Americans. The U.S. Census Bureau (2004b, 2005) projects that the number of Hispanic Americans, currently the largest U.S. minority, will more than double during the next 50 years. At the same time, the number of white Americans (currently the majority culture) is estimated to decrease by approximately 25%, whereas the number of African Americans should remain approximately the same. Furthermore, by that same time, the number of white Americans will be about the same as the combined number of all "minority" populations (U.S. Census Bureau, 2004b).

Such changes are likely to have important influences on all aspects of what is perceived as "American" culture. They also will force U.S. society to examine and redefine the meaning of "majority" and "minority" (Table 6.1).

Assimilation

Throughout most of the 20th century, assimilation was the predominant U.S. attitude toward culture. **Assimilation** is the process of immigrants and minority groups becoming more like the majority culture. U.S. immigrants were expected to abandon native languages and customs and conform to

TABLE 6.1 Trends in U.S. Demographics

Group	2010 (%)	2050 (%)
African American/Non-Latino	12.6	13.6
Asian and Pacific Islander	4.8	8.2
American Indian (AI)/Alaska Native (AN)	0.7	0.9
Hispanic/Latino	16.4	24.5
White/Non-Latino	72.4	52.8

Source: U.S. Bureau of the Census, 2010.

dominant norms, including the adoption of Western technology and medicine. In many cases, success for these groups was rooted in achieving a status similar to and accepted by the dominant culture.

Unmodifiable characteristics (race, age, sex) made assimilation more difficult for nonwhites, the very old, and women. Such groups faced and continue to struggle with significant barriers to full participation in mainstream society. Assimilation also fostered a sense of **ethnocentrism**, or the belief that one's own cultural practices and values are inherently correct or superior to those of others. Ethnocentric attitudes can lead to the following problems:

- **Prejudice**—Negative preconceived opinions about other people or groups based on hearsay, perception, or emotion
- **Stereotyping**—Beliefs that one member of a cultural group will display certain behaviors or hold certain attitudes (usually negative) simply because he or she is a member of that cultural group
- **Discrimination**—Differential treatment based on race, class, sex, or other variables rather than on individual merit
- **Stigmatization**—Attribution of negative characteristics or identity to one person or group, causing feelings of rejection, alienation, and ostracization from society

In the health care industry, traces of racism and discrimination continue in practices ranging across the continuum of diagnosis, treatment, prescribing, and referrals (Ard et al., 2005; Burnes Bolton et al., 2004; Ezenwa et al., 2006; Franks et al., 2005; Lin & Larson, 2005; U.S. Department of Health and Human Services [USDHHS], 2001a). Stereotyping, discrimination, stigmatization, prejudice, and racism are clearly stressful for clients and can affect both physical and mental health adversely. Within the context of discrimination models, the causal mechanisms linking racial/ethnic minority status and health disadvantage lie in the harmful effects of chronic experiences with actual and/ or perceived race-based discrimination. These experiences are thought to contribute to physiologic responses (eg, high blood pressure, increased cortisol, hypervigilance) that eventually lead to disease and higher mortality rates (Mays et al., 2007). The USDHHS (2001a) suggests three general areas of research to assess the role of racism in the mental health of minorities:

- *Self-worth:* Racial stereotypes and negative images resulting in internalization and denigration can affect self-worth, thereby adversely affecting social and psychological functioning.
- *Institutional racism and discrimination:* Persistent stressors (eg, poverty, crime, violence) affecting mental health result in the overrepresentation of minority populations in lower socioeconomic brackets and poorer living conditions.

- *Stressful events:* Racism and discrimination are stressful events that can affect mental health both psychologically and physiologically.

Evidence is being compiled indicating differences in stress factors based on assimilation. For example, U.S. immigrants from conflict-ridden native areas may have more trauma-related symptoms (Jamil et al., 2007; Marshall et al., 2005; Robertson et al., 2006; USDHHS, 2001a). People who have been forced to migrate because of persecution, human rights violations, repression, torture, conflict, and natural and human-made disasters share a traumatic past. Escape may increase such trauma as a result of exposure to physical danger, attack, and violence during the escape.

Further compounding these traumas are issues of unauthorized status and risk of removal. Even when immigrants obtain legal status, they face such difficulties as chronic unemployment, poverty, discrimination, lack of access to care and housing, high levels of crime, and absence of networks (Dey & Lucas, 2006). Assimilation also is connected with education and economic levels.

Thus, the level of assimilation is important to evaluate. Recent immigrants still adapting to U.S. culture face different stressors than do long-term residents. Further complicating this picture are differences in diagnosis based on place of birth. For example, U.S.-born Mexican Americans report higher rates of depression and phobias than do U.S. immigrants from Mexico (USDHHS, 2001a). Lifetime disorders for all Mexican Americans are lower than those for whites, whereas prevalence rates for Puerto Ricans and other Hispanics are not different from those of whites (USDHHS, 2001a). Nurses must consider such findings when evaluating a client's help-seeking behaviors to avoid stereotyping a client or group. Considering another example, black Americans with low incomes tend to wait until a mental health problem is severe before seeking help. Contributing factors to this behavior include suspicion, viewing problems as external, and lacking funds, insurance, or access to services. In contrast, U.S. immigrants from the Caribbean Islands, who also are black, tend to value medical institutions but are reluctant to express their feelings. Therefore, they tend to consider therapy as positive when it is presented as self-change or intellectual improvement (Fernandez & Fernandez, 2005a; USDHHS, 2001b).

Implications for Health Care

Overall, international demographics indicate that the majority populations of most countries consist of people of color. However, Western (European) medicine, which is rooted in a high-technology, intervention-focused approach, continues to dominate the thinking of many practitioners. Consequently, Western medical practitioners often disregard, supersede, or fail to recognize traditional healing methods found in non-European cultures. They often forget that humanity is a composite of cultural beings with different beliefs, values, and constructs.

Changes in North American ethnic populations will continue to challenge the capabilities of mental health care systems. Furthermore, growing numbers of providers from non-Western orientations increasingly will influence the nursing and mental health care professions. With more North Americans coming from non-Western cultures, health care providers will need to operate in ways that respect different traditions and behaviors while providing optimal care. Therefore, nurses and other mental health care providers must understand and appreciate cultural diversity as something to celebrate. Practicing and student nurses cannot ignore or be complacent about the cultural needs of their clients. Knowledge of cultural diversity and the influence of culture on health care is vital to providing effective interventions needed to meet changing demographics.

> **Checkpoint Questions**
>
> 1. Why is culture such an important factor to consider when working with clients who have mental health problems?
> 2. What are four negative consequences of ethnocentric attitudes?

Culturally Competent Health Care

Cultural competence means having the skills, both academic and interpersonal, to understand and appreciate cultural differences and similarities within, between, and among groups to meet the social, cultural, and linguistic needs of an individual. In this dynamic process, health care providers (or systems) find the specific delivery strategy that is meaningful and useful to each client based on their knowledge of cultural heritage, beliefs, attitudes, and behavior. Cultural competence is the foundation for mutual respect and understanding between client and caregiver.

Skills in cultural competence are relevant for all variables to which differences may apply. Examples include gender, race, ethnicity, language, country of origin, acculturation, age, religious and spiritual beliefs, sexual orientation, socioeconomic class, and disabilities. The culturally competent provider is willing and able to draw on community-based values, traditions, and customs and to work with knowledgeable people from the community to formulate appropriate interventions and supports for clients according to the aforementioned variables (Markova & Broome, 2007).

To deliver care that is culturally competent, nurses require ways of systematically ensuring that culture is a factor in assessment and delivery of intervention. The Cultural Formulation is described in the *Diagnostic and Statistical Manual of Mental Disorders,* 4th edition, text revision (American Psychiatric Association [APA], 2000), enhancing the biopsychosocial approach by highlighting how culture influences disease presentation and symptoms. The Cultural Formulation begins with a review of aspects of client's cultural identity, including ethnicity, language, age, gender, socioeconomic status, sexual orientation, religious and spiritual beliefs, disabilities, political orientation, and health literacy. Next the formulation explores the role of culture in the expression and assessment of a client's illness. Cultural factors related to psychosocial stressors, social supports, and levels of function or disability are also assessed, focusing on the roles of family systems, religion, and spirituality in providing support. The Cultural Formulation also includes specific consideration of cultural elements that influence the relationship between the individual and nurse. It concludes with an overall assessment of the ways in which these varied cultural considerations apply to mental health diagnosis and treatment planning (Mezzich et al., 2009).

In 2003 the National Organization of Nurse Practitioner Faculties recommended a structured approach to cultural competence as an entry-level competence for all mental health nurses (Mahoney et al., 2006). The Mental Health Services Oversight and Accountability Commission (2007) has adopted a work plan to address cultural competency, including cultural and linguistic competence. The commission's intent is to build on the December 2000 report of the Centers for Disease Control and Prevention's Office of Minority Health and Health Disparities (MHSOAC, 2007), which identified 14 standards for measurement of cultural competence. See Box 6.1.

Cultural Congruence

In a culturally competent health care system, care delivery is culturally congruent. **Cultural congruence** means that clients receive an overall message, conveyed both verbally and nonverbally, of personal and cultural validation. In culturally congruent mental health care, providers integrate the client's value system, life experiences, and expectations about treatment into the therapeutic process, even when the client is not fully aware that it is happening. As a result, the full weight of the client's cultural system can help support healing.

For mental health services to be culturally congruent, providers from all aspects of the delivery system must respond to diverse cultural values consistent with the client's specific context. Theoretical approaches encompassing such values, while remaining flexible and adaptable, have been long in coming and difficult to define. Since the 1950s, Dr. Madeleine Leininger has consistently urged that, as societies throughout the world become increasingly multicultural, cultural competence in human relationships should be a major concern for nursing and other health disciplines (Leininger & McFarland, 2002). However, the health professions traditionally have lacked culture-specific interventions that recognize the unique combinations of disorders found in groups not embraced by Western society. Such disorders (eg, traumatic losses, soul loss, culture shock, cultural isolation, somatoform and anxiety disorders, and unique culture-bound syndromes) require specific culturally oriented treatments.

Cultural competence is a broad-based approach to transform the organization and delivery of all services to meet the diverse needs of all clients. Studies indicate that tailoring services to needs makes such services more inviting and therefore improves use and outcomes (Sue & Sue, 2008).

Standard 1: Health care organizations should ensure that patients/consumers receive from all staff members effective, understandable, and respectful care that is provided in a manner compatible with their cultural health beliefs and practices and preferred language.

Standard 2: Health care organizations should implement strategies to recruit, retain, and promote at all levels of the organization a diverse staff and leadership that are representative of the demographic characteristics of the service area.

Standard 3: Health care organizations should ensure that staff at all levels and across all disciplines receive ongoing education and training in CLAS.

Standard 4: Health care organizations must offer and provide language assistance services, including bilingual staff and interpreter services, at no cost to each patient/consumer with limited English proficiency at all points of contact, in a timely manner during all hours of operation.

Standard 5: Health care organizations must provide to patients/consumers in their preferred language both verbal offers and written notices informing them of their right to receive language assistance services.

Standard 6: Health care organizations must assure the competence of language assistance provided to limited English proficient patients/consumers by interpreters and bilingual staff. Family and friends should not be used to provide interpretation services (except on request by the patient/consumer).

Standard 7: Health care organizations must make available easily understood patient-related materials and post signage in the languages of the commonly encountered groups and/or groups represented in the service area.

Standard 8: Health care organizations should develop, implement, and promote a written strategic plan that outlines clear goals, policies, operational plans, and management accountability/oversight mechanisms to provide CLAS.

Standard 9: Health care organizations should conduct initial and ongoing organizational self-assessments of CLAS-related activities and are encouraged to integrate cultural and linguistic competence-related measures into their internal audits, performance improvement programs, patient satisfaction assessments, and outcomes-based evaluations.

Standard 10: Health care organizations should ensure that data on the individual patient's/consumer's race, ethnicity, and spoken and written language are collected in health records, integrated into the organization's management information systems, and periodically updated.

Standard 11: Health care organizations should maintain a current demographic, cultural, and epidemiological profile of the community as well as a needs assessment to accurately plan for and implement services that respond to the cultural and linguistic characteristics of the service area.

Standard 12: Health care organizations should develop participatory, collaborative partnerships with communities and use a variety of formal and informal mechanisms to facilitate community and patient/consumer involvement in designing and implementing CLAS-related activities.

Standard 13: Health care organizations should ensure that conflict and grievance resolution processes are culturally and linguistically sensitive and capable of identifying, preventing, and resolving cross-cultural conflicts or complaints by patients/consumers.

Standard 14: Health care organizations are encouraged to regularly make available to the public information about their progress and successful innovations in implementing the CLAS standards and to provide public notice in their communities about the availability of this information.

Retrieved from http://www.minorityhealth.hhs.gov.

The responsibility for such competence lies with the system or practitioner, not the client.

Health Literacy

Low health literacy, cultural barriers, and limited English proficiency have been coined the "triple threat" to effective health communication by The Joint Commission (Schyve, 2007). **Health literacy** is defined as "the degree to which individuals have the capacity to obtain, process, and understand basic health information and services needed to make appropriate health decisions" (Institute of Medicine, 2004, p. 32). It is estimated that more than one third of American adults don't have the knowledge needed to make medical decisions. Moreover, with more than 43% of American adults unable to read above a sixth-grade level, it is easy to see how written words may be a barrier to the client's recovery.

Culture and language have a large impact on skills necessary for health literacy. Reading, writing, speaking, and listening in English, critical thinking, and decision making are all affected by an individual's culture and primary language (Singleton & Krause, 2009). In addition to the ability to read and speak English, other factors can affect health literacy, such as age, disability, complexity of information, experience with the health care system, emotional responses, and cultural views of the client's mental health condition and health system. All client communication is dependent on how well the health professional delivers information, then ensures and confirms that the client understands. As the diversity of the U.S. population changes and increases, all health professionals must actively learn and grow in areas of diversity and cultural competence.

Models of Transcultural Nursing

Learning how to explore the worldview and social structure of clients from different cultures assists providers to provide culturally congruent care. How to provide care stems from the client's cultural context as part of an extended family, group, and community. Without this vital information, providers are apt to misdiagnose, mismanage, and misunderstand clients.

Various ethnographic and culturally sensitive instruments have been developed to assist in interviewing people from diverse cultures. These can involve multiple in-depth questions regarding family, religion, gender, food, and health care values. Using self-awareness and ethnographic instruments is critical in preparing nurses in the development of appropriate treatment plans. Even with knowledge, cultural bumps may occur. *Cultural bumps* are those times when an action is incongruent within the cultural context, despite prior knowledge of that cultural context. An example is a woman using her left hand to reach out to touch a man from Afghanistan, even though she knows that use of the left hand for greetings is impolite in Islamic countries and that Afghan men do not touch women in public.

During the past few years, various theorists have developed models of transcultural nursing. Tortumluoglu (2006) evaluated four of the most prominent:

- Leininger's sunrise model
- Campinha-Bacote's model of cultural competence in health care delivery
- Purnell's model for cultural competence
- Giger and Davidhizer's transcultural assessment model

Full citations for the most recent works representing these models are found in the references. Each model is described briefly here.

SUNRISE MODEL. Leininger's culture care theory, the sunrise model, emphasizes learning principles related to culture care, cultural assessments, the universality of cultural diversity, and the importance of fit between the client's health care values and services provided. According to this model, health professionals are bound ethically to explore their own culture first to evaluate, acknowledge, and respect cultural differences in their own worldviews and then attempt to understand the culture of clients. Self-awareness assessments can vary from multipage questionnaires to 1-page exercises to assist nurses to identify personal experiences that helped shape their values and thoughts. See Assessment Tool 6.1 for an example.

CULTURAL COMPETENCE IN HEALTH CARE DELIVERY. Campinha-Bacote's model (2007b) looks at cultural competence as a process of building toward cultural awareness, knowledge, and skills. Such development gradually helps nurses to change attitudes and thus eventually leads to competence. Professionals learn to collect relevant cultural data while doing the health history. This model is depicted as a process that erupts into a volcano as the nurse becomes more competent (Figure 6.1).

CULTURAL COMPETENCE. Purnell's model categorizes cultural characteristics as primary and secondary. *Primary characteristics* are age, nationality, race, color, gender, and religion. *Secondary characteristics* are educational and socioeconomic status, occupation, military status, political beliefs, residential status (ie, urban vs. rural), marital and parental status, physical characteristics, sexual orientation/gender, and reason for migration (as applicable). This model is depicted as a circle with person, family, and community/global society surrounding the various characteristics. It was originally developed as a framework or tool by which nurses could organize a cultural assessment. The model also can be used as a tool for assessment, strategic planning,

---

▲ ASSESSMENT TOOL 6.1 ▲

Fostering Cultural Self-Awareness

To deliver culturally competent care, nurses first must evaluate the influence of their own culture on beliefs and attitudes. Answering the following questions can help nurses acknowledge the influence of their cultural heritage on behavior.

1. Where and when were you born?
2. Where did you grow up? What about your parents? Grandparents? Great grandparents?
3. What is your earliest family memory? School memory?
4. As a family, what events did you celebrate?
5. As an adult, what events or holidays do you celebrate?
6. Did you travel or move as a child? What about as an adult?
7. With what ethnic group(s), socioeconomic class, religion, age group, and communities do you currently identify?
8. Identify one positive and one negative experience that you have had with people from the groups listed above.

9. Identify one positive and one negative experience that you have had with people from outside the groups you listed above. What did you learn about people who are different from you?
10. Do you find anything about your ethnic group, socioeconomic class, religion, or age embarrassing or needing change? Why?
11. What cultural factors might contribute to you being misunderstood or rejected by members of other cultures?
12. What training or educational programs have you undertaken to enhance knowledge and skills in the provision of services to culturally, ethnically, racially, and linguistically diverse groups?
13. Name two ways in which you are responsive to the needs of diverse groups.

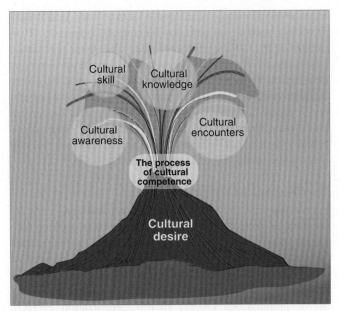

FIGURE 6.1 Campinha-Bacote's model of cultural competence depicts the process as erupting into a volcano as the nurse develops skills. (Source: Campinha-Bacote, J. [2007]. *The process of cultural competence in the delivery of healthcare services. A culturally competent model of care* [5th ed.]. Cincinnati, OH: Transcultural CARE Association.)

and individual interventions; thus, it is useful for clinicians, managers, and researchers (Purnell, 2002; Purnell & Paulanka, 2008).

TRANSCULTURAL ASSESSMENT MODEL. This model is based on an assessment that assists nurses to develop an awareness and knowledge of each client's needs. Training is necessary to properly assess the health and well-being of people from various cultures (Giger & Davidhizar, 2008).

> **Think About It 6.1**
>
> A 60-year-old Hispanic American woman is brought to the mental health clinic by her son and daughter for evaluation. The client speaks some English but talks to her children primarily in Spanish. During the past several months, the children have noticed that their mother has been staying in bed most of the day and not getting dressed or eating. Her son reports that she used to go to church every morning but has stopped. The client's husband died approximately 1 year ago. How would the nurse provide culturally competent care?

Disparities in Mental Health and Barriers to Effective Treatment

Many studies document major disparities in key health indicators between nonwhite and white populations. People of color, particularly in inner cities, have major health disparities in neonatal mortality rates, cardiovascular problems, and mental health compared with those of white people (Purnell,

2002; Purnell & Paulanka, 2008). Such disparities negatively affect health outcomes and explain why minorities are among those most in need of high-quality health care.

Historically, many members of ethnically and racially diverse populations have avoided the mental health care delivery system. This avoidance arose from fear of being institutionalized, diagnosed incorrectly, or labeled "abnormal" because of culturally ingrained differences. Other reasons minority groups may display resistance to, and feel uncomfortable about, seeking mental health services include the following:

- Stress experienced from forced migration, dislocation, or immigration
- Inability to speak or comprehend the dominant language and distrust of culturally inappropriate interpreter services
- Differences in religious beliefs and practices
- Environmental stress as a result of poverty or lack of equal access to education, employment, housing, or medical care
- Culture-specific beliefs about seeking help (eg, history, fear of being labeled or controlled by medications, shame, basic belief about illness)
- Use of traditional healers and alternative medicines for specific culture-bound situations
- Differing values and attitudes
- Misinterpretation of behaviors (eg, lateness, sense of bewilderment, codependence, assimilation, distrust, quietness)

Variability and Vulnerability

Variability in the incidence of mental illnesses among different cultural groups may be related to differences in genetic vulnerability (including variances among Native American tribes). For example, Native Americans collectively have increased rates of alcoholism, depression, anxiety, violence, and suicide; they are at higher risk for mental illness than most other U.S. ethnic groups (APA, n.d.; Substance Abuse and Mental Health Services Administration, 2004). In addition, many tribes have maintained sovereign status, adding to the necessity for practitioners to understand mental health services within each tribe's historical, geographic, and educational context.

Unfortunately, many people of color face issues related to poverty, which providers must consider when assessing for vulnerabilities such as increased rates of illness, homicide, alcohol abuse, and infant mortality. Infant mortality rates, a primary indicator of a nation's or culture's health, range from slightly higher for Asian Pacific Island groups to twice as high for African Americans when compared with those of nonminority infants (OMHD, 2007a). The health gap between minority populations and whites is emphasized when reviewing other major causes of death, such as cancer, AIDS, diabetes, heart disease, homicide, and suicide.

Ethnopharmacology

Substantial racial and ethnic differences, which reflect both genetics and environment, influence responses to medications. This issue also can influence the quality and quantity of care given to minorities (Burroughs et al., 2002; Campinha-Bacote, 2007b). In the past, individualized attention to medications was virtually ignored. Today, individualized therapy according to age, sex, culture, ethnicity, and other life circumstances is the recognized standard of practice (Figure 6.2).

Furthermore, providers must understand how racial and ethnic differences can affect metabolism of prescribed medications, which can influence a drug's safety and effectiveness with a particular client. Clinical effectiveness and side effects have been shown to vary among racial and ethnic groups. Generally, African American and Asian American clients are considered slow metabolizers of antipsychotic and antidepressive drugs. Asians also may experience toxic side effects at lower levels of antipsychotic medications than do whites. Use of antipsychotic medications is higher in black Americans (including higher dosages). Researchers have found that clozapine has been associated with agranulocytosis in clients of Jewish ancestry at a rate of 20% versus 1% in the general population (Burroughs et al., 2002). Few studies have included Native Americans. Repercussions could be serious if clinicians fail to consider such variations and prescribe all clients the "normal dose," which generally was developed for whites. People with slow metabolism may experience increased side effects, nonadherence, and increased long-term risks (eg, tardive dyskinesia) if they receive doses higher than needed.

Other environmental, psychosocial, and genetic factors can influence cultural responses to medications. For example, different characteristics in generic substitutes for brand-name drugs may lead to problems with effectiveness and toxicity, particularly among slow metabolizers. This makes it inherently important for nurses to monitor drug levels and to recommend dosage adjustments as necessary. Health care providers need to be alert for unexpected responses (Burroughs et al., 2002). However, they also need to balance consideration of such variations to avoid racial profiling and treatment stereotyping. Race or ethnicity cannot stand alone. Another complication is that many clients have a mixed ethnic or racial heritage. Clients who initially may be considered "nonresponders" to certain psychotropic drugs could actually have a genetic basis for the lack of response. Careful individualized dosing and treatment are critical.

Traditional Medicine

People from all parts of the world use traditional, complementary, or alternative medical practices. When working with clients, nurses must be aware that clients may be using such "treatments." For example, 80% of the African population uses traditional medicine for primary health care, whereas 30% to 50% of the Chinese population consumes traditional herbal preparations (World Health Organization [WHO], 2003). Less well known is that 158 million U.S. adults and more than 50% of the industrialized world has used alternative modalities at least once (WHO, 2003). Thus, it is imperative to question all clients about alternative therapies used.

Clinicians must document use of herbs in clients taking psychotropic medications to avoid negative events such as overdose, toxicity, and interactions. Unregulated or inappropriate use of traditional medicines can be dangerous. For example, St. John's wort (an herb commonly used to treat depression) can interact with antidepressants and may potentiate the effects of treatment with monoamine oxidase inhibitors (Campinha-Bacote, 2007a).

Accessibility

The Americans with Disabilities Act of 1990 and Title VI of the Civil Rights Act of 1964 mandate accessibility to health care services and facilities for all U.S. citizens. Historically, however, mainstream mental health services have failed to meet the needs of people of color adequately. Native Americans, refugees, and illegal immigrants underuse health services, including preventive services, and delay care until conditions become serious. Failure to use such services may be related to cost, language, cultural barriers, fear, or apprehension (OMHD, 2007b; Trujillo, 2008).

Cultural barriers to treatment range from cultural insensitivity to obstacles such as difficulty understanding appointment procedures, lack of public transportation, signs written in a language not understood by the client, and formidable-looking buildings (Singleton & Krause, 2009) (Figure 6.3). In addition, many services are inaccessible because of location (eg, Indian Health Services [IHS] are primarily on reservations) or hours of service (eg, 9 to 5 Monday through Friday only). These institutional structures combine to preclude a culturally inviting environment. Cultural barriers also may be related to historical circumstances that have led to a group's economic, social, and political status in the community. Health care providers must be aware of the

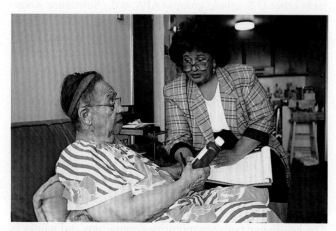

FIGURE 6.2 Nurses must work carefully with clients to ensure that their medication regimens are consistent with parameters such as age, sex, culture, ethnicity, and other life circumstances. (Photo © K. Sloane.)

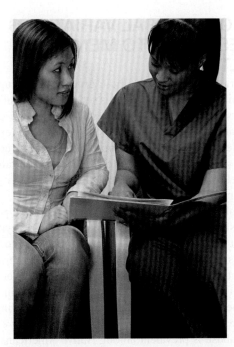

FIGURE 6.3 Barriers to treatment can include difficulties with language and understanding instructions. Nurses should work diligently with each client, especially those with identified language barriers and cultural differences, to enhance their understanding and ensure they are receiving the care they need.

group's underlying history and how it influenced the psychological well-being of its members (Betancourt et al., 2003; Campinha-Bacote, 2007a).

Racial Bias

Clients from nonwhite populations are institutionalized more frequently than are whites. This finding includes admissions to hospitals, involuntary commitments, and incarcerations. Racial bias affects such factors as definition of dangerousness, severity of diagnostic labels, and choice of treatments. Data indicate that African Americans are more frequently diagnosed as having serious and persistent mental illness than are other ethnic or racial populations admitted to psychiatric facilities (Burroughs et al., 2002). Furthermore, compared with whites, people of African descent:

• Drop out of services at a significantly higher rate
• Use fewer treatment sessions for their mental health problems
• Enter mental health treatment services at a later stage of illness
• Overuse inpatient psychiatric care in state hospitals
• Underuse community mental health services of all kinds
• Are misdiagnosed more often by mental health practitioners
• Are diagnosed more often as having a severe mental illness

To underscore the influence of racial bias on mental health care delivery to people of color, Box 6.2 discusses the

---

BOX 6.2 Diagnosis and Race: The Case of Junius Wilson

In 1925, Junius Wilson, a 17-year-old black man, was charged with attempted rape in the New Hanover community of Castle Hayne, North Carolina. In court, he was found incompetent to stand trial. The charges were dropped after he arrived at Cherry State Hospital, a state mental institution. Junius was castrated and remained in a locked mental ward for 69 years. In the 1920s, castration was a standard procedure for black men accused of rape. John Badgett, deputy director of the state Division of Mental Health, states that Wilson "has been the victim of social politics that we look back on now and are deeply troubled by." In 1992, after a review of Wilson's medical records, a social worker discovered that Wilson was deaf, not mentally ill. This discovery, with legal assistance, led to the release of Mr. Wilson and compensation by the state for the abuse and years of imprisonment.

Swofford, S. (1995, December 28). News and Record, pp. B1–B2.

---

case of Junius Wilson. This incident is neither isolated nor exclusive to African American history. Thousands of Native Americans experienced terrible social isolation as the result of a U.S. government policy of forcibly removing children from their families and placing them in boarding schools to indoctrinate them into European American practices. Forced relocation caused deaths and problems such as dealing with being conquered, shame, forced dependency on the government, and loss of traditional roles. Native Americans have dealt with broken treaties, restriction to reservations, poverty, and consequences of not relocating. These issues of historical trauma (discussed later) continue to affect tribes today.

Religious and Spiritual Influences

Many clients from minority populations interpret symptoms or signs of mental illness as spiritual. Consequently, they may choose to seek help from trusted spiritual leaders. Clients, families, and spiritual leaders may not identify signs or symptoms as a mental health problem, or clients may be diagnosed with a mental health problem only after traditional healing methods have failed. For example, folk medicine is integral to routine health care for many Mexican Americans. Use of traditional healers may include *curanderas* (female folk healers believed to be chosen by God), herbalists, *sobadoras* (female healers who use massage and manipulation), *brujos* (male witches), or *brujas* (female witches) (Lopez, 2005). Other traditional healers also may be involved, such as burn doctors, traiteurs, or wise women. They may use laying-on of hands, prayer, cupping, or other methods. Dr. Alberto Quezada, director of research at Cuenca University, is an expert in traditional medicine. He underscores the importance of understanding various indigenous population's use of traditional medicine, indicating that this understanding is a prerequisite for indigenous people to accept modern medicine. Furthermore, success in treatment follows the combination of traditional and modern medicine (Chelali, 2007).

In many cases, clients do not share with Western providers that they are seeing folk healers (Lopez, 2005). Nurses must understand that, in many cases, spiritual beliefs provide the structure by which some ethnic groups explain disease. Because Western medicine is technologically focused and emphasizes biophysical aspects, its providers often consider a group's characteristic response as "abnormal" when it differs from the response of the dominant culture. Awareness of cultural factors that influence client behavior is essential to avoid labeling clients as difficult, abnormal, or both.

This problem is glaringly evident in a retrospective assessment of a Hmong child named Lia described by Anne Fadiman (1998) in *The Spirit Catches You and You Fall Down: A Hmong Child, Her American Doctors, and the Collision of Two Cultures*. Lia had a seizure disorder. Providers asked what caused it, and Lia's family indicated "soul loss," which began when an older sister slammed the door and scared the soul from the child's body. However, when providers attempted to administer traditional healing methods, the family expressed reluctance:

> You should give Lia medicine to take for a week but no longer. After she is well, she should stop taking the medicine. You should not treat her by taking her blood or the fluid from her backbone. Lia should also be treated at home with our Hmong medicines and by sacrificing pigs and chickens. We hope Lia will be healthy, but we are not sure we want her to stop shaking forever because it makes her noble in our culture, and when she grows up she might become a shaman.

In this circumstance, everyone involved was concerned for Lia's health care, yet no one explored the family's perception of the illness (ie, "shaking" was a blessing with Lia's potential to become a shaman). This exploration of the cultural misunderstanding between the medical community and the Laotian refugee family underscores how well-meaning families and well-meaning health care providers can fail to understand each other. Although everyone had good intentions, the inability of the medical community to understand or to communicate with Lia's family, and their inability to understand and to communicate with her physicians resulted in tragic consequences. Undermedication and sporadic treatment resulted in Lia suffering from status epilepticus and subsequently sustaining severe brain damage. Lia is "still alive and still lovingly cared for by her mother and siblings. Her medical condition has not changed" (Fadiman, 2003). Many times culture challenges are perceived as culture clashes, making it difficult to understand behavior different from that of the established culture (Trujillo, 2008).

Checkpoint Questions

3. What is ethnopharmacology?
4. What do some ethnic groups use as a basis for explaining disease?

SOCIOCULTURAL VARIATIONS IN RESPONSE TO MENTAL HEALTH CARE

Each person belongs to multiple groups (eg, occupational, community, religious), so various sets of values, beliefs, and behaviors are influential. Belief systems include concepts such as attitudes toward methods of stress relief (eg, use of drugs, alcohol, yoga) and use of home remedies (eg, eating chicken soup for the common cold). These culturally influenced belief systems can shape a client's receptivity to different types of interventions.

Problems such as alcoholism, delinquency, violence, and physical illness can mask acute psychiatric symptoms. Different cultural values and symptom patterns complicate diagnosis in non-Western groups. Diagnosis of serious and persistent mental illness is underrepresented or not represented in several nonwhite groups because of reinterpretation of behaviors (eg, spiritual issues) or mislabeling of the symptom as the disease (eg, use of alcohol). For example, alcohol abuse is prevalent among Native Americans experiencing mental illness, but this community often sees drinking as the cause of the problem. This interpretation is more acceptable to the community because they believe that there is a "cure" for drinking. Thus, accurate diagnosis is difficult because alcohol use or abuse masks symptoms. Treatment approaches must be redefined to provide for comorbidity to address simultaneously mental illness and chemical use (Szlemko et al., 2006).

Mental health programs that provide culturally congruent services integrate prevention and stress reduction through a holistic approach that emphasizes the environment, living arrangements, medical care and health care, job availability, and use of traditional healers and alternative health practices. Effective programs use culturally appropriate assessment tools and develop culturally and ethnically appropriate clinical standards. These include terminology that reflects the client's system.

Hispanic and Latino(a) Clients

The Hispanic population is the fastest growing in the United States. Projections are that by 2050 nearly 25% of the U.S. population will be Hispanic (U.S. Census Bureau, 2004b). Hispanic and Latino(a) clients comprise a large, diverse group that includes Puerto Ricans, South Americans, Central Americans, Dominicans, Cubans, people from the Caribbean, people of Spanish descent, and Mexicans, who comprise approximately one third of this entire group. Most Latino(a)s live in the Southwest (approximately 60%). States with fast Hispanic growth rates are Arkansas, North Carolina, Georgia, Nebraska, and Tennessee.

Academic achievement varies among this population: high school graduation rates vary from 79% of Cuban Americans, to 64% of Puerto Ricans, to 5% of Mexican Americans (USDHHS, 2000). Hispanics are underrepresented in the homeless population and in child foster care.

However, they are highly represented among the incarcerated (particularly men), Vietnam veterans with post-traumatic stress disorder (PTSD), refugees from Central America with PTSD, and substance abusers, particularly Latino men and Mexican Americans (compared to Mexican-born immigrants, particularly women). The following are concerns for the Hispanic population:

- Mental illness among Mexican Americans is higher than among Mexican immigrants.
- Depression is higher for Puerto Ricans living on the U.S. mainland than those living in Puerto Rico.
- Lack of employment has resulted in many Hispanics having no health insurance (USDHHS, 2001a).

Research shows that Latino(a)s are most likely to use formal mental health services during crises. Fewer than 1 in 11 contact mental health specialists; fewer than 1 in 5 contact general health providers; and, among Hispanic immigrants, fewer than 1 in 20 use mental health services, and fewer than 1 in 10 use general health (USDHHS, 2001a). In each identified group, the family is the first source of assistance.

Hispanic groups tend to revere elders for their wisdom. Elders may recommend wearing of religious medals, visiting shrines, or offering prayers as methods of dealing with stress or illness. Men are considered the heads of the house, but women are considered sacred. Personal matters are considered to be family problems. Families usually seek help through recommendations from priests and are unlikely to turn to mental health services until all other options (eg, counseling from clergy) have failed. Generally, Hispanic people do not seek professional assistance, particularly for prevention. They are expressive and expect that they will be taken care of as an expression of family love (Figure 6.4).

Health care providers working with Hispanic consumers should consider the importance of the Catholic Church, prayers, herbs, and the strong influence of hot-and-cold or good-and-evil imbalances in promoting well-being. Latino(a)s often maintain two systems of beliefs regarding illness and health (McGoldrick & Giordano, 2005) and may think that psychiatric problems are punishment for sin. In these instances, clients may be more likely to follow medication regimens and recover if spiritual leaders are involved with treatment.

Curanderismo is the preferred medical system in many cases. Study findings vary on the use of folk medicine, with reports of those using such measures ranging from 4% to 44% (WHO, 2003). Health care providers should become familiar with culture-bound syndromes such as *susto* (fright), *nervios* (nerves), *mal do ojo* (evil eye), and *ataque de nervios* (uncontrolled screaming, crying, trembling, aggression, dissociation, seizure, fainting, or suicidal gestures). The prevalence rate of mental illness is comparable to that of the U.S. population except for Latino youths, who experience higher rates of anxiety, depression, and drug use. The rate of suicide attempts in young Latinas is also rising within an overall Latino suicide rate that is 50% of that of the U.S.

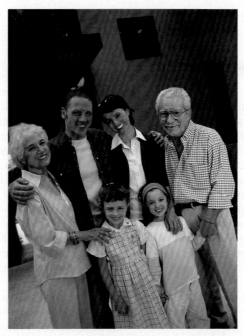

FIGURE 6.4 The family unit is of paramount importance to the Hispanic culture. Some people from this culture may consider that their health problems are to be dealt with only within the family itself, which may cause delays in treatment.

population (Trujillo, 2008). Few studies are available regarding Latino response to mental health care. One randomized study conducted with Spanish-speaking families found that low-income members were more likely to have an exacerbation of schizophrenia if they were in highly structured family therapy, instead of case management. Misdiagnosis between schizophrenia and bipolar disorder has been reported to occur (Trujillo, 2008). Furthermore, bilingual clients are evaluated differently when they are assessed in their native language.

Black Americans

Approximately 13% of the U.S. population identifies as African American (Ratogi et al., 2011). Most members of the black community have descended from people who came to America as slaves from the West Coast of Africa. Some members trace their origins to the West Indies, Dominican Republic, Haiti, and Jamaica. They, too, may be descendants of slaves but themselves primarily came to the United States voluntarily and relatively recently. People from African countries continue to move to the United States.

This large, diverse group has wide and varied attitudes and beliefs influenced by factors such as occupation, religion, country of origin, social class, and time spent in the United States. For example, culture views vary greatly between black people whose families have lived in the United States for hundreds of years versus blacks living in the United States who have immigrated recently from Somalia (Case Vignette 6.1). The recent immigrants do not identify

Case Vignette 6.1

Somalia is a hot, semiarid African land that continues to experience instability and the challenging consequences of decades of civil war, famine, and disease. Somalia's large extended family clans are subdivided into lineage units, which are further subdivided into kinship alliances. These kinship alliances are important to how Somalis address one another. Until recently, the Somali language was unwritten, with three main oral dialects. Songs and poetry are important vehicles for passing oral traditions.

Somali women generally do not eat with or touch men when greeting them. They socialize at home or the market. Most Somalis are Sunni Muslims, who cleanse their bodies and pray five times a day. They also abstain from alcohol and pork. Muslims observe Ramadan, the ninth month of the Muslim year, by fasting from sunrise to sunset.

All this information was important in the case of a 35-year-old Somali woman with schizophrenia who relocated to Chicago. The client had never been diagnosed with mental illness in her home country. Health care providers were not sure if the stress of conditions at home and relocation precipitated schizophrenia or if she had a history of the illness. The client attended a Psychosocial Rehabilitation Center for 4 years. No one there understood her dialect, and she knew no English. A Muslim Somali man from a neighboring program provided some translation for client and staff; however, this situation was uncomfortable for the client because the translator was not only male, but also not of her lineage. Other problems were as follows:

- The client had stopped taking psychotropic medications, and her condition was deteriorating. Rehospitalization appeared imminent.
- She locked herself in the program's only female restroom two or three times a day for long periods. When she was finished, she would leave water all over the floor, creating a hazard for others. Other participants complained of the client's lengthy uses of the bathroom as well as the "mess" she left behind.
- The client refused to eat several meals. Because the program served the most substantial meal of the day for its participants, her nutritional status was of increasing concern.

A nurse from the program was assigned to help create a culturally specific support plan to address these issues and try to stabilize the client in the community. The nurse sought assistance from a trained female interpreter and a Muslim elder in the community. Together, this group worked with the client and health care staff to reach the following conclusions:

- The client's crisis point occurred during Ramadan, when Muslims are required to fast from sunrise to sunset. While the client was at the center, the program served food during lunch and dinner hours only. These were periods when the client could ingest nothing but water. Because she had no money, the client had nothing at home to eat. Furthermore, because she was supposed to take medications with meals, she had stopped using them during Ramadan. The nurse found that this client had the same pattern of difficulty and rehospitalization during Ramadan since starting the program 3 years ago. The team created a plan for the client to take medications and eat meals after sunset and before sunrise. Staff members arranged to send food home with the client for meals.
- The client was using the restroom for ritual cleansing before prayer. Staff members assigned the client to a quiet place away from the bathroom for prayers. They instructed other participants to respect the client's privacy during this time. The nurse also asked the client to remove as much of the water overflow as possible so that it would no longer be a hazard.
- Meals that the client was refusing during times other than Ramadan contained pork. Thus, the team arranged to provide alternatives when pork was on the menu, and also for the client to assist in the kitchen with other participants. This decision helped to foster socialization by letting the client practice skills within a familiar context.
- Finally, the nurse designed educational opportunities for staff members and participants to learn about Somalia. Speakers originally from there came to the center to give presentations about their country of origin, which helped the client feel accepted and "at home." This Somali woman has not been rehospitalized at any time, including Ramadan, for the past 2 years. She regularly takes her psychotropic medications and is involved in the program.

Reflection and Critical Thinking

- How do you think cultural stereotyping influences the delivery of psychiatric care? Can you find evidence of stereotyping in the case? How might such problems have been prevented?
- What future issues could emerge in the care of this client?
- What role should health care providers assume when clients do not have supportive family or community?

▲

immediately or necessarily with the African American experience. More than 50% of black Americans live in the South. As a whole, they remain relatively poor, with approximately 25% at or below poverty level (U.S. Census Bureau, 2004a).

Religions, which vary, are an essential part of life for many black Americans. Whatever the denomination, the influence of the religious community, as well as of elders, is strong for black Americans born in the United States and those born in Caribbean-speaking islands (Drayton-Brooks & White, 2004;

Ohm, 2003). The latter group also may be more comfortable with a spiritual approach and use of rituals (McGoldrick & Giordano, 2005). Some Caribbean-born blacks may have remaining ties to voodoo.

Studies have shown that thriving black families and communities tend to be strength focused (Drayton-Brooks & White, 2004; Murry & Brody, 2004). Therefore, a successful intervention strategy may be to identify the strengths of the family or community and incorporate them into treatment planning.

Prevention and treatment practices may have roots in Africa. Treatment methods may not distinguish among mind, body, and spirit and include laying-on of hands and prayer. Psychosocial programming is particularly adaptable for black Americans. Communities tend to hold elders in high esteem because of their knowledge and wisdom (Figure 6.5). Death is referred to as "passing on" to another state and may be celebrated as such (Fernandez & Fernandez, 2005a).

Rates of mental illness appear to be similar to those of non-Hispanic whites; however, prevalence indicates significant differences. Black Americans are at increased risk for phobias; somatization; major depression; culture-bound syndromes such as *falling out* (sudden collapse sometimes preceded by dizziness) or *sleep paralysis* (inability to move while falling asleep or waking up); suicide (particularly among black men and those 10 to 14 years old); homelessness; incarceration; juvenile custody; foster care; and exposure to violence (OMHD, 2007b).

Many black Americans are uninsured, with nearly 21% using Medicaid (U.S. Census Bureau, 2004a). Nearly 60% of older black Americans fail to receive needed services, with only one third of clients with mental health issues receiving care (USDHHS, 2001b). They are more likely to go to emergency departments, family doctors, or alternative practitioners. They are overrepresented in publicly funded inpatient facilities and residential centers (USDHHS, 2001b).

In terms of evidence-based clinical treatment trials, few have been evaluated. Data show that black Americans respond favorably to treatment. Stereotyping in diagnosis results in having more blacks diagnosed with schizophrenia and fewer with affective disorders. Other ramifications are as follows:

* 27% of blacks compared with 44% of whites receive antidepressants.
* Fewer prescriptions of the newer SSRI medications (with fewer side effects) are given to blacks (USDHHS, 2001b).

As discussed in the section on ethnopharmacology, studies have shown that blacks are slow metabolizers. Despite this, they often are prescribed higher dosages of drugs and experience more severe side effects than do whites. This leads to noncompliance, with many clients stopping their medications because of their discomfort.

Native Americans

American Indian and Alaska Natives comprise approximately 0.7% of the U.S. population, representing more than 560 different tribes with federal recognition. (Many other tribes have not been officially recognized and continue to fight for this distinction.) Across these groups are more than 200 indigenous languages. Many AI/ANs continue to speak their native tongues when at home.

Most of these clients reside in the western United States, primarily in rural areas (42%), living on reservations or trust lands. The trend toward moving to urban and suburban areas has increased, so currently 50% of AI/ANs live in urban, suburban, or rural non-Indian lands (Zerger, 2004).

These clients are more than twice as likely to be unemployed as the general population; approximately 25% live in poverty. They are over-represented in high-needs populations, including those who are homeless, incarcerated, or residing in foster care; those with substance use disorders; and those who have been the victims of trauma (Zerger, 2004). Factors contributing to problems among AI/ANs, who experience the most severe health disparities of any U.S. group, include history, demographics, urbanization and housing problems, low income, unemployment, limited education, unsafe water, inadequate disposal facilities, proximity to toxic waste sites, discrimination, lack of or inadequate health care (particularly prevention and psychiatric), and government policies. All these elements combine to define a population at extremely high risk (Zerger, 2004).

Successful care of Native American families requires mutual understanding and knowledge between practitioner and client (Grandbois, 2005; Zerger, 2004). Without such an approach, poor diagnosis and one-sided assessment are unavoidable. Another consideration is the client's

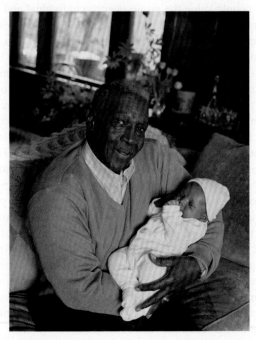

FIGURE 6.5 Many black communities hold high regard for their elders, respecting them for their life experience and knowledge.

particular tribe. All North American tribes do not share the same worldview.

Globally, adequate access to quality care is a challenge for indigenous populations (Marrone, 2007). AI/ANs have higher rates of high blood pressure, obesity, type 2 diabetes, cardiovascular disease, and cancer. Suicide rates among indigenous young adult men are 2 to 5 times that of the general population (Marrone, 2007). These chronic diseases and other factors (eg, smoking, poverty, living conditions) culminate in decreased lifespans and increased mortality rates.

Very little to no research has been documented regarding health service access for AI/ANs, including in the area of ethnopharmacology. Available information is primarily anecdotal and does not investigate causes or solutions. It also does not meet the criteria for evidence-based practice.

Several treaties gave the U.S. federal government primary responsibility for Native health care. The IHS has primary responsibility for IHS hospitals and clinics. Public Law 93-638 provides funding for tribal-run facilities and, more recently, some limited funds for the few Urban Indian programs that have been developed. Most of these services are on or near reservations in rural locations. Thus, only 20% of eligible recipients can access IHS programs (Zerger, 2004). Medicaid, Medicare, and private insurances are available to help with access to services when clients meet their qualifications. Access to services is further complicated by reluctance to participate, distrust of organizations (especially those that are government run), shortage of providers, and cultural and socioeconomic factors (Grandbois, 2005). Delays in access often lead clients to receive care from emergency departments, causing "log jams" in such departments that could have been avoided if more appropriate services were available or had been used.

Sensitivity to issues confronting Native people is paramount when developing culturally congruent services. Native American clients demonstrate a need for cultural maintenance or preservation when they express a desire to use traditional herbs or to participate in a sweat lodge or pipe ceremony to aid in healing. These people use oral tradition, exploration of dreams, and spirituality to express their beliefs (Figure 6.6). One study found that 70% of Native respondents in Washington State used traditional medicine such as smudging, herbs, and specialized healing ceremonies (Marrone, 2007). Health care providers who communicate sensitivity to, interest in, and even rudimentary knowledge about traditional healing practices are more likely to learn from clients about the full range of their health-related beliefs and behaviors. Conversely, clients are more likely to comply with an approach that allows them to preserve familiar practices. Because belief can play a major part in healing outcomes, it follows that effort should be made to support whatever clients believe will help—unless strong evidence shows that a practice is harmful (O'Connor, 1995).

Clients may be suspicious of the role of service providers (eg, social workers, police) out of fear (based on historical fact) that children will be removed. Majority health

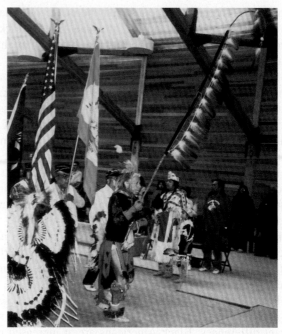

FIGURE 6.6 Native American clients may use traditions and spirituality, including use of regalia and dances, to express their beliefs.

care providers symbolize oppression, power, and invalidation of traditional beliefs (United Way of Minneapolis Area and Gray Hill, 1994). Having one's experience discredited or made to seem unimportant is painful. The key to involvement with AI/ANs is understanding the role of extended families (which may include friends and neighbors), respect for elders, and community responsibility for children's safety. Native people value the group over the individual and focus on harmony with nature. Thus, explanations for sickness and treatments should focus on balance and its restoration.

No discussion of Native people and their mental health issues is complete without examining the effects of historical trauma. **Historical trauma** is defined as "a constellation of symptoms that occur as a result of cumulative emotional and psychological trauma, which is transmitted across the life span of generations as a result of colonization and genocide" (Yellow Horse Brave Heart, 2003). The key ideas in this definition are *across the lifespan* and *generational*. This trauma results from government policies focused on the colonization and elimination of Native people and directly relates to health. Some related issues include the forced rapid shift from a cooperative clan-based society to a nuclear family-based system, the marginalization of native language, and the outlawing of spiritual practices. Assimilation was forced on the ancestors of AI/ANs in many ways, including the death of millions resulting from infectious European diseases and the destruction and loss of ability to use land. Other examples are as follows:

- *Illness/murder:* forcing relocations and moves to reservations; withholding food; disallowing traditional means of survival (hunting, fishing, gathering); generating disease without treatment; imprisoning resistors

- *Boarding schools:* kidnapping; personal humiliation; renaming; blocking familiar clan contact; abuse; survivor syndrome; failure to fit; intergenerational breakdown of family bond
- *Urbanization relocation:* lack of promised jobs, housing, and financial support; failure to fit upon returning to the reservation
- *Terminations and allotments:* land signed over without consent; termination of tribal rights; internal conflicts; destroyed land base
- *Genealogy-Dawes Act of 1887:* identification by blood quantum (Struthers & Lowe, 2003)

Historical trauma directly links past atrocities with unresolved grief for entire generations. It has devastating physical and mental effects, including tuberculosis, culture loss, alcoholism, drug dependency, diabetes, overeating, suicide, and abuse. Traditional spiritual resources are being used to assist communities to begin discussing their collective past and moving toward recovery. Struthers and Lowe (2003) use a talking circle to help people deal with these issues. Extensive research regarding historical trauma is needed. To date, Native Americans are just beginning to explore their experiences with historical trauma.

Asian and Pacific Islanders

Many Asian Americans live in the western United States, although the population is significant across the entire country and is expected to double during the next 25 years. Immigration from China, India, the Philippines, Korea, Vietnam, and all of Southeast Asia has grown rapidly. Most Asian Americans were born outside the United States; however, most Pacific Islanders are not immigrants. These clients are the "descendants of the original inhabitants of land taken over by the United States" (USDHHS, 2001a).

Asian and Pacific Islanders include more than 43 different ethnic groups with various levels of language proficiency and education. They include Japanese Americans whose families were held in U.S. internment camps during World War II and those displaced by war in their homelands (eg, Korea, Laos). Poverty rates range from 6% among Filipino Americans to 64% among Hmong Americans. Thus, nurses must assess clients carefully to discern their particular circumstances, influences, and cultural expectations.

Subjective evidence indicates that Asian and Pacific Islander clients tend to endure distress for long periods before seeking mental health services. However, epidemiologic studies have included few Asian Americans, Pacific Islanders, and people with limited English proficiency (USDHHS, 2001a). When Asian and Pacific Islander clients finally enter the service delivery system, their health tends to be poorer, with more severe or chronic problems (Cultural Spotlight 6.1). Language barriers and problems accessing culturally congruent services pose challenges related to

---

Cultural *Spotlight* 6.1

Post-Traumatic Stress Disorder and Culture-Bound Syndromes Among Asian Groups

Southeast Asian refugees disproportionately experience higher levels of depressive symptoms, somatic complaints, and PTSD. This diagnostic "label" also is found in other dislocated ethnic groups (eg, Somalis). However, many states exclude PTSD as a serious mental illness, blocking access of affected clients to the public service system. These factors contribute to the likelihood that Southeast Asian refugees will come to the attention of the mental health system only during acute stress or crisis.

In addition to PTSD, nurses should be familiar with the following culture-bound syndromes common to some Asian populations:

- *Neurasthenia:* characterized by fatigue, weakness, poor concentration, memory loss, irritability, aches and pains, and sleep disturbances
- *Hwa-byung* (suppressed anger syndrome): characterized by constriction in the chest, palpitations, flushing, headache, dysphoria, anxiety, and poor concentration (USDHHS, 2001a)

---

shame and stigma. Some of these clients may mistakenly believe that enrollment in Medicaid may jeopardize their citizenship, contributing to a reluctance to access services.

When working with Asian/Pacific Islander families, recognizing the role of the father is important. These men historically have had total authority over family decisions. Acculturation of the family has led to generational differences as children (and in some cases wives) assume Western roles and expectations. Acknowledging vital family resources is essential. Use of a cultural consultant may be necessary. However, nurses must take care to remember the diversity within this group (both group to group and generational) to limit misunderstandings. Not all Asian/Pacific Islander clients are refugees, although most specialized services focus on this segment of the population (Tseng, 2004).

Some clients believe that health is a state of spiritual and physical harmony with nature, and that illnesses are an imbalance between *yin* and *yang* (hot and cold). They believe that their body is not their own property and therefore must be taken care of (balanced). Asians may tend not to complain. Nurses must be ready to read other signs, such as untouched food or withdrawal, to discern the status of these clients. Clients may consult herbalists and acupuncturists (Figure 6.7). Asian Americans and Pacific Islanders tend to use alternative medications at a higher rate than do other groups. Families respect therapists as authority figures who give concrete, realistic advice. They expect nurses to develop a personal human relationship before giving advice (McGoldrick & Giordano, 2005).

Few studies have examined the response of Asian Americans to treatment. Higher dropout rates and lower satisfaction with care have been reported. Both can be mitigated by

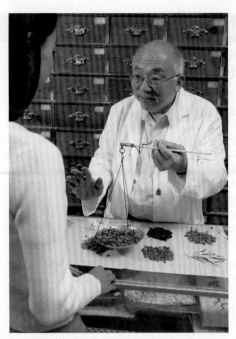

FIGURE 6.7 Use of alternative treatments such as herbal remedies may be more common among Asian American and Pacific Islander clients.

employing ethnically matched health care providers (Trujillo, 2008). Ethnopharmacologic studies have shown Asians to be slow metabolizers and therefore in need of lower doses of medications than are people of other races and ethnicities.

Middle Eastern Clients

The Middle Eastern community consists of 22 countries spanning the Middle East and North Africa. Iranians, Afghans, Saudi Arabians, and other Middle Easterners tend to view the heart as the seat of all emotions. They describe problems as heart distress, weak or tired nerves, general body pain or exhaustion, or upper gastric pain and discomfort. Usually they discuss these problems with same-sex and same-age friends whom they swear to secrecy (McGoldrick & Giordano, 2005). Privacy is very important, especially for Saudi Arabians.

Various religions are practiced throughout the Middle East. Many Arab Christians live in Lebanon, Palestine, Iraq, and Egypt. However, Islam is the dominant religion and greatly influences the view that Allah controls everything according to his will. Ramadan is a month in the Islam calendar that requires fasting during the day. Muslims tend to be conservative and do not eat pork or drink alcohol. A healthy diet and good hygiene are of primary importance.

Practitioners of Islam consider it impolite to point, signal a person with the hand, or use the left hand to gesture. They use the right hand to pass objects. In some cases, they use both hands, but never the left hand alone. Insults include pointing the bottom of the foot at another person and crossing one ankle over the knee. Most Middle Eastern men do not shake hands with or touch women in public. If the woman is

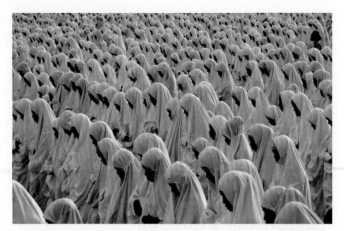

FIGURE 6.8 Islam is an influential element in Middle Eastern culture. For religious Muslims, prayer and ritual play important roles in their daily lives.

wearing a veil, it is not expected that she will be introduced. Middle Easterners may use amulets for protection or burn incense to avoid illness and harm. Saying prayers five times a day is very important to Muslims (Fernandez & Fernandez, 2005b) (Figure 6.8).

Arab clients tend not to wait to seek help for illness and expect relief immediately. They may not continue treatment after symptoms improve. Trust and confidence are important to establish before moving into a relationship. Those of Middle Eastern descent may be very conscious of personal and family honor. They can be offended easily by perceived insults to that honor. Additional common cultural traits are piety and stoicism. Health care providers need to focus on quick results and tangible assistance to be viewed positively (eg, offering vitamins, prescriptions, and quick interventions) (McGoldrick & Giordano, 2005). Other positive interventions include honoring the family by providing an environment where they feel understood. Relatives and close friends are a significant part of their support system.

Except during gynecologic examinations, both men and women prefer male health care providers and family members to stay with clients during a session. This culture reveres its elders for their experience. Death is considered to be a destiny decided by Allah (Fernandez & Fernandez, 2005b).

Eastern Europeans

The countries found in Eastern Europe reflect incredible diversity and differences. Racially, they usually consistently identify as white. Other commonalities include the shared experience of life under Communist rule and that most of their populations grew up in industrialized societies. Identification of immigrants from these countries as white and industrialized makes their adaptation to the United States easier than for some other groups.

Following the fall of the Soviet Union in 1991, many countries of the Eastern Bloc reverted to their original states. For example, Yugoslavia divided into separate nations, including Bosnia, Croatia, and Serbia. Historically, Bosnians,

Serbs, and Croats descend from Slavic tribes that arrived in the Balkans from 500 to 600 AD. This region has been conquered many times and absorbed into many different empires, for example, Byzantine, Roman, Austro-Hungarian, Ottoman (Snyder et al., 2005). Dissolution of the Soviet Union enabled old conflicts that had been controlled under Soviet rule to again fester. Civil war and "ethnic cleansing" (eg, by the Serbian military against Bosnian Muslims) included such atrocities as mass murders and rapes. A recent study of Muslim war refugees from Kosovo and Bosnia indicated that the use of private prayer was an important method of coping (Ai et al., 2005). Many older Bosnians believe that they will be able to return someday to their native land because they are still land owners. Others lost everything, had to leave Bosnia, and have started over with nothing (the Bosnian retirement age is 55 years). War trauma has led to PTSD and culture shock for many of these people (Snyder et al., 2005).

Overall, formal religion is not a strong influence in Eastern Europe. Religion and language divide Bosnians. Although Serbo-Croatia is their traditional language, some of these immigrants speak German or English. Serbo-Croatian is similar to English in terms of alphabet and syntax, facilitating the transfer of language skills. In addition, Islam is the predominant religion of Bosnia. Islam in Eastern Europe is less strict than in some other areas, but it still influences health practices (see earlier discussion on Middle Eastern people) (Guilford Center, 2006). Serbs have the predominant religion of Orthodox Christianity and speak Serbian. Croats predominantly follow Catholicism and speak Croatian. Albanians are largely Muslim, with some people identifying as Catholic or Orthodox or evangelical Christian. Many Russians belong to the Russian Orthodox Church or are Jewish. Although some Russians learned English in school, the predominant language is Russian.

Class status may be less important than level of education for Eastern European immigrants. Education can often be a source of stress because many of these people worked hard for degrees in their native lands only to come to the United States where those degrees might not be recognized as legitimate (Guilford Center, 2006).

Many Eastern European immigrants live in nuclear families with closely knit family ties. Two to three generations might live together in one household. It is generally undesirable for women older than 25 years to remain unmarried. Marriage gives women social status; their careers are considered less important than men's (Guilford Center, 2006).

Health care in the former Soviet Union and Eastern Bloc nations was socialized (free) and emphasized prevention, factors that can make the U.S. health care system especially confusing and challenging for these clients (Figure 6.9). Although some tests were unavailable and care was provided under poor conditions in Eastern Europe, the inaccessibility of U.S. health care is a disappointment to them. In Eastern Europe, there were no insurance plans to deal with,

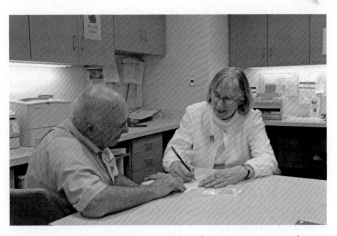

FIGURE 6.9 Clients from countries that once were under Communist rule may have difficulty navigating the U.S. health care system. Nurses can play an important role in providing explanations and helping clients understand differences.

care was accessible, and medications were given out in small doses (Grabbe, 2000).

Common psychiatric issues among Eastern European immigrants include PTSD, depression, obsessive-compulsive disorder, schizophrenia, and dementia. A study comparing British and Russian attitudes toward mental illnesses found that Russians were unlikely to identify dementia as a mental illness, preferring informal services as treatment (Shulman & Adams, 2002). Other treatment preferences include psychosocial rehabilitation, case management, psychoeducation, normalization, and, in some cases, cognitive–behavioral therapy. Nurses can play a huge role in "keeping it real," teaching coping skills, discussing disturbing thoughts, identifying trauma triggers, teaching cognitive strategies that connect the thoughts to feelings, and making home visits.

During home visits, nurses should remember to remove their shoes as a sign of respect. In addition, families may offer a nurse a strong cup of coffee; drinking it will be appreciated by the family and can help the relationship between the nurse and family members. Sensitivity to body language and speech tone is essential. Restoration to psychological health and dignity, establishment of a positive self-image, and development of a positive network of supportive services are essential to assisting Eastern European refugees to establish a solid foothold (Snyder et al., 2005).

Alcohol is a real problem aggravated by social traditions, culture shock, and PTSD. Many Eastern European immigrants use alcohol as a coping mechanism. Culturally appropriate services that include interpreters or culture guides are needed to address this issue. Other substance use issues are nicotine and caffeine addiction, as well as medication abuse. These clients with substance use disorders generally do not seek treatment early. In many cases, these disorders are not identified until the client needs hospitalization or family members or an employer intervenes (Shulman & Adams, 2002).

Certain culture-bound illnesses are unique. An example is intracranial hypertension, characterized by a large head circumference and bulging fontanels. Children with this condition are irritable and have problems in school. Causes of illness are thought to be naturalistic and are explained in impersonal, systemic terms (eg, cold drinks cause sore throats; clean air and rest are essential to health) (Grabbe, 2000). Superstitions and magical curing (znakharstvo) are also prevalent. Folk medicines and home remedies, including the use of vodka, are believed to have many advantages. Furthermore, it is important that nurses recognize the differences in the various countries that comprised the former Soviet Union. It is important to be respectful of each client's unique experiences.

> ### Checkpoint Questions
> **5.** What is a common problem associated with mental illness and treatment in African American clients?
> **6.** When working with Asian/Pacific Islander families, which family member's role is especially important to consider?
> **7.** What are two traits common to the Middle Eastern culture?

CULTURALLY COMPETENT AND CONGRUENT NURSING CARE

Nurses in mental health care settings are critical to the promotion and practice of culturally congruent care. Given that there are hundreds of different cultures, innumerable additional categories of diversity, and as many ways to interpret human experience as there are people, nurses must be reasonable about what they expect to know. Understanding everything about cultural beliefs and health care is impossible. Nevertheless, it is possible to develop and communicate attitudes that express sincere interest, willingness to learn, and respect for other viewpoints.

To provide culturally congruent care, nurses must possess knowledge about cultural illnesses and healing practices and intercultural communication skills. They must develop self-awareness, flexibility, and working relationships that cross the lines of difference. They must become aware of their own cultural heritage and anticipate the culture shock of working outside their comfort zone (Koskinen & Tossavainen, 2004). In face-to-face intercultural exposure, stereotyping is less likely (Campinha-Bacote, 2007b). Findings from a study of Finnish nurses who were required to study abroad identified three ethnocategories:

- Transition from one culture to another
- Adjustment to the difference
- Gain of intercultural sensitivity

Further, it was found that a period for "reentry debriefing" was important. The program also emphasized the exploration of the individual's own cultural beliefs (as do many authors), the importance of face-to-face encounters, and assessment

of the other country's health care system (Koskinen & Tossavainen, 2004).

Providers who are not **culture bound** (limited by the parameters of their own culture) are more likely to have a broader worldview and work with clients in a nonjudgmental, accepting way (Wilson, 2010). Nurses also must learn what clients and their families identify as "normal" and "abnormal" within the cultural context. Such identification applies not only to defining health problems, but also to outlining expectations for care, cure, or both. In this context, the client's culture and subcultures influence the expression, presentation, recognition, labeling, explanations for, and distribution of mental illness.

When assessing and intervening with ethnic minorities, nurses must consider the following (Giger & Davidhizar, 2008):

- Communication, including written and oral language, gestures, facial expressions, and body language
- Personal space, including both the space itself and the items sharing the designated space
- Social organization, including patterns of behavior during life events, such as births, puberty, childbearing, illness, and death
- Time, both concrete and abstract
- Environment, including perceptions regarding control of the environment
- Biologic variations among racial groups

However, holistic care recognizes and incorporates family care with religious values and cultural beliefs (Leininger & McFarland, 2002; Wilson, 2010). When determining a client's explanation for illness, nurses must listen carefully to the client's story. Several factors, including spiritual beliefs, cultural values, and food preference, are closely related to the healing process.

Within a transcultural focus, nurses think "about differences and similarities among people and their beliefs, practices, and life ways" while learning to "value understanding people regarding their special needs and concerns" (Leininger & McFarland, 2002). Thus, nurses develop different culturally appropriate ways to help by assessing each client's particular cultural orientation. By doing so, they learn from clients how best to provide sensitive, compassionate, and competent care (Box 6.3).

Essential Skills

The nursing profession is rooted in a sense of caring. Nurses are expected to possess the personal characteristics of genuineness, empathy, warmth, and objectivity. As nurses develop a transcultural focus, they learn to incorporate additional skills in care delivery. Four critical skills that nurses must acquire to provide culturally competent care are as follows (Battaglia, 1992):

1. *Cross-cultural understanding* means knowledge about how and why people of different cultures behave in

> **BOX 6.3** Treatment Strategies for Cultural Competence in Mental Health care Delivery
>
> - Determine your own cultural heritage and behavior patterns.
> - Recognize coexisting belief systems about mental health and illness.
> - Assess client's personal beliefs, concerns, and fears about the illness.
> - Assess and consider family history and search for generational patterns.
> - Explain, negotiate, and, when indicated, collaborate on a treatment plan that considers the client's cultural beliefs. Discuss the client's expectations of the treatment regimen. Preserve helpful beliefs or repattern acknowledged harmful beliefs or practices.
> - Recognize informal caregivers as allies in the treatment process.
> - Read documented information about specific cultural groups.
> - Determine if the client is seeking Western health care in conjunction with, or exclusive of, any personal cultural beliefs about mental illness.
> - Collaborate with key informants and others who are adept at interpreting meanings of language and behaviors of specific cultures.
> - Demonstrate patience, a nonjudgmental attitude, and genuine respect for the client no matter what behavior he or she exhibits.

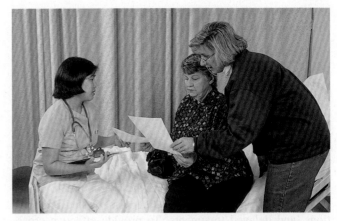

FIGURE 6.10 Interpreters may sometimes be necessary to explain and communicate information to clients whose primary language differs from that of health care providers. (Photo © B. Proud.)

certain ways. For nurses to develop cross-cultural understanding, they might study the relevant culture or identify a colleague from that culture and learn about the culture's values, norms, and mores. However, nurses should not use this strategy in isolation. Doing so may cause them to begin to overgeneralize that they should treat all members of a specific group exactly the same.

2. *Intercultural communication* is essential because communication is at the center of cross-cultural psychiatric–mental health nursing. Some differences in communication are readily apparent; others are harder to discern, such as degree of openness, self-disclosure, emotional expression, insight, and even talkativeness. Intercultural communication requires nurses to develop listening skills, including learning to decipher nonverbal behavior and detect barriers that interfere with communication. Psychiatric–mental health nurses should excel in this area; any unidentified intrapersonal stereotypes and biases would hinder their communicative skills. If a nurse recognizes that he or she has a different communication style than a client, the nurse should spend additional time with that client to improve understanding and ensure culturally competent care. If a nurse speaks a different language than the client, he or she should design strategies to minimize problems during interviews. The nurse and client may need an interpreter to communicate effectively (Figure 6.10).

3. *Facilitation skills* focus primarily on conflict resolution and the ability to negotiate interactions potentially inconsistent with the value and belief system of a client or family from a culture that differs from that of the nurse.

4. *Flexibility* means the ability to embrace change by modifying expectations, readjusting old operating norms and stereotypes, and trying new behavior (see Chap. 13).

> **Think About It 6.2**
> Consider the 60-year-old Hispanic American woman described in Think About It 6.1. How would the nurse use the four critical skills of cross-cultural understanding, intercultural communication, facilitation, and flexibility to provide culturally competent care?

Phases of Transcultural Nursing Knowledge

Leininger and McFarland (2002) describe three phases in the development of transcultural nursing knowledge:

1. *Phase I*—Becoming aware of and sensitive to culture care differences and similarities (cultural awareness)
2. *Phase II*—Using theories to discover and explain transcultural nursing phenomena (use of theories to guide research and explain)
3. *Phase III*—Using transcultural research findings to improve care of people (use of knowledge in practice for congruent care)

Transcultural Assessment

To determine the factors that influence a client's basic beliefs about illness and wellness, nurses must ensure that the assessment is transculturally focused. Data from the transcultural assessment can help nurses to identify cultural factors pertinent to the client's health, ranging from views on religion to folk medicine. Basic beliefs of clients about health and disease vary greatly among cultures in relation to the following (McGoldrick & Giordano, 2005):

- The experience of pain
- What a culture labels as a symptom
- How people communicate pain or symptoms
- Beliefs about the cause of pain or symptoms
- Attitudes toward helpers (doctors and hospitals)
- Desired or expected treatment

Although some providers believe that assessing a person's cultural perception is too costly and time consuming, when this assessment is not done, the cost is much greater in terms of misperceptions, misdiagnosis, wasted interventions, and delayed treatments. To provide effective cross-cultural services, nurses should ask the following questions, developed by Dr. Arthur Kleinman of Harvard, to elicit the client's explanation of the illness (Fadiman, 1998):

- What is the problem?
- What do you think has caused the problem?
- Why do you think it started when it did?
- What do you think the sickness does? How does it work?
- How severe is the sickness? Will it have a short or long course?
- What kind of treatment do you think the client should receive? What are the most important results you hope he or she receives from this treatment?
- What are the chief problems the sickness has caused?
- What do you fear most about the sickness?

Building Cultural Awareness

Nursing's unique advantage is the opportunity to help clients tell their stories while receiving care. Leininger and McFarland (2002) describe a conceptual picture of the components of cultural care that can help nurses understand the multiple factors influencing an effective transcultural interaction:

- Attend to gender differences, communication modes (eg, stories, use of silence), special language terms, interpersonal relationships, and use of space and food.
- Show genuine interest in the client while maintaining a learning and respectful attitude.
- Keep alert to whatever the client shares about cultural care values, religion, and kinship relationships.
- Discover and remain aware of your own cultural biases and prejudices.
- Be aware of subcultures or special groups to which the client may belong (eg, homeless, gay).
- Know the strengths, variabilities, and assets of your own culture.
- Clarify that the purpose is to focus on helping the client.
- Maintain a holistic view of the client's world and environmental context.

While hearing the stories of clients, nurses maintain the role of active listener and keep interventions focused on the client's constructs for health and wellness. Encouraging

expressions of culture is important, particularly in the areas of dress and adornment, eating rituals and foods, care activities, sleep rituals, and healing rituals wherever these can be compatible and therapeutic. When nurses display an empathetic and caring attitude, remain flexible, and listen, they are participating in culturally competent care.

Cultural Self-Awareness

Some authors have defined the final stage of human development as coming to terms with one's own cultural identity. Using a cultural lens to look inward, nurses can better understand the values associated with belonging to a group and identify with others. The realization of multiple perspectives becomes a reality. A multicultural approach may cause nurses to question formerly held "truths" about health care delivery. Nurses must first identify their own "baggage" to then discard it or set it aside. This struggle is essential for awareness and elimination of biases, stereotypes, and prejudices. Health care providers should learn to change perspectives and view situations based on a specific ethnic or cultural group to modify interventions in ways that are culturally compatible. In this way, providers can "walk in the shoes of others without tripping. They can see the world through many cultural perspectives. Each of us lives in a cultural bubble; a multiculturalist can enter another cultural bubble without bursting it" (United States Psychosocial Association, 2007).

Most current mental health treatment modalities have evolved from a Western mind-set. The emphasis on technology and distancing often is incompatible with the traditional beliefs of many cultures. Nurses must examine the belief system of their own culture to ascertain if there is compatibility between their worldview and the client's worldview. Flexibility and adaptability are crucial to accepting this challenge.

> **Checkpoint Questions**
> 8. What are the three phases in Leininger's development of transcultural nursing knowledge?
> 9. What are six areas in which basic beliefs of clients about health and disease vary greatly among cultures?
> 10. Why should nurses examine the belief system of their own culture?

EVIDENCE-BASED PRACTICE

To date, very few studies related to culture rise to meet the standards of evidence-based practice. Many research projects have been important and illuminating, but findings generally have been anecdotal. However, a recent research project focusing on children examines the advantages and disadvantages of implementing an evidence-based parenting model in community settings in large multicultural North American cities. Outcomes from this study may be illustrative for health care providers who work with diverse families (Stern et al., 2007).

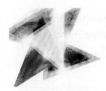

Reviewing and Applying Your Knowledge

Chapter Summary

- Culture is a main ingredient of personality.

- The more stress a person experiences, the greater the manifestation of his or her culturally based perceptions, beliefs, and behaviors.

- Self-knowledge facilitates personal comfort and understanding of others when caring for culturally diverse clients in a variety of psychiatric–mental health settings.

- To provide effective, individualized mental health services, nurses must view consumers through a cultural lens that includes the context of their cultural group and their individual experiences from being a part of that group.

- Nursing staff development programs are beneficial to improve outcomes of care for culturally diverse psychiatric clients.

- Although diverse cultural groups may have various responses with respect to the evaluation and treatment of mental illness, culturally competent care is maximized by the nurse's open, honest, and accepting attitude.

- Recognition of generational patterns within one's own culture can assist the nurse to assess and recognize generational patterns in other cultures.

- Specific stressors, including war, trauma, violence, migration patterns, economic status, racism, discrimination, cultural values and beliefs, and survival tactics, need to be addressed in providing mental health services.

- The nurse can ascertain how the aforementioned factors relate to the individual and his or her perception of mental health.

- Nurses' self-knowledge, viewing position, and preparation as culturally competent providers greatly affect the care of diverse clients.

Study Questions

1. During an interview, a client of Polish heritage states, "My ancestors used to speak Polish in the house all the time, but then everybody learned to speak English." The nurse would interpret this as indicative of which of the following?

   a. Flexibility

   b. Culture

   c. Assimilation

   d. Cultural competence

2. When developing a plan to promote the use of mental health services by minority groups in a community, which of the following would be most important for the nurse to address?

   a. Similarities in religious beliefs

   b. Use of traditional healers

   c. Equality in access to housing

   d. Consistent interpretation of behavior

3. A group of nursing students is assigned to lead a discussion group comparing approaches to mental health services between black and white Americans. Which of the following statements about black Americans would be most accurate for students to include?

   a. Clients typically engage mental health services at an earlier stage.

   b. They commonly use more treatment services at earlier stages.

   c. There is a significantly higher rate of use for continuing services.

   d. Mental health practitioners frequently misdiagnose these clients.

4. To provide culturally competent care, which of the following would the nurse consider incorporating into the plan of care for a Native American client?

   a. Participation in a sweat lodge ceremony

   b. Influence of hot-and-cold imbalances

   c. Knowledge of increased incidence of PTSD

   d. Balance of good and evil

5. The nurse is explaining cross-cultural understanding to a group of students. Which of the following descriptions would be most appropriate to include?

   a. Conflict resolution with the ability to negotiate

   b. Listening skills with learning how to decipher nonverbal behavior

   c. Ability to embrace change by modifying expectations

   d. Knowledge about how and why people of different cultures behave

(continues on page 114)

Critical Thinking Questions

1. What roles might be culturally defined for family members? How can such roles hinder or facilitate a client's mental health treatment?

2. How do your own experiences affect your thoughts and feelings toward clients with a cultural frame of reference that differs from your own?

References

Ai, A. L., Tice, T. N., Huang, B., & Ishrsaka, A. (2005). Wartime faith-based reactions among traumatized Kosovar and Bosnian refugees in the United States. *Mental Health, Religion and Culture, 8*(4), 291–308.

American Psychiatric Association. (n.d.). Ask a psychiatrist: An APA expert answers common questions about the mental health of American Indian and Alaska Natives. Retrieved from http://healthyminds.org/expertopinion06.cfm

American Psychiatric Association. (2000). *Diagnostic and statistical manual of mental disorders* (4th ed., text rev.). Washington, DC: Author.

Ard, J. D., Durant, R. W., Edwards, L. C., & Svetkey, L. P. (2005). Perceptions of African-American culture and implications for clinical trial design. *Ethnicity and Disease, 15*(2), 292–299.

Battaglia, B. (1992). Skills for managing multicultural teams. *Cultural Diversity at Work, 4*(3), 4.

Betancourt, J. R., Green, A. R., Carrillo, J. E., & Ananeh-Firempong, O. (2003). Defining cultural competence: A practical framework for addressing racial/ethnic disparities in health and health care. *Public Health Report, 118*(4), 293–302.

Burnes Bolton, L., Giger, J. N., & Georges, C. A. (2004). Structural and racial barriers to health care. *Annual Review of Nursing Research, 22,* 39–58.

Burroughs, V. J., Maxey, R. W., & Levy, R. A. (2002). Racial and ethnic differences in response to medicines: Towards individualized pharmaceutical treatment. *Journal of the National Medical Association, 94*(10), 1–26.

Campinha-Bacote, J. (2007a). Becoming culturally competent in ethnic psychopharmacology. *Journal of Psychosocial Nursing, 45,* 26–33.

Campinha-Bacote, J. (2007b). *The process of cultural competence in the delivery of healthcare services. A culturally competent model of care* (5th ed.). Cincinnati, OH: Transcultural CARE Association.

Chelali, C. (2007). *Health in the Andes.* Retrieved from http://www.Americas.oas.org

Dey, A. N., & Lucas, J. W. (2006). Physical and mental health characteristics of U.S.- and foreign-born adults: United States, 1998–2003. *Advanced Data, 369,* 1–19.

Drayton-Brooks, S., & White, N. (2004). Health promoting behaviors among African American women with faith-based support. *ABNF Journal, 15*(5), 84–90.

Ezenwa, M. O., Ameringer, S., Ward, S. E., & Serlin, R. C. (2006). Racial and ethnic disparities in pain management in the United States. *Journal of Nursing Scholarship, 39*(1), 225–233.

Fadiman, A. (1998). *The spirit catches you and you fall down: A Hmong child, her American doctors, and the collision of two cultures.* New York, NY: Noonday.

Fadiman, A. (2003). *The spirit catches you and you fall down: Updates.* Retrieved from http://www.spiritcatchesyou.com/update

Fernandez, V. M., & Fernandez, K. M. (2005a). *Transcultural nursing: The Black-American community.* Retrieved from http://culturediversity.org/afro.htm

Fernandez, V. M., & Fernandez, K. M. (2005b). *Transcultural nursing: The Middle Eastern community.* Retrieved from http://culture-diversity.org/mide.htm

Franks, P., Fiscella, K., & Meldrum, S. (2005). Racial disparities in the content of primary care office visits. *Journal of General Internal Medicine, 20*(7), 599–603.

Giger, J., & Davidhizar, R. (2008). *Transcultural nursing: Assessment and intervention* (5th ed.). St. Louis, MO: Mosby.

Grabbe, L. (2000). Understanding patients from the Soviet Union. *Family Medicine, 32*(3), 201–206.

Grandbois, D. (2005). Stigma of mental illness among American Indian and Alaska Native nations: Historical and contemporary perspectives. *Issues in Mental Health Nursing, 26*(10), 1001–1024.

Guilford Center. (2006). *Kaleidoscope: Tips for working with Eastern Europeans.* Retrieved from http://www.guilfordcenter.com/resources/kaleidoscope/18_e_europeans.pdf

Hofstede, G., & Hofstede, G. J. (2004). *Cultures and organizations: Software of the mind* (2nd ed.). New York, NY: McGraw-Hill.

Institute of Medicine (2004). Health literacy: A prescription to end confusion. Washington, DC: National Academy of Sciences.

Jamil, H., Nassar-McMillan, S. C., & Lambert, R. G. (2007). Immigration and attendant psychological sequelae: A comparison of three waves of Iraqi immigrants. *American Journal of Orthopsychiatry, 77*(2), 199–205.

Koskinen, L., & Tossavainen, K. (2004). Study abroad as a process of learning intercultural competence in nursing. *International Journal of Nursing Practice, 10,* 111–120.

Leininger, M., & McFarland, M. R. (2002). *Transcultural nursing concepts, theories, research & practice* (3rd ed.). New York, NY: McGraw-Hill Medical.

Lin, S. X., & Larson, E. (2005). Does provision of health counseling differ by patient race? *Family Medicine, 37*(9), 650–654.

Lopez, R. A. (2005). Use of alternative folk medicine by Mexican American women. *Journal of Immigrant Health, 7*(1), 23–31.

Mahoney, J. S., Carlson, E., & Engelbretson, J. (2006). A framework for cultural competence in advanced practice psychiatric and mental health education. *Perspectives in Psychiatric Care, 42*(4), 227–237.

Markova, T., & Broome, B. (2007). Effective communication and delivery of culturally competent health care. *Urologic Nursing, 27*(3), 239–242.

Marrone, S. (2007). Understanding barriers to health care: A review of disparities in health care services among indigenous populations. *International Journal of Circumpolar Health, 66*(3), 188–198.

Marshall, G. N., Schell, T. L., Elliott, M. N., Berthold, S. M., & Chun, C. A. (2005). Mental health of Cambodian refugees 2 decades after resettlement in the United States. *Journal of the American Medical Association, 294*(5), 571–579.

Mays, V. M., Cochran, S. D., & Barnes, N. W. (2007). Race, race-based discrimination, and health outcomes among African Americans. *Annual Review in Psychology, 58,* 24.1–24.25.

McGoldrick, M., & Giordano, J. (2005). *Ethnicity and family therapy* (3rd ed.). New York, NY: Guilford Press.

Mental Health Services Oversight and Accountability Commission. (2007). *Cultural and Linguistic Competence Resource Group (CLCTRG) draft workplan.* Washington, DC: Author.

Mezzich, J. E., Caracci, F., Fabrega, H., & Kirmayer, L. J. (2009). Cultural formulation guidelines. *Transcultural Psychiatry, 46,* 383–405.

Murry, V. M., & Brody, G. H. (2004). Partnering with community stakeholders: Engaging rural African American families in basic research and the Strong African American Families Preventive Intervention Program. *Journal of Marital and Family Therapy, 30*(3), 271–283.

O'Connor, B. B. (1995). *Healing traditions: Alternative medicine and the health professions.* Philadelphia, PA: University of Pennsylvania Press.

Office of Minority Health and Health Disparities, Centers for Disease Control and Prevention (OMHD). (2007a). *Eliminate disparities in infant mortality.* Retrieved from http://www.cdc.gov/omhd/AMH/factsheets/infant.htm

Office of Minority Health and Health Disparities, Centers for Disease Control and Prevention (OMHD). (2007b). *Eliminating racial and ethnic health disparities.* Retrieved from http://www.cdc.gov/omh/AboutUs/disparities.htm.

Ohm, R. (2003). The African American experience in the Islamic faith. *Public Health Nursing, 20*(6), 478–486.

Purnell, L. (2002). The Purnell model for cultural competence. *Journal of Transcultural Nursing, 13*(3), 193–196.

Purnell, L. D., & Paulanka, B. J. (2008). *Transcultural health care: A culturally competent approach* (3rd ed.). Philadelphia, PA: F. A. Davis Company.

Ratogi, S., Johnson, T. D., Hoeffel, E. M., & Drewery, M. P. (2011). The black population: 2010. Retrieved from http://www.census.gov/prod/cen2010/briefs/c2010br-06.pdf

Robertson, C. L., Halcon, L., Savik, K., Johnson, D., Spring, M., Butcher, J., … Jaranson, J. (2006). Somali and Oromo refugee women: Trauma and associated factors. *Journal of Advanced Nursing, 56*(6), 577–587.

Schyve, P. (2007). Language differences as a barrier to quality and safety in health care: The Joint Commission perspective. *Journal of General Internal Medicine, 22*(S2), 360–361.

Shulman, N., & Adams, B. (2002). A comparison of Russian and British attitudes towards mental health problems in the community. *International Journal of Social Psychiatry, 48*(4), 226–278.

Singleton, D., & Krause, E. M. S. (2009). Understanding cultural and linguistic barriers to health literacy. *Online Journal of Issues in Nursing,14*(3). Retrieved from http://web.ebscohost.com/ehost/detail?vid=3&hid=112&sid=ee56b191-76a0-493e-94ce-54b2df79e394%40sessionmgr110&bdata=JnNpdGU9ZWhvc3QtbGl2ZQ%3d%3d#db=rzh&AN=2010587440

Snyder, C. S., May, J. D., Zulcic, N. N., & Gabbard, W. J. (2005). Social work with Bosnian Muslim refugee children and families: A review of the literature. *Child Welfare League of America,* 607–630.

Stern, S., Alaggia, R., Watson, K., & Morton, T. (2007). Transporting evidence-based parenting program to multicultural prevention settings. Retrieved from http://sswr.confex.com/sswr/2007/techprogram/P7343.HTM

Struthers, R., & Lowe, J. (2003). Nursing in the Native American culture and historical trauma. *Issues in Mental Health Nursing, 24*(3), 257–272.

Substance Abuse and Mental Health Services Administration. (2004). Risk and protective factors for substance use among American Indian or Alaska Native youths. Retrieved from http://www.oas.samhsa.gov/

Sue, D. W., & Sue, D. (2008). *Counseling the culturally diverse: Theory and practice* (5th ed.). New York, NY: Wiley.

Szlemko, W. J., Wood, J. W., & Thurman, P. J. (2006). Native Americans and alcohol: Past, present, and future. *Journal of General Psychology, 133*(4), 435–451.

Tortumluoglu, G. (2006). The implications of transcultural nursing models in the provision of culturally competent care. *ICUS Nursing Journal, 25*(Jan–Apr), 1–11.

Trujillo, M. (2008). Multicultural aspects of mental health. *Primary Psychiatry, 15*(4), 65–71, 77–84.

Tseng, W. (2004). Culture and psychotherapy: Asian perspectives. *Journal of Mental Health, 13,* 151–161.

U.S. Census Bureau. (2004a). *Current population survey, annual social and economic supplement, 2004, racial statistics branch, population division.* Retrieved from http://www.census.gov/

U.S. Census Bureau. (2004b). *U.S. interim projections by age, sex, race, and Hispanic origin.* Retrieved from http://www.census.gov/

U.S. Census Bureau. (2005). *Facts for features: Hispanic Heritage Month.* Retrieved from http://www.census.gov/

U.S. Department of Health and Human Services (USDHHS). (2000). *Revised CLAS standards from the Office of Minority Health.* Retrieved from http://www.omhrc.gov/

U.S. Department of Health and Human Services (USDHHS). (2001a). *Mental health: Culture, race, and ethnicity—A supplement to* Mental health: A Report of the Surgeon General. Rockville, MD: Author.

U.S. Department of Health and Human Services (USDHHS). (2001b). *Mental health: Culture, race, and ethnicity fact sheets: African Americans.* Retrieved from http://mentalhealth.samhsa.gov/cre/fact1.asp

U.S. Department of Homeland Security. (2007). *2006 yearbook of immigration statistics.* Retrieved from http://www.dhs.gov/

United States Psychosocial Association. (2007). *Multicultural principles.* Linthicum, MD: Author.

Wilson, D. W. (2010). Culturally competent psychiatric nursing care. *Journal of Psychiatric and Mental Health Nursing, 17,* 715–724.

World Health Organization (WHO). (2003). *Fact sheet No. 134: Traditional medication.* Retrieved from http://www.who.int/

Yellow Horse Brave Heart, M. (2003). The historical trauma response among natives and its relationship with substance abuse: A Lakota illustration. *Journal of Psychoactive Drugs, 35*(1), 7–13.

Zerger, S. (2004). *Health care of homeless Native Americans.* Retrieved from http://www.nhchc.org

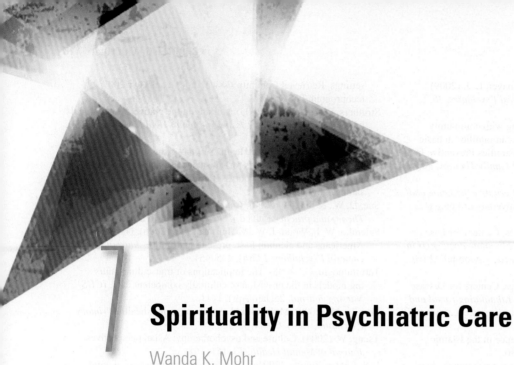

7

Spirituality in Psychiatric Care

Wanda K. Mohr

KEY TERMS

bibliotherapy
contemplation and meditation
prayer
religion
rituals
spirituality
values
worship

LEARNING OBJECTIVES

On completion of this chapter, you should be able to accomplish the following:

- Discuss the concepts of spirituality and religion.
- Explore reasons for the resurgence of interest in the spiritual aspects of health care.
- Analyze the strengths and weaknesses of the research findings related to spirituality, religion, and health.
- Describe how religious and spiritual themes may be manifested in mental illnesses.
- Debate the importance of clarifying values and becoming self-aware in relation to implementing spiritual and religious interventions.
- Examine the role of clergy in mental health care.
- Discuss the components of spiritual assessment.
- List several spiritual coping practices and interventions that nurses might use when working with clients.
- Evaluate the importance of ethical considerations while attending to a client's spiritual and religious needs.

Psychiatric–mental health nurses concern themselves with suffering and its alleviation. Within this context, suffering is uniquely multilayered and multileveled, involving body, mind, and spirit. Often, such distress challenges personal meaning systems for both nurses and clients. Indeed, because nursing as a profession espouses a holistic (body–mind–spirit) view of humanity, nurses are obligated to acknowledge and appreciate the physical, emotional, and spiritual uniqueness of each client under their care (Burkhardt & Nathaniel, 2008).

Research has shown that clients want to be seen and treated as whole people, not as disease states (Astrow et al., 2001; Koenig, 2009). Being whole implies having physical, emotional, social, and spiritual dimensions. Ignoring any of these human aspects may leave clients feeling incomplete and may even interfere with healing (Koenig, 2009).

For many clients, spirituality is an important part of wholeness. When providing all types of care, including psychiatric, nurses cannot ignore that component of personhood. Spirituality also represents a foundational value for many clients. Effective care demands that nurses understand their clients and the values they consider most important. It also requires nurses to know themselves, develop awareness of their own values (see Chap. 8), and establish competence in recognizing and addressing clients' spiritual needs.

This chapter discusses spirituality and religion and their importance within the context of mental health and illness. It presents religious and spiritual interventions in mental health care and the specific role of the nurse. The chapter also reviews some ethical considerations involved in meeting clients' unique spiritual needs.

SPIRITUALITY, RELIGION, AND MENTAL HEALTH

Despite millennia of debate, there is little consensus about the meanings of spirituality and religion. These terms often are used interchangeably; however, there are important differences.

Definitions

Spirituality outside the context of religion is amorphous and difficult to define and explore. **Spirituality** has been described as a person's experience of, or belief in, a power apart from his or her own existence. It also has been described as an individual search for meaning (Beckman et al., 2007; Koenig et al., 2001). Spirituality may exist within, but is ultimately apart from, a single person. It is the individual's sense of relationship or connection with a power or force, which may or may not be a deity. Although intangible, spirituality has been conceptualized as a component of a person's wholeness that carries implications throughout one's life (Ameling & Povilonis, 2001; Cavendish et al., 2004). Spirituality may incorporate a sense of relationship with oneself, others, or a higher "power" (Beckman et al., 2007) (Figure 7.1). Broad associations include belief in a power greater than oneself, a system of ethics, a purpose in life, the ability to forgive, gratitude for life, the ability to find meaning in suffering, trust in providence, and faith (Emmons, 2003).

Not every person who professes to be spiritual is religious or even believes in a deity. Agnostics (who doubt the existence of God) and atheists (who deny the existence of God) can have rich spiritual lives. At its core, spirituality consists of all the beliefs and activities by which people

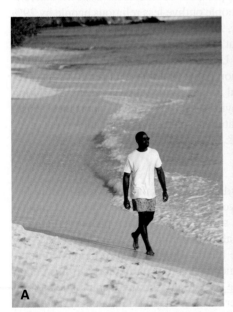
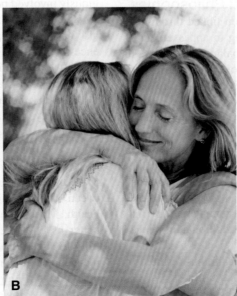
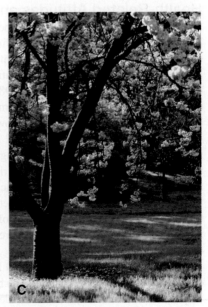

FIGURE 7.1 A sense of spirituality can be manifested through a relationship with (**A**) oneself, (**B**) other people, or (**C**) transcendent forces, such as God or nature.

attempt to relate their lives to God, a divine being, or some other conception of transcendence. Spirituality is not an individual creation; it is shaped by larger social circumstances and by the beliefs and values of the wider culture. Spirituality is unique to an individual and may be influenced through social interaction. In societies as complex as those of the United States and Canada, people express spirituality in many different ways.

Religion is the outward practice of a spiritual system of beliefs, values, codes of conduct, and rituals (Koenig et al., 2001). Religion serves as a platform for the expression of spirituality through an organized system of practices and beliefs.

Importance of Spirituality and Religion in North America

Population surveys consistently have established the centrality of religion in the lives of many Americans . The United States is generally a religious nation, with more than 9 out of 10 Americans (92%) believing in the existence of God or a universal spirit, although the degree of this religiosity varies across states and regions of the country (Gallup, 2009). The *U.S. Religious Landscape Survey* conducted in 2009 by the Pew Foundation shows that more than half of Americans rank the importance of religion very high in their lives, attend religious services regularly, and pray daily. A robust 65% of the U.S. population reported in 2008 that religion was important in their daily lives. Americans are also overwhelmingly sure there's a God who answers prayers.

Religion seems to be equally important to Canadians as well, although recent surveys show that public religious behavior, religious affiliation, and attendance have been declining among much of the Canadian population, and the share of Canadians ages 15 and older reporting no religious affiliation has been increasing (Clark & Schellenberg, 2006).

Health-Related Attitudes and Philosophies

Spiritual care and health care have been linked throughout history. Past societies attributed healing to appeasement of spirits or gods or equilibration of an imbalanced life force. In some current cultures, the same practitioner dispenses health care and spiritual care (Fadiman, 1998). In the West, as scientific advances made medical care more effective, spiritualism and medicine drifted apart. However, during the past few decades, interest in the spiritual aspects of health has surged. Reasons for this reawakening range from research findings that suggest benefits of a spiritual life to health, acknowledgment of the limits of medical care, and "a sense that something is missing" (Astrow et al., 2001). Multiculturalism and heightened awareness of complementary and alternative medicine (see Chap. 17) are additional influences (Richards & Bergin, 2005).

Research on religion and mental health has resulted in challenges to assumptions about psychiatric illness. For example, scholars recently have discarded simplistic formulas based on descriptions of phenomena as the basis for distinguishing among religious beliefs, overvalued ideas, and delusions. Controversy continues, however. Some scholars, after careful phenomenologic enquiry, regard pathologic and spiritual phenomena as indistinguishable (Fulford, 1997; Jackson & Fulford, 1997; Shorto, 2001). Others have conceptualized both psychotic and spiritual phenomena as cultural ascriptions (Littlewood, 1997) or as complex fields produced by neural activity (Fenwick, 1997), with no "out there" existence.

Whatever the view, after many years of neglect, the field of psychiatry has recognized the importance of spirituality. In 1994 the American Psychiatric Association (APA) included the new category "religious or spiritual problem" as one of a variety of conditions that may be the focus of clinical attention, on par with acculturation and phase-of-life problems (APA, 2000).

Positive Effects of Spirituality and Religion

Much research about spirituality and its relationship to health is rooted in measurements of religious beliefs and practices. This is because of the difficulties described earlier in differentiating spirituality from religion.

Religion provides many clients with social support as well as a clinically effective cognitive scheme (McIntosh et al., 1993). Such benefits may serve to enhance well-being and decrease distress. Religious involvement predicts successful coping with physical illness and more rapid remission of depression, an association particularly strong in clients whose physical function is not improving.

Research has generally found a positive relationship between religiosity and good physical and mental health (Koenig et al., 2001). Studies have found that religious people are physically healthier, lead healthier lifestyles, and require fewer health services than do those who are not religious (Koenig, 2009). During the past three decades, several carefully controlled prospective studies have shown that religiously involved people outlive less religious people by 29% (McCullough et al., 2000; Mueller et al., 2001). Researchers also have found that religious practices may positively influence the health of U.S. teens. Studies consistently indicate a positive association between adolescent religious involvement and prosocial values, with religious teens exhibiting fewer at-risk behaviors, such as suicide, substance abuse, delinquency, premature sexual activity, and adolescent pregnancy (Marcovitz & Snyder, 2004).

Mental Health

More than 850 studies have examined the relationship between religious involvement and various aspects of mental health. Most have shown that religious people experience better psychological functioning and adapt more successfully to stress. The relationship between religious commitment and positive mental health is particularly strong among older adults (Figure 7.2). Many seniors who practice a faith tradition have lower levels of depression, anxiety, and alcoholism; experience higher life satisfaction and greater well-being; and adapt better to the rigors of personal loss, physical

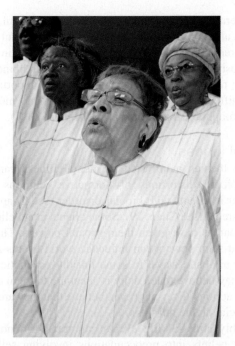

FIGURE 7.2 Involvement in religion and religious activities may help promote health and well-being for older adults.

illness, and disability than do their nonreligious counterparts (Koenig et al., 2001).

Religious commitment may be related to a lower incidence of substance abuse. Studies link abuse of alcohol and other drugs with a lack of purpose, which often is associated with minimal religious involvement (Beitel et al., 2007; Heinz et al., 2007). Michalak et al. (2007) found a strong association between religion variables and abstention. Research by Heinz et al. (2007) suggests that spirituality and religion play a significant role in recovery from substance abuse.

Religious involvement has been associated with decreased anxiety and reduced incidence of major depression. Koenig (2007) found that using religious belief as a coping resource was related to a reduced likelihood of major depression. The link between religious coping and depression was maintained even after controlling for other predictors of depression, such as social support, functional status, history of psychiatric problems, and age. Among outpatients with heart failure, greater spiritual well-being, particularly meaning/peace, was strongly associated with less depression. This result suggests that enhanced spiritual well-being might reduce or prevent depression and thus improve quality of life and other outcomes (Bekelman et al., 2007). Research also demonstrates that, in addition to protecting against depression, higher levels of religious commitment may afford protection against one of the most severe outcomes of depression—suicide. The inverse relationship between religious involvement and suicide was first reported in 1897 and has been confirmed several times since (Case Vignette 7.1).

Case Vignette 7.1

Marilyn, 64 years old, comes to the community mental health center with her daughter. The daughter states that Marilyn seems depressed. "All she wants to do is stay in bed and sleep all day, and she isn't eating or taking care of herself like she should." Marilyn sits in the chair, somewhat withdrawn and distant. She is dressed neatly, but her hair is uncombed. Further inquiry reveals that Marilyn's husband died about 1 year ago after a lengthy illness during which Marilyn was the primary caregiver. Before her husband's illness and death, they would get up early every morning and go to church. They also were active in helping at church-sponsored activities. The daughter states, "They did everything together, and the church was a big part of their lives. Now she won't even go out to the grocery store, let alone to church."

Reflection and Critical Thinking

- What additional information would you consider exploring with Marilyn and her daughter? Explain your answer.
- How would you assess the spiritual aspects of Marilyn's life? What types of questions would you ask?
- How would you determine if spiritual interventions would be an appropriate component of Marilyn's plan of care? What ethical issues might arise from these interventions? Explain why.

Critiques and Criticisms of Available Research

Several different types of spiritual or religious therapies have been shown to be helpful for clients with different types of psychological problems, but the body of research is very small at present. For example, in a review of religious and spiritual psychotherapies, Hook and his colleagues (2010) found Muslim psychotherapy for depression to be an efficacious treatment when combined with medication.

However, despite the aforementioned finding and those correlating well-being and spirituality or religion, some researchers have criticized the methodology of published work on religion and health. Three main areas of critique involve construct measurement, study design, and data analysis. Thus, readers must use caution when evaluating studies of spirituality and health because significant disputes exist regarding the quality of research (Berry, 2005; Post et al., 2000).

Some researchers have failed to control for confounding variables and other covariates and for multiple comparisons using multiple statistical procedures. Confounders such as behavioral and genetic differences and stratification variables such as age, sex, education, ethnicity, socioeconomic status, and health status may play important roles in the association between religion and health. Failure to control for them can lead to biased estimations. Likewise, many studies on religion and health fail to adjust for the greater likelihood of finding a statistically significant result when conducting multiple statistical tests.

Research findings have lacked consistency, even among well-conducted studies (Hook et al., 2010). For example, while one study found some effects of religious attendance on functional capacity in older adults, it failed to associate health outcomes with measures of "religious involvement." In two other large studies (House et al., 1992; Strawbridge et al., 1997), church attendance was associated with lower mortality, but only in women. To some degree, lack of consistency is characteristic of an evolving field and may be the product of differences in study design, definitions of religious and spiritual variables, and outcome variables. The absence of specific definitions of religious and spiritual activity is important because many studies define these activities differently. Better definitions would enhance research substantially. For now, the empirical literature suggests the positive benefits of spirituality and religious involvement. However, empirical inconsistencies make it difficult to support recommendations for clinical interventions.

Negative Effects of Religion and Spirituality

Few systematic studies have shown an association between religious involvement and negative physical or mental health outcomes. However, like any other lifestyle choice, religion can have adverse consequences. For example, religious beliefs may encourage avoidance or discontinuance of traditional treatments or lead to a delay in seeking timely medical care or a failure to do so. In some cases, religious beliefs may contribute to the physical abuse of children. A consistent pattern of physical abuse in some families generally begins with corporal punishment that progressively gets out of control. Such families may justify punishment on religious grounds (Straus & Donnelley, 2001). The Bible contains verses that, taken literally, support physical punishment of children. An example is Proverbs 23:13–14: "Withhold not correction from the child: for if thou beatest him with the rod, he shall not die. Thou shalt beat him with the rod, and shalt deliver his soul from hell." Another is Proverbs 20:30: "The blueness of a wound cleanseth away evil: so do stripes the inward parts of the belly." And Proverbs 13:24 seems to advise a quick resort to such punishments: "He that spareth his rod hateth his son: but he that loveth him chasteneth him betimes." The danger of such literal interpretations is represented by the case of an Oregon man who severely and frequently beat his 6-year-old daughter, who experienced brain damage and became comatose. Investigations revealed that the man had marked the cited passages in his Bible as a rationale for his behavior (Straus & Donnelley, 2001).

People preoccupied with religion may have unrealistically high expectations for themselves. This characteristic can lead to isolation or alienation from those who do not share their beliefs. Unhealthy, fanatical belief systems can adversely affect physical and mental health (Mueller et al., 2001).

Several studies have implicated religion, particularly of a theologically conservative orientation, as a powerful predictor of homophobia (Finlay & Walther, 2003). Certain aspects of religiosity may mediate ethnic differences in homophobic attitudes; religion's effect may be even more important than gender differences, which have generally found men to be more homophobic than women (Rosik et al., 2007).

Mental Illness

Spiritual themes manifested in mental illness vary. Psychopathologic distortions of normative religious beliefs can occur in clients with bipolar disorder (see Chap. 27) or schizophrenia (see Chap. 29). Some clients may believe that divine sources have given them special powers. They may think that such powers can influence world events in wondrous or nihilistic ways. In some floridly psychotic stages, clients may believe that a deity is speaking to them or guiding their actions. They may even believe that they are deities with special divine missions.

Highly stressful life events can transform normative religious beliefs into preoccupations involving self-blame and guilt over real or imagined transgressions (Figure 7.3). Without relief from this type of stress, clients may exhibit psychotic distortions with religious themes. For example, a severely depressed client may see himself or herself as damned, with no hope of salvation and in need of punishment by God. Those who believe that their transgressions are so severe that they cannot be saved or forgiven may become suicidal (see Chap. 34).

Nurses must use caution when approaching clients whose mental illnesses have strong religious overtones. Richards and Bergin (2005), scholars committed to spiritual strategies in psychotherapy, counsel that spiritual intervention and exploration can be relied on more readily with "less disturbed" clients. By "less disturbed," they mean people with moderate

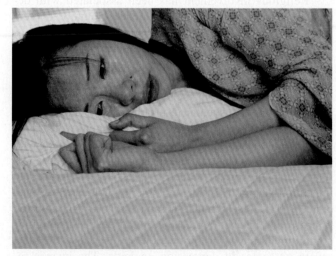

FIGURE 7.3 Guilt and sadness over real or imagined transgressions can evolve into psychological problems and risk for depression and suicide, particularly if these feelings also contain an element of spiritual despair.

anxiety and depression, self-esteem problems, adjustment difficulties, and interpersonal, family, or marital challenges. As the severity of a disorder increases, technical and somatic interventions (eg, hospitalization, electroconvulsive therapy, medications) are more appropriate. Although spiritual interventions can become components of treatment after somatic therapies have been instituted, spiritual interventions are contraindicated for delusional or psychotic clients (Richards & Bergin, 2005).

Checkpoint Questions

1. What is the meant by the term *spirituality*?
2. What is the major difficulty associated with recommending the incorporation of spirituality and religious involvement with clinical interventions?
3. Based on research, for which clients would spiritual interventions most likely be contraindicated?

RELIGIOUS AND SPIRITUAL INTERVENTIONS IN MENTAL HEALTH CARE

No responsible practitioner would advocate the abandonment of somatic treatments for mental illness. Clearly, clients who become destructive or so religiously preoccupied that it interferes with their day-to-day functioning need mainstream psychiatric care. However, because research suggests that believers may use religion as a way to cope with illness, ethical practice requires nurses and other professionals to stay abreast of debate and research findings related to clinically useful interventions, including those of a spiritual nature. Professional organizations, including the American Psychological Association, the Accreditation Council of Graduate Medical Education, the Council on Social Work Education, the Academy of Family Physicians, the Joint Commission, and the Commission on Accreditation of Rehabilitation Facilities, have all mandated that clinicians be able to recognize, respect, and address the spiritual issues of clients (Joint Commission, 2009).

Clarifying Values

Values are ideals or beliefs of importance to people that greatly determine how they act and behave. Family background, peer interaction throughout the lifespan, and secular and religious education influence values and ways of thinking (Boehnlein, 2000). Values help people make decisions and influence behavior.

Nurses and other health care providers do not enter clinical situations as blank slates. Rather, they come with assumptions, preconceived ideas, and worldviews that make them most comfortable within prescribed boundaries and familiar surroundings. Although values can influence behaviors in important and helpful ways, they also can be unproductive and sometimes damaging when they result in intolerance, prejudice, bigotry, or demonization of those who do not

share them. Cultural anthropology provides ample evidence of the human tendency to view those who are different as "others" (O'Connell, 2000). Thus, nurses and other health care providers must develop an awareness of the influence of their values on their identity and professional life.

Clarifying values helps nurses discover what they believe and what matters to them. It also involves becoming conscious of what clients regard as important and how such priorities might influence their attitudes and behaviors in clinical settings. Values clarification and self-awareness go hand in hand. When working with clients, nurses and other health care providers must become aware of their own personal values, their clients' values, and the differences between them. Self-awareness allows health care providers to act from their own spiritual or cultural perspectives, while taking care not to impose those values on others (Figure 7.4). Chapter 8 explores the importance of values clarification and self-awareness in more detail.

The Role of Clergy in Mental Health Care

The multidisciplinary treatment team is fundamental to the care of clients with serious psychiatric problems (see Chap. 12). Because health care is provided in complex institutional and community settings to clients with multisystemic problems, a collaborative approach reduces fragmentation and results in better-informed treatment.

Clergy, although not traditionally members of interdisciplinary treatment teams, can give needed support to clinicians, providing a context for and insight into the lives and worldviews of clients (Figure 7.5). Many clients turn to clergy for help, and some consider their clergy to be their primary mental health care provider (Larson et al., 2000).

Currently, clinicians are not well prepared to deal with psychiatric clients' spiritual concerns. Psychiatric nursing curricula and texts devote little content to spirituality. Yet clients clearly want this aspect of their lives to be considered in their care. Nurses are encouraged to build collaborative relationships with clergy and chaplains to learn more about

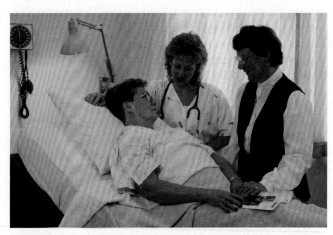

FIGURE 7.4 Nurses and clergy can work with clients as desired to provide spiritual assistance. (Photo copyright © Mark Gibson.)

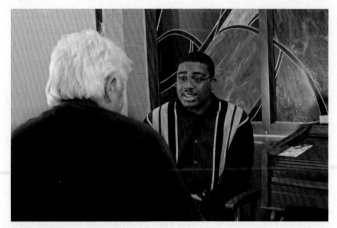

FIGURE 7.5 A key component to being able to provide nursing care related to the spiritual dimension of clients is for nurses to clarify their own values and beliefs. Speaking with clergy, nursing supervisors, or other trusted colleagues may help nurses identify their views and become more self-aware.

spiritual interventions and the rich diversity of spiritual and religious views. They are encouraged to invite clergy to consult and to be members of clients' treatment teams. As clients express a desire for greater attention to spiritual issues in their care, structured collaborations can assist in providing those with mental health problems the balanced and holistic approach they seek but which is not always available to them.

The Role of the Nurse in Mental Health Care

The nursing literature contains many different views on spiritual assessment and intervention. Nursing theorists such as Jean Watson (1985) and Sister Calista Roy (Roy & Andrews, 1999) clearly identify spiritual care as a nursing responsibility and provision for clients' spiritual needs as part of the nursing role. The second edition of *Nursing's Social Policy Statement* emphasizes that the goal of nursing activities is to help clients, families, and communities to improve, correct, or adjust to physical, emotional, psychosocial, spiritual, cultural, and environmental conditions for which they seek assistance (American Nurses Association [ANA], 2003). Both the ANA's *Code of Ethics for Nurses With Interpretive Statements* (2001) and the International Council of Nurses' *Code of Ethics for Nurses* (2006) advise nurses to provide care in an environment that respects the values, cultures, and spiritual beliefs of the individual. *Psychiatric–Mental Health Nursing: Scope and Standards of Practice* identifies the spiritual dimension as an area of focus for nursing assessment (ANA, American Psychiatric Nurses Association, & International Society of Psychiatric–Mental Health Nurses, 2007).

As mentioned, the research literature on the benefits of spiritual and religious involvement is inconclusive. Nursing studies substantiating the validity of nursing interventions related to spirituality are sparse. Moreover, student nurses may feel inadequately trained to intervene, or even to do a spiritual assessment (Hoffert et al., 2007; McSherry, Cash & Ross, 2004). What should nurses do? They certainly should approach clients holistically as beings who are more than the sum of their parts. They also should acknowledge and respect the spiritual lives of clients and always keep interventions client centered.

> **Think About It 7.1**
> Review the defining characteristics associated with the nursing diagnosis of Spiritual Distress. Then consider Marilyn, the 64-year-old woman described in Case Vignette 7.1. Propose possible defining characteristics that might be applicable for this client.

Spiritual Assessment

Acknowledging the spiritual lives of clients may involve asking about that aspect when taking a health history. A spiritual history is not appropriate for every client. Four simple questions might be asked of clients with serious illness or in distress:

1. Is faith (religion, spirituality) important to you in this illness?
2. Has faith been important to you at other times in your life?
3. Do you have someone to talk to about religious matters?
4. Would you like to explore religious matters with someone?

Nurses can preface these questions by explaining that such information helps with planning for support services should clients develop complications or other serious health problems (Astrow et al., 2001).

In addition, open-ended questions that allow clients to tell nurses about how they view relationships, the meaning of their illness, or what kinds of coping have helped them in the past can yield information about spiritual concerns and practices that nurses might include in plans of care (Burkhardt & Nathaniel, 2008). Clients who are less comfortable talking about this private and personal aspect of their lives may drop hints about spirituality. Therefore, attention to their interactions and conversation with their families, other clients, and staff members is vital. Conducting a brief spiritual assessment can help nurses better understand their clients' worldviews and help determine whether clients' religious and spiritual beliefs and community could be a useful resource to help them cope, heal, and grow. See Therapeutic Communication 7.1.

Spiritual Coping Practices and Interventions

The nursing literature on spiritual coping strategies used by clients in illness is limited and focuses mostly on religious coping mechanisms (Baldacchino & Draper, 2001). Knowledge of spiritual and religious coping practices can inform client intervention. Nursing Spotlight 7.1 organizes current

Therapeutic Communication 7.1

Spiritual Dialogue

Desmond Grant is a 23-year-old man who has been attending regular outpatient therapy at a clinic for assistance with stress management and anxiety. He is waiting for his session with a therapist to begin. The nurse, Lila Ward, checks in to do a routine preliminary assessment.

LESS EFFECTIVE DIALOGUE	MORE EFFECTIVE DIALOGUE
LILA: "How are you today, Desmond?"	LILA: "How are you today, Desmond?"
DESMOND: "OK. I had a good week last week, but watching the news made me feel a little down."	DESMOND: "OK. I had a good week last week, but watching the news made me feel a little down."
LILA: "What do you mean by 'down'?"	LILA: "What do you mean by 'down'?"
DESMOND: "Oh, just upset about the state of the world and wondering if there's any meaning in this. Wondering if this is all there is." (*Smiles*)	DESMOND: "Oh, just upset about the state of the world and wondering if there's any meaning in this. Wondering if this is all there is." (*Smiles*)
LILA: "Well, when I start to get overwhelmed by the outside world, I just rely on my faith. I feel very strongly that someone (*points to the sky*) watches over us and cares for us."	LILA: "Have you been discussing these issues with the doctor or anyone else up to now?"
DESMOND: (*Shrugs his shoulders*) "I wish I could have that reassurance. I'm not religious."	DESMOND: "A little bit. Dr. Leonard always asks me when I have anxious or stressful feelings what things I think will help. My family was never religious, but I've been wondering lately if some faith exploration would be useful."
LILA: "Maybe you should discuss this with the doctor today."	LILA: "Do you know anyone with whom you might be able to explore such matters?"
DESMOND: "It's just more of the same. Everything is really OK."	DESMOND: "I have a friend whose father is a minister. I was thinking about consulting with him—he's always been kind to me."
	LILA: "It's good you have a potential resource with whom you feel comfortable. I will make a note of what we've talked about for Dr. Leonard—perhaps you can explore this further with her today."
	DESMOND: "Thank you. That makes sense."

Reflection and Critical Thinking

- What approaches by the nurse in the first scenario might have caused Desmond to shut down and halt the discussion?
- What elements of spiritual assessment did the nurse in the second scenario use? Could she have done anything differently?
- Analyze what the nurse in the second scenario helped the client to do.

diagnoses, outcomes, and interventions related to the spiritual domain.

Richards and Bergin (2005) differentiate between religious and spiritual interventions on the basis of structure. They consider religious interventions more denominational, external, cognitive, ritualistic, and public, and spiritual interventions more ecumenical, cross-cultural, internal, affective, transcendent, and experiential. However, because religion and spirituality are interrelated so closely in the health care literature, this section makes no distinction between the two. Moreover, all strategies discussed can be ecumenical or denominational. The nature of delivery should be based on agreement with clients. Nurses should tailor interventions to

clients' worldviews and unique coping mechanisms, particularly those reported by clients to have helped them during past illnesses or crises.

In several situations, spiritual interventions are contraindicated:

- When clients are psychotic or delusional
- When clients have made it clear that they do not want to participate in these interventions
- With minors whose parents are unaware that their children are participating in activity contrary to their denomination and faith (this can result in unwanted legal repercussions)

NURSING SPOTLIGHT 7.1

NANDA, NOC, and NIC Related to Spirituality

NANDA Diagnoses

Decisional Conflict (specify)
Impaired Religiosity
Moral Distress
Noncompliance (specify)
Readiness for Enhanced Decision Making
Readiness for Enhanced Hope
Readiness for Enhanced Religiosity
Readiness for Enhanced Spiritual Well-Being
Risk for Impaired Religiosity
Risk for Spiritual Distress
Spiritual Distress

NOC Labels

Client Satisfaction: Cultural Needs Fulfillment
Client Satisfaction: Protection of Rights
Coping
Decision Making
Dignified Life Closure
Grief Resolution
Hope
Information Processing
Participation: Health Care Decisions
Personal Well-being
Quality of Life
Spiritual Health

NIC Labels

Abuse Protection Support: Religious
Decision-Making Support
Dying Care
Forgiveness Facilitation
Grief Work Facilitation
Hope Instillation
Learning Facilitation
Referral
Religious Addiction Prevention
Religious Ritual Enhancement
Self-Awareness Enhancement
Self-Esteem Enhancement
Self-Modification Assistance
Self-Responsibility Facilitation
Spiritual Growth Facilitation
Spiritual Support
Values Clarification

From: Bulechek, G. M., Butcher, H. K., & McCloskey
Dochterman, J. (2008). *Nursing interventions classification (NIC)*
(5th ed.). St. Louis, MO: Mosby; Moorhead, S., Johnson, M.,
Maas, M. L., & Swanson, E. (2008). *Nursing outcomes classification (NOC)* (4th ed.). St. Louis, MO: Mosby; NANDA International.
(2007). *NANDA International nursing diagnoses: Definitions and classification, 2007–2008.* Philadelphia, PA: Author.

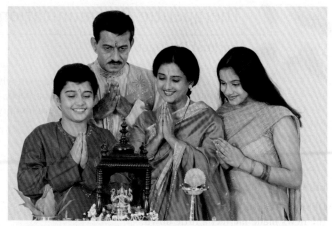

FIGURE 7.6 **Prayer is an activity found in most theistic traditions. This Hindu family is praying together.**

PRAYER. Prayer can be a powerful form of coping that helps people physically and mentally. **Prayer** is a kind of communication or conversation with a power that clients recognize as divine (Figure 7.6). All Western theistic religions and several Eastern traditions (eg, Hinduism, Buddhism, Shinto, Tao) practice prayer, although the form and content may vary for each. Different kinds of prayer (ie, group versus solitary) may have different effects on well-being and satisfaction. Polls and studies have shown that some Americans want their physicians to pray with them, with a majority of Americans thinking that physicians should join in prayer with clients if asked (MacLean et al., 2003).

Whether nurses should join clients in prayer if asked is a personal choice. The nursing literature has addressed the subject of nurses praying with clients in terms of ethical or legal implications. One nursing scholar cautions that prayer should be led by an identified religious leader distinct from the medical team whenever possible so as to avoid even an appearance of religious coercion (Becker, 2009). Koenig (2000) counsels that prayer as an adjunct to appropriate treatment might seem innocuous but that praying with clients could create a new source of liability if clients see themselves as being influenced unduly by practitioners.

BIBLIOTHERAPY WITH SACRED WRITINGS.
Bibliotherapy involves the use of literature to help clients gain insight into feelings and behavior and learn new ways to cope with difficulties. It is a process of interaction between the personality of the reader and the literature, which may be used for personality assessment, adjustment, or growth (Alpers, 1995; Finnegan & McNally, 1995). All major world religions have some type of text or writing that their followers view as holy and that they use as a source of comfort, insight, wisdom, and guidance (Nigosian, 2008). Western theistic traditions generally teach that God has revealed himself and his word to humanity through these writings. Major Eastern religions view their sacred writings as a

source of wisdom but not one necessarily revealed by a deity. The stories and narratives in these writings can provide solace and inspiration for clients. Spiritual reading is a significant part of 12-step programs (see Chap. 30). Before recommending any literature to clients, nurses should consult with the treatment team and the clients' family and clergy.

CONTEMPLATION AND MEDITATION. **Contemplation and meditation** are mental exercises that involve calmly limiting thought and attention. Meditative traditions include Zen, vipassana, visualization, transcendental, and devotional (National Center for Complementary and Alternative Medicine, 2007). Many forms of contemplation and meditation have their origins in Eastern traditions, most notably Hinduism and Buddhism. All forms involve isolation from distracting environmental noise, active focusing or repetition of thoughts or a word (mantra), muscle relaxation, release, and surrender of control. Guided imagery, a popular form of meditation, uses visualization and can be augmented with music and voice instruction (Figure 7.7).

Caution is urged when using contemplation and meditation as an intervention without knowledge of a client's denomination, preferences, or views. Contemplation and meditation are likely inappropriate interventions for clients with paranoid ideation (belief that their minds are being controlled).

REPENTANCE AND FORGIVENESS. All major theistic religions teach that people should forgive those who have harmed them and seek forgiveness from those whom they have harmed (Richards & Bergin, 2005). From a religious perspective, repentance and forgiveness are acts with important spiritual consequences. In addition, clients themselves may associate personal growth with admitting and making restitution for shortcomings and failings. Lifting of "the weight of the past" may release spiritual, emotional, and psychological pain.

Forgiveness and repentance are integral parts of 12-step programs (see Chap. 30). The process of repentance can be intensely painful for clients. Forgiveness and repentance in psychiatric settings should be interventions within the purview of a pastoral counselor or clergyperson (Becker, 2009).

WORSHIP AND RITUALS. All major religions encourage their followers to engage in private and public acts of worship. **Worship** is the devotion accorded to a higher power or deity, and **rituals** are the ceremonies, rites, or acts such as prayer; singing hymns; fasting or abstaining from food, water, or sex; and partaking of sacramental emblems. Acts of worship and ritual serve to express peoples' devotion to a deity. They facilitate their commitment or recommitment to a spiritual or moral life, offer penitence, offer settings and opportunities for solidarity with others, and provide for spiritual enlightenment (Smart, 2000). Benson (1997) suggests that worship services are full of "potentially therapeutic elements such as music, aesthetic surroundings, familiar rituals, distraction from everyday tension, prayer and contemplation, and opportunities for socializing and fellowship with others" (p. 176). Nurses should make certain that clients who wish to worship have the opportunity to do so (Figure 7.8). Professional service providers should be careful about participating with clients in worship or ritual because of potential confusion over role boundaries (Richards & Bergin, 2005).

FELLOWSHIP AND ALTRUISTIC SERVICE. The basic need for mutual support and connection with others is universal among humans. All religions encourage fellowship and provide opportunities for its expression and fulfillment (Richards & Bergin, 2005). Altruistic service can take many

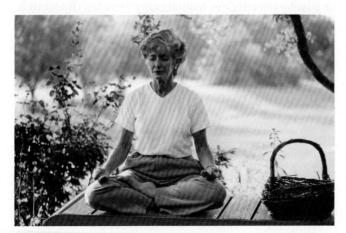

FIGURE 7.7 Contemplation and meditation may be useful for clients to help manage stress, anxiety, and other psychological challenges.

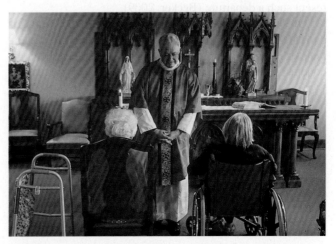

FIGURE 7.8 A key intervention for clients is to help them attend religious services if desired. Doing so may be difficult for clients who are hospitalized or living in assisted living or long-term care environments. Many health care facilities have chapels or similar settings to enable participation in religious activities.

forms, such as providing emotional support to discouraged people, taking clothes or food to the needy, or visiting the sick. Fellowship and altruism provide ways to reduce alienation and self-preoccupation and may be particularly helpful for clients who are socially isolated, lonely, depressed, suicidal, or experiencing major life crises (Richards & Bergin, 2005).

JOURNAL WRITING. Nurses can encourage clients to keep journals concerning their spiritual struggles, insights, and experiences.

Checkpoint Questions

4. When collecting a spiritual history, what type of questions would be most appropriate for nurses to use?
5. What do acts of worship and rituals express?
6. What three coping practices or interventions are important components of 12-step programs?

ETHICAL CONCERNS

Spiritual interventions and the incorporation of clients' religious beliefs in their treatment have several enthusiasts and devout practitioners (Richards & Bergin, 2005). However, some professionals have raised ethical concerns. All mental health professionals have a privileged status by virtue of the specialized knowledge they have attained through years of study and practice (Parsons, 2001). Thus, they are in positions of great influence with respect to clients. When they depart from areas of established expertise to promote a personal agenda or enter an area in which they are not expert, they abuse their professional status. Inquiries into a client's spiritual life with the intent of making recommendations that link religious practice with better health outcomes may represent such a departure (Becker, 2009).

A second ethical consideration involves the limits of current research. As mentioned, findings related to the effects of religious or spiritual factors on health have been inconclusive, largely because of questions related to research design, construct, and methodology. Nurses must take care not to misrepresent the state of research, lest suggestible clients abandon allopathic treatment for spiritual interventions to the detriment of their health.

A third ethical consideration has to do with the danger of imposing one's own values on clients. Devout nurses may view their work as an extension of their religious beliefs. Although there is no moral objection to discussing faith issues, intrusive and unethical practices include preaching, teaching, or otherwise attempting to persuade clients to the nurse's religious or spiritual viewpoint (Richards & Bergin, 2005). Such behavior clearly violates boundaries and roles and may harm vulnerable clients. For example, a nurse should never convey that he or she regards a client as spiritually deficient or immoral because of a choice with which the nurse does not agree (eg, abortion). Religious proselytizing is another clear boundary violation. Examples of proselytizing include giving clients literature from the nurses' spiritual tradition or denomination or teaching clients about religious beliefs when they have not requested such information or it is irrelevant to treatment goals.

Another ethical consideration raised by Richards and Bergin (2005) is that clinicians should pursue religious or spiritual goals and interventions only when clients have expressed explicitly their desire for them. They also recommend that clinicians using spiritual or religious interventions should always obtain informed consent from clients (or clients' parents).

A final ethical pitfall involves the possibility of violating work-setting (church–state) boundaries. Professionals who work in civic settings should be sure that they understand and adhere to work-setting policies regarding the separation of church and state. In light of legal rulings about school prayer and devotional scriptural readings (Staver, 1995), caution is especially important related to spiritual interventions for children and adolescents. Indeed, clinicians working in schools or other civic settings should avoid praying with children and teens, reading scriptures with them, or passing out religious bibliotherapy literature (Richards & Bergin, 2005).

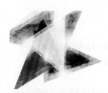

Reviewing and Applying Your Knowledge

Chapter Summary

- Spirituality has been described as a person's experience of, or belief in, a power apart from his or her own existence. It also has been described as an individual search for meaning. Religion is the outward practice of a spiritual system of beliefs, values, codes of conduct, and rituals. It is an organized system of practices and beliefs.

- Various reasons for the resurgence of interest in spiritual aspects of health care include the potential health benefits of a spiritual life, an acknowledgment of the limits of medical care, and research findings about religion and mental health.

- Research findings to document the beneficial effects of spirituality and religion on health show interesting results but remain inconclusive.

- Religious and spiritual themes may be manifested as psychopathologic distortions of normal religious beliefs in clients with schizophrenia or bipolar disorder. In addition, clients with normal religious beliefs who experience stress may become excessively preoccupied with self-blame or guilt over real or imagined transgressions.

- Nurses and other health care providers must become aware of their own personal values, their clients' values, and the differences between them. This will help professionals to act from their own perspectives without imposing their values on others.

- Clergy can play a large role in mental health care. They can provide needed support to clinicians by providing context and insight into clients' lives and worldviews. In addition, clients often turn to clergy for help and often consider their clergy to be their primary mental health care providers.

- In-depth spiritual assessment is not appropriate for every client. Some simple questions might explore the importance of spirituality or religion to the client now or at other times, whether he or she has someone with whom to discuss such matters, and whether the client wants to explore the topic. Other open-ended questions might be about how clients view relationships, the meaning of their illness, and past methods of coping.

- Examples of spiritual interventions for clients who desire them and for whom they are not contraindicated include prayer, bibliotherapy with sacred writings, contemplation and meditation, repentance and forgiveness, worship and rituals, fellowship and altruistic service, and journal writing.

- The role of nurses in terms of spirituality and religion is fraught with ethical concerns. Nurses can conduct brief spiritual assessments, but in the absence of special training, spiritual interventions are best implemented with help from clergy or spiritual healers of the client's choice.

Study Questions

1. During assessment a client states, "I believe in a power bigger than all of us." The nurse interprets this statement as indicative of which of the following?

   a. Religion

   b. Spirituality

   c. Values

   d. Worship

2. While interviewing a client, the nurse asks, "What is important to you?" The nurse is attempting to do which of the following?

   a. Clarify the client's values

   b. Determine client rituals

   c. Assist with meditation

   d. Use bibliotherapy

3. Which of the following questions would be most helpful to use when attempting to elicit information about a client's spiritual concerns?

   a. "Do you go to church regularly?"

   b. "What religion do you practice?"

   c. "What does being ill mean to you?"

   d. "Do you participate in any special rituals?"

4. After teaching a group of students about rituals, which of the following, if stated by the group as an appropriate example, would indicate successful teaching?

   a. Fasting on the eve of a holiday

   b. Providing food to the needy in a soup kitchen

   c. Practicing guided imagery

   d. Reading Bible stories for insight

(continues on page 128)

5. When developing a plan of care for a client, which of the following would be most important to keep in mind in relation to spiritual interventions?

a. Religious practice is highly and positively correlated with better health outcomes.

b. Giving clients literature about the nurse's religion is an appropriate teaching strategy.

c. Obtaining informed consent is essential before implementing any spiritual intervention.

d. Spiritual interventions are appropriate for use with any client, regardless of age.

Critical Thinking Questions

1. What ethical considerations or principles should guide nurses whose clients request them to pray with them?

2. What actions should a nurse take in the event that a client is actively trying to convert other clients within a health care setting to his or her religious beliefs?

3. Do you believe that it is ever appropriate to discuss your religious beliefs with psychiatric clients who are experiencing religious delusions or hallucinations?

References

Alpers, R. J. (1995). Spiritual reading as bibliotherapy. *Journal of Chemical Dependency, 5*(2), 49–63.

Ameling, A., & Povilonis, M. (2001). Spirituality, meaning, mental health, and nursing. *Journal of Psycho-Social Nursing and Mental Health Services*, 39(4), 14, 16–20.

American Nurses Association (ANA). (2001). *Code of ethics for nurses with interpretive statements*. Silver Spring, MD: American Nurses Publishing.

American Nurses Association (ANA). (2003). *Nursing's social policy statement* (2nd ed.). Silver Spring, MD: Author.

American Nurses Association, American Psychiatric Nurses Association, & International Society of Psychiatric–Mental Health Nurses. (2007). *Psychiatric–mental health nursing: Scope and standards of practice*. Silver Spring, MD: American Nurses Publishing.

American Psychiatric Association (APA). (2000). *Diagnostic and statistical manual of mental disorders* (4th ed., text rev.). Washington, DC: Author.

Astrow, A. B., Puchalski, C. M., & Sulmasy, D. P. (2001). Religion, spirituality, and health care: Social, ethical, and practical considerations. *American Journal of Medicine, 110*(4), 283–287.

Baldacchino, D., & Draper, P. (2001). Spiritual coping strategies: A review of the nursing literature. *Journal of Advanced Nursing, 34*(6), 833–841.

Becker, A. L. (2009). Ethical considerations of teaching spirituality in the academy. *Nursing Ethics, 16*(6), 697–706.

Beckman, S., Boxley-Harges, S., Bruick-Sorge, C., & Salmon, B. (2007). Five strategies that heighten nurses' awareness of spirituality to impact client care. *Holistic Nursing Practice, 21*(3), 135–139.

Beitel, M., Genova, M., Schuman-Olivier, Z., Arnold, R., Avants, S. K., & Margolin, A. (2007). Reflections by inner-city drug users on a Buddhist-based spirituality-focused therapy: A qualitative study. *American Journal of Orthopsychiatry, 77*(1), 1–9.

Bekelman, D. B., Dy, S. M., Becker, D. M., Wittstein, I. S., Hendricks, D. E., Yamashita, T. E., & Gottlieb, S. H. (2007). Spiritual well-being and depression in patients with heart failure. *Journal of General Internal Medicine, 22*, 470–477.

Benson, H. (1997). *Timeless healing: The power and biology of belief*. New York, NY: Gale Group.

Berry, D. (2005). Methodological pitfalls in the study of religiosity and spirituality. *Western Journal of Nursing Research, 27*(5), 628–647.

Boehnlein, J. K. (2000). *Psychiatry and religion: The convergence of mind and spirit*. Washington, DC: American Psychiatric Press.

Burkhardt, M. A., & Nathaniel, A. K. (2008). *Ethics and issues in contemporary nursing* (3rd ed.). Albany, NY: Delmar Publishers.

Cavendish, R., Luise, B. K., Russo, D., Mitzeliotis, C., Bauer, M., McPartlan Bajo, M. A.,... Medefindt, J. (2004). Spiritual perspectives of nurses in the U.S. relevant for education and practice. *Western Journal of Nursing Research, 26*, 196–212.

Clark, W., & Schellenberg, G. (2006). Who's religious? Retrieved from http://www.statcan.gc.ca/pub/11-008-x/2006001/9181-eng.htm

Emmons, R. A. (2003). *The psychology of ultimate concerns: Motivation and spirituality in personality*. New York, NY: Simon & Schuster.

Fadiman, A. (1998). *The spirit catches you and you fall down*. New York, NY: Strauss & Giroux.

Fenwick, P. (1997). Neurophysiology of religious experience. In D. Bhugra (Ed.), *Psychiatry and religion: Context, consensus and controversies* (pp. 167–177). London, UK: Routledge.

Finlay, B., & Walther, C. S. (2003). The relation of religious affiliation, service attendance, and other factors to homophobic attitudes among university students. *Review of Religious Research, 44*, 370–393.

Finnegan, D. G., & McNally, E. B. (1995). Defining God or a higher power: The spiritual center of recovery. In R. J. Kus (Ed.), *Spirituality and chemical dependency* (pp. 39–48). Binghamton, NY: Haworth Press.

Fulford, K. W. M. (1997). Religion and psychiatry: Extending the limits of tolerance. In D. Bhugra (Ed.), *Psychiatry and religion: Context, consensus and controversies* (pp. 5–22). London, UK: Routledge.

Gallup, G. (2009). *Religion in America*. Princeton, NJ: Princeton Religious Research Center. Retrieved from http://www.gallup.com/poll/114022/state-states-importance-religion.aspx

Heinz, A., Epstein, D. H., & Preston, K. L. (2007). Spiritual/religious experiences and in-treatment outcome in an inner-city program for heroin and cocaine dependence. *Journal of Psychoactive Drugs, 39*(1), 41–49.

Hoffert, D. H., Henshaw, C., & Nyaradzo, M. (2007). Enhancing the ability of nursing students to perform a spiritual assessment. *Nurse Educator, 7*, 66–72.

Hook, J. N., Worthington, E. L., Davis, D. E., Jennings, D. J., Gartner, A. L., & Hook, J. P. (2010). Empirically supported religious and spiritual therapies. *Journal of Clinical Psychology, 66*(1), 46–72.

House, J. S., Robbins, C., & Metzner, H. L. (1992). The association of social relationships and activities with mortality: Prospective evidence from the Tecumseh Community Health Study. *American Journal of Epidemiology, 116,* 123–140.

International Council of Nurses. (2006). *The ICN code of ethics for nurses.* Geneva, Switzerland: Author.

Jackson, M., & Fulford, K. W. M. (1997). Spiritual experience and psychopathology. *Philosophy Psychiatry and Psychology, 4,* 41–65.

Joint Commission. (2009). *Accreditation guidelines: The 2009 accreditation standards and requirements.* Retrieved from http://www.jointcommission.org/AccreditationPrograms/Home Care/Standards/09 FAQs/PC/Spiritual Assessment

Koenig, H. G. (2001). Religion, spirituality and medicine: How are they related and what does it mean? *Mayo Clinic Proceedings, 76*(12), 1189–1191.

Koenig, H. G. (2007). Religion and depression in older medical inpatients. *American Journal of Geriatric Psychiatry, 15*(4), 282–291.

Koenig, H. G. (2009). Research on religion, spirituality, and mental health: A review. *Canadian Journal of Psychiatry, 54*(5), 283–291.

Koenig, H. G., McCullough, M. E., & Larson, D. B. (2001). *Handbook of religion and health.* New York, NY: Oxford University Press.

Larson, D. B., Milano, M. G., Weaver, A. J., & McCullough, M. E. (2000). The role of clergy in mental health care. In J. K. Boehnlein (Ed.), *Psychiatry & religion: The convergence of mind and spirit* (pp. 125–144). Washington, DC: American Psychiatric Press.

Littlewood, R. (1997). Commentary on "spiritual experience and psychopathology." *Philosophy Psychiatry and Psychology, 4,* 66–77.

MacLean, C. D., Susi, B., Phifer, N., Schultz, L., Bynum, D., Franco, M., ... Cykert, S. (2003). Patient preference for physician discussion and practice of spirituality. *Journal of General Internal Medicine, 18*(1), 38–43.

Marcovitz, H., & Snyder, G. (2004). *Gallup youth survey: Major issues and trends.* Broomall, PA: Mason Crest Publishers.

McCullough, M. E., Hoyt, W. T., Larson, D. B., Koenig, H. G., & Toresen, C. (2000). Religious involvement and mortality: A meta-analytic review. *Health Psychology, 19,* 211–222.

McIntosh, D. N., Silver, R. C., & Wortman, C. B. (1993). Religious role in adjustment to a negative life event. *Journal of Personality and Social Psychology, 6,* 812–821.

McSherry, W., Cash, K., & Ross, L. (2004). Meaning of spirituality: Implications for nursing practice. *Journal of Clinical Nursing, 13*(8), 934–941.

Michalak, L., Trocki, K., & Bond, J. (2007). Religion and alcohol in the U.S. National Alcohol Survey: How important is religion for abstention and drinking? *Drug & Alcohol Dependence, 87*(2–3), 268–280.

Mueller, P. S., Plevak, D. J., & Rummans, T. A. (2001). Religious involvement, spirituality and medicine: Implications for clinical practice. *Mayo Clinic Proceedings, 76*(12), 1225–1235.

National Center for Complementary and Alternative Medicine. (2007). *Meditation for health purposes.* Retrieved from http://nccam.nih.gov/health/meditation

Nigosian, S. A. (2008). *World religions: A historical approach* (4th ed.). New York, NY: St. Martin's Press.

O'Connell, L. J. (2000). The worlds of psychiatry and religion: Bioethics as an arbiter of mutual respect. In J. K. Boehnlein (Ed.), *Psychiatry and religion: The convergence of mind and spirit* (pp. 145–157). Washington, DC: American Psychiatric Press.

Parsons, R. D. (2001). *The ethics of professional practice.* Boston, MA: Allyn & Bacon.

Pew Foundation Forum on Religion and Public Life. (2009). Retrieved from http://religions.pewforum.org/reports# Post, S. G., Puchalski, C. M., & Larson, D. B. (2000). Physicians and patient spirituality: Professional boundaries, competency, and ethics. *Annals of Internal Medicine, 132*(7), 578–583.

Richards, P. S., & Bergin, A. E. (2005). *A spiritual strategy for counseling and psychotherapy* (2nd ed.). Washington, DC: American Psychological Association Press.

Rosik, C. H., Griffith, L. K., & Cruz, Z. (2007). Homophobia and conservative religion: Toward a more nuanced understanding. *American Journal of Orthopsychiatry, 77*(1), 10–19.

Roy, C., & Andrews, H. A. (1999). *The Roy adaptation model* (2nd ed.). Upper Saddle River, NJ: Prentice Hall.

Shorto, R. (2001). *Saints and madmen: How pioneering psychiatrists are creating a new science of the soul.* New York, NY: Henry Holt.

Smart, N. (2000). *Worldviews: Cross-cultural explorations of human beliefs* (3rd ed.). Upper Saddle River, NJ: Prentice Hall.

Staver, M. D. (1995). *Faith and freedom.* Wheaton, IL: Crossway Books.

Straus, M., & Donnelley, D. A. (2001). *Beating the devil out of them: Corporal punishment in American children* (2nd ed.). San Francisco, CA: Transaction.

Strawbridge, W. J., Cohen, R. D., Shema, S. J., & Kaplan, G. A. (1997). Frequent attendance at religious services and mortality over 28 years. *American Journal of Public Health, 87,* 957–961.

Watson, J. (1985). *Nursing: The philosophy and science of caring.* Boulder, CO: University of Colorado Press.

THREE

The Nurse–Client Relationship

8

Nursing Values, Attitudes, and Self-Awareness

Wanda K. Mohr

LEARNING OBJECTIVES

On completion of this chapter, you should be able to accomplish the following:

- Identify sources of stigma that influence public perceptions of and behaviors toward people with mental illness.
- Distinguish between situational and dispositional factors affecting attributions that people make about phenomena in the environment.
- Discuss how situational factors can potentially influence the behavior of health care professionals toward clients with mental illness.
- Explain *horizontal violence* and its effects on professionals in work settings, including nursing and health care environments.
- Identify signs of professional burnout.
- List potential ways for nurses to cope with burnout.

The field of psychiatric–mental health nursing is rich, with many nuances requiring awareness from student and practicing nurses. This chapter is different from, but no less important than, others in this book. It is designed to present to students facts about mental illness, reduce uncertainty and fear, and foster self-awareness.

Recognition of personal values and behaviors and of the client's needs allows professionals to focus on those receiving care, accurately assess them, appropriately intervene, and evaluate outcomes (see Chap. 9). However, such awareness is neither straightforward nor automatic. Self-awareness involves reflection and the ability to observe one's own behavior and understand the attitudes, values, assumptions, and beliefs underpinning it. It also requires evaluation of the effects of behavior on others. This is particularly important when health care professionals are entrusted with the care of exceedingly vulnerable and challenging people, as is frequently the case in psychiatric–mental health nursing (Figure 8.1).

Prevailing approaches in teaching nursing values involve discussing the philosophical bases for and tenets of codes of ethics, as well as analyzing related cases. Chapter 5 of this book follows a similar model. While this approach is valid and important, it generally underestimates the powerful influences of situational factors, attitudes, roles, and language on ethical actions and practice. The literature of disciplines such as sociology and social psychology offers relevant concepts and experiments that can broaden discussions of ethics and values to help future nurses understand more fully the influence of situational contexts and role expectations in ethical analysis. Nursing does not happen in isolation but in a larger context. For this reason, this chapter presents several classic studies with concepts not widely discussed in nursing but that have important implications for self-awareness and, ultimately, client care. It also stresses how environmental influences can affect and shape professional behavior, even when nurses have a strong and well-grounded moral compass and a clear sense of values.

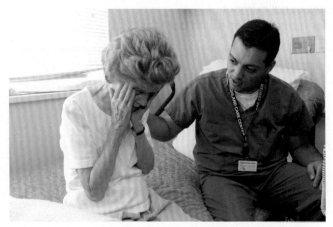

FIGURE 8.1 Self-awareness is critical to providing quality and humane care to clients with challenging and difficult mental health problems.

FEAR OF MENTAL ILLNESS: STIGMA AT WORK

It is normal to dislike uncertainty and to feel some fear or apprehension as a result. Many students new to psychiatric–mental health nursing are afraid because they do not know what they will encounter or because they have preconceived ideas about mental illness. It is human nature to fear what we do not understand, and many people fear those with psychiatric problems. Unfortunately, despite contributions made by researchers and the efforts of advocacy groups, mental illnesses still carry **stigma** (widespread fear and misunderstanding of mental illness; see Chap. 1). In some cases, the phrase "mental illness" conjures images of people tortured by demons that only they can hear or see.

Stigma is a major clinical and public health issue that worsens the course and outcome of mental illness and is a tremendous burden on many people with mental illness (Corrigan, 2005; Hinshaw, 2007). Studies continue to reveal that people with mental illness are often exposed to social rejection from friends and the public due to prejudices and stigma. The most common experience is to be treated differently, or as less competent, after being a client in mental health care (Lundberg et al., 2009).

Persons with mental illness face discrimination in all areas, the most common being discrimination in employment. Moreover, according to recent research, despite anti-stigma campaigns, stigma and discrimination remain largely as strong, damaging, and enduring as they were a decade ago (Lyons et al., 2009).

Not only do stigmatized individuals face public discrimination and become targets of negative stereotypes, but sadly they also often agree with these stereotypes and apply them to themselves, resulting in low self-esteem, which affects their situation adversely (Corrigan & Watson, 2002). In fact, research confirms that this self-stigma predicts poor quality of life (Rusch et al., 2010), suggesting that interventions to ameliorate these negative cognitions and the stigma that gives rise to them are important curative measures that nurses can apply as part of their work with clients who have mental illnesses.

Dramatic, and not always accurate, depictions in movies and literature have fostered common mistaken beliefs about mental illness. Films and books often rely on extraordinary symptoms of psychotic illnesses (eg, schizophrenia), or they draw on outmoded descriptions, rooted in theories or methodologies that experts no longer consider valid or accurate. In some cases, the movies or stories were created in a different time and continue to be viewed or read because they have an essential story or message that is valuable, but they depict beliefs, treatments, or ideas from the past that may be confusing to the public.

An example of misrepresentation of the symptoms of mental illness involves visual hallucinations, which are the most dramatic manifestation of psychosis and a symptom that may be overportrayed in films and television. Visual hallucinations alone are not characteristic of a mental disorder.

BOX 8.1 Visual Hallucinations in Charles Bonnet Syndrome

The ocular condition Charles Bonnet syndrome occurs in people with eye diseases that prevent normal nerve impulses from reaching the brain. The brain may generate spontaneous nerve activity, leading to visual hallucinations. The syndrome is more common in women than men and more likely if disease affects both eyes. The subsequent hallucinations are complex and fully formed images, usually of animals, people, faces, or scenery. Unlike many clients with psychoses, clients with Charles Bonnet syndrome know that the hallucinations are not real. No other sensory hallucinations develop, nor are delusions a feature. The hallucinations may last for seconds or for most of the day. They tend to disappear when people close their eyes. The syndrome may be experienced for days to years. For most people with macular degeneration, the condition is managed by educating clients and their families and reassuring them that they are not "going insane" or experiencing a psychotic disorder (Adachi, 1996; Jacob et al., 2004).

They can be common among people other than those with mental disorders. Examples of alternative causes include macular degeneration, Parkinson's disease, Lewy body dementia, leprosy (Hansen's disease), ingestion of hallucinogens, alcohol withdrawal, temporal lobe epilepsy, Charles Bonnet syndrome, and vertebro artery basilar syndrome (see Chap. 39). (Box 8.1)

Visual hallucinations in schizophrenia usually occur in people with a severe form of the illness and are accompanied by other symptoms, such as auditory or command hallucinations and delusions (see Chap. 29). The book and film *A Beautiful Mind* (Nasar, 2001) presents one of the most accurate and moving portrayals of the internal world of someone with schizophrenia, including showing what the experience of visual hallucinations can be like for such clients.

Intense media coverage of tragedies such as those that occurred at Columbine High School in Colorado and Virginia Tech focuses on the mental state of the violent perpetrators, which also contributes to negative reactions toward and stigmatization of people with mental illness. Those who have seen or read sensational characterizations and dramatic news reports do not realize that people with even the most severe mental illnesses are in touch with reality as often as they are disabled. Few mental illnesses have hallucinations as symptoms. For example, most people with phobic disorder do not have hallucinations or delusions, and neither do those with obsessive-compulsive disorder (see Chaps. 23 and 36). Most people with depression are not so seriously ill that they act on bizarre sensory perceptions or thought processes (see Chap. 28). However, psychiatric illnesses do have challenging emotions that may be hard for others to comprehend, such as the unrelenting hopelessness, helplessness, and suicidal thoughts of depression, or the despair brought on by alcoholism or drug abuse. These symptoms are not hallucinations or delusions but a painful reality.

MYTHS AND MENTAL ILLNESS

Critical examination of any accepted belief in a practice discipline must involve exploring whether any underlying assumptions, preconceived ideas, or myths support the belief. Myths must be made explicit, and the assumptions based on those myths should be evaluated as appropriate, inappropriate, or in need of further review. In other words, it is important for nurses to know why they do what they do. Likewise, it is important for nursing practices to be based on sound research and to be free from myths of the past. See Chapters 3 and 4.

Myths are erroneous beliefs held by groups to stimulate, rationalize, and organize actions about certain phenomena. Myths are often adhered to against all evidence, and they can be very strong. Frequently, they are rooted in cultural values. Often myths arise from *ideologies,* which are shared values, norms, or beliefs that bind groups together and help them make sense of the world (Mohr, 1995). These ideologies often guide behavior and responses. For example, an ideology of the United States promotes individualism, competition, and rewards for performance (ie., only the strong survive) (Trice & Beyer, 1993). This ideology values achievement and has helped to make the United States a world power. Conversely, this ideology works against the interests of those with serious mental illnesses, whose performance often is "out of sync" with mainstream values.

Myths serve as explanations and resolve oppositions and contradictions. Unfortunately, they also can misguide human actions. Throughout this text we have discussed some common myths versus truths about mental illness. Widespread assumptions and myths related to mental illness neglect the fact that as many as 8 in 10 people with psychiatric problems can effectively return to normal, productive lives if they receive appropriate treatment—treatment that is readily available (National Alliance for the Mentally Ill [NAMI], 2007).

The stigmatization of the mentally ill is well established. Unfortunately, health care personnel, including nurses, are considered by consumers to be primary contributors to stigma and discrimination against those with mental illness (Sartorius, 2007). Nurses need to fight this stigma as part of their professional advocacy role. To improve negative attitudes among the general public, nurses need to identify the myths underpinning those attitudes and improve the mental health literacy of themselves and the public.

UNDERSTANDING MENTAL ILLNESS: CLIENTS IN THEIR OWN WORDS

The fields of psychiatry and psychiatric nursing have long passed the point of believing that mental illness is the result of possession by evil spirits. The understanding of certain truths of human experience, such as pain and anguish, is central to nursing, and people with mental illness experience pain from the illness. Often if clients are to be deeply understood, detached observations or consultations of the *Diagnostic and Statistical Manual* may be insufficient.

Obviously students cannot directly experience all the conditions that can plague clients. Many people with mental illnesses have written eloquent books that communicate what their experiences are like. Textbooks, including this one, are full of facts about biology, the brain, and evidence-based interventions. Equally important, however, is trying to convey to students the kinds of challenges that clients with psychiatric illness face.

One of the most moving descriptions of mental illness comes from Kate Millett, who in 1990 published her memoir *The Loony-Bin Trip*. Millet suffered from bipolar disorder for many years. She describes her experience with depression:

> During depression the world disappears. Language itself. One has nothing to say. Nothing. No small talk, no anecdotes. Nothing can be risked on the board of talk. Because the inner voice is so urgent in its own discourse: How shall I live? How shall I manage in the future? Why should I go on? There is nothing ahead, my powers are failing, I am aging. I do not want to continue into the future as I see it.…
>
> The loss of language is so crucial, such a bereavement. Language does not really go away, it goes inward. Downward. Shriveling in the process, becoming repetitious, as one facing great peril repeats the same protective formulas. Yet one mourns language, sociability, camaraderie, needing it now more than ever. And how necessary it becomes just as one observes its superficiality; the wavering of friends, the coldness of strangers, the essential uncaring of life itself, its monstrosity. And in the face of this evil—not even to have words to protect one from the vacuum. To grow mute as well as helpless. (Millett, 1990, pp. 283–284)

This passage is not just splendidly written, but also conveys the struggle of someone so profoundly depressed that she has disappeared into herself. She has lost the will and ability to communicate, yet she has not lost the desire for human contact. This description also evokes the stigma of what the writer is suffering and the sorrow over the struggle of friends who are unsure of what to do or say. Millett's words may help students reflect on how they feel when a client is noncommunicative and seems amotivational, and what is reasonable to expect of someone with this depth of sorrow.

Another magnificent piece about the experience of mental illness is Dr. Kay Redfield Jamison's description of her manic episodes. Dr. Jamison, a professor of psychology at Johns Hopkins Medical School, is an important figure in the advocacy movement to bring parity and justice to people with mental illness. She writes:

> People go mad in idiosyncratic ways. Perhaps it was not surprising that as a meteorologist's daughter, I found myself in that glorious illusion of high summer days, gliding, flying, now and again lurching through cloudbanks and ethers, past stars, and across fields of ice crystals. Even now, I can see in my mind's rather peculiar eye, an extraordinary shattering and shifting of light, inconsistent but ravishing colors laid out across miles of circling rings; and the almost imperceptible, somehow surprisingly pallid moons of this Catherine wheel of a planet. I remember singing "Fly me to the moons" as I swept past those of Saturn, and thinking myself terribly funny. I saw and experienced that which had been only dreams or fitful fragments of aspiration.
>
> Was it real? Well, of course not, not in any meaningful sense of the word real. But did it stay with me: Absolutely. Long after my psychosis cleared, and the medications took hold, it became part of what one remembers forever, surrounded by an almost Proustian melancholy. Long since that extended voyage of my mind and soul, Saturn and its icy rings took on an elegiac beauty, and I don't see Saturn's image now without feeling an acute sadness at its being so far away. (Jamison, 1995, preface)

In this passage, Jamison describes the intensity of a manic experience. Again this description is a brilliant piece of writing that conveys not only the exuberance of mania, but also the sadness felt by the person from whom such experiences are removed. Thus, it is little wonder that clients are reluctant to take medications that would dull such feelings, even though they know that it is necessary to clear their psychosis. Students might remember this passage when evaluating a client's nonadherence to a medication regimen.

Both of these pieces of literature were chosen for their beauty and expressiveness to raise the consciousness of students who may fear (or judge) clients whose behavior is different. It is an attempt at what the philosopher Martin Buber (1958) called "a bold swing…into the life of the other." This swing involves empathy. Empathy can be curative, or at least helpful, for clients with the "existential pain" that comes from the troubles of living with mental illnesses. Their complaints will be relieved by medications, but also through catharsis and talking. But, for that, nurses must be ready to hear the words of pain, be aware of those that will bring relief, and they must take the time to listen. Listening can create empathy—if nurses remain open to be moved by the stories they hear.

> ### Checkpoint Questions
> 1. From where do myths frequently arise?
> 2. What can nurses do to help improve the general public's negative attitudes about mental illness?

HURTFUL LANGUAGE

Words can hurt. Words like *crazy, cuckoo, psycho, wacko,* and *nutso* are just a few examples of terms that keep the stigma of mental illness alive. These words belittle and offend people with mental health problems. Many people use them without intending any harm. But just as nurses would never deride someone for having a physical illness (eg., cancer, heart disease), it is cruel to mock someone with a mental illness.

But these are not the only ways that words can hurt clients. The medical record and the manner in which professionals speak about clients in clinical settings also can be hurtful and create negative attributions of certain clients that are then passed among staff members. Mohr and colleagues conducted a study in which they coded more than 4,000 entries made by registered nurses in psychiatric medical records. Pejorative adjectives used to describe clients outnumbered nonpejorative adjectives by 3 to 1. Examples of pejorative descriptors included *manipulative, argumentative, disruptive, defiant, whiny, superficial,* and *attention-seeking* (Mohr & Noone, 1997). In a second study, Mohr (1999a) examined more than 500 medical records and described nine categories of entries made by registered nurses or other staff members. Only 1% of entries reflected any kind of positive assessment of clients. An example of a judgmental, critical, or even biased entry reads "is controlling and engages in power plays with staff." Such discussion can affect how staff members act toward certain clients; staff members may make assumptions that are, in fact, incorrect.

The other "take-home point" is that documentation and discussion of clients' actions must be objective, with concrete examples given to show evidence of what one means by a label (eg., aggressive) (Figure 8.2). In the event of litigation, the presence of substandard, judgmental, and biased charting is often a "red flag" signal to astute attorneys that a client's civil rights may have been violated (Mohr, 2006). See Chapter 5.

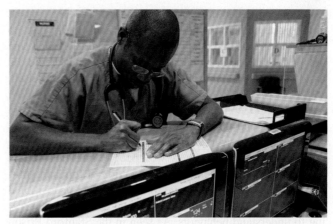

FIGURE 8.2 Nurses must take care to ensure that their documentation of client care and encounters is objective. Any descriptions of behaviors require concrete supporting examples.

Think About It 8.1

A small group of nursing students is sitting around the table at the campus coffee shop talking about their upcoming mental health clinical rotation. One student says, "We had a neighbor down the street who had a mental illness. Boy, everybody said that he was really crazy. He was always arguing with everyone, screaming, yelling, and upsetting the neighborhood. One time he even threw a rock at someone. We were all really afraid of him. I think they finally took him to the nut house." How do the student's statements promote the stigma associated with mental illness? Give an example of a situation that you feel reinforced the stigma of mental illness.

SITUATIONAL AND DISPOSITIONAL FACTORS IN CLINICAL SETTINGS

One of the most amazing features of human beings is that they can explain anything. No matter the cause, people have a strong need to understand and explain what is going on in the world. A simple theory about how people explain things is called **attribution theory.** (Think of the term *explanation* as a synonym.) Attributions often arise from assumptions. Assumptions consist of mind-sets so firmly established that they create powerful incentives within people or groups to act in certain ways and to explain things (or make attributions).

Two kinds of attributions are mentioned in the social psychology literature: *dispositional* and *situational* (Carlson et al., 2004). The celebrated social psychologist Philip Zimbardo (2007) has studied what he calls dispositional and situational phenomena for many years, and his work has significant implications for psychiatric nurses. Dispositional factors are those that people attribute as inherent personal qualities that lead to an action: character, free will, genetic makeup. It is a traditional explanation, especially in individualistic societies such as the United States, which attributes blame and fame to personal characteristics, rather than to external forces. Situational factors are those thought to be the vectors or transmitters of certain actions. To further clarify, dispositional factors are considered the elements within a person that account for or explain his or her actions or qualities. Situational factors involve the social phenomena or outside elements (eg., peer pressure) that influence a person's or a group's behavior.

Zimbardo conducted his now famous Stanford Prison Experiment in 1972. Along with colleagues, Zimbardo constructed a mock prison within the basement of Stanford University. Although no hypothesis was tested, the general purpose of the study was to explore the interpersonal dynamics of a prison environment by simulating a prison in which no prior dispositional differences existed among prisoners.

Twenty-four thoroughly screened young and healthy subjects volunteered to be randomly assigned into one of two groups for the study. One group would play the role of "prisoner"; the other would play the role of "prison guard." Within just 2 days of the experiment, four of the "prisoners" were released because of severe emotional reactions, such as rage, depression, crying, and severe anxiety. A fifth prisoner was released after he manifested a severe "psychosomatic rash." Meanwhile, most of the "guards" appeared to be enjoying their part in the proceedings and clearly had no intention of quitting. They kept up their harassment, some behaving sadistically and "delighting in what could be called the ultimate aphrodisiac of power" (Zimbardo et al., 1973, p. 44).

Zimbardo commented that strong social forces were in operation and that people fell into their respective roles very quickly. The lack of people "just quitting" attests to the power of obedience and how well people will stick to "the rules" presented to them. The implication of this and similar studies is that humans tend to overestimate dispositional factors and to underestimate situational qualities when trying to understand behaviors. As seen in the Stanford Prison Experiment and in other examples (eg., Abu Ghraib in Iraq), otherwise good people are capable of great cruelty toward others. Moreover, hierarchies and peers tend to tolerate and even reinforce such actions.

How do such findings apply to psychiatric nursing? In mental health settings, clients are vulnerable. Nurses and clinical staff, for all the emphasis on collaboration with clients and families, remain in positions of power. This power derives from their status as members of a profession with specialized knowledge that clients and their families may not have. The power differential is even greater in locked units to which clients have been involuntarily committed.

Despite progress that has been made in the past several decades, the history of psychiatry has not always been pretty. Clients have been unnecessarily incarcerated simply because they have lucrative insurance policies (Mohr, 1997), they have been subjected to capricious punishment by staff members (Mohr, 1997), they have been treated poorly, they have been secluded for hours, and they have been killed proximal to restraint use that may not have been necessary (Nunno et al., 2006) (see Chap. 32). In 1998, the NAMI asked its members to share their experiences with the use of seclusion and restraint. The grassroots response was overwhelming. Fifty-eight horror stories, including six deaths in 24 states, were shared with the public in NAMI's *Cries of Anguish* report (NAMI, 2000).

Those working in institutions in which atrocities against clients were committed were not evil people. Rather, they were immersed in situations that unleashed powerful situational forces that transformed normal behavior. The importance of Zimbardo's research to student nurses is that, although we may think of ourselves as having a consistent and stable personality across time and space, we are not always the same people working alone as we are working in a group (Zimbardo, 2007). The American Nurses Association's *Code of Ethics for Nurses* is specific about the principles of beneficence, nonmaleficence, and justice. Nurses must be aware of the cultures in which they find themselves and be prepared to deal with these powerful forces.

Checkpoint Questions
3. What is *attribution theory?*
4. What are dispositional factors?

LABELING AND SOCIAL PERCEPTION

Labeling theory focuses on the reaction of other people and the subsequent effects of those reactions, which create deviance. When others become aware that a person has engaged in acts that society considers deviant, that person is segregated and assigned labels. Examples include terms such as *crazy, trash,* and *junkie* (Mohr, 1999a, 1999b). Central to this labeling is **social perception,** which refers to the processes through which people use available information to form impressions of and assess others. Social perceptions can be flawed—even skilled observers can misperceive, misjudge, and reach the wrong conclusions.

Professor David Rosenhan (1973) conducted one of the most famous studies of the power of labeling and flawed social perception. His research design examined the difficulty that people have shedding the "mentally ill" label. He was particularly interested in how staff members in mental institutions process information about clients. He decided that the best way to get this information was from the inside through a participant observation study.

Rosenhan and seven associates had themselves committed to different mental hospitals by complaining that they were hearing voices. The other pseudo-patients came from varied backgrounds. All used pseudonyms. During their admission interviews, the pseudo-patients said that they heard an unfamiliar voice of the same sex as themselves that said "empty," "hollow," and "thud." The three women and five men were admitted; staff did not know the pseudo-patients were actually part of a field experiment. They assumed they were patients like any others and had no reason to believe the reported symptoms were bogus.

Beyond the alleged symptoms and falsification of names and occupations, the important events of the pseudo-patients' life histories were presented as they had actually occurred. Furthermore, prior to the study, Rosenhan instructed the pseudo-patients to act completely normal upon admission into the hospital. That is, they were not to act "crazy" in any way.

Despite doing nothing out of the ordinary, the pseudo-patients remained hospitalized for an average of 19 days. Their sanity was never detected except, ironically, by actual patients in the hospitals. At no time during their hospital stay did staff members ever question the legitimacy of the pseudo-patients' schizophrenic label. They simply assumed that the pseudo-patients were schizophrenic. Staff members perceived everything the pseudo-patients did and said while institutionalized from this premise. Consequently, they overlooked entirely or greatly misinterpreted normal behaviors. Minor disagreements became deep-seated indicators of emotional instability. Staff interpreted boredom as nervousness or anxiety. They even viewed the act of writing on a notepad as a sign of some deeper psychological disturbance.

Even though there was nothing "pathologic" about the pseudo-patients' histories, their records were reinterpreted to be consistent with the schizophrenic label. For instance, one pseudo-patient reported to the psychiatrist that he had a close relationship with his mother but a remote one with his father during early childhood. He added that as he matured, he became closer to his father, whereas his relationship with his mother became more distant. He had a warm and loving relationship with his wife and children, although there were occasional fights and friction. In short, there was nothing particularly unusual about this person's history. However, the attending psychiatrist translated this history into something troubled and psychopathologic: "This white 39-year-old male...manifests a long history of considerable ambivalence in close relationships, which began in early childhood" (Rosenhan, 1973, p. 253). The pseudo-patients took extensive notes recording the daily events on the ward. The staff members interpreted this note taking as part of a pathologic symptomatology, describing in the medical records that the pseudo-patients were "engaging in writing behavior."

Staff members consistently interpreted normal behavior as abnormal. A pacing pseudo-patient was asked if he was nervous; he was bored. Patients had little to look forward to and sometimes lined up outside the cafeteria half an hour before food was to be served. One psychiatrist described this behavior as demonstrating the "oral-acquisitive nature of their syndromes."

Rosenhan's work has other far-reaching implications. The pseudo-patient experiment offered a rare opportunity to study firsthand how psychiatric patients were treated. For example, the pseudo-patients were administered a total of 2,100 pills. The average contact with psychiatrists, psychologists, residents, and physicians combined was timed at 6.8 minutes a day.

The label of schizophrenia was so powerful that many of the pseudo-patients' normal behaviors were overlooked entirely or profoundly misinterpreted. Patient-initiated encounters frequently took the following form:

Pseudo-patient: "Pardon me, Dr. X. Could you tell me when I am eligible for grounds privileges?"
Physician: "Good morning Dave. How are you today?" (Moves off without waiting for a response.)

Rosenhan and his confederates recorded and collated numerous interactions with staff members. In 88% of encounters with nurses or attendants and in 71% of encounters with psychiatrists, staff members ignored questions and physically avoided having to interact with patients. Consider the following:

Neither anecdotal nor "hard" data can convey the overwhelming sense of powerlessness which invades the individual as he is continually exposed to the depersonalization of the psychiatric hospital....At times, depersonalization reached such proportions that pseudo-patients had the sense that they were invisible, or at least unworthy of account. (Rosenhan, 1973, p. 256)

Rosenhan's study also painted an unflattering picture of the quality of care provided. Staff members spent relatively little time with patients, and this was especially true of senior staff. Likewise, the pseudo-patients documented a number of unethical and abusive staff behaviors.

Student readers might ask what this could possibly have to do with them. Rosenhan's study conducted so many years ago is a stunning example of how labels affect those who are labeled and those who are doing the labeling. It also suggests that wrong first impressions are likely to persist. Rosenhan reached several conclusions about labeling effects. For example, he claimed that "psychiatric diagnoses...carry with them personal, legal, and social stigmas" (Rosenhan, 1973, p. 252). He stated that "the data speak to the massive role of labeling in psychiatric assessment. Having once been labeled schizophrenic, there is nothing the pseudo-patient can do to overcome the tag. The tag profoundly colors others' perceptions of him and his behavior" (pp. 252–253). Because "the sane are not 'sane' all the time...the insane are not always insane." Rosenhan reasoned that psychiatric problems can cast people in a hopeless light, as "the label sticks, a mask of inadequacy forever" (p. 257).

The implications for those who work with clients who have mental illness is that they must always be cognizant that the person who has schizophrenia is not a schizophrenic. That is, he or she is not his or her label. Moreover, just because a person is in a psychiatric setting, his or her status should not be what identifies him or her. First and foremost, the client's status should be that of human being.

Students may ask why these studies, which are quite old, are used as examples in this chapter. There are several reasons. One is that they are seminal—they broke new ground in terms of the science in this area (much as Peplau was a classic pioneer in psychiatric nursing). The second is that there have been no actual empirical replication studies conducted that are more current. The third has to do with the second, in that it would be unethical under current rules of research integrity to conduct such studies. The fourth is that the necessity of getting full informed consent in the way that health care providers and researchers currently must do would seriously bias any study that would seek to affirm the results achieved by Rosenhan and Zimbardo. The fifth is that in today's litigious society, it is highly unlikely that administrators would permit a study such as the one conducted by Rosenhan. As far as how little things may have changed in institutions despite dramatic changes in science, one need look no further than the for-profit psychiatric hospital scandal of the 1980s and 1990s to affirm that we have a long road to travel before optimum attitudes and care of people with mental illness are achieved (Mohr, 1994a, 1994b, 1995, 1996, 1996b, 1997; Mohr & Mahon, 1996; *Sixty Minutes II*, 1999).

> **Checkpoint Questions**
> **5.** How does social perception affect our views of mental illness?
> **6.** What did the results of Rosenhan's study show?

REALITY AND MENTAL HEALTH CARE: CHALLENGES FOR NURSING

Clients seeking mental health care are often frightened, relieved, or anxious about what will happen to them. They may fear that treatment will dehumanize them or that providers will overmedicate or not listen to them. They may be suspicious about the process of receiving mental health care. They may believe that nurses and other mental health professionals will solve their problems for them and may expect to play a passive role while an "expert" cures them. Nurses and other health care providers are responsible for clarifying these misconceptions and providing straightforward information about the importance of participation from clients and their families.

Recommendations for Working with Clients

Students new to this field should consider the following suggestions and observations:

- Just as people rarely welcome physical illness, having a mental health problem can be distressing. However, the person with a psychiatric, rather than physical, illness also must cope with the burden of other people's attitudes toward him or her.
- You may wonder if your attempts at therapeutic intervention will ever produce therapeutic effects. Know that your energy, enthusiasm, and openness to learning and exploring issues are exactly what most clients need and are refreshing to other staff members.
- You may learn from your classes and readings to use certain interventions in certain situations. However, in real practice, things may be done differently. Be open minded, discuss these differences with your instructor, and realize that clinical practice is not black or white but many shades of gray (Figure 8.3).
- You may wonder what to discuss with clients. Try to focus on something fairly concrete at first, such as what led the client to seek treatment, what he or she expects to gain

from treatment, and what progress the client has made in treatment. These discussions will help the client view various circumstances, gains, and expectations from new perspectives.

- The client may ask you not to repeat some information he or she has revealed to you. Nurses must never promise clients that they will not reveal such information. Rather, they should review with the client the meaning and purposes of confidentiality. Remind clients that you will share pertinent information with other members of the treatment team so that they can provide optimal care.
- The client may want to become friends with you or maintain a relationship after your clinical experience ends. Personal relationships with clients are never appropriate or wise. Clients must learn the boundaries of relationships and that a professional relationship helps the client learn valuable skills and develop strengths. If a client asks you to be his or her friend or indicates a desire for a personal relationship, discuss this development immediately with your instructor to turn this situation into a professional, therapeutic relationship.
- A client may or may not make progress or get well. Do not take a client's lack of progress personally or feel like a failure. Mental illness has many causes. Clients get better or well through many kinds of treatments: therapy, medications, structured environments, skill development, and social supports. Your participation in a client's care is never a sole determinant in his or her progress or lack of it.

Managing Stress and Burnout

Many nurses who enter the psychiatric field frequently are motivated by a sense of **altruism;** that is, they are working from a desire to contribute something valuable to society. Although the work has an innately humanitarian purpose, it also has stressors that induce nurses to feel fearful, anxious, offended, helpless, repulsed, pitying, embarrassed, hopeless, angry, or all of these (Figure 8.4). The behaviors of clients represent the range of human disturbance—from violent, hostile, or aggressive to bizarre, regressed, or dependent. How nurses deal with these behaviors reflects their personal values and experiences, as well as their success in the field.

Nurses may feel ashamed of their reactions to disturbances in clients or feel that their responses are unprofessional and hide or deny their feelings. Learning to acknowledge, express, and deal with feelings is as important for nurses and other mental health professionals as it is for their clients. In fact, nurses model for clients how to cope with feelings in a positive way.

The stressors that psychiatric–mental health nurses experience are considerable, exact a heavy price, and require enormous personal and professional resources. Nurses should be alert to the warning signs of increasing job-related stress. Such signs may take the form of **horizontal violence.** Horizontal violence refers to a variety of unkind, discourteous, and antagonistic interactions that occur between people at the same organizational hierarchy (Longo, 2007). It is often

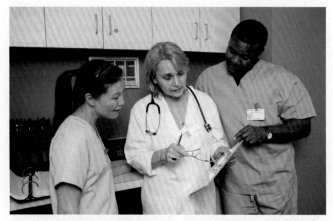

FIGURE 8.3 Students should review with their supervisors and teams practices that differ from what they learned in class and textbooks.

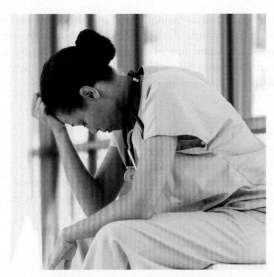

FIGURE 8.4 Nurses must find ways to manage the stress and emotions that accompany humanitarian work in a helping profession. Their ability to manage their feelings and responses directly influences their professional success.

described as divisive, infighting, backbiting, and off-putting. Horizontal violence can manifest as the anger or negativity that a nurse directs at another nurse. Or it may take the form of *passive-aggressive behavior,* which undermines the effectiveness of other nurses' work. An example of passive-aggressive behavior is when a nurse resists requests for adequate daily performance but expresses this resistance "indirectly," thus the description as "passive." Such resistance might take the form of procrastination, calling in sick, dawdling, intentional inefficiency, or "forgetfulness" (Mohr, 1996).

Horizontal violence may be conveyed in various forms that denigrate a clinician's professional dignity. Several nurse scholars have suggested that horizontal violence has its roots in the phenomenon of oppressed group behavior (Hedin, 1992; Roberts, 1983). An oppressed group tends to develop low self-esteem and hatred of their own culture because the powerful, dominant group mandates that their own attributes (eg, skin color, clothing, gender, language) are to be valued and rewarded above any others; thus, members of the oppressed group attack "their own" (Freire, 1971). These nurses believe that oppressed group behavior results from a culture in which physicians are valued over nurses. Using this logic, one could extrapolate that nurses are valued over clients; therefore, clients should be engaging with each other in the same way. But this is not true; clients are often supportive of each other in treatment settings. Although there may be a kernel of truth in these scholars' arguments, like many facile explanations, it undoubtedly is too simplistic. The behavior called horizontal violence is multifactorial in nature.

Another significant issue for psychiatric nurses is the attitudes of their colleagues. There is considerable evidence that the subspecialty of psychiatry is devalued within the profession of nursing. Part of this trend may be due to the devaluation of relational practice, and the prizing of technological skills. It may be perpetuated by the segregation of psychiatric client populations from general medical settings, thereby segregating the staff as well (Lauber & Sartorius, 2007).

Some client behaviors are more stressful to deal with than others, including suicidal threats or actions, violence, and passive-aggressive behavior. Some agencies and institutions are toxic environments that expect nurses to be overinvolved in their work or extremely self-sacrificing. These unhealthy environments do not promote high-quality care. Rather, they drain nurses, leaving them personally and professionally depleted, especially when dealing with acutely ill clients and challenging behaviors (Mohr & Mahon, 1996). Many chapters in this text include examples of such challenging behaviors and potential interventions and approaches to them. Thus, **burnout** (an emotional state characterized by exhaustion, a diminished sense of personal accomplishment, and cynicism) is a problem in nursing. Indeed, it is a problem in all of the helping and other professions, including medicine, social work, psychology, and teaching.

Warning signs of burnout are loss of energy and enthusiasm, fatigue, insomnia, and alcohol and drug use. Increasing burnout leads to more severe symptoms: physical illness or exhaustion, withdrawal, mood changes, depression, hopelessness, and increased use of alcohol and drugs.

Positive coping with job-related stress and burnout requires a concerted effort (Box 8.2). Support systems at home and work allow nurses to express feelings and keep situations in perspective. Nurses need to cultivate realistic expectations

---

BOX 8.2 Managing Work-Related Stress

Staying energized in the face of multiple demands and stressors requires psychiatric–mental health nurses to attend to self-care needs and activities. To do so, they can draw on strategies that promote coping with and managing stress optimally. Some of these strategies are as follows:

- Do physical activity. Engaging in some form of aerobic exercise (eg., walking, running) for 30 minutes three times per week contributes to cardiopulmonary fitness, aids in weight control, improves mood, and fosters a sense of well-being. Strength-training exercises can build endurance, power, and flexibility.
- Eat nutritiously. Follow a diet that contains a variety of foods that are low in fat and saturated fat. Choose plenty of vegetables, fruits, and grains.
- Do not use tobacco, alcohol, and other drugs.
- Explore the use of meditation and other relaxation techniques.
- Learn the value of planning. Anxiety and poor coping can result from feeling overwhelmed. Plan a realistic schedule that includes personal activities and pleasures.
- If necessary, seek help. Never think that because you are a nurse you won't need help from others. Communicate needs to family, friends, and coworkers. If you are feeling especially overwhelmed, obtain assistance from a professional.

from the job and from themselves. Frequent, brief vacations may be more relaxing and refreshing than infrequent, longer ones. Paying attention to one's health needs brings great returns in stress reduction and increased satisfaction with life.

In addition, nurses need to evaluate their work environment honestly to determine whether they are being forced to lower their standards of care or prevented from providing high-quality care (situations likely to result in burnout). To stay healthy and happy, nurses should refuse to accept responsibility for others' problems; manage client care according to priorities; keep priorities for family, friends, and personal goals in order; search for creative ways to express excellence at work; and never stop learning. Lifelong learning is needed to address the changing issues and problems

faced by psychiatric–mental health nurses. Stress and burnout in the psychiatric nursing workplace can be minimized through early detection of stress symptoms and by using self-care measures, being involved in nonnursing activities, and setting and maintaining priorities.

Checkpoint Questions

7. What is the motivation that frequently leads nurses to enter the psychiatric field?

8. How might increasing job-related stress be manifested?

9. What are two ways to minimize stress and burnout in the psychiatric nursing workplace?

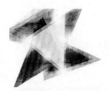

Reviewing and Applying Your Knowledge

Chapter Summary

- Mental illness carries a stigma. This stigma is often fostered by erroneous beliefs about mental illness through dramatic, and not always accurate, depictions in movies and literature and intense media coverage of tragedies. Myths, arising from ideologies, and hurtful language also promote the stigma.

- People have a strong need to understand and explain what is going on in the world. According to the attribution theory, attributions arise from assumptions. These assumptions consist of mind-sets so firmly established that they create powerful incentives within people or groups to act in certain ways and to explain things (make attributions). Two types of attributions are dispositional factors (inherent personal qualities that lead to action) and situational factors (social phenomena or outside elements) that influence a person's or group's behavior.

- Many nurses entering the psychiatric field frequently are motivated by a sense of altruism, working from a desire to contribute something valuable to society. The stressors that psychiatric–mental health nurses experience are considerable, exact a heavy toll, and require enormous personal and professional resources.

- Signs of increasing job-related stress may take the form of horizontal violence (unkind, discourteous, antagonistic interactions between people at the same organizational hierarchy often described as divisive, infighting, back-biting, or off-putting) or passive-aggressive behavior (eg, resistance demonstrated indirectly to requests or demands).

- Warning signs of burnout include loss of energy and enthusiasm; fatigue; insomnia; and alcohol and drug use. Increasing burnout leads to more severe symptoms, such as physical illness or exhaustion, withdrawal, mood changes, depression, hopelessness, and increased use of alcohol and drugs.

- Stress and burnout in the psychiatric nursing workplace can be minimized through early detection of stress symptoms and by using self-care measures, being involved in nonnursing activities, and setting and maintaining priorities.

Study Questions

1. When preparing a class discussion on attribution theory and dispositional and situational factors, which of the following would the instructor describe as an example of a situational factor?

   a. Genetic makeup

   b. Personal values

   c. View of right and wrong

   d. Views of a peer group

2. After a nurse teaches a local community group about mental health and illness, which statement from the group would indicate a need for additional instruction?

   a. "Most mentally ill people have average or above-average intelligence."

   b. "People with mental illness are more likely to be violent than other groups."

   c. "Mental illness has nothing to do with being weak or lacking willpower."

   d. "People with mental illness cannot just snap out of it."

3. A client with a psychiatric illness asks the nurse not to repeat his statements to anyone else. Which action by the nurse would be most appropriate?

   a. Tell the client that the nurse cannot promise not to reveal this information.

   b. Maintain the client's confidentiality by not revealing the information.

   c. Immediately tell the client's primary care provider of the client's request.

   d. Ask the client to provide more information before making a decision.

4. A nurse is meeting with a colleague who works at a psychiatric–mental health clinic. During their visit, the nurse becomes concerned that the colleague is experiencing burnout. Which of the following statements by the colleague would lead the nurse to suspect burnout?

   a. "Sometimes it's hard for me to get to the gym after work."

   b. "I've been working overtime lately because money is tight."

   c. "I just wish I could get a good night's sleep these days."

   d. "I'm going to Hawaii next week. I can't wait."

(continues on page 142)

5. On the last day of the clinical experience, a client states to a student nurse, "I hope we can be friends after you leave. I've really enjoyed talking with you." How should the student respond?

   a. Give the client a phone number that he can use to reach the student.

   b. Tell the client forcefully that this would never be possible.

   c. Talk with the instructor about how to deal with this situation.

   d. Keep the client's request private and confidential.

Critical Thinking Questions

1. Think about how you respond to stress. Describe the measures that you use to cope with stress and determine if these measures are positive or negative.

2. As part of a community education program, a nurse is asked to develop a presentation about mental health and illness. Outline the issues that the nurse would need to address to help reduce the stigma associated with mental illness.

3. What are your biases? Share your thoughts and feelings of mental health and mental illness.

References

Adachi, N. (1996). Charles Bonnet syndrome in leprosy: Prevalence and clinical characteristics. *Acta Psychiatrica Scandinavica, 93*(4), 279–281.

Buber, M. (1958). *I and thou.* Translated by R. G. Smith. New York, NY: Charles Scribner's Sons.

Carlson, D. S., Kacmar, K. M., & Bratton, V. K. (2004). Situational and dispositional factors as antecedents of ingratiatory behaviors in organizational settings. *Journal of Vocational Behavior, 65,* 309–331.

Corrigan, P. W. (2005) *On the stigma of mental illness: Practical strategies for research and social change.* Washington, DC: American Psychological Association.

Corrigan, P., & Watson, A. (2002). The paradox of self-stigma and mental illness. *Clinical Psychology: Science and Practice, 9*(1), 35–53.

Freire, P. (1971). *Pedagogy of the oppressed.* New York, NY: Herder & Herder.

Hedin, B. (1992). A case study of oppressed group behavior in nursing. *Image: Journal of Nursing Scholarship, 18*(2), 53–57.

Hinshaw, S. P. (2007). *The mark of shame: Stigma of mental illness and an agenda for change.* Oxford, UK: Oxford University Press.

Jacob, A., Prasad, S., Boggild, M., & Chandratre, S. (2004). Charles Bonnet syndrome—Elderly people and visual hallucinations. *British Medical Journal, 328,* 1552–1554.

Jamison, K. R. (1995). *An unquiet mind: A memoir of mood and madness.* New York, NY: Random House Inc.

Lauber, C., & Sartorius N. (2007). At issue: Anti-stigma endeavours. *International Review of Psychiatry 19,* 103–106.

Longo, J. (2007). Horizontal violence among nursing students. *Archives of Psychiatric Nursing, 21*(3), 177–178.

Lundberg, B., Hansson, L., Wentz, E., & Bjorkman, T. (2009). Are stigma experiences among persons with mental illness related to perceptions of self-esteem, empowerment and sense of coherence? *Journal of Psychiatric and Mental Health Nursing, 16,* 516–522.

Lyons, C., Hopley, P., & Horrocks, J. (2009). A decade of stigma and discrimination in mental health: Plus ça change, plus c'est la même chose (the more things change, the more they stay the same). *Journal of Psychiatric and Mental Health Nursing, 16,* 501–507.

Millett, K. (1990). *The loony-bin trip.* Chicago, IL: University of Chicago Press.

Mohr, W. K. (1994a). The private psychiatric hospital scandal: A critical social approach. *Archives of Psychiatric Nursing, 8*(1), 4–8.

Mohr, W. K. (1994b). The uneasy values fit between nursing and the for-profit hospital care industry. *Journal of Nursing Administration, 24*(3), 12–16.

Mohr, W. K. (1995). Values, ideologies and dilemmas: A discussion of professional and occupational contradictions in a changing health care environment. *Journal of Psychosocial Nursing, 23*(1), 29–35.

Mohr, W. K. (1996). Psychiatric nurses work experiences in troubled environmental contexts. *Archives of Psychiatric Nursing, 10*(4), 197–206.

Mohr, W. K. (1997). The outcomes of corporate greed. *Image: Journal of Nursing Scholarship, 29*(1), 39–47.

Mohr, W. K. (1999a). Deconstructing the language of psychiatric hospitals. *Journal of Advanced Nursing, 29*(5), 1052–1059.

Mohr, W. K. (1999b). Discovering a dialectic of care. *Western Journal of Nursing Research, 21*(2), 224–243.

Mohr, W. K. (2006). Psychiatric records. In P. Iyer, B. J. Levin, & M. A. Shea (Eds.), *Medical legal aspects of medical records* (pp. 691–707). Tucson, AZ: Lawyers & Judges Publishing.

Mohr, W. K., & Mahon, M. M. (1996). Dirty hands: The underside of marketplace medicine. *Advances in Nursing Science, 19*(1), 28–38.

Mohr, W. K., & Noone, M. J. (1997). Deconstructing progress notes in psychiatric settings. *Archives of Psychiatric Nursing, 11*(6), 325–332.

Nasar, S. (2001). *A beautiful mind.* New York, NY: Simon & Schuster.

National Alliance for the Mentally Ill (NAMI). (2000). *Cries of anguish: A summary of reports of restraints and seclusion abuse received since the October 1998 investigation by the* Hartford Courant. Alexandria, VA: Author.

National Alliance for the Mentally Ill (NAMI). (2007). *Inform yourself about mental illness.* Retrieved from http://www.nami.org/content/NavigationMentu/Inform_Yourself/About_Mental_Illness/Inform_Yourself/About_Mental_Illness/htm

Nunno, M., Holden, M., & Tollar, A. (2006). Learning from tragedy: A survey of child and adolescent restraint fatalities. *Child Abuse & Neglect, 30*(12), 1333–1342.

Roberts, S. J. (1983). Oppressed group behavior: Implications for nursing. *Advances in Nursing Science, 3,* 21–30.

Rosenhan, D. L. (1973). On being sane in insane places. *Science, 179,* 250–258.

Rusch, N., Corrigan, P. W., Todd, A. R., & Bodenhausen, G. V. (2010). Implicit self-stigma in people with mental illness. *Journal of Nervous and Mental Disorders, 198,* 150–153.

Sartorius N. (2007). Stigma and mental health. *The Lancet, 370,* 810–811.

Sixty Minutes II (1999, March). Unsafe haven. Retrieved from http://www.cbsnews.com/stories/1999/04/15/60II/main43232.shtml

Trice, H., & Beyer, J. (1993). *The culture of work organizations.* Englewood Cliffs, NJ: Prentice Hall.

Zimbardo, P. (2007). *The Lucifer effect: Understanding how good people turn evil.* New York, NY: Random House.

Zimbardo, P. G., Haney, C., Banks, W. C., & Jaffe, D. (1973, April 8). A Pirandellian prison: The mind is a formidable jailer. *New York Times Magazine,* pp. 38–60.

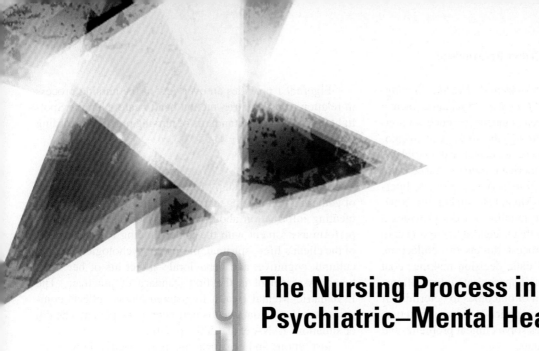

9

The Nursing Process in Psychiatric–Mental Health Care

Suzanne Perraud and Susan Breitenstein

KEY TERMS

assessment
behavioral statement
mental status examination (MSE)
nursing diagnosis
nursing process
psychosocial assessment
taxonomy
variance

LEARNING OBJECTIVES

On completion of this chapter, you should be able to accomplish the following:

- Apply the nursing process to psychiatric–mental health nursing.
- Explain components of a psychosocial assessment.
- List some nursing diagnoses that may apply to clients with psychiatric disorders.
- Explain the use of the multiaxial diagnostic system in the *Diagnostic and Statistical Manual of Mental Disorders,* 4th edition, text revision.
- Discuss how to organize and use psychosocial assessment data in formulating nursing care plans.
- Explain the use of standardized nursing care plans and clinical pathways in mental health care.
- Describe the critical thinking process that shapes moment-to-moment interventions with clients.
- Explain how evaluation relates to the other phases of the nursing process.
- Accurately document the application of the nursing process in the care of clients with psychiatric disorders.

According to *Psychiatric–Mental Health Nursing: Scope and Standards of Practice,* "Psychiatric–mental health nursing is a specialized area of nursing practice committed to promoting mental health through the assessment, diagnosis and treatment of human responses to mental health problems and psychiatric disorders" (American Nurses Association [ANA], American Psychiatric Nurses Association, & International Society of Psychiatric–Mental Health Nurses, 2007, p. 1). The methodology of the nursing process provides a framework for critical thinking that is central to nursing care (ANA, 2010). The nursing process directs the collection, analysis, and interpretation of data; decision making; goal setting; prioritization; selection of appropriate interventions; implementation; and evaluation of outcomes to determine if a plan has been effective. When applied to nursing practice, the nursing process helps nurses solve clinical problems and plan systematic care for all clients.

STEPS OF THE NURSING PROCESS

The **nursing process** is an organized approach for providing quality psychiatric–mental health nursing care. The steps involved are the same as those used in other nursing specialties (eg, maternal–newborn, medical–surgical). However, differences for psychiatric nursing exist in terms of the manner and focus of the nurse's observations, the particulars of interviewing during data collection, and the types of interventions used for identified problems.

The steps of the nursing process are as follows:

1. *Assessment,* or gathering data
2. *Diagnosis,* or identifying a problem
3. *Planning,* or creating strategies to achieve desired outcomes
4. *Implementation,* or enacting the plan
5. *Evaluation,* or determining the effectiveness of the plan

These steps provide a convenient way to organize and implement nursing practice in various settings, circumstances, and time frames. Envisioning each part of the nursing process as a step is useful because doing so implies sequencing, or passage through time. However, each step depends on and is related to the others. For example, an accurate diagnosis is impossible without careful assessment, and interventions will prove ineffective without a correct diagnosis and appropriate plan for guidance.

In addition, nurses may return to a step in the nursing process at any time in a client's care. In other words, assessment becomes reassessment with the revelation of new data or information. For example, a client may reveal more as his or her trust in the nurse–client relationship increases. Or a change in the client's status may necessitate reassessment. The information obtained from reassessment may be significant enough to change the focus of care or the nursing diagnosis. Similarly, information that nurses obtain during evaluation may lead to an adjustment in intervention planning and implementation to achieve the desired outcome.

Figure 9.1 provides an overview of the nursing process in relation to psychiatric–mental health care. Nursing Spotlight 9.1 presents the standards of nursing practice according to each step.

Assessment

Assessment, the first step of the nursing process, is the act of gathering, classifying, categorizing, analyzing, and documenting information about a client's health status. Nurses perform assessment with the understanding that all aspects of the client's life—spiritual, biologic, psychological, social, cultural, cognitive, and behavioral—affect his or her well-being. Assessment is the first standard of practice: "The Psychiatric–Mental Health Registered Nurse collects comprehensive health data that is pertinent to the patient's health or situation" (ANA et al., 2007, p. 29).

Institutions and organizations may specify, through assessment forms and electronic health record (EHR) systems, which data nurses are to collect. In addition, nurses may use their judgment to determine what data to gather based on the setting. For instance, on an inpatient unit where the nurse is one of several treatment team members, he or she may combine data gathered by different professionals to form a complete picture of the client's functioning. In a home care setting, where the psychiatric–mental health nurse may be the sole practitioner, he or she conducts a more extensive, autonomous assessment of client and family to develop the plan of care.

Nurses obtain assessment data from several sources:

- Interview with clients and their families
- History and physical examination
- Mental status examination
- Medical record review
- Review of records from other health care facilities or prior treatments
- Laboratory and psychological tests
- Assessments by other professionals and paraprofessionals

Chapter 10 is devoted to assessment and interviewing, a critical component of psychiatric nursing. The following paragraphs briefly review important components within the context of the overall nursing process.

Interview

The interview is perhaps the most important method of gathering data about the client's health because it allows the nurse to hear the client's perspective on the problem (Figure 9.2) and to begin building an alliance with the client (Rhoads, 2011). Clients provide *subjective data,* or information that depends on their report, ranging from the reason for seeking help, to why they think the problem or illness occurred, to what they expect as an outcome of treatment.

Astute observation and attentive listening are hallmarks of effective interviewers. Nurses must be sensitive to verbal and nonverbal cues. For example, if a client nervously taps a pencil throughout a discussion, quickly looks away in response to

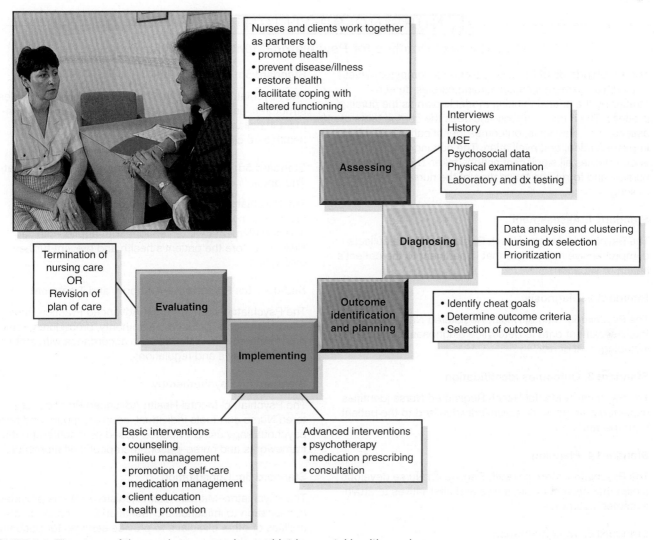

Nurses and clients work together as partners to
• promote health
• prevent disease/illness
• restore health
• facilitate coping with altered functioning

Assessing

Interviews
History
MSE
Psychosocial data
Physical examination
Laboratory and dx testing

Diagnosing

Data analysis and clustering
Nursing dx selection
Prioritization

Outcome identification and planning

• Identify cheat goals
• Determine outcome criteria
• Selection of outcome

Termination of nursing care OR Revision of plan of care

Evaluating

Implementing

Basic interventions
• counseling
• milieu management
• promotion of self-care
• medication management
• client education
• health promotion

Advanced interventions
• psychotherapy
• medication prescribing
• consultation

FIGURE 9.1 The steps of the nursing process in psychiatric–mental health nursing.

a particular question, or suddenly slumps the shoulders when asked about an issue, the effective nurse would use these cues to focus the interview. An example might be "When I asked you about your relationship with your husband, you seemed upset. Is there something more you'd like to tell me?" More information on interviewing and therapeutic communication is found in Chapters 10 and 11.

Health History

Nurses collect the historical health data of clients during holistic assessment. Such information helps nurses describe adaptive and maladaptive behaviors, formulate priorities, identify problems, predict probable responses to potential interventions, and analyze client perceptions.

A nursing health history is focused on the client's problems and needs and is used to gather information to help plan nursing care in both health and illness. Often clinicians use standardized tools to provide a basis for making treatment decisions and measuring change in behavior or function. Nurses may use assessment forms as vehicles to organize and record client information before, during, and after the interview. They should use these tools only as guides—they do not replace the need to follow cues and focus on areas that clients reveal as particularly or potentially troubling. See Chapter 10.

Mental Status Examination

The **mental status examination (MSE)** helps identify whether clients are experiencing abnormalities in thinking and reasoning, feelings, or behavior. It is part of the "tool kit" for gathering objective and observational data. The MSE includes questions and techniques related to the client's appearance, behavior and speech, thoughts, mood and affect, abstract reasoning, memory, intelligence, concentration, orientation, and judgment and insight.

Chapter 10 outlines the components of the MSE in detail. The MSE is particularly useful when clients are experiencing disruptions in cognition, memory, attention, and concentration. Congruence or discrepancies in thought and affect apparent during the interview may uncover important

NURSING SPOTLIGHT 9.1

Standards of Practice for Psychiatric–Mental Health Nursing

The six Standards of Practice describe a competent level of psychiatric–mental health nursing care as demonstrated by the critical thinking model known as the nursing process. The nursing process includes the components of assessment, diagnosis, outcomes identification, planning, implementation, and evaluation. The nursing process encompasses all significant actions taken by registered nurses, and forms the foundation of the nurse's decision making.

Standard 1. Assessment

The Psychiatric–Mental Health Registered Nurse collects comprehensive health data that is pertinent to the patient's health or situation.

Standard 2. Diagnosis

The Psychiatric–Mental Health Registered Nurse analyzes the assessment data to determine diagnoses or problems, including level of risk.

Standard 3. Outcomes Identification

The Psychiatric–Mental Health Registered Nurse identifies expected outcomes for a plan individualized to the patient or to the situation.

Standard 4. Planning

The Psychiatric–Mental Health Registered Nurse develops a plan that prescribes strategies and alternatives to attain expected outcomes.

Standard 5. Implementation

The Psychiatric–Mental Health Registered Nurse implements the identified plan

Standard 5a: Coordination of Care

The Psychiatric–Mental Health Registered Nurse coordinates care delivery.

Standard 5b: Health Teaching and Health Promotion

The Psychiatric–Mental Health Registered Nurse employs strategies to promote health and a safe environment.

Standard 5c: Milieu Therapy

The Psychiatric–Mental Health Registered Nurse provides, structures, and maintains a safe and therapeutic environment in collaboration with patients, families, and other health care clinicians.

Standard 5d: Pharmacological, Biological, and Integrative Therapies

The Psychiatric–Mental Health Registered Nurse incorporates knowledge of pharmacological, biological, and complementary interventions with applied clinical skills to restore the patient's health and prevent further disability.

Standard 5e: Prescriptive Authority and Treatment

The Psychiatric–Mental Health Advanced Practice Registered Nurse uses prescriptive authority, procedures, referrals, treatments, and therapies in accordance with state and federal laws and regulations.

Standard 5f: Psychotherapy

The Psychiatric–Mental Health Advanced Practice Registered Nurse conducts individual, couples, group, and family psychotherapy using evidence-based psychotherapeutic frameworks and nurse–patient therapeutic relationships.

Standard 5g: Consultation

The Psychiatric–Mental Health Registered Nurse provides consultation to influence the identified plan, enhance the abilities of other clinicians to provide services for patients, and effect change.

Standard 6. Evaluation

The Psychiatric–Mental Health Registered Nurse evaluates progress toward attainment of expected outcomes.

Source: American Nurses Association, American Psychiatric Nurses Association, & International Society of Psychiatric–Mental Health Nurses (2007). *Psychiatric–mental health nursing: Scope and standards of practice.* Silver Spring, MD: American Nurses Publishing.

© 2007 ANA, APNA, and ISPN

---

information and may be as revealing as clients' responses to the questions themselves.

Psychosocial Assessment

A **psychosocial assessment** focuses on dimensions of the client's life, such as occupation, sexuality, hobbies, spirituality, activity and exercise, coping, roles and relationships, and lifestyle. Such areas can exert vast influences over health;

often, information in these areas becomes the main focal points of nursing care. See Chapter 10.

Physical Examination and Laboratory and Diagnostic Testing

Clients experiencing mental illness frequently undergo an overall physical examination and pertinent laboratory and diagnostic testing. Such investigation helps identify whether

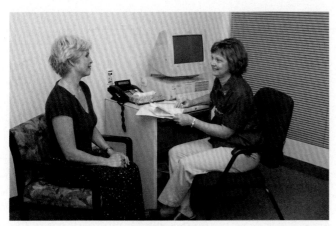

FIGURE 9.2 During the interview with the client, the nurse has the opportunity to hear the client's perspective on his or her problems.

other underlying systemic problems are contributing to or resulting from psychiatric illness and helps establish the client's overall health status (see Chaps. 10 and 39).

Checkpoint Questions

1. What is the single most important source of information for assessment?

2. What is the rationale for performing an MSE?

Nursing Diagnosis

The second step of the nursing process includes analysis of data collected during assessment, which leads to *diagnosis,* or identification of the clinical problem to address. Standard 2 of *Psychiatric–Mental Health Nursing: Scope and Standards of Practice* states "The Psychiatric–Mental Health Registered Nurse analyzes the assessment data to determine diagnoses or problems, including level of risk" (ANA et al., 2007, p. 31).

Defining client problems using accepted nursing terminology and definitions about what the diagnosis represents results in a clear diagnostic statement. The rationale for clarity and conciseness is that accurate nursing diagnoses guide the selection of effective interventions that help clients meet their health care needs and achieve desired health outcomes.

Nurses treat conditions that may not be found in medical or psychiatric diagnostic categories. For example, the nursing diagnosis Spiritual Distress related to inability to practice faith as a result of hospitalization, as evidenced by the comment "I feel so lost," likely has no medical or psychiatric equivalent. Nevertheless, nurses unquestionably can assist clients with and formulate interventions for this condition (see Chap. 7).

Articulating what nurses do that makes up their independent domain of care is a challenge for the nursing profession and has resulted in the creation of the concept of a nursing diagnosis and the formation of the North American Nursing Diagnosis Association (NANDA), now called NANDA International. This group defines **nursing diagnosis** as a "clinical judgment about individual, family, or community responses to actual or potential health problems/life processes" (1991, p. 65). This clinical judgment forms the basis for treatment and leads to the achievement of outcomes for which nurses are accountable (NANDA, 1991). NANDA is responsible for the creation, testing, and validation of existing and new nursing diagnoses. Its standardized taxonomy (classification system) and diagnostic labels are the most widely used resources for nursing diagnosis, establishing it as an important adjunct to other diagnostic systems (Gulanick & Myers, 2011).

The NANDA Taxonomy

Taxonomy means the organization of objects into related groups based on some common factor. The current NANDA Taxonomy II includes 13 domains subdivided into classes and further sorted into diagnoses (Figure 9.3). Having these different domains and classes allows nurses to logically group clinically related diagnoses. Taxonomy II revisions are in compliance with the National Library of Medicine regulations related to health care terminology codes, as well as many other national and international standards for health care terminology (NANDA International, 2009).

Seven concepts, called *axes,* are considered when creating a nursing diagnosis. These axes help nurses to limit and focus a diagnosis, thereby increasing its applicability and the ability of nurses to suggest appropriate interventions. The axes are as follows:

1. The *diagnostic concept*—the fundamental concept being addressed, including such things as denial, attachment, body image, hopelessness, and grieving—in other words, all realms of human responses.
2. *Subject*—the person or people for whom the diagnosis is intended. The values may include individual, family, group, or community.
3. *Judgment*—a word that modifies the meaning of the diagnosis. Modifiers include words like *compromised, decreased, deficient,* and *excessive.*
4. *Location*—describes part of the body or function affected. Examples include auditory, cerebral, mucous membranes, oral, or peripheral vascular.
5. *Age*—can range from fetus to older adult.
6. *Time*—the period during which a condition will last, such as acute, chronic, intermittent, or continuous.
7. *Status*—status of the diagnosis reflects whether the problem is actual or potential (at risk for), or whether it can be categorized as associated with wellness/health promotion (NANDA International, 2009).

Although nurses do not use all axes in all diagnostic statements, combinations can result in precise diagnostic statements, such as "acute interrupted development, adolescent." The flexibility that the axes afford also enables modifications. Although creating unique diagnoses is possible,

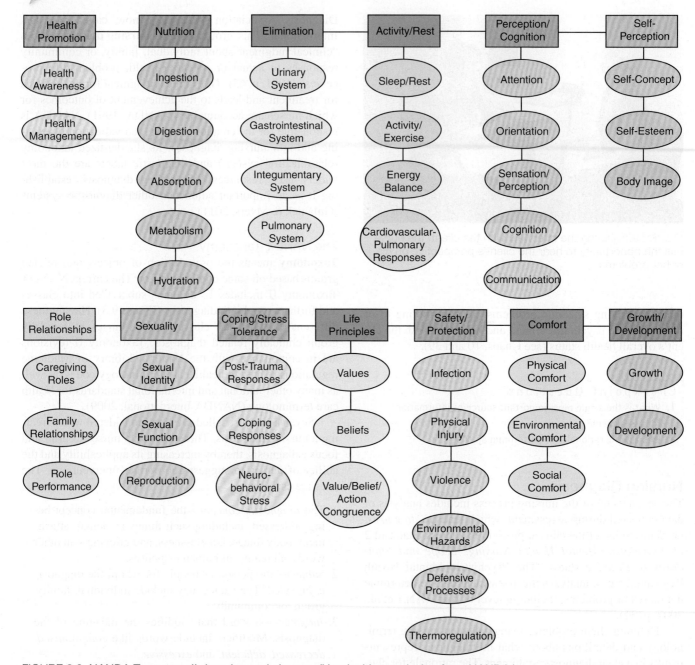

FIGURE 9.3 **NANDA Taxonomy II domains and classes.** (Used with permission from NANDA.)

NANDA recommends that clinicians use only approved and tested nursing diagnoses. By doing so, psychiatric–mental health nurses can communicate the focus of care using accepted and standardized language to other nurses.

Choosing and Formulating the Nursing Diagnosis

Nurses identify the diagnostic concept from the approved NANDA list that fits the assessment data by examining definitions for those concepts and considering additional information such as risk factors. They then combine Axis I (the diagnostic concept) with Axis II (the subject if other than an individual) and Axis III (judgment) if needed, along with values from the other axes if added clarity is important (NANDA International, 2009). For example, following

assessment of an adolescent with a history of self-mutilation, the diagnostic concept might be "risk for self-mutilation." The subject "individual" does not need to be stated because it is implied. A descriptor for Axis III (judgment) might be "enhanced." Because the subject is a teenager, an Axis 5 descriptor would be appropriate. Thus, the final nursing diagnosis is "enhanced risk for self-mutilation, adolescent" (NANDA International, 2009).

NANDA definition lists include some combination of definitions, defining characteristics, related factors, and risk factors. These lists include the subjective and objective data that substantiate use of the diagnosis. In other words, if a client exhibits no signs or symptoms that NANDA lists in the defining characteristics for a specific diagnosis, then using that diagnosis

TABLE 9.1 Writing the Diagnostic Statement: Examples of Incorrect and Correct Diagnoses

Incorrect	Correct	Rationale
Depression related to loss of spouse	Dysfunctional Grieving related to lack of adequate support secondary to death of spouse, as evidenced by the statement "I have nothing to live for" and weepy affect	Depression is a psychiatric diagnosis, not a nursing diagnosis. The complete nursing diagnosis includes an etiology that, in most cases, nursing can change through appropriate interventions. Interventions will focus on development of support. Defining characteristics are usually included from the assessment data (as evidenced by) to justify the diagnosis from the client's behavior.
Ineffective Coping related to lack of adequate ability to cope	Ineffective Coping related to overuse of denial, rationalization, and projection secondary to alcoholism, as evidenced by euphoric affect and blaming of problems on wife	Etiology (related to) should not repeat the main idea of the nursing diagnosis.
Disturbed Sleep Pattern related to noise on the unit and lack of adequate supervision	Disturbed Sleep Pattern related to sensitivity to environmental stimuli	Avoid any statements implying poor nursing judgment or poor staffing that may have legal implications.

would most likely be inaccurate. Table 9.1 contains examples of correctly and incorrectly written nursing diagnoses.

Once nurses identify all problems or needs related to a particular client, they document them in the plan of care in order of priority. Although it is preferable for clients to review and validate the problems, nurses must be sure to identify those problems related to client safety, regardless of whether clients believe such concerns are relevant.

Nursing Diagnosis and Psychiatric Diagnosis

As discussed in Chapter 1, the taxonomy of *psychiatric diagnosis* is found in the *Diagnostic and Statistical Manual of Mental Disorders,* 4th edition, text revision (*DSM-IV-TR*) (American Psychiatric Association, 2000). This criteria-based diagnostic system specifies the type, intensity, duration, and effects of various behaviors and symptoms required for clients to qualify as having a specific psychiatric disorder. Guidelines represent the clinical judgments of experts in psychiatry.

Nurses assist with psychiatric diagnosis by sharing important information about clients gathered during the nursing history, MSE, and daily observations. Thus, a nurse's working knowledge of the *DSM-IV-TR* maximizes efforts by interdisciplinary teams to help clients. Knowledge about the criteria for varying psychiatric diagnoses from the *DSM-IV-TR* also may help nurses make accurate clinical decisions relative to nursing diagnoses. For example, nurses cannot cure schizophrenia within their nursing role, but they can design interventions for problems within the domain of nursing practice related to the symptoms or sequelae of schizophrenia. Such problems would include anxiety, self-care deficits, and attention and concentration deficits. Later chapters of this book include foci of care or nursing diagnoses

associated with specific *DSM-IV-TR* diagnoses, along with nursing care designed to address those problems.

> **Checkpoint Questions**
> 3. What do the defining characteristics of a nursing diagnosis statement reflect?
> 4. How do nursing diagnoses differ from those in the *DSM-IV-TR*?

Planning

The third step of the nursing process is *planning,* which involves outcome identification and intervention selection. "The Psychiatric–Mental Health Registered Nurse develops a plan that prescribes strategies and alternatives to attain expected outcomes" (ANA et al., 2007, p. 33). Planning requires use of evidence-based interventions to attain expected outcomes. The plan of care results from collaboration among client, family, nurse, and other health care team members. EHR systems have the potential to become invaluable in the creation of collaborative and relevant multidisciplinary plans of care due to their ability to store and provide access to data input by multiple practitioners (Heerman Langford et al., 2010). Some computerized plans must be carefully individualized so that they are relevant for each client.

Identifying Outcomes

Standard 3 of *Psychiatric–Mental Health Nursing: Scope and Standards of Practice* states, "The Psychiatric–Mental Health Registered Nurse identifies expected outcomes for a plan individualized to the patient or to the situation" (ANA et al., 2007, p. 32). During *outcome identification,* nurses identify realistic, measurable outcomes that are expected as a result of care and establish a realistic timeline for their accomplishment. The nursing diagnosis drives the selection of interventions to achieve a particular outcome or outcomes (Moorhead et al., 2008). The SMART acronym is a useful way to guide nurses in outcome identification. Outcomes should be S (specific), M (measurable), A (achievable and realistic), R (relevant), and T (time specific). SMART outcomes serve as the basis for evaluating the effectiveness of nursing interventions. Table 9.2 contains examples of SMART outcome indicators.

The Nursing Outcomes Classification (NOC) research team at the University of Iowa developed a classification of outcomes linked to nursing care (Johnson et al., 2006; Moorhead et al., 2008). Such outcomes are measurable in terms of the response of an individual, family, or community to an intervention. NOC outcomes reflect client behaviors or states (Wilkinson, 2007). An example is Self-Care: Bathing.

Indicators accompany NOC outcomes. They are specific, stated in behavioral terms, and used to set goals. In turn, goals are used to evaluate outcomes and consist of measurable (observable) client and family behavioral statements (Wilkinson, 2007). A **behavioral statement** describes an action that can be observed. A clear and measurable behavioral statement usually starts with an action verb that focuses on some aspect of client behavior. Examples linked with client outcome indicators in psychiatric nursing are as follows:

- The client will bathe daily and wash hair without needing reminders from staff.
- The client will describe situations that trigger increased anxiety.
- The client will demonstrate respect for authority and obey school rules.
- The client will refrain from binge eating and purging.

Outcome indicators should be realistic, meaning that clients should have a good chance of achieving them. To determine whether indicators meet this criterion, nurses consider the nature of the problem, the efficacy of the treatment, the client's contextual resources, and any barriers. For example, attending therapy at the community health clinic may be an inappropriate outcome for a client with obsessive-compulsive disorder (OCD) whose ritualistic behaviors prevent him from dressing completely before leaving the apartment (see Chap. 23). A more realistic outcome indicator may be to reduce the frequency or intensity of ritualistic behavior.

Another aid to the development of realistic outcomes is the establishment of short-term outcomes that lead incrementally to a long-term outcome. For example, a long-term outcome for a person with agoraphobia and panic disorder would be the ability to function outside the home without panic. A step in that direction might be the ability to stand outside the front door without panic. Once the client successfully achieves the first short-term outcome, then the nurse can plan another, such as walking to the end of the driveway (see Chap. 23).

A related aspect of care planning that nurses should address as early as possible is *discharge planning* or posttreatment follow-up care. Once the interdisciplinary team defines the expected outcomes for each phase of treatment, referrals should begin that target issues relevant to continuity of care. Discharge planning helps ensure that when leaving a specific treatment environment, clients have a plan in place that matches the intensity of follow-up services with the intensity of the client's needs and will aid in achieving desired outcomes.

Selecting Interventions

After establishing behavioral outcomes, nurses select appropriate nursing actions, or *interventions,* to help clients achieve them. Wide arrays of nursing interventions exist. Nurses have a unique opportunity to identify and utilize evidence-based practices within their clinical setting. Psychiatric–mental health nurses select them according to their levels of practice (see Chap. 13). Examples of common psychiatric–mental health nursing interventions include the following:

- Assisting a client with depression to decide what to wear
- Providing finger foods and a water bottle to a client with mania who cannot slow down to eat or drink
- Offering to listen to an adolescent who is not getting along with her parents (Figure 9.4)
- Suggesting alternatives for handling problems to a suicidal client
- Removing an aggressive client from a group setting in which he or she has threatened others

TABLE 9.2 Examples of SMART Outcome Indicators

Outcome	SMART Outcome Indicators
Improved organization. Client will:	1. Prepare individual daily schedules including tasks and appointments with the assistance of the psychiatric home health nurse, on a weekly basis. 2. After 1 month, independently prepare individual daily schedules, including tasks and appointments.
Increased adherence to medication regimen. Client will:	1. Each Monday, fill weekly medication organizer, which will be checked by home health nurse weekly. 2. Complete medication adherence checklist daily after she takes medication. 3. Talk to the nurse about how she feels about the medication each week. 4. Agree to take medication even when feeling better and will review this agreement with the nurse each week.

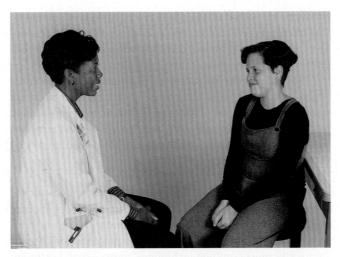

FIGURE 9.4 Interventions in psychiatric–mental health nursing can involve several different domains of care. Often, just listening to the client provides therapeutic help.

The Nursing Interventions Classification (NIC), another comprehensive standardized classification system, was developed by another research team at the University of Iowa. The NIC focuses on nurse, rather than on client, behavior (Bulechek et al., 2008; Johnson et al., 2006). The NIC group defines a nursing intervention as a judgment- and knowledge-based treatment provided by a nurse to enhance client outcomes.

When planning interventions, nurses can refer to resource materials, such as standardized care plans and clinical pathways. Increasingly, facilities house interventions in EHR systems. Such systems often include, but are not limited to, the ANA-approved NIC interventions (Dochterman & Jones, 2003).

NANDA and the NOC and NIC Taxonomies

Not long ago, NANDA, NOC, and NIC formed an alliance with the goal of creating a common, unifying structure (taxonomy) across the three classification systems. In other words, they linked nursing diagnoses with expected outcomes, and with appropriate major, suggested, and optional interventions leading to those outcomes. Available texts provide the unified language of NANDA, NOC, and NIC for care planning and evaluation (Wilkinson, 2007). In addition, many computerized documentation systems have been updated to reflect the integration of the language of nursing diagnosis, intervention, and outcomes.

STANDARDIZED CARE PLANS. As a result of the proliferation of computerized information systems, efforts to standardize and validate nursing diagnoses, interventions, and outcomes have intensified during the past few years (Moorhead et al., 2008). Standardized care plans typically list nursing actions and interventions with rationales and expected outcomes. They are organized according to the problem areas of a specific diagnostic category or nursing diagnosis. Their purpose is to achieve consistent care of specific clients within an organization. In other words, a standardized care plan reflects the facility's goal that all clients

with a specific health problem, regardless of context of care (such as shift, nursing skill, or day of the week), will receive the same care. Standardized care plans for a wide range of diagnostic categories can be found in reference texts and computerized information systems.

CLINICAL OR CRITICAL PATHWAYS. Clinical pathways are similar to standardized nursing care plans, but they are designed for the entire treatment team. Clinical pathways, also known as critical pathways, care maps, clinical maps, and clinical trajectories, have been developed to ensure that the health care team meets a standard of quality in providing care during this time of scarce health resources. Clinical pathways also provide a map for interdisciplinary teams to follow when they deliver essential clinical services to clients with a particular condition. There have been very few studies on the efficacy of clinical pathways in psychiatry, and they have been used less often in psychiatry than elsewhere in the health care system. As reimbursement structures change, we may see a renewed interest in the value of clinical pathways in psychiatry because of their potential to improve the efficiency and quality of mental health care and to identify outcomes of interventions for potential reimbursement (Evans-Lacko et al., 2008). Common components of clinical/critical pathways include consultations, diagnostic tests, assessments (all disciplines), activity level, medications, diets, therapies, client education, discharge planning, outcomes, and variances.

A **variance** is anything that alters the client's progress through the normal pathway. It can be related to clinician behavior, unexpected client response, or unusual systems issues. The study of variances can yield important information about quality of care and best practices. Significant variances may signal the need for a change in the plan or in policies and procedures.

Think About It 9.1

A client with OCD engages in frequent, persistent, and excessive hand washing. Assessment reveals a disheveled appearance and matted, tangled, and uncombed hair. Her hands are extremely dry, red, and chapped, with small cracks on the palms. Among the nursing diagnoses on her plan of care are Impaired Skin Integrity related to persistent and excessive hand washing as evidenced by reddened, dry, chapped hands; and Bathing and Hygiene Self-Care Deficit related to excessive time spent on hand washing as evidenced by disheveled appearance and tangled, matted hair. Develop appropriate short-term outcomes for the nursing diagnoses listed.

Implementation

Standard 5 of *Psychiatric–Mental Health Nursing: Scope and Standards of Practice* states, "The Psychiatric–Mental Health Registered Nurse implements the identified plan" (ANA et al., 2007, p. 35). *Implementation* occurs when nurses perform planned nursing actions. All nursing shifts perform all identified interventions. Continuity in carrying out specific interventions is critical to achieving desired outcomes. In most institutions, nurses are expected to document that they carried out interventions and the clients' responses to them. Quality care occurs only through careful and ongoing observation of its effects. For clients with psychiatric disorders, as for clients with other medical problems, the incremental responses to each intervention and nurse–client interaction serve as the building blocks for the full achievement of desired outcomes.

For nursing students, interactions with clients may be awkward and anxiety provoking. Although students will have communicated with many clients through various clinical experiences, they confront an important difference in psychiatric–mental health nursing. When preparing for a planned interchange with a client, the focus is no longer on performing a psychomotor skill correctly, but rather on verbal and nonverbal behavior. The therapeutic intent of words and actions takes center stage (Figure 9.5).

Typically, clients make statements or exhibit behaviors, and nursing students understand that a response is required. Students have read the client's chart and plan of care. Now they must combine this knowledge of the client's history with what is happening at the moment to formulate a therapeutic response. Consider, as an example, the therapeutic principle of empathy (see Chap. 11). It is not enough to understand the concept of empathy and its use in supporting clients and recognizing the human meaning of illness. During face-to-face discussion with clients who are in distress or facing a challenging recovery, nurses must use words to forge a mutual understanding of that experience.

The first few attempts at conveying empathy, combining a natural act such as talking with intent, may be awkward.

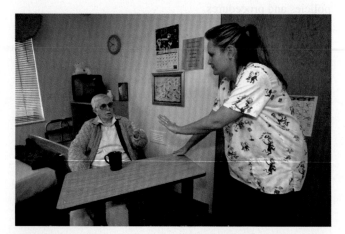

FIGURE 9.5 Nursing students and beginning practitioners may find interactions with clients awkward and anxiety provoking. Especially in psychiatric care, emotions can be challenging and intense. Nurses need to be aware of their own verbal and nonverbal behavior in their interactions. They must focus on the therapeutic intent of their words and actions and make sure not to convey behaviors or body language that clients could perceive as aggressive or disrespectful.

Students are aware of the pressure to frame a statement so that clients experience nurses as understanding and responsive. After some practice, demonstrating empathy with clients will probably come naturally.

The same internalization of principles to frame statements with intent must occur with psychiatric–mental health nursing interventions. However, internalizing intervention principles is more complicated because the process demands that nurses keep several considerations in focus while crafting the response.

Intervention Strategies for Beginning Practitioners

Intervention strategies for beginning practitioners include counseling interventions: problem solving, crisis intervention, stress management, and behavior modification. Nurses frequently must combine techniques across several different domains to achieve their purposes. Consider a nurse working with a client who has depression. Using problem solving, the nurse might focus on reinforcing some thought-stopping techniques that the client learned in a cognitive therapy group. With a psychoeducational approach, the nurse would teach the client more about depression, perhaps explaining how and why negative thoughts often accompany it. A biologic approach might point toward monitoring the client's response to psychotropic medication. This book details the conceptual framework for various intervention strategies specific to various mental disorders.

The basic approach nurses use in moment-to-moment interactions depends on the care plan and the particulars of the situation. For instance, if it were late in the day and a client were about to travel home, the nurse might talk about behavioral techniques the client could use in the evening hours to cope with negative thoughts. There is no one "right" approach. It is crucial that nurses have a clear theoretical rationale for an intervention and that the intervention is consistent with assessment and nursing care plan data.

Supervision

Supervision is the process by which psychiatric–mental health nurses obtain feedback about their interventions and analyze the emotions particular clients generated in them. This process helps nurses and other mental health professionals learn to be objective about their reactions and to "bracket off" emotions. In subsequent interactions, these emotions are then less likely to interfere with moment-to-moment interventions.

This skill develops during interventions with clients when professionals learn to maintain at least a partial awareness of their own reactions and emotions. This awareness should not interfere with the nurse's focus on what the client is communicating. On the contrary, this self-awareness is essential so that the nurse's own emotional reactions do not intrude on processing and understanding the client's communication.

A particular challenge for beginning nurses is to control their own anxiety during initial client interactions. In

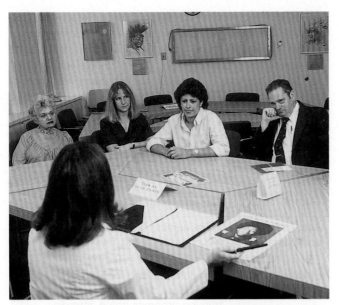

FIGURE 9.6 Postclinical conferences provide a mechanism for nursing students to discuss and receive feedback about their interactions with clients.

postclinical conferences, nursing students should recall the feelings and reactions that arose while talking with clients because training oneself to recall interactions and accompanying emotions is the essence of supervision, which, in turn, is central to the work of psychiatric nursing (Figure 9.6).

Checkpoint Questions
5. When using a psychoeducational approach, the nurse would focus on what area?
6. What is the purpose of clinical supervision?

Evaluation

Standard 6 states, "The Psychiatric–Mental Health Registered Nurse evaluates progress toward attainment of expected outcomes" (ANA et al., 2007, p. 44). *Evaluation* means determining the value of each intervention or the attainment of desired outcomes. Evaluation is essential because of professional accountability and the nursing profession's commitment to clients and families. This commitment demands that nurses continually monitor interventions to determine if they are effective and serve the needs of individuals and families. The nursing process is cyclical, so evaluation is the catalyst for modifying other components of the care plan.

Evaluation of a client's care is twofold. It centers on the changes experienced by clients and the quality or the effectiveness of the nursing care. For example, the nurse may assess a withdrawn client as disoriented and specify as an outcome of nursing care, "The client will verbalize awareness of time and place." Nursing interventions to achieve that goal might include visual cues placed in the client's environment (calendars and clocks) and verbal reinforcement of time and place.

Nurses evaluate the effects of interventions by observing client behaviors. In the previous example, the nurse may ask the following questions: Is the client present at activities that he or she is expected to attend? How did the client respond to periodic checks of orientation to time, person, and place? If the client's behavior does not change, the nurse must review and modify the care plan by modifying the outcomes or devising new interventions (Figure 9.7).

Review of the care plan also provides information relevant to evaluating nursing care. Was the initial assessment of the client complete? Were goals realistic, specific, and measurable? Did other nurses who intervened follow the care plan consistently? Did care plan modifications sufficiently

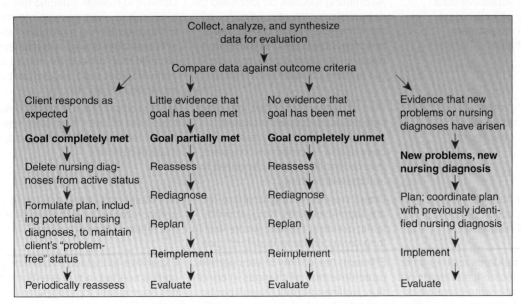

FIGURE 9.7 Flowchart to identify actions to take after judging how interventions have affected achievement of client goals.

address unanticipated complications in the client's response? Seeking the answers to these and related questions engages nurses in problem solving, which is essential to the evaluation and improvement of nursing care. Furthermore, as we move into the digital age in health care, our ability to evaluate outcomes over time and across large numbers of clients will be vastly improved and will allow rapid development and dissemination of evidence-based (best) practices.

DOCUMENTATION

The nursing process provides a framework for managing the care of clients. Documentation of the nursing process is a key component of communicating the nursing care provided in each step (Table 9.3). Documenting in the care record is necessary to (1) communicate important details related to the client's care and status, (2) communicate with all members of the treatment team to establish continuity of care, and (3) provide information used for evaluation and reimbursement for care (Wilkinson, 2007). The advent of EHRs has presented unique opportunities to reduce redundancies often found in paper records and to identify data useful for case finding and care planning, but is not without challenges related to identifying relevant and useful structures that will adequately capture the nursing process (Kim et al., 2011).

Table 9.4 compares the different types of documentation notes currently in use; Figure 9.8 provides examples of types commonly used in psychiatric–mental health care. Documentation methods might differ among settings and may be in electronic or paper format; however, components of the nursing process are reflected in the record of

TABLE 9.3 Documentation of the Nursing Process

Components	Documentation Methods
Assessment and diagnosis	Initial nursing database, MSE, nursing progress notes, flow sheets, treatment and discharge summaries
Planning and implementation	Standardized and individualized care plans, clinical/critical pathways, nursing progress notes, interdisciplinary treatment plans, client education forms
Evaluation	Nursing progress notes communicating the client's response to interventions, flow sheets, clinical/critical pathways, client education forms

TABLE 9.4 Comparing Documentation Notes

	Format	Advantages	Disadvantages
Narrative	Information provided in written sentences or phrases; usually time sequenced.	Easy to learn; easy to adjust length as needed; can explain in detail.	Time consuming; difficult to retrieve information; irrelevant information often included; possibly unfocused and disorganized.
SOAP	S subjective data O objective data A assessment P plan	All charting focuses on identified client problems; interdisciplinary—all team members chart on the same progress notes; easy to track progress for identified problem; steps in the nursing process are mirrored.	Difficult to master. Specific focus makes it difficult to chart general information without identifying a problem; lengthy and time consuming; assessment identification difficult for nurses and confusing because assessment data are provided in S and O.
PIE	P problem I interventions E evaluations	Plan of care incorporated into progress notes; outcomes included, which increases quality assurance; daily review to determine progress; less redundancy; easily adapted to automated charting.	Must read progress notes to determine plan of care; if problem has not been identified, difficult to chart; not multidisciplinary.
FOCUS	D data A action R response	Broad view permitting charting on any significant area, not just problems; concise, flexible; works well in long-term care or ambulatory care.	Not multidisciplinary; difficult to identify chronologic order; progress notes may not relate to the care plan.
Charting by exception (CBE)	Standards met—sign or check off; standards not met—write narrative or SOAP note	Efficient; use of flow sheets permits rapid detection of changes in condition; outlines normal assessments; can take the place of plan of care.	Expensive to institute; inservicing of staff is needed; not prevention focused; not appropriate for long-term or ambulatory care.

3/15/09	0730 Client awake, alert, denies com-
	plaints, sitting up in bed watching TV, VS
	taken, 0830 100% of full liquid breakfast
	taken 600 mg lithium PO. 0900 Partial
	bath at bedside, pt tolerated sitting in
	chair ✕30 min without fatigue. 1200 Reg
	lunch taken 100%
	————————————— MS Gorski RN

A

Problem #1	3/15/09 0900	"S" My head hurts right in the back of my eyes. Client describes pain worse bending over, like sinus headaches in past.
		"O" Eyes closed, lights dim, hesitant to move head when questioned. HR80 R20 BP140/90 T98.6
		"A" HA probable 2° sinus pressure.
		"P" 1. Decongestant prn as ordered
		2. Warm wash cloth to eyes
		3. Monitor temp q 4°
		4. Assess pain after med and contact physician as indicated
		————————————— MS Gorski RN

B

3/15/09 0400	Problem #1	Caregiver role strain related to chronically ill spouse, lack of immediate family support, and financial stress.
	Intervention for P(#1)	IP(#1): Acknowledge and talk with caregiver about stress involved with 24-hour care for loved one.
		IP(#1): Allow caregiver to express feelings.
		IP(#1): Help caregiver identify possible supports within the family and community.
	Evaluation for P(#1)	EP(#1): Caregiver discussed the strain of caring for her husband; crying and demonstrating signs of anxiety
		eg. "I just don't think I will be able to do this for long and then what is going to happen to us all? Sometimes it seems so hopeless." Stated she felt her children were supportive but they lived in another state and could not help with the day-to-day problems. —R. Wolfe, RN
		Note: as additional data are charted for the problem of caregiver role strain, Problem #1 is used to identify the problem.

C

FIGURE 9.8 Institutions use various methods for documenting and recording client data. Examples here include (**A**) narrative notes, (**B**) SOAP notes, and (**C**) PIE charting.

the client's status, nursing care plan, and client's response to intervention.

When documenting the nursing process, key components and principles remain consistent:

- Nursing documentation becomes part of the client's permanent record.

- Nurses document objective and subjective data.
- Written documentation should be clear and legible.
- Nurses should avoid including inferences or judgments regarding the data or the client in documentation.
- Nurses avoid general statements such as *good, fine,* or *tolerated well.* Instead, they use concrete and specific terms to describe data (Wilkinson, 2007).

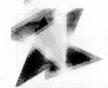

Reviewing and Applying Your Knowledge

Chapter Summary

- Nursing assessment involves gathering data and exploring the needs, problems, and adaptive resources of clients. Through the holistic approach to assessment, the nurse–interviewer explores functioning in psychological, social, biologic, behavioral, cognitive, cultural, and spiritual areas.

- The nursing diagnosis is a statement of a client's response pattern to a health disruption and guides the planning and intervention phases of the nursing process.

- The *DSM-IV-TR* classification system fosters a holistic approach to clients; it includes specific behavioral criteria for each psychiatric diagnosis.

- Nursing care plans define the goals or outcomes of care and the methods to achieve them.

- Standardized care plans provide nurses with documented standards of practice for clients with particular conditions.

- Intervention requires nurses to combine data from plans of care with information from what is occurring at the moment, prioritize client needs, and then match this information with an appropriate therapeutic strategy.

- Evaluation is the final phase of the nursing process in which nurses determine the effectiveness of an intervention or the attainment of a preset goal.

Study Questions

1. A client admitted for severe depression is brought to the inpatient unit. Applying the nursing process, which action would the nurse do first?

   a. Develop relevant diagnoses.

   b. Assess mental and physical health status.

   c. Establish outcomes such as "The client will not express suicidal thoughts."

   d. Offer to teach the client stress management techniques.

2. A 44-year-old woman is in the outpatient mental health clinic for anorexia nervosa. The nurse performs a thorough psychosocial and physical assessment, which reveals, among other things, that the 5′6″ client weighs 95 lb (43.1 kg). The client also describes severely ritualistic behaviors, such as cutting food into ½-inch pieces and eating only certain foods on certain days. When planning the client's care, the nurse and the client identify outcomes. Which of the following would be most appropriate for this client?

   a. The client will gain 4 lb (1.8 kg) per week until she reaches her goal weight of 130 lb (58.9 kg).

   b. The client will eliminate ritualistic behaviors within 1 month of initiating therapy.

   c. The client will learn to identify situations that trigger anxiety.

   d. The client will acknowledge that she is emaciated and looks very ill.

3. A 70-year-old client has been referred to the mental health clinic by his primary care provider. The client's wife died suddenly 3 months ago, and he has been severely depressed since. He states that he cries all the time and can't sleep or eat well. Based on these data, which of the following nursing diagnostic categories is most appropriate?

   a. Hopelessness

   b. Dysfunctional grieving

   c. Spiritual distress

   d. Ineffective coping

4. A nurse diagnoses her client with Impaired Social Interaction related to self-concept disturbance, as evidenced by the client's verbalized inability to experience satisfying relationships with peers or family. When choosing interventions to address this problem, the nurse designs interventions to accomplish which of the following?

   a. Improve the client's social environment.

   b. Help the family cope with the client.

   c. Address the client's self-concept.

   d. Help the client make new friends.

5. The nurse is evaluating a client's plan of care 5 days after his admission to a closed unit. The client, a 15-year-old boy, has a history of inflicting daily self-injury by cutting himself. The plan included the outcome that the client would stop injuring himself. The nurse contracted with the client that he would seek out a staff member whenever he felt like hurting himself and would gain privileges for making that admission.

Which of the following would be the best indicator that the plan is effective and the outcome is being met?

a. The client reports that he has not cut himself in 3 days.

b. No fresh cuts are on the client's body, and staff members report that he has been seeking them out for help.

c. The client has only one new cut in 3 days and has been able to refrain from cutting without the staff's help.

d. The client reports that when he feels like hurting himself, he begins exercising instead.

Critical Thinking Questions

1. How would different treatment settings influence the prioritization of the client's needs?

2. Describe how you would explain "nursing diagnosis" to someone from a social work background.

3. Plan three nursing interventions for a client with depression.

References

American Nurses Association (ANA). (2010). *Nursing: Scope and standards of practice.* Silver Spring, MD: American Nurses Publishing.

American Nurses Association (ANA), American Psychiatric Nurses Association, & International Society of Psychiatric–Mental Health Nurses. (2007). *Psychiatric–mental health nursing: Scope and standards of practice.* Silver Spring, MD: American Nurses Publishing.

American Psychiatric Association. (2000). *Diagnostic and statistical manual of mental disorders* (4th ed., text rev.). Washington, DC: Author.

Bulechek, G. M., Butcher, H. K., & McCloskey Dochterman, J. (2008). *Nursing interventions classification (NIC)* (5th ed.). St. Louis, MO: Mosby.

Evans-Lacko, S. E., Jarrett, M., McCrone, P., & Thornicroft, G. (2008). Clinical pathways in psychiatry. *British Journal of Psychiatry, 193,* 4–5.

Dochterman, J. M., & Jones, D. A. (Eds.). (2003). *Unifying nursing languages: The harmonization of NANDA, NIC, and NOC.* Silver Spring, MD: American Nurses Publishing.

Gulanick, M., & Myers, J. L. (2011). *Nursing care plans: Diagnoses, interventions, and outcomes.* St. Louis, MO: Elsevier Mosby.

Heermann Langford, L. K., Tinker, A., & Martial, M. (2010). A new life for the care plan? *Nursing Management, 41*(12), 22–24.

Johnson, M., Bulechek, G., Butcher, H., Dochterman, J. M., Maas, M., Moorhead, S., & Swanson, E. (Eds.). (2006). *NANDA, NOC, and NIC linkages: Nursing diagnoses, outcomes and interventions* (2nd ed.). St. Louis, MO: Mosby.

Kim, H., Dykes, P. C., Thomas, D., Winfield, L. A., & Rocha, R. A. (2011). A closer look at nursing documentation on paper forms: Preparation for computerizing a nursing documentation system. *Computers in Biology & Medicine, 41*(4), 182–189.

Moorhead, S., Johnson, M., Maas, M. L., & Swanson, E. (2008). *Nursing outcomes classification (NOC)* (4th ed.). St. Louis, MO: Mosby.

NANDA International. (2009). *NANDA International nursing diagnoses: Definitions and classification, 2009–2011.* Philadelphia, PA: Wiley-Blackwell.

North American Nursing Diagnosis Association (NANDA). (1991). The NANDA definition of nursing diagnosis. In R. M. Carroll-Johnson (Ed.), *Classifications of nursing diagnosis: Proceedings of the Ninth Conference* (pp. 65–71). Philadelphia, PA: Lippincott.

Rhoads, J. (2011). *Clinical consult to psychiatric mental health care.* New York, NY: Springer.

Wilkinson, J. M. (2007). *Nursing process and critical thinking* (4th ed.). Upper Saddle River, NJ: Pearson Prentice Hall.

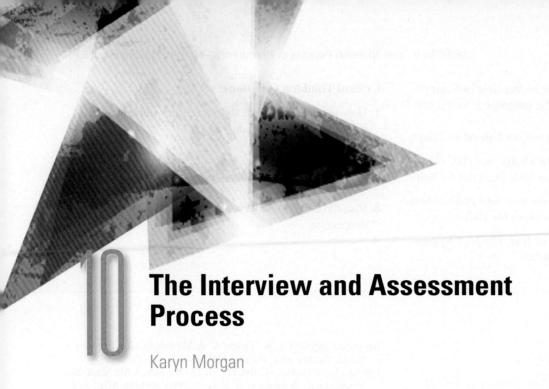

10

The Interview and Assessment Process

Karyn Morgan

KEY TERMS

affect
assessment
data collection
homicidal ideation
mental status examination (MSE)
mood
process recording

LEARNING OBJECTIVES

On completion of this chapter, you should be able to accomplish the following:

- Recognize variables to consider when preparing to interview clients in mental health treatment settings.
- Describe essential elements to include in psychiatric interviews and the assessment process.
- Identify selected standardized tools that health care providers may use to support their clinical observations and assessments.
- Conduct an assessment process with consideration for cultural, spiritual, and other individualized needs of clients.
- Apply critical thinking skills in analyzing psychiatric assessment data.

As noted in *Psychiatric–Mental Health Nursing: Scope and Standards of Practice* (American Nurses Association [ANA], American Psychiatric Nurses Association, & International Society of Psychiatric–Mental Health Nurses, 2007), nurses are committed to promoting mental health through assessment, diagnosis, and treatment of human responses to mental health problems and psychiatric disorders. The psychiatric interview and assessment process are critical elements for appropriate intervention and referral for clients seeking mental health services.

Pursuing this process thoroughly and efficaciously requires not only identification of *what* information to collect but also thoughtful understanding of *how* to establish trust, formulate inquiries, and evaluate the reliability of collected data. This chapter explores variables to consider and elements to include in interviewing, data collection, and identification of health problems requiring nursing intervention.

PREPARATION

Preparation for the psychiatric interview and mental health assessment can influence outcomes significantly. A basic understanding of the difference between data collection and assessment is helpful. **Data collection** refers to the objective data that nurses observe and the subjective data that clients report. **Assessment** more specifically refers to a health care provider's interpretation and prioritization of collected data. Recognizing the difference helps interviewers to avoid drawing premature conclusions or making unsubstantiated claims about a client's health problems. For example, statements such as "the client is depressed" or "the client has poor insight" are interpretations or inferences. Their accuracy depends on supportive data, such as "the client manifests a sad affect, *reports* feeling depressed, and has stopped participating in usual activities" or "the client states he takes his medications even though he doesn't know what they are for," respectively. Other factors that can influence outcomes of psychiatric interviews include the nurse's awareness of his or her own communication style and personal values/beliefs, prior knowledge of the client's health history, and setting for the interview.

Self-Awareness

Currently, no laboratory tests or diagnostic studies can diagnose mental illnesses definitively. Although research continues to explore and make advances in identifying biologic markers that may be diagnostic, at present, clinician interview and assessment remain the most reliable tools (Frances, 2010). The process of interviewing and assessment is a complex interaction of the nurse's communication and behavior with the client's. As nursing theorist Hildegard Peplau advanced more than 50 years ago, the interpersonal relationship between the nurse and the client is the foundation of all therapeutic intervention. This concept remains relevant today and suggests, with regard to assessment, that the nurse's knowledge of self is a critical attribute in conducting interviews that encourage clients to share personal information (see Chap. 8).

In the assessment process, the nurse's knowledge of self requires incorporating self-reflection in addition to analyzing the client's responses to questions and observing the client's behavior. All these elements are interconnected (Forchuk, 1993). For example, anxiety on the nurse's part is one of many factors that can influence outcomes. Often, assessment interviews occur during the orientation phase of the interpersonal relationship (see Chap. 11). Because the nurse and client are new to one another, anxiety may be higher than usual. It is widely recognized that as anxiety increases, the person's ability to focus narrows (Forchuk, 1993). Nurses who begin interviews in a highly anxious state may find it difficult to focus on thorough data collection or interpretation. In addition, because anxiety can be transmitted interpersonally (Forchuk, 1993), an unaware nurse may not consider whether the client's anxiety level appears worse because the nurse's anxiety is contributory (Figure 10.1). Awareness of one's own emotions as well as other factors that influence interpersonal relationships is influential in ongoing personal and professional development and essential to effective client assessment.

Many options and tools for developing self-awareness are available (Freshwater, 2002; Ghaye & Lillyman, 2009; Kuiper & Pesut, 2004). The **process recording** provides a written analysis of each interactional exchange with clients to assist nurses to recognize the effects of their communication style. Videotaping or audiotaping (done only with proper written consents from clients) can assist the nurse's recall and evaluation. Ultimately, self-review and self-awareness aid in exploring *alternative* communication and behaviors for improving interactions. One example is that of a student who couldn't understand why a client seemed to "shut down" and not want to communicate further during an assessment interview. In writing the process recording, the student recognized that the client could have interpreted several of the nurse's statements as judgmental. She recognized that she

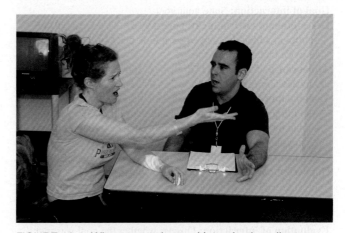

FIGURE 10.1 When assessing and interviewing clients, nurses must remain self-aware about how their own reactions and levels of anxiety may be contributing negatively to interactions. An unaware nurse may compound a client's emotional reaction.

was imposing her values and beliefs on the client and that this may have contributed to the client's unwillingness to continue the interaction. This new awareness enabled the student to explore alternative responses to improve nonjudgmental communication. Similarly, a review of literature about physician–client interactions identified that communication training improved the ability of clinicians to encourage disclosure from clients, as well as to identify their cues and concerns (Zimmerman et al., 2007). Such research lends support to the idea that self-awareness and strong communication skills not only may encourage clients to share information, but also are critical to adequate assessment (Box 10.1).

Supervision by a more experienced clinician is also beneficial in helping nurses to develop self-awareness. This process involves nurses seeking and accepting feedback based on someone else's interpretation of their behavior and communication. It can be difficult sometimes because it requires a measure of vulnerability to explore the viewpoint of others about personal relational skills. In many cases, nurses may have little insight about the impressions they make or how they appear to others. The supervisory process is an expected part of a student nurse's education (between instructor and student), but practicing professionals also can benefit from ongoing supervision and feedback.

Use of various expressive arts such as music, poetry, drawing/painting, or journaling may also serve as tools for self-reflection. The ideal outcome of all self-awareness tools is to identify and manage personal variables that may affect the nurse's ability to relate to, collect information from, and effectively determine the client's health care needs. See also Chapter 8.

BOX 10.1 Process Recording Format

Client's initials:
Age:

Nursing diagnosis:
Goal of interaction: State your goal.
Description of environment: Give a visual description of the setting in which the conversation took place, including noise level and odors.
Appearance of the client: Give a description of the client's physical appearance.
Verbal communication: State the communication verbatim, including what the client states and your responses. List in sequential order and identify therapeutic and nontherapeutic techniques used during the conversation. Identify any defense mechanisms used by the client.
Nonverbal communication: Include your thoughts and feelings, as well as any facial expressions, gestures, position changes, or changes in eye contact, voice quality, and voice tone by the client or yourself.
Evaluation of interaction: Discuss whether the goal was met. What changes would you make, if any, after evaluating this interaction?

Review of the Client's History

Nurses may conduct assessment interviews at different points of service during a client's treatment. When they encounter clients during a triage assessment (eg, in an emergency department), they may have little background or historical information. In other circumstances, nurses conduct assessments of clients whom other health care professionals from various settings have already seen and treated. In these circumstances, nurses may have access (with the client's written consent) to a wealth of information about the client's history that they can use as a foundation for comparison and further assessment. Nurses need to be familiar with current laws as established in the Health Insurance Portability and Accountability Act, because these address legal parameters for sharing and receiving information from resources other than clients.

In all circumstances, the nurse's understanding of the client's health history is helpful in preparing the interview setting, guiding the interview, and making recommendations for further care. Previous medical or surgical problems, psychiatric hospitalizations, psychotropic medications, and counseling interventions are just a few key components that can provide clues about which interventions have been successful or unsuccessful. Information about any family history of mental illness and suicidal tendencies can provide valuable information in assessing current risks. Historical data about the client's behavioral responses to intervention (eg, past verbal or physical aggression) can serve as important considerations when making decisions about where and how to conduct the interview in a way that minimizes risks for nurses and clients.

Think About It 10.1
Police bring a woman to the emergency department because she was shouting and screaming threateningly at people walking in and out of a local coffee shop. The woman is dressed in torn, ragged, and stained clothing. Dirt and soot cover her hands and face. She wears mismatched shoes and socks, both of which have numerous tears. How might the nurse's degree of self-awareness affect assessment of this client?

Setting Preparation

As noted, assessment interviews can produce anxiety because they often occur during the orientation phase of the nurse–client relationship (see Chap. 11). Thus, it is beneficial for nurses to consider the environment and other variables that may minimize stress for both parties.

The client's right to privacy is an essential setting consideration. It is an ethical responsibility of the nurse and a legal right of the client (see Chap. 5). Nurses must make critical clinical judgments about the optimal setting that maintains privacy while also ensuring safety. A small conference room may provide excellent privacy but may be threatening to clients with paranoia. In such a case, options may include leaving the door open, choosing a larger room, or interviewing the client in a private day lounge area. For comfort and safety, nurses should always sit in a location with easy access to an exit.

Another aspect to consider is seating arrangements. It is generally accepted that the least threatening arrangement is to sit at an angle to the client, rather than face to face (MacKinnon et al., 2006; Shea, 1998; Sommers-Flanagan & Sommers-Flanagan, 2009). This position enables but does not force eye contact (at eye level). Nurses also must consider whether they need to work at a desk during the interview and, if so, the most appropriate placement. Clinicians vary on their recommendations. Some clinicians feel that sitting behind a desk conveys that the nurse is an authority figure, whereas sitting beside the desk at an angle to the client conveys more intimacy (Shea, 1998) (Figure 10.2).

Proximity to the client is also a consideration. Although in general, 4 to 5 feet apart is what most clinician trainees identify as a comfortable seating arrangement (Shea, 1998), nurses may also arrange a few different seating options (that are comfortable for nurses) and allow clients to choose among them. This provides some insight into the client's comfort level with regard to proxemics.

Lighting that is too bright and objects of distraction (eg, paintings, colorful curtains) can interfere with the conduct of the interview. For some clients (eg, those with anxiety, mania, or cognitive disorders), these otherwise pleasant focal points can become monumental distractions. As noted, access to the client's history or presenting symptoms prior to the interview can be useful in preparing a setting tailored to the client's individual needs.

Checkpoint Questions

1. What is the foundation of all therapeutic intervention?
2. What is the purpose of a process recording?

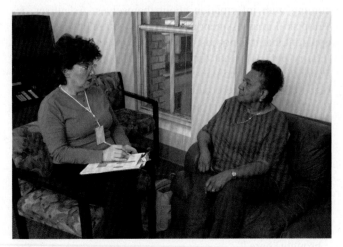

FIGURE 10.2 **Nurses arrange seating arrangements for interviews and assessments that consider the purpose of the discussion, the client's condition and level of comfort, and setting.**

CONTENT OF THE ASSESSMENT

Little evidence-based research within the nursing literature supports a single "best practice" for identifying and structuring the content to collect in a psychiatric–mental health assessment. While research from physicians and psychologists may be more prevalent, such studies are primarily for the purpose of ensuring that the content and process of assessment lead to an accurate *medical* diagnosis (Calinoiu & McClellan, 2004; Thibault & Prassad Steiner, 2004). Within the scope of *nursing* practice (ANA et al., 2007), assessment is geared toward identifying not only manifestations of mental health problems, but also unhealthy responses to actual or potential psychiatric illness. Although professionals from different disciplines may collect the same or similar data, it is the focus on accurate assessment of unhealthy client responses that more specifically defines nursing's purpose.

Variables to consider when structuring the content of the nursing assessment include structured versus semistructured formats, the client's ability and reliability in responding to questions, and clinician skill in identifying relevant information. Of course the less structured the interview, the more reliance there is on the nurse's skill in determining what information to collect and how best to formulate relevant questions. Further, when the reliability of the client's responses is questionable, various tools, including standardized psychological tests, also may be valuable. Although student nurses often express anxiety about wanting to know "the right way to ask something" or "the right thing to say" to clients, there are many equally acceptable options for how to formulate assessment questions. The details and suggestions provided here assume a novice practitioner (Benner, 2000). As such, nurses can modify them as they develop knowledge, skill, experience in the assessment process, and their own communication style.

The PERSONS acronym is one framework for identifying essential data to collect during the initial interview (Assessment Tool 10.1).

Although additional information may be necessary, depending on the treatment setting and the client's individual needs, the aspects of the PERSONS tool provide a basic foundation for identifying issues related to presenting problems, client safety, and areas needing further assessment. The order in which nurses collect these data is often a matter of preference and style, but nurses should consider which aspects might be most threatening for clients and discuss such aspects with clients later in the assessment process, allowing time for the orientation phase of the relationship to progress.

Figure 10.3 provides a sample structure for the psychiatric interview form completed for a client with depression. Each aspect of data collection reviewed in the following sections gives attention to describing what kinds of data nurses need to collect, sample questions, and the rationale for collecting this information to complete a nursing assessment.

▲ A S S E S S M E N T   T O O L   1 0 . 1 ▲

PERSONS Acronym for Identifying Major Aspects of Psychiatric–Mental Health Nursing Assessment

P—Perceptions of the client, Presenting symptoms, Previous psychiatric treatment, Previous medication, Previous medical illness, Precipitating events, Physical Assessment

E—Educational background, Employment background, Environment of home life

R—Relationships (with family, significant others, support systems), Review of systems

S—Substance use and abuse

O—Objective observations (of thought content, thought processes, mood/affect and behavior, physical examination), Obstacles to treatment (including financial and environmental)

N—Needs that are specialized (language, hearing, reading/writing, cultural, spiritual)

S—Safety assessment (suicide potential, homicidal ideation, victimization issues such as abuse or neglect)

Copyright © 2007 by K. I. Morgan. Used by permission of the author.

Health History

Even when nurses have access to previous health history documents, it is wise to explore the client's perspective on these issues in each initial assessment. Because clients subjectively report much of the data collected in the health history, their recall of events may differ over time, their perspective may change, or both. When it is possible (within the limits of privacy laws) to obtain information from family members or other secondary sources, nurses should ask these questions of them as well. This can be an important opportunity to check the accuracy and reliability of information obtained from clients. For clients with thought disturbances, psychotic features, or both, secondary sources can be pivotal in accurate interpretation of responses.

Initial Information

Orienting clients to the purposes of the interview provides nurses with an opportunity to begin establishing trust and can provide insight about clients' reactions to being interviewed (Box 10.2).

An example might be to say, *"I'm going to ask you several questions about your background and current concerns so you and I can determine your health care needs."* Notice the nurse's message that the determination of the client's health care needs is a collaborative process. It may also be helpful to encourage clients to feel free to share any information that they think would be beneficial for nurses to know about their health concerns. This, too, offers clients an initial opportunity to identify their important concerns and to reassure them that they are active participants in this assessment.

Obtaining information about the client's medical diagnosis prior to the assessment may help in some respects. However, some consider this controversial, suggesting that it may bias the interviewer's perception about how to interpret current behaviors and responses of the client (Scheff, 1975). In a classic study, Rosenhan (1973) demonstrated that when eight people were admitted to a treatment setting with a fabricated diagnosis, health professionals' subsequent

assessments supported the existence of that diagnosis (see Chap. 8). Many classic writings on the topic of psychiatric labels suggest that health professionals at least need to be aware of the potential for bias so that they continually focus efforts on ensuring objectivity in data collection.

Reason for Seeking Health Care

The client's perception about primary concerns and needs for health care intervention is important information to collect initially in the interview process. Some suggested questions about this issue include the following:

- "Tell me about your most important, current concerns."
- "Tell me about your reasons for seeking health care at this time."
- "What's been happening in the recent past that brings you here?"

The rationale for including these data is to help nurses begin to understand the perspective of clients, their insight into illness-related events, and their willingness to be forthcoming with information about themselves. As nurses develop skill in assessment and communication, it will become apparent that it is not just what clients *say* in response to this inquiry but also what their verbal and nonverbal responses *imply* that guide the nurse's follow-up questions. For example, a client may respond that she doesn't believe she needs to be in this treatment setting or doesn't have any current illnesses. This is sometimes the case with clients who have paranoia. It is almost always the case when someone has been admitted involuntarily for treatment. Never challenge the client's response to this inquiry. Remember that it *is* the client's perspective. Some options for response that convey concern without challenging the client's perspective are as follows:

- "What was happening right before you arrived (or were brought) here?"
- "I'd like to ask some more questions about recent events so we can figure out what led to your being brought here and how I can best help you."

Name Jane Doe   **Age** 30   **Date** 3/10/09   **Marital Status** Recently divorced

Referred by Dr. R. Morgan, primary care physician   **Release signed for contact** Yes

Client's Perception of Main Problem "I've been feeling depressed ever since my husband left, and I told my doctor I don't want to live anymore."

Current Symptoms Reports sleeping 12–14 hours/day for past 3 weeks, doesn't "feel like doing anything," reports feeling hopeless and had stolen sister's antidepressant with intent to take a lethal dose, decreased appetite, lost 15 lb (6.8 kg) in 1 month

Precipitating Factors Divorce was finalized 4 weeks ago after a 10-year marriage

Current Treatment Denies prescription medications or other treatments

Allergies No known allergies

Substance Use Denies illicit drug use, reports drinking three 12 oz (354.8 mL) cans of beer/day for past week c. last alcohol consumption 3 hours ago, smokes cigarettes ½ ppd for 15 years, reports taking OTC diet pills "can't remember the name or dose," CAGE score +2

PAST ILLNESS

Psychiatric Denies previous hospitalization, reports saw a counselor 10 years ago while in college r/t depression after a relationship break–up

Medical Appendectomy 1996, DVT, 2003- hospitalized and treated with Coumadin

Family History Father died in 1995 from liver failure secondary to alcoholism, mother has a history of depression, sister currently on antidepressant therapy for depression, denies any family history of suicide attempts, denies awareness of other medical illness in family members

Personal History Reports father was physically and verbally abusive toward her mother through most of her childhood. States she feels close to her sister and to her mother but "can't expect them to help now because they have their own problems." States her ex-husband is also an alcoholic and was verbally abusive throughout their marriage. Denies history of physical abuse, currently lives alone, identifies no other friends or support systems, currently employed for past 8 years at User Friendly, Inc where she does computer programming, denies problems at work but recently has lost interest in her job.

REVIEW OF SYSTEMS

Respiratory Reports shortness of breath on exertion which she attributes to smoking

Cardiovascular History of deep vein thrombosis, denies current symptoms

Gastrointestinal Reports loss of appetite and weight loss over the past month, recent constipation

Urogenital Denies complaints

Sexuality Reports not sexually active in the last 4 years of marriage, no children, never pregnant, denies history of STDs, denies history of sexual abuse

Sleep and Rest Reports 12–14 h of sleep per day for past 3 weeks, "always feel tired," "wake up early and can't go back to sleep"

MENTAL STATUS

Appearance and Behavior Tearful throughout the interview, sighing, hair is uncombed and matted, little eye contact maintained, slouched posture, clothing is wrinkled and stained, appears thin, weighs 100 lb (45.3 kg) and is 5'4" tall

Level of Consciousness Alert and Oriented X 3

Mood Reports feeling sad, depressed, and hopeless

Affect: Flat ___ **Blunted** ___ **Sad** X **Happy** ___ **Elated** ___ **Anxious** ___ **Angry** ___ **Incongruent with verbal content** ___

Speech Slow and at times barely audible with little variation in tone

Thought Processes Coherent but pt. is slow to respond

Thought Content Expresses hopelessness and helplessness, no evidence of delusions

Perceptions Reports c/o pain that moves to different locations but currently in her neck and rates the pain as "5" on a scale of 1–10, denies any other unusual sensations, self medicating for pain with aspirin

Insight and Judgment States " I know I need help" and "I gave the medication back to my sister," but also reports this was after her sister confronted her about the missing pills

Cognitive Functions Recent and remote memory intact, completed college degree in Computer Science, denies learning disabilities, enies difficulty reading or writing

FIGURE 10.3 An assessment form completed for a client with depression admitted to an inpatient psychiatric unit.

(continued)

SUICIDE POTENTIAL

Ideas Y_____ **Current** Yes_____ **Past** Denies_____

Plans Y_____ **If yes, specify** Overdose on antidepressants_____

Intentions States "I don't think I would do it because I believe it's a sin" but states "I might feel differently tomorrow."_____

Access to Means Reports sister took all medication away from pt._____

Attempts N_____ **Recent** Denies_____ **Past** Denies_____

Alcohol/ Drugs Yes_____

Panic Attacks Denies_____

Family History Denies_____

Dangerousness or Homicidal Ideation No known history of aggressive or violent behavior, denies homicidal ideas_____

Cultural Issues States that she is uncomfortable with touch and that she doesn't like people to "get too close," sitting 4 feet from interviewer and states this is a comfortable distance_____

Spiritual Issues Reports belief in God and historically has found comfort in prayer but "lately I can't even do that"_____

ASSESSMENT

The presenting problem is depression with suicidal ideation and a plan but no attempt. This is supported by subjective report and objective evaluation of clinical presentation. Jane expresses hopelessness and helplessness although she identifies that she knows she needs help. Her continued ideation, lack of identified support systems, and expressed hopelessness and helplessness warrant close observation and suicide precautions.

Recent increase in alcohol consumption, CAGE score of +2, and family history of alcoholism warrant further screening, education and referral for CD consult.

Refer to dietician for nutritional consult r/t recent weight loss.

Physical assessment issues requiring further evaluation:

Current SOB with history of DVT, and 15 year history of smoking cigarettes.

Pain Assessment for complaints of "shifting pain"; currently 5 on a 10 point scale.

FIGURE 10.3 *(continued)*

> ### BOX 10.2 Tips for Interviewing Clients With Psychiatric Disorders
>
> • Find a quiet and private place for the interview where both you and the client can sit, if possible.
> • Introduce yourself with your name and title. Ask the client how he or she wants to be addressed.
> • Let the client know how much time you have before beginning. If your time is limited, obtain priority information first and return later for the remainder of information.
> • Avoid the use of diagnostic labels or jargon if possible. For instance, "When did you first notice that you had become more active?" is better than "When did you first become manic?"
> • Allow the client to tell his or her "story" without interrupting or trying to structure the information.
> • Use active listening; show that you are hearing what is being said. Link your questions to what the client just said. For example, "Just now you mentioned that no one is there for you and that you are feeling hopeless. How long have you felt this way?"
> • Use open-ended questions such as "Tell me more..." or "How did that happen?"
> • If there are cues that something is wrong, ask about them. For example, "I can see that you seem uncomfortable when we talk about your girlfriend. What can you tell me about your relationship with her?"

Other clients may have insight about their primary concern. An example is the client who responds, "I'm here because I've been depressed for several years and lately it's gotten worse. I've been thinking a lot about wanting to die." This provides a logical segue to explore further the client's *present illness*.

Present Illness

Encouraging clients to describe the present illness includes identifying current symptoms, precipitating factors, the client's perception of how these symptoms are affecting the current situation, and current treatments. It is helpful to use focused questions to collect this information. Examples include the following:

• "What kinds of changes in your thoughts, emotions, or behavior have you been concerned about?"
• "Are you aware of any recent events that may have triggered these symptoms?"
• "Tell me about any recent events that may have triggered these symptoms."
• "How are these changes affecting your ability to function in your usual activities?"
• "What medications are you currently taking?"
• "What other things have you been doing to try to combat these symptoms?"

Focused, present-oriented questions encourage clients to discuss what's happening now, rather than in the remote past. The nurse's awareness of the need to ask present-oriented questions is critical to obtaining data and to recognizing the need to refocus clients who begin to dwell on remote history. Present-oriented data provide nurses with key information about unhealthy responses to actual or potential problems. Such findings provide the foundation for determining nursing diagnoses.

Medications

When collecting data about current medications, nurses should inquire not only about prescribed drugs but also over-the-counter (OTC) and alternative remedies such as herbal supplements. Clients may not list these without prompting because they lack awareness of the potential for these remedies to interfere with or potentiate their prescribed medications. A thorough list of all ingested substances is critical for physicians and advanced practice nurses when decisions are being made about which medications and dosages to prescribe and in evaluating the effectiveness of current treatments.

Nurses should make every effort to ensure that data they collect about medications are accurate and thorough. Asking clients if they have pill bottles or a list of their current medications with them provides nurses with information to validate client reports (Figure 10.4). Clients who are presenting with anxiety, difficulty concentrating, or memory deficits are especially at risk for not being able to recall these details. Obtaining written consent from clients to allow nurses to talk to family members, other prescribing health professionals, or both can be helpful in filling in information gaps.

Drug Allergies

Collecting information about a client's drug allergies is basic to safe nursing practice and is a standard aspect of data collection in any initial nursing assessment. However, clients don't always recognize which of their responses to medications may indicate allergies. Clients also may experience symptoms that they refer to as "allergic" reactions, which

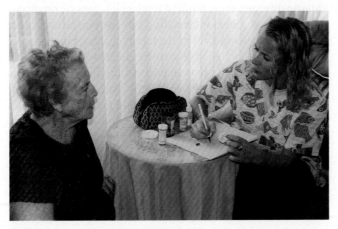

FIGURE 10.4 It is helpful for clients to bring their current pill bottles or a list of current medications with them to the initial assessment.

in fact are idiosyncratic or adverse reactions to a medication. For these reasons it is beneficial, in addition to asking if clients have any known drug allergies, to inquire about how they are responding to the medication and if they've had any troubling symptoms since they began taking particular drugs. For example, consider a client who reports he is "allergic to haloperidol." When the nurse asks him to describe his symptoms, the client reports that he stopped taking it because it made him sleepy. The nurse now has information that disconfirms an allergic response, but does confirm a troubling symptom and provides the fact that the client has stopped taking his prescribed medication. It is well understood that nonadherence to psychotropic medication regimens is a common contributing factor to recidivism or relapse. Thus, collecting information about allergies, troubling symptoms, and compliance issues is critical to safe practice (to identify true allergies or adverse reactions) and to assessing the client's need for medication education.

Substance Use

In addition to inquiring about prescribed medication, OTC drugs, and alternative or herbal remedies, nurses assess for the use of other mood-altering substances, which include alcohol, illicit drugs, tobacco, and caffeine. They can advance various questions to obtain information about current use and associated risks. Some examples include the following:

- "How often do you drink alcohol (take drugs, smoke tobacco, etc.)?"
- "How much do you drink (use, smoke, etc.) in a typical day?"
- "When was your last drink (use)?"

Nurses should be cautious about accepting the responses of clients to these questions at face value. Clients who are abusing or addicted to substances may experience guilt, shame, or fear of consequences associated with their use. For these reasons they may minimize or deny their use. MacKinnon and colleagues (2006) add that those with substance use disorders often deceive health care professionals because they are seeking more drugs. Standardized screening tools and drug tests (ie, of urine, breath, or serum) are especially helpful in clarifying issues.

Collecting information about substance use is certainly useful for the purpose of identifying substances that may interfere with prescribed mood-altering medications. However, an even more critical reason is related to the potentially fatal consequences of untreated alcohol or drug withdrawal. A short screening tool such as the CAGE screening questionnaire can be useful at the outset to identify whether alcohol use is problematic (see Chap. 30). Asking clients with suspected alcohol abuse when they had their last drink gives nurses the opportunity to identify how soon to expect withdrawal symptoms to appear (early symptoms may become apparent as early as 6 to 12 hours after the last drink), initiate further assessment if withdrawal symptoms are an imminent concern, or intervene as soon as this concern becomes apparent.

Once alcohol withdrawal is suspected, a screening tool such as the Clinical Institute Withdrawal Assessment of Alcohol Scale Revised (CIWA-R) can assist nurses to identify the severity of symptoms (see Chap. 30). Many other options for screening tools to assist in such data collection are available, but it is critical in the initial assessment to identify alcohol use and potential for withdrawal. Identified abuse issues also may warrant referral to specialists in chemical dependence education and treatment.

A third rationale for collecting data about substance use in the initial assessment is that many drugs may precipitate psychosis, either during acute intoxication or during withdrawal. In withdrawal states, alcohol and sedative/hypnotic drugs may precipitate psychotic features. During acute intoxication, PCP and amphetamines may manifest these symptoms. Recent research connects marijuana use to psychotic episodes and suggests that genetically predisposed people may be at increased risk for manifestations of schizophrenia (Rey, 2007). Considering all the listed rationales, it should be apparent that collecting information about substance use is critical to accurate diagnosis and to identifying critical safety issues. It is also important in identifying comorbidity (eg, concurrent substance use and bipolar disorders) that may require education, specialized intervention, or both.

Checkpoint Questions

3. What is the focus of a nursing assessment?

4. Why is obtaining information from family members and secondary sources important?

5. What is one reason to collect information about substance use during the initial assessment?

Past Illnesses

Collecting data about past illnesses includes past episodes of psychiatric and medical–surgical illnesses. It is helpful when inquiring about historical information to ask not only about the illnesses but also about previous treatments (including medications), treatment settings, and outcomes. Because this history is a "who, what, where, when" summary, details can become cumbersome and difficult to organize without a very structured approach. Nurses may wish to visually represent these data in a chronologic timeline format (see Figure 10.3).

Sample inquiries include the following:

- "Tell me when you were last treated for (a mental health problem)."
- "What treatment did you receive?"
- "How effective was this treatment?"
- "When did you first get treatment for (a mental health problem)?"
- "Tell me about any medical or surgical problems you've experienced."

Some health care settings have structured forms for clients to self-report this information; nurses can then focus inquiries on clarifying and filling in any information gaps.

The obvious rationale for collecting this information in an initial assessment is to determine what treatments have been implemented and the client's perception about effectiveness. Nurses also use this information to assess the appropriate level of care needed currently. For example, if a client has had several episodes of outpatient counseling without effective outcomes, these data can support the need for a higher level of care (eg, partial hospitalization, intensive outpatient counseling).

In addition, looking at medical and psychiatric history concurrently can provide important cues about the dynamic interaction between these aspects of well-being (see Chap. 39). Many medical illnesses can manifest with psychiatric symptoms. Examples include thyroid disorders, diabetes, stroke, or traumatic head injuries. Likewise, psychiatric illness may significantly affect physical health. Some psychotropic medications can increase risks for diabetes or blood dyscrasias. Further, current research supports that in geriatric populations anxiety is more likely to be expressed as medical rather than psychiatric symptoms (Bassil et al., 2011). The complex interaction of physical and psychiatric disorders makes a thorough physical examination with appropriate diagnostic testing essential to care.

Family History

Collecting information about the family history includes a review of significant medical and psychiatric issues. Sample inquiries include the following:

- "Have any family members been diagnosed with a mental illness?"
- "Tell me about any significant medical illnesses among your immediate family members."
- "Is there anyone in your immediate or extended family who has attempted or successfully completed a suicide?"

The primary rationale for collecting this information is to assess risks of illness or suicide for *this* client. Many psychiatric illnesses show familial tendencies, genetic predispositions, or both. Such information can cue nurses to explore symptoms further in light of the family history. For example, a client reports to the nurse that she is feeling depressed and manifests symptoms that support depression. However, as the nurse explores the client's family history, he learns that the client's mother, maternal aunt, and a cousin have been diagnosed with bipolar disorder. This information prompts the nurse to explore in more detail whether the client has any history of mood swings and to note this family history as a significant positive finding.

With regard to assessing family history of suicidal behavior, Shea (1998) notes that family members can model suicidal behavior and that when this occurs, the client may be at greater risk of similar behaviors. Consequently, a positive family history should alert nurses to be thorough in asking clients specific questions about their own history of suicidal ideas.

Personal and Social History

Review of the client's personal and social history provides an opportunity for discussion of significant *past* events. Some clinicians prefer to ask general questions that allow clients to address those issues significant from their perspective. For example, a nurse may inquire "Tell me about your background" or "How would you describe your life growing up?" Often clients start by describing issues that stand out for them. Nurses can encourage further description by asking more focused questions, such as "Were you close with your siblings?" or "Tell me more about who you feel closest to among your family or friends." At a minimum, this aspect of data collection should include educational background, work history, and significant relationships/support systems.

Such information is important because it can signal how significantly individual and family illnesses have affected a client's general functioning in work, school, and relationships. Exploring educational background can reveal previously undisclosed information about learning disabilities or intellectual limitations. Background information on social relationships and support systems can provide information about whether the client has ever had close bonds with specific people or if significant events interfered with interpersonal relationships. Knowing the client's previous functional ability in these important areas is basic to assessing adaptations needed in care planning and the need for referral. In the current health care environment, clients may be involved with a particular level of care for only a few days, so collecting data about the client's resources for functioning and support can be critical in assessing and deciding about safety when referring clients to a less restrictive level of care.

On a deeper level, personal and social information can be used to better understand a client's personality development. Knowledge about the frameworks of developmental theorists (such as Erikson, Maher, Piaget, and Peplau) can help nurses identify issues related to unfulfilled developmental tasks that may be pursued further in a therapy setting.

Review of Systems

The review of systems is a structured series of interview questions that encourage clients to report system-specific symptoms that may be connected to their mental health and physical well-being. One approach is to methodically ask the client about each system. Examples include the following:

- "Do you have any cuts, bruises or scars?" (Integumentary)
- "Do you have any heart conditions? High blood pressure? Palpitations?" (Cardiovascular)
- "Do you have any breathing problems? Shortness of breath?" (Respiratory)
- "Have you had any recent constipation, diarrhea, or weight changes?" (Gastrointestinal)

MacKinnon and colleagues (2006) note that every review of systems for psychiatric clients should include statements about sleep patterns, appetite and weight changes, bowel functioning, and sexual functioning. Disruptions in these areas are common among people with mental and emotional illness. For example, sleep disruption can be symptomatic of some mental illnesses; it also can interfere with treatment response (Assessment Tool 10.2).

Other physical signs may raise suspicion of specific disorders. Appetite and weight changes are common in clients with depression, anxiety, and eating disorders. Constipation often accompanies depression or may be a side effect of psychotropic medication. Diarrhea may accompany anxiety disorders. Sexual functioning may be disrupted in clients with histories of sexual trauma or abuse.

Note that nurses collect these and all data described thus far based on client report. Some health care settings have preprinted forms that pose these questions and that clients complete independently. In other settings, nurses may collect this information through interview. It is most important to recognize that data collection does not replace the objective evaluation of systems obtained through physical examination; rather, it is adjunctive. Its importance in the initial assessment is to identify immediate concerns requiring attention and as a screening tool.

Checkpoint Questions

6. What is the most important reason for collecting information about the client's family history?

7. What part of the initial health history provides information to aid in understanding a person's personality development?

ASSESSMENT TOOL 10.2

Brief Review of Sleep Patterns

1. Average hours/night _____
2. Routine times _____ Variable routine _____ No routine _____
3. Difficulty Falling Asleep _____ Staying Asleep _____ Early AM wakening _____
4. Nightmares _____ Night Terrors _____ Sleepwalking _____
5. Sleep Apnea _____ Snoring _____
6. Sedative/Hypnotic Medications (name, dose, duration of use, effectiveness):
   _____
   _____

Physical Examination

Typically, physicians or nurse practitioners complete a physical examination. However, psychiatric nurses still assume a critical role in basic physical examination to identify immediate problems and apparent physical symptoms. Several symptoms could be manifestations of psychiatric illness, other medical illnesses, or both (Table 10.1) (see Chap. 39). Thus, clear, objective report of examination findings provides a foundation for further assessment and diagnostic testing.

TABLE 10.1 Physical Assessment Findings That May Be Psychiatric or Medical in Origin

Common Physical Examination Findings	Associated Psychiatric Conditions	Medical Conditions with Similar Symptoms
Neurologic		
Tremors	Somatoform disorders Alcohol use Alcohol withdrawal Delirium tremens Anxiety	Hyperthyroidism Hypoglycemia Multiple sclerosis Parkinson's disease
Agitation	Alcohol use Alcohol withdrawal Anxiety disorders Attention deficit hyperactivity disorder (ADHD) Manic episode Schizophrenia	Asthma COPD Hypertension Pulmonary edema Salicylate poisoning
Short-term memory loss	Alcohol use ADHD Depression Somatoform disorders	Alzheimer's disease Hypothyroidism Obstructive sleep apnea Postconcussion syndrome Parkinson's disease Seizure disorders
Integumentary		
Cuts, bruises, scars	Self-inflicted wounds Abuse High-risk behavior	Bleeding disorders Blood dyscrasias
Hair thinning or loss	Anorexia nervosa Trichotillomania	Hypothyroidism Cirrhosis of the liver
Head, Eyes, Ears, Nose, Throat		
Dilated pupils	CNS stimulants Hallucinogens Alcohol use	Stroke Ventricular fibrillation Hypothermia
Constricted pupils	Narcotics	Stroke
Nosebleeds	Cocaine snorting	Common colds Sinusitis Hypertension Leukemia
Dental caries	Bulimia nervosa	Sialadenitis
Vital Signs		
Increased blood pressure	Anxiety	Angina
Increased pulse	Alcohol withdrawal	Hypertension Stroke
Elevated temperature		Neuroleptic malignant syndrome
Shortness of breath	Anxiety	Asthma Myocardial infarction Allergic reactions

Common Physical Examination Findings	Associated Psychiatric Conditions	Medical Conditions with Similar Symptoms
Gastrointestinal		
Loss of appetite	Depression	Cholecystitis Appendicitis
Weight loss	Anorexia nervosa Depression	Diabetes Hepatitis Hodgkin's disease Hyperthyroidism Intestinal parasites
Weight gain	Bulimia nervosa Depression	Hypothyroidism Congestive heart failure Acute renal failure
Nausea and vomiting	Alcohol use Anxiety Anorexia nervosa	Appendicitis Cholecystitis Irritable bowel syndrome Gastroenteritis Myocardial infarction
Diarrhea	Alcohol use Anorexia nervosa Anxiety	Hyperthyroidism Irritable bowel syndrome Intestinal parasites Pancreatitis
Constipation	Anorexia nervosa (laxative abuse) Depression	Hypothyroidism Irritable bowel syndrome Ulcerative colitis Parkinson's disease
Genitourinary		
Erectile dysfunction	Alcohol use	Diabetes Arteriosclerosis Hypothyroidism Adverse drug reactions
Difficulty with intercourse	Post-traumatic stress disorder Somatoform disorder	Chronic fatigue syndrome Sexually transmitted infection Endometriosis

Note that physical examination relies heavily on inspection, palpation, percussion, and auscultation (Estes, 2009). Subsequently, it is critical for nurses to be sensitive to the client's comfort level with procedures that require physical contact. Orienting clients to the procedure and asking their permission before approaching or touching them are advised. If a client refuses any aspect of assessment, the nurse should document this and reattempt later when the client may be more amenable.

Current research has focused on increased mortality rates in clients with mental illness related to weight gain, smoking, cardiovascular disease, and diabetes. One study notes that people with major mental illness typically lose between 13 and 30 years of normal lifespan, and that approximately 60% of premature deaths are related to natural causes, rather than suicide or injury (Colton & Manderscheid, 2006). These staggering statistics highlight the importance of intertwining physical and mental health care. Parameters such as blood pressure, waist circumference screening, monitoring of weight change, and serum levels for cholesterol, triglycerides, and glucose are critical indicators (Figure 10.5).

The importance of careful questioning about physical symptoms and physical assessment cannot be overemphasized. Consider the following examples:

- A client frequently reports to an emergency department and is known as a homeless person with chronic schizophrenia. On this visit his speech is garbled, and he "appears to be hallucinating." On the surface, it appears to be an acute exacerbation of schizophrenia, but careful physical assessment reveals that he has had a stroke.
- A client who has been diagnosed with undifferentiated schizophrenia expresses frequent delusions and hallucinations that a "rock band" rehearses in her head. Later she

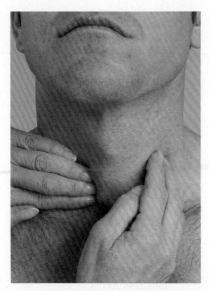

FIGURE 10.5 Because of the common overlap between physical and mental illnesses, thorough physical examinations of clients are necessary to ensure appropriate diagnosis and optimal treatment. For example, the nurse would check the client's thyroid gland to detect any preliminary abnormalities that might point to a physical or medical cause for psychiatric symptoms.

reports to the nurse that the band has moved to her chest and the drummer is pounding hard. Physical assessment reveals that the client has had a heart attack.

In each example, health care providers could easily mistake the symptoms of life-threatening emergency as psychiatric manifestations. These examples also speak to the concern that when clients have a known psychiatric illness, they may be at risk for inaccurate assumptions about the nature of their complaints. Careful physical examination not only promotes accurate assessment but also protects clients by combating the stigmatizing (and false) notion that all symptoms for clients with mental illness are psychiatric in nature.

Mental Status Examination

The **mental status examination (MSE)** is a central aspect of the psychiatric assessment process that assesses current cognitive and affective functioning through data collection on appearance, behavior, level of consciousness, speech, thought content and processes, cognitive ability, mood and affect, insight, and judgment. This assessment relies almost exclusively on observation, rather than inquiry, and is expected to change during treatment. Despite the central importance of this aspect in understanding the client's mental functions, there is a general lack of standardization for what to include and how to conduct this evaluation. MacKinnon and colleagues (2006) note that this has led to increased reliance on formal rating scales. One such widely used standardized tool is Folstein's Mini-Mental Status Examination, which focuses on assessing cognitive functions through a series of 11 cognitive tasks assigned to the client (Folstein

et al., 1975). This tool, which measures cognitive function in several domains, including time orientation, short-term memory recall, serial sevens, reading, writing, drawing, and verbal/motor comprehension, is most useful in screening for cognitive impairments seen in dementia and delirium (see Chap. 31).

Although nurses often use standardized tools as adjuncts to assessment, they still rely heavily on general communication and observation skills in practice. To adequately screen for various mental health problems, psychiatric nurses need to recognize the significance of the client's verbal/nonverbal communication, behavior, appearance, and cognitive abilities to assess how he or she is thinking or feeling. They must also recognize certain behaviors and communication patterns that are common symptoms of thought or affect disturbance. As such, they are collecting and observing these data throughout the interview, rather than in a separate interview section.

Note again the distinction between data collection and assessment. If nurses document opinions and inferences rather than objective observations when conducting a MSE, their assessment conclusions are not reliable. The following sections explore each aspect of the MSE to describe what to look for (data) and possible interpretations (assessment).

Appearance and Behavior

From the first moment of interaction with clients, nurses observe appearance and behavior that can signal disturbances in mental status. Nurses should document crying, twitching, scratching or picking at one's skin, clenched fists, or repeated behaviors (Figure 10.6). They should consider "What am I seeing?" and develop awareness about "What do I expect to see?" Exploring both questions encourages them to reflect on how their own expectations may affect their powers of observation.

For example, the nurse is interviewing a young Hispanic woman who appears to be timid, obedient, and

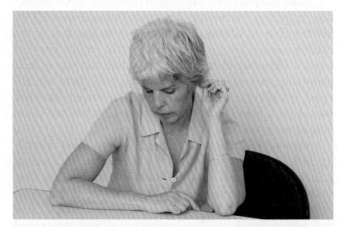

FIGURE 10.6 When documenting a client's appearance and behavior, the nurse would note this client's repeated playing with her hair.

submissive in response to her husband. This appearance might raise suspicions of spousal abuse or passive dependent personality traits. However, in Hispanic culture, the concepts of men as the dominant authority in the family and women as submissive and obedient are cultural norms (Paniagua, 2000). Understanding cultural differences with regard to dress, eye contact, and modes of expression can sensitize nurses to be thoughtful about the significance of what they are observing and to be steadfast in efforts to state observations objectively. In any case, nurses rarely can use single pieces of data alone to draw an inference. Rather, they consider each observation a springboard for further evaluation and inquiry so that they can firmly support inferences and subsequent interventions with adequate and culturally screened data.

LEVEL OF CONSCIOUSNESS. Nurses note initial observations about wakefulness and awareness. Is the client *alert* and aware of the interview being conducted? Is there a disturbance such as *hyperawareness/watchfulness, sedation,* or *catatonia?* Hyperawareness or watchfulness might warrant further assessment for anxiety, mania, or paranoia. Sedation or catatonia may warrant further assessment for depression, drug use, or schizophrenia.

POSTURE AND MOTOR MOVEMENTS. Nurses observe posture—how the client sits or stands as well as movement (Figure 10.7). Is the client *relaxed* and *focused* on the interview? Or is the client *tense/rigid, slumped,* or *focused* elsewhere? Tense or rigid postures may signal anxiety, paranoia, or agitation. Slumped posture may signal depression. When the client's posture and awareness focus on something other than the interview, the nurse may assess further for anxiety, attention problems, or hallucinations.

Motor movements may be described as *slow* or *retarded,* which are common findings with depression. Nurses may observe movements that are *rapid* or *pacing* or *restlessness*

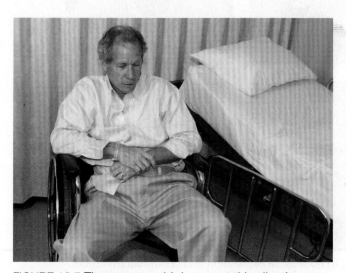

FIGURE 10.7 **The nurse would document this client's slumped and downcast posture.**

with anxiety or during manic episodes. Echopraxic motor movements (mimicking those of the interviewer) are sometimes seen in people with thought disorders such as schizophrenia.

DRESS, GROOMING, AND HYGIENE. Initial observations about dress, grooming, and hygiene can provide clues about a client's ability to manage self-care and activities of daily living. Is clothing *clean* or *dirty?* Does attire seem *odd* or *excessive?* Is the client's hair *groomed* or *disheveled?* Are there any *obvious body odors?*

Often, clients experiencing depression, schizophrenia, or both lack energy or motivation to complete basic grooming. During manic episodes, clients may present with clothing that seems excessive in color and amount or appears sexually provocative. Any of these observations should prompt nurses to further explore a client's self-care management. Note again that because dress and grooming practices vary widely and can be culturally influenced, nurses should be cautious about making premature inferences about symptomatic significance in this area.

Mood and Affect

Mood is assessed by client report (verbal responses), but **affect** refers to the physical manifestations of the client's mood and is assessed by observing the client's facial expression in conjunction with other nonverbal clues. Nurses must evaluate the appearance of the affect and the congruence among facial expressions, nonverbal cues, and verbal responses. It is generally expected that people in interactions would express a full range of facial expressions and nonverbal behaviors congruent with verbal statements about their mood (although cultural norms also should be considered).

When verbal responses are consistently high and exceptionally positive, the mood is described as *elated* or *euphoric.* This symptom may warrant further assessment for mania. On the other hand, if the client's responses are downcast and negative, the mood may be described as *depressed, dysphoric,* or *dysthymic.* In this case the nurse assesses for other indications of depression or other mood disturbances. At times, the client may report mood swings or frequently changing moods. This mood is described as *labile* or *cyclothymic.*

Many terms describe the facial expression/nonverbal manifestations of mood as noted in the sample assessment form (see Figure 10.3). Psychiatric nurses need to be familiar with these descriptors to document accurately any observations made about the client's affect. Perhaps a most unsettling experience for a novice practitioner in mental health nursing is the observation that affect and mood don't seem to go together or that there seems to be no visual or verbal evidence of the client's mood and affect. The first scenario would be described as *incongruent mood and affect.* The second scenario can be described only with regard to the affect (because it assumes the client is not reporting clear statements about mood) and it is described as a *flat affect.* Both may be symptoms of a thought disorder (see Chap. 29). At times, clients with profound depression also present with such a poverty of affect that it appears flat, rather than sad or blunted. Clients may present with symptoms of a mood and thought disorder at the same time. The meaning or diagnostic implications of these symptoms are interpreted after review and collation of all data. During data collection, it is most important for nurses to describe only what they are observing. See Figure 10.8.

Speech and Language

The nature of speech and language can provide important clues to thought processes, thought content, and emotional responses. Nurses document general observations about the character, rate, and volume of speech. Does the client articulate words clearly or is speech *slurred, stuttering,* or *pressured?* Is rate of speech *rapid, slow,* or *impoverished?* Is a client speaking audibly, or is the volume *loud, soft,* or *barely audible?* Stuttering, rapid, loud, and pressured speech may signal anxiety, agitation, mania, or all of these responses. Clients who present with slow speech or seem to be having trouble expressing thoughts may have depression or a thought disturbance.

Clients with thought disorders (eg, schizophrenia) may rhyme (*clang associations*) or use made-up words (*neologisms*). Nurses always should document these symptoms. Some neurologic disturbances such as cerebrovascular

accidents or Parkinson's disease also may affect speech and language, so medical etiology should always be ruled out.

Nurses continue throughout the interview to listen to *what* clients are saying and *how* they are expressing themselves. Nurses then can make more specific observations about the organization or disorganization of thought content, processes, and perceptions.

Thought and Perception

As noted earlier, no diagnostic or laboratory tests assess for thought disorders, so nurses must rely on speech patterns and content implications. Five main aspects of data collection related to thoughts and perceptions include thought content, thought processes, perceptions, insight, and judgment.

THOUGHT CONTENT. Thought content describes what clients are saying. It would be impossible to document everything clients say during an interview, so nurses must develop skill in identifying content *themes* and detecting modes of expression that may be associated with mental health problems. For example, a nurse documents that the client repeatedly made derogatory comments such as "I'm worthless" or "I don't deserve to be alive." This theme in the client's expressed thoughts may signal unhealthy responses to depression.

Some expressions of thought content, referred to as *delusions* (false beliefs), are common with thought disorders and sometimes occur in mania. It is not always easy to determine whether a client's statements are delusional. For

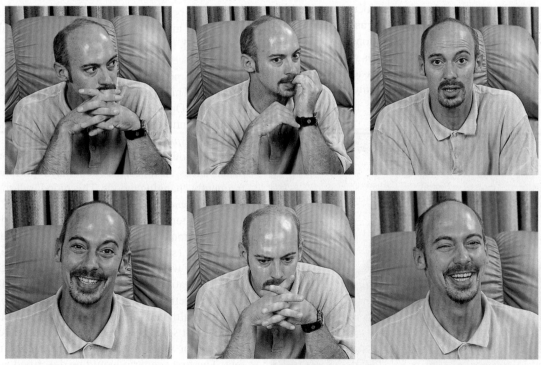

FIGURE 10.8 An important area of assessment is to note facial expression and nonverbal behaviors. Nurses also should observe the congruence between such expression and verbal communication the client offers. What messages do these different photos reflect to you?

example, consider the client who reports to the nurse that he has four college degrees in business and psychology and has written textbooks on organizational psychology. It might be a grandiose delusion (a false belief of inflated self-importance), but it is feasible that it could be true. The nurse must be thoughtful about inferences and make every possible effort to validate the reliability of information before drawing conclusions.

In other circumstances, it may be immediately clear that a client's thoughts are delusional. For example, a client who states he is the one and only President of the Universe is obviously exhibiting disturbed thoughts. Other common examples of thought content disturbances are listed in Table 10.2.

THOUGHT PROCESSES. This aspect refers to data about how thoughts connect to one another. Often when a nurse feels confused about how to interpret communication, it is a signal that thoughts are not flowing smoothly. In some cases the client presents several thoughts that don't make sense in conjunction with one another. This is often seen in clients with acute exacerbations of schizophrenia and is described as *loose association*. Other clients may express several thoughts that when carefully evaluated do have a connection but are hard to follow because the client's thoughts are racing. This symptom is referred to as *flight of ideas* and is common in clients during an acute manic episode. Clients may be able to validate that their thoughts are racing, so it is beneficial to ask this question when suspected. Thought process disturbances are explained in more detail in Chapter 29.

PERCEPTIONS. Observation about perceptions involves an attempt by clients to describe their sensory experiences. A client may tilt the head, look elsewhere, or appear to be paying attention to something unknown to the interviewer. When the nurse notices these behaviors, he or she may pose the question, "Are you hearing (seeing) someone or something besides me right now?" It is not advisable to ask clients if they are hallucinating because this implies that their experience is not real, and they may deny it based on that premise alone. Primarily, nurses must rely on what clients report, although clients may present with behaviors that raise suspicion. In psychotic illness, clients may have sensory experiences of seeing, hearing, feeling, tasting, or smelling things with no evidence in objective reality. The most common descriptor is to state that the client is experiencing "hallucinations" and to specify which sense is affected. Another common descriptor is to report that the client is "internally stimulated." This is different from illusions, which are misinterpretations of real sensory experiences.

Collecting data about the character of sensory experiences is beneficial for two reasons. First is safety. If a client is experiencing command hallucinations (ie, voices direct the client to take some action such as to hurt self or others), the nurse may need to initiate interventions to protect the safety of the client or others should the client be inclined to respond to those directives. Recent studies have highlighted the importance of assessing whether voices in an auditory hallucination are familiar to the client and whether the client believes the voices to be real. When these characteristics are present, the likelihood is increased that the client will comply with command hallucinations (Buccheri et al., 2007; Erkwoh et al., 2002). Nurses can pose questions about command hallucinations directly:

- "Do you recognize the voices you describe?"
- "Can you distinguish these voices from my voice?"

The second reason for assessing the character of hallucinations is that the feelings being symbolically represented

TABLE 10.2 **Thought Content Disturbances**

Symptom	Definition	Example
Delusion, grandiose	False belief of inflated self-importance	"I am known in all the universe as the smartest person."
Delusion, paranoid	False suspicions	"They are poisoning my food through telepathy."
Delusion, erotomanic	False belief of being loved by a celebrity	"The president secretly wants to marry me."
Delusion, somatic	False belief about bodily functions	"The bugs crawl under my skin and eat my brain."
Ideas of reference	Belief that external events have personal significance	"The newscaster sent me a message on TV last night."
Magical thinking	Belief that thinking about something will make it happen	"I'm thinking about a sunny day so you won't need a raincoat."
Thought broadcasting	Belief that thoughts are known by others	"Well, you know what I'm thinking, so why don't you just say it?"
Obsessions	Unwanted repetitive thoughts	"I can't stop thinking that I'm in mortal danger."

in the client's hallucinations may provide an opportunity for nurses to engage clients in an assessment of their feeling states. For example, a client reports that "The military police are trying to wipe out my memories because I know too much. They'd kill me but they don't want a scandal." The nurse responds, "That sounds like it must be frightening. Is that how you feel?"

On a cautionary note, clients with active psychoses tend to experience increased intensity of symptoms when anxious. Nurses must develop skill at assessing verbal and nonverbal behaviors that could signal anxiety or agitation. They never attempt to "force" clients to discuss thoughts or feelings if it appears that doing so is increasing anxiety or agitation. Increased behaviors such as pacing, fist clenching, or loud or angry shouting may signal the need for the nurse to move to less threatening topics, assist the client with anxiety reduction, or both.

INSIGHT. Insight is a cognitive process of understanding. Assessment of insight attempts to glean the client's awareness and understanding of current circumstances, illness, and treatment. For example, when a client states that "the cause of my condition is the aliens infiltrating my brain," the nurse would document insight as *poor* or *impaired*. On the other hand, the nurse could describe a client who states "I understand this antidepressant may not have full effects for several weeks" as having *good insight*.

JUDGMENT. Judgment may be viewed as the action-oriented counterpart to insight.

Decisions that clients make and the actions they take reflect whether judgment is *intact* or *impaired*. A client who reports that he struck his boss because his vacation time was too short is manifesting poor or impaired judgment. Conversely, a client who reports that he decided to seek help because he needs to learn how to manage his anger before it causes problems is manifesting good or intact judgment.

It is useful to also assess the impulsivity of judgments from clients' descriptions of events. For example, clients during a manic episode may report impulsive spending sprees. Assessing for this may have implications for protective interventions. Similarly, for clients with anger management problems, assessing their impulsivity may have safety implications. Because the terms to describe judgment and insight are relative and open to misinterpretation, nurses must clearly state data to support inferences that insight and judgment are good, poor, intact, or impaired.

Cognitive Functions

Assessment of cognitive functions involves collecting data to evaluate the client's abilities in orientation, memory, attention/concentration, intelligence, and abstract reasoning. As noted earlier, Folstein's Mini-Mental Status Examination is a standardized tool that evaluates several areas of cognitive ability and, as such, provides an efficient framework for this assessment.

Disruptions and changes in cognitive function are commonly associated with dementia but also with depression (especially in older adults). Difficulty with memory, attention, and abstract reasoning are also common with schizophrenia. General assessment of intelligence deficits can have implications for which treatment modalities to use. Therefore, it is important for nurses to develop skill in screening each aspect of cognitive function.

ORIENTATION. One of the most basic assessments of cognitive function is the client's orientation to *person, place,* and *time*. Nurses ask clients direct questions about themselves and their situation to assess orientation. Examples such as "What is the name of the place you are in right now?" or "Can you recall where you were right before you came here?" assess for orientation to place. To assess for time orientation, nurses can ask "Do you recall what month and year this is?" or "What is today's date?"

When clients are oriented in all spheres, nurses typically document "oriented × 3." When there is a deficit in one or more areas, nurses should document specific concrete statements to describe the problems noted. An example is "The client is oriented to person but cannot provide the day, month, or year or her current location."

MEMORY. Collecting data about the client's memory entails three domains: immediate, recent, and remote. Immediate memory refers to the ability to retain information presented within the past several minutes. Nurses may ask clients to repeat three words and then recall those three words several minutes later. Recent memory refers to the client's ability to recall information from within the past few weeks, whereas remote memory involves recall of events from many years ago. It is sometimes difficult to validate the accuracy of the client's recall, but efforts to stick to questions about widely known events can improve the nurse's confidence in the reliability of this information.

How well *anyone* remembers events and details is a subject of some debate. To some extent, fabrication or distortion of remembered details (confabulation) may be considered normal (Loftus, 2001). Thus, nurses must look for consistent patterns of memory impairment in one or more of these domains to identify actual or potential risks associated with deficits.

ATTENTION/CONCENTRATION. Perhaps the most common method to assess attention and the ability to concentrate is testing of calculation by adding or subtracting several items. An example is the serial sevens test, in which examiners ask clients to start from 100 and recite the subtraction of 7s sequentially ($100 - 7 = 93$, $93 - 7 = 86$, etc.). However, this test generally is difficult for clients who are medically compromised or elderly; interviewers may switch to a serial threes calculation or ask clients to recite the months backward (MacKinnon et al., 2006). In addition, Paniagua (2000) notes the potential for cultural bias in these tests. Thus, nurses should exercise caution when making inferences about attention and concentration abilities based on calculation ability in clients from different cultural backgrounds.

INTELLIGENCE. Assessment of intelligence is one of the most controversial aspects of the process. Researchers have widely debated the potential for cultural bias, and few people agree on a single definition of intelligence. Still, intelligence is sometimes inferred from education level, from an assessment of a client's vocabulary and fund of knowledge, and from the various observations made about orientation, consciousness, and memory (Sommers-Flanagan & Sommers-Flanagan, 2009). Because nurses often are conducting screening assessments, they need to take extra caution not to make specific statements about a person's intelligence too hastily. Noting a client's scope of *vocabulary, ability to read and write,* and any *previously diagnosed learning disabilities* can have important implications for treatment planning. Nurses should document findings in such areas without making inferences about the client's overall intelligence.

ABSTRACT REASONING. Clients with schizophrenia often have a disrupted ability to employ abstract reasoning. Commonly this manifests as *concrete thinking.* To assess for this disruption, nurses may ask clients to describe the meaning of well-known proverbs, such as "People who live in glass houses should not throw stones." A client who is thinking very concretely might say, "They shouldn't throw stones because the glass will break." It is important to assess for this symptom because it has implications for treatment modalities and communication approaches. For example, colloquial phrases such as "What's the buzz?" or "You kill me!" require abstract reasoning to interpret correctly. Much humor is also rooted in abstract thinking (as well as being culturally defined). Nurses should avoid both colloquial and humorous approaches in clients with disrupted abstract reasoning.

> **Think About It 10.2**
> A client is admitted to the psychiatric unit stating "I am a famous rock 'n' roll star. I've traveled all over the world singing everywhere." She has incurred numerous debts from spending sprees and states that "men just can't keep their hands off me." She speaks very rapidly and changes topics frequently. What areas of the MSE would be most important for the nurse to assess?

Safety Assessments

The most important priority in conducting a mental health assessment interview is determination of the client's safety toward self (*suicide potential*), toward others (*homicidal ideation*), and from others (*victimization through abuse or neglect*). Adequate assessment of these aspects requires the establishment of a therapeutic relationship (see Chap. 11). The nurse's skill in conveying genuine concern and empathy is essential to this relationship.

Some clients have difficulty establishing trust or choose not to be forthcoming with information despite the best efforts of nurses. Consequently, decisions about the reliability of client reports and whether clients need hospitalization for close observation require complex critical thinking skills and judgment. Key to these safety assessments is the nurse's skill in examining the congruence or incongruence of verbal and nonverbal communication. Nurses should consider hesitation, evasiveness, inconsistency, or nonchalance from clients as potential safety concerns. Novice psychiatric nurses will profit from gaining experience and supervision in safety assessment to develop these skills.

> **Checkpoint Questions**
> **8.** What is meant by the term *loose associations?*
> **9.** What areas are assessed when evaluating a client's cognitive function?

Suicide Assessment

Many myths about suicide and suicidal behavior contribute to apprehension when approaching this topic with clients. One is the fear of "planting" the idea of suicide in a client's mind simply by discussing it. In fact, it is critical for nurses to ask direct questions to protect the safety of clients. Use of closed-ended questions is particularly beneficial during this inquiry because they require specific responses.

When completing an assessment of suicide potential, nurses should attempt to differentiate between the desire to hurt versus the desire to kill oneself. Some clients desire to inflict pain or to injure themselves but do not have the desire or intention to die. Other clients may want to die but would deny their desire to "hurt" themselves. Making this distinction can have different implications for inferences made, as well as for determining appropriate nursing interventions.

When assessing suicide potential, nurses may become aware that clients have agreed to a safety contract (an agreement to discuss suicidal ideas before taking action). This finding may be adjunctive to report but should never be considered an indication that suicide potential is no longer a concern. Contracts are never a substitute for other safety interventions (eg, hospitalization, close observation) when other risk factors are present. See also Chapter 34.

Dangerousness to Others and Homicide Assessment

When investigating dangerousness toward others or **homicidal ideation**, it is important to collect supporting evidence from family, other health care professionals, and legal authorities, rather than relying solely on the client's report. Formulating questions that focus on facts rather than client interpretations is also an important skill. For example, asking "Did you hurt anyone?" allows clients to interpret and possibly to minimize the seriousness of their violent behavior (Shea, 1998). A better alternative is "Did you physically hit anyone?" which attempts to solicit a factual response. See Chapter 32.

Psychiatric nurses also must be familiar with laws and agency policies related to reporting threats of violence from clients against specific individuals. Many states have laws that establish the duty of psychiatric clinicians to warn and take measures to protect potential victims.

Victimization Through Abuse or Neglect

Collecting data about abuse or neglect requires nurses to collate information from the interview and findings of the physical examination. They also must minimize variables that could interfere with accurate reports, such as the presence of a spouse or someone who answers for the client during the interview. It is critical for nurses to be familiar with state laws that govern reporting of actual or suspected abuse or neglect and to pursue this process without delay when findings are of concern. Reporting requirements may vary based on the client's age and circumstances.

This topic is highly sensitive for clients to disclose. It may involve history related to domestic abuse, childhood trauma, or violent crime (eg, rape). Although direct inquiry about these issues is important, nurses must develop skill in timing questions, keen awareness of the client's tolerance for discussing details, and readiness to provide needed support. See also Chapter 33.

Individualized Needs

Collecting data about individualized needs includes focusing on the client's perception of his or her state of wellness.

It also involves examination of the client's strengths and weaknesses, cultural needs, spiritual needs, and preferred methods of coping or stress management.

Wellness

Clients can benefit from a general review of their overall state of wellness or well-being. A key component of nursing's scope of practice is health promotion for all clients. In addition, health and health needs can greatly influence adherence to treatment regimens as well as the pharmacokinetics of psychotropic medications (see Chap. 16). Assessment Tool 10.3 provides a sample form for reviewing a client's state of wellness.

Nurses must summarize and document findings in a clear, readable format useful for other providers.

Strengths and Weaknesses

Some clients have difficulty identifying their own strengths. This finding alone can be significant in drawing inferences about the client's self-concept and self-esteem. One method for inquiry is "Tell me what you think are your greatest assets (weaknesses)." The answers to both of these questions contribute to recognizing unhealthy responses to actual or potential problems and to the development of interventions that are specific to the client's perceived needs.

Cultural Needs

Assessing cultural needs requires an understanding of the client's values and behaviors within the context of cultural norms (see Chap. 6). It may be a universal phenomenon that people desire to belong to a group with common behaviors and beliefs; however, the diversity that exists from

---

▲ ASSESSMENT TOOL 10.3 ▲

Wellness Evaluation

Instructions and key: Circle the number below that most applies. **1** = less than 25% of the time, **2** = 25–49% of the time, **3** = 50–74% of the time, **4** = 75–100% of the time.

Health

1 2 3 4	1.	I exercise for 30–60 minutes a day.
1 2 3 4	2.	I eat a nutritious diet (minimum five servings fresh vegetables and fruit a day) and avoid chemicals, high fat content, and refined sugar.
1 2 3 4	3.	I try to keep all my body systems in balance. I take care of my hygiene every day.
1 2 3 4	4.	I get 6–8 hours of undisturbed sleep a night.
1 2 3 4	5.	I do not use caffeine, alcohol, street drugs, or ephedrine.
1 2 3 4	6.	It is easy for me to remember and to understand what I hear and read (my brain works right).
1 2 3 4	7.	I am free from infections/illness.
1 2 3 4	8.	My hearing, seeing, feeling (touch), smelling, and tasting work right.
1 2 3 4	9.	I have the energy to do the things I want to do.
1 2 3 4	10.	I use prescription drugs as prescribed.

HEALTH SCORE _____ (Total possible is 40)

Environment/Interpersonal Relationships

1 2 3 4	11.	I am satisfied with my performance at work/school.
1 2 3 4	12.	I try to learn something new every day.

ASSESSMENT TOOL 10.3   Wellness Evaluation (continued)

1 2 3 4   13.   I live in pleasant surroundings.
1 2 3 4   14.   Life skills (survival skills) are easy for me. (This includes personal hygiene, care of residence, financial management, and meal preparation.)
1 2 3 4   15.   I have a positive, satisfying relationship with all members of my family.
1 2 3 4   16.   I am able to negotiate with important others in ways that satisfy all our needs.
1 2 3 4   17.   I am satisfied with my income and ability to manage finances.
1 2 3 4   18.   I have at least three people who will help me out at any time.
1 2 3 4   19.   The services I need are easily available to me.
1 2 3 4   20.   I do something nice for at least one person every day.

ENVIRONMENT/INTERPERSONAL RELATIONSHIPS SCORE _____ (40 possible)

Spiritual

1 2 3 4   21.   I pray or meditate daily.
1 2 3 4   22.   I seek after truth.
1 2 3 4   23.   I am able to forgive myself and others.
1 2 3 4   24.   I acknowledge God as I understand Him to be.
1 2 3 4   25.   I express thanks for each new day.
1 2 3 4   26.   I spend at least 5 minutes a day reviewing how my faith affects my life.
1 2 3 4   27.   I am able to express and receive love from others.
1 2 3 4   28.   I spend at least 10 minutes a day reading and/or listening to spiritual material.
1 2 3 4   29.   My spiritual/religious practices are a source of strength to me.
1 2 3 4   30.   I am satisfied with my level of spiritual health.

SPIRITUAL SCORE _____ (Possible 40)

Attitudes/Behavior

1 2 3 4   31.   I look forward to the new day.
1 2 3 4   32.   I have a successful program I follow to manage my wellness.
1 2 3 4   33.   I can deal effectively with the pain and pleasure in my life.
1 2 3 4   34.   I enjoy life.
1 2 3 4   35.   I feel I make a worthwhile contribution to society.
1 2 3 4   36.   I am able to express my love to others.
1 2 3 4   37.   I accept responsibility for my own behavior.
1 2 3 4   38.   I have a working action plan for success.
1 2 3 4   39.   I allow others to make their own choices.
1 2 3 4   40.   My life is in balance.

ATTITUDES/BEHAVIOR SCORE _____ (Total possible 40)

TOTAL SCORE _____ (Total possible = 160)

ITEM TO WORK ON:

PLAN:

group to group is vast. Because group norms influence perceptions of mental health and mental illness (and what is considered a healthy versus an unhealthy response), nurses must develop skill in assessing how cultural norms (the nurse's and the client's) are affecting the nurse–client relationship and the client's perception of treatment needs. The client's cultural affiliation may be within the context of a religious group, an ethnic group, a gay or lesbian group, or some other group. It may also be a blend of several group norms.

Nurses need to recognize that identification of a client's affiliation is inadequate information from which to draw inferences about a client's individual cultural needs. For example, nurses should not assume that an Asian American client necessarily follows traditional Asian cultural values. Nurses must develop skill in asking questions that define cultural variables with regard to communication, touch, proximity to others, family roles, and social roles. Sample questions include the following:

- "How do you typically respond when people touch you?"
- "What is a comfortable distance between you and a stranger? Between you and a close friend?"
- "What is your role in your family? In social relationships?"
- "Are there any routines or other usual activities that you believe are important to consider when planning your treatment?"

Developing a fund of knowledge about traditional cultural variables helps nurses to develop skill in culturally sensitive interpretation of behavior and communication. Asking clients to identify any cultural practices that may affect their treatment respects their collaboration with their treatment and the nurse's concern for their culturally specific needs.

Spiritual Assessment

The aspect of spiritual assessment, although difficult to define, generally attempts to reveal information about the client's belief systems, connectedness to the universe, and religion (Miller, 2003). It may be intimately linked to cultural values and is often misunderstood as simply a function of a person's religious affiliation. To assess a client's spirituality requires nurses to develop awareness of their own spirituality and their comfort level when discussing spiritual issues. Some authors caution that psychiatry has had a tendency to view spirituality from two extreme vantage points: either as pathologic or as something that should not be discussed (Lukoff et al., 1995). Current standards consider spirituality to be an essential element of nursing assessment because it respects individualized needs and may be an important part of the experience of health and illness. In addition, it provides the opportunity to draw inferences about healthy or unhealthy responses, needs for support or referral, and the prominence of these needs in the counseling relationship (Richards & Bergin, 2005).

Sample questions include the following:

- "How would you describe your spiritual life?"
- "Who or what is your greatest source of comfort? Greatest source of support?"
- "Do you have religious beliefs? A relationship with a higher power?"
- "Is prayer something you find helpful?"
- "Are there any spiritual needs of yours that you think should be considered in planning your treatment?"

See Chapter 7 for more in-depth discussion.

Coping and Stress Management

Asking questions about the client's usual methods for coping and stress management can provide information about the client's values, perceived effectiveness in managing stress, and unhealthy responses to stress. Sample inquiries are as follows:

- "What do you do when you need to relax? What works? What hasn't worked?"
- "What kinds of activities do you do in your spare time?"

Appreciating the client's perceptions about what works, what hasn't worked, and the reasons can be pivotal in the nurse's determination of whether alternative coping and stress management skills are needed, whether the client needs education, or both.

Checkpoint Questions

10. What is a safety contract?

11. What data are collected when assessing a client's individualized needs?

RATING SCALES

Several standardized rating scales are available to clinicians for identifying illness symptoms, functional ability, or both. One resource identifies and reviews more than 80 rating scales to evaluate various aspects of mental health and mental illness (Sajatovic & Ramirez, 2003). Some examples include the following:

- The *Beck Depression Inventory* is a scale that assesses the *client's report* of various degrees of depression symptoms (see Chap. 27).
- The *Abnormal Involuntary Movement Scale* relies on *clinician observation* to identify abnormal movements associated with adverse effects from antipsychotic medication (see Chap. 16).
- *Folstein's Mini-Mental Status Examination* has been identified as a common tool used to assess cognitive functions (see Chap. 31).
- A widely used scale for assessing overall functional ability is the *Global Assessment of Functioning Scale (GAF)* incorporated in the *Diagnostic and Statistical Manual of Mental Disorders* multiaxial diagnostic system. See Appendix A.

These many and varied scales are available for purchase or general use and are supportive in initial diagnosis, for comparing the client's progress over time, and for evaluating outcomes of treatment. They should always be used as an adjunct to the clinical interview, rather than alone. Some studies identified that depression screening tools were far more reliable when a client was already suspected of having depression and that general screening (regardless of risk) yielded high false-positive results (Thibault & Prassad Steiner, 2004). This research reinforces that the interview and clinical judgments made by experienced clinicians continue to have central importance.

SPECIAL CHALLENGES

Some special challenges require nurses to modify or adapt interviewing and the assessment process. Examples involve point in the lifespan and clients with challenging communication issues.

Age Group

Assessing children and older adults requires age-specific competencies from nurses. This includes recognizing developmental tasks associated with specific age groups and modifying interviewing techniques accordingly. For example, when assessing children, nurses may find interactive play, drawing, or both to be more effective information-gathering strategies than direct inquiry (Figure 10.9). For older adults, life review is an important developmental task. Nurses who are sensitive to the importance of appreciating the experiences of elders recognize that assessment and interviewing may require more time to complete for them.

Communication Challenges

Many clients who seek mental health services present with some type of communication impairment or problem. Nurses must develop tolerance as well as skill in responding appropriately to these challenges. For example, clients with severe depression or those experiencing thought disturbances may be slow to respond to questions. In these cases, nurses must develop skill in patient, silent attending, rather than reframing or posing different questions.

For clients who are very talkative or tangential in communication, a nurse's skill in refocusing techniques and closed-ended questioning may assist clients to respond more appropriately. However, at times the nurse's best efforts to refocus clients can be unsuccessful. This finding is important to document. Nurses must recognize that there are no "quick fix" responses to these clinical symptoms.

Experienced clinical interviewers also need to recognize and address literacy, language, and sensory barriers to

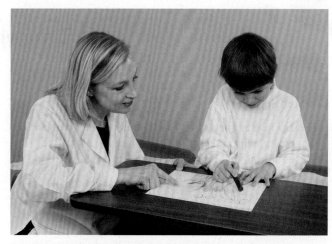

FIGURE 10.9 This nurse practitioner is working with a pediatric client to understand family relationships through pictures, rather than inquiry alone, based on the child's developmental level.

communication. Having a repertoire of resources, including interpreters, Braille screening tools, visual and audio response options, and other adaptations, is essential to the conduct of interviewing and assessment that accommodate these needs.

NURSE'S FOLLOW-UP

With the current practices of brief inpatient hospital stays (see Chap. 19) and multiple levels of care, the nurse's assessment skills move to the forefront of importance. The primary concerns of assessment are first and foremost to identify the need to protect clients from self-harm, harm to others, and victimization through abuse or neglect to the extent of current laws. In addition to identifying needs requiring immediate attention, nurses need to develop knowledge and skill in areas that require referral, as well as how to access services expeditiously.

Reviewing and Applying Your Knowledge

Chapter Summary

• In every interaction with a client, the nurse must consider variables that promote information sharing as well as safety for both the nurse and the client.

• The interviewing and assessment process for the psychiatric mental health client is a complex set of skills that requires knowledge of symptoms of mental health problems within a culturally defined context, appropriate physical assessment skills, the ability to critically synthesize observation and listening skills, and skill in relationship building with clients who may have impairments in their ability to relate to others.

• Recognizing appropriate avenues for obtaining information from secondary sources such as the family, other health care providers, and local authorities can contribute greatly to the fund of information needed to make accurate and timely decisions about treatment needs as well as needs for referral.

• Identifying and incorporating appropriate adjunctive resources (psychological testing, laboratory and diagnostic testing, and standardized rating scales) also assures that multiple sources are compared to support assessment findings. All of these skills revolve around the nurse's awareness and critical thinking about the impact of the nurse's own emotions, values, beliefs, and behaviors on his or her communication and interpretation of assessment findings.

Study Questions

1. Which of the following statements by the client is an example of a precipitating factor?

 a. "I had a fight with my husband and said I was going to kill myself."

 b. "My father left us when I was 3."

 c. "I go to a special classroom in school for the 'trouble-makers.' "

 d. "My husband is an alcoholic."

2. A client reports to the emergency department with complaints of depression and an increase in obsessive hand washing since he filed for bankruptcy. His hands appear reddened with some areas of broken skin. He appears tremulous, diaphoretic, and agitated. He denies taking any prescription medication for anxiety or depression. He admits to drinking a gallon of wine daily for the past 10 years but states he never gets drunk. His last alcohol consumption was about 24 hours ago. Which of these assessment findings requires immediate intervention?

 a. Complaints of depression

 b. Impaired skin integrity

 c. Bankruptcy

 d. Alcohol withdrawal

3. A client is admitted to the inpatient psychiatric unit after a suicide attempt in which she cut both wrists and required sutures. When the nurse approaches her to conduct an initial assessment, her husband states, "I need to be in the room during the assessment because my wife gets very upset and won't be able to answer your questions." His wife is slouched over and not making eye contact with the nurse or her husband. Which of these is the best response by the nurse?

 a. "That's fine; thanks for being so supportive."

 b. "Please come in but let your wife answer the questions."

 c. "I'll need to conduct this part of the assessment with only your wife. Perhaps we can talk after that."

 d. "I'm not allowed to talk to you."

4. An 80-year-old man is admitted to the gero-psychiatry unit after his daughter brings him to the emergency department reporting that he is confused and having trouble remembering things. She adds that he has been having trouble ever since his wife of 60 years died 3 months ago. Which of the following facts should the nurse consider while conducting an assessment?

 a. Depression may mimic signs of dementia in the elderly.

 b. Based on the client's age, he is suffering from dementia.

 c. It is normal for people of the client's age to experience confusion and memory loss.

 d. Confusion and memory loss are normal components of grief and mourning.

5. A client reports during assessment, "I don't feel like living anymore now that my husband left me. I feel so ugly

and small. His new girlfriend is half my age." Which is the best response by the nurse?

a. "Tell me about why your husband left you."

b. "You're not ugly or small."

c. "Are you having thoughts of killing yourself?"

d. "Tell me about your feelings."

Critical Thinking Questions

1. A client walks into the community mental health agency stating, "The bugs are winning, grinning, sinning." His clothes appear dirty, are in ill repair, and smell strongly of urine and feces. He asks to talk to the nurse about his "lobetrics." When the nurse asks the client to have a seat and discuss what's been bothering him, he replies, "I've been seeing naked little children."

a. What are your immediate thoughts about this client?

b. What feelings does this client's presentation generate in you?

c. What symptoms of a mental health problem or problems are suggested?

d. How will you structure the environment to conduct an assessment of this client?

e. How will you begin your assessment of this client?

f. Write down two statements or questions you would use to explore this client's statement about seeing naked little children.

2. How would you react and respond differently if the client from Question 1 presented as a well-educated, neatly dressed man who states "I came in because my pain medication isn't working and I think I need stronger sleeping pills"?

References

American Nurses Association (ANA), American Psychiatric Nurse's Association, & International Society of Psychiatric–Mental Health Nurses. (2007). *Psychiatric–mental health nursing: Scope and standards of practice.* Silver Spring, MD: American Nurses Publishing.

Bassil, N., Ghandour, A., & Grossberg, G. (2011). How anxiety presents differently in older adults. *Current Psychiatry, 10*(3), 65–70.

Benner, P. (2000). *From novice to expert: Excellence and power in clinical nursing practice.* Menlo Park, CA: Addison-Wesley.

Buccheri, R., Trygstad, L., & Dowling, G. (2007). Behavioral management of command hallucinations to harm in schizophrenia. *Journal of Psychosocial Nursing, 45*(9), 47–54.

Calinoiu, I., & McClellan, J. (2004). Diagnostic interviewing. *Current Psychiatry Reports, 6,* 88–95.

Colton, C. W., & Manderscheid, R. W. (2006). Congruencies in increased mortality rate, years of potential life lost, and causes of death among public mental health clients in eight states. *Preventing Chronic Disease, 3*(2), A42.

Erkwoh, R., Willmes, K., Eming-Erdman, A., & Kunert, H. (2002). Command hallucinations: Who obeys and who resists when? *Psychopathology, 35,* 272–279.

Estes, M. (2009). *Health assessment and physical examination* (4th ed.). Clifton Park, NY: Thomson Delmar Learning.

Folstein, M. E., Folstein, S. E., & McHugh, P. R. (1975). "Mini-mental state": A practical method for grading the cognitive state of patients for the clinician. *Journal of Psychiatric Research, 12,* 189–198.

Forchuk, C. (1993). *Hildegard Peplau: Interpersonal nursing theory.* Newbury Park, CA: Sage.

Frances, A. (2010, July 14). Understanding mental disorders. *Psychiatric Times.* Retrieved from http//www.psychiatrictimes.com/dsm-5/content/article/10168/1607874

Freshwater, D. (Ed.). (2002). *Therapeutic nursing: Improving patient care through reflection.* London, UK: Sage.

Ghaye, T., & Lillyman, S. (2009). *Reflection principles and practices for health care professionals.* London, UK: Quay Books.

Kuiper, R., & Pesut, D. (2004). Promoting cognitive and metacognitive reflective reasoning skills in nursing practice: Self-regulated learning theory. *Journal of Advanced Nursing, 45*(4), 381–391.

Loftus, E. F. (2001). Imagining the past. *Psychologist, 14,* 584–587.

Lukoff, D., Lu, F. G., & Turner, R. (1995). Cultural considerations in the assessment and treatment of religious and spiritual problems. *Cultural Psychiatry, 18,* 467–485.

MacKinnon, R., Michels, R., & Buckley, P. (2006). *The psychiatric interview in clinical practice* (2nd ed.). Washington, DC: American Psychiatric Publishing.

Miller, G. (2003). *Incorporating spirituality in counseling and psychotherapy.* Hoboken, NJ: John Wiley & Sons.

Paniagua, F. (2000). *Diagnosis in a multicultural context: A casebook for mental health professionals.* Thousand Oaks, CA: Sage.

Rey, J. (2007). Does marijuana contribute to psychotic illness? *Current Psychiatry, 6,* 36–46.

Richards, P. S., & Bergin, A. E. (2005). *A spiritual strategy for counseling and psychotherapy* (2nd ed.). Washington, DC: American Psychological Association.

Rosenhan, D. (1973). On being sane in insane places. *Science, 179*(1), 250–258.

Sajatovic, M., & Ramirez, L. (2003). *Rating scales in mental health* (2nd ed.). Hudson, OH: Lexi Comp.

Scheff, T. (Ed.). (1975). *Labeling madness.* Englewood Cliffs, NJ: Prentice Hall.

Shea, S. (1998). *Psychiatric interviewing: The art of understanding* (2nd ed.). Philadelphia, PA: W. B. Saunders.

Sommers-Flanagan, J., & Sommers-Flanagan, R. (2009). *Clinical interviewing* (4th ed.). Hoboken, NJ: John Wiley & Sons.

Thibault, J. M., & Prassad Steiner, R. W. (2004). Efficient identification of adults with depression and dementia. *American Family Physician, 70*(6), 1101–1110.

Zimmerman, C., Del Piccolo, L., & Finset, A. (2007). Cues and concerns by patients in medical consultations: A literature review. *Psychological Bulletin, 133*(3), 438–463.

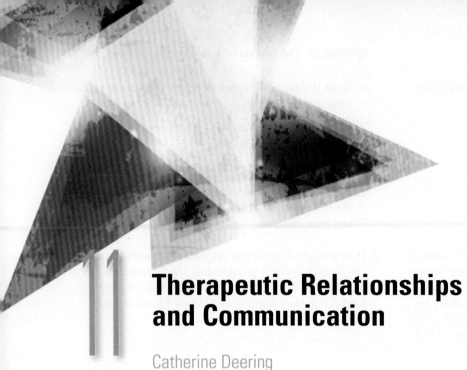

11

Therapeutic Relationships and Communication

Catherine Deering

KEY TERMS

aggressiveness
apathy
assertiveness
caring
channel
communication
communicator
confrontation
countertransference
décoding
empathy
encoding
environment
external noise
feedback
genuineness
listening
maturity
noise
nontherapeutic communication
passive-aggressive communication
perception check
physiologic noise
positive reframing
professional
psychological noise
therapeutic communication
transactional analysis (TA)
trust
unconditional positive regard

LEARNING OBJECTIVES

On completion of this chapter, you should be able to accomplish the following:

- List the key ingredients of therapeutic relationships.
- Identify some potential obstacles to therapeutic relationships.
- Describe the three phases of therapeutic relationships.
- Apply a theoretical model to explain the process of nurse–client communication.
- Describe effective listening skills to use with clients.
- Contrast effective and ineffective communication techniques with clients.
- Identify ways to use confrontation and self-assertion with clients.
- Discuss the appropriateness of different levels of self-disclosure with clients.
- Describe the role of family and loved ones in the client's care.

People experiencing mental health problems are vulnerable and usually afraid. Building relationships and communicating with them pose challenges that require skill, knowledge, and perceptiveness to discern what will be most helpful. At the same time, working with those in emotional distress can be highly rewarding when nurses know that clients and families feel understood, cared for, and better able to cope with their unique situations.

This chapter focuses on how to create therapeutic relationships and communicate effectively with clients and families. It explores attitudes and behaviors that foster positive encounters with recipients of health care services. Therapeutic relationships progress through several predictable phases. This chapter examines the key tasks of each phase and how nurses can facilitate progress toward healthy change and growth. It differentiates effective from ineffective communication skills and provides specific guidelines for confrontation, assertiveness, and self-disclosure. The overarching purpose is to provide a guide for productive interactions with clients and families.

THERAPEUTIC RELATIONSHIPS

The foundation of all nursing care is the *therapeutic relationship*—a close, helping relationship based on trust, which fosters collaboration. The purpose of the therapeutic relationship in psychiatric–mental health nursing is to help clients solve problems, cope more effectively, and achieve developmental goals.

Despite significant progress in biotechnology that holds the promise for treatment, and possibly even cure, of mental disorders, the therapeutic relationship remains the central medium through which all psychiatric care is provided (Evidence-Based Practice Spotlight 11.1). In the midst of

---

△ EVIDENCE-BASED PRACTICE SPOTLIGHT 11.1 △

The Primacy of the Therapeutic Relationship in Psychiatric Treatment

Overview of Effective Treatment: Based on decades of research and meta-analyses of treatment outcome studies, the therapeutic relationship is a crucial component in the change process in psychiatric settings. Regardless of the clinical problem or the treatment modality being used, studies show that a positive therapeutic relationship robustly predicts a positive response to treatment. Consensus across studies shows that the key components of a therapeutic relationship include warmth, flexibility, accurate empathy, congruence, and positive regard for the client. Without these elements of the relationship, treatment is more likely to prematurely terminate and less likely to produce positive change. The quality of the therapeutic relationship is particularly predictive of treatment outcome when measured early in treatment. One study of clients with severe and persistent mental illness found that they viewed the therapeutic relationship with their community psychiatric nurses as "life sustaining and suggested that their survival in the community depended on it" (O'Brien, 2001).

What Has Not Been Shown Effective: Mental health professionals who are rigid, critical, hostile, and lacking in self-awareness, and who use inappropriate self-disclosure are more likely to form negative therapeutic relationships and to experience premature dropout from treatment.

Studies also show that when faced with misunderstandings or "ruptures" in the therapeutic relationship, professionals who continue to adhere to rigid approaches, as opposed to adjusting to clients' needs and perceptions, are unable to repair the relationship and may even exacerbate conflict with clients.

Implications for Practice: Nurses and other mental health professionals should focus on fostering a therapeutic relationship with clients from the moment treatment begins. Objective measures of the therapeutic alliance are widely available and can be used to assess the client's perceptions of the relationship and in conjunction with research on treatment outcomes. Nurses should not assume that their own perceptions of the relationship are valid indicators of the client's experience because studies show that their client's perceptions may significantly differ. Because most research on the therapeutic relationship in nursing has been imported from psychotherapy studies, additional investigation of the unique aspects of the therapeutic relationship in psychiatric nursing is needed. Because the therapeutic relationship is arguably the most robust predictor of change in psychiatric treatment, greater focus should be placed on training professionals to foster a positive alliance and to attend to problems or ruptures in the relationship in a timely, flexible manner.

References

Castonguay, L. G., Constantino, M. J., & Holtforth, M. G. (2006). The working alliance: Where are we and where should we go? *Psychotherapy: Theory, Research, Practice, Training, 43*(3), 271–279.

Finfgeld-Connett, D. (2009). Model of therapeutic and non-therapeutic responses to patient aggression. *Issues in Mental Health Nursing, 30*(9), 530–537.

Haugh, S., & Paul, S. (2008). Is the relationship the therapy? *Therapy Today, 19*(10), 34–37.

Hewitt, J., & Coffey, M. (2005). Therapeutic working relationships with people with schizophrenia: A literature review. *Journal of Advanced Nursing. 52*(5), 561–570.

Priebe, S., & McCabe, R. (2006). The therapeutic relationship in psychiatric settings. *Acta Psychiatrica Scandinavica, 113*(Suppl. 429), 67–72.

Welch, M. (2005). Pivotal moments in the therapeutic relationship. *International Journal of Mental Health Nursing, 14,* 161–165.

Zuroff, D. C., & Blatt, S. J. (2006). The therapeutic relationship in the brief treatment of depression: Contributions to clinical improvement and enhance adaptive capacities. *Journal of Consulting and Clinical Psychology, 74*(1), 130–140.

rapid advances in psychopharmacology and brief treatments, many psychiatric nursing leaders view the primacy of the therapeutic relationship as an endangered concept and are calling for a renewed emphasis on teaching the skills and values needed to preserve this key context that underlies nursing care (Foster & Hawkins, 2005; Perraud et al., 2006). No matter what techniques we use, nurses still need to establish therapeutic relationships to ensure that clients will actually utilize and benefit from our mental health services.

Essential Elements

Every human relationship is unique. The backgrounds, beliefs, and personalities of both nurse and client influence their work together. However, certain key elements must exist for a therapeutic relationship to develop. They include trust, professionalism, mutual respect, caring, and partnership.

Trust

The foundation of all close relationships is trust. **Trust** involves taking the risk of sharing oneself with another, knowing that there is a chance of being hurt, embarrassed, judged, and disappointed. People with mental health problems may be particularly reluctant to trust others because they are in emotional pain and fear being misunderstood. Nurses must earn clients' trust through caring presence and sensitive interactions.

Behaviors that foster trust include predictability, consistency, and clear expectations. Nurses need to explain what clients can expect to prevent feelings of fear, betrayal, and helplessness (Figure 11.1). For example, hospitalized clients need to know if and when they can have visitors and phone calls. Community mental health nurses who visit families must communicate clearly that nurses are mandated to report cases of child or elder abuse. Nurses working in outpatient settings should provide clients with information about how and when to reach them during crises. Thoughtful and

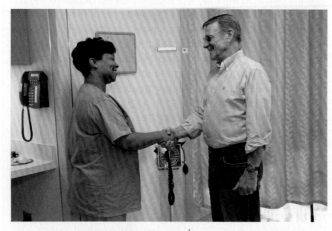

FIGURE 11.1 When establishing a therapeutic relationship with a client, the nurse must clearly outline expectations and then behave with predictability and consistency to role model correct actions and to foster trust.

consistent interactions demonstrate that nurses are reliable, honest, and available. Even small actions, such as indicating how much time a nurse has available to talk, may help clients gauge their level of self-disclosure.

Another important component of trust is *confidentiality*. Mental health providers must reassure clients that they will not share details of clients' lives outside the professional environment. In this context, confidentiality also includes the right for clients to conceal that they are receiving treatment. For example, it would be a major breach of trust and a violation of confidentiality for nursing students to mention to their family that they saw someone the family knew on a psychiatric unit and to reveal that person's identity.

Trust is also based on acceptance without judgment. Many clients with psychiatric problems are ashamed of socially alienating symptoms (eg, hallucinations, flashbacks, withdrawal) or difficulties in managing relationships. Clients need to know that nurses will not blame, fear, or look down on them. This means that nurses must be comfortable with psychiatric symptoms so that they can fully accept clients, regardless of level of functioning (see Chap. 8).

Professionalism

In the therapeutic relationship, the nurse acts as a **professional**, a person who applies a specific background of knowledge and skills. The purpose of the professional relationship is to promote the client's mental health. The professional role can be contrasted with a social relationship designed to meet the friendship needs of both parties (Table 11.1). Nurses demonstrate professionalism through their knowledge of psychiatric problems and their ability to intervene effectively. Thus, nurses must learn about their clients' conditions, medications, and treatments so they can provide current information and accurate insight. The nurse may need to seek out opportunities to assess and educate clients despite limited time and competing demands. For example, an observational study of nurses administering medication on three psychiatric units found that although the nurses were warm and caring, they did not initiate an exchange of information about the medication with their clients, thereby reducing the therapeutic value of their interactions (Duxbury et al., 2010). In short, nurses must make an effort to help clients both emotionally and pragmatically for a relationship to be therapeutic.

Mutual Respect

A therapeutic relationship is based on mutual respect. Although stigma surrounding mental disorders has decreased with greater awareness of contributing biologic and genetic factors and wider use of treatment services, clients and families still encounter negative and condescending attitudes (Shattell et al., 2007). People with mental illness are no less human or deserving of respect than anyone else. In fact, nurses working with clients and families who have faced psychiatric challenges often feel more respect for them when

TABLE 11.1 Social Versus Therapeutic Relationships

Aspect	Social Relationships	Therapeutic Relationships
Purpose	Interactions provide companionship, recreation, and support for both parties.	The focus is health promotion, behavior change, and growth for the client.
Basis	Parties share equal give and take.	The nurse cares for the client; the client is not expected to respond to the nurse's personal needs.
Superficial discussions	Exploration of topics such as the weather, sports, and television programs is normal.	Such talk blurs boundaries by introducing the nurse's background and personal preferences and distracting from the task of therapeutic change.
Self-disclosure	Both parties engage in increasingly free and revealing exchanges as the relationship develops.	The nurse facilitates the client's self-disclosure to promote change and growth. Nurses use self-disclosure only when it serves the client's needs.
Conflict	Both parties may argue freely, with relatively few constraints on words and emotions.	The nurse uses therapeutic communication skills to listen, confront, and set limits with clients while remaining calm, professional, and respectful. Even when clients are out of control, rude, or inappropriate, the nurse models appropriate communication.
Termination	Relationship may gradually fade or abruptly end if dissatisfaction or distance develops. Conversely, the relationship may be lifelong.	The nurse initiates and encourages discussion of any problems or behaviors that disrupt or inhibit the relationship. Termination is expected once the client resolves the presenting problem or moves to another therapeutic setting. Termination is planned and deliberate with therapeutic value.

they realize how they have struggled with extraordinary events and disabling symptoms. A sense of reverence for the human spirit and wonder at the uniqueness of each person develops as nurses get to know those who have overcome mental health problems.

Studies show that clients hospitalized both voluntarily and involuntarily on psychiatric units are more likely to report feeling disrespected and coerced when they perceive the quality of their therapeutic relationships to be poor (Sheehan & Burns, 2011).

Families of people with mental illnesses often fear criticism or blame for their loved one's problems. This worry stems from a long history of psychological theories that attributed disorders to childhood traumas and family dynamics. Although family difficulties sometimes contribute to mental health problems, biologic, genetic, and environmental stressors outside the family unit (eg, poverty, traumatic events, relationships with peers) are also involved (see Chap. 3). Mental illness greatly strains families who cope daily with such problems as mood swings, unpredictable behavior, and continual dependence on others. Nurses must

show respect for families who are doing the best they can to help their loved ones while also coping with their own, often challenging circumstances (see Chap. 15).

Nurses must be sensitive to cultural backgrounds (see Chap. 6). An awareness of cultural influences on values, family function, and worldviews helps nurses to interact effectively and to avoid offending others. For example, acknowledging the father as the head of the family is important in many traditional Hispanic families. Asian American families may delay mental health treatment as a result of stigma and shame, often mistaking psychiatric symptoms for physical problems (eg, fatigue, sleep disturbance, memory loss) (Barrett, 2006). In many African American families, extended family members such as grandparents and aunts are key figures, viewed as central to the family's everyday life (Figure 11.2). Nurses should attempt to set aside their personal concepts of family structure and learn more about how each client's family relates so that they do not exclude or minimize people who can influence the client's recovery and assist with planning care in the community.

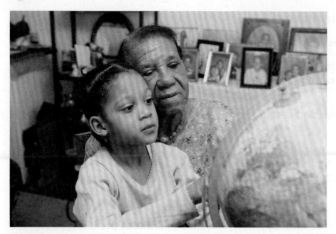

FIGURE 11.2 Older women play key roles in several African American families, which can be an essential cultural parameter to assess when working with clients facing mental health challenges.

In addition, religious beliefs are an important resource for many clients coping with emotional problems (see Chap. 7). In some cases, they serve as the most important source of strength for clients, who need to be able to share their beliefs without fear of offending the nurse or provoking judgment. If clients are afraid that their feelings or behaviors conflict with their religious faith or that they have alienated themselves from their religions, a referral to a chaplain may be helpful.

In a therapeutic relationship, respect must be both given and received. Nurses need to set limits when clients are disrespectful so that the boundaries of the relationship remain intact. For example, if a client with mania is hypersexual and making seductive remarks, the nurse should make it clear that this behavior is unwelcome and needs to stop. Calmly stating, "This is not a time for sexual talk. Tell me about how you are doing, Mr. Jones" should be sufficient. If an intoxicated client insults or swears at a nurse, the nurse should set firm limits by saying, "Lower your voice, stop swearing, and let's talk about what you need, Mrs. Smith." A calm, nondefensive, and respectful demeanor eventually helps set the tone for the interaction and reduces the client's emotional escalation. If problematic behavior persists, the nurse should simply repeat the limit-setting statements calmly and firmly, leave the room for a period of time, or request help if the client appears about to lose control. In most cases, the establishment of a therapeutic relationship based on genuine respect, careful listening, responsiveness, and limit setting can prevent escalation of verbal and physical aggression (Cowin et al., 2003). A study comparing nurses' and clients' perceptions of precursors to aggression on three inpatient psychiatric units found that whereas the nurses perceived the main cause of aggression to be the clients' mental illness, the clients reported that environmental conditions (feeling like "prisoners") and disrespectful communication by the nurses were the most common precursors (Duxbury & Whittington,

2005). Another observational study of inpatient psychiatric nurses showed that simply acknowledging the client and engaging in a "dialogue of wondering reflection" about the client's concerns was often more effective than direct limit setting (Vatne & Fagermoen, 2007).

Think About It 11.1

The police bring Mr. Greene to the emergency department for treatment of lacerations after an arrest for drunken and disorderly conduct. He has experienced a relapse after completing three treatment programs in the past 5 years for substance use disorder. His wife and adult daughter are in the waiting room, hoping to take him home. Mr. Greene shouts at the nurse, "You tell those (expletive) women that they can get the hell out of here. You can get lost, too!" He then urinates on the floor. What specific actions would be most helpful to establish a basis for communication with this client?

Caring

Caring, one of nursing's core values, consists of three primary behaviors: (1) giving of the self, (2) meeting the needs of clients in a timely manner, and (3) providing comfort measures for clients and family. Creating a therapeutic relationship involves time and energy. Nurses must be genuinely invested in clients' welfare and willing to do what it takes to reduce suffering, anxiety, and uncertainty as much as possible. The opposite of caring is **apathy**, a sense of detachment and the belief that nothing one does makes any difference, which leads to a lack of concern about the problem or outcome. Many clients experience apathy when they struggle with chronic psychiatric symptoms and are tempted to give up trying to cope. Caring involves having the energy and optimism to keep working with clients, despite discouragement. One study of therapists working with substance-abusing clients found that helping clients find hope and remaining connected to them despite setbacks were key components to effective therapeutic relationships (Kothari et al., 2010). Another study of hospitalized clients with depression found that after nurses provided an initially nurturing and comforting presence during admission, clients perceived them as distancing themselves and focusing mainly on physical symptoms (Moyle, 2003). The study also showed that clients reported a "yearning" for closeness to nursing staff, and especially a need for continued reassurance that they would recover.

Caring also involves showing empathy by listening to clients' viewpoints and trying to understand their experiences (Figure 11.3).Carl Rogers (1952), a psychologist who wrote extensively about effective therapeutic relationships, identified three major ingredients:

1. **Empathy**. Emotionally knowing another person goes beyond just having facts about his or her history. It means feeling what it must be like to be that person. Extensive

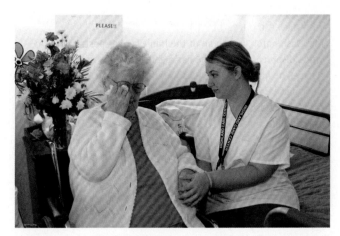

FIGURE 11.3 Empathy, or fully appreciating the experience of another person, is a core element of the nursing value of caring.

research has shown that both nurses and clients value empathy and understanding as primary components of the therapeutic relationship (Dziopa & Ahern, 2009b). Empathy involves listening carefully, being in tune with what clients are saying, and having insight into the meaning of their thoughts, feelings, and behaviors. A recent study found that professionals' interest, willingness, and desire to understand were more critical to people with mental illness than actually understanding their experience (Shattell et al., 2006). Clients said that being understood was a physical, somatic "gut" feeling they could sense in their bodies. In addition, all the clients reported painful feelings of being misunderstood by professionals.

2. **Genuineness**. Being "real" means true engagement in knowing and interacting with clients in open, human exchanges. Obviously, genuineness cannot be fake, and comes through as an attitude that arises from deep concern. It also means being able to relax and resist trying to impress others.

3. **Unconditional positive regard**. This third key component means being able to give to clients with "no strings attached." From this position, clients are worthy of respect and attention, regardless of their behavior and despite their flaws and setbacks.

Partnership

Historically, relationships between health care providers and clients were unequal. Professionals were seen as healers, and clients were viewed as relatively passive recipients of treatment. However, current approaches emphasize the role of clients and families as active partners in care. Collaborative, client-centered approaches focus on mutually solving problems, jointly planning treatments, and empowering clients to care for themselves (Adams & Drake, 2006). Partnership involves power sharing and negotiation (Gallant et al., 2002). One study investigating how psychiatric nurses

develop high-quality therapeutic relationships found that partnership was a key component, even though nurses varied in their styles of partnership, with some emphasizing equality and others seeing themselves more as protectors or senior guides (Dziopa & Ahern, 2009a). Another study of nursing care in home settings found that clients and their caregivers who had effective therapeutic relationships attempted to cocreate their care and establish a "professional friendship" that valued the knowledge and opinions of family members (Lindahl et al., 2011).

Families and loved ones are invaluable resources for clients, who are now cared for mostly in community settings and often depend on relatives for daily support. If loved ones are not treated as partners in care, they may feel alienated, judged, and devalued. All efforts must work to integrate their unparalleled knowledge of the client's situation and insights about how various interventions may work.

Checkpoint Questions

1. What are five essential elements of a therapeutic relationship?
2. What are nurses displaying when they demonstrate detachment and the belief that nothing they do makes any difference?

Obstacles to Therapeutic Relationships

Nurses entering psychiatric–mental health settings bring with them values, beliefs, and perspectives that influence their interactions with clients. At the same time, these clients usually have intense emotions and complex behaviors. Their care can pose unique challenges for nurses to control their own emotional reactions and check their social biases (Case Vignette 11.1).

Attitudes and behaviors that may block effective interaction with clients experiencing mental health problems include judgmental attitudes, excessive probing, and lack of self-awareness. Nurses need to approach each client with unbiased perspectives. During discussions, nurses need to make sure they remain focused on essential problems and avoid explorations unrelated to the issue or challenge of concern. Additionally, nurses must be able to monitor and contain their own responses when clients discuss frightening incidents or relate tragedies that generate feelings of hopelessness, despair, anxiety, disgust, fear, anger, or distress. Chapter 8 discusses nursing values, attitudes, and self-awareness in detail.

Confronting Judgmental Attitudes

Judgmental attitudes from nurses are an obvious problem. Before working in psychiatric settings, nurses need to ask themselves the following questions:

• Do I believe that mental illness is as real as any physical illness (eg, diabetes, asthma)?

Case Vignette 11.1

Mr. Smith, a 38-year-old man with bipolar disorder, has taken an overdose of antidepressants and been admitted for his eighth psychiatric hospitalization. Stressors leading to this hospitalization include stopping his medications 4 months ago, losing his job, and recently alienating his 14-year-old daughter.

Although they have been divorced for 3 years, Mr. Smith's ex-wife continues to provide emotional and financial support for the client. Before the divorce, the family experienced severe financial difficulties when Mr. Smith went on spending sprees during manic episodes. Erratic behavior, sleeplessness, and sudden prolonged disappearances distressed his family.

Currently, Mr. Smith expresses remorse about the problems he has caused. He says he wishes he could reunite with his wife but understands that the relationship seems irreparable. His greatest worry is that his daughter may never forgive him for hurtful things he said during their most recent argument. He continues to have suicidal thoughts, but he has no immediate intention to harm himself.

The nurse approaches Mr. Smith to ask him how he is feeling. He replies, "How do you think I'm feeling? I have no family, no job, no future. … I'm just one big screwup. And here I am, doped up in the hospital. What's the point?"

Reflection and Critical Thinking

- If you were the nurse, how would you initially respond?
- What challenges will the nurse face in building a relationship with Mr. Smith?
- What challenges will the nurse face in communicating with Mr. Smith?
- How can nurses learn to modify their emotions and reactions when dealing with clients?

▲

- Do I suspect that clients are overdramatizing their symptoms or using them as a crutch to avoid work and social responsibility?
- Do I view mental illness as a sign of a weak character?
- Do I find myself asking, "Why doesn't this person just snap out of it, put his or her problems in perspective, or focus on something else?"

If nurses have these thoughts when working with clients with psychiatric disorders, they require more education and exposure to the reality of mental illness. Psychiatric symptoms are every bit as real and disabling as any physical disease and often more devastating to quality of life. Although a nurse may feel critical of a client who slashes her wrists for the fourth time in what seems to be a bid for attention, the nurse must be aware that anyone who would use this method of coping must feel desperate and see no other alternative. Remembering that clients in psychiatric settings are doing the best they can with limited coping skills is helpful.

Enhancing Self-Awareness

Interacting with clients in emotional pain requires maturity and self-awareness (Eckroth-Bucher, 2010) (see Chap. 8). Psychiatric nurses consider self-awareness a precondition for establishing therapeutic relationships (Dziopa & Ahern, 2009b). Nurses must be able to monitor and contain their own anxiety when clients discuss frightening incidents or relate tragic events that generate feelings of hopelessness and despair. Listening to clients without mentally or physically fleeing from the situation or offering impersonal platitudes is key to the therapeutic relationship. Clients must feel safe with the nurse. They must be able to sense that the nurse can handle what they are saying without becoming overwhelmed by the nurse's reactions. One study of nursing students' first professional encounter with clients on a psychiatric unit found that students preoccupied with their own needs felt more helpless and were more rejecting than their peers. In this instance, lack of willingness by clients to engage in a therapeutic relationship met the students' own negative expectations (Granskar et al., 2001). In contrast, students who could put aside their own anxieties and focus on client needs were more confident, more able to see each client as a unique person, and ultimately proud when clients wanted to establish a relationship with them. For this reason, nurses must appreciate the importance of taking care of their own mental health.

Developing self-awareness is a lifelong process that requires continual work (see Chap. 8). It necessitates disciplined attention to one's own needs, as well as insight about how to meet them. Nurses also go through ups and downs, rendering them more or less able to respond flexibly and easily to others' demands. Knowing one's own limits, detecting signs of becoming exhausted or less tolerant, and being able to nourish oneself physically, mentally, and spiritually are essential to becoming a therapeutic agent for others. For some nurses, being critical or defensive with clients is a warning signal that it is time to take a rest or seek support. Other important warning signals include the following:

- Worrying about clients when off duty
- Becoming overinvolved with clients in inappropriate ways (eg, making extra visits when time does not allow for them, calling clients when off duty)

- Believing that you are the only person who can help a client; that is, having "rescue fantasies"

Both negative, rejecting attitudes and overprotective, rescuing behaviors may be indicators of what are called **countertransference** reactions in nurses and mental health professionals (Jones, 2005). Determining the appropriate level of involvement with clients that maximizes therapeutic relationships while protecting one's energy and mental health is something most nurses learn with experience.

Maturity is another important quality linked with self-awareness. Of course, maturity is not just a function of age. Some middle-aged people behave immaturely, whereas some young people are wise beyond their years. **Maturity** involves being able to integrate aspects of life into a whole and find balance in one's outlook and attitudes toward others. This important factor allows nurses to feel empathy. Whereas nurses who lack maturity cannot see the similarities between themselves and others, more mature nurses can see and imagine the smallest of similarities because they feel a oneness with all human beings. One study of psychiatric nurses' perceptions of the therapeutic relationship found that knowledge and skill were inadequate for understanding clients unless the nurses were able to utilize insights from their own life experiences (Scanlon, 2010).

Excessive Probing

Clients in the mental health system typically must tell their stories to many different professionals. Technically, professionals have the right to ask any questions they deem necessary. However, they should recognize that the goal is to help clients cope with their current situation. Asking clients to relate painful details of their childhood or to recount the embarrassing circumstances leading to their hospitalization (eg, being arrested, going on a manic spending spree, being found in a regressed psychotic state) may place an unfair burden on them. This is especially true when the relationship is short term.

Nurses must ask themselves whether their questions are designed to satisfy their own curiosity or to meet the client's current needs. Are the nurse and client embarking on a long-term relationship in which the client can fully discuss experiences from childhood to achieve some kind of resolution? Or is the nurse unearthing sensitive aspects of the client's history and then proceeding as if nothing happened? Being in a therapeutic relationship does not give nurses unlimited permission to invade a client's privacy. Communication with clients should follow their lead.

Maslow's hierarchy of needs may provide a useful guide for determining the kinds of questions to ask clients (Figure 11.4). When basic needs such as safety and physical health are not met, probing into the client's history to discover the roots of poor self-image is irrelevant. Concrete help with referrals to social services and education about self-care will be vastly more useful to the client than an exploration of family dynamics, particularly in the brief treatment settings that pervade most of the current health care system.

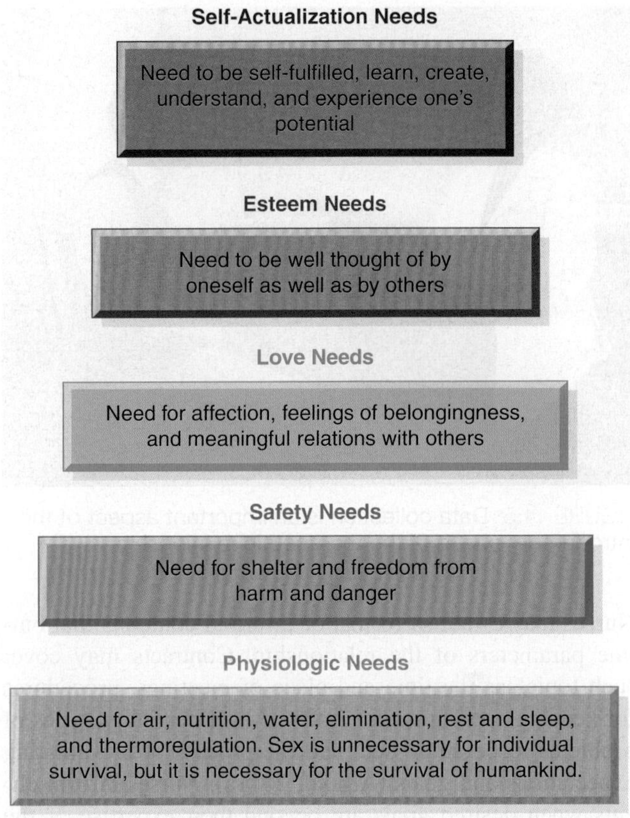

Self-Actualization Needs

Need to be self-fulfilled, learn, create, understand, and experience one's potential

Esteem Needs

Need to be well thought of by oneself as well as by others

Love Needs

Need for affection, feelings of belongingness, and meaningful relations with others

Safety Needs

Need for shelter and freedom from harm and danger

Physiologic Needs

Need for air, nutrition, water, elimination, rest and sleep, and thermoregulation. Sex is unnecessary for individual survival, but it is necessary for the survival of humankind.

FIGURE 11.4 **Maslow's hierarchy.**

Nurses should view their access to the private thoughts and feelings of clients as a delicate privilege to handle with the utmost care.

Phases of the Therapeutic Relationship

Each phase of the therapeutic relationship has predictable behaviors, dynamics, and challenges. Studies show that the nurse–client relationship passes through three distinct phases that build upon each other (Coatsworth-Puspoky et al., 2006). This discussion enumerates the key tasks of each phase and describes how the relationship moves forward from introduction to termination.

Introductory Phase

Therapeutic relationships are not instantaneous; they take time. The goal of the introductory phase is to establish rapport and build a foundation for further work. Nurses focus on the following:

- Introducing themselves and greeting clients by name
- Communicating interest in clients
- Responding to any immediate concerns, such as questions, comfort needs, or emergency issues
- Setting the parameters for nurse–client interactions
- Gathering data (Figure 11.5)
- Discerning the focal problem, setting goals, and beginning to plan interventions
- Reducing client anxieties

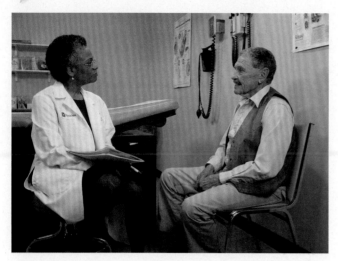

FIGURE 11.5 Data collection is an important aspect of the introductory phase of the therapeutic relationship.

Nurses may establish formal or informal contracts that outline parameters of the relationship. Contracts may cover such topics as the time and place of meetings, procedures for keeping appointments, limits of confidentiality, types of problems to be addressed, and the process of reevaluating expectations and goals (Arnold, 2011a). Nurses inform clients when desired goals are beyond their expertise or the duration of the interaction. For example, if a client wants a nurse to help find housing and this is beyond the scope of the nurse's role, the nurse makes an appropriate referral so that the client does not feel frustrated with the nurse's apparent lack of attention to his or her needs.

During the introductory phase, clients commonly test the nurse's commitment by acting-out or missing appointments. They may show their worst behavior (eg, challenging, withdrawing) to see whether the nurse can handle the intensity of their problems (Challenging Behaviors 11.1). After all, if the client's symptoms and coping patterns scare off the nurse, the relationship may be unsafe or there may be no point in investing energy in it. Clients may wonder whether nurses are just doing their job or really care. One study of clients hospitalized on psychiatric units showed that during the first phase of the therapeutic relationship, if nurses seemed to retreat to their work stations and withhold support and comfort, the clients responded with avoidance that led to a spiraling deterioration through the subsequent phases of the relationship (Coatsworth-Puspoky et al., 2006). Particularly when the relationship is new and vulnerable, nurses must demonstrate that they are consistently available, caring, and respectful. Gently confronting or questioning acting-out behaviors sets the stage for open discussion throughout the relationship, indicating that nurses can tolerate conflict and help clients explore their own ambivalence about treatment and behavior change.

In the therapeutic relationship, nurses exercise some power over clients through language, persuasive techniques, and control of the agenda. However, the aim is to create a collaborative and open relationship in which clients feel free to identify needs, desires, and goals. Use of professional jargon can impede understanding, create distance, and alienate clients. An important focus is the nurse's sincere attempt to learn about the client's cultural background and perspectives, especially because they may differ from the nurse's own worldview. The relationship is under way when nurse and client progress beyond exchanging information to exploring deeper feelings and issues of pressing concern to the client.

Many clients in today's health care environment are discharged or transferred from psychiatric units while still in the orientation or introductory phase of the nurse–client relationship. For this reason, a preponderance of the research on the phases of the therapeutic nurse–client relationship has been done in Canada and the United Kingdom, where constraints on the length of mental health treatment are fewer (Stockmann, 2005). Whereas negative preconceptions by both clients and nurses have been associated with a prolonged

Challenging Behaviors 11.1

The Withdrawn Client

Situation: Mr. Boswell has a diagnosis of major depression. When you approach him, he says, "I don't want to talk with anyone right now. I'm too tired."

Your Potential Feelings: Frustration, rejection, helplessness.

What Is Going On? Mr. Boswell is experiencing symptoms that create barriers to communication. He may be concerned that the nurse will try to cheer him up or lecture him, rather than listen to his feelings. Feelings of worthlessness may cause Mr. Boswell to believe he does not deserve the nurse's time. He may be testing the nurse.

Strategy: Gently encourage Mr. Boswell to describe his experience with depression and express his feelings. Make thoughtful observations about his mood and behavior to demonstrate caring, affirm his uniqueness, and facilitate further dialogue. Allow silence and remain present, showing respect for Mr. Boswell's need to move slowly and to be understood. If this strategy fails, allow Mr. Boswell some privacy and attempt the process again later.

Nurse Action/Communication: "You do look tired. It must be discouraging. . . . I noticed that your wife was here earlier. How are you feeling about the visit?"

introductory phase, longer interactions with clients (eg, one 30-minute interaction instead of several 10-minute "check-ins") have been found to predict faster movement to the working phase (Forchuk, 1994, 1995).

Before moving to the next phase of the relationship, the nurse and client evaluate whether they have met the following goals of the pivotal introductory stage:

* Trust is established, and both parties perceive the relationship as safe.
* The client can verbalize thoughts and feelings.
* Both the nurse and client have identified and agreed upon a focal problem or purpose for the relationship.
* The client's strengths, weaknesses, and priorities for intervention are becoming clear.
* The nurse has explained his or her role.

Working (Middle) Phase

In the working phase, clients are involved actively in achieving goals set during the initial phase. They make progress by testing new behaviors, identifying resources, and discovering avenues for change. For example, a client with schizophrenia may try new strategies for dealing with hallucinations. Success in coping with hallucinations may allow the client to function better in family or community settings, cultivate a more hopeful attitude toward the illness, and find new opportunities, such as supervised employment and friendships. As clients achieve goals, nurses provide feedback and support. This support is especially important for clients who may not notice or take credit for their own gradual improvements. Behaviors do not change easily. Energy, practice, and willingness to risk failure are essential for any significant progress. In addition, nurses need to remain sensitive to clients' daily sociocultural context (eg, poverty, lack of family and other social support, traditional gender role constraints), which may cause them to view change as difficult, if not impossible or even undesirable (Russell et al., 2003).

Of course, many clients go through periods of resisting change. This development is normal during the working phase of the therapeutic relationship. Change is usually not linear; rather, it tends to happen in "stops and starts," with periods of regression to old patterns. Some clients demonstrate so much resistance to change that it seems they are making no progress. Examples include the following:

* Clients who have repeated psychotic episodes because they stop taking their medications
* People who have made multiple suicide attempts
* Adolescents with anorexia who lose the weight they gained each time they leave the hospital
* Clients recovering from substance use disorders who relapse

Nurses must maintain hope and optimism that change will occur when the time is right, clients have learned what they need to know and have developed new coping skills, adequate support systems are in place, and circumstances have

facilitated a major shift in thinking. It may help if nurses reflect on a bad habit or personality trait that they themselves have been trying to change and note how slow and difficult the process has been.

When working with clients who are highly resistant to change, mental health professionals may feel so frustrated that they become critical and blaming. Although confrontation and education are part of the therapeutic relationship, criticism and blame can destroy it. Hoff and colleagues (2009) refer to the *victim–rescuer–persecutor syndrome*. In this familiar cycle:

1. The client is vulnerable and requests help.
2. Mental health professionals offer help.
3. The client has difficulty changing well-established behavior patterns.
4. The professional feels frustrated with the "treatment failure."
5. The professional "persecutes" the client (victim) for failing to respond.
6. Finally, the victim becomes the persecutor and punishes the professional for well-intended but inappropriate efforts to help.

To avoid this destructive pattern, nurses need to be aware of countertransference reactions (see Chap. 3); monitor their levels of patience, empathy, and flexibility in dealing with persistent behavioral patterns that resist change; and seek support and supervision when they become frustrated with clients (Figure 11.6).

For some clients, the working phase is a period of major life reorganization. An adolescent may stop acting out and find a way to communicate with parents; a homeless person may find employment; a depressed mother may begin to enjoy her family again. Nevertheless, many clients with chronic conditions revisit their problems throughout their lives, focusing on different layers of difficulties and new challenges. For those clients, the goal may be to reduce the

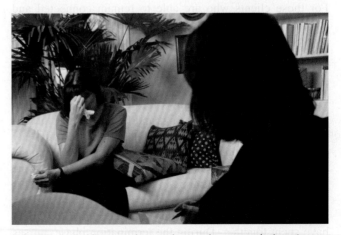

FIGURE 11.6 Nurses who are becoming overwhelmed by their work with clients need to seek support and supervision from trusted mentors and colleagues. In some cases, they themselves may need to seek mental health interventions.

impact of their symptoms, improve their level of functioning, and enhance the quality of their lives.

Before moving to the next phase of the relationship, the nurse and client evaluate whether they have met the following goals of the working stage:

- The client has identified past behaviors that have been ineffective for coping with the focal problem.
- The client has developed a plan of action, practiced implementing it, and evaluated its effectiveness.
- The client has integrated a new self-concept, worldview, or attitude toward the illness as a result of changes in behavior and circumstances.
- The client and family express increased hopefulness for the future and ability to function independently.

Termination Phase

Whether a therapeutic relationship is brief or long term, nurses must pay attention to the termination phase and ensure that clients know the termination date well in advance. Termination always involves loss. If substantial work has been done, both nurse and client may feel the loss of the helping relationship. If goals have not been realized because of time constraints or limitations in the relationship, termination may seem less significant.

Clients often regress during the termination phase. Examples include evidencing original symptoms or testing the nurse's belief in the client's abilities to function independently. Most likely, clients are worried about the loss of a relationship that has provided a source of support. Now clients will have to handle problems on their own. Anxiety contributes to reverting to previous bad habits. Considering that loss is a universal human experience, the client's historical way of dealing with it may manifest itself during the termination phase. Some clients feel rejected, others withdraw prematurely to protect against the pain of grieving, and others try to end the relationship angrily and abruptly. For those clients who are able to remain connected and tolerate the mixed feelings involved in termination, this phase can offer an opportunity to make meaning of their illness experience, perhaps discovering that they have grown or learned to take more responsibility for their own lives (Schon, 2009).

As the relationship draws to a close, the nurse's job is to remain consistent, caring, and hopeful about the client's progress. This is the time to review work, discuss any remaining questions, clear up misconceptions, and applaud the client's progress. On a more human level, it is a time to remember the high points in the relationship (moments of laughter or insight), acknowledge and let go of the low points, and appreciate the time that the nurse and client have spent together. During the termination phase, nurses should feel free to share their positive feelings and admiration for clients, as well as to express enjoyment of the relationship.

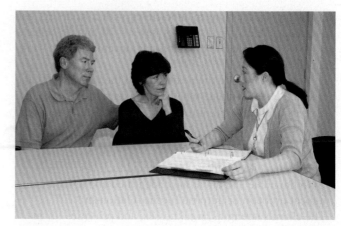

FIGURE 11.7 In the termination phase, nurses spend time teaching family members important aspects of follow-up care for clients.

At this time, nurses educate families about the client's condition, advise them of the potential for symptom recurrence, and inform them about signs of relapse (Figure 11.7). They make specific recommendations regarding how to help clients maintain their improved functioning. Studies show that careful discharge planning, including the establishment of a safety net of professional and peer (mental health consumer) support, significantly lowers the chance of relapse and readmission (Forchuk et al., 2007).

Before concluding treatment, the nurse and client evaluate whether they have met the following goals of the termination stage:

- Contacts between nurse and client are spaced further apart or appointments are shorter to allow for increased independence.
- Both parties have expressed feelings about the loss of the relationship.
- Interactions are more relaxed, less intense, and focused on the future.
- The nurse discourages cues that lead to new areas of exploration.
- The nurse provides necessary referrals and links with community resources.

> ### Checkpoint Questions
> 3. How can nurses facilitate movement from the introductory phase into the working phase of the therapeutic relationship?
> 4. During which phase of the therapeutic relationship does the client commonly regress?

THERAPEUTIC COMMUNICATION

Communication is the process of conveying information through various complex verbal and nonverbal behaviors. This process can be broken into several components.

Communicators are people who simultaneously send and receive messages through words and nonverbal actions (eg, nodding, eye contact, facial expressions, posture). **Encoding** is the process by which a communicator puts into words or behaviors the ideas or feelings that he or she is trying to convey. Examples of encoding include shouting, crying, looking away, and choosing particular words. **Decoding** is the process by which a communicator discerns or interprets what another is saying. The **channel** is the route or method a communicator chooses to convey a message. Channels include writing, talking, looking, e-mailing, and phoning. **Feedback** is the discernible response that a receiver makes to a sender's message. All behaviors, including silence and ignoring, are forms of feedback.

Environment refers to the personal experiences and cultural background that each communicator brings to the interaction. Environmental variables include age, socio-economic status, race, and life events such as death, divorce, and illness. Whereas similarities in environmental experiences can lead to common understanding, coming from different environments can create communication gaps (Adler & Proctor, 2010). Another factor that can influence the effectiveness of communication is **noise**, which consists of any force that interferes with effective communication:

- **External noise** refers to any factor outside a communicator that creates distractions. Examples include other people talking, a cold or hot room, and background noise.
- **Physiologic noise** is any factor within the communicator that detracts from effective communication. Some examples are hearing loss, tiredness, sedating medication, or physical pain.
- **Psychological noise** refers to any force within a communicator that interferes with the ability to accurately express or understand a message. Possibilities include anger, defensiveness, paranoia, apathy, and fear. A recent literature review cites studies showing that inpatient psychiatric nurses spend less than half their working day with clients, mainly because of heavy workloads and staff shortages (Sharac et al., 2010). Such situations create potent psychological noise that distracts nurses from interacting with clients, despite their best intentions

Therapeutic communication occurs when the nurse demonstrates empathy, uses effective communication skills, and responds to the client's thoughts, needs, and concerns. This planned process allows nurse and client to build a trusting relationship in which the client is free to express thoughts, feelings, and options without fear of judgment. It is based on specific skills that nurses learn to implement through careful practice and experience. It does not just arise naturally. Therapeutic communication also involves nurses carefully encoding communication to make it

understandable to clients of different cultural backgrounds and ages. By the same token, client messages must be understood and decoded in the context of the cultural background or environment in which the client lives. For example, if an Asian client does not make eye contact or initiate interactions, this may be a sign of deference to authority, rather than a lack of interest or energy.

Therapeutic (or effective) communication techniques include giving broad openings, paraphrasing, offering general leads, reflecting feelings, focusing, voicing doubt, clarifying, sequencing events, giving information, encouraging formulation of a plan, and testing discrepancies. Purposes and examples are found in Table 11.2.

Nontherapeutic communication develops when nurses respond in ways that cause clients to feel defensive, misunderstood, controlled, minimized, alienated, or discouraged from expressing thoughts and feelings. Types include responding socially, using closed-ended questions, changing the subject, belittling, making stereotyped comments, offering false reassurance, moralizing, interpreting, advising, challenging, and defending. Although most people use nontherapeutic responses in everyday communication, it is important to be aware of how these responses deter open discussion and increase the likelihood of withdrawal by clients. Learning the labels for nontherapeutic approaches helps nurses to recognize and avoid them. Reasons for and examples of them are found in Table 11.3.

Theoretical Framework and Communication Model

A communication model can help explain interactions between people, including nurses and clients (Figure 11.8). Within this model, nurse–client communication consists of many interrelated components, giving rise to highly unique interactions depending on the backgrounds, moods, and circumstances of each situation. In this sense, no two interactions are the same, and predicting how an encounter will unfold is impossible. The wonder of human communication is that it generates the variety and spontaneity that make nursing challenging and ever-changing work.

External, physical, and physiologic noise can occur at any point in the nurse–client interaction and disrupt accurate communication. Insufficient overlap in the environments of the communicators (eg, nurses using professional jargon that clients do not understand, clients trying to convey their financial desperation to nurses who have never known hunger or homelessness) may block the process before it begins. The subtle and obvious nonverbal reactions of both nurse and client continually shape each interaction in a complex way, creating a unique climate or tone for each relationship. Thus, to become effective communicators, nurses must practice the art of carefully observing their clients' messages and consistently monitoring their own words and behaviors. Even the nurses' manner of dress communicates messages that affect others' perceptions.

TABLE 11.2 Therapeutic Communication Techniques

Technique	Purpose	Example
Giving broad openings	Communicates a desire to begin a meaningful interaction Allows the client to define the problem or issue	"What would you like to discuss today?" "Tell me about how you have been doing."
Paraphrasing	Reflects the meaning of the client's message in the nurse's words Allows for clarification Lets the client know that the nurse has understood the message	"So you're saying that your husband is unwilling to work on the marriage any more."
Offering general leads	Encourages client to continue elaborating Communicates the nurse's interest in listening	"I see." "Uh-huh."
Reflecting feelings	Reflects the emotion underlying the client's message Conveys empathy	"It sounds like you're feeling hopeless about the situation."
Focusing	Encourages the client to expand upon one part of a statement Concentrates on a single issue Useful technique with clients who are confused or overwhelmed by many issues at the same time	"Can you give me an example of how that typically happens for you?" "Let's go back to _____ because I'm not sure I follow you." "What is it about _____ that bothers you?"
Voicing doubt	Gentle way of challenging the client's perceptions Encourages reconsideration	"Really?" "Are you sure that your parents will never accept your decision?"
Clarifying	Makes clear that which is vague or not meaningful May help clients clarify their own understanding	"I'm not sure what you mean by _____."
Placing events in time sequence	Allows the client to organize thoughts Provides clues to recurring patterns Helps the nurse follow the client's train of thought and understand what is happening	"So how did this start?" "What happened next?"
Giving information	Allows for teaching and clarification	"Several halfway houses have work programs."
Encouraging formulation of a plan	Encourages client to think about solutions without the nurse giving advice Helps the client problem solve	"What do you think you should do about this problem?" "What are your options, as you see them?"
Testing discrepancies	Helps the client become aware of inconsistencies in statements versus behaviors Allows for gentle confrontation	"You say that you want to participate in this group, but I notice that you have missed the past three meetings."

Listening

Listening, or focusing on all behaviors that clients express, is the foundation of therapeutic communication. Listening requires energy, concentration, and specific skills in asking questions, while allowing clients to determine the content and level of disclosure. This active process focuses objective, empathic attention on clients. Characteristics of active listening are as follows:

- Maintaining eye contact
- Facilitating proximity (if this is not threatening to the client)
- Projecting a relaxed physical orientation
- Speaking calmly

Nurses set the stage for listening by removing environmental distractions, such as television or the presence of others; preventing interruptions; and attending to the client's physical comfort. Another key component is a

TABLE 11.3 Nontherapeutic Communication Techniques

Technique	Detrimental Consequence	Example
Social responding	Engaging in superficial conversation that is not client centered	Client: "I'm glad I'm being discharged today." Nurse: "Are you going to watch the football game tonight?"
Asking closed-ended questions	Questions that elicit a "yes" or "no" answer instead of allowing for wider exploration of the client's thoughts and feelings	Nurse: "Do you understand everything I've told you about electroconvulsive therapy?"
Changing the subject	Introducing an unrelated or peripherally related topic (usually to avoid sensitive issues or reduce the nurse's anxiety)	Client: "I don't think my husband finds me attractive since I had the mastectomy." Nurse: "I didn't realize you had breast cancer. Does it run in your family?"
Belittling	Discounting the client's feelings or making comparisons that imply the client's problems are smaller than he or she perceives	Client: "My home was totally destroyed in the fire." Nurse: "At least you are alive."
Making stereotyped comments	Offering platitudes or wise sayings that seem automatic or contrived	Client: "I can't get over the loss of my mother." Nurse: "Time heals all wounds. Everything happens for a reason."
Offering false reassurance	Attempting to cheer up the client by suggesting there is no real problem	Client: "I'm afraid my boss will fire me if he finds out I have a substance abuse problem." Nurse: "Don't worry. He wouldn't do that."
Moralizing	Passing judgment by imposing one's own values on the client and implying that the client's thinking is wrong	Client: "I want a divorce." Nurse: "Don't you think you owe it to your children to give the marriage another try?"
Interpreting	Making intrusive comments in an attempt to overanalyze or "psychoanalyze" clients' statements	Client: "I don't want to take this medication." Nurse: "I think you're in denial about your illness."
Advising	Making specific suggestions instead of offering information and asking clients what they think is most likely to work	Client: "I feel depressed." Nurse: "You should do some volunteer work to take your mind off things."
Challenging	Denying or diminishing the client's perceptions, forcing the client to prove what he or she is saying	Client: "Nobody cares about me." Nurse: "What about your sister? I saw her visiting yesterday."
Defending	Arguing or justifying your position rather than attempting to hear the client's concerns	Client: "I can't get any help with this problem." Nurse: "We are doing our best to help you but we are very busy."

nonjudgmental stance that allows for supportive, objective feedback.

Nurses note congruence (agreement) or incongruence between verbal and nonverbal communication and validate observations with clients. An example of incongruence would be a client experiencing psychosis who says he is willing to talk but projects nonverbal cues of fear and withdrawal. Nurses must attend to their own feelings and thoughts that may provoke nontherapeutic reactions, such as changing the subject because of anxiety, becoming annoyed or critical, or feeling overwhelmed by sadness or helplessness over the client's situation.

For examples of how nurses can use effective listening skills in interactions with clients, see Therapeutic Communication 11.1.

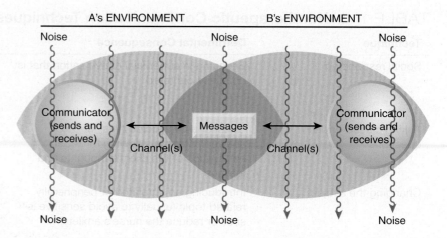

FIGURE 11.8 A transactional communication model. (Source: Adler, R. B., & Proctor, R. F. [2010]. *Looking out/looking in* [13th ed.]. Belmont, CA: Thomson\Wadsworth.)

Therapeutic Communication 11.1

Encouraging Formulation of a Plan

Rosa Rodriguez has just had her second child and is suffering from postpartum depression. The home health care nurse is making a follow-up visit.

INEFFECTIVE DIALOGUE

CLIENT: "The clinic told me you were coming. Come on in. The house is a mess."

NURSE: "Oh, you should see my house." *(Using inappropriate self-disclosure and social responding)*

CLIENT: "I bet yours isn't this bad. I just can't get anything done with the new baby."

NURSE: "Don't worry. Things will be back to normal soon." *(Giving false reassurance)*

CLIENT: "I don't know what normal is anymore. I can't get any sleep. The baby cries all the time."

NURSE: "All the time? Are you sure you're not exaggerating?" *(Challenging)*

CLIENT: "Maybe not every minute. But he's not like my Maria was. She let me sleep."

NURSE: "It's not right to compare one child to another. Every child is different. The baby is small, and he can't help it when he cries." *(Moralizing)*

CLIENT: "Well, I guess I'm just not a good mother because I can't handle it. Maybe I never should have had this baby."

NURSE: "Don't say that. Let's talk about your medication." *(Changing the subject)*

CLIENT: "That medication doesn't work."

NURSE: "Antidepressants can be highly effective if you give them a chance." *(Defending)*

CLIENT: "I took them for a few days, but they didn't help me sleep, so I figured there wasn't any point. Besides, they have side effects."

NURSE: "You have to take the medication for about 10 days or 2 weeks to get the full effect. It doesn't work right away. And

EFFECTIVE DIALOGUE

CLIENT: "The clinic told me you were coming. Come on in. The house is a mess."

NURSE: "Nice to see you, Mrs. Rodriguez. How are things with the baby?" *(Broad opening)*

CLIENT: "He's not easy—not like my Maria was."

NURSE: "So it's been rough for you." *(Paraphrasing)*

CLIENT: "He's a screamer. And he never sleeps, especially at night."

NURSE: "You must be really tired." *(Reflecting feelings)*

CLIENT: "Yeah. I don't know how I can keep going."

NURSE: "You sound discouraged. How is your depression at this point?" *(Reflecting feelings, focusing)*

CLIENT: "It's coming back. Sometimes I forget to take the pills. I don't know if they really would help anyway."

NURSE: "What do you mean?" *(Clarifying)*

CLIENT: "I took them for the first 3 days, but they didn't really do anything, so I stopped. I thought they would help me stop crying, but they didn't."

NURSE: "I can see how you would be frustrated that you didn't get any immediate relief from your depression. The medicine you were taking doesn't begin to have its full effect until about a week or so after you start taking it, but it can be very effective if you take it regularly. *(Giving information)*

CLIENT: "That seems like forever right now. I just want one good night's sleep."

NURSE: "Well, I'll talk to the doctor today about restarting your medication, but in the meantime, what do you think could help with sleep?" *(Encouraging formulation of a plan)*

with the side effects, remember—"no pain, no gain." You have to give a little to get a little." *(Making stereotyped comments)*

CLIENT: "Well I'm not getting anything—especially sleep."

NURSE: "Why don't you try a nice cup of herbal tea before going to sleep?" *(Advising)*

CLIENT: "I don't like herbal tea, and I'm too tired to make myself anything. I haven't even been eating much."

NURSE: "Well, that's not good. Didn't you get the pamphlet about nutrition at the hospital?" *(Moralizing, using a closed-ended question)*

CLIENT: "Yeah."

NURSE: "I think you'll feel better once you get back on your medication and get some sleep. Remember, infancy doesn't last forever. Before you know it, he'll be sleeping through the night." *(Giving false reassurance, belittling feelings)*

CLIENT: "If you say so. I find it hard to believe right now."

CLIENT: "I guess I could ask my sister to take care of the children so I could have a nap."

NURSE: "That's one option. Anything else?" *(Encouraging formulation of a plan)*

CLIENT: "Oh, I guess I can handle it if I have to."

NURSE: "You say you can handle it, but I can tell you are tired, and your depression seems to be returning." *(Testing discrepancies)*

CLIENT: "Yeah. I just don't have the energy to even think about it."

NURSE: "Well, let's think this through and come up with a plan. It's hard enough to take care of small children when you have some energy, but when you're depressed, it really becomes difficult. I'm concerned about you." *(Encouraging formulation of a plan, reflecting feelings)*

Reflection and Critical Thinking

- What do you think the mother in this example needed most from the nurse?
- According to the transactional analysis model discussed in this chapter, what were the positions taken by the nurse and client in the ineffective dialogue (ie, adult, parent, or child)?
- Why do we often feel the need to cheer up people or minimize their problems when they are depressed? What is the effect of these attitudes, and how do they contribute to clients feeling misunderstood?
- How can nurses find a balance between encouraging clients to solve their problems while also validating their feelings of discouragement?

Assertiveness

Assertiveness, means saying what one thinks, feels, or wants directly and respectfully. Nurses can teach and model assertive behavior to clients. Assertiveness can be contrasted with **aggressiveness**, which is belittling, threatening, moralizing, coercing, or communicating in a condescending way, and with **passive-aggressive communication**, which is indirect aggression through backstabbing, sabotage, ignoring, or "forgetting" things.

One theoretical model for understanding assertive communication comes from **transactional analysis (TA)**. According to TA, people function from three ego states: parent, adult, and child (Hough, 2010). Communication patterns reflect these ego states and may either be crossed (eg, controlling parent to adult) or complementary (eg, parent to child, adult to adult). Assertive communication means speaking from one's own adult ego state to another's adult ego state.

The following is a simple formula for making an assertive statement based on adult–adult communication, as opposed to talking down to clients (ie, parent–child communication):

- "I understand/know/can see…." *(Show empathy; acknowledge other's viewpoint.)*
- "But I think/feel…." *(Express the conflict from a personal view or experience.)*
- "So I suggest/prefer/would like…." *(Make a specific plan or proposal.)*

For example, a client with alcohol addiction complains that she does not think much of Alcoholics Anonymous. A nurse using the previous formula would respond as follows: "I know that you don't like Alcoholics Anonymous, but I am concerned about the seriousness of your drinking. So I'd like you to attend the meeting and give it a try." In another scenario, a client expresses anger and frustration about being admitted to a psychiatric hospital. The nurse can be assertive by responding, "I understand that you are upset about being admitted, but I can't talk with you when you are shouting, so I suggest that we sit down and discuss this calmly."

Assertiveness is marked by the use of "I statements," as opposed to "you statements" that blame or attack the other person. A person communicating assertively may restate the message, say "no," refocus the content of the interaction, or reflect the other person's feelings without losing his or her own stance.

Confrontation and Limit Setting

Confrontation is the skill of pointing out, in a caring way, the discrepancies between what clients say and do (Balzer-Riley, 2008). A three-step formula for confrontation is called a **perception check:**

1. Describe the inconsistent or confusing behavior.
2. Offer at least two possible interpretations of that behavior.
3. Ask for feedback (Adler & Proctor, 2010).

or example, at the end of a bulimia group therapy session, a client goes to use the bathroom and comes out crying. The next time the nurse sees the client, he or she uses a perception check and says, "I noticed that you went into the bathroom after our bulimia group ended last week and came out looking upset. I was thinking that maybe you were distressed about something we discussed or possibly you felt the need to vomit. Can you tell me what happened?"

In another example, a client misses two appointments in a row. When the client attends the next scheduled visit, the nurse says, "You haven't kept your last two appointments. I was wondering if you were getting more depressed and reluctant to leave your house or if you were having second thoughts about our work together. Can you explain what's happening?"

A perception check has the advantage of not accusing clients or making assumptions about them because nurses offer at least two possible interpretations. By giving alternatives, nurses make the message tentative and leave the situation open for clients to provide feedback.

Learning to set limits in a matter-of-fact, nonattacking way is an important skill that nurses need to develop to maximize the effectiveness of their relationships with clients. It requires the ability to be firm without being demeaning, bossy, or critical. For example, when clients make sexual or aggressive comments, simply saying, "I don't want you to talk to me that way" is usually sufficient.

When limits must be set on a client's behavior, specifically stating the desired changes is more effective than criticizing the negative behavior. This technique is called **positive reframing** (Deering, 1993). Examples are found in Table 11.4.

Checkpoint Questions

5. What are four therapeutic communication techniques?
6. How is assertiveness different from aggressiveness?
7. What is positive reframing?

TABLE 11.4 Examples of Positive Reframing

Negative or Ineffective Criticism	Positive Reframing
"That behavior is inappropriate, Mr. Jones."	"I want you to keep your clothes on and focus on what I am asking you."
"You're going into seclusion if you keep acting that way."	"Calm down and show me that you can keep yourself under control."
"Stop complaining and feeling sorry for yourself."	"Let's discuss what your options are and make some decisions about where to start."

Self-Disclosure

In therapeutic relationships, clients always are the focus of communication. Thus, the general principle is that nurses do not talk about themselves unless clients ask them a direct question or sharing personal information has a specific therapeutic purpose. Occasionally, however, clients ask nurses personal questions in an effort to establish rapport, show interest, or just to pass time while waiting for a procedure or meeting to begin (eg, "Are you new here?" "I see you have a ring on your finger; are you married?" "Where are you from?"). Usually, the best response is to provide a brief reply and then deflect the question back to clients, keeping the focus on them (eg, "I'm from Puerto Rico. Did you grow up here?").

Views about self-disclosure in nurse–client relationships have changed during the past several years (Deering, 1999). In the past, nurses were cautioned never to answer any personal questions, even briefly. However, current clinical writings and research have revealed that small amounts of self-disclosure by nurses can sometimes be therapeutic (Welch, 2005). For example, a nurse who reveals that her child had colic and cried a lot during infancy but grew out of it may comfort a client feeling frustrated and hopeless about his or her parenting skills. In this case, simply deflecting the client's question about whether the nurse has children (eg, "I'd rather not get into that...tell me about yours.") might seem rigid and insensitive. Other therapeutic reasons to use limited self-disclosure with clients are to enhance trust, decrease role distancing, facilitate the client's self-disclosure, convey support, or normalize the client's experience (eg, "I remember yearning for the company of other adults when my children were small. Do you have any friends with young children?").

Nurses use self-disclosure in the nurse–client relationship only with careful consideration of its therapeutic benefits. The following guidelines may be helpful:

- Use self-disclosure to help clients open up to you—not to meet your own needs.
- Keep your disclosures brief.
- Be careful not to imply that your experience is exactly the same as the client's. (Every situation is unique.)
- Disclose only those situations that you have mastered (eg, overcoming a physical limitation, adapting well to a life change).
- Do not use self-disclosure to discuss painful situations from which you have not recovered because this reverses the nurse–client roles.
- If you have a tendency to talk too much about yourself, work on trying to curb this and listen more to clients.
- Bear in mind that the amount of self-disclosure considered appropriate or comfortable varies according to culture.
- Monitor the client's nonverbal behavior to determine whether he or she is receptive to your self-disclosure, and respect the client's need for privacy (Deering, 1999).

Therapeutic Communication in Special Situations

Certain situations in psychiatric nursing pose particular challenges and call for variations in communication techniques. One example, clients who are angry or frustrated, is discussed in Challenging Behaviors 11.2. The following section discusses how to modify communication to help clients who are anxious or psychotic and how to interact with families involved in the mental health treatment planning process.

Clients With Anxiety

Clients in settings such as emergency departments, crisis centers, and disaster situations may be experiencing great anxiety that interferes with communication (Stanton, 2007). When interacting with such clients, nurses must determine the level of anxiety by noting nonverbal behavior (eg, pressured speech, shaking, wringing hands, frightened facial expressions). When clients are experiencing panic, effective communication may be impossible because such clients cannot process information.

The initial steps in reducing high anxiety are to provide for physical comfort needs and give realistic reassurance of safety. Providing accurate information about what has happened or what is about to occur often reduces anxiety. Explanations should be brief because too much information can be overwhelming. Depending on the client's level of functioning, nurses may need to be directive (eg, "Sit down here. Take a deep breath. Focus on what I'm saying."). Because anxiety is contagious, nurses focus on conveying a calm presence to clients (Figure 11.9). On a positive note, when anxieties are relieved, clients are usually very grateful (see Chap. 23).

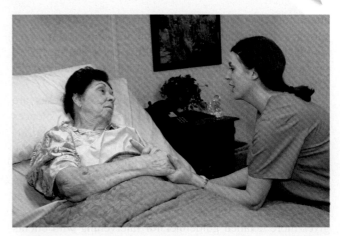

FIGURE 11.9 **The nurse's calming presence can help clients manage escalating anxiety.**

Clients With Psychoses

Clients experiencing psychoses pose challenges to communication because their thinking is not based in reality. Furthermore, their speech may be disorganized. Nurses must be able to decode themes within the content of psychotic speech to discern the underlying message and respond helpfully. For example, a client says, "I feel and believe that there are people dinking and chinking me into thinking, and that's why you must go." The nurse should not clarify the nonsense speech but say something like, "Are you afraid people can control your thoughts? I am here to ask you how you are doing." The focus of the interaction is on reducing anxiety and providing reality testing without reinforcing the psychotic thoughts. A recent study of expert psychiatric nurses working with clients experiencing psychosis found that allowing clients to explain their symptoms and

---

Challenging Behaviors 11.2

The Angry Client

Situation: Mrs. Clark was admitted 5 days ago for a suicide attempt. She is scheduled for discharge tomorrow and is angry that she cannot stay longer in the hospital.

Your Potential Feelings: Defensiveness, helplessness, frustration.

What Is Going On? Mrs. Clark is frightened about returning home in view of her history of suicidal thoughts and depression. She fears that the same stressors she encountered before admission will pose problems when she returns. Her depression and sensitivity to rejection are causing her to personalize the discharge. Trends toward decreased funding for hospital stays prevent the nurse from negotiating for extra time, increasing feelings of helplessness.

Strategy: Acknowledge Mrs. Clark's frustration with the short length of stay. Ask her to explain her concerns about returning home and expectations for her recovery. Explore Mrs. Clark's resources for support after discharge, helping her problem solve regarding ways to cope with suicidal feelings and depression while at home. Identify professionals, family, and friends available for continued support. Avoid becoming defensive about the short hospital stay, lecturing, or belittling Mrs. Clark's fears.

Nurse Action/Communication: "You have only been here a short time. I can see how frustrating it must be to return home without everything being resolved. What are you concerned might happen when you get home? Whom can you call if you are feeling overwhelmed?"

mpting to accept and understand their experiences in a caring way were the most important elements of communication (Bowers et al., 2010). Seeking out opportunities to interact with the clients while also respecting their privacy is another key intervention.

Interactions with clients experiencing psychoses are generally brief to prevent overstimulation, but long silences may increase anxiety and lead to regression or paranoia. Attention to personal boundaries is important because these clients may feel threatened. Providing adequate interpersonal space and a nonthreatening environment (eg, keeping the door open, sitting at eye level instead of standing over the client, using a calm tone of voice) is helpful. Chapter 29 gives more detailed guidelines for intervening with clients experiencing psychoses.

Families

Interviewing and working with families may seem more challenging than communicating with clients alone because the group interaction is more intense, with many cues and styles. The first task is to establish rapport with the family as a unit by conveying warmth and comfort. Nurses should note the rules governing the family system by observing interactions (Arnold, 2011b). For example, if the grandmother takes the lead in discussing the problem, acknowledging her first would be appropriate. At the same time, giving each person the opportunity to share his or her perceptions

is important, particularly if one relative has said something about another's behavior, thoughts, or feelings. This includes children and adolescents, whose views of events are unique and related to their developmental levels (see Chap. 36). The use of communication strategies with pediatric clients requires specific skills and accommodations (Deering & Cody, 2002). For example, nurses take care not to discuss frightening or serious situations (eg, a parent's serious health problems or drug abuse) in front of young children who are unprepared to comprehend what is happening and to tolerate the adults' reactions. A general principle of communication with families is to address each member directly, without allowing individuals to speak for one another (Arnold, 2011b). Nurses assess families' perceptions of the client's problems and strengths, enlist their support, and educate them about symptom management. Further discussion about families is provided in Chapter 15.

Checkpoint Questions

8. When would it be appropriate for the nurse to use self-disclosure?
9. What are the priorities when communicating with a highly anxious client?
10. What is the first task to accomplish when communicating with families?

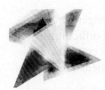

Reviewing and Applying Your Knowledge

Chapter Summary

- Trust, professionalism, mutual respect, caring, and partnership are key elements of a therapeutic nurse–client relationship.

- Obstacles to effective nurse–client relationships in the psychiatric setting include the nurse's judgmental attitudes, excessive probing, and lack of self-awareness.

- The phases of the therapeutic relationship are the introductory phase, working phase, and termination phase.

- Each phase of the therapeutic relationship has a unique set of characteristics and goals.

- A theoretical model of communication can be used to analyze the components of the nurse–client dialogue.

- The nurse uses a specific set of listening skills to facilitate communication with clients, while avoiding ineffective listening techniques.

- Assertiveness and confrontation skills are necessary for communicating effectively and respectfully with psychiatric clients who are in distress.

- The focus of the therapeutic relationship is on the client's needs, and the nurse should follow strict guidelines for using self-disclosure with clients.

- Building a therapeutic relationship with the client's family and loved ones is a key component of effective nursing care.

- Continued self-examination and practice are required to become a skilled, effective, and caring professional nurse.

Study Questions

1. The mother of a 17-year-old girl with a history of several hospitalizations for depression seems guarded and defensive during the interview. She states, "We really are a loving family." The nurse interprets this statement as indicative of the mother's defensiveness, which may be related to which of the following?

   a. Perceived blame from others for her daughter's illness

   b. The mother's own dysfunctional behavior

   c. A feeling of mutual disrespect by the nurse and mother

   d. The mother's desire to cover her own sense of failure

2. A mental health nurse, on her weekend off, arranges to meet a client with depression. The nurse is worried that the client will be lonely over the weekend because her family is away on vacation. The nurse is demonstrating which of the following?

   a. Conscientious caring

   b. Continuation of a therapeutic relationship

   c. Countertransference

   d. Judgmental attitude

3. A client has failed to show up for her second appointment with the nurse. She calls later, sounding intoxicated, claiming she forgot the appointment. The nurse understands that testing behavior is common in the introductory phase of relationship development. Which response would be most appropriate?

   a. Rescheduling the appointment without discussing the behavior

   b. Gently questioning the client about her acting-out behavior

   c. Firmly establishing boundaries for acceptable and unacceptable behavior

   d. Referring the client to another therapist

4. A client in the open psychiatric unit tells the nurse he doesn't love his wife and has had many extramarital affairs. After this discussion, the client avoids further talks with the nurse by not meeting scheduled appointments. Which of the following approaches by the nurse would be most helpful to the therapeutic relationship?

   a. "I understand that you think that you were possibly too open with me at the last session, but I feel like you're trying to avoid me now. I would like to schedule a meeting with you to discuss this matter."

   b. "You missed our last two appointments. I thought maybe you were sorry you revealed your feelings about your wife or that possibly my response was not helpful. Can you tell me more about what you're feeling?"

   c. "We haven't talked in a few days. That's a problem. Would you like to talk more about your feelings toward your wife?"

   d. "When we spoke on Monday, you said that you didn't love your wife. Now it seems as though you are holding back. Is there more going on than what you have told me?"

(continues on page 202)

While interviewing a family for the first time, the nurse notes that the mother takes charge of introducing everyone, relating that they've come to therapy because of the older son's acting-out behavior. The father and the three children nod but do not say anything. Which response would be most appropriate by the nurse immediately?

a. Acknowledge the older son first, because his behavior has been mentioned as problematic.

b. Acknowledge the father first, because he is the other parent.

c. Acknowledge the children first, because they may feel left out of the situation.

d. Acknowledge the mother first, because she seems to take the lead.

Critical Thinking Questions

1. Talk with your peers about the essential elements of therapeutic relationships discussed in this chapter (eg, trust, professionalism, respect, caring, partnership). Which elements do you think your peers embody? Why?

2. Reflect on your own background and development to consider which obstacles to establishing therapeutic relationships might pose particular challenges for you. What situations or clients would be most difficult for you to work with and why? How can you cultivate self-awareness to become more sensitive to clients, regardless of the setting where you practice?

3. Recall a helping relationship in your life with a teacher, clergy person, counselor, or other community resource person. How did the phases of the therapeutic relationship mirror those described in this chapter? Which tasks were most difficult to achieve? How did the helper build an effective therapeutic relationship and facilitate your movement through the phases?

4. After an interaction with a client, write down a verbatim account of what was said to the best of your recollection. Which therapeutic and nontherapeutic communication techniques did you use? What were the effects of these techniques on the therapeutic relationship? How can you improve your listening skills?

5. Practice the assertiveness, perception checking, and positive reframing techniques described in this chapter. How difficult were they to use? What was the outcome? How did these techniques differ from your usual mode of communication?

References

Adams, J. R., & Drake, E. (2006). Shared decision-making and evidence-based practice. *Community Mental Health Journal, 42*(1), 87–105.

Adler, R. B., & Proctor, R. F. (2010). *Looking out/looking in* (13th ed.). Belmont, CA: Thomson\Wadsworth.

Arnold, E. C. (2011a). Communicating with families. In E. C. Arnold & K. U. Boggs (Eds.), *Interpersonal relationships: Professional communication skills for nurses* (6th ed.). Philadelphia: W. B. Saunders.

Arnold, E. C. (2011b). Structuring the relationship. In E. C. Arnold & K. U. Boggs (Eds.), *Interpersonal relationships: Professional communication skills for nurses* (6th ed.). Philadelphia: W. B. Saunders.

Balzer-Riley, J. (2008). *Communication in nursing* (6th ed.). St. Louis, MO: Mosby.

Barrett, S. (2006). Interviewing techniques for the Asian-American population. *Journal of Psychosocial Nursing, 44*(5), 29–34.

Bowers, L., Brennan, G., Winship, G., & Theodoridou, C. (2010). How expert nurses communicate with acutely psychotic patients. *Mental Health Practice, 13* (7), 25–26.

Coatsworth-Puspoky, R., Forchuck, C., & Ward-Griffiths, C. (2006). Nurse–client processes in mental health: Recipients' perspectives. *Journal of Psychiatric and Mental Health Nursing, 13,* 347–355.

Cowin, L., Davies, R., Estall, G., Berlin, T., Fitzgerald, M., & Hoot, S. (2003). De-escalating aggression and violence in the mental health setting. *International Journal of Mental Health Nursing, 12*(10), 64–73.

Deering, C. G. (1993). Giving and taking criticism. *American Journal of Nursing, 93,* 56–61.

Deering, C. G. (1999). To speak or not to speak: Self-disclosure with clients. *American Journal of Nursing, 99,* 34–38.

Deering, C. G., & Cody, D. J. (2002). Communicating effectively with children and adolescents. *American Journal of Nursing, 102*(3), 34–42.

Duxbury, J., & Whittington, R. (2005). Causes and management of patient aggression and violence: Staff and patient perspectives. *Journal of Advanced Nursing, 50* (5), 467–478.

Duxbury, J. A., Wright, K. M., Hart, A., Bradley, D., Roach, P., Harris, N., & Carter, B. (2010). A structured observation of the interaction between nurses and patients during the administration of medication in an acute mental health unit. *Journal of Clinical Nursing, 19,* 2481–2492.

Dziopa, F., & Ahern, K. (2009a). Three different ways mental health nurses develop quality therapeutic relationships. *Issues in Mental Health Nursing, 30,* 14–22.

Dziopa, F., & Ahern, K. (2009b). What makes a quality therapeutic relationship in psychiatric/mental health nursing: A review of the research literature. *Internet Journal of Advanced Nursing Practice, 10*(1), 1–19.

Eckroth-Bucher, M. (2010). Self-awareness: A review and analysis of a basic nursing concept. *Advances in Nursing Science, 33*(4), 297–309.

Forchuk, C. (1994). The orientation phase of the nurse–client relationship: Testing Peplau's theory. *Journal of Advanced Nursing, 20,* 532–537.

Forchuk, C. (1995). Development of nurse–client relationships: What helps? *Journal of the American Psychiatric Nurses Association, 1,* 146–153.

Forchuk, C., Reynolds, W., Sharkey, S., Martin, M. L., & Jensen, E. (2007). Transitional discharge based on therapeutic relationships: State of the art. *Archives of Psychiatric Nursing, 21*(2), 80–86.

Foster, T., & Hawkins, J. (2005). The therapeutic relationship: Dead or merely impeded by technology? *British Journal of Nursing, 14*(13), 698–702.

Gallant, M. H., Beaulieu, M. C., & Carnevale, F. A. (2002). Partnership: An analysis of the concept within the nurse–client relationship. *Journal of Advanced Nursing, 40*(2), 149–157.

Granskar, M., Edberg, A., & Fridlund, B. (2001). Nursing students' experience of their first professional encounter with people having mental disorders. *Journal of Psychiatric & Mental Health Nursing, 8*(3), 249–256.

Hoff, L. A., Hallisey, B. J., & Hoff, M. (2009). *People in crisis: Clinical and diversity perspectives* (6th ed.). New York, NY: Routledge.

Hough, M. (2010). *Counseling skills and theory* (3rd ed.). New York, NY: Oxford University Press.

Jones, A. C. (2005). Transference, countertransference and repetition: Some implications for nursing practice. *Journal of Clinical Nursing, 14*(10), 1177–1184.

Kothari, G., Hardy, G. & Rouse, G. (2010). The therapeutic relationship between therapists and substance-using clients: A qualitative exploration. *Journal of Substance Abuse, 15*(4): 257–271.

Lindahl, B., Liden, E., & Lindblad, B. (2011). A meta-synthesis describing the relationships between patients, informal caregivers, and health professionals in home-care settings. *Journal of Clinical Nursing, 20*(3/4): 454–463.

Moyle, W. (2003). Nurse–patient relationship: A dichotomy of expectations. *International Journal of Mental Health Nursing, 12,* 103–109.

O' Brien, A. J. (2001). The therapeutic relationship: Historical development and contemporary significance. *Journal of Psychiatric and Mental Health Nursing, 8*(2), 129–137.

Perraud, S., Delaney, K. R., Carlson-Sabelli, L., Johnson, M. E., & Shephard, R. (2006). Advanced practice psychiatric mental health nursing, finding our core: The therapeutic relationship in the 21st century. *Perspectives in Psychiatric Care, 42*(4), 215–226."

Rogers, C. R. (1952). *Client-centered therapy.* Boston, MA: Houghton Mifflin.

Russell, S., Daly, J., Hughes, E., & Hoog, C. O. (2003). Nurses and "difficult" patients: Negotiating non-compliance. *Journal of Advanced Nursing, 43*(3), 281–287.

Scanlon, A. (2010). *Psychiatric nurses perceptions of the constituents of the therapeutic relationship.* New York, NY: Nova Science.

Schon, U. K. (2009). How men and women in recovery give meaning to severe mental illness. *Journal of Mental Health, 18* (5), 433–440.

Sharac, J., McCrone, P., Sabes-Figuera, R., Cspike, E., Wood, A., & Wykes, T. (2010). Nurse and patient activities and interaction on psychiatric inpatient wards: A literature review. *International Journal of Nursing Studies, 47*(7), 909–917.

Shattell, M. M., McAllister, S., Hogan, B., & Thomas, S. P. (2006). "She took the time to make sure she understood": Mental health patients' experiences of being understood. *Archives of Psychiatric Nursing, 20*(5), 234–241.

Shattell, M., Starr, S. S., & Thomas, S. P. (2007). Take my hand, help me out: Mental health service recipients' experience of the therapeutic relationship. *International Journal of Mental Health Nursing, 16,* 274–284.

Sheehan, K. A., & Burns, T. (2011). Perceived coercion and the therapeutic relationship: A neglected association? *Psychiatric Services, 62*(5), 471–476.

Stanton, K. (2007). Emergency: Communicating with ED patients who have chronic mental illnesses. *American Journal of Nursing, 107*(2), 61–65.

Stockmann, C. (2005). A literature review of the progress of the psychiatric nurse–patient relationship as described by Peplau. *Issues in Mental Health Nursing, 26,* 911–919.

Vatne, S., & Fagermoen, M. S. (2007). To correct and acknowledge: Two simultaneous and conflicting perspectives of limit-setting in mental health nursing. *Journal of Psychiatric and Mental Health Nursing, 14,* 41–48.

Welch, M. (2005). Pivotal moments in the therapeutic relationship. *International Journal of Mental Health Nursing, 14,* 161–165.

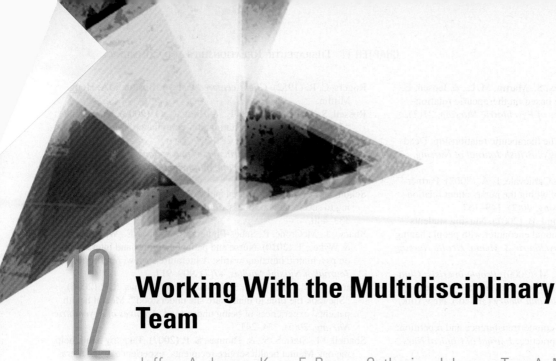

Working With the Multidisciplinary Team

Jeffrey Anderson, Kerry E. Brown, Catherine Johnson, Tara A. Mohr,
Theodore A. Petti, Scott M. Reid, and Patricia A. Troyanowski

KEY TERMS

art therapists
enabler
friendly visiting
functional behavioral
    assessment (FBA)
Individualized Education
    Program (IEP)
multidisciplinary teams
occupational therapist (OT)
psychiatrist
psychologist
recreation therapist (RT)
registered dietitian (RD)
sensory integration
service coordination
social broker/advocate
social worker
special education law
strengths-based philosophy

LEARNING OBJECTIVES

On completion of this chapter, you should be able to accomplish the following:

- Discuss the role of multidisciplinary teams in the care of clients.
- Discuss specific skills that psychologists, occupational therapists, social workers, psychiatrists, and registered dietitians bring to the treatment and management of clients.
- Identify how each professional reviewed in this chapter interacts with psychiatric nurses in the assessment and treatment of clients.
- Describe treatment modalities for each profession discussed in this chapter.

Multidisciplinary teams consist of professionals from diverse disciplines who collaborate to provide comprehensive assessments of clients, establish and perform interventions, and regularly consult with one another about progress. Clients and their families are also members of such teams. The primary purpose of multidisciplinary teams is to help resolve challenging cases; however, they provide various additional functions. For example, they can promote coordination among agencies or between professionals and families. They can also identify service gaps or challenges to communication between agencies and people. They can enhance the professional skills and knowledge of individual team members by providing a forum for learning more about the strategies, resources, and approaches that different disciplines use.

Each discipline has its own perspective, jargon, mandates, mores, and resources. When professionals fail to understand existing variations, misunderstandings or "turf" conflicts may develop. Conversely, when professionals learn about the approaches, resources, and perspectives of colleagues from other disciplines, they can expand their repertoire of skills, increase available resources for clients, and enhance understanding of various problems. Collaboration and interaction can facilitate interagency coordination, resulting in more and improved services for clients. As a result, the likelihood increases that clients will not "fall through the cracks" of the service network and that wasteful overlap will be reduced.

Professional disciplines typically represented in psychiatric–mental health settings include nurses, psychologists, occupational therapists, social workers, psychiatrists, art therapists, recreation therapists, and registered dietitians. However, actual team compositions are as diverse as are the settings for care and the individual strengths and needs of clients. In this chapter, several professionals discuss their roles and unique contributions. In their narratives, they describe the specific skills they bring to the care of clients with mental health problems and their families, as well as how they interact with other professionals. In addition, these professionals discuss their common cooperation with nurses and how collaboration can promote effective management of client problems. Case vignettes illustrate how collaborative efforts can achieve integrated and successful caregiving.

PSYCHOLOGISTS

By Jeffrey Anderson, PhD
Indiana University, School of Education, Bloomington, Indiana
Psychology is a science-based profession that studies how people think, act, react, and interact. It is concerned with all aspects of behavior, including underlying thoughts and feelings (see Chap. 3). **Psychologists** deal with how the mind works, and with motivation.

Educational Background and Training

Psychologists can specialize in various areas, including mental health, education, and occupational psychology. Licensed psychologists must have a doctoral degree. Most psychologists

work in five broad employment categories: (1) research, (2) teaching, (3) service provider, (4) administrator, or (5) consultant. Many psychologists combine two or more of these categories. For example, a university-based psychologist may teach, conduct research, and engage in clinical practice. Another psychologist may work as an administrator and in the clinic. A counseling psychologist with a master's degree may be a service provider and teach at a local college.

Psychologists work in many different settings. Primary employment sites include universities, colleges, elementary and secondary schools, independent practices, hospitals, clinics, businesses, and government and other human services. Other possibilities include advertising, criminal justice, consumer relations and products, telecommunications, armed forces, entertainment, and sports. More than 50 areas of specialization in psychology at the master's or doctoral level exist. Most have subspecialties for teaching, research, practice, or some combination.

Although psychologists often work with clients in hospitals, most interactions are community based. For children and families, school psychologists play a major role in treatment planning and intervention because children spend most of their time in school. The following discussion focuses on school-based treatment and intervention.

> **Checkpoint Questions**
> 1. What educational preparation is required to become a licensed psychologist?
> 2. In which setting do most psychologists care for clients with psychiatric problems?

The Role of School Psychologists

School psychologists have advanced professional training in child and adolescent development, counseling, learning theory, academic and behavioral interventions, consultation, and assessment. Their role varies according to the school's specific needs. Generally, school psychologists provide essential services to students, faculty and other staff, and parents. This includes designing interventions to address and prevent academic and behavioral difficulties. When necessary, they may also provide crisis intervention and individual or group counseling to address behaviors that interfere with learning (see Chap. 35). They are active in efforts to prevent suicide and violence and can act as liaisons between schools and community mental health professionals.

After the family, schools are the primary stakeholders in the lives of youth with emotional and behavioral challenges. The Individuals With Disabilities Education Improvement Act of 2004 (IDEIA), often referred to as the **"special education law,"** requires school districts to provide free and appropriate education to all children with disabilities (Friend & Bursuck, 2008). Despite this law, young people with emotional and behavioral disabilities struggle in school. Research shows that they fail more courses, miss more school, receive lower grades, experience significant social difficulties with peers and adults, and are retained and drop out at higher rates than any other group with a disability (U.S. Department of Education, 2007). In mathematics and reading, these children are approximately 18 months behind peers without disabilities, a disparity that increases with time (Anderson et al., 2001).

When a school identifies students in need of special education services and develops appropriate plans for them, a school-based multidisciplinary team is formed. Members of the team include school psychologists, school nurses, social workers, teachers, physical and occupational therapists, school administrators, speech/language therapists, mental health counselors, and, most importantly, family members. Youth also usually participate (Figure 12.1).

Individualized Education Programs

Multidisciplinary teams develop and monitor **Individualized Education Programs (IEPs),** which become legal documents. IEPs outline the educational, social, and behavioral goals and objectives of students with disabilities, providing school-based plans to meet them. IEPs drive what occurs in schools for students with disabilities. The purposes of the IEP process are to identify the child's specific disability and to detail the supports and services needed for success in school. Each IEP includes necessary curricular, instructional, and environmental modifications; target behaviors for interventions; and related services (e.g., mental health counseling) to provide. In addition, most IEPs also include information about the child's strengths. Teams meet at least annually to monitor overall progress and update the program. During the school year, a special education teacher is responsible for implementing and monitoring the IEP. For children and youth with emotional and behavioral challenges, IEPs include assessments and support planning that focus on increasing behaviors associated with academic success (e.g., getting along with peers, following instructions).

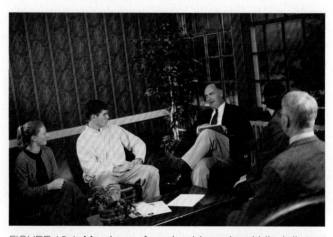

FIGURE 12.1 Members of a school-based multidisciplinary team are meeting with you to discuss appropriate service for special education needs.

Similar to the tools that clinicians use to make mental health diagnoses, assessments that schools use to evaluate for emotional and behavioral disabilities include behavioral rating scales, self-report scales, interviews with parents and teachers, intellectual and achievement tests, and direct observation (Whelan, 1995). A technique called **functional behavioral assessment (FBA)** provides more thorough information about challenging behaviors and their likely environmental contexts (Sugai et al., 1999). The FBA is generally considered a problem-solving process; the focus is on identifying significant, pupil-specific social, affective, cognitive, and environmental factors associated with challenging behaviors. The goal is to understand what is causing and reinforcing them. The IDEIA requires schools to use FBAs to support the development and implementation of behavioral support plans (BSPs).

Each BSP outlines strategies for classroom and school success. The goal is to replace challenging behaviors with appropriate ones that elicit similar consequences from the environment. For example, a child has a history of acting aggressively when angry with peers. His BSP focuses on teaching and providing him with support in using conflict resolution instead of aggression. When developed and implemented thoughtfully, BSPs can greatly increase a student's academic success. Focus can then shift to helping school personnel understand the child's mental health challenges and develop *proactive* responses to them. During this process, the team fully assesses both the assets and the challenges of the school environment for the student. Members consider such factors as (1) peers' understanding of the child's potential challenging behaviors and strengths; (2) expertise among staff in implementing BSPs and adapting curricula and instruction; (3) aspects of the environment that can be modified to support the child (e.g., increased positive reinforcement from teachers); and (4) the potential for crisis and the development of prevention and contingency plans.

Together, FBAs and BSPs require practitioners to focus not only on the child with an emotional or behavioral issue, but also on the environmental events that evoke and maintain challenging behaviors. In turn, practitioners use such information to implement more effective classroom interventions. Consider the work of an IEP team to return a child to an inclusive classroom after a lengthy stay in a residential setting. When team members focus assessment efforts only on challenging behaviors, they may overlook competencies or resiliencies that might help the child succeed in the classroom. Conversely, when assessment considers the child's ecologies across domains, team members may discover that the child has strong interpersonal skills and performs well during activities with little structure.

Multidisciplinary Service Coordination Plans in Communities

The IEP focuses primarily on educational needs. Multidisciplinary service coordination teams are for children and

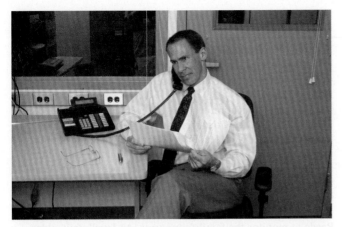

FIGURE 12.2 This care coordinator is making arrangements for a family to receive needed assistance from a community service organization following a child's return from residential placement.

youth with serious and complex needs that extend beyond the capacity of a single school, organization, or system (Anderson, 2000). **Service coordination** connects the various systems, agencies, and people (including family members) participating in care, while ensuring effective, ongoing communication among all involved so that services and interventions are consistent and directed toward common goals (Stroul, 1996). Often, service or care coordinators manage this process; their role is to guide the multiagency service coordination (child and family) team and ensure that it meets regularly (Figure 12.2).

They must organize and manage all services a child receives, not just those related to education (Anderson & Matthews, 2001).

TEAM COMPOSITION. Child and family teams consist of people who will be involved with the student and family over time. They include parents or caregivers, the child or teen (as appropriate), the service coordinator, service providers, school psychologist, teachers, and other family or community members. Other participants may include a probation officer, a child welfare case worker, a nurse or other health care provider, and therapists or counselors. Primary members have ongoing relationships with the child and family and attend all team meetings. Others attend as required, such as religious advisors, neighbors, extended family, and people who work intermittently with the family (e.g., academic tutor, swim coach). Team composition varies based on the family's unique social and support networks. Minimum membership is the immediate family and their supports (Anderson & Matthews, 2001).

TEAM FUNCTIONING. Child and family teams create, implement, and monitor multisystem service coordination plans. For schools, such plans do not replace IEPs. Because multisystem service coordination plans encompass multiple domains (home, school, and community), they may incorporate and integrate various aspects of IEPs. Unlike IEPs, service coordination teams are concerned with children in and out of school (Anderson et al., 2007). They require authentic and permanent involvement from the child's family. The concept of *family-driven service provision* evolved from the principle of family centeredness in contemporary approaches to multisystem service coordination for children and youth (Stroul & Friedman, 1986).

Development of the comprehensive, multisystem plan begins when the family and care coordinator bring team members together to discuss and document the strengths, concerns, and needs of a child and family. Key to this process is when the team conducts a strengths-based assessment to identify skills, resources, and abilities, as well as available assets in the home, school, and community (Anderson & Mohr, 2003). **Strengths-based philosophy** recognizes that all children, families, and environments possess assets that can be used to overcome challenges and to meet needs. A strengths assessment produces necessary information for developing effective interventions. Such approaches are fundamentally different from perspectives that blame families and communities for problems (Anderson, 2000).

Multidisciplinary teams adhere to the principle that services should be individualized, coordinated, and community based by supporting families as being best able to achieve success and independence at home and in the community as opposed to in restrictive settings (e.g., residential placement). This goal is comparable with the least restrictive environment requirement of IDEIA. A core value for these teams is the presence of a family member at every team meeting. Teams do not meet without family representation, and meetings do not disenfranchise families by excluding them from professional or "expert" discourse. Furthermore, the team removes any barriers to family involvement, including "turf" issues, transportation challenges, time and work conflicts, and child care needs.

Although school IEP teams typically meet once a year, child and family teams meet monthly and at other times necessary for consultation, monitoring, or problem solving. Members share information honestly and openly about both successes and concerns so they can update or modify the plan as necessary (Friesen & Poertner, 1995). When team members differ in opinions, they actively work to find resolution (Wright et al., 2006).

Teams also focus on helping families develop and use natural supports (e.g., involving extended family members to help with interventions). The goal for those who need traditional services is to use community services (i.e., in-home family therapy, not residential placement). Desired outcomes include reduced reliance on out-of-home and out-of-community placements, increased family independence, and improved functioning for the child or youth in the home, school, and community (Anderson & Matthews, 2001). See Case Vignette 12.1.

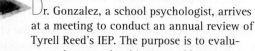

Case Vignette 12.1

Dr. Gonzalez, a school psychologist, arrives at a meeting to conduct an annual review of Tyrell Reed's IEP. The purpose is to evaluate Tyrell's progress and ensure that his team addresses any areas of concern. Dr. Gonzalez believes the meeting will be routine because Tyrell, now in ninth grade, is doing well in all his classes.

To prepare, Dr. Gonzalez worked closely with Tyrell and his family. She assessed Tyrell's academic achievements and thoroughly reviewed his special education records. She was pleased that during the 6 years since being diagnosed with a learning disability, Tyrell had closed the gap between his academic ability and reading performance. Moreover, she saw that all of Tyrell's teachers reported he was doing well. Although Tyrell continued to struggle with reading, Dr. Gonzalez noted that accommodations and modifications to curriculum and instruction implemented in previous IEP team meetings appeared to be working. Even in history and biology, both of which required much reading, Tyrell was maintaining a low B average.

A special education teacher, Lakeisha Price, supported Tyrell's teachers. Dr. Gonzalez and Ms. Price had gotten to know each other well. Ms. Price was responsible for monitoring Tyrell's IEP by helping teachers individualize curriculum and instruction, focusing on the changes necessary for Tyrell to learn successfully. Such support also helped other students struggling with the material.

Ms. Price and Dr. Gonzalez met periodically with the Reeds to monitor the family's progress. As Tyrell grew older, he, too, was starting to attend these meetings. Dr. Gonzalez thought that regular communication had led to a strong connection between home and school, which helped decrease overall problems and increase successes.

Psychologists, Nurses, and Multidisciplinary Teams

School psychologists interact with physicians, school nurses, families, and, importantly, teachers, who spend the most time with students and have the best opportunity to evaluate and observe them. School nurses, who specialize in advancing the well-being and academic success of students, collaborate actively with psychologists and teachers to build student and family capacity for healthy adaptation, self-management, self-advocacy, and learning. They promote safety and provide case management so that children can excel academically. They are responsible not only for the physical care of students with chronic illnesses, but also for responding to and counseling students on social and health issues. For students with medical needs, they also serve as liaisons with physicians and other health care providers.

Teachers know their students well academically, socially, and behaviorally. As such, they bring important perspectives to multidisciplinary service coordination teams. Indeed, such teams are incomplete without their participation. Nevertheless, traditional classroom teachers tend to work alone. When they first participate on child and family teams, the process may seem demanding. The challenges of collaborating with people from different disciplines can seem burdensome. However, the benefits are numerous. Initially, teachers learn they are not alone in trying to help children with emotional and behavioral challenges achieve success (Anderson & Matthews, 2001).

Multidisciplinary team participation allows members to understand children from both school and nonschool perspectives and to connect better with families and service providers. For example, if a student struggles with reading, his or her team could develop a plan to work on language development in nonschool environments. Members might arrange for a tutor or find academic materials for the family to work on in the evenings. They could ensure that the child's after-school program at a community center includes computer-based reading instruction.

Checkpoint Questions

3. What are the two purposes of an IEP?
4. Which team members are essential for a multidisciplinary service coordination team?

OCCUPATIONAL THERAPISTS

By Catherine Johnson, OTRIL
La Vida Felicidad, Los Lunas, New Mexico

An **occupational therapist (OT)** provides treatment that helps people achieve independence in all facets of their lives. They help clients develop necessary skills for satisfying lives. Every day, children and adults live with or develop health conditions that significantly affect their ability to manage. With the help of OTs, many of these people can achieve or regain independence. When clients cannot develop or improve their skills and strength, OTs offer creative solutions and alternatives for performing daily activities.

Typical services that OTs provide include the following:

- Performance skills assessment and treatment
- Comprehensive home and job-site evaluations with adaptation recommendations
- Customized treatment programs designed to improve daily activities
- Recommendations for adaptive equipment and training in correct use (Figure 12.3)
- Guidance to family members, caregivers, and other professionals

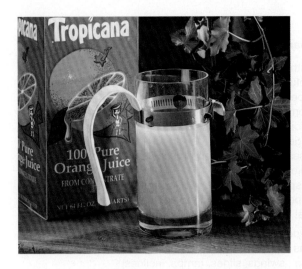

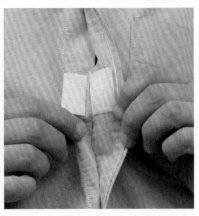

FIGURE 12.3 Occupational therapists may help make recommendations for adaptive equipment and training related to fine motor skills. For example, they may help ensure that clients with coordination challenges have special tools and devices for feeding and dressing independently.

Educational Background and Training

OTs are professionals whose education includes the study of human growth and development, with specific emphasis on the social, emotional, and physiologic effects of illness and injury. They have a bachelor's, master's, or doctoral degree; most OTs have a master's degree. They must complete a supervised internship in various health care settings and pass a national examination. Typically, students do fieldwork in hospitals or schools that coordinates with their course work. Clinicals include practice in general rehabilitation or physical disability and then progress to a specialty, such as pediatrics or mental health. OTs have their own professional organization, and most states regulate their practice.

The Role of Occupational Therapists

Like physical therapists, OTs are concerned with rehabilitation. In contrast to physical therapists, who focus on gross motor and gait training, OTs are concerned with visual and fine motor skill development. Gross motor skills involve major muscle groups and require balance and coordination (e.g., jumping, running). By contrast, fine motor skills involve small muscle movements: those in the finger, coordinated with the eyes. They allow people to do such things as write and manipulate small objects.

Sensory integration, an innate neurobiologic process, refers to the brain's integration and interpretation of sensory stimulation from the environment. It focuses primarily on three basic domains: tactile, vestibular, and proprioceptive. The interconnections of these realms start forming before birth and continue to develop as people mature and interact with the environment. These three are not only interconnected but also linked with other systems in the brain. Although these sensory systems are less familiar than vision and hearing, they are critical to basic survival (Table 12.1). Basically, they allow people to experience, interpret, and respond to different environmental stimuli.

Sensory integration dysfunction manifests in many ways. Children may be overresponsive or underresponsive to sensory input; activity may be unusually high or low;

children may be in constant motion or fatigue easily. In addition, some children fluctuate between extremes. Problems with gross motor coordination, fine motor coordination, or both may result in speech/language delays and academic underachievement. Behaviorally, children may be impulsive or easily distracted and show a general lack of planning. Some children also have difficulty adjusting to new situations and may react with frustration, aggression, or withdrawal.

Goals of OTs in evaluation and treatment of basic sensory integrative processes are as follows:

1. To provide sensory information that helps organize the central nervous system
2. To assist clients to inhibit or modulate sensory information
3. To assist clients to process a more organized response to sensory stimuli

OTs work with people of all ages who have a disability or a physical or mental illness. They use individually selected and graded activities to help clients restore, develop, or maintain skills. They assess and treat people from a client-centered perspective, encouraging them to identify their own needs or difficulties and collaborating on realistic treatment programs. Box 12.1 lists people whose conditions can benefit from occupational therapy.

Typical work activities vary greatly depending on whether the OT works in physical health or mental health and also in a hospital or the community. A typical day for a hospital-based therapist working on a stroke ward might include the following activities:

- Discussing the progress of clients in a morning meeting with other health care professionals
- Assessing clients' physical and cognitive skills in activities such as washing and dressing, preparing meals, and getting in and out of the bath safely
- Working with the clients' families and staff members from other services to plan for clients' discharge from hospital

TABLE 12.1 Systems in Sensory Integration

System and Purpose	Components	Manifestations of Dysfunction
Tactile system Communicates light touch, pain, temperature, and pressure, all of which contribute to environmental perception Assists with protective reactions for survival	Nerves under the skin surface that send information to the brain	Withdraws from being touched Refuses to eat "textured" foods or to wear certain types of clothing Complains about having hair or face washed Avoids getting hands dirty (e.g., glue, sand, mud, finger-paint) Uses fingertips rather than entire hands to manipulate objects Misperceives touch, pain, or both (hypersensitive or hyposensitive), leading to self-imposed isolation, general irritability, distractibility, and hyperactivity
Vestibular system Detects movement and changes in head position (e.g., tells when the head is upright or tilted, even with the eyes closed)	Structures within the inner ear (semicircular canals)	*Hypersensitivity* Has fearful reactions to ordinary movement activities (e.g., swings, slides, ramps, inclines) Has trouble learning to climb or descend stairs or hills Shows apprehension when walking or crawling on uneven or unstable surfaces *Hyposensitivity* Actively pursues very intense sensory experiences (e.g., excessive body whirling, jumping, spinning) Shows signs of trying to stimulate the vestibular system continuously
Proprioceptive system Helps body position automatically adjust in different situations (e.g., provides the necessary signals that allow a person to sit properly in a chair or to step off a curb smoothly) Enables object manipulation that relies on fine motor movements (e.g., writing with a pencil, using a soup spoon, buttoning a shirt) Contributes to praxis or motor planning, which means the ability to plan and execute different motor tasks	Components of the muscles, joints, and tendons that provide a subconscious awareness of body position	Is clumsy Tends to fall Lacks awareness of body position in space Shows odd body posturing Crawls minimally when young Has difficulty manipulating small objects (buttons, snaps) Eats sloppily Resists new motor movement activities

---

BOX 12.1	Client Groups That Benefit from Occupational Therapy

People who can benefit from occupational therapy include, but are not limited to, those with:
- Work-related injuries
- Stroke or myocardial infarction
- Serious chronic conditions (e.g., arthritis, multiple sclerosis)
- Birth injuries, developmental delays, or learning disabilities
- Mental health or behavioral problems, including dementia, substance abuse, and eating disorders
- Spinal cord injuries, amputations, burns, fractures, or other injuries from falls, sports injuries, or accidents

The working day of a community-based therapist working with people with learning disabilities might include the following activities:

- Visiting a client to assess his or her progress
- Attending a multiprofessional case conference to plan and review ongoing treatment of a client
- Assessing the accessibility of a potential new home for a client who uses a wheelchair

Occupational Therapists, Nurses, and Multidisciplinary Teams

OTs work with other professionals in health and social services such as physicians, physiotherapists, nurses, speech/language therapists, social workers, and counselors. Multidisciplinary team efforts are always geared toward the client. Like other professionals, OTs document all their work. They keep others working with the same client up to date about the client's progress from their unique perspective.

Interactions with nurses are particularly important in several ways. In institutions or partial hospitalization facilities, nurses observe clients in multiple venues and contexts. Whereas other professionals spend discrete times with clients, nurses spend several hours with them over time. They communicate to other team members how therapies are generalizing and how clients are applying new skills in different situations. These observations provide valuable feedback for OTs, who can tailor interventions with specific contexts in mind (Case Vignette 12.2).

PROFESSIONAL SOCIAL WORKERS

By Tara A. Mohr, MSW

City of Philadelphia Homeless Services, Philadelphia, Pennsylvania

Of approximately 600,000 U.S. social workers, nearly 40% work in state, county, or municipal government agencies, primarily in departments of human resources, social services, child welfare, mental health, health, housing, education, and corrections. Most employment opportunities in the private sector are in voluntary social service agencies, community and religious organizations, hospitals, nursing homes, and home health agencies. Increasingly, social workers are in private practice. Employment for social workers is expected to increase faster than the average for all occupations.

Social work requires knowledge of human development and behavior; social, economic, and cultural institutions; and how all these factors interact. It is driven by the application of the following values, principles, and techniques:

- Helping people obtain tangible services
- Providing counseling and psychotherapy with individuals, families, and groups
- Helping communities or groups provide or improve social and health services
- Participating in legislative processes

Educational Background and Training

For many years, careers in social service did not require specialized education. Students with bachelor's degrees in psychology, sociology, education, philosophy, and urban affairs (among other fields) could consider a career in social services. Today, the social service field is becoming more stringent in its requirements, focusing on those with specialized education. The social work profession encourages employers to hire educated and licensed social workers exclusively to help maintain accountability and professionalism.

Social work education has three levels: the bachelor of social work (BSW), the master of social work (MSW), and the doctorate of social work (DSW or PhD). Offered in many large universities, the BSW instructs college students in direct practice, preparing them for entry-level counseling

Case Vignette 12.2

Matt was 11 years old when a drunk driver struck the car in which he was riding with his mother and brother. His mother was killed. His brother suffered extensive internal injuries. Matt lay sprawled on a cold, deserted rural road with a catastrophic open head injury.

Matt eventually arrived at a local medical center, where he remained for 7 weeks. When he finally revived, he was more alert than expected. Hope soared when he scored high on his first standardized test. But Matt was not back to normal. He had weakness on the left side of his body, vision problems, visual-spatial difficulties, and organizational deficits. The psychological stress of losing his mother and returning to a family dealing with the crises resulting from the accident compounded his physical problems.

The key to Matt's successful transition back into the community was the commitment to his recovery from everyone involved. The acute care therapist, who lived in Matt's community, contacted the local public school and an occupational therapist who worked exclusively in schools. By doing so, he helped ensure that Matt's therapy continued smoothly after discharge from the medical center.

The school created an environment of care and support. Matt wore a baseball cap to hide his scar and noticeable skull depression. The day he returned to classes, all the students wore baseball caps to show support. Matt brought a different classmate with him to therapy every week. This kept his peers interested in Matt's recovery.

For the first 6 months after the accident, occupational therapy included self-care, neurodevelopmental therapy, and functional approaches to rehabilitation. This therapy also helped Matt emotionally. He asked many questions about brain injury and talked with the OTs about loss and the future.

As Matt regained strength and his motor control improved, he was referred to another OT for biofeedback therapy to enhance his schoolwork. Biofeedback helped Matt with postural control, relaxation of the shoulder, and movement of the left arm.

Matt had 2 years of trials and victories. The three OTs he worked with educated teachers, family, and Matt himself. They also rehabilitated his arm, assisted in classroom modifications to compensate for organizational and visual-spatial deficits, and took an active role in meeting his psychosocial needs. Today Matt is on the honor roll and the recipient of an award for outstanding achievement in science.

or case management. The MSW expands on the BSW by improving and refining direct service skills. These graduate programs place students in social service agencies for internships under practicing social workers. In general, student placements target areas that represent particular interests, such as homeless agencies, children's shelters, and juvenile justice facilities. The MSW also introduces broad concepts, such as supervision, administration, research, and policy analysis. Finally, the DSW and PhD further instruct students to become experts in social work research, counseling, and agency administration.

The BSW is the minimum requirement for most positions. An MSW is usually necessary for positions in health and mental health settings. Jobs in some private agencies also require an MSW.

Social workers can take additional course work toward professional certification in certain areas. Examples are advanced practice with children, youth, and families; school social worker; specialist in case management; advanced practice in health care social work; advanced practice in alcohol, tobacco, and other drugs; and certification in palliative and end-of-life care.

The Role of Social Workers

A degree in social work provides great career versatility. Roles include services such as counseling, psychotherapy, and mediation. Social workers are involved in policy and program development, policy analysis, and policy planning and implementation.

Social workers help clients and families cope with mental illness and problems such as inadequate housing, unemployment, lack of job skills, financial mismanagement, serious illness, disability, substance abuse, unwanted pregnancy, and antisocial behavior. They also work with families who have serious conflicts, including those involving domestic violence (see Chap. 33).

The philosophy and role of social work have changed over the years. For many years, society considered people in need as somehow deficient in personal responsibility or their desire to help themselves. As a result, responses were characterized by the concept of **friendly visiting**. Friendly visitors were members of the upper classes who regularly "visited" the lower classes in hopes that discrete glimpses of people with a better life would motivate the lower classes to change their conditions. This charity work was based on the assumption that all problems were inherent. It ignored the systematic forces that thwart people's abilities to respond and to adjust to the vagaries of reality.

As social work emerged as a profession, attitudes shifted from blaming and attempting to change people. Rather, the profession began considering a larger picture. Instead of focusing on a client's innate faults and deficiencies, modern social workers strive to address the interrelationships between the clients and the surrounding environment (Zastrow et al., 2002). When a person faces difficulty, social workers conceptualize the problems as arising from a change within

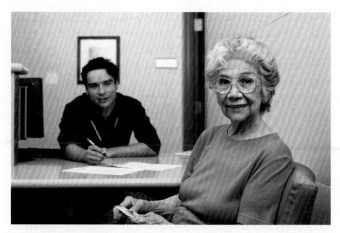

FIGURE 12.4 Social workers help clients of all ages and backgrounds to solve practical challenges and access needed resources and support.

the person, his or her environment, or the person–environment interrelationship. They help clients work through presenting problems, with the intent of minimizing adverse consequences so that lives continue with little disruption (Figure 12.4).

Social work interventions have one or more of the following goals:

- Promoting and enhancing clients' coping and problem-solving abilities
- Establishing connections between resources or services and clients
- Facilitating and maximizing the benefits provided by resources on behalf of clients
- Strengthening interactive relationships between resources and clients so that seeking assistance becomes an accepted behavior

Empowered by the overarching desire to "meet the client where he or she is," social workers assume different roles when working directly with clients. The **enabler** improves social functioning by helping clients resolve their own issues. The **social broker/advocate** connects clients with resources and services and acts as an intermediary representing the clients' interests. The *teacher* promotes clients' abilities to cope and adapt to changes in their environments.

Typical social work activities across settings and specialties include the following:

- Conducting and recording assessments (often with other disciplines) that meet specified standards and time scales
- Conducting interviews with clients and their families to assess and to review their situation
- Organizing and managing packages of client support activities
- Recommending and sometimes making decisions about the best course of action for a particular client
- Liaising with and making referrals to other agencies
- Participating in multidisciplinary teams and meetings (e.g., child protection, mental health)

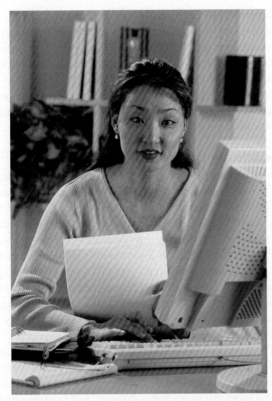

FIGURE 12.5 A social worker often must complete extensive paperwork and documentation to facilitate effective care management for clients.

- Offering information and counseling support to clients and their families
- Maintaining accurate records and preparing evidence and reports for legal action and court cases (Figure 12.5)
- Participating in training, supervision, and team meetings

Working in various settings and within a framework of relevant legislation and procedures, social workers support individuals, families, and groups in the community. Settings include clients' homes, schools, hospitals, and other public sector and voluntary organizations. Social work assistants often provide support and work closely with other health and social care staff.

Social workers must maintain a friendly but professional relationship with clients. Their clients often are in crisis or socially excluded. Social workers aim to offer support that enables people to help themselves by developing their skills and abilities to use their own and community resources to resolve problems.

Characteristics of an effective social worker are based on good interpersonal skills. These professionals must be empathic, genuine, warm, and culturally competent. They must have good "intuitive whiskers" and constantly hone and refine their ability to win the trust and respect of clients by being attuned to their verbal and nonverbal expressions.

Clients often refer to the central role that good social workers have played in their lives. They mention the closeness of the relationships built with social workers, frequently

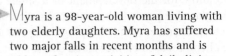

Case Vignette 12.3

Myra is a 98-year-old woman living with two elderly daughters. Myra has suffered two major falls in recent months and is having serious trouble performing activities of daily living. A team of professionals meets with the family to discuss the case. Members include social workers from a housing agency, mental health agency, older adult agency, and faith-based organization.

Because of the client's age and reliance on her daughters, the team understands the benefits of Myra not moving to a nursing home. The group works to divide tasks so that all three women can live independently. In the following weeks, the team arranges to move the family from a dilapidated three-story home to a new one-floor apartment. They also arrange for each woman to undergo a mental health assessment, to ensure that they all are capable of living independently. The team also offers legal assistance to foreclose their prior home and to set up an ongoing financial assistance plan.

as a result of the client and open approaches adopted (Ribner & Knei-Paz, 2002). Maintaining an honest atmosphere and treating clients as equals are essential. By downplaying a position of authority and emphasizing collaboration, social workers appear generally interested in helping clients. Making sure to keep in touch, meeting the client at the most convenient location and time, and generally being approachable and accessible are crucial elements of successful social work. Other professions may encourage members to develop these characteristics or aspire to achieve the intimacy and trust that social workers regularly elicit (Case Vignette 12.3) (Zastrow et al., 2002).

Social Workers, Nurses, and Multidisciplinary Teams

Social workers provide services to clients not only on a one-to-one basis, but also as members of multidisciplinary teams. Their duties vary depending on setting. In hospitals, social workers link the treatment team and family to community resources. They contribute to the care, treatment, and rehabilitation of older adults and clients who are physically or mentally ill or who have disabilities. In health and community services centers, social workers collaborate with other disciplines to provide counseling to clients and families and services to older adults. Those who work as community developers help citizens identify needs and propose ways to meet them.

As an intervention model, the interdisciplinary approach to client service benefits not only the client, but also various team members. Having different professionals come together to work on a client's case integrates expertise and knowledge that can lead to the formation of strong and effective strategies to address problems. This system offers team members an opportunity to explore alternative explanations for problems that a member of a single discipline would not otherwise have considered. Integration and collaboration also allow for the development of a single comprehensive care plan that poses little conflict for the client and among the team members while keeping the entire team, including the client, focused on the shared goals.

The team approach further benefits all involved by protecting fragile clients from repeating traumatic stories endlessly while preventing manipulative clients from pitting workers against one another. Teams permit different workers to assume roles that are necessary for progress but potentially conflicting (e,g,, being a friend and advocate versus an enforcer). Finally, from a systems perspective, interdisciplinary teams improve coordination and prevent duplication of services while increasing the quality and quantity of solutions generated.

Social workers provide individual, relationship, and family assessments and interventions in collaboration with other team members. They must interact closely with psychiatric nurses. As the team members who have the most contact with clients, nurses can provide observations of family interactions that can inform the social workers' interventions. For example, a social worker may be unaware of specific family disagreements or tensions. A reluctance to discuss or display significant behaviors, such as verbal or emotional abuse, may sabotage social workers' efforts with families. Nurses may observe such interactions during family visiting, thus providing valuable input to the professional social worker in developing a successful treatment plan. Nurses also serve as valuable sources of referral for social workers. They can refer clients to social services if there are problems with finances (including benefits), child care, and housing.

Because social workers have honed their skills as relationship builders and resource managers, they often are appointed as team leaders, serving as primary liaisons between team members and clients. Thus, social workers have a unique opportunity to benefit from and contribute to teams. As more of them experience the utility and advantages of teams, they increasingly will help clients navigate the complex problems and issues of today's world.

Checkpoint Questions

5. Modern social workers focus on what aspects of the client?

6. What roles is the social worker assuming when he or she connects the client with resources and services?

PSYCHIATRISTS

By Theodore A. Petti, MD, MPH
Robert Wood Johnson Medical School, University of Medicine and Dentistry of New Jersey, Piscataway, New Jersey

A **psychiatrist** is a physician who specializes in the prevention, diagnosis, and treatment of mental illnesses and emotional problems. Because they receive a medical education before specializing in psychiatry, psychiatrists understand the complex relationship between emotional illness and other

health problems. They can specialize in fields such as substance abuse psychiatry, geriatric psychiatry, forensic psychiatry, mental retardation psychiatry, community psychiatry, and consultation liaison psychiatry. Child and adolescent psychiatrists (CAPs) have special training to understand and to work with children and adolescents who suffer from or are at risk for psychiatric disorders, their families, and the professionals in systems from which they receive services.

Educational Background and Training

Psychiatrists possess an undergraduate degree and a degree from medical school. They pass a written examination for a state license to practice medicine and do 1 year of residency, caring for clients with a wide range of medical illnesses. After completing this preparation, they spend at least 3 additional years in a psychiatric residency, learning about the diagnosis and treatment of mental illnesses, psychotherapies, and use of psychiatric medications and other treatments. They are then eligible to take a certification examination given by the American Board of Psychiatry and Neurology, to become "board certified."

The education and training of the CAP includes all of the aforementioned steps as well as 2 additional years of training in child and adolescent psychiatry. This training includes working in multidisciplinary and interdisciplinary teams, understanding normal and abnormal child development and associated underlying theories and concepts, being exposed to intensive and extensive service settings, and gaining practical experience in consultation and liaison activities with pediatric hospitals/clinics and community settings such as schools, child care, welfare, and juvenile justice.

Critical dimensions of psychiatric training include the following:

- Learning to conduct and report a biopsychosocial assessment
- Learning to develop and implement a treatment plan within a multifactor universe that comprises contributions from multiple disciplines and data sources (Figure 12.6)
- Learning to address the identified factors

The Role of Psychiatrists

Psychiatrists bring several unique skills to client care. They include a perspective influenced by the medical model, which demands the development of hypotheses (diagnoses) tested through treatments. These treatments are expected to lead to specified results or changes. If no treatments are known to have a positive effect, the medical model promotes the observation of the course of illness. Knowledge and administration of psychopharmacologic remedies have become of prime importance to practice, as are knowledge and understanding of systems issues as related to the three levels of prevention (primary, secondary, and tertiary). These elements involve evidence-based and rational prescribing of a wide array of psychotropic medications to treat psychiatric disorders.

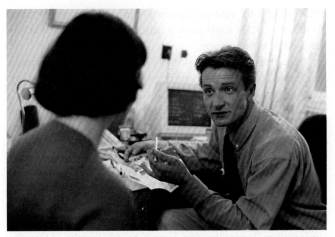

FIGURE 12.6 Psychiatrists are physicians with prescriptive authority. Their knowledge and administration of psycho-pharmacologic remedies is of prime importance to current psychiatric practice.

Psychiatrists, Nurses, and Multidisciplinary Teams

Advanced practice nurses are independent medication prescribers in many states. They work in close partnership with psychiatrists, often as key workers for clients, which means that they are the first point of contact for clients or their caregivers. They stay in regular contact with clients and are responsible for ensuring that care planned for them is delivered. Psychiatric nurses are trained to assess the client's mental state and decide whether he or she should see a psychiatrist for review of medication or other treatment.

In the team setting, psychiatrists have a wide perspective on assessment/evaluation tools and procedures, diagnosis and formulation of psychopathology, protective factors,

family and individual dynamics and related interventions, systems issues, and the role of health status on the individual client and family. The team effort is of tremendous value to effective and quality client care (CaseVignette 12.4).

> **Checkpoint Questions**
> **7.** After graduation from medical school, how many additional years of training are required of a CAP?
> **8.** Who is often the first point of contact for the client or caregiver and works in close partnership with psychiatrists?

REGISTERED DIETITIANS
By Patricia A. Troyanowski, BS, MS, RD
Speciality Hospital, Albuquerque, New Mexico

Food and water are essential to life. The humanistic psychologist Abraham Maslow asserted that unless these basic physiologic needs were met, people could not achieve higher functioning (see Chap. 3). Food and drink are so fundamental to health and well-being, and nutrition is so vital to healing, that the care of clients calls for health care professionals who can assess and meet these most basic physiologic needs. Their skills provide a basis for other types of interventions to meet higher-level needs.

A **registered dietitian (RD)** is a health care provider whose overall goal is to improve the nutritional health of clients, households, and communities by addressing the social, psychological, and environmental causes of nutrition problems. RDs are experts in food and nutrition. They assess nutrient needs and provide dietetic interventions for clients with disabilities and across the continuum of care (Figure 12.7).

Case Vignette 12.4

Christa, 16 years old, presents to an intermediate-term state psychiatric hospital for dangerously impulsive behavior. Referral material suggests possible psychosis or borderline personality disorder. Christa sometimes makes bizarre statements. She reports that over the past 2 years, intrusive thoughts that later made no sense led her to engage in risky behaviors like unprotected sex. She is taking neuroleptic medication at a dosage sufficient to control psychotic symptoms; the drugs, however, have no positive effects. A review of previous outpatient testing with an electroencephalogram (EEG) shows no evidence of seizures or related activity. Projective testing reveals no signs of a psychotic disorder.

A social worker conducts individual therapy with Christa and provides her parents supportive family work and parenting skill training. Although the working diagnoses are conduct disorder and parent–child problems, the social worker thinks

Christa might have dissociative identity disorder (see Chap. 25). In the hospital school, Christa's performance is erratic. Male teachers report occasional seductive behavior toward them.

The CAP remains concerned that an underlying medical condition is the cause. During discussions with Christa, he learns that she sometimes claims to detect unusual odors before problematic episodes. Further EEG testing reveals paroxysmal activity in the temporal region, a finding consistent with a partial-complex seizure disorder. The CAP shares with Christa and her parents that this finding might explain her behavior. Christa begins taking an anticonvulsant medication.

After a brief drug trial, Christa's behavior markedly improves. She is soon discharged. The CAP's understanding of biologic factors that can cause psychopathology and knowledge of adequate tools for diagnosis allowed for a satisfactory resolution of the client's major problems.

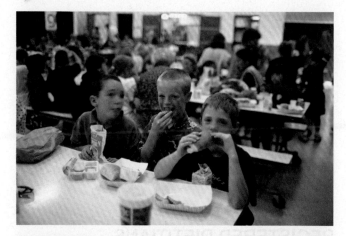

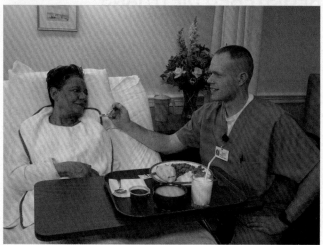

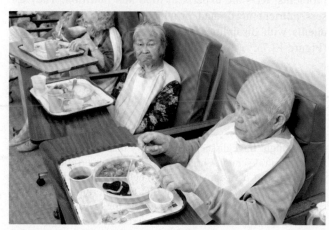

FIGURE 12.7 Registered dietitians work with clients from all age groups and in various settings. Schools, hospitals, and long-term residential care facilities all may employ their services to ensure optimal nutritional health for clients.

Educational Background and Training

Being a "food expert" (although everyone is a food expert in a certain sense!) involves more than knowing nutritional requirements and basic food groups. Dietitians must take courses in physiology, chemistry, and biochemistry, all of which are necessary to understand fully the science of nutrition and to separate erroneous information from facts. To practice, RDs must pass a national examination that ensures basic competence.

At a minimum, RDs possess a bachelor's degree from a regionally accredited university or college, with course work approved by the Commission on Accreditation for Dietetics Education (CADE) of the American Dietetic Association (ADA). Because of the complexity of medical care and concurrent high acuity of clients needing nutritional interventions, many facilities, especially research programs, require RDs also to have entry-level master's degrees.

Part of the minimum education requirement is a supervised internship or practice program in a CADE-accredited health care facility, community agency, or food service corporation. Typically, this lasts 6 to 12 months. After the didactic and practice course work, the dietitian must pass a national examination administered by the Commission on Dietetic Registration (CDR). To maintain registration, the RD must complete continuing professional educational requirements.

Some RDs hold additional certifications in specialized areas, such as pediatric or renal nutrition, nutrition support, and diabetes education. These certifications are awarded through CDR, the credentialing agency for the ADA, or other medical and nutrition organizations. They are recognized within the profession but not required for practice.

The Role of Registered Dietitians

The goal of dietetics is to try to help people improve their quality of life. RDs have hospital privileges and write orders under the supervision of a physician. They carry malpractice insurance and work in hospitals, inpatient rehabilitation centers, home health settings, and privately.

RDs care for the whole client—not just the nutritional component. To succeed, RDs examine each client's social, cultural, psychological, and physical aspects. In this way, they can make good assessments relative to nutritional status (Case Vignette 12.5). The various contributions of RDs to treatment plans are described in Box 12.2.

Registered Dietitians, Nurses, and Multidisciplinary Teams

Food and nutrition have enormous psychological implications. The most striking example is when a client has an eating disorder (see Chap. 26). Certainly, RDs play a major role when a client faces starvation or is beginning rehabilitation. However, such clients must also face their underlying psychological issues before nutritional therapy can succeed. The treatment of eating disorders not only illustrates how RDs can greatly help clients and families, but also exemplifies a situation requiring extensive teamwork and coordinated communication.

Professional dietetics is not about paperwork or 2-hour lectures. It is about putting clients first and meeting them as equal and unique partners in the plan of care. It is also about providing individualized care.

Case Vignette 12.5

An older adult resident at a long-term care facility is losing weight and diagnosed with depression. Despite treatment for the psychiatric disorder, she refuses to eat solid foods. The activities director notes that the client no longer attends social activities or goes to the dining room for meals. The client's family members demand intervention by a social worker.

The social worker calls a chaplain, who speaks with the client and learns that she does not want to eat because she wants to die. Family members are shocked by this revelation, saying that the client never previously showed suicidal inclinations. The client's living will specifies that she wants no nutritional care. The facility's policies do not allow forced feeding. In this instance, the client's wishes directly conflict with the family's.

The dietitian meets with the client and assures her that the facility will not pressure or force her to eat. After several discussions, the dietitian persuades the client to try some nutritional formulas. Improvements in nutrition and appropriate weight gain eventually help the client gain the strength needed to deal better with her depression.

▲

BOX 12.2   Role of the Registered Dietitian in Treatment Plans

- Assesses ideal body weight and caloric and dietary needs.
- Recommends foods that help facilitate swallowing.
- Develops special diets.
- Recommends dietary modifications to accommodate a disability (e.g., tube feeding formulas and schedules for clients who cannot swallow).
- Provides client and family education on nutrition topics related to diseases (e.g., diabetes).
- Recommends appropriate food choices.
- Develops verbal and written guidelines to assist people in making continuing individualized, healthy selections to nourish their bodies and minds, and to give them better quality of life and longevity.

ART THERAPISTS

By Scott M. Reid, MA
Alzheimer's Association Delaware Valley Chapter, Philadelphia, Pennsylvania

Art therapy is a mental health profession that uses the creative process of art-making as a primary part of treatment. Creating artwork can help clients acquire new skills, identify and use effective coping strategies, aid in emotional expression or containment, increase social engagement, bolster self-esteem and self-awareness, and aid in developing insight (American Art Therapy Association, 2011). **Art therapists** use a wide range of art media and different art tasks to help achieve these therapeutic goals, aid psychological and physical healing, and enhance the general well-being of their clients.

Art therapists can be found in hospitals, schools, mental health clinics and community centers, long-term care, respite services, hospice and palliative care, and in private practice. Clients may receive art therapy as part of a group or individually, depending on the setting, the treatment plan, and the needs of the client. Art therapy may also be used in the context of family therapy, to help resolve problems in the family unit that extend beyond the identified client.

The field of art therapy encompasses work with a broad range of clients. However, individual art therapists tend to specialize in areas based on their professional experience and expertise. Populations that can benefit from art therapy include those with psychiatric disorders, learning or developmental disorders, substance abuse, eating disorders, trauma, and medical conditions or diseases. The process of making art is an incredibly adaptable tool, which can be made accessible and meaningful for any individual with a chief complaint.

Educational Background and Training

Art therapists usually have an eclectic background in the humanities and/or the arts. Professional art therapists have received a master's level education from a school certified by the American Art Therapy Association (AATA). Before admission to an AATA program, students must have completed extensive course work in both psychology and studio art. An understanding of both abnormal and developmental psychology, as well as the use of various art materials, is foundational knowledge for art therapists because it will inform their practice of art therapy on a daily basis.

During a master's program, students develop proficiency in the application of art therapy for various clinical settings and populations. Typically this includes client assessment, individual therapy, and group therapy. Required courses include the study of psychopathology, human growth and development, counseling and psychological theory, cultural and social diversity, clinical assessment, research, and studio art (AATA, 2007). Students must also complete an internship with a minimum of 700 clinical hours.

Postgraduate credentialing as a registered art therapist (ATR) and as a board-certified art therapist (ATR-BC) can be obtained after a certain number of clinical hours. The ATR-BC also requires an additional examination, which is issued independently by the Art Therapy Credentials Board. Some art therapists may also hold the title of licensed practicing counselor, which can be obtained in certain states after the requirements for that credential are met. Art therapists may also have a doctorate in a related field, and some may have a doctorate in art therapy specifically.

Role of the Art Therapist

Most professional art therapists operate in one of two modalities: art as therapy or art psychotherapy. Art as therapy primarily relies on the art-making process to help clients explore self-expression and self-understanding. Art therapists who take this approach believe that clients benefit from the art-making process itself, without the need for further, verbal elaboration. Art psychotherapists, on the other hand, work with clients, their art process, and the art product to provide therapy within a psychoanalytic framework. Psychoanalysis relies heavily on discussion of internal thoughts and feelings, which may be unknown to the client or difficult to address. The theoretical approach of using art in therapy is determined by the individual therapist, the setting, and the population; however, in practice, aspects of both theoretical approaches are used with clients.

Art therapists have the same goals in working with their clients as any other therapists would. These include developing a therapeutic relationship with the client to establish a sense of trust and safety, known as the holding environment, which is also provided by the physical space of the art room. Art therapists are also trained in theories of transference and countertransference to help moderate and build these relationships. This helps the art therapist avoid reenacting previous and unhealthy relationship dynamics with clients, which would be counterproductive to treatment. Art therapists may also offer support and guidance to clients through unconditional positive regard.

Clients may uncover or share thoughts and feelings that are difficult to express to others. Therefore, making and sharing art can reveal a person's internal thoughts and feelings about past or present. Working with an art therapist can help clients resolve these issues through the recapitulation of past events or relationships, and relate them to current events or relationships. What is seen and discussed through the artwork often parallels the experience of the individual creating it, because of art's isomorphic property of representing the self through symbolism. Discussing the chief complaint through the metaphor of the artwork may feel more acceptable to the client, because of the objectivity of the artwork and its perceived separation from the artist (Wadeson, 1980).

In clinical settings, many art therapists work with groups to facilitate interactions among group members. Groups are used to examine and understand an individual's awareness of self and of his or her relationships with others. Art therapists explore this through observation and discussion of the actions of a client in a group setting or among group members as dyadic or triadic relationships, and of the group dynamic as a whole. The art therapist also uses the art produced by clients in a group to help explore these dynamics by, for example, discussing similarities and differences in art, the experience of creating art in a group, and common themes represented by the group.

Providing an outlet for socialization is a key goal for many art therapists. Preventing isolation and increasing social engagement with others can have several beneficial effects for clients. Creating art in a group decreases depression and anxiety by promoting universality (Yalom, 1983) and may help clients identify creative ways of coping. Clients often comment that knowing others who are struggling with the same issues they are is a source of great comfort. Making and sharing art with others acts as a catalyst for this connection. For those who suffer from chronic psychiatric problems, illness or disease, or developmental impairment, creating art as a group can also provide a sense of normalcy and belonging.

One of the most powerful aspects of art therapy is affect management. Art therapists use art materials to encourage the expression, or containment, of affect along the expressive therapies continuum (Lusebrink, 1990). Encouraging self-expression can have a cathartic effect, which can help clients become more in touch with their emotions and also relieve stress and create energy. For clients who have poor affective management, art therapists can provide more structured tasks and media to help these clients deal with their emotions in a more productive way. Self-expression and emotional release and/or control are primary objectives for the art therapist.

Art Therapists, Nurses, and Multidisciplinary Teams

Art therapists choose art tasks that highlight and support therapeutic goals established by the treatment team. Doctors, nurses, and social workers may all consult with the art therapist about the client's progress during the course of treatment. Information provided by the art therapist to the clinical team may include an initial and periodic art assessments, daily progress notes, and routine recommendations based on client observation in group or individual therapy. Having the art therapist sit in on treatment meetings, consult charts and client records, and be in regular communication with doctors, nurses, primary therapists, and social workers should be encouraged.

By engaging in the art process, clients lower their defense mechanisms, which may inform the therapist of factors such as psychotic or delusional thinking, suicidal ideation, drug abuse, self-injury, or other issues of concern. Therefore, clients may also be more inclined to share thoughts and feelings they may not be comfortable sharing with the doctors or nurses. If so, it is imperative that the art therapist inform the rest of the treatment team. Nurses have an especially important role in relaying and acting on information provided by the art therapist, because it can lead to more supervision and monitoring on the unit, increase communication and education about use and abuse of pharmaceuticals, and contribute to a better understanding of the psychological needs of the client in general.

Similarly, if the nursing staff or treatment team has information about the client—from allergies to presenting symptoms to events that occur on the unit—they should share it with the art therapist whenever possible. This will help the art therapist determine the most appropriate tasks and materials for the client. If a client suffers from severe asthma attacks, for example, the art therapist would not choose a project involving chalk pastels, which might exacerbate or even cause an asthma attack. Or, if a nurse were to report a client's self-injurious behavior in the form of cutting, the therapist would restrict the use of sharps and do a scissor-count at the end of the day.

Nurses and art therapists can be great allies for the betterment of the client's treatment by being advocates for their care. Adverse side effects from changes in medication, traumatic triggers, and other general health concerns can all be addressed and confirmed by both the art therapist and the nursing staff, and can then be communicated to doctors or administration. Nurses and art therapists are also both integral in identifying clients who may be at high risk for suicide or homicide, self-injury, relapse, acting out, or other behaviors. Communicating these red flags to the appropriate members of the treatment team can help save lives.

PROFESSIONAL CERTIFIED THERAPEUTIC RECREATION SPECIALISTS

By Kerry E. Brown, CTRS

Alzheimer's Association Delaware Valley Chapter, Philadelphia, Pennsylvania

Of the 30,000 U.S. and Canadian certified therapeutic recreation specialists (CTRs), the majority, 52%, work in nongovernment agencies, 9% in federal gove rnment agencies, 29% in local government agencies, 6% in private practice, and 5% as consultants. Employment opportunities for CTRs are found in the areas of corrections, parks and recreation, outpatient and day treatment, hospitals, skilled nursing facilities, human services, adult day programs, residential settings, and disability organizations. CTRs serve the geriatric population and clients with behavioral or mental health problems, physical disabilities, and developmental disabilities (National Council for Therapeutic Recreation, 2009).

A **recreation therapist (RT)** provides treatment in a systematic way that uses activity-centered interventions based on an assessment of the client's needs. The purpose of the RT process is to improve or maintain physical, cognitive, social, emotional, and spiritual functioning in order to facilitate full participation in life. RT is a unique profession because it makes treatment enjoyable and fun by using activities of purpose that are also areas of interest for the individual, thereby leading to increased motivation and success. Typical outcomes of recreational therapy include improvement in a client's physical health, cognitive and psychosocial status, ability to use community resources, and motivation to follow preventive health strategies.

Educational Background and Training

RTs are professionals who have earned a bachelor's degree or higher from an accredited university and completed course work that emphasizes the physical, biologic, and behavioral sciences as well as leisure theory. RTs also need to complete a formal 12-week (480-hour) internship under the supervision of a Certified Therapeutic Recreation Specialist and pass the national certification exam. Qualified professionals are certified through the National Council for Therapeutic Recreation Certification (NCTRC), and the certification standards require that candidates gain exposure to the following job analysis task domains during their internships: (1) professional roles and responsibilities; (2) assessment; (3) planning interventions and/or programs; (4) implementing interventions and/or programs; (5) evaluating outcomes of interventions and/or programs; (6) documenting intervention services; (7) working with treatment and/or service teams; (8) organizing programs; (9) managing TR/RT services; and (10) public awareness and advocacy. CTRs must maintain their credentials every 5 years through the NCTRC recertification process. In 2010, NCTRC also began offering specialty certifications that require more continuing education credits in a 5-year period, in the areas of physical medicine/rehabilitation, geriatrics, developmental disabilities, behavioral health, and community inclusion services.

The Role of Recreational Therapists

Like other therapists, RTs are concerned with treatment goals as part of the rehabilitation process, but the difference lies in how the goals are achieved and the professional point of view. The primary purpose of treatment services, according to the American Therapeutic Recreation Association (ATRA), is to restore, remediate, and rehabilitate in order to improve functioning and independence, as well as to reduce or eliminate the effects of illness or disability. The primary purpose of recreational services is to provide recreational resources and opportunities in order to improve health and well-being (ATRA, 1986).

Like OTs, RTs work with people of all ages who have a disability or a physical or mental illness. They use individually selected activities, often from the client's past leisure repertoire, to help restore, develop, or maintain skills. Assessment and treatment is from a client-centered perspective, encouraging clients to identify their own needs or difficulties and collaborate on realistic treatment programs.

Although an RT's job can look very different from setting to setting, the following job duties are commonly performed by RTs in a typical day working in the field:

- Attending a multidisciplinary team meeting to discuss the progress of current clients or set goals for newly admitted clients
- Assessing clients' physical, cognitive, social, emotional, and spiritual skills through activities of daily living, meal preparation, money management, and community outings
- Working with clients and their social networks to plan and implement their safe discharge from the program, or setting quarterly goals for long-term clients
- Spending one-on-one time with a client to assess progress in the setting or community
- Attending care conferences with clients and family members to plan and review ongoing treatment
- Assessing the environment and skills needed for a potential leisure program that a client wants to return to or initiate
- Identifying ways to adapt activities for individuals using techniques such as task analysis (breaking activities down to the smallest possible step) or using strengths-based programming (based on the individual's abilities, interests, and strengths, rather than on problems, weaknesses, or loss)

Recreational Therapists, Nurses, and Multidisciplinary Teams

RTs work with professionals in all health care environments, such as physicians; registered nurses; physical, occupational, and speech therapists; social workers; and the clients themselves and their family members. The multidisciplinary team works together closely to develop highly personalized, coordinated therapy plans that help clients achieve the greatest level of leisure independence. From nursing care to daily routines, treatment approaches, and therapy goals, each client's unique needs are incorporated into care plans that involve the skills of the entire care team.

BENEFITS OF THE MULTIDISCIPLINARY APPROACH

Clients with chronic mental illness and complex psychiatric disorders require the care of a well-coordinated multidisciplinary team. Members with significant contributions include not only general practitioners and medical specialists (e.g., neurologists, gerontologists, rehabilitation staff) but also, ideally, a wide range of other health professionals, including physiotherapists, OTs, speech therapists, RDs, psychologists, art therapists, RTs, and nurses. From the beginning, clients are not only the focus of teams, but their most important members. The relationship is reciprocal because clients are a team's reason for existing. Clients cannot be cared for adequately without a fully functioning and communicating team.

Nurses are pivotal to collaborative teams. They plan interventions to help clients achieve goals established by various members. They ensure that goals are not in conflict. Nurses gather contributions, input, and feedback from clients themselves, as well as their family members and other caregivers (Figure 12.8).

The many complex and often closely intertwined problems that clients with mental illness face underscore the

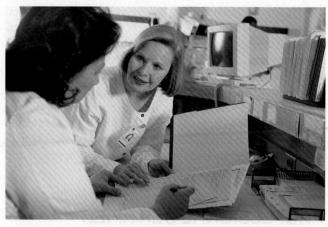

FIGURE 12.8 A nurse confers with a colleague from another field about care issues related to a client.

urgent need for a multidisciplinary approach. It is impossible for a single provider or specialist to manage such problems. First, one person cannot be available to a client at all times. Standard medical management alone often ignores important domains of functioning. In fact, some medical interventions, such as drug therapy, may contribute to new problems or exacerbate established conditions.

Multidisciplinary teams are not there only for clients with "complex" problems. They can also be helpful during early or acute stages of illness. They can address possible worries about the future or prevent problems before they arise.

> **Think About It 12.1**
> An older adult being treated for dementia and depression has a stroke and experiences right-sided weakness; his ability to swallow is also affected. He lives at home with his wife, who has diabetes and cataracts. Examine how the multidisciplinary team would care for this client, including examples of care that each member would provide.

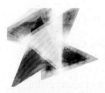

Reviewing and Applying Your Knowledge

Chapter Summary

• Multidisciplinary teams consist of groups of professionals from diverse disciplines who come together to provide comprehensive assessments of clients, establish and carry out interventions for them, and engage in regular consultations about clients' progress.

• Each discipline has its own perspective, jargon, mandates, and resources.

• When professionals fail to understand differences, barriers, misunderstandings, or "turf" conflicts may develop. On the other hand, when professionals learn about the approaches, resources, and perspectives of colleagues from other disciplines, they can expand their repertoire of skills, increase their available resources for clients, and enhance their understanding of various problems.

• The need for a multidisciplinary approach is crucial in the care of clients with complex psychiatric problems that a single provider or specialist cannot manage.

• Multidisciplinary teams can be helpful during early or acute stages of illness and can address possible worries about the future or prevent problems before they arise.

Study Questions

1. After working as a member of a multidisciplinary team developing an IEP for a child with a learning disability, the nurse expects to review the IEP

   a. every 30 days.

   b. every 60 days.

   c. twice a year.

   d. yearly.

2. A client demonstrates clumsiness and a tendency to fall, appearing unaware of his body position in space. The nurse identifies a sensory integration dysfunction in which system?

   a. Tactile

   b. Proprioceptive

   c. Visual

   d. Vestibular

3. Which team member often acts as the primary liaison between the team and the client?

   a. Social worker

   b. Professional dietitian

   c. Psychiatrist

   d. Occupational therapist

4. A class is taught about the various disciplines within psychology. Successful teaching has occurred if the class identifies which discipline as being involved with understanding how psychology relates to the law and clinical settings?

   a. Environmental psychology

   b. Counseling psychology

   c. Forensic psychology

   d. Clinical psychology

5. Services coordination teams differ from IEPs in which of the following ways? Select all that apply.

   a. Based on the concept of family-driven service provision

   b. Concerned with the child in and out of school and with the family

   c. Primarily limited to the child in the home-based setting

   d. Implemented by a special education teacher

   e. Require presence of a family member at each team meeting

References

American Art Therapy Association (AATA). (2007). *Masters educational standards*. Retrieved from http://www.americanarttherapyassociation.org/upload/masterseducationstandards.pdf.

American Art Therapy Association (AATA). (2011). *AATA about us: Art therapy*. Retrieved from http://www.americanarttherapyassociation.org/aata-aboutus.html.

American Therapeutic Recreation Association. (1987). *Definition statement for therapeutic recreation*. Hattiesburg, MS: Author.

Anderson, J. A. (2000). The need for interagency collaboration for children with emotional and behavioral disabilities and their families. *Families in Society: The Journal of Contemporary Human Services, 5,* 484–493.

Anderson, J. A., Kutash, K., & Duchnowski, A. J. (2001). A comparison of the academic progress of students with emotional and behavioral disorders and students with learning disabilities. *Journal of Emotional and Behavioral Disorders, 9,* 106–115.

Anderson, J. A., & Matthews, B. (2001). We care for students with emotional and behavioral disabilities and their families. *Teaching Exceptional Children, 33*(5), 34–39.

Anderson, J. A., & Mohr, W. K. (2003). A developmental ecological perspective in systems of care for children with serious emotional disturbances and their families. *Education and Treatment of Children, 26*(1), 52–74.

Anderson, J. A., Wright, E. R., Smith, J. S., & Kooreman, H. E. (2007). Educational profiles of students at enrollment in a system of care. *Remedial and Special Education, 28*(1), 9–20.

Friend, M., & Bursuck, W. D. (2008). *Including students with special needs: A practical guide for classroom teachers* (5th ed.). Boston, MA: Allyn and Bacon.

Friesen, B. J., & Poertner, J. (1995). *From case management to service coordination for children with emotional, behavioral, or mental disorders*. Baltimore, MD: Paul H. Brookes.

Lusebrink, V. J. (1990). *Imagery and visual expression in therapy*. New York, NY: Plenum Press.

National Council for Therapeutic Recreation. (2009). *Certified Therapeutic Recreation Specialists* [Brochure]. New York, NY: Author.

Ribner, D. S., & Knei-Paz, C. (2002). Client's view of a successful helping relationship. *Social Work, 47*(4), 379–387.

Stroul, B. A. (1996). Service coordination in systems of care. In B. A. Stroul (Ed.), *Children's mental health: Creating systems of care in a changing society* (pp. 265–280). Baltimore, MD: Paul H. Brookes.

Stroul, B., & Friedman, R. M. (1986). *A system of care for children and youth with severe emotional disturbances* (rev. ed.). Washington, DC: Georgetown University Child Development Center, CASSP Technical Assistance Center.

Sugai, G., Horner, R. H., & Sprague, J. R. (1999). Functional assessment-based behavior support planning: Research-to-practice-to-research. *Behavioral Disorders, 24,* 223–227.

U.S. Department of Education. (2007). *27th annual report to Congress on the implementation of the Individuals with Disabilities Education Act, 2005,* Vol. 1. Washington, DC: Author.

Wadeson, H. (1980). *Art psychotherapy*. New York, NY: John Wiley & Sons.

Whelan, R. J. (1995). Emotional disturbance. In E. L. Meyen & T. M. Skrtic (Eds.), *Special education & student disability, an introduction: Traditional, emerging, and alternative perspectives* (pp. 271–338). Denver, CO: Love.

Wright, E. R., Wright, D. E., Kooreman, H. E., & Anderson, J. A. (2006). The nature and impact of conflict within service coordination teams for children and adolescents with serious emotional and behavioral challenges. *Administration and Policy in Mental Health and Mental Health Services Research, 33*(3), 302–315.

Yalom, I. D. (1983). *Inpatient group psychotherapy*. New York, NY: Basic Books.

Zastrow, C. H., Gebo, L., & Concilla, C. (2002). *Practice of social work* (7th ed.). Belmont, CA: Wadsworth.

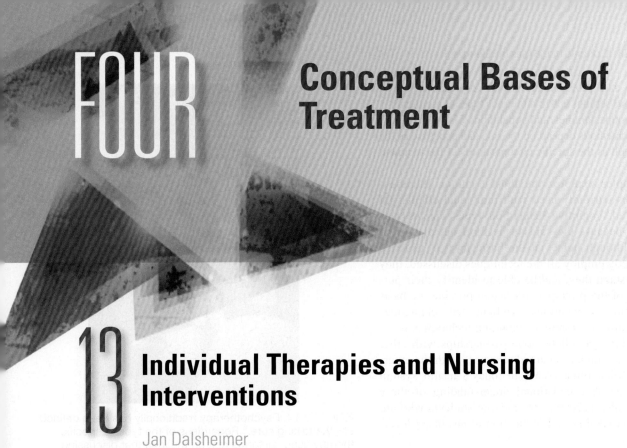

FOUR

Conceptual Bases of Treatment

13 Individual Therapies and Nursing Interventions

Jan Dalsheimer

KEY TERMS

cognitions
cognitive distortion
cognitive triad
countertransference
invalidating environment
mindfulness
positive reinforcement
psychotherapy
schema (core beliefs)
unconditional positive regard

LEARNING OBJECTIVES

On completion of this chapter, you should be able to accomplish the following:

- Define psychotherapy.
- Discuss the goals of therapeutic modalities used with individual clients.
- Identify current trends influencing choice of therapies.
- Describe various approaches to psychotherapy and key techniques within each.
- Discuss basic level therapeutic nursing interventions for clients with psychiatric problems.
- Explain advanced practice functions for clients with psychiatric problems.
- Compare and contrast the roles of the RN-PMH and the APRN-PMH in individual psychiatric care.

Health care professionals provide psychiatric care in various settings and to numerous types of recipients—individuals, groups, families, and populations. Use and delivery of the specific methods depend on the role and expertise of the provider, as well as the specific circumstances of the recipient or recipients.

This chapter explores the most common therapeutic approaches currently used with individual clients. Of those reviewed, cognitive–behavioral types receive particular focus because they are at the forefront of current treatment. Although nurses at the basic level of practice may not directly employ all the techniques discussed, they should understand them and be able to identify their purposes. Many of the principles presented provide the basis for core nursing interventions for clients with challenges to mental health. Awareness of common techniques is integral to working in collaborative partnerships with other team members, which has gained relevance with the emergence of interdisciplinary care in today's health system (see Chap. 12). A foundational understanding of these techniques is also necessary for nursing students who are considering expanding their education to advanced levels of practice.

In addition to outlining common therapeutic techniques, the chapter explains the general approaches and common skills used by psychiatric–mental health nurses who work with individual clients. It differentiates the role of basic level psychiatric–mental health nursing specialists from that of advanced practice nurses in the discipline. It also provides examples of interventions associated with both levels of practice, settings for their application, and rationales for their implementation.

THERAPIES FOR INDIVIDUAL CLIENTS

An understanding of the concepts of individual therapy is essential for all those who work with people in the psychiatric arena, including nurses. Historically, individual psychotherapy has been defined as "the talking cure." This vague definition embraces the essence that people who seek therapy describe. Namely, talking and sharing pain with a trusted person leads to psychological healing (Figure 13.1). A more specific definition of **psychotherapy** is a process by which a person with professional skills uses evidenced-based procedures rooted in empirically supported theories to help clients make adaptive changes in their lives. These changes are expressed in behaviors and in ways of thinking. Although the support of family or friends may be helpful and even have a therapeutic quality, only trained professionals provide psychotherapy. Information or other contact about medication is not considered psychotherapy, though it may be important for the process (Andersson & Cuijpers, 2009; Schnyder, 2009).

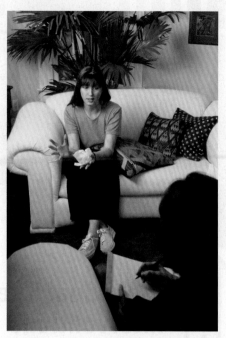

FIGURE 13.1 Psychotherapy traditionally has been defined as "the talking cure." Regardless of the type of specific therapy used, all forms rest on the idea that discussing problems with a trusted professional can improve psychological health.

Goals of Individual Therapy

The overall goals of individual therapy are for the client to experience less psychological distress, increase self-awareness and self-esteem, and learn new, more functional ways to cope. The therapist–client relationship is the vehicle through which insight as well as cognitive and behavioral change occurs.

Some researchers believe that it is the unique meeting between the therapist and the client that is the driving force behind the client's success (Andersson & Cuijpers, 2009). The quality of the therapist's presence as well as the expression of verbal and nonverbal behaviors impacts the quality of treatment (Bacal & Carlton, 2010). Even in modalities that do not emphasize the importance of this relationship, the client needs to be comfortable with the therapist. Chapter 11 provides details about key elements of therapeutic relationships and communication.

Practitioners of Psychotherapy

Trained professionals who offer psychotherapy include psychiatrists (MD), clinical psychologists (PhD), social workers (LMSW), licensed professional counselors (LPC), and psychiatric–mental health advanced practice registered nurses (APRN-PMH). While styles of practice vary with discipline, the one commonality is the importance of the therapist–client relationship. For the client's therapy to have a successful outcome, the therapist must be able to relate to the client in order to decrease suffering and promote client growth (Bruce et al., 2010).

Current Trends

Probably the most influential trend in current psychotherapy modalities used for individual treatment has been the advent of managed mental health care. Insurance companies no longer reimburse clients for long-term, insight-oriented therapy that was the hallmark of care during the 1960s through the 1980s. The shorter-term focus of "how" to change thoughts, feelings, and behaviors has superseded extended investigations of the "why" behind a person's problems. For this reason, cognitive–behavioral therapies (CBT) and strategies, which are most conducive to achieving quick results, have become preferred. With inpatient stays limited to 3 to 5 days and outpatient therapy capped at 4 to 10 sessions in 6 to 12 months, therapists increasingly have felt the pressure to find creative ways to make their treatment as efficacious as possible within these constraints. Computer-based cognitive–behavioral focused treatments as well as CBT integrated with other therapies are trends that are beginning to emerge.

An additional demand in current practice is the need to choose a therapy that research has validated as effective for the client's psychiatric diagnosis. Combining clinical expertise with research-based information and doing so in the context of the client are the principles that guide practice (Wilson et al., 2009). The question being asked is "What treatment is most effective for which disorder?" A quantitative method such as the randomized controlled trial (RCT) is an example of evidence development that has become the standard for estimating treatment effects (Fisher & Happell, 2009). Explanations of such trials and more details about evidence-based practice are found throughout this chapter and book. See also Chapter 4.

Common Modalities

The following sections review eight psychotherapeutic approaches: psychoanalysis/psychodynamic; cognitive–behavioral, with the subtypes of cognitive, rational emotive behavior, and dialectical behavior; behavioral; client centered; and solution focused. See also Table 13.1.

Psychoanalysis/Psychodynamic Therapies

Sigmund Freud (1856–1939) pioneered *psychoanalysis,* a form of therapy that explores the client's conscious and unconscious conflicts with past coping patterns. Freud postulated that conflicts among three personality parts (id, ego, and superego) cause mental illness. The goal of psychoanalysis is to promote insight and integrate repressed conflicts into the personality so that the person can be happier and enjoy improved functioning (see Chap. 3).

Psychodynamic psychotherapy shares similar philosophical and theoretical foundations with psychoanalysis. Therapy sessions may be less frequent than in psychoanalysis, however, with once or twice per week being the norm. The treatment time frame may be limited or open ended. The essence of treatment is similar to that of psychoanalysis in that the client explores parts of the self that are not fully known. Central to the therapy is the relationship with the therapist and the dynamic of *transference.*

A great benefit of psychodynamic psychotherapy is its potential for providing lasting effects that extend beyond symptom remission (Shedler, 2010). Bateman and Fonagy (2008) reported that 5 years after treatment, 13% of patients who received psychodynamic psychotherapy for treatment of borderline personality disorder no longer met diagnostic criteria, compared with 87% who received other treatment. Ryum and colleagues (2010) found in their study of 49 clients with Cluster C diagnoses that low doses of the transference may be beneficial for reducing interpersonal problems, if alliance with the therapist is lacking. Sarnat (2010) noted that qualities of psychoanalytic practitioners include helpfulness to the client in balancing emotional and intellectual understanding, effectiveness in timing interventions, and appropriate use of the transference.

Because of their cost, lack of insurance reimbursement, and time commitment from clients, psychoanalysis and long-term psychodynamic psychotherapy often are not practical choices in today's era of managed mental health care. Also, RCTs for other forms of psychotherapy, particularly CBT, exist in greater numbers. While it can be a highly effective type of therapy that provides depth and fullness to sessions (Pesale & Hilsenroth, 2009), one that CBT needs to be measured against, more research to determine its methodological rigorousness needs to done for psychodynamic psychotherapy (Shedler, 2010, 2011).

Currently emerging are some studies on the combination of CBT and psychodynamic therapy. According to Kush (2009), CBT and brief psychodynamic psychotherapy, either in their pure forms or combined, appear to be the most commonly used psychotherapies. Lawson (2010) reported that the integration of these therapies resulted in a significant decrease in recidivism rate and partner violence in men with a history of abusive behaviors.

Important psychoanalytic/psychodynamic concepts for psychiatric nurses include transference, countertransference, and defense mechanisms (see Chap. 3). Because repetitive themes from a person's relationships are often brought into therapeutic relationships (Shedler, 2010), nurses need to be aware of these concepts. When working with clients, nurses should be alert to any extreme emotional response that clients direct toward them. Warm feelings, even affection, from clients are common; conversely, clients may become annoyed with nurses. Expressed feelings may not always have a basis in current events or realities. For example, a client who is irritated because a nurse is late for a meeting is expressing a legitimate emotion over easily identifiable circumstances. However, when feelings, either positive or negative, seem extreme or disproportionate to the circumstances, nurses should consider whether a *transferential* reaction has occurred. In other words, the current relationship with the nurse has ignited something in the client's past from an old relationship, usually one involving an authority figure, such as a parent. Clients may need help to identify such

TABLE 13.1 Selected Approaches to Psychotherapy

Approach	Focus	Key Points for Nurses	Desired Outcome
Psychoanalysis Psychodynamic psychotherapy	Client's conscious and unconscious conflicts	Transference Countertransference Defense mechanisms (see Chap. 3)	Insight into repressed conflicts Restructuring of the personality
Cognitive–behavioral therapy	Changing distorted thoughts, with the result being positive behavioral change	Identification of situations involving undesirable thoughts and actions Homework assignments	New skills
Cognitive therapy	*Client's perception of self, world, and future (cognitive triad)* *Exploration of client's thought processes*	*Development of problem lists* *Session agendas* *Homework* *Evaluation of successes and failures*	*Recognition of self-defeating thought patterns* *Release of self-blame* *Enhancement of `responses*
Rational emotive behavior therapy	*Exploration of irrational thinking*	*Identification of activating situations and negative emotions, leading to irrational beliefs*	*Client control of behavior and thinking* *Change in thinking leading to positive change in behavior*
Dialectical behavior therapy	*Acceptance of emotions fused with acknowledgment of need for behavior change*	*Empathy* *Reflection of feelings* *Exploration of perceptual distortions and dysfunctional behaviors*	*Client's embracing of intense emotions (living in the moment)* *Self-acceptance* *Change in cognitions leading to more functional coping patterns*
Behavior therapy	Promoting desirable behaviors Extinguishing undesirable behaviors	Token economies Reinforcements	Reshaping of behavior with elimination of negative behaviors
Client-centered therapy	Relationship with therapist Self-acceptance leading to insight	Unconditional positive regard Empathy Reflection of feelings	Increased self-esteem Positive foundation so that client sees self and situations more clearly
Solution-focused therapy	Problems result from mishandling life's events	Joint partnership between therapist and client Client development of alternate views of situation based on identification of past successes and factors maintaining the problem	Satisfactory life adjustments and ability to change, interact, and reach goals through solutions

transference. Nurses are most beneficial to clients in this event by remaining compassionate, not becoming defensive, and assisting clients to identify the feelings and possible past reasons for them.

Countertransference occurs when nurses have extreme emotional responses (positive or negative) to clients. Although these responses are not uncommon, nurses need to understand and closely monitor countertransference. Analysis of its causes may require assistance from a mental health colleague or the treatment team. Nursing students must also be aware of possible countertransference responses and be open to discussing their feelings with instructors and peers in supervised clinical conferences.

> ### Checkpoint Questions
> 1. What are three overall goals of individual therapy?
> 2. What are two main reasons that psychoanalysis is not currently the therapy of choice?
> 3. How can a nurse best work with a client experiencing transference?

Cognitive–Behavioral Therapies

Cognitive therapy focuses on how clients think about themselves and their world; *behavioral therapy* assumes that human responses are learned and therefore can be unlearned.

Cognitive–behavioral therapy (CBT) fuses cognitive and behavioral techniques. It does not explore how a person became a certain way; instead, it focuses on changing current thinking and behavior. It is results oriented and defines goals so that progress toward them can be monitored. The therapist acts as a coach and teacher for the client learning new skills. He or she may help the client identify situations that trigger undesired thoughts and actions and then assist with the development of alternatives (Dowd et al., 2010). The behavioral part involves homework that the therapist assigns to the client to complete before the next appointment.

Two major CBT modalities are cognitive therapy, developed by Aaron Beck in 1963, and rational emotive behavioral therapy, developed by Albert Ellis in 1955. A third type is dialectical behavior therapy, developed by Marsha Linehan in 1993 specifically for clients with borderline personality disorder (see Chap. 25).

All cognitive–behavioral models share some fundamental assumptions:

- **Cognitions** (thoughts) influence a person's responses and affect the degree of adjustment or maladjustment.
- Cognitions can be monitored and altered, and new behaviors can be consciously chosen.
- CBTs are time limited, and most applications are for specific problems. They help to develop skills applicable to other problems.

CBT is supported by evidenced-based research as a treatment for various psychiatric diagnoses (Evidence-Based Practice Spotlight 13.1).

In an RCT of clients with intermittent explosive disorder, CBT was administered in 12-week group and individual sessions. Results indicated that both modes of delivery were effective in reducing anger, aggression, hostile thinking, and depressive symptoms. Anger control was also improved (McCloskey et al., 2008). In their study of 86 veterans with post-traumatic stress disorder (PTSD), Marshall et al. (2010) found that CBT used in an anger management group decreased anger not associated with personality disorder traits. Sobell and colleagues (2009) found that both group and individual treatments using CBT were effective for substance use. No difference between formats was found.

CBT has also been found useful for the treatment of children. Ollendick and associates (2009) found that one-session treatment using CBT techniques resulted in a decrease in phobic responses in children ages 7 to 11 years. In an RTC of children ages 4 to 7 with anxiety disorders, a developmentally appropriate parent–child CBT protocol was effective for social phobia/avoidant disorder, separation anxiety disorder, and specific phobia (Hirshfeld-Becker et al., 2010).

CBT is also appropriate for anxiety disorders in adults. Hien and colleagues (2009) found, in an RTC with 353 women, that CBT was effective in reducing PTSD symptoms. In a study of 43 clients, 70% of whom were female, a 12-week CBT treatment for panic disorder was effective. A change in catastrophic misinterpretations resulted in reductions in panic attacks (Teachman et al., 2010). CBT, both cognitive therapy and rational emotive therapy, as well as pharmacotherapy, has been found to decrease symptoms associated with depression (Sava et al., 2009). Simons and colleagues (2010) also indicated that CBT is useful in decreasing depression. While other treatment was also effective, only CBT helped to decrease additional symptoms of

---

EVIDENCE-BASED PRACTICE SPOTLIGHT 13.1

Cognitive Behavioral Therapy

- In an RCT of 150 women diagnosed with post-traumatic stress disorder (PTSD) and depression subsequent to intimate partner violence (IPV), results of Cognitive behavioral therapy (CBT) treatment revealed reductions in depressive and PTSD symptoms. Patients were exposed to different forms of CBT with assessments done at nine time points, which included a 6-month follow-up. Because women with PTSD and depression resulting from IPV are at high risk for continuing abuse in relationships, a decrease in these symptoms as a result of CBT directly decreases the likelihood of IPV victimization (Iverson et al., 2011).
- Three hundred forty-one high school students at risk for depression were randomized to the following groups: group cognitive behavioral (CB) intervention, group supportive expressive intervention, CB bibliotherapy, or an educational brochure control condition. One-year and 2-year follow-ups were done. While the supportive expressive participants showed greater symptom reduction than the CB bibliotherapy group at the 2-year follow-up, both group CB intervention and CB bibliotherapy were more effective than the brochure control. Group CB intervention, CB bibliotherapy, and supportive expressive therapy were all found to produce intervention effects that are long term (Stice et al., 2010).

References

Iverson, K. M., Gradus, J. L., Resick, P. A., Suvak, M. K., Smith, K. F., & Monson, C. M. (2011, February 21). Cognitive-behavioral therapy for PTSD and depression symptoms reduces risk for future intimate partner violence among interpersonal trauma survivors. *Journal of Consulting and Clinical Psychology, 79*(2), 193–202. doi:10.1037/0022512

Stice, E., Rohde, P., Gau, J. M., & Wade, E. (2010). Efficacy trial of a brief cognitive-behavioral depression prevention program for high-risk adolescents: Effects at 1- and 2-year follow-up. *Journal of Consulting and Clinical Psychology, 78*(6), 856–867. doi:10.1037/a0020544

anxiety. In a study of 36 university students with test anxiety, cognitive–behavioral test-anxiety interventions that included positive self-statements and self-hypnosis were effective. Students used the interventions provided and then created their own to use when other strategies did not work. A benefit was that students perceived their own strategies as consistently being within their control (Dundas et al., 2009).

A criticism of CBT is that, although it is considered helpful for people with fairly rigid patterns of viewing themselves and the world, some clients may find it too simplistic. For example, a client undergoing intensive psychodynamic therapy may believe that the concept of "changing thinking leading to behavior change" does not leave room for exploring the self that is not definite. CBT is useful for challenging "all-or-nothing" thinking but may be less useful when the client's thinking falls into a more "gray" zone (Craddy, 2006). CBT therapies rarely focus on the therapeutic relationship or on the therapy process; only about 30% focus on the present moment (Kanter et al., 2009). For clients who value the depth of processing that exploring the transference can give, CBT may be experienced as superficial.

> **Think About It 13.1**
> A client with obsessive-compulsive disorder who repeatedly rearranges items in the bathroom medicine cabinet is to receive CBT. What techniques would you expect the treatment team to employ to help this client?

COGNITIVE THERAPY. Cognitive therapy (CT) focuses on how clients think about themselves and their world. Addressing cognitions, CT posits that how a person perceives an event, rather than the event itself, determines its relevance and the emotional response to it. CT helps clients recognize the process and results of their thinking. This model is short term (10 to 20 sessions), active, collaborative, and psychoeducational. A trusting relationship between client and therapist is important but not the main mechanism of change. In CT, clients learn to use their skill comprehension and then take credit for their own efforts at change (Jarrett et al., 2011; Leichsenring et al., 2006). The overall goal is increased self-efficacy or proficiency and a sense of self-control. The client must participate actively and be committed to change. The goal-oriented collaborative partnership between therapist and client has a beginning, a middle, and an end.

Because it focuses on process (how) rather than content (what), CT strategies are appropriate for many clients, problems, and therapeutic contexts. It is effective in reducing symptoms and relapse rates in a wide variety of psychiatric disorders (Beck, 2005). For example, CT is part of treatment for anxiety, eating disorders, personality disorders, depression, and sexual disorders; it is used in individual, family,

and group settings. Dobson and associates (2008) found in an RCT that CT and behavioral activation were effective in the treatment of depression. A 2-year follow-up showed that patients exposed to both therapies did as well as those patients who had continued medication. Dozois and colleagues (2009) also found CT to be effective in treating depression. In their study of 42 clients, 21 were assigned to medications, and 21 were assigned to medication plus CT. Both groups had significant and similar reductions of depression, automatic thoughts, and dysfunctional attitudes. Regarding cognitive organization, however, the combination of CT with medication indicated better results.

Core Issues. According to CT, three issues result in the formation and maintenance of common psychological disorders (Beck, 2005):

- **Cognitive triad.** Beck (1979) developed the triad to help explain the interaction of the client's negative view of self, the world, and the future. He believed that all issues and problems can be subsumed under one or a combination of these three areas. These issues vary in intensity; one client may be more concerned about self (Can I do this?), while another may be worried about the future (Will there be a job for me?). In anxiety, this triad represents the client's concern about a threat to the self from the world or a future experience.
- **Cognitive distortion.** Clients may apply distortions to self, experiences, or expectations of others. They may distort positively or negatively. Positive distortions may lead people to take chances that others would avoid (eg, risky investments) or be unrealistically positive about life-threatening conditions (eg, chest pains, breast lumps). Negative distortions include beliefs such as "I always do it wrong," "Nobody likes me," or "It's all his fault!" Usually, negative distortions are maladaptive and become the focus of treatment, which involves identification of the effects of the distortion on the client's life. Examples of distortions appear in Table 13.2.
- **Schema or (core beliefs) (basic rules of life). Schema or core beliefs** are an accumulation of the person's learning and experience within the family, religion, ethnicity, gender, regional subgroups, and broader society. They begin at birth and are well fixed by middle childhood. The client's ability to change these core beliefs depends on:
  - Whether there is a powerfully associated belief that something cannot be changed no matter what (eg, "My father said this is the only way.")
  - Whether significant others have reinforced the belief continuously
  - Whether there has been reinforcement for a positive contrary belief (an ignoring of one's sense of self-worth); parents or significant others often offer opposition to the developing positive image by saying "It's not nice to brag," instead of "I'm glad you're feeling better about yourself."

TABLE 13.2 Cognitive Distortions

Distortion	Example	Commonly Associated Psychiatric Diagnoses
All-or-nothing thinking	"I'm either a success or a failure."	Borderline personality disorder
	"The world is either black or white."	Obsessive-compulsive personality disorder
Mind reading	"They probably think that I'm incompetent."	Avoidant personality disorder
	"I just know that he disapproves."	Paranoid personality disorder
Emotional reasoning	"Because I feel inadequate, I am inadequate."	Anxiety disorders
	"Because I feel uncomfortable, the world is dangerous."	
Overgeneralization	"Everything I do turns out wrong."	Depression
	"My choices are always wrong."	
Catastrophizing	"If I ____, there will be terrible consequences."	Social anxiety
	"If I ____, it always fails."	Social phobia
		Panic disorders
Control fallacies	"If I'm not in complete control all the time, I will go out of control."	Obsessive-compulsive disorder
	"I must control all things in my life."	Obsessive-compulsive personality disorder
Disqualifying the positive	"This success was only a fluke."	Depression
Perfectionism	"I must do everything perfectly or I will be criticized and a failure."	Anxiety disorders
Selective abstraction	"The rest of the information doesn't matter."	Depression
	"I must focus on negative details and ignore all the positive aspects of this."	
Externalization of self-worth	"My worth depends on what others think of me."	Depression
	"They think/believe _____, therefore I am ____."	
Should/shouldn't/must/ought statements	"I should visit my family every time they want me to."	Obsessive-compulsive disorders
	"You/They should do whatever I say because it is right."	
Jumping to conclusions	"I know they will not let me join."	Depression
Fallacy of change	"You should change your behavior because I want you to."	Narcissistic personality disorder
	"They should act differently because I expect it."	
Fallacy of worrying	"If I worry about it enough, it will be resolved."	Anxiety disorders
	"One cannot be too concerned."	
Fallacy of ignoring	"If I ignore it maybe it'll go away."	Depression
	"If I don't pay attention, I won't be responsible."	Anxiety disorders
Fallacy of fairness	"Life should be fair."	Avoidant personality disorder
	"People should be fair."	Social anxiety disorder
Fallacy of attachment	"I can't live without a man."	Depression
	"If I were in a relationship, all my problems would be gone."	Anxiety disorders
Being right	"I must prove that I am right, as being wrong is unthinkable."	Obsessive-compulsive personality disorder
	"To be wrong is to be a bad person."	Narcissistic personality disorder

Treatment Approach. A general CT treatment approach includes the following (Table 13.3):

1. Building trust, active listening, and having empathy (see Chap. 3)
2. Turning data into goals or a working problem list to identify the client's direction and when to assess his or her progress
3. Reviewing the past week and successes and problems the client has with homework assigned by the therapist
4. Deciding on an agenda for each session (may include previous problem, dysfunctional thinking, or a new desired skill)
5. Working on an agenda
6. Reviewing the session. Approximately 5 minutes before a session ends, the client should review the interaction, state feelings about it, and explain what he or she has gained from it. The therapist then can clarify, note accomplishments, and assign homework for the next session.

The therapist questions the thinking distortions and underlying schema to help the client respond in more functional ways and recognize irrational thinking patterns. Sometimes, the client may seem noncompliant during a session or with assigned homework. There could be many reasons for this, including

TABLE 13.3 Therapeutic Techniques of Cognitive Therapy

Technique	Description	Examples
Look for idiosyncratic meaning	Ask the client directly about what words and thoughts mean to him or her.	"What does that mean to you?" "Give me an example."
Question the evidence	Examine the source of data and recognize that the client may be overlooking parts.	"That sounds like what your mother would say." "It also might mean ___." What evidence do you have that that is true?"
Reattribute	Distribute responsibility among all relevant parties, not just the client.	"Your brother and sister were also part of that." "As a child you could not know ___."
Decatastrophize	Recognize that the client is overestimating the catastrophic nature of the situation.	"What is the worst that can happen?" "If it does occur, what would be so terrible?"
Fantasize consequences	Ask the client to describe the situation. Often, he or she can see the irrationality of his or her ideas. If the problem remains real, then help the client develop coping strategies.	"What might be the effects in 10 years?"
Weigh advantages and disadvantages	Ask the client to look at all sides of the issue before defining a reasonable course of action. Writing helps concretize thoughts.	"What are the pros and cons?"
Examine options and alternatives	Ask the client to generate additional options. This is especially difficult for the suicidal client. Don't discount his or her feelings.	"You may be right, something may be wrong with you. What other conclusion might there be?"
Turn adversity to advantage	Present opportunities that stem from challenges.	"Losing this job may be an entry point to a new career."
Use thought-stopping	Stopping dysfunctional thoughts is best at the beginning, not the middle. Dysfunctional thoughts can have a snowball effect. Encourage the client to use devices to stop negative thoughts as they arise.	Examples include snapping fingers, popping a rubber band around the wrist, or tapping on the knee.
Use distraction	Distraction is especially helpful with anxiety problems because it is difficult to maintain two thoughts at the same time. Anxious thoughts generally preclude more adaptive thinking. A focused thought distracts the anxiogenic thought.	Have the client count to 200 by 13s (not by 2, 5, 10, or 11); count people wearing yellow or count only small trucks. Have the client do a physical activity such as walking, focusing on the in and out of breathing, or counting every other step; it works best when using a complex activity.

headache, hunger, new difficulties, or just not wanting to do it. Any of these may indicate the need for change in assignments or goals. The therapist must recognize the client's anxiety and concerns as well as progress made. The client defines progress; current goals may no longer fit and need to be reset. The therapist must find some way to compliment the client, even if only recognizing that he or she is "surviving a terrible situation."

RATIONAL EMOTIVE BEHAVIOR THERAPY. Albert Ellis developed rational emotive therapy (RET) in 1955 after becoming dissatisfied with psychoanalysis. In 1993, the therapy was renamed rational emotive behavior therapy (REBT) to encompass a behavioral component (Ellis, 2004).

Ellis believed that people are disturbed not by things or events, but by their view of them. REBT posits that rational beliefs are evaluative and nonabsolute cognitions. They are expressed as wishes, likes, and dislikes that may or may not be attained. Irrational beliefs tend to be dogmatic and are expressed in a rigid form: "must," "should," "ought," or "have to." They lead to negative emotions that interfere with goal pursuit and attainment (Dryden & David, 2008; Szentagotai et al., 2008). Healthy beliefs underlie functional behaviors, whereas unhealthy beliefs underlie dysfunctional behaviors, such as procrastination and substance abuse.

REBT rests on the client's realization that he or she is the creator of the psychological disturbance and that he or she can change it. Crucial to this recognition is the understanding that such disturbance primarily results from irrational beliefs. Once identified, the client can dispute and philosophically restructure these beliefs, ultimately leading to change. Change means moving from absolutes to "preferences" (ie, what the client would like to happen). The primary goal of REBT is to replace irrational beliefs with rational ones (Vaida et al., 2008).

The "ABC" approach is the method of resolving irrational beliefs (see Chap. 3). The client must realize that the activating event (A) does not directly cause emotional and behavioral consequences (C). Rather, the client's beliefs (B) about the activating event (A) contribute primarily to the consequences (C). In other words, irrational beliefs about events lead to inappropriate consequences (Dryden & David, 2008; Szentagotai et al., 2008).

Unconditional self-acceptance, no matter what one's professional or personal failings may be, is an important principle of REBT. Acceptance of others as people, not necessarily of their behaviors, is also part of the REBT philosophy. Finally, acceptance of life and a high frustration tolerance assist a person to live a functional life (Ellis, 2005).

REBT is used in a variety of settings, such as counseling and education. Vaida et al. (2008) reported on a model for education in which high school students were exposed to REBT with the goal of decreasing students' irrationality and offering them the opportunity to develop a life philosophy by changing the way they see and perceive things. Changes were seen in belief systems, emotions, and behaviors. Wilde (2008) reported that REBT techniques and rational coping statements, in combination with relaxation and thought-stopping, were effective in decreasing anxiety problems in children.

Dryden and David (2008) noted that while Ellis was an enthusiastic practitioner of psychotherapy and believed REBT to be effective for a wide range of clinical problems, rigorous research historically has not supported Ellis's beliefs. In 2008, a 6-month follow-up comparison of CT, REBT, and use of an antidepressant medication (fluoxetine) revealed that REBT significantly improved scores on the Hamilton Rating Scale for Depression. The study included 170 outpatients with major depressive disorder who had been randomly assigned to one of the three treatments (David et al., 2008).

DIALECTICAL BEHAVIOR THERAPY. Marsha Linehan (1993) developed dialectical behavior therapy (DBT) specifically for treatment of borderline personality disorder (BPD). BPD, one of most serious personality disorders, occurs in approximately 10% of outpatients and 20% of inpatients (Salsman & Linehan, 2006). The premise of DBT is that BPD is a disorder of the emotion-regulation system. When an emotionally vulnerable child is paired with an invalidating environment, the result over time is pervasive dysfunction in regulating emotions. An **invalidating environment** is one in which children receive the message that what they feel is invalid, and that if they were more effective, they wouldn't have such feelings. Examples of invalidation include punishing, ignoring, or contradicting children.

Results of brain-imaging studies show enhanced frontolimbic activation to environmental or interpersonal cues that are upsetting (Smoski et al., 2011). Strong emotion is part of the client profile; over time, clients with BPD have learned not to trust their feelings. When they experience strong feelings, their cognitive, behavioral, and emotional systems break down. Internal confusion results in outward manifestations of BPD—impulsive actions such as substance abuse, binge eating, gambling, and reckless driving (see Chap. 25).

Shortcomings of standard CBTs for BPD are that they focus solely on change without validating the client's emotions. Because clients with BPD are highly sensitive to nonacceptance, suggestions of change by the therapist are often interpreted as invalidation and criticism (Goldfried, 2007). Several components of DBT make it different and particularly effective. A cornerstone of DBT is weaving acceptance of the client into treatment, with an additional goal of the client accepting himself or herself, his or her emotions, thoughts, environment, and others (Swales, 2009). A core strategy of DBT is "validation," which involves active listening and accurately reflecting the client's spoken and unspoken thoughts, feelings, and behaviors. Expressing that the client's dysfunctional behavior is logical within his or her past or current context and interacting with the client in a genuine manner are crucial. However, focusing entirely on acceptance invalidates the seriousness of the client's suffering and the real need for change (Lynch et al., 2006). The balance between acceptance and change of emotions is the central dialectic of DBT (Swales, 2009).

DBT is extensive and involves individual therapy, group therapy, and a therapist consultation team to enact the five functions of treatment, which are as follows (Swales, 2009):

1. **Enhancing the client's capabilities.** Examples include helping the client to regulate emotions and pay attention to the present. **Mindfulness** helps the client accept and attend to what is currently happening. Rather than running away from or ignoring a feeling, the therapist encourages the client to embrace it while attending to one thing at a time, thereby focusing on effective behavior. This component usually requires a weekly skills group session, with assigned homework so that the client can practice skills between sessions. Stepp and colleagues (2008) found that DBT was effective in increasing individual skills related to mindfulness, tolerance of distressful feelings, relationship effectiveness, and emotional regulation.

2. **Generalizing treatment skills to the client's environment.** This often is practiced in individual sessions so that the client can anticipate difficult situations. In addition, the therapist is available by phone between sessions to help the client apply skills should a crisis arise (Figure 13.2).

3. **Improving motivation and decreasing dysfunctional behaviors.** The therapist asks the client to complete a self-monitoring form called a "diary card" on which he or she will track treatment targets, such as self-harm or emotional distress. The therapist then will prioritize session time, focusing first on any life-threatening behaviors, followed by behaviors that interfere with therapy or quality of life. The therapist and client will examine antecedent events leading to the behavior, possible consequences, and more effective future behaviors and emotions.

4. **Maintaining the therapist's capabilities and motivation.** In weekly therapist consultation-team meetings, therapists support one another, assist with problem-solving involving challenging clients, encourage a compassionate attitude toward clients, and sometimes provide structured training for skill-building.

5. **Structuring the environment.** The primary therapist ensures that the five functions are being met and elements of effective treatment are in place. This may also mean helping the client find ways to modify his or her environment (eg, finding new friends).

DBT has been found to decrease suicide attempts in women with BPD (Neacsiu et al., 2010) and to decrease deliberate self-harm in female adolescents (James et al., 2008). DBT in combination with modules for daily self-monitoring, weekly weighing, and weekly education about weight and eating was found to be effective for eating disorders (Kroger et al., 2010). Chen and colleagues (2008) found DBT to be effective for binge-eating disorder and bulimia nervosa as well as BPD. Iverson and associates (2009) found that DBT resulted in a reduction of depression, hopelessness, and psychiatric distress as well as an increase in social adjustment in female victims of domestic violence. DBT was effective with clients with Axis I substance dependence disorders who also had BPD (Harned et al., 2008).

Results of DBT include retention in therapy (Herschell et al., 2009) and fewer psychiatric hospitalizations (Moran, 2007). Despite its effectiveness, however, access to a DBT-trained therapist can be challenging. Although used increasingly in community mental health settings, offering DBT can be challenging for agencies due to reimbursement issues, time commitment, and staff training. Possible solutions may include streamlining training, supporting staff who undergo training, and careful planning of financial issues (Herschell et al., 2009).

An encouraging finding reported by McMain and colleagues (2009) centered on the result of a single-blind study in which 180 clients diagnosed with BPD were randomly assigned either to 1 year of DBT or 1 year of general psychiatric management. General psychiatric management included psychodynamically based psychotherapy and symptom-focused medication management. Both groups improved in BPD symptoms, and there were no significant differences in outcomes between the groups. While CBT has limitations for effectiveness with BPD clients, psychodynamically based psychotherapy may be indicated, especially in the absence of access to a DBT-trained therapist.

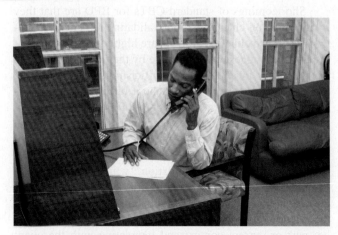

FIGURE 13.2 An important provision of dialectical behavioral therapy is that the therapist is available by phone between sessions to help clients apply skills during a crisis.

Checkpoint Questions

4. For which client population is CBT most effective?

5. What are the goals of REBT?

6. What is an "invalidating environment," and how does it contribute to BPD?

7. How does dialectical behavior therapy differ from traditional CBT?

Behavioral Theory

B. F. Skinner (1904–1990), a leading behaviorist of the 20th century, conceptualized several principles to explain how behaviors can be developed and altered. His principles of positive and negative reinforcement (see Chap. 3) are still used in psychiatric treatment.

An example of behavioral intervention is the "token economy," which relies on positive reinforcement. Initially developed in the middle of the 20th century, token economies were mainstays of long-term inpatient treatment. Health care providers might give clients a token (or coin) as a reward for positive behaviors, in other words provide **positive reinforcement** so the desired behaviors will increase and be maintained. Clients can then use tokens to "buy" privileges or special treats. Examples include supervised walks on hospital grounds and candy from the hospital store. Today, token economies are still used for clients with chronic conditions such as mental retardation and autism.

When using behavioral techniques with clients, health care personnel, including nurses, need to be consistent in implementing the treatment plan. Communication, verbal or written, among personnel of varying shifts is necessary to ensure that staff members provide appropriate reinforcement for clients. Inconsistencies are disruptive to the client's treatment and progress. The client's psychological safety and ability to make improvements depend on staff consistency. It should be stressed, however, that consistency should not be confused with rigidity. At times it may be more therapeutic not to insist on following rules if those prescribed rules serve to agitate clients and lead to conflict.

Treatment plans are negotiated between the treatment team members and the individual clients and/or their families. They are adapted to clients' specific problems and the goals should be measureable and attainable. In addition, rather than stating that the client will "not" do something, the plan states what the client will do instead—*instead* being the key word. For example, a plan might state that the client will "sit quietly for 10 minutes when Aunt Pat is here." While the overall goal is to increase or decrease a particular behavior when confronted with similar situations in the future, this approach does not have the added dimension of assisting clients with explorations of thoughts and feelings.

Some research has been conducted using behavior therapy as the treatment modality. Bickel and associates (2008) reported using a computer-based behavioral therapy intervention, both therapist delivered and computer assisted, for opioid dependence. One hundred thirty-five volunteer adult outpatients were randomly assigned to the intervention group and treatment as usual group and to a "standard treatment" group receiving only counseling at a methadone treatment clinic. The behavioral intervention groups produced comparable results with clients maintaining significantly more weeks of abstinence than the standard treatment group.

Client-Centered Therapy

Carl Rogers (1902–1987) was a humanistic psychologist whose approach emphasized the therapeutic relationship and empathetic responding to clients. He believed that people have the ability to grow psychologically and that all a therapist needs to do is provide the conditions for change to occur, that the quality of the client–therapist relationship alone has healing potential (Goldfried, 2007). Several of his principles are foundational in the nurse–client relationship and are reviewed in detail in Chapter 11.

Rogers explained *empathy* as the ability to enter into and appreciate the client's experience, without losing the "as if" quality. In this way, nurses can feel deeply for the client while also maintaining an emotional boundary that enables true helpfulness to the client. Being empathetic is an active process that requires careful listening and attending to the client. Direct eye contact, a concerned expression, occasional head nods, and leaning forward while listening are nonverbal communication skills that convey empathy (Figure 13.3). Empathy can help a person feel valued and accepted as a person (Stuart, 2009). Empathetic responses, such as "you're going through a difficult time" can provide clients with an opportunity to listen to themselves and gain self-awareness. Reflecting feelings, clarifying, and paraphrasing are therapeutic communication techniques that verbally indicate empathy. Bruce and colleagues (2010) noted that forming an empathetic relationship with the client can lead to the client's ability to be attuned to self. This attunement can then result in less client suffering and greater well-being.

Unconditional positive regard means consistently considering the client in a positive way, not having conditions for acceptance or evaluating the client negatively. A client who senses acceptance from the nurse will likely feel safe in the therapeutic relationship. This client will have an increased capacity for honesty and openness, a willingness

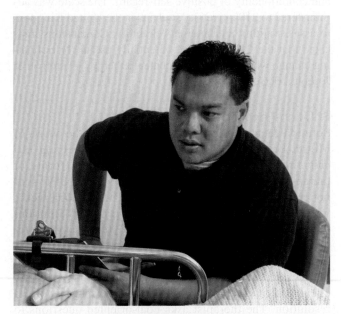

FIGURE 13.3 The therapist's nonverbal behaviors are important during interactions with clients. Some examples of appropriate strategies include careful listening, direct eye contact, a concerned expression, occasional nods, and leaning forward while listening.

to self-explore, and a greater likelihood of thriving in the therapeutic environment (Stuart, 2009).

Psychiatric nurses often use the client-centered philosophy as a foundation for practice. The therapeutic use of "self" is a basic principle of psychiatric nursing. The relational components with clients lead to positive change. The therapeutic relationship begins with the belief that the client is competent and capable and that the client and nurse will identify solutions jointly.

Because client-centered therapy focuses on the whole person and not just specific symptoms, producing clinical evidence showing its effectiveness is difficult. In fact, Rogers' approach has been so widely adopted that it is now sometimes difficult to find client-centered theory cited as a separate therapy (Goldfried, 2007). In a survey of 2,400 psychotherapists, Rogers was picked as the theorist who had the most impact on therapists' practices (Cook et al., 2009). The theory itself predicts that the core relationship between client and therapist ensures a positive therapeutic change in the client. The theory predicts that the client's increase in unconditional positive self-regard and decrease in conditions related to negative self-worth lead to greater autonomy and congruence. Miller and Rose (2009) credited Rogers' contribution of the therapist–client relationship in their development of motivational interviewing. Motivational interviewing involves an interview format in which the therapist empathizes, accepts, and validates a resistant client's experience while gradually leading the client toward realizing negative consequences of behavior.

The need for evidence-based research, however, has led to a study focusing on the Unconditional Positive Self-Regard (UPSR) Scale, a 12-item scale measuring self-regard and conditionality of positive self-regard. The scale was administered to 210 university students in the United Kingdom to assess validity and internal reliability. Conclusions indicated that the UPSR may be potentially useful for evaluating change when using client-centered therapy (Patterson & Joseph, 2006).

Solution-Focused Therapy

Solution-focused therapy (SFT), based on the work of Milton Erickson (1901–1980), emphasizes helping clients find solutions to their problems. Many forms of therapy (eg, CBT) work toward solutions, but SFT does not employ predetermined solutions. The therapist works with the client as he or she solves the problem. Solution-focused therapists use the word "we" (client and therapist), suggesting a joint experience. In the SFT process, there may be some initial discussion of the problem, but the therapist then focuses on change. The therapist and client determine a central issue and concentrate on its resolution. The therapist asks goal-oriented questions to further facilitate movement toward an effective solution (Box 13.1). He or she looks for times when the problem was not in evidence or when, even for a short time, there was a solution to the problem (De Jong & Berg, 2008;

Langdridge, 2006). The entire solution-focused process concentrates on goals and the resulting positive expression of behavior (Nims, 2007).

Usually, the therapist and client take a break toward the end of a therapy session, during which the therapist composes some constructive feedback that conveys a positive message to the client about his or her work and competence. Sometimes the therapist asks the client to perform a task away from the session, such as thinking about something differently or engaging in a specified action. However, the therapist does not take a psychoeducational role. Instead, he or she continues to encourage the client's work (De Jong & Berg, 2008; Langdridge, 2006).

Checkpoint Questions

8. How is behavioral therapy used on an inpatient psychiatric unit?

9. What qualities does the client-centered nurse convey to clients?

10. How would a solution-focused therapist explain the origin of a client's problems?

11. What is the role of the solution-focused therapist?

Integrative Approaches to Psychotherapy

Current studies reflect a trend toward examining the use of two or more therapies for the treatment of various psychiatric disorders. Newman and associates (2008) found that CBT alone was less effective for generalized anxiety disorder (GAD) than the use of CBT plus interpersonal therapy or supportive listening. This combination was effective in decreasing GAD symptomatology for up to 1 year following treatment.

In an RCT of 22 depressed adults assigned to either treatment with CT or integrative CT, the clients receiving integrative CT had a more positive relationship with the therapist after addressing difficulties in the relationship. An integrative approach, not usually used with CT, involved discussing present thoughts and feelings about difficulties in the therapeutic relationship. Therapists who empathized with their clients after such disclosures—and even found some truth in the clients' criticisms—saw improvement in the therapeutic relationship. With a repaired relationship and resumption of standard CT, clients had higher alliance toward the therapist (Constantino et al., 2008).

Kanter and colleagues (2009) noted that several approaches recommend combining a present-focused approach with CBT. A present-focused approach addresses problems as they occur in the therapeutic relationship. They found, however, that no more than 30% of CBT approaches focus on the therapy process or the relationship and that they rarely focus on the present moment. Harrington and Pickles (2009) argued against the use of "mindfulness" in CBT, maintaining that to use mindfulness with CBT necessitates a paradigm shift. Kuyken and colleagues (2008) found that

BOX 13.1 Process of Solution-Focused Therapy

1. **Set the agenda.** Why are you here today? What would be helpful for us to discuss? What would be helpful for me to know about you and your situation? What would be more helpful? Tell me why.

2. **Understand the effects of the problem.** How has this problem affected your life? How is it still affecting you? How has this problem kept you from moving forward in the way you would like? How has it gotten in the way of your life? How would your best friend, teacher, mother, or spouse say this problem has affected your life? Do you agree? How do you feel about that?

3. **Identify exceptions.** Are there times when you would expect the problem to happen, but it does not? How do you get that to happen? (A focus on client competency.) What are you doing differently when you're standing up to the problem? Tell me about a time when you were even a little successful in standing up to the problem. Would your family or friends say there are times when the problem is less of a problem? What's going on when they say that?

4. **Make sense of the exceptions.** How do you account for your ability to do this (the exception)? Is this something that surprised you about yourself? What about you helped you to do this? Did you know before you did ___ that you would be able to do it? If yes: How did you know this about yourself? What was different about this situation compared with a situation when the problem was more in charge? What was different about you? What would your family, friends, mate, teacher, or boss say if I were to ask them how they think you did this?

5. **Use future orientation.** Create the expectation of noticeable change. Expecting change implies that the client has the power to change.

6. **Ask the "miracle question."** If a miracle happened tonight while you were asleep and tomorrow you awoke to find that this problem no longer existed, what would be different?

How would you know the miracle had happened? How would others know without you telling them? What would your feelings be when ___ is not controlling your behavior or thinking? (Keep increasing the level and amount of details.)

7. **Ask for a "video description."** If I had two videotapes, one of you when you are standing up to the problem and another when the problem is getting the best of you, what would I notice about when you are in charge? What's different? If one tape is in the past and one is in the future, what's most noticeable in the future tape that tells us that things are better for you?

8. **Reinforce small steps.** What will be a small sign, something you'll likely notice in the next few days, that will tell you that things are better for you? What will indicate to you there's reason to be hopeful?

9. **Scale questions.** On a scale from 1 to 10, with 1 being "pretty bad" and 10 being "pretty good," how would you rate how you are doing now? When you can move 1 or 2 points toward 10, what will be happening differently? What's the highest you've ever been? When was that? How were you able to do that?

10. **Continue to work toward solutions.** Instruct the client to observe and take note of things that go well in the next week; look for examples of exceptions. Then, tell the client to pretend that the solution or miracle has happened, or that he or she has reached a higher point on the scale. This may involve picking particular days to pretend or a daily coin toss with the pretending to be done on "heads" days. If others are involved in the therapy, they may be asked to pretend also or to try to "guess" when the client is pretending. The client should then "practice" particular steps and behaviors that have been identified, such as making a phone call to say ___ or talking out loud to himself/herself in the mirror. Ask the client, "What is the most far-fetched explanation for this problem you can think of?"

---

mindfulness-based cognitive therapy (MBCT) resulted in a reduction of depressive symptoms and was more effective than antidepressants alone. Of 61 clients receiving MBCT and support to taper or discontinue medication, 46 patients were able to discontinue medication.

Internet-based treatment protocols are being developed and tested against more traditional therapies. De Graaf and associates (2010) compared unsupported online computerized CBT (CCBT), usual care by a primary physician that includes medication as needed, and CCBT with usual care. In this study, 303 depressed patients were randomly assigned to the three groups. Results indicated that CCBT was most effective for clients with the least impairment. More depressed clients responded more favorably to CCBT with usual care. Usual care alone was least effective. Khanna and Kendall (2010) studied 49 children ages 7 to 13 with an anxiety disorder. The clients were randomly assigned to computer-assisted CBT for anxiety in youth, individual CBT, or a computer-assisted education method. Results indicated significant improvement in anxiety

for clients who received individual CBT and the computer-assisted CBT. Bickel and colleagues (2008) found that therapist-delivered computer-based behavioral therapy intervention and computer-assisted intervention were both effective methods for treating opioid dependence. Standard treatment, that is, counseling at methadone treatment clinics, was found to be less effective for these 135 volunteer adult outpatients. In an RCT of 77 patients, Sugarman and colleagues (2010) also found that computer-based CBT increased coping strategies, which then decreased drug use.

Cultural Considerations in Psychotherapy

Psychotherapies are generally products of Western philosophies and ways of thinking. Thus, their assumptions are culturally specific. The implicit foundations of the various forms of psychotherapy reflect the notions of Western societies. For example, a value placed on extraversion leads practitioners to pay more attention to what is said, rather than what remains unsaid. A regard for individualism emphasizes development of the inner self and a strong sense of self-direction. Individual therapies require a client to use explicit talk about thoughts and feelings to effect change.

For clients from cultures that avoid negative or unduly intense emotions, or even view such expressions as immature, Western psychotherapy may conflict with their values. Such clients may view the catharsis that therapy encourages as burdensome or of little help. Some cultures value acceptance of difficult situations and being able to relate to a natural world that is larger than oneself (Kirmayer, 2007). For example, the Buddhist approach to change differs greatly from that espoused by proponents of cognitive therapy (Figure 13.4). Buddhism focuses on changing expectations and desires, whereas cognitive therapy emphasizes changing evaluations of life events. The difference is letting go versus changing (Dowd & McCleery, 2007). Santiago-Rivera and associates (2008) found that Latinos responded more positively to motivational techniques for change than to CBT when dealing with depression. Taking action is more prized than understanding beliefs and underlying attitudes.

Because of these differences in culturally influenced or determined values, it is imperative for health care providers to consider a client's background, beliefs, and concerns when choosing therapies and interventions (see Chap. 6). Culturally sensitive psychotherapy is the tailoring of psychotherapy to specific cultural groups so that values of those groups can be addressed (La Roche & Christopher, 2009). Understanding how culture enhances the meaning of the client's life history, the impact of culture on illness and help-seeking, and

the client's expectations of treatment will deeply impact the client–therapist relationship (Schnyder, 2009).

PSYCHIATRIC NURSING ROLES AND STRATEGIES FOR INDIVIDUAL CLIENTS

All registered nurses who have completed a nursing program and passed their state's licensing certification examination are likely to work with clients who have psychiatric diagnoses. Nurses in all practice areas are bound to find clients struggling with psychosocial issues who are receiving care for other primary problems. For example, nurses who specialize in maternal–newborn care need to understand the signs and symptoms of postpartum depression and ways to assist new families to adapt to the changes childbirth necessitates. Medical–surgical nurses need to be prepared to help clients cope emotionally with life-threatening illnesses or invasive treatments (see Chap. 39). Similar examples can be found across all practice areas.

A nurse who specializes in psychiatric–mental health is designated as either a *psychiatric–mental health registered nurse* (RN-PMH) or a *psychiatric–mental health advanced practice registered nurse* (APRN-PMH). The specific title depends on the nurse's education and certification.

Basic-Level Psychiatric Nursing Care

RN-PMHs hold a baccalaureate degree in nursing and have worked in psychiatric–mental health nursing for at least 2 years. They use the nursing process to help clients cope with actual or potential mental health problems and psychiatric disorders, as well as maximize their strengths and minimize disabilities. RN-PMHs work in a wide variety of clinical inpatient and outpatient settings (American Nurses Association [ANA], American Psychiatric Nurses Association [APNA], & International Society of Psychiatric–Mental Health Nurses [ISPN], 2007). Skills and practices may include assessing and recording behavior, administering and evaluating the effectiveness of medications, communicating with other team members, and being in charge of the psychiatric milieu.

RN-PMHs may incorporate principles from the different psychotherapeutic techniques previously discussed into their general interactions with clients. However, they do not function as individual therapists. For example, they can learn and incorporate SFT into most nursing interactions. Nurses who use techniques from this therapy must consciously change their orientation from the "whys" of the past to focus on previous successes and then to define specific behaviors and future goals. Practicing the questions and techniques increases the nurse's comfort level and effectiveness when working with clients. However, using the techniques and approaches within the scope of their interventions is different from fully designing, implementing, and evaluating actual psychotherapies. Nurses need to define and use techniques that seem to make the most sense to them, but a particular treatment program may have a defined focus, and nurses should use techniques compatible with it.

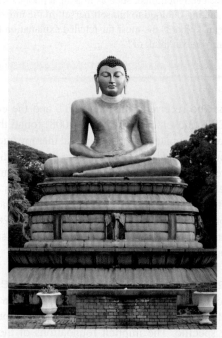

FIGURE 13.4 The Buddhist religion is just one example of a cultural perspective that may be in conflict with Western psychotherapy. Practitioners of Buddhism may believe that it is more important to let go of expectations, desires, and emphasis on worldly problems.

According to *Psychiatric–Mental Health Nursing: Scope and Standards* (ANA et al., 2007), basic psychiatric nursing interventions include health promotion and health maintenance, intake screening and evaluation, case management, provision of a therapeutic environment (milieu), tracking clients and assisting them with self-care activities, administering and monitoring psychobiologic treatment regimens, health teaching, counseling and crisis intervention, psychiatric rehabilitation, community-based care, outreach activities, and advocacy. These interventions are discussed briefly in the following sections and in other chapters in the text. They are compatible with therapeutic interventions in nursing, pioneered in the 1950s by Hildegard Peplau (1988) with her interpersonal theory and its emphasis on the nurse–client relationship. Development of the therapeutic relationship is primary, requires intensive work, and includes skillful application of learned information and activities. It is also objective, goal directed, and client centered and must include the development of boundaries, trust, and safety (see Chap. 11).

Health Promotion and Health Maintenance

The goals of health promotion and health maintenance related to psychiatric nursing involve helping clients understand, accept, and integrate suggested changes in lifestyle, activities, and interpersonal interactions that will lead to a more functional life. Examples of interventions related to psychiatric health promotion and health maintenance include the following:

- Scheduling routine follow-up appointments with health care providers
- Instructing clients about early signs and symptoms of psychiatric problems
- Teaching stress-reduction techniques (see Chap. 23)
- Providing literature about or referring clients to substance abuse awareness programs (Figure 13.5)

- Educating clients that positive mental health is a direct function of choices; clients may not want to pursue treatment; however, that may be the only way to achieve a desired goal

Intake Screening and Evaluation

When clients enter the mental health system for psychiatric care, nurses perform activities related to intake screening and evaluation. They use their education and experience in understanding human behavior and applying the principles of assessment and interviewing (see Chap. 10) to observe and investigate the circumstances applicable to each client. Examples of activities may include the following (ANA et al., 2007):

- Assessing the client's physical and psychosocial state (Figure 13.6)
- Making diagnostic judgments
- Facilitating the client's movement into appropriate services
- Considering the client's biophysical, psychological, social, cultural, economic, and environmental aspects to appreciate his or her experience of the problem and the type of assistance he or she requires
- Referring the client for additional testing

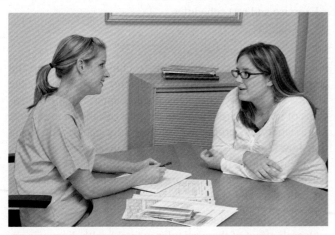

FIGURE 13.5 Basic-level psychiatric nurses work with clients to review literature related to mental illnesses, including substance abuse disorders.

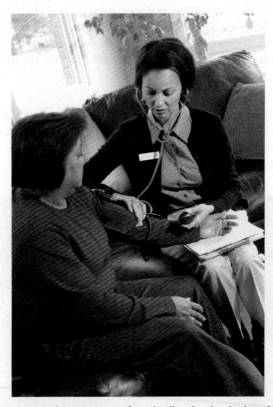

FIGURE 13.6 Assessment of each client's physical and psychosocial health is a key intervention for all levels of nurses working in psychiatric practice.

Case Management

Case managers help clients achieve their highest level of functioning so that they become more self-sufficient and progress toward optimal health (ANA et al., 2007). The case management role occurs in both inpatient and outpatient practice settings. Specific nursing interventions related to case management include the following:

- Assessing risk
- Counseling
- Problem solving
- Teaching
- Monitoring medication and health status (Figure 13.7)
- Providing care planning
- Identifying and coordinating with other health care services

Milieu Therapy

Basic-level nurses use institutional and community resources to help clients acquire or regain abilities and skills (ANA et al., 2007). A basic tenet of milieu therapy is that the setting or environment can greatly influence a person's behavior, positively or negatively. As a result, when working with clients, the psychiatric nurse is aware of and attends to environmental factors, including the physical environmental.

Promoting Self-Care Activities

When working with clients therapeutically, teaching and promoting self-care and activities of daily living (ADLs) are significant components of direct nursing care. The focus is on educating clients in key areas so that they can move from dependent to interdependent and independent behaviors. Examples of interventions in this category include the following (ANA et al., 2007):

- Developing recreational activities
- Helping the client improve practical life skills, including cooking, hygiene measures, shopping, and using public transportation (Figure 13.8)
- Teaching medication and symptom management

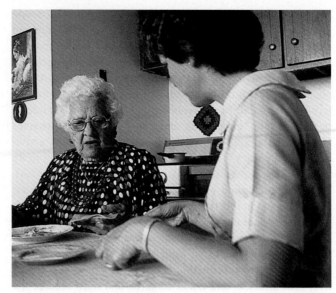

FIGURE 13.8 Clients living in the community frequently benefit from the assistance of nurses who teach ways to enhance life skills and ADL.

Implementing Psychobiologic Interventions

Nurses play a key role in implementing psychobiologic interventions because of their ability to assess the client holistically and to treat the clients' responses to actual and potential health problems (ANA et al., 2007). A major focus of this area involves overseeing and monitoring the client's compliance with his or her medication regimen. Nurses often are the professionals who first identify side effects or problems with medications and report on such developments to physicians. They conduct extensive teaching for clients and their families about psychopharmacologic drugs. Key roles in this area also involve assessment, management, and oversight related to over-the-counter drugs, supplements, and integrative therapies.

Other interventions may include (but are not limited to) the following:

- Relaxation techniques
- Nutrition and diet management
- Exercise and rest schedules

Health Teaching

Nurses incorporate basic health teaching into the specific care of each client. Such teaching must be tailored to the client's specific circumstances and encompass all the dimensions of holistic care. Such teaching assists clients to achieve more satisfying, productive, and healthy patterns of living (eg, how increased levels of stress can affect the client's health condition). It also involves family and others who will participate in the client's care. Health teaching focuses on the following key areas:

- Psychobiologic effects of medication
- Overall effect of the particular mental health diagnosis on interactions within the identified family, work, and school situation

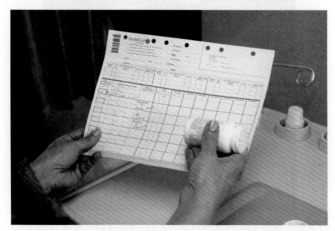

FIGURE 13.7 Ongoing monitoring of medications and their effects on clients is integral to quality psychiatric nursing.

- How to deal with stress and anxiety
- Relaxation techniques and imagery

One example of individualized teaching would be educating the client with major depression about antidepressants, maintenance of adequate nutrition, sleep measures, ways to enhance self-care management, goal setting and effective problem solving, and social interaction skills. Another example would be educating the client with obsessive-compulsive disorder about psychopharmacologic therapy, skin care measures, appropriate alternative activities for ritualistic behaviors, thought-stopping and relaxation techniques, and appropriate follow-up and available community resources.

Counseling and Crisis Intervention

The nurse uses counseling interventions to help clients improve or regain previous coping abilities. Counseling interventions also foster mental health and prevent mental illness and disability. A closely related technique is crisis management for clients who have faced traumatic personal situations (eg, loss of job, bodily function, family member, role status), natural or national disasters (eg, fires, floods, terrorist attacks), or both.

When providing crisis management for clients, it is essential that nurses

- Understand that the person's experience of the crisis is his or hers alone (not the nurse's)
- Become self-aware (eg, knowledgeable of their own anxiety levels during crises and how they demonstrate these signs)
- Recognize and respond to the person's experience with compassion and understanding
- Actively listen, provide empathy, and develop therapeutic communication techniques such as acceptance, reflection, validation, and use of open-ended statements.

Chapter 35 explores crisis intervention in detail.

Psychiatric Rehabilitation

The focus of psychiatric rehabilitation is strengthening self-care and promoting and improving quality of life through relapse prevention. Areas of focus for psychiatric nurses include the following (ANA et al., 2007):

- Consumer empowerment
- Recognition of the role of the family and larger social network
- Focus on accountable programming, cost effectiveness, and outcomes
- Stronger collaborative relationships with treatment services
- Emphasis on recovery of hope and development of functional competencies (see Chap. 20)

Advanced-Level Therapeutic Nursing Interventions

APRN-PMHs are licensed registered nurses who have also been prepared at the master's or doctoral level in psychiatric–mental health nursing and hold advanced

practice specialty certification from the American Nurses Credentialing Center (ANCC). Their role is complex and autonomous. These nurses can perform all the interventions and roles outlined for the basic-level nurse; they also demonstrate a greater depth and breadth of knowledge, more data synthesis, and interventions of higher complexity.

Although many mental health practitioners treat some of the symptoms of psychiatric disorders, APRN-PMHs provide comprehensive services that make up primary psychiatric care and treatment (ANA et al., 2007). They work with clients seeking mental health services and professional colleagues in various settings:

- **Psychotherapy (individual, group, family).** Examples include all common forms of brief or long-term therapy. The therapist role that the APRN-PMH assumes is formal and structured and often involves contracts (verbal, written, or both) with clients.
- **Psychopharmacologic interventions (as defined by state laws).** In addition to the teaching and monitoring role that basic-level nurses assume, APRN-PMHs also have prescriptive authority in many states and can order and interpret laboratory and diagnostic tests.
- **Case management.** This intervention is expanded for APRN-PMHs to include population-specific knowledge and research.
- **Program development and management.** APRN-PMHs work directly in communities to focus on mental health issues and psychiatric disorders that are affecting entire populations.
- **Consultation and liaison.** Nurses at the advanced level often serve in this capacity in health care settings such as hospitals, rehabilitation centers, schools, extended care facilities, and outpatient clinics (Figure 13.9).
- **Clinical supervision.** As a result of their education and experience, APRN-PMHs can provide clinical supervision to clinicians at lower levels of practice or qualification. Within this role, they provide direct client care, as well as mentoring, role modeling, and clinical consulting for others.

> **Think About It 13.2**
> The parents of a client with schizophrenia bring their son to the emergency department because of increasingly strange behavior. "He's hardly slept or eaten and he's been isolating himself in his room over the last few days. He's been pacing all over the house. We've noticed that it seems like he is talking to someone, but nobody is there." Further assessment reveals that the client stopped taking his antipsychotic medication 2½ weeks ago. The client is admitted to the inpatient unit. How would the roles and functions of an RN-PMH compare with those of an APRN-PMH for this client?

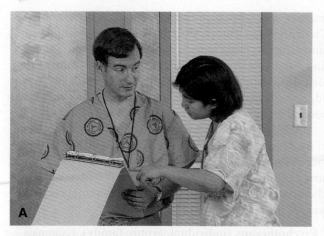
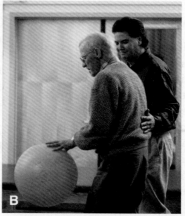
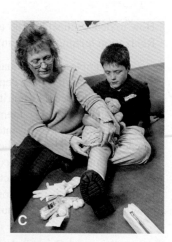
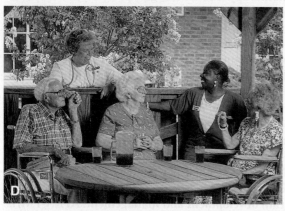
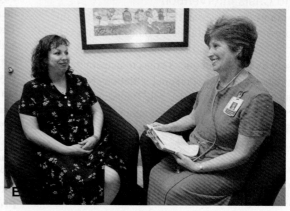

FIGURE 13.9 Advance practice nurses frequently provide consultation in various settings, including (**A**) hospitals, (**B**) rehabilitation centers, (**C**) schools, (**D**) extended care facilities, and (**E**) outpatient clinics. (Part D: Copyright © Will & Deni McIntyre/Photo Researchers, Inc.)

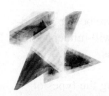

Reviewing and Applying Your Knowledge

Chapter Summary

- The client in individual therapy often works with a team consisting of nurses, a social worker, a psychologist, a psychiatrist, and other professionals. All members of the team, including the client, have the same overall goals: for the client to experience more satisfying relationships with a resultant increase in self-esteem and self-worth, integrate himself or herself with self-chosen work activities, and find greater meaning in his or her life.

- Psychotherapy approaches mental and emotional disorders using the psychoeducational methods of support, reeducation, and insight to alter maladaptive patterns of coping and to encourage personality growth. The general trend of psychotherapy has moved from long-term analysis of the causes of dysfunction to a shorter-term focus on changing thoughts, feelings, and behaviors.

- The many different types of individual psychotherapy include psychoanalytic/psychodynamic; cognitive–behavioral, behavioral, client centered, and solution focused. Subtypes of cognitive–behavioral therapy include cognitive therapy, REBT, and dialectical behavior therapy.

- There are basically two types of psychiatric nurses: RN-PMHs and APRN-PMHs. RN-PMHs work with individuals, families, groups, and communities to assess mental health needs; develop diagnoses; and plan, implement, and evaluate nursing care. APRN-PMHs have all the basic-level knowledge, as well as expertise in psychotherapy and psychobiologic interventions.

- In addition to listening and observing nonjudgmentally to understand the client's life experience, basic therapeutic nursing interventions in individual psychiatric nursing care include health promotion and health maintenance, intake screening and evaluation, case management, provision of a therapeutic environment (milieu), tracking clients and assisting them with self-care activities, administering and monitoring psychobiologic treatment regimens, health teaching, counseling and crisis intervention, psychiatric rehabilitation, community-based care, outreach activities, and advocacy.

Study Questions

1. When beginning a therapeutic relationship with a client, the nurse would assume that the client

   a. plays a passive, dependent role.

   b. demonstrates incompetence.

   c. has the necessary capabilities.

   d. develops solutions on his or her own.

2. During an interview, the client states, "Whenever I try something new, I always make a fool of myself because I fail." The nurse interprets this statement as which of the following?

   a. Catastrophizing

   b. Absolute thinking

   c. Perfectionism

   d. Overgeneralization

3. A nurse is implementing a token economy system for a client. The nurse understands that this system involves which type of therapy?

   a. Psychodynamic therapy

   b. Behavioral therapy

   c. Rational emotive behavior therapy

   d. Solution-focused therapy

4. Which of the following statements might be made by a dialectical behavior therapist?

   a. "During our time together, we will explore the influence of your relationship with your mother."

   b. "Your work with me will include homework assignments and rewards for behavior changes."

   c. "Given your past experiences with relationships, I can understand why you're making some current choices."

   d. "Your irrational thoughts are causing you to make some unhealthy choices. We'll work together on your thought processes."

5. Which of the following questions would be most appropriate to use when setting the agenda for a client who is to undergo solution-focused therapy?

   a. "In what ways is the problem still interfering with your life?"

   b. "Are there times when you expect the problem to happen and it doesn't?"

   c. "What would be helpful for me to know about you and your situation?"

   d. "How does your spouse say this problem is affecting your life?"

(continues on page 242)

Critical Thinking Questions

1. Smoking cessation programs often use behavior modification. Explore how such programs apply this behavioral technique.

2. Describe how a nurse would incorporate the techniques of solution-focused therapy into interactions with a client who is unhappy about how he or she communicates with a spouse.

3. Discuss how the RN-PMH should prepare before providing counseling to a client and how this will influence the effectiveness of the nursing interventions.

4. Develop a health teaching plan detailing the types of information you would want to include for a client and his or her family about ways to deal with stress and anxiety.

References

American Nurses Association (ANA), American Psychiatric Nurses Association (APNA), and International Society of Psychiatric–Mental Health Nurses (ISPN). (2007). *Psychiatric–mental health nursing: Scope and standards of practice.* Washington, DC: Author.

Andersson, G., & Cuijpers, P. (2009). "Psychological treatment" as an umbrella term for evidenced-based psychotherapies? *Nordic Psychology, 61*(2), 4–15. doi:10.1027/1901-2276.61.2.4

Bacal, H., & Carlton, L. (2010). Who can do what, therapeutically, with whom, in what way? *Journal of Psychotherapy Integration, 20*(1), 46–50. doi:10.1037/a0018817

Bateman, A., & Fonagy, P. (2008). 8-year follow-up of patients treated for borderline personality disorder: Mentalization-based treatment versus treatment as usual. *American Journal of Psychiatry, 165*(5), 631–638.

Beck, A. T. (1979). *Cognitive therapy and the emotional disorders.* New York, NY: Penguin Books, International Universities Press.

Beck, A. T. (2005). The current state of cognitive therapy: A 40 year retrospective. *Archives of General Psychiatry, 62*(9), 953–959.

Bickel, W. K., Marsch, L. A., Buchhalter, A. R., & Badger, G. J. (2008). Computerized behavior therapy for opioid-dependent outpatients: A randomized controlled trial. *Experimental and Clinical Psychopharmacology, 16*(2), 132–143. doi:10.1037/1064-1297.16.2.132

Bruce, N. G., Manber, R., Shapiro, S. L., & Constantino, M. J. (2010). Psychotherapist mindfulness and the psychotherapy process. *Psychotherapy: Theory, Research, Practice, Training, 47*(1), 83–97. doi:10.1037/a0018842

Chen, E. Y., Matthews, L., Allen, C., Kuo, J. R., & Linehan, M. M. (2008). Dialectical behavior therapy for clients with binge-eating disorder or bulimia nervosa and borderline personality disorder. *International Journal of Eating Disorders, 41*(6), 505–512.

Constantino, M. J., Marnell, M. E., Haile, A. J., Kanther-Sista, S. N., Wolman, K., Zappert, L., & Arnow, B. A. (2008). Integrative cognitive therapy for depression: A randomized pilot comparison. *Psychotherapy: Theory, Research, Practice, Training, 45*(2), 122–134. doi:10.1037/0033-3204.45.2.122

Cook, J. M., Biyanova, T., & Coyne, J. C. (2009). Influential psychotherapy figures, authors, and books: An Internet survey of over 2,000 psychotherapists. *Psychotherapy: Theory, Research, Practice, Training, 46*(1), 42–51. doi:10.1037/a0015152

Craddy, C. (2006). A place for CBT... and CBT in its place. *Therapy Today, 17*(10), 28–29.

David, D., Szentagotai, A., Lupu, V, & Cosman, D. (2008). Rational emotive behavior therapy, cognitive therapy, and medication in the treatment of major depressive disorder: A randomized clinical trial, posttreatment outcomes, and six-month follow-up. *Journal of Clinical Psychology, 64*(6), 728–746. doi:10.1002/jclp.20487

De Graaf, L. E., Hollon, S. D., & Huibers, M. J. H. (2010). Predicting outcome in computerized cognitive behavioral therapy for depression in primary care: A randomized trial. *Journal of Consulting and Clinical Psychology, 78*(2), 184–189. doi:10.1037/a0018324

De Jong, P., & Berg, I. K. (2008). *Interviewing for solutions* (3rd ed.). Belmont, CA: Thomson Higher Education.

Dobson, K. S., Hollon, S. D., Dimidjian, S., Schmaling, K. B., Kohlenberg, R. J., Gallop, R. J., ... Jacobson, N. S. (2008). Randomized trial of behavioral activation, cognitive therapy, and antidepressant medication in the prevention of relapse and recurrence in major depression. *Journal of Consulting and Clinical Psychology, 76*(3), 468–477. doi:10.1037/0022-006X.76.3.468

Dowd, E. T., Clen, S. L., & Arnold, K. D. (2010). The specialty practice of cognitive and behavioral psychology. *Professional Psychology: Research and Practice, 41*(1), 89–95. doi:10.1037/a0018321

Dowd, T., & McCleery, A. (2007). Elements of Buddhist philosophy in cognitive psychotherapy: The role of cultural specifics and universals. *Journal of Cognitive and Behavioral Psychotherapies, 7*(1), 67–79.

Dozois, D. J. A., Bieling, P. J., Patelis-Siotis, I., Hoar, L., Chudzik, S., McCabe, K., & Westra, H. A. (2009). Changes in self-schema structure in cognitive therapy for major depressive disorder: A randomized clinical trial. *Journal of Consulting and Clinical Psychology, 77*(6), 1078–1088. doi:10.1037/a0016886

Dryden, W., & David, D. (2008). Rational emotive behavior therapy: Current status. *Journal of Cognitive Psychotherapy, 22*(3), 195–209. doi:10.1891/0889-8391.22.3.195

Dundas, I., Wormnes, B., & Hauge, H. (2009). Making exams a manageable task. *Nordic Psychology, 61*(1), 26–41. doi:10.1027/1901-2276.61.1.26

Ellis, A. (2004). How my theory and practice of psychotherapy has influenced and changed other psychotherapies. *Journal of Rational-Emotive & Cognitive-Behavior Therapy, 22*(2), 79–83.

Ellis, A. (2005). Why I (really) became a therapist. *JCLP/In Session, 61*(8), 945–948. doi:10.1002/jclp.20166

Fisher, J. E., & Happell, B. (2009). Implications of evidence-based practice for mental health nursing. *International Journal of Mental Health Nursing, 18*, 179–185. doi:10.1111/j.1447-0349.2009.00607.x

Goldfried, M. R. (2007). What has psychotherapy inherited from Carl Rogers? *Psychotherapy: Theory, Research, Practice, Training, 44*(3), 249–252. doi:10.1037/0033-3204.44.3.249

Harned, M. S., Chapman, A. L., Dexter-Mazza, E. T., Murray, A., Comtois, K. A., & Linehan, M. M. (2008) Treating co-occurring Axis I disorders in recurrently suicidal women with borderline personality disorder: A 2-year randomized trial of dialectical behavior therapy versus community treatment by experts. *Journal of Consulting and Clinical Psychology, 76*(6), 1068–1075. doi:10.1037/a0014044

Harrington, N., & Pickles, C. (2009). Mindfulness and cognitive behavioral therapy: Are they compatible concepts? *Journal of Cognitive Psychotherapy, 23*(4), 315–323. doi:10.1891/0889-8391.23.4.315

Herschell, A. D., Kogan, J. N., Celedonia, K. L., Gavin, J. G., & Stein, B. D. (2009). Understanding community mental health administrators' perspectives on dialectical behavior therapy implementation. *Psychiatric Services, 60*(7), 989–992.

Hien, D. A., Wells, E. A., Jiang, H., Suarez-Morales, L., Campbell, A. N. C., Cohen, L. R., ... Nunes, E. V. (2009). Multisite randomized trial of behavioral interventions for women with co-occurring PTSD and substance use disorders. *Journal of Consulting and Clinical Psychology, 77*(4), 607–619. doi:10.1037/a0016227

Hirshfeld-Becker, D. R., Masek, B., Henin, A., Blakely, L. R., Pollack-Wurman, R. A., McQuade, J., & Biederman, J. (2010). Cognitive behavioral therapy for 4- to 7-year-old children with anxiety disorders: A randomized clinical trial. *Journal of Consulting and Clinical Psychology, 78*(4), 498–510. doi:10.1037/a0019055

Iverson, K. M., Gradus, J. L., Resick, P. A., Suvak, M. K., Smith, K. F., & Monson, C. M. (2011). Cognitive-behavioral therapy for PTSD and depression symptoms reduces risk for future intimate partner violence among interpersonal trauma survivors. *Journal of Consulting and Clinical Psychology, 79*(2), 193–202. doi:10.1037/a0022512

Iverson, K. M., Shenk, C., & Fruzzetti, A. E. (2009). Dialectical behavior therapy for women victims of domestic abuse: A pilot study. *Professional Psychology: Research and Practice, 40*(3), 242–248. doi:10.1037/a0013476

James, A. C., Taylor, A., Winmill, L., & Alfoadari, K. (2008). A preliminary community study of dialectical behaviour therapy (DBT) with adolescent females demonstrating persistent, deliberate self-harm (DSH). *Child and Adolescent Mental Health, 13*(3), 148–152. doi:10.1111/j.1475-3588.2007.00470.x

Jarrett, R. B., Vittengl, J. R., Clark, L. A., & Thase, M. E. (2011). Skills of cognitive therapy (SoCT): A new measure of patients' comprehension and use. *Psychological Assessment, 23*(3), 578–586. doi:10.1037/a0022485

Kanter, J. W., Rusch, L. C., Landes, S. J., Holman, G. I., Whiteside, U., & Sedivy, S. K. (2009). The use and nature of present-focused interventions in cognitive and behavioral therapies for depression. *Psychotherapy: Theory, Research, Practice, Training, 46*(2), 220–232. doi:10.1037/a0016083

Khanna, M. S., & Kendall, P. C. (2010). Computer-assisted cognitive behavioral therapy for child anxiety: Results of a randomized clinical trial. *Journal of Consulting and Clinical Psychology, 78*(5), 737–745. doi:10.1037/a0019739

Kirmayer, L. J. (2007). Psychotherapy and the cultural concept of the person. *Transcultural Psychiatry, 44*(2), 232–257. doi:10.1177/1363461506070794

Kroger, C., Schweiger, U., Sipos, V., Kliem, S., Arnold, R., Schunert, T., & Reinecker, H. (2010). Dialectical behaviour therapy and an added cognitive behavioural treatment module for eating disorders in women with borderline personality disorder and anorexia nervosa or bulimia nervosa who failed to respond to previous treatments. An open trial with a 15-month follow-up. *Journal of Behavior Therapy and Experimental Psychiatry, 41*, 381–388. doi:10.1016/j.jbtep.2010.04.001

Kush, F. R. (2009). Brief psychodynamic and cognitive therapy regarding acute treatment. *Journal of Psychotherapy Integration, 19*(2), 158–172. doi:10.1037/a0016069

Kuyken, W., Byford, S., Taylor, R. S., Watkins, E., Holden, E., White, K., ... Teasdale, J. D. (2008). Mindfulness-based cognitive therapy to prevent relapse in recurrent depression. *Journal of Consulting and Clinical Psychology, 76*(6), 966–978. doi:10.1037/a0013786

La Roche, M. J., & Christopher, M. S. (2009). Changing paradigms from empirically supported treatment to evidence-based practice: A cultural perspective. *Professional Psychology: Research and Practice, 40*(4), 396–402. doi:10.1037/a0015240

Langdridge, D. (2006). Solution focused therapy: A way forward for brief existential therapy? *Existential Analysis, 17*(2), 359–370.

Lawson, D. M. (2010). Comparing cognitive behavioral therapy and integrated cognitive behavioral therapy/psychodynamic therapy in group treatment for partner violent men. *Psychotherapy: Theory, Research, Practice, Training, 47*(1), 122–133.

Leichsenring, F., Hiller, W., Weissberg, M., & Leibing, E. (2006). Cognitive-behavioral therapy and psychodynamic psychotherapy: Techniques, efficacy, and indication. *American Journal of Psychotherapy, 60*(3), 233–259.

Linehan, M. M. (1993). *Cognitive-behavioral treatment of borderline personality disorder.* New York, NY: Guilford Press.

Lynch, T. R., Chapman, A. L., Rosenthal, M. Z., Kuo, J. R., & Linehan, M. M. (2006). Mechanisms of change in dialectical behavior therapy: Theoretical and empirical observations. *Journal of Clinical Psychology, 62*(4), 459–480.

Marshall, A. D., Martin, E. K., Warfield, G. A., Doron-Lamarca, S., Niles, B. L., & Taft, C. T. (2010). *Psychological Trauma: Theory, Research, Practice, and Policy, 2*(3), 224–231.

McCloskey, M. S., Noblett, K. L., Deffenbacher, J. L., Gollan, J. K., & Coccaro, E. F. (2008). Cognitive-behavioral therapy for intermittent explosive disorder: A pilot randomized clinical trial. *Journal of Consulting and Clinical Psychology, 76*(5), 876–886.

McMain, S. F., Links, P. S., Gnam, W. H., Guimond, T., Cardish, R. J., Korman, L., & Streiner D. L. (2009). A randomized trial of dialectical behavior therapy versus general psychiatric management for borderline personality disorder. *American Journal of Psychiatry, 166*(12), 1365–1374.

Miller, W. R., & Rose, G. S. (2009). Toward a theory of motivational interviewing. *American Psychologist, 64*(6), 527–537.

Moran, M. (2007, June). Psychotherapies combat prominent BPD symptoms. *Psychiatric News, 42*(11), 13.

Neacsiu, A. D., Rizvi, S. L., & Linehan, M. M. (2010). Dialectical behavior therapy skills use as a mediator and outcome of treatment for borderline personality disorder. *Behaviour Research and Therapy, 48*, 832–839.

Newman, M. G., Castonguay, L. G., Borkovec, T. D., Fisher, A. J., & Nordberg, S. S. (2008). An open trial of integrative therapy for generalized anxiety disorder. *Psychotherapy: Theory, Research, Practice, Theory, 45*(2), 135–147. doi:10.1037/0033-3204.45.2.135

Nims, D. R. (2007). Integrating play therapy techniques into solution-focused therapy. *International Journal of Play Therapy, 16*(1), 54–68. doi:10.1037/1555-6824.16.1.54

Ollendick, T. H., Ost, L. G., Reuterskiold, L., Costa, N., Cederlund, R., & Sirbu, C., ... Jarrett. M. A. (2009). One-session treatment of specific phobias in youth: A randomized clinical trial in the United States and Sweden. *Journal of Consulting and Clinical Psychology, 77*(3), 504–516. doi:10.1037/a0015158

Patterson, T. G., & Joseph, S. (2006). Development of a self-report measure of unconditional positive self-regard. *Psychology and Psychotherapy: Theory, Research and Practice, 79*, 557–570. doi:10.1348/147608305X89414

Peplau, H. E. (1988). *Interpersonal relations in nursing* (9th ed.). New York, NY: Springer.

Pesale, F. P., & Hilsenroth, M. J. (2009). Patient and therapist perspectives on session depth in relation to technique during psychodynamic psychotherapy. *Psychotherapy: Theory, Research, Practice, Training, 46*(3), 390–396. doi:10.1037/a0016999

Ryum, T., Stiles, T. C., Svartberg, M., & McCullough, L. (2010). The role of transference work, the therapeutic alliance, and their interaction in reducing interpersonal problems among psychotherapy patients with Cluster C personality disorders.

Psychotherapy: Theory, Research, Practice, Training, 47(4), 442–453. doi:10.1037/a0021183

Salsman, N. L., & Linehan, M. M. (2006). Dialectical-behavioral therapy for borderline personality disorder [Abstract]. *Primary Psychiatry, 13*(5), 51–58.

Santiago-Rivera, A., Kanter, J., Benson, G., Derose, T., Illes, R., & Reyes, W. (2008). Behavioral activation as an alternative treatment approach for Latinos with depression. *Psychotherapy: Theory, Research, Practice, Training, 45*(2), 173–185. doi:10.1037/0033-3204.45.2.173

Sarnat, J. (2010). Key competencies of the psychodynamic psychotherapist and how to teach them in supervision. *Psychotherapy: Theory, Research, Practice, Training, 47*(1), 20–27. doi:10.1037/a0018846

Sava, F. A., Yates, B. T., Lupu, V., Szentagotai, A., & David, D. (2009). Cost-effectiveness and cost-utility of cognitive therapy, rational emotive behavioral therapy, and fluoxetine (Prozac) in treating depression: A randomized clinical trial. *Journal of Clinical Psychology, 65*(1), 36–52. doi:10.1002/jclp.20550

Schnyder, U. (2009). Future perspectives in psychotherapy. *European Archives of Psychiatry and Clinical Neuroscience, 259* (Suppl. 2), 123–128. doi:10.1007/s00406-009-0051-z

Shedler, J. (2010). The efficacy of psychodynamic psychotherapy. *American Psychologist, 65*(2), 98–109. doi:10.1037/a0018378

Shedler, J. (2011). Science or ideology? *American Psychologist 66*(2), 152–154. doi:10.1037/a0022242

Simons, A. D., Padesky, C. A., Montemarano, J., Lewis, C. C., Murakami, J., Lamb, K., ... Beck, A. T. (2010). Training and dissemination of cognitive behavior therapy for depression in adults: A preliminary examination of therapist competence and client outcomes. *Journal of Consulting and Clinical Psychology, 78*(5), 751–756. doi:10.1037/a0020569

Smoski, M. J., Salsman, N., Wang, L., Smith, V., Lynch, T. R., Dager, S. R., ... Linehan, M. M. (2011). Functional imaging of emotion reactivity in opiate-dependent borderline personality disorder. *Personality Disorders: Theory, Research, and Treatment, 2*, 230–241. doi:10.1037/a0022228

Sobell, L. C., Sobell, M. B., & Agrawal, S. (2009). Randomized controlled trial of a cognitive-behavioral motivational intervention in a group versus individual format for substance use disorders.

Psychology of Addictive Behaviors, 23(4), 672–683. doi:10.1037/a0016636

Stepp, S. D., Epler, A. J., Jahng, S., & Trull, T. J. (2008). The effect of dialectical behavior therapy skills use on borderline personality disorder features. *Journal of Personality Disorders, 22*(6), 549–563.

Stice, E., Rohde, P., Gau, J. M., & Wade, E. (2010). Efficacy trial of a brief cognitive-behavioral depression prevention program for high-risk adolescents: Effects at 1- and 2-year follow-up. *Journal of Consulting and Clinical Psychology, 78*(6), 856–867. doi:10.1037/a0020544

Stuart, G. W. (2009). Therapeutic nurse–patient relationship. In G. W. Stuart (Ed.), *Principles and practice of psychiatric nursing* (9th ed., pp. 13–43). St. Louis, MO: Mosby Elsevier.

Sugarman, D. E., Nich, C., & Carroll, K. M. (2010). Coping strategy use following computerized cognitive-behavioral therapy for substance use disorders. *Psychology of Addictive Behaviors, 24*(4), 689–695. doi:10.1037/a0021584

Swales, M. (2009). Dialectical behaviour therapy. *Healthcare Counselling & Psychotherapy Journal, 9*(4), 25–27.

Szentagotai, A., David, D., Lupu, A., & Cosman, D. (2008). Rational emotive behavior therapy versus cognitive therapy versus pharmacotherapy in the treatment of major depressive disorder: Mechanisms of change analysis. *Psychotherapy: Theory, Research, Practice, Training, 45*(4), 523–538. doi:10.1037/a0014332

Teachman, B. A., Marker, C. D., & Clerkin, E. M. (2010). Catastrophic misinterpretations as a predictor of symptom change during treatment for panic disorder. *Journal of Consulting and Clinical Psychology, 78*(6), 964–973. doi:10.1037/a0021067

Vaida, S., Kallay, E., & Opre, A. (2008). Counseling in schools. A rational emotive behavior therapy (REBT) based intervention. *Cognition, Brain, Behavior, 12*(1), 57–69.

Wilde, J. (2008). Rational-emotive behavioral interventions for children with anxiety problems. *Journal of Cognitive and Behavioral Psychotherapies, 8*(1), 133–141.

Wilson, J. L., Armoutliev, E., Yakunina, E., & Werth, J. L. (2009). Practicing psychologists' reflections on evidence-based practice in psychology. *Professional Psychology: Research and Practice, 40*(4), 403–409. doi:10.1037/a0016247

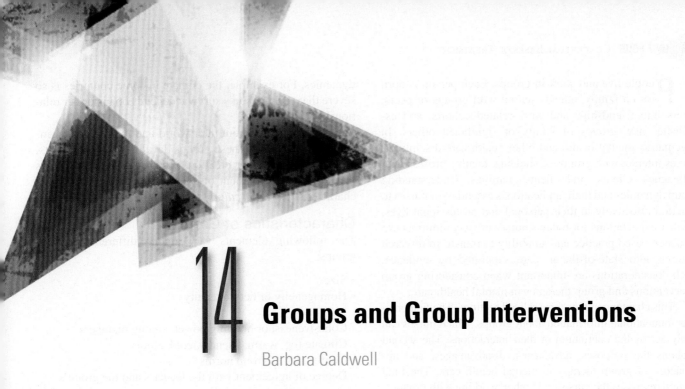

14 Groups and Group Interventions

Barbara Caldwell

LEARNING OBJECTIVES

On completion of this chapter, you should be able to accomplish the following:

- Identify the characteristics of a group.
- Explain group norms.
- Compare styles of group leadership.
- Define three major categories of group roles.
- Identify communication processes within groups.
- Describe the stages of group development.
- Discuss the advantages of group therapy.
- Discuss therapeutic factors that influence group therapy.
- Compare the various types of group therapy.
- Discuss the nurse's role in working with groups.

Peple live and work in groups. Each person is born into a family, attends school with groups of peers, enters into friendships and work-related cohorts, and establishes new groups of family or significant others. In psychiatric–mental health and other health care disciplines, nurses interact with groups of students, faculty, professional colleagues, clients, and clients' families. Understanding group dynamics and their application is essential for nurses to function effectively in their personal and professional lives. Further expectations for today's nurses are a commitment to evidence-based practice and an ability to transform research findings into state-of-the-art care supported by evidence. Such considerations are important when considering group interventions and group therapies in mental health care.

This chapter contains three related sections. The first presents foundational information about groups, which nurses can apply across the continuum of their interactions. The second explains the purposes, advantages, disadvantages, and approaches of group therapy in mental health care. The final section discusses the nurse's role when working with groups.

GROUP PROCESS

A **group** is three or more people with related goals. Factors that influence these goals include interpersonal and intrapersonal needs, physical environment, and unique group dynamics. For example, the climate in some countries is so severe that each person's survival depends on his or her relationships with others.

Humans learn about their world and themselves by interacting in groups. These groups develop structures, traits, and roles. The further creation of systems and subsystems leads to the development of complex societies that display characteristics called *culture* (see Chap. 6).

Characteristics of Groups

The following elements vary among different types of groups:

- Size
- Homogeneity or heterogeneity
- Stability
- Cohesiveness, or bonding power, among members
- Climate (eg, warm, friendly, cold, aloof)
- Conformity to group norms
- Degree of agreement with the leader's and the group's norms
- Ability to deal with members' infractions
- Goal-directedness and task orientation of work

Types of Groups

Groups may be primary or secondary, formal or informal (Figure 14.1).

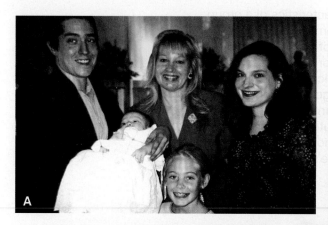
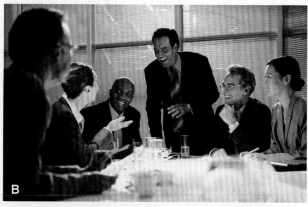
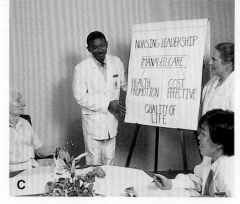
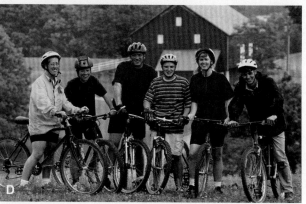

FIGURE 14.1 (**A**) A family is a primary group because it has face-to-face contact, boundaries, norms, and explicit and implicit interdependent roles. (**B**) Secondary groups (eg, business departments) usually do not have emotional ties. (**C**) Formal groups, like that of a faculty meeting, have structure, and authority. (**D**) Informal groups, such as a bike club, contribute to personal values and education.

Members of **primary groups** have face-to-face contact, boundaries, norms, and explicit and implicit interdependent roles. An example is a family. **Secondary groups** are usually larger and more impersonal than primary groups. Members do not have emotional ties. An example is a political party or business. A **formal group** has limited interaction, structure, and authority, which usually emanates from above. A faculty meeting is an example. **Informal groups** provide much of a person's education and contribute greatly to his or her values. In informal groups, such as friendships or hobby groups, members do not depend on one another.

Group Norms

A **group norm** is the development, over time, of a pattern of interaction with certain attached behavioral expectations. Group norms affect scope and functioning. They also help structure role expectations and provide sanctions, taboos, and reference power.

Consider a nursing team meeting designed to discuss client care and staff communication. *Role expectation* norms are for the team leader to chair the meeting and for members to arrive on time and possibly sit in assigned places. A *formalized norm,* such as a meeting agenda, might state that nursing staff will communicate before the discussion to plan client care. Other group norms may be *universal* with regard to the task role of one member, such as the secretary who records the minutes. Members who present their clients' history and assessment accurately, clearly, and with organization receive *sanction*. A group *taboo* is to fall asleep and snore while someone else is talking! Such behavior, especially if it recurs, leads others to view the member as deviant.

Norms exert a controlling element by setting boundaries. To promote growth and stimulation, group members must learn to change norms that no longer function or apply. A group is more creative if each member becomes a "change agent" for outmoded norms.

Group Leadership

The concepts of power, influence, and authority affect leadership. **Power** is the perceived ability to control appropriate reward, therefore lending influence to the leader. Nurse leaders gain authority through such influence and through having knowledge, and expertise. They also understand effective ways to use authority and decide to what extent they will expand or limit it.

Effective leaders also determine whether authority should be *autocratic* (centralized) or *democratic* (decentralized) (Figure 14.2). They reach this decision, in part, according to the type of group. For example, leaders may readily relinquish authority in a training group (T group), whose purpose is to improve members' ability to communicate or relate to others. Members of groups generally possess certain knowledge and experience and therefore can impart skills to others. In groups in which members are likely to have personality disorganization and faulty communication and interpersonal skills, leaders may exercise centralized authority. In other therapy groups, distribution of power may depend on the age and emotional maturity of members.

Styles of Group Leadership

Several factors influence leadership style, including philosophy of treatment; personality of the leader; traits, characteristics, and purpose of the group; and degree of mental, emotional, or cognitive impairment of group members. Nurses alter leadership style according to the situation. The three basic leadership styles are autocratic, democratic, and laissez-faire. See Table 14.1.

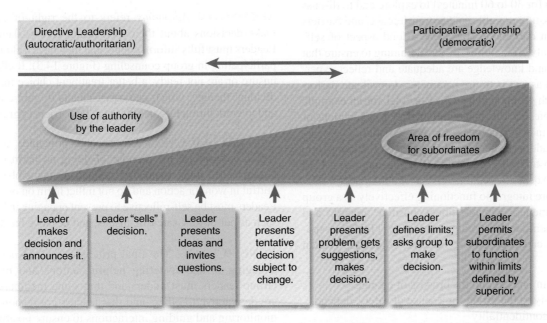

FIGURE 14.2 Leadership style can vary from directive or *autocratic* to participative or *democratic*. (Adapted by permission of *Harvard Business Review*. An exhibit from "How to choose a leadership pattern" by R. Tannenbaum & W. H. Schmidt [May/June 1973]. Copyright © 1973 by the Presidents and Fellows of Harvard College; all rights reserved.)

TABLE 14.1 Leadership Styles

Style	Characteristics	Advantages	Disadvantages
Autocratic	The leader exercises significant authority and control over group members. He or she rarely seeks or uses input from members and does not encourage their participation or interaction.	Autocratic leadership may be most effective during emergencies because it conserves time and energy and dictates roles and responsibilities to members.	Constant use of autocratic leadership may cause hostility, scapegoat behavior, dependence on the leader, and limitation of growth potential for group members.
Democratic	The leader encourages group interaction, problem solving, and decision making.	The leader values input and feedback from each member, seeks spontaneous and honest interaction among the group, and creates an atmosphere that rewards contributions. The leader solicits opinions and tailors the group's work to common goals.	The group may need significant time and effort to accomplish its goals. This style is not ideal when quick or immediate action is needed.
Laissez-faire	Group members are free to operate as they choose.	This style may be effective if members are highly knowledgeable, task oriented, and motivated.	The laissez-faire approach is time consuming and often inefficient in the accomplishment of group tasks.

Leadership Qualities for Effective Groups

Group leadership is a dynamic and highly challenging process requiring training and education in the principles of group therapy. Leaders should also embrace specific professional attributes to ensure effective client outcomes. They need to perform ongoing self-evaluation, which entails both concrete and self-reflective activities.

The first aspect of self-evaluation is clinical supervision from a more experienced group therapist. This step helps ensure that group leaders are cognizant of potential problems inherent in group experiences. Supervision can be regular (eg, twice a month for 30 to 60 minutes) to explore and to discuss major group issues, possible countertransference, and barriers encountered in current sessions. The second aspect of self-evaluation involves obtaining advanced training to ensure that current skills and knowledge are adequate and reflect expertise. The third aspect is to use parameters to evaluate performance for each group activity. See Box 14.1 for an example of an evaluation checklist that highlights key role functions of group leaders in different types of group activities.

Group leaders are responsible for creating a therapeutic milieu that fosters alliances with all group members. Carl Rogers (1985) describes characteristics of a therapeutic relationship that are integral to functioning effectively as a group leader: genuineness, unconditional positive regard, and accurate empathic understanding (see Chap. 11). Other specific qualities can contribute to effective leadership (Rutan et al., 2007):

- Confidence in oneself and the process of change
- Responsibility to the group for a sense of safety, dependability, and confidentiality
- Attentiveness and capacity to engage in effective listening

- Warmth and respect
- Flexibility
- Creativity and spontaneity
- Enthusiasm
- Constructive humor

Ethical Principles in Group Counseling

Three ethical principles are important when discussing group counseling and the role of the leader: autonomy, nonmaleficence, and beneficence (see Chap. 5). In addition, confidentiality and informed consent are paramount concerns.

AUTONOMY. *Autonomy* refers to the right of clients to make decisions about their own health care (Aiken, 2004). Leaders must fully inform clients that they have a choice about participating in group counseling (Figure 14.3). If clients feel unsure or are not ready, a better treatment choice may be individual therapy, which can assist clients to gain confidence and to work through issues that may be barriers to group work.

NONMALEFICENCE. The second principle, *nonmaleficence*, is based on the premise of doing no harm to others. Group leaders must ensure that they and group members are not hurtful in word or action and do not inflict harm on one another. Leaders must be self-reflective to prevent engaging in behaviors such as put-downs, sarcasm, insults, and negative feedback.

BENEFICENCE. The final principle, *beneficence*, means engaging in and fostering helpful actions and behaviors. Group leaders must understand that some members' words are destructive to others and that leaders are responsible for monitoring and guiding interactions to ensure positive experiences. A group leader who believes that the group process

BOX 14.1 Role Function Areas for Evaluation of a Group Leader

Introduction

- Explains purpose of the group/topic/focus for the session
- Uses warm-up exercise
- Reviews rules and time frame

Activity/Topic

- Prepares for group members
- Provides direction to members
- Manages time
- Asks for feedback from members

Sharing

- Invites each member to share thoughts
- Uses appropriate verbal and nonverbal communication
- Acknowledges members' feelings
- Limits inappropriate behaviors

Processing

- Elicits members' feelings and thoughts about the experience, one another, and the leader

- Works with group to process difficult issues
- Focuses on similar issues of members
- Summarizes themes and significance to group members
- Attempts to apply group learning to daily activities

Group Motivation

- Shares with group sense of hopefulness and confidence
- Encourages members to take on new experiences and behaviors
- Encourages members to actively participate

Termination of Group

- Summarizes the most salient issues discussed
- Reinforces learning that took place
- Acknowledges contribution of each member
- Ensures that all problematic issues are resolved or followed up
- Ensures that the group ends on time

Source: Cole, M. (2005). *Group dynamics in occupational therapy: The theoretical basis and practice application of group intervention.* Thorofare, NJ: SLACK Incorporated.

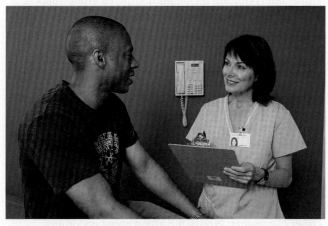

FIGURE 14.3 The leader must engage in careful discussion and evaluation with a potential team member before that person begins group therapy.

format is not meeting a member's treatment goals should find alternative settings or strategies for that client. In many cases, clients need to start with individual therapy and then progress to group therapy. Such clients may have frightening or shameful issues. After time in individual therapy, they can transition to group therapy.

CONFIDENTIALITY. The American Nurses Association's *Code of Ethics for Nurses* (2001) emphasizes that nurses must protect confidential information judiciously. A primary goal for group leaders is to protect each client's right to privacy. Confidentiality is the key building block

for group therapy. The major issue related to confidentiality among groups is protection of the anonymity of individual members. Leaders normally introduce maintenance of confidentiality as a primary group rule. They inform members not to reveal any shared information to people outside the group.

Group leaders are responsible for ensuring that members understand that the rule of confidentiality must be broken if one member reveals to another that he or she is considering serious harm to self or others. For instance, a client may report to a fellow member that he or she feels like "walking in front of a bus to take away all my pain." The person hearing this information would be obligated to alert the leader or another party to prevent a possible suicide.

INFORMED CONSENT. Ethical guidelines from the American Group Psychotherapy Association (2007) support the use of *informed consent,* a process of communicating essential information about group treatment to clients during the preparation process so that they are apprised of their risks, rights, and obligations as members. Using informed consent confers four benefits: it increases client autonomy, reduces risk of member dependency, enhances the working relationship between the group leader and the potential member, and increases the practitioner's accountability (Fallon, 2006). Potential members receive information on purpose and goals, other treatments that may be available, risks of participating, expected length of time, what to do if they believe the group is not helping, and fees. Nurses can incorporate this into the process of assessing the eligibility of clients for a particular group.

Documentation

A key responsibility of group leaders is documentation. Leaders initiate documentation during the evaluation stage of group development, in which they provide a diagnosis and formulate short-term goals. Spitz (2001) has developed both an individual and a group progress note form to assist group therapists to record clients' progress (Figure 14.4). Documentation follows each session and reflects goal progression. The individual progress note contains a working diagnosis or other indications for treatment, such as anger management, major problem areas, group behaviors, treatment goals, progress toward goals, plans toward treatment, and a statement of evaluation of progress to date. The group note includes the names of the group leader and members, date of the session, and session number. In addition, it addresses group goals, barriers to group progress, interventions, plans for next session, changes in membership, and comments.

Client: Gary Sweeny **Group** 4 **Date of session** 10/09/08

Working Diagnosis: *309.24-Adjustment Disorder with anxious mood*

Major Symptoms: *Social isolation, physical complaints–sweating, stomach pains; discomfort in new social situations*

In-Group Behavior (level of participation, prevailing mood, main interpersonal posture adopted in sessions, attitude and behavior toward the therapist): *Gary remains on the periphery of the group and contributes infrequently. He gives monosyllabic responses and says he is afraid to "expose" himself in front of others.*

Individual Treatment Goals: *Work on interpersonal anxiety using the support elements present in group. Gently encourage more active participation and self-disclosure by modeling this with other group members and by judicious use of therapist self-disclosure in selected areas.*

Progress Toward Goal Attainment: *Gary remains aloof, but seems to have developed the beginnings of a bond with the other male group members. He described taking the same bus home from group with Felix after last week's session.*

Treatment Plan: *Therapist will sit next to Gary to concretize issues of support. Next group meeting will be theme-focused in order to take the pressure off Gary and to help him participate in group discussions around a shared group issue. Possibility of antianxiety medication will be considered if his progress continues to be slow or if he shows signs of regressing to earlier withdrawn behavior.*

Prognosis (some informal estimate of patient's capacity for change based on group participation to date): *Gary appears to be "coming out of his shell" and if this trend continues it appears that the group will be of great value to him.*

Group Leader: Jason Difazio **Date** 10/19/08
Members Present: All **Session #** 3

Group Goals: Social skills training

Focus of Current Session: Group discussed anxieties connected with meeting new people or being in unfamiliar situations.

Any Specific Problems Impeding Group Progress: Mr. L. mentioned that he was thinking of dropping out of the group.

Major Interventions/Techniques: Utilized group support and universalization to reassure Mr. L. and encourage him to remain in group. Also did brief role-playing exercise addressed at learning techniques for how to manage when meeting new people.

Therapist Factors: Co-therapy issues; practical matters such as leader vacation schedule; need for consultation/supervision about a specific leadership or membership problem.

Any Changes in Group Composition: Dropouts from group; addition of new members.

Other Comments: Notify the group about upcoming holiday and discuss the possibilities for changing the meeting to another day of the week in order not to lose the continuity of the sessions.

Plans for Next Session: Try to get Mr. L. to begin the group discussion; discuss his reaction and those of the other group members to today's session. Assign "homework" outside of group in which each member has to introduce themselves to a new person or "stranger" and report the experience back to the group.

FIGURE 14.4 **(left)** Example of an individual note form. **(right)** Example of a group note.

Decision Making

Decision making is a necessary component of leadership, power, influence, authority, and delegation. In formal groups, specific guidelines determine which decisions the leader will make and which decisions will be decentralized or delegated to group members. The ability to make effective decisions depends on the group's knowledge of the subject, its ability to choose appropriate methods to solve problems, its ability to test and evaluate problem solving and decision making, and its maturity and ability to reverse or modify a decision that has proven unwise, unfair, or otherwise unacceptable.

Decisions may be made by consensus, majority vote, or minority decision. In *consensus,* all members agree. Although consensus can be time consuming and costly to achieve, especially in a large group, it optimizes overall satisfaction. The democratic leader uses consensus whenever possible. In *majority vote,* the largest number of group members decides the issue. Democratic leaders often use this method when reaching consensus is impossible. A *minority decision* may occur when a self-delegated subgroup or a group appointed as a subcommittee to explore a situation in greater depth reaches a decision.

Structuring the Group

Leaders are instrumental in establishing and maintaining group cohesiveness. They also select and orient new members in beginning and continuing groups. For new groups, careful selection of members is important to encourage rapid induction and cohesion. The following are personal strengths that leaders should observe for when initially interviewing clients to determine appropriate "fit" for a group (Rutan et al., 2007):

- Ability to give and receive feedback
- Self-reflective capacity
- Role flexibility
- Empathic ability
- Frustration tolerance
- Ability to acknowledge the needs of others
- Interpersonal strengths and weaknesses
- Well-considered rationale for placement
- Similar target treatment goals

Effective leaders ensure that the structuring process defines group norms, sets realistic expectations (which may be clarified), sets standards for performance, and maintains cohesiveness as new members are introduced. They discuss some of these issues with new members before introducing them. An example of such a discussion follows:

Leader: Jane, welcome. I am Ms. C., the group leader. I always meet with new members to share with them the group's goals and expectations. *(pause)* The group will have eight members, including you. We will meet from 1 to 2 PM each day in the blue room. Members will enter and leave the group as their behavior and needs change. *(pause)*

Jane: What are we expected to do?

Leader: Group members are expected to share their problems and their feelings about those problems with other members.

Jane: Is that all?

Leader: No. I also expect group members to discover techniques of problem solving by exploring their problems and feelings. Eventually, when members learn to relate more effectively to one another, my expectation is for them to transfer newly acquired skills to other relationships.

Jane: That sounds difficult and frightening.

Leader: Change and growth involve a certain amount of pain (anxiety).

Leaders structure groups by determining size, homogeneity, and leadership style. The purpose and goals define a group's scope, limitations, and desired accomplishments. Responsibilities of a leader to members include ensuring psychological safety, establishing and maintaining group norms, role modeling relationship skills, and commenting on group processes. To receive gratification, members must participate through introspection, self-disclosure, nurturing others, expressing feelings, and contributing to the maintenance of the group.

Checkpoint Questions

1. What are group norms? How do they affect a group?
2. Which type of leadership would likely be the most effective in an emergency?
3. What three characteristics of a therapeutic relationship are integral to effective functioning of a group leader?
4. What are three methods for decision making in a group?

Group Roles

Group leaders and members have interdependent functions. Member roles can enhance the effectiveness of a group leader and vice versa. Roles observed in groups are categorized as task, building and maintenance, and individual. Individually oriented behavior, which often stems from anxiety, distracts from and temporarily stymies the group and its progress. Conversely, task, building, and maintenance roles promote group growth and productivity.

Task Roles

Task roles help groups identify problems and methods of solving them. Problem solving helps a group reach its goal or mission. Examples of task roles include the following:

- *Initiator–contributor:* suggests or proposes new ideas or different ways of regarding the problem or goal
- *Information seeker:* asks for clarification (Figure 14.5)
- *Information giver:* offers facts or generalizations considered authoritative or shares relevant personal experiences
- *Coordinator:* shows or clarifies how ideas can work
- *Orienteer:* keeps the group on target by defining its current state compared to its goal
- *Recorder:* writes down productive discussions and decisions

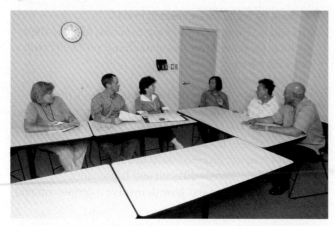

FIGURE 14.5 An important task role in groups is that of *information seeker*, who asks for clarification about issues or questions under discussion.

Building and Maintenance Roles

Group building and maintenance roles are oriented toward overall functioning. They alter or maintain the way of working to strengthen, regulate, and perpetuate the group. Examples include the following:

- *Encourager:* gives acceptance to the contributions of others
- *Harmonizer:* reconciles differences among members
- *Gatekeeper:* facilitates and encourages the contributions of others, thereby keeping communication open
- *Group observer:* notes and reports what is occurring to the group with an evaluation or interpretation of the group's procedure
- *Follower:* goes along with the ideas of others, assuming an audience role

Individual Roles

Individual roles meet the needs of only one group member. They hamper, rather than enhance, group functioning. Examples include the following:

- *Aggressor:* deflates the status of individual and group accomplishment
- *Blocker:* resists progress by arguing or disagreeing beyond reason
- *Recognition seeker:* calls attention to himself or herself through boasting and pointing out achievements
- *Play person:* horses around, demonstrating lack of involvement
- *Dominator:* asserts authority and superiority by manipulating the group or certain members

> **Think About It 14.1**
> Consider the students in your clinical rotation group. Analyze the roles that they assume, categorizing them as task, building and maintenance, and individual.

Group Communication

Nurses use various therapeutic communication techniques with clients. Examples are included in Table 14.2.

Latent and Manifest Communication

The content of *latent communication* is not discussed, occurs on an emotional level, and seldom is verbalized (eg, hidden agendas). *Manifest communication* involves spoken words. Groups are most effective when latent and manifest content match. The further apart these levels are, the more the group experiences communication problems.

TABLE 14.2 Group Communication Techniques

Technique	Description	Examples
Approval	Condoning or encouraging an attitude, feeling, or action	Frank: "I decided to move to a new apartment." Nurse: "You made a wise decision."
Acceptance	Conveying an attitude or a relationship that recognizes an individual's worth without implying approval of behaviors or personal affection	Marty: "Nurse, I was angry at you for not cancelling the session." Nurse: "It's all right for you to get angry at me, Marty."
Clarification	Restating of the substance of what the client has said	Abel: "I feel hopeless, no way out." Nurse: "You feel you have no way out?"
Exploration	Shifting from considering one aspect of a situation to considering another	Frank: "My son decided to leave the business." Nurse: "Tell me how that came about."
Identification	Delineating specific factors for the purposes of understanding or clarifying	Frank: "I often do favors for others, like my father did. He said it is rewarding and makes us better people." Nurse: "Sounds like you had respect for your father's opinions and judgment."
Interpretation	Finding or explaining the meaning or significance of the information	Mr. B.: "All this talking is really a pain in the neck." Nurse: "Mr. B., you seem annoyed at all the talking." *or* Abel: "I feel hopeless, no way out." Nurse: "You sound suicidal."

Technique	Description	Examples
Information giving	Stating facts about a problem	Marty: "All the staff write notes in the charts after the group meeting and put their own interpretation on what we say, don't they?" Nurse: "I can only speak for myself. I write notes in the chart, but I try hard not to misinterpret what members state in the group."
Encouraging expression of feelings or ideas	Indicating in some way that it is permissible or desirable to talk about feelings or ideas	Mr. W.: "It takes me 10 or 15 minutes to get oriented in the morning and then I'm all right." Nurse: "Are there others who feel this way?" Ms. S.: "I always get up to eat and have some coffee. Then I feel more like facing others."
Reassurance	Offering the client confidence about a favorable outcome through suggestion, persuasive arguments, or comparing similar situations	Frank: "I was afraid to move at first." Nurse: "Frank, we are always here to listen to your fears and try and help you work them out."
Support	Giving comfort, approval, or acceptance	Marty: "My busted arm has played heck with me. Getting anything for it has been a federal case. And I'm not one who shows pain easily." Nurse: "This must be pretty infuriating." Marty: "Well, it really bugs me."
Intervention	Performing an action that directs or influences the client's behavior	Nurse: "Frank, you've been silent, inattentive, and haven't shared with the group since your weekend pass. Will you tell us what is going on with you?" Frank: "I had a horrible weekend. I don't know how to share what happened, but I'll try."
Understanding	Indicating verbally or nonverbally that the feelings being communicated by the client are comprehended	Marty: "Nurse, I feel frightened about discharge." Nurse: "I can understand your feeling frightened. Leaving the hospital is not always easy."
Reflection	Repeating to clients what they said; mirroring their statement	Mr. B.: "All this talking is really a pain in the neck." Nurse: "This talking is a pain in the neck."
Listening	Concentrating on the client's communication without interrupting	Nurse listens and attends to client.
Teaching	Helping the client learn specifics in relation to events and behavior	Abel (to the nurse): "You were irritated at me, weren't you, but we were able to talk about it and work it out." Nurse: "Yes, we did. I was irritated because I felt you were not listening, and we did talk about it."
Silence	Using no verbal or spoken words	Nurse is silent while attending to client.
Structuring	Shaping the content of the group meeting	Frank: "I'm going home soon." Mrs. C.: "Really?" Nurse: "Maybe you would like to talk about it?"
Limit setting	Deciding how far group members and the group may go before the therapist ceases or restricts to a point the behavior, activity, or verbal expression of members	Marty: "I feel we need to cancel our therapy session next week because the next day is a holiday and we need a long weekend to travel." Nurse: "Holiday weekends are difficult; however, we will not cancel our group session."

A group may not solve problems readily because of interference from latent content. Hidden agendas hinder group communication. For example, if a group member believes that he or she would be punished for verbalizing an opinion, especially one that differs from that of the leader, his or her latent communication would influence overt behavior and interfere with group growth.

Content and Process Communication

Content and process are important concepts. What is being said during discussion is the *content*. How the group handles its communication is *process*. Who talks to whom, what is said, and what is left unspoken are examples of process.

Transference and Countertransference

Transference occurs when a client attributes characteristics and behavior of a family member or significant other to the therapist, thereby responding to the therapist in a certain manner. Clarification of this distortion with clients helps create a therapeutic process of learning. Countertransference occurs when the therapist responds negatively to the client's transference, further complicating communication. See Chapters 3 and 13 for more discussion.

Communication Themes

Leaders observe for themes in group communication that relate one session to another and then explore the meanings of these themes. Through therapeutic communication, leaders may help groups uncover and solve problems. Leaders also evaluate group functioning by observing changes in members' behavior, such as their ability to apply new techniques to solving problems.

Highly functioning groups and groups with mild to moderate psychopathology have few hidden agendas and minimal use of symbolic language. Therapists encourage these groups to deal with here-and-now material and to manage anxiety more readily than they do with groups that communicate on a symbolic level. They identify group themes and use appropriate communication techniques (see Chap. 11) to help the group solve the problem.

Stages of Group Development

Initial Stage

The initial stage of group development is likely to involve superficial, rather than open and trusting, communication. Members are becoming acquainted and searching for similarity between themselves and others. They may be unclear about the purposes or goals of the group. Some structuring of group norms, roles, and responsibilities takes place during this stage (Box 14.2).

Working Stage

The group accomplishes its real work during the working stage. Because members are already familiar with one another, the leader, and the group's rules, they are free to approach and attempt to solve their problems. Conflict and cooperation surface during the group's work.

Mature Stage

The mature group demonstrates such positive characteristics as empathy, effective communication, and a definite, inclusive group culture.

However, even if a group reaches a mature stage, individual members, or even the whole group, can regress. This change may result from the addition or loss of a member or a new and stressful group problem (see Table 14.3). The more serious the disturbance is, the greater the potential for regression. The more experience the group has in applying problem-solving skills, the more it can be resilient in the face of difficulties and return to its former mature stage. A group "image" of "problem solver" also facilitates group functioning.

BOX 14.2 Stages of Group Development

Initial

1. Works on getting acquainted with group leader and members
2. Depends on the leader for direction
3. Searches for meaning and purpose of the group
4. Restricts content and communication style
5. Searches for similarity among members
6. Gives advice

Working

1. Solves selected problems of working together
2. Handles conflicts between members or between members and leader
3. Works on issues of dominance, control, and power within group
4. Cooperates to accomplish the group's work

Mature

1. Develops workable norms and a group culture
2. Resolves conflict when it occurs; conflict arises from issues of importance, not emotional issues
3. Evaluates own work and individuals assume responsibility for their work
4. Accepts each others' differences without placing value judgments on them
5. Sanctions role assignment by members of the group
6. Discusses topics and makes decisions by means of rational behavior, such as sharing information and open discussion
7. Provides a feeling of "we" for the leader and members
8. Demonstrates cohesion
9. Validates itself; has a group image

Termination

1. Evaluates and summarizes the group experience
2. Explores positive and negative feelings about the group experience

---

Leadership is also important in sustaining the group and returning it to mature functioning after crisis or change.

Termination Stage

During termination, the group evaluates the experience and explores members' feelings about it and the impending separation. Group termination may help members who have difficulty with separation to learn to deal more realistically and comfortably with this normal human experience.

Checkpoint Questions

5. Which category of group roles identifies group problems and selects methods to solve them?
6. How does content communication differ from process communication?
7. During which stage of group development would members accept one another's differences without placing value judgments on them?

TABLE 14.3 Common Problems Affecting Group Therapy and Process

Group Problem	Goal	Nursing Intervention	Rationale
Fear of authority resulting in timid, hostile, aggressive, or withdrawn behavior	Group members will deal with authority directly and openly discuss their views and feelings about authority.	Use nonverbal and verbal communication techniques; listen to and encourage client to share and explore feelings. Respond in an understanding manner when the client expresses feelings (even when they are hostile). Reassure client that the nurse-therapist will not respond punitively to the expression of feelings.	The nurse-therapist functions as a role model of healthy communication. Acceptance of feelings allows group members to acknowledge and own their feelings.
Initial anxiety in a group, displayed by silence, fidgeting, nervous movement, and selective hearing	Group members' anxiety will be lessened so they can function more effectively in a group. Group members will respond to leader and other members in a productive manner.	Give "strokes" for positive interaction. Help client establish a role in the group, one related to the client's skills. Share with client that discomfort in the initial state of group development is common. Meet client's dependency needs.	Reinforcing group members' interaction increases their continuing interaction and promotes the development of group roles. Reassurance and meeting group members' dependency needs allows them to feel safe in the group.
Hidden agenda	Group members will communicate and act openly. Group members will express their feelings about the issues being discussed.	Identify the source of individual and group anxiety causing the hidden agenda. Explore the hidden agenda with the group and its meaning and effect on the group's functioning.	Hidden agendas sabotage the group's progress, create anxiety in members, and may cause members to form subgroups or leave the group.
Subgrouping	Unproductive subgroups will be eliminated. Members will discuss content related to group topics in the group.	Establish clarifying goals and purpose of the group (thereby lessening the group's anxiety and aiding in elimination of subgroups). Direct subgroup interest toward the goals of the group, thereby lessening subgroup preoccupation with outside themes.	Clarification allows group members to establish their group roles, which aids in problem solving. A sense of belonging to the group increases members' participation and furthers their comfort in role taking.
Deviant behavior—behavior that meets personal needs and undermines the group	Members' deviant behavior will be modified. Group members will function comfortably and effectively in an independent fashion; group will not disintegrate in leader's absence.	Identify deviant behavior and discuss it with the client. Identify sources of discomfort in the environment that affect the client. Explore with the client whether he or she identifies the behavior as deviant. Help members of the group identify deviant behavior. Help the client explore how this behavior affects his or her relationship in the group. Use group pressure to help the deviant member change or conform to group norms.	Dealing directly with deviant behavior helps the group learn effective ways to problem solve. Giving the client an independent role in the group allows the client to explore, achieve, and receive reinforcement.
Resistance to therapy (eg, grunting, moaning, staring into space, overresponding to situations, changing the subject, absence from group)	Members will demonstrate increased acceptance of, and participation in, therapy. Members will discuss problems and feelings in place of acting out.	Explore resistance behavior with client. Confront the client with his or her actions and behavior, using an understanding approach.	Some degree of resistance is common in every group. To promote individual and group progress, resistance must be confronted.

(continues on page 256)

TABLE 14.3 Common Problems Affecting Group Therapy and Process (continued)

Group Problem	Goal	Nursing Intervention	Rationale
Termination of the group, resulting in increased anxiety and self-defeating behavior	Members will accept group termination and learn from termination experience. Members will explore achievements accomplished in the group and feelings related to termination.	Help the client identify what he or she has accomplished while a member of the group. Help the client work through feelings of loss during termination (ie, feelings of anger, depression, euphoria, rejection). Help the client express both positive and negative feelings about the group and evaluate the group experience realistically. Plan a termination activity that allows expression of group members' feelings. Lessen intensity of group interaction as group nears termination.	Learning process in the group depends on the ability to express feelings and evaluate members' achievements at termination.

GROUP THERAPY

One purpose of group psychotherapy is to intervene in mentally disordered behavior, thinking, and feeling. Group therapy offers multiple stimuli to reveal, examine, and resolve distortions in interpersonal relationships. The purpose of each group is related to its goals and expected outcomes. For example, T groups help members improve their styles of relating to others. Interpersonal groups foster the development of intellectual understanding known as *insight*. Insight occurs on different levels, such as clients gaining understanding of how others see them or what clients are doing in various relationships (Yalom & Leszcz, 2005). Some insight is necessary for change. Thus, a person needing to develop or heighten skills in relating would join a T group, whereas a person needing assistance with achieving insight would join an interpersonal psychotherapy group.

Advantages and Disadvantages

Group psychiatric therapy has advantages and disadvantages. Advantages include the following:

- More clients can be treated at once, fostering cost effectiveness.
- Members benefit by hearing others discuss similar problems; feelings of isolation, alienation, and uniqueness often decrease, encouraging members to share problems.
- Group therapy allows clients to explore their specific styles of communication in a safe atmosphere where they can receive feedback and undergo change.
- Members learn from others multiple ways to solve problems, and group exploration may help them discover new ways.
- Members learn about the functional roles of individuals in a group. Sometimes, a member shares the responsibility as the co-therapist. Members become culture carriers.

- The group provides for its members understanding, confrontation, and identification with more than one person. The members gain a reference group.

Disadvantages of group therapy include the following:

- A member's privacy may be violated, such as when a conversation is shared outside the group. This behavior obstructs confidentiality and hampers complete and honest participation.
- Clients from various diagnostic groups may differ based on neurobiologic functioning. For instance, a client with schizophrenia may have multiple deficits in information processing, such as attention, learning, and memory. Because of these possible deficits, the group leader must be cognizant of the limitations and adjust the group process accordingly.
- Clients may experience difficulty exposing themselves to a group or believe that they lack the skills to communicate effectively. Some clients may use these factors as resistance; others may be reluctant to expose themselves because they do not want to change (see Table 14.3).
- Group therapy is not helpful if the therapist conducts the group as if it is individual therapy. Such a therapist may see dynamics and group processes as incidental or antagonistic to the therapeutic process. The effective group leader must be skilled in techniques and interventions that foster group interaction and shape group behavior and growth.

Therapeutic Factors of Group Therapy

Various authors have researched and described the therapeutic factors in group therapy, which are *interdependent* (do not operate separately). Different factors are more functional and helpful to group process at different stages. Although the same therapeutic factors operate in all therapy groups, their emphasis and importance vary according to the type of group.

1. Interpersonal learning
2. Catharsis
3. Group cohesiveness
4. Self-understanding
5. Development of socializing techniques
6. Existential factors
7. Universality
8. Instillation of hope
9. Altruism
10. Corrective family reenactment
11. Guidance
12. Identification/imitative behavior

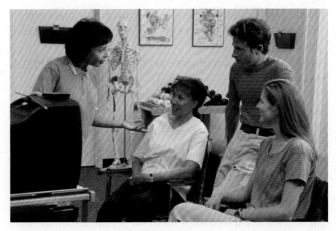

FIGURE 14.6 Groups may watch videos or other electronic media that impart pertinent information.

Yalom and Leszcz (2005) describe 12 curative (therapeutic) factors of group therapy, which could also be called healing factors or factors responsible for therapeutic change (Box 14.3).

These factors relate to different parts of the change process and are necessary for change to occur (Yalom & Leszcz, 2005). Several are described in more detail in the following sections.

Instillation of Hope

Instillation of hope helps clients maintain faith in the therapy. Clients are optimistic and believe that they will get better. Instillation of hope is important in pretherapy and can be correlated with a positive outcome. Inpatient groups have selected instillation of hope as a therapeutic factor, one that affects outcome more than in outpatient groups.

Universality

Universality prevents clients from feeling "different" in a negative way. Within the group, clients begin to feel less isolated and more like others. Learning that others have similar problems, thoughts, and feelings strengthens this feeling. Universality limits the fears that clients have about being alone with unacceptable thoughts, impulses, and fantasies; it provides more consensual validation than individual therapy (Yalom & Leszcz, 2005).

Imparting of Information

Imparting of information is use of data in a planned, structured manner, such as didactic instruction given in a lecture format. Audiovisual and other teaching aids may accompany these lectures (Figure 14.6). The topic of the didactic presentation is clear (Yalom & Leszcz, 2005).

Group Cohesiveness

Group cohesiveness relates to bonding and solidarity, the feeling of "we" instead of "I." Cohesiveness is demonstrated through group attendance and the group's ability to communicate positive and negative expressions without disintegrating. In cohesive groups, members try hard to impress one another, are accepting, and enter and leave with minimal disruption.

Norms are protected, and members who deviate from them are not tolerated. The client's role in a cohesive group greatly influences his or her self-esteem. Cohesive groups produce positive client outcomes (Yalom & Leszcz, 2005).

Catharsis

Catharsis is the expression of feelings, especially those involving deep emotions. It is a particularly important therapeutic factor. Catharsis is effective in group therapy when insight and cognitive learning follow (Yalom & Leszcz, 2005).

Existential Factors

Existential factors emphasize quality and content of experience, subjective awareness, freedom of choice, and state of being. They are important in boundary situations as clients work through impending death and inevitable developmental experiences, such as retirement and aging—that is, things that "are." Existential factors such as responsibility, capriciousness of existence, and recognition of mortality are factors with therapeutic value explored in group therapy (Yalom & Leszcz, 2005).

> **Checkpoint Questions**
> 8. What is the purpose of interpersonal group psychotherapy?
> 9. How is group cohesiveness demonstrated?
> 10. What do existential factors emphasize?

Types of Therapy Groups

Most types of group therapy can be categorized as psychotherapeutic or growth oriented. Factors for each member that determine the maximal therapeutic benefit of a psychotherapy or growth group include the following:

- Extent of personality disorganization and its effects on interpersonal functioning as a family member, provider, and productive citizen
- Degree of functional ability and role success or failure

- Ability to harness impulses in stressful group situations
- Purpose in joining a group, including both articulated and hidden agendas
- Ability to share and support others in problem-solving tasks
- Ability to use the material produced in a group to solve unique problems

Psychotherapeutic Groups

Group psychotherapy has many different theoretical approaches, including psychoanalysis, transactional analysis, cognitive, rational-emotive, humanistic, gestalt, and interpersonal (see Chaps. 3 and 13). In addition, psychodrama can be used to explore the truth through dramatic methods.

Leaders of psychotherapy groups assume more responsibility than they would in growth groups. In psychotherapy groups, members or clients may have limiting, maladaptive, or severe emotional disorders. They may be referred to groups from individual therapy. Clients do not become the therapist, and the therapist never assumes the client's role. Leaders also provide more support for members who may have less tolerance for stress.

Psychotherapeutic groups can be inpatient or outpatient. The type of setting influences group goals and aims. Clients in inpatient environments routinely are assigned to an array of groups to foster increased functioning toward discharge and resumption of community living. In outpatient modalities, clients are assigned based on individual needs, such as grief and anger management. Specific illness and level of functioning are determining factors for the selection of group assignment (Evidence-Based Practice Spotlight 14.1).

Medication management groups can be targeted to specific types of drugs. For instance, a group of clients taking Clozaril, which has serious side effects, can be managed better in a group format that allows for monitoring of their physical and psychological status.

INPATIENT PSYCHOTHERAPEUTIC GROUPS. Inpatient groups involve meetings in which all clients and staff members on the unit discuss and address a continuum of issues related to rehabilitation. Particular areas of attention are gaining skills and knowledge to support recovery and eventual discharge from the hospital, as well as issues in community living that they may encounter. In a typical day, clients may participate in groups focusing on social skills, conversation, assertiveness, community living, health management, or coping (Bellack et al., 2005). Each group meets daily for 45 to 60 minutes. Membership is transient and may change with each meeting. The main focus is working in the present with the issues that each client brings, with the ultimate goal of discharge to the community. The active leader structures, supports, and encourages participation from others. Inpatient groups support a client's ability to improve functional level and to gain greater skills toward community living.

One example is a specifically targeted type of group therapy for clients with schizophrenia called cognitive enhancement therapy (Lewandowski et al., 2011). This type of therapy is based on a theoretical model that assumes that schizophrenia is characterized by deficits in information processing and memory, which interfere with interpersonal communication. This therapy begins with individual assessment, rapport building, and treatment planning. There is a component of computer

---

▲ EVIDENCE-BASED PRACTICE SPOTLIGHT 14.1 ▲

Reminiscence Therapy for Dementia

Overview of Effective Treatment: Reminiscence therapy (RT) refers to discussion of past events, experiences, and actions with other people or groups, using the assistance of actual objects, such as photographs, personal items, music, or literature. Groups meet and are encouraged to discuss the past at least once per week. Four randomized studies support that RT improves cognition, mood, and general behavioral functioning, in addition to reducing strain for caregivers. Some limited evidence shows that behavior therapy–pleasant events and behavior therapy–problem solving reduce depressive symptoms, whereas psychomotor therapy groups seem to reduce aggression in dementia.

What Has Not Been Shown Effective: Social contact intervention groups and communication groups have no solid support.

Implications for Practice: RT involves person-centered care. Involvement from family caregivers would certainly add an important dimension to outcomes. Furthermore, health care providers must consider the severity of dementia in group members during design and implementation.

References

Stinson, C., & Kirk, E. (2006). Structured reminiscence: An intervention to decrease depression and increase self-transcendence in older women. *Journal of Clinical Nursing, 15*(2), 208–218.

Wang, J. (2005). The effects of reminiscence on depressive symptoms and mood status of older institutionalized adults in Taiwan. *International Journal of Geriatric Psychiatry, 20*(1), 57–62.

Woods, B., Spector, A., Jones, C., Orrell, M., & Davies, S. (2005). Reminiscence therapy for dementia. *Cochrane Database of Systematic Review, 2005*(2). CD001120.DOI:002/14651858. CD001120.pub2.

Wu, L., Chou, C., Lu, S., & Tseng, H. (2006). Developing practical guidelines for group reminiscence therapy. *Journal of Evidenced-Based Nursing, 2*(3), 173–179.

training and social cognitive group sessions. Another recent development in psychiatric rehabilitation is evidence-based practices, in particular, illness management and recovery (IMR). Based on a group format, IMR incorporates five empirically supported interventions: psychoeducation, cognitive–behavioral approaches to medication adherence, relapse prevention, social skills training, and coping skills training. IMR is being further tested; preliminary studies support its effectiveness (Mueser et al., 2006). Its modules focus on recovery strategies, practical facts about mental illness, the stress–vulnerability model, building social supports, using medication effectively, reducing relapses, coping with stress, coping with problems and symptoms, and getting needs met in the mental health system. This structured curriculum can be used for both inpatient and outpatient settings. Cultural sensitivity must be considered in the implementation of IMR.

OUTPATIENT PSYCHOTHERAPEUTIC GROUPS. Outpatient groups are usually conducted in community behavioral health settings with various goals and aims. They are time limited (60 to 90 minutes). Clients are usually recommended by primary therapists to attend specific groups based on behavioral or psychological deficits. These groups are usually developed based on the needs of the client population. For example, one group may be for psychological trauma associated with severe mental illness. The trauma may also be from multiple areas: childhood abuse, spousal abuse, abuse experienced as a result of previous hospitalization, or living in unsafe conditions.

A new multifamily group intervention for families exposed to severe and chronic psychological trauma, including family violence, drug activity, incarceration, and interpersonal violence, has been developed to support recovery (Kiser et al., 2010). Normally, psychological trauma treatment is individual, but new research is demonstrating that families can experience significant improvement in parenting skills and increased feelings of competency and support in a family group process. For veterans experiencing post-traumatic stress disorder (PTSD), group-based interpersonal therapy that focuses on interpersonal sensitivity, interpersonal disputes, role transitions, and grief and loss has been found to be successful (Ray & Webster, 2010). Group work involves attention to problematic attachment styles, reduction of PTSD symptoms, development of new and supportive relationships, and coping skills. Another type of group therapy is supportive–expressive for women with metastatic breast cancer, which can improve quality of life and protect against depression (Kissane et al., 2007).

Another dimension of outpatient group psychotherapy is the construction of groups based on the ethnic background of the population serviced by the community behavioral health center. Gater and colleagues (2010) developed a social group intervention for Pakistani women with depression. The intervention addressed social difficulties, isolation, and poor access to primary care in order to treat ongoing depressive symptoms. A taxi service was used to increase compliance in coming for treatment and was a key factor in successful outcomes for this group (see Chap. 6). In another successful group intervention for reduction of alcohol and cocaine use for HIV-positive adults with childhood sexual abuse histories, baseline assessment data were collected and "Living in the Face of Trauma" (LIFT) was used as a treatment intervention. This intervention focused on current stressors, use of substances, other health behaviors, and the development of effective coping strategies.

Growth Groups

In the past three decades, numerous growth groups, including self-help groups and group counseling, have been developed. In a growth or self-help group (eg, T group), the leader and members have attained emotional stability, and there is not a great discrepancy between their functioning at the beginning and at the end of the experience. The group initially uses the leader for guidance and clarification. However, toward the end, the leader becomes part of the group, and members may perform several leadership functions. In a growth group, members may receive less support from the leader while dealing with anxiety, but there is conflict resolution by the end. Three types of growth groups include encounter groups, T groups, and community support groups.

ENCOUNTER GROUPS. The purpose of an encounter group is personal change, often as a result of deeply felt experiences (Figure 14.7). The differences between marathon and encounter groups are minimal, and the theoretical orientations of group leaders are diverse. The term *marathon group* refers to the amount of concentrated time the participants spend together. Examples of themes are "The Challenge of Change, Danger, and Fulfillment," "Closeness: Can It Hurt?" and "Marriage: How to Survive It."

TRAINING GROUPS. The T group is the oldest and best-known therapeutic method coming out of the sensitivity T-group movement. The first T-group conference was held in Bethel, Maine, in 1946. The goal of each T-group conference is to verify experimentally the T-group method. This

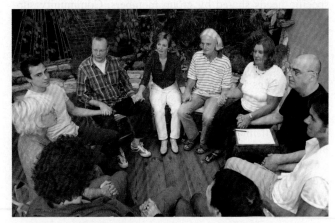

FIGURE 14.7 Encounter groups focus on personal change through shared, deeply felt experiences.

TABLE 14.4 Community Support Groups

Type of Group	Target Members	Examples
Victims of violence	Clients and families who have been physically or emotionally abused	Safe house, rape trauma, battered children
Birth anomaly	Clients and families dealing with birth defects and congenital anomalies	Down syndrome, cerebral palsy
Acquired diseases	Those coping with, and adjusting to, diseases originating after birth that are not inherited or innate	Leukemia, AIDS, diabetes
Chronic illness	Clients and families in which there is an illness of long-term duration, slow progression, and, often, little change in the symptomatology	Chronic obstructive pulmonary disease, cancer, arthritis
Developmental adjustment	Clients and families with physical or emotional development that deviates from the norm	Autistic children, runaway teens
Grief education and resolution	Clients and families with physical and emotional loss	Loss because of death of a significant person, sudden infant death syndrome
Interracial and biracial	Clients and families of interracial siblings, children, spouses, parents, and neighborhoods	Asian American families
Self-help and improvement	Perspectives on behavior and attitude change	Assertiveness, Weight Watchers, Alcoholics Anonymous
Family structure	Clients and families of non-traditional (non-nuclear) family structure	Step-parenting, Parents without Partners, Lucky Mother's Club
Work related	Workers who experience job-related stress	Burnout groups, Friday evening groups

involves the study of group norms, roles, communication distortions, and effects of authority on behavior patterns, personality, and coping mechanisms. Members receive feedback by exposing their inner selves to others in the group, and they experiment with new and more productive behavior.

COMMUNITY SUPPORT GROUPS. Numerous support groups have emerged under the category of community mental health psychiatry. Some were founded to lend continued or added support to previously hospitalized psychiatric clients. Others have resulted from the needs of people in the community. Lay people have developed self-help groups to address specific needs shared by group members. Community support groups, of which there are more than 500 examples, may be classified in various ways (Table 14.4).

The main purpose of community support groups is to provide identification, clarification, understanding, role modeling, feelings of togetherness, and group cohesion. They help prevent a person from feeling lonely and isolated. Some groups evolve into educational models that enhance communication, self-image, body image, problem solving, decision making, and growth processes.

Most community support groups help their members decrease levels of stress and increase levels of self-acceptance. With group help, the member can better deal with problems that he or she brought to the group. The outcome of this process is rewarding; the member develops new or more effective patterns of behavior.

Although community support groups have structures similar to those of other groups, they may be larger than therapy groups. Members may share leadership; that is, leadership is a process. Senior members are expected to provide direction and structure and help establish norms.

Think About It 14.2
Investigate the local community for available support groups. Attend one or two meetings. Analyze the group for its type, target members, purpose, goals, and structure.

NURSES AND GROUP PROCESS AND THERAPY

Nurses have used groups and the group process in hospitals and other health care settings. As nursing progressed from functional assignments to the team approach, many studies were undertaken to discover ways to enhance task and maintenance roles. Nurses have collaborated with colleagues in examining group theory, group dynamics, and group functioning in various health care delivery systems. Psychiatric–mental health nurses have explored specifically the use of groups as a teaching method and as a therapeutic tool with clients.

Group Process and Therapy in Nursing Education

Nurse educators use group seminars as part of the teaching–learning process to enable students to participate in groups, learn group roles, and learn the function and dynamics of the student–participator role. Instructors delegate some authority to the students, yet serve as democratic leaders who structure the course and define class expectations. This experiential learning sparks an exciting way to learn group theory, enabling students to transfer their knowledge of, and experience in, group dynamics to other arenas, such as milieu therapy, client groups, and supervision groups. Often, these seminars are prerequisites for advanced courses in group therapy in graduate nursing programs.

In addition to group seminars, the use of groups in nursing education has increased in the form of study, special project, and testing groups. The following example is from the Front Range Community College nursing program, which formed student groups to help their students learn about groups and group theory. With increased challenges, the nursing faculty formed additional groups with the following objectives:

- Initiate brainstorming among the members to enhance critical thinking.
- Foster "bonding" of group members.
- Help students increase their survival skills.
- Help students learn conflict resolution and assertiveness and become change agents.
- Practice collaboration in the student role to apply this process on the job after graduation and thus prevent unhealthy competition.
- Build self-esteem.
- Learn how to teach clients and families by teaching one another.
- Learn decision making and its accompanying responsibility.
- Foster achievement of peers—for example, an "A" student helping students with lower grades.

Study groups developed their own operational rules and norms. They established tolerance, limit setting, and group problem solving. Student group members learned group dynamics and how to reach out for help through the group. Groups sponsored individual growth through imitative behavior. Students learned about the change process by developing these skills in their groups and discovered that diversity of group members fosters strength.

Evaluation of these nursing student groups revealed a positive experience. Members gained knowledge about group functioning through their participation and expressed individual growth. Identified problems were group meeting times that conflicted with family schedules and finding a mutually convenient meeting time for all group members.

Group Process and Therapy in Nursing Practice
Historical Perspective
Past psychiatric–mental health nurses learned group therapist and co-therapist roles and responsibilities. Hildegard Peplau, an early authority on psychiatric nursing specialist

programs, augmented nurses' involvement in group therapy through what is known as *experiential learning*. Nurses developed increasing skills in the techniques of group therapy; psychiatric nursing clinical specialists became highly skilled in group intervention.

The mental health revolution, sponsored by President John F. Kennedy in the 1960s, demanded that more health professionals administer formal and informal group therapy in community mental health centers. Responding to this need, psychiatric clinical nurse specialists have become more active in group leader or co-leader roles in many formal and informal psychotherapeutic and growth group therapies in therapeutic communities, outpatient settings, and private settings. They have also become active as liaison psychiatric nursing consultants in general hospitals.

Contemporary Nursing Groups
Reassessing the need for change in individuals, groups, and environments has led nurses to seek alternative ways to improve communication. Economics and expanded collaborative and cooperative nursing practice have encouraged innovation in group work. Because computer networks are interactive media, computer groups have been established to diminish the problems of distance, time, and need for speedy feedback. Economic currents have also fostered the creation of short-term, solution-focused crisis groups, encouraging the use of more "open–open" groups. Members can enter or leave at any time, which also provides a richer medium of information that can lead to problem solving.

Social and societal needs influence contemporary nursing groups. An important nursing role in relation to group therapy is referral of clients to various community-based support groups, including the National Alliance on Mental Illness, Alcoholics Anonymous, Narcotics Anonymous, Overeaters Anonymous, and other eating disorder groups. These support groups are free or inexpensive and more effective for clients needing long-term approaches, compared with ongoing psychotherapy.

Nurses use various methods and approaches when working with groups (Evidence-Based Practice Spotlight 14.2). Examples include didactic and experiential learning; cognitive–behavioral training (panic disorder and agoraphobia); solution-focused group therapy; directive therapist approach (in clinical gerontology); and validation therapy (for those with dementia). Contemporary nursing groups include those that focus on the following:

- Intergenerational relationships: one example is youths from local schools interacting with senior citizens (Figure 14.8)
- High-risk populations (incarcerated women's and men's groups)
- Victims of violence (gangs, school violence, domestic violence)
- Medication noncompliance (clients whose noncompliance may lead to socially deviant behavior)

⚠ EVIDENCE-BASED PRACTICE SPOTLIGHT 14.2 ⚠

Group Behavior Therapy for Smoking Cessation

Overview of Effective Treatment: Group therapy can be more effective than individual modalities in assisting clients to stop smoking. Group approaches provide the necessary setting to learn behavioral techniques and strategies to stop smoking within a therapeutic milieu of mutual support and encouragement. Furthermore, inclusion of a component of relapse prevention enhances treatment effectiveness. Also effective is advice from both doctors and nurses with structured interventions and individual treatment. Nicotine replacement in all forms is also effective.

What Has Not Been Shown Effective? Brief advice from a health professional, casual care, aversive stimuli treatment

with the use of silver acetate, anxiolytics, acupuncture, exercise, and hypnotherapy are approaches without proven support.

Implications for Practice: Although evidence supports group treatment, many people struggling with nicotine dependence do not consider or participate in this approach. Therefore, the use of the techniques involved in group treatment would need to be applied within the individual counseling model.

References

Lancaster, T., Stead, L., Silagy, C., Sowden, A., & Cochrane Tobacco Addiction Review Group. (2000). Effectiveness of interventions to help people stop smoking: Findings from the Cochrane Library. *British Medical Journal, 321*(7257), 355–358.

Stead, L., & Lancaster, T. (2007). Group behavior therapy programmes for smoking cessation. *Cochrane Database of Systematic Reviews, 2007*(2). CD001007.DOI:10.1002/14651858. CD001007.pub2.

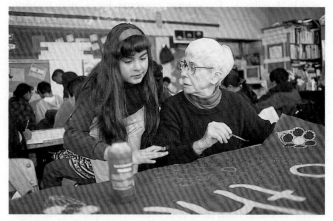

FIGURE 14.8 Some groups involve intergenerational activities and relationships. This older adult volunteer participates in a support group for preteens living in an at-risk community. (Photo © Kathy Sloane.)

- Alzheimer disease—these groups bond, emphasizing what they remember and supporting one another in their loss, and learn and accept what they have lost
- Disabilities (caused by work, industrial injury, and other trauma)

- Senior counseling to help prevent and work with depression
- Behavior patterns, which are feelings-oriented programs that teach children, in a school setting, how to manage their emotions
- Creativity, in which psychiatric nurses lead groups to focus on creative expression rather than psychotherapy; activities promote acceptance of self and by the group
- Coping skills, in which clients with a chronic disability or disease learn to deal with fear, live with chronic pain, and cope with loss, anger, and depression
- Reminiscence therapy (nursing homes)
- Smoking cessation (work and school settings)
- Culturally similar people: focus on acculturation, adjustment, and other specific issues (eg, recovery from torture or other strife in war-torn areas)

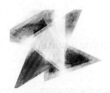

Reviewing and Applying Your Knowledge

Chapter Summary

- A group is three or more people with related goals; groups vary according to their size, homogeneity of membership, climate, norms, and goal-directedness.

- Group norms are the patterns of interaction that develop within a group.

- Three styles of group leadership are autocratic, democratic, and laissez-faire.

- Roles in groups are categorized as task, building and maintenance, and individual.

- Important concepts of group communication include latent and manifest communication, content and process communication, transference and countertransference, and communication themes.

- The three stages of group development are the initial, working, and termination stages.

- The advantages of group therapy include its effectiveness and efficiency in time and cost.

- There are 12 therapeutic factors observed in group therapy, including instillation of hope, universality, imparting of information, altruism, corrective recapitulation of the primary family group, development of socializing techniques, imitative behavior, interpersonal learning, group cohesiveness, catharsis, and existential factors.

- Most therapeutic group experiences can be categorized as psychotherapy or growth groups.

- Nurses participate as leaders and co-leaders in multiple formal and informal groups; contemporary nursing groups are influenced by social and societal needs. Examples include intergenerational groups, medication noncompliance groups, and coping skills groups.

Study Questions

1. When developing a presentation about group types, which of the following would the nursing instructor include as characteristics of a primary group?

   a. High degree of structure and authority

   b. Explicit and implicit interdependent roles, boundaries, and group norms

   c. Large size and impersonal

   d. Provision of education and cultural values

2. The nursing department of a psychiatric hospital has organized a group of nurses to develop a continuing education program in psychiatric–mental health nursing research and ethics. The group leader develops a list of tasks to be completed and assigns a task to each group member. The nurse is using which leadership style?

   a. Laissez-faire

   b. Democratic

   c. Autocratic

   d. Egalitarian

3. A group is meeting to develop a plan for a rural community outreach program. The group learns that funding for the program has been cut by 40%. Which of the following suggests that the group is in the mature stage of development?

   a. Group members are unsure how to proceed and look to the leader for direction.

   b. Group members suggest solutions with conflict, but attempt to cooperate.

   c. Group members are upset, but supportive. After a period of disorganization, the group begins problem solving.

   d. Group members, supportive of one another and trying to solve the problem, cannot reach a decision about how to proceed and inform the group leader.

4. A group of women recovering from alcoholism meets weekly. One member has been sharing about how her in-laws have been aloof and distant from her since she started treatment. She feels ashamed and tongue-tied around them. Which of the following responses by the group suggests a highly functioning, therapeutic group?

   a. The group can share their experiences with their in-laws.

   b. A group member can accompany her to the next family function for support.

   c. The group can give feedback about developing effective communication with her in-laws.

   d. The group can confront her about her passive personality and offer advice.

(continues on page 264)

5. After teaching a group of students about the advantages and disadvantages of group therapy, which of the following statements, if identified by the students as an advantage, indicates effective teaching? Select all that apply.

   a. Group members can be confronted with negative feedback.

   b. Group therapy can work as individual therapy.

   c. Group members may be expected to function as co-therapists.

   d. Group members are exposed to the problems of others.

   e. Group members readily expose themselves to other members.

Critical Thinking Questions

1. How does a client in a therapy group become a culture carrier?

2. How does a leader affect the initial stage of a group? Give an example.

3. What are the stages of a group? List a characteristic of each stage.

4. Discuss six characteristics of a mature group.

5. What are the six advantages of group therapy?

6. Discuss five therapeutic factors observed in group therapy.

7. Describe treatment interventions that can be accomplished by the use of group therapy.

References

Aiken, T. (2004). *Legal, ethical, and political issues in nursing.* Philadelphia, PA: F. A. Davis.

American Group Psychotherapy Association Science to Service Task Force. (2007). Practice guidelines for group psychotherapy. Retrieved from http://www.agpa.org

American Nurses Association. (2001). *Code of ethics for nurses with interpretive statements.* Silver Spring, MD: American Nurses Publishing.

Bellack, A., Mueser, K., Gingerich, S., & Agresta, J. (2005). *Social skills training for schizophrenia: A step-by-step guide.* New York, NY: Guilford Press.

Fallon, A. (2006). Informed consent in the practice of group psychotherapy. *International Journal of Group Psychotherapy, 56*(4), 431–450.

Gater, R., Waheed, W., Husain, N., Tomenson, B. Aseem, S., & Creed, F. (2010). Social intervention for British Pakistani women with depression: Randomized controlled trial. The *British Journal of Psychiatry, 197*, 227–233.

Kiser, L., Dohohue, A., Hodgkinson, S., Medoff, D., & Black, M. (2010). Strengthening family coping resources: The feasibility of a multifamily group intervention for families exposed to trauma. *Journal of Traumatic Stress, 23*(6), 802–806.

Kissane, D., Garbsch, B., Clarke, D., Smith, G., Bloch, A., Snyker, S., & Li, Y. (2007). Supportive-expressive group therapy for women with metastatic breast cancer: Survival and psychosocial outcome from a randomized control trial. *Psycho-Oncology, 16*(4), 277–286.

Lewandowski, K., Eack, S., Hogarty, S., Greenwald, D., & Keshavan, M. (2011). Is cognitive enhancement therapy equally effective for patients with schizophrenia and schizoaffective disorder. *Schizophrenia Research, 125*, 291–294.

Mueser, K. Meyer, T., Penn, D., Clancy, R., Clancy, D., & Salyers, M. (2006). The illness management and recovery program: Rationale, development, and preliminary findings. *Schizophrenia Bulletin, 32*(1), 32–43.

Ray, R., & Webster, R. (2010). Group interpersonal psychotherapy for veterans with posttraumatic stress disorder: A pilot study. *International Journal of Group Psychotherapy, 60*(1), 131–140.

Rogers, C. (1985). *A way of being.* Boston, MA: Mariner.

Rutan, J. S., Stone, W. N., & Shay, J. J. (2007). *Psychodynamic group psychotherapy.* New York, NY: Guilford Publications.

Spitz, H. (2001). Brief group therapy. In S. R. Sauber (Ed.), *Managed mental health care* (pp. 103–132). London, UK: Brunner/Mazel.

Yalom, I., & Leszcz, M. (2005). *Theory and practice of group psychotherapy* (4th ed.). New York, NY: Basic Books.

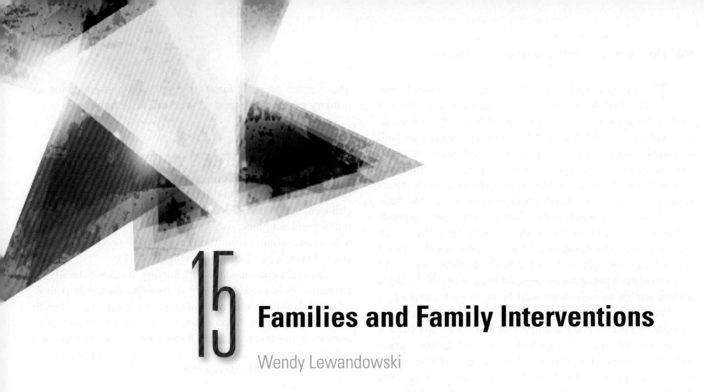

15

Families and Family Interventions

Wendy Lewandowski

KEY TERMS

adaptation
dyad
ecomap
family
family burden
family consultation
family education
family empowerment
family interventions
first-order change
genogram
iatrogenic burden
multigenerational
negative feedback
objective burden
positive feedback
secondary prevention
second-order change
serious and persistent mental
   illness (SPMI)
subjective burden
triad

LEARNING OBJECTIVES

On completion of this chapter, you should be able to accomplish the following:

- Describe the family as a system adapting to change.
- Identify the components of a family assessment.
- Give examples of cognitive, affective, and behavioral psychiatric nursing interventions applied to the care of families.
- Explain the rationale for involving families in the treatment of clients.
- Define *family burden.*
- Differentiate among objective, subjective, and iatrogenic burden.
- Explain secondary prevention and its relevance to families who have relatives with mental illness.
- Explain *family consultation* and how it differs from family therapy.
- Provide examples of how nurses can function as family consultants.

This chapter focuses on the family as the unit of care. The first section discusses important theories and models for nurses to understand when working with families dealing with short-term psychiatric challenges, as well as those facing serious and persistent mental illness in one or more members. The chapter reviews techniques of family assessment and introduces family interventions. **Family interventions** include both health promotion measures and steps to improve family functionality. Their effectiveness depends on the readiness of families to adapt and change. Often, such readiness depends on the relationship a nurse has developed with a family (Wright & Leahey, 2005). Building a positive relationship is a powerful strategy for improving the family's holistic health, as well as the well-being of each member.

Family interventions differ from *family therapy,* which consists of specialized techniques to modify family behavior. Advanced practice psychiatric–mental health nurses and other advanced mental health professionals implement family therapy using evidence-based therapies for specific family issues and/or problems. However, nurses at all levels can conduct effective family interventions that are also evidence based.

The second part of this chapter focuses on care and assistance for families when one or more members have chronic, serious psychiatric illness. Such families face many struggles and need assistance to manage care, reduce stress, and work together to facilitate treatment for their members.

The chapter presents family consultation and education as primary nursing roles and services for such families.

FAMILY THEORIES AND MODELS

The contemporary definition of **family** is the unit that defines itself as such. This unit can be a mother, father, and children; an unmarried couple with no children; a single mother and daughter; two same-sex partners; children living with grandparents; or any other group of people who consider themselves a family unit (Figure 15.1).

In psychiatric–mental health nursing, models of family intervention have moved away from focusing on family pathology and dysfunction to recognizing the importance of health in the whole family. Approaches to care emphasize strengths, competencies, and resources. Today's nurses are partners and collaborators with families to achieve and maintain family health (Marsh, 2001; Moore, 2005).

Family as a System

A *system* is a complex of interacting elements. It represents a set of parts, with relationships between the parts and between properties of the parts. In *family systems theory,* the family is a "total interlocking system, with each member a subsystem influencing all other members and further existing within a larger social system" (Jackson, 1967, p. 45).

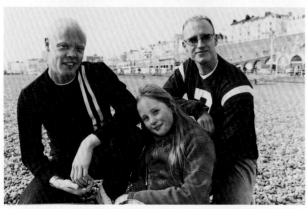
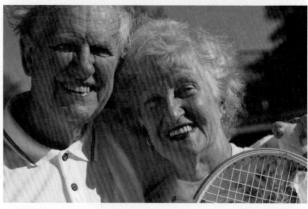
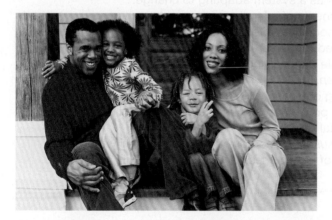
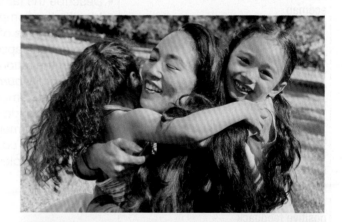

FIGURE 15.1 A family consists of those members who identify themselves as belonging to it. These photos reflect different family configurations.

The following concepts and propositions of family systems theory are helpful in assessing and working with families receiving psychiatric care:

1. *Family systems have interacting parts (subsystems).* Family subsystems include individual members, **dyads** (relationships between two members), and **triads** (relationships among three members). An example of a dyad is a father and son. An example of a triad is two parents and a child.

2. *The system and subsystems are interdependent.* The family also belongs to larger systems, such as its neighborhood of residence, and interacts with still other systems, such as the local school, church community, work settings, and health care system.

3. *A change in one part (subsystem) affects the whole system.* When a family is affected in some way, its dynamics shift to a new balance. The family reorganizes or begins functioning at a different level than it did before the change, disturbance, or intervention. A change in one member affects all members. A frequent analogy is to liken a family system to a mobile hanging over an infant's crib. When one part of the mobile is touched, the other parts of the mobile move to a new configuration (Figure 15.2).

4. *Family systems have boundaries.* Boundaries in family systems serve as structural frames to keep family members cohesively together. Family systems are characterized as either *open* or *closed,* based on the permeability of their boundaries. Such permeability plays a vital role in a family's growth and development. For example, in a closed family system, boundaries maintain family secrets (e.g., sexual abuse, substance abuse, chronic psychiatric illness). The more closed or impermeable a family is to new information and resources, the less likely it will be to have the energy and knowledge to meet its expanding needs (Nichols, 2010). The clarity of boundaries within a family is a useful parameter for evaluating family functioning. Rigid, overly restrictive

boundaries inhibit interpersonal contact and result in *disengagement.* Boundaries characterized by a heightened sense of support, but at the expense of independence and autonomy, lead to *enmeshment.* A family system characterized by clear boundaries—in which each subsystem has interpersonal contact with another without undue interference—can adapt and change under stressful conditions (Nichols, 2010).

5. *Family systems are adaptable.* The family can adapt to both inside and outside influences. Although the family often tries to maintain itself and its boundaries, it is capable of change. There are two levels of change (Wright & Leahey, 2005). A change that does not affect family functioning is called a **first-order change**. An example is a father preparing dinner because the mother, who usually cooks, is ill with a cold. A **second-order change** has greater effects. An example is a mother who develops depression and no longer wants to leave the house. Her inability to leave her home causes ripple effects in the family system, which necessitate that other family members assume new and different roles. The reorganization necessary after a divorce or the death of a family member also results in second-order change. Likewise, nursing interventions can cause second-order change, assisting families to reach a higher level of functioning.

6. *Family systems experience circularity.* Family systems have mechanisms of *feedback,* a circular process whereby part of a system's output is monitored and fed back as input. Feedback enables self-regulation and is categorized as negative or positive. **Negative feedback** maintains the system's homeostasis, whereas **positive feedback** allows the system to change, grow, and innovate. An example of negative feedback is demonstrated in a mother and father's response to their teenage daughter's increasingly disordered eating. The worried parents become critical, hostile, and overly controlling, resulting in protracted arguments with the daughter in an attempt to make her eat. The child entrenches further in anorectic behavior to avoid difficult interpersonal situations with her parents and to maintain her safety. Nurturing this family's capacity to tolerate and resolve interpersonal conflict and express feelings is an example of positive feedback.

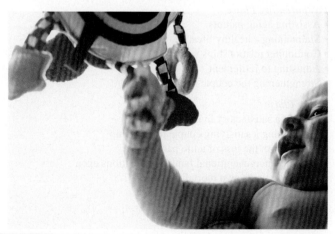

FIGURE 15.2 **The family as a system can be compared to an infant mobile—when one part is moved, the whole structure changes.**

Checkpoint Questions

1. What term describes family subsystems with rigid, overly restrictive interpersonal boundaries?
2. What type of change does not affect family functioning?
3. What is an example of positive feedback in a family system?

Family Development

Social scientist Ruben Hill (1970) laid the descriptive foundation for family development by outlining families as **multigenerational**, with beliefs and traditions handed down from one generation to the next. One of the most influential models of family growth and development is Duvall's

(1977) *family development theory,* which incorporates eight chronological stages and predictable tasks that families must master before proceeding to the next stage. The eight stages are beginning family, childbearing family, family with preschoolers, family with teenagers, family launching, young adults, family with middle-aged parents, and family in retirement. Because Duvall based these stages on a very traditional, white, middle-class model, more recent theorists have expanded their models to include different stages and tasks. Examples include divorce/postdivorce families and remarried families (McGoldrick et al., 2010).

McGoldrick and Carter (2007) refer to family development as the *family life cycle.* In their model, stages include joining families in marriage, families with young children, families with adolescents, families at midlife, and families in later life. They also revolve their stages around the traditional role of families, which involves having and launching children.

Recent family development theorists have focused on the importance of sociocultural factors and changes in the role of women, which have dramatically influenced the predictable stages of the family life cycle. A family's life cycle greatly depends on its particular sociocultural context. Factors such as poverty and discrimination can greatly influence the shared futures of relatives. Many families face disruptions, such as job insecurity, homelessness, and violence (Walsh, 2007). Today's families do not necessarily include children, and for those that do, the role of women working outside the home or being the primary or sole household provider has caused major changes in the predictable family life cycle. For instance, single-parent families account for 25% of U.S. households, with more than 50% of children spending some time in a single-parent home as a result of divorce (Walsh, 2007).

Despite these realities, the traditional stages of family development are still the standard against which many families measure themselves. Developmental tasks at the different stages of the family life cycle affect the family system. Because similar developmental tasks influence most families, knowledge of the family life cycle remains a useful road map in most cases. See Box 15.1 for a review of family developmental stages and tasks.

Role of the Family

Family serves as a personal care system that molds health and mobilizes health care. The roles of the "energized" or healthy family are to (1) respond to family members' needs, (2) cope actively with life's problems and stresses, (3) accomplish family tasks with equal distribution of power, (4) encourage interaction among family members and the community, and (5) promote positive personal health practices. Healthy families assume the role of socializing children while preserving cultural values and traditions.

Members, who play different roles within the family, also have roles in the community. A parent may provide financial resources for the family. Thus, he or she may have the role of

---

BOX 15.1 Family Development Stages and Tasks

Transitional Stage

- Separating from one's family of origin
- Developing intimate relationships
- Establishing independence in work and finances

Expanding Family Stage

Establishment Phase
- Building a mutually satisfying relationship
- Incorporating spouse/partner into relationships with extended family
- Setting up a household and delineating household responsibilities for each partner
- Planning for own family

Childbearing Phase
- Integrating an infant into the family
- Maintaining a satisfying couple relationship
- Expanding relationships with extended family by adding the parenting and grandparenting roles

Child rearing Phase
- Meeting basic physical needs of all family members
- Socializing children (peers, school, community)
- Integrating new child members while meeting needs of other children
- Maintaining a satisfying couple relationship

Contracting Family Stage

Child Launching Phase
- Releasing young adults to work, college, military service, and marriage with appropriate assistance
- Adjusting the couple relationship as children leave the family home
- Expanding the family circle with the marriage or relationships of children

Postparenting Phase
- Assisting aging parents
- Maintaining a healthy lifestyle
- Continuing relationships with children and parents
- Adjusting to retirement
- Strengthening the couple relationship

Aging Phase
- Finding a satisfactory living arrangement
- Maintaining a satisfying couple relationship
- Coping with the loss of a life partner
- Keeping intergenerational family connections open
- Accepting one's own mortality

teacher or attorney outside the home and the role of cook or rule setter for children inside the home. A child may also have outside roles such as student and inside roles such as table setter or baby-sitter for younger children. Roles vary with different families and situations. For example, many grandparents have active roles in providing child care. Healthy families can share, trade, and be flexible about roles. This flexibility allows for adaptation as situations demand. Unhealthy families tend to have rigid roles that do not allow for adaptation. Alternatively, they may be too flexible, which can lead to chaos (Walsh, 2007).

Family and Stress

The ABCX family crisis model can be used to describe how stress affects families (Hill, 1958). A (stress) interacts with B (the family's coping skills), and C (the family's perception of the stress) produces X (the crisis). McCubbin and Patterson used this model to create the Typology Model of Family Adjustment and Adaptation (McCubbin, 1995). Outlined in Figure 15.3, this model demonstrates how the family's circumstances, resources, perceptions, and level of stress interact to create outcomes.

Families, especially those dealing with chronic illness (eg, schizophrenia), face many stresses over time. Just as stressors may grow, resources for coping can also accumulate. Those who have faced chronic health problems may have past experiences or resources to use for assistance. They may have help from friends and the community, including the health care system and nurses. **Adaptation** is the outcome of adjusting to stress and is achieved through reciprocal relationships between family and community (McCubbin et al., 1999).

Models of family resiliency emphasize family adaptation to stress or crisis (Boss, 2006; Greff et al., 2006). While adjusting to stress, families try to maintain their usual interactions and roles. The only changes are first-order changes. The resiliency model suggests that families must make second-order changes during adaptation. They need to substantially change their patterns of interaction and roles if they are to cope with chronic illness or major trauma (e.g., divorce, death). To adapt successfully, they must draw on internal and community strengths and resources. Nurses can assist families to develop additional strengths and can connect members with appropriate community resources.

The circumplex model of marital and family systems identifies three dimensions of family behavior that help resilient families maneuver through adaptation (Olson & DeFrain, 2007). The first dimension, called *family cohesion,* refers to the solidity of the family system and ranges from separated and connected to disengaged and enmeshed. The second dimension, *family adaptability,* refers to the family's ability to be flexible and to change. It ranges from rigid and structured to flexible and chaotic. The third dimension, *family communication,* focuses on communication among family members and is considered critical to help them alter their levels of cohesion and flexibility to meet developmental or situational demands (Olson & DeFrain, 2007). The circumplex model represents the family as a dynamic, changing system, with second-order change as beneficial to functioning. It emphasizes the importance of second-order change as a family moves through stages of its development (life cycle). For example, a family may be cohesive when children are small, but become more disengaged as children leave home to establish their own residence. On the other hand, if a child has a chronic illness, the family may be more flexible and draw on respite services or support groups to maintain adaptation.

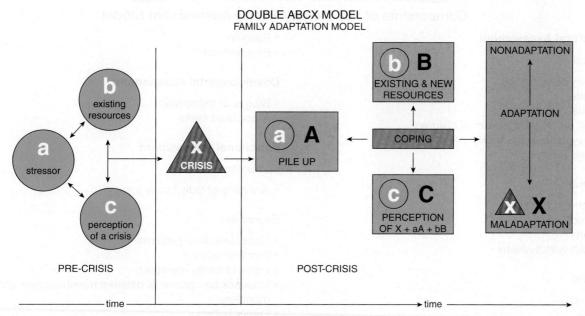

FIGURE 15.3 In the Typology Model of Family Adjustment and Adaptation, the accumulation of the family's historic and current circumstances, resources, perceptions, and level of stress interact and overlap to create outcomes. Such outcomes can include nonadaptation, maladaptation, and adaptation.

Strengths Perspective With Families

The family strength model focuses on the resilience of the family and resources in the environment (Early & Glen-Maye, 2000). It is based on a collaborative approach in which nurses form partnerships with families to achieve goals and outcomes. The emphasis is on the results that families, not nurses, desire. Together, they access resources, learn skills, and practice behaviors that they decide will improve family functioning. Families may need referral to counseling or other health care services to improve strengths and functioning. Nurses also may need to mobilize community resources such as respite care or transportation to and from health care.

Checkpoint Questions

4. How would one describe family roles in unhealthy families?
5. According to the resiliency model, during which phase would a family make second-order changes?
6. What are the three dimensions of family behavior identified by the circumplex model?
7. What is the emphasis of the family strength model?

NURSING ASSESSMENT WITH FAMILIES

The Calgary Family Assessment Model (CFAM) provides a guide that nurses can use to conduct assessments with families (Wright & Leahey, 2005). The CFAM has three major categories: structural, developmental, and functional assessment. Nurses proceed through the CFAM with the family, discussing the parts that seem appropriate for the particular circumstances of the individual members and family as a whole. Assessment Tool 15.1 reviews key components of each of the three categories of the CFAM.

Structural Assessment

Structural assessment includes subcategories of internal, external, and context. The *internal* subcategory involves family composition, gender and sexual orientation of members, rank or birth order of children, subsystems (e.g., mother and father, mother and daughter), and boundaries. *External* structure includes the extended family (e.g., grandparents, aunts, uncles, cousins) and larger systems such as school, church, and health care systems. *Context* includes ethnicity, race, social class, religion, and environment (e.g., housing, shopping, day care).

Two tools that can be helpful when doing a structural family assessment are the genogram and the ecomap. The **genogram** illustrates the family tree to show genetic connections; family transitions such as marriages, births, and deaths; and health conditions (Wright & Leahey, 2005) (Figure 15.4). It is most helpful if nurses actually draw genograms with families so that members can explain connections and transitions.

The **ecomap** illustrates the family's interaction with larger external systems (Figure 15.5). Again, nurses should construct these directly with families when possible. The

---

ASSESSMENT TOOL 15.1

Components of the Calgary Family Assessment Model

Structural Assessment

Internal

- Family composition
- Gender
- Sexual orientation
- Rank order or birth order of children
- Subsystems in the family
- Boundaries

External

- Extended family
- School
- Church
- Health care systems

Context

- Ethnicity
- Race
- Social class
- Religion
- Environment

Developmental Assessment

- Stages of the family
- Associated tasks

Functional Assessment

Instrumental

- Activities of daily family living

Expressive

- Communication patterns
- Problem solving
- Roles of family members
- Influence and power of different members over other members
- Family beliefs
- Alliances

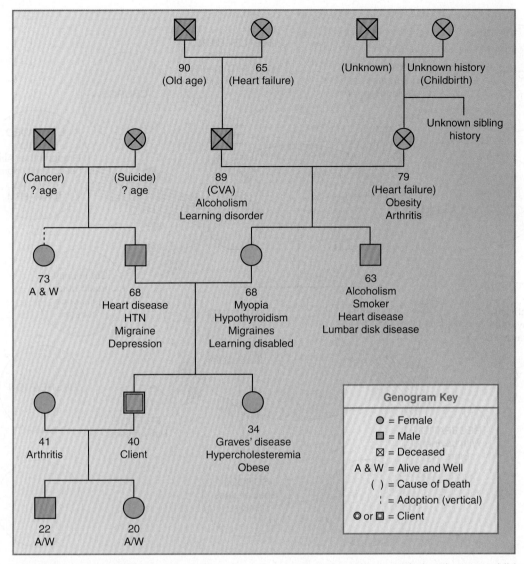

FIGURE 15.4 A genogram is a useful tool with which to identify genetic connections, marital and parent–child relationships, and health factors over time in a family.

ecomap starts with a circle that includes the family unit. Outside the circle are lines from each family member to the larger systems with which he or she interacts. The type of line depicts the nature of the family's relationship with external agencies and groups. The diagram can also show the strength and positive or conflicting nature of the relationships. For example, double or triple lines can denote positive attachment, whereas a train track can denote a troubled connection.

Developmental Assessment

The large category of developmental assessment includes an assessment of the family's capacity to complete important life-cycle tasks. For example, a family with young children has the task of socializing children to value kindness and learning. Questions and investigations depend on the particular stage and structure of the family in question. Refer to Box 15.1 for common tasks in different stages.

Functional Assessment

Functional assessment includes the subcategories of instrumental and expressive. The *instrumental* subcategory involves activities of daily living. Examples to review are each member's chores and responsibilities. The *expressive* subcategory includes interaction between and among family members: communication patterns (including nonverbal), problem solving, roles of family members, influence and power of different members over others, family beliefs, and alliances.

Cultural Considerations

Nurses must remember that ethnicity and culture play a large role in communication patterns, roles of the family, and family beliefs (Lynch & Hanson, 2004). They explore the family's ethnicity and cultural roots and are aware of the influences that these roots may have on family functioning.

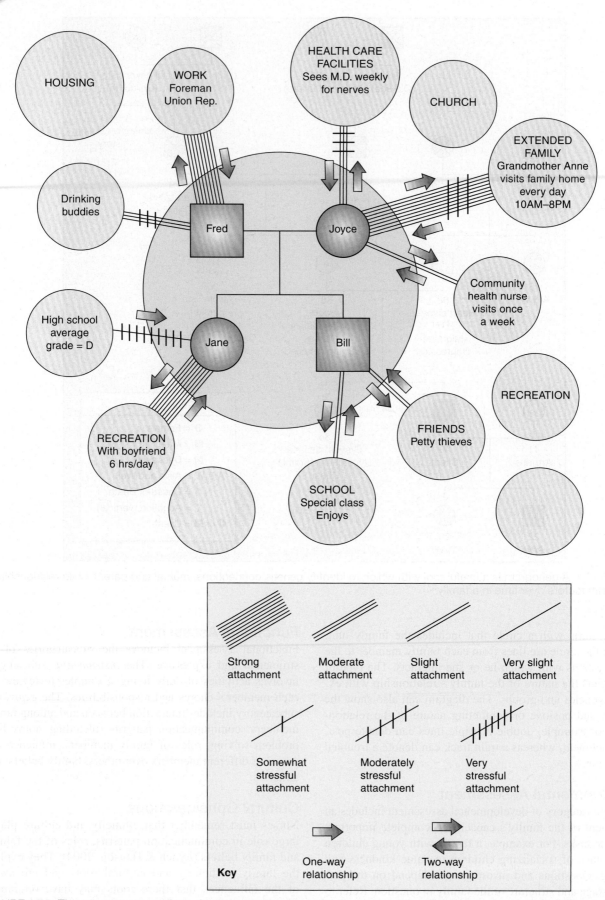

FIGURE 15.5 The ecomap can outline a family's relationships with its surrounding neighborhood and community.

NURSING INTERVENTIONS

Nursing Spotlight 15.1 reviews diagnoses, outcomes, and interventions commonly applicable to families.Such labels are wide ranging and depend on the specific issues or problems that each unit is facing. It is up to the family to accept suggested interventions when ready and to move through change at a pace that works for them.

Changing established patterns, boundaries, and roles is difficult and must involve all family members, who may accept change at different paces. Prochaska and colleagues (1992) established stages to better understand the continuum of change:

1. *Precontemplation:* No intention to change and perhaps no awareness of a problem
2. *Contemplation:* Awareness of a problem and thinking about change
3. *Preparation:* Getting ready to change
4. *Action:* Modifying behavior
5. *Maintenance:* Working to prevent relapse

Nurses may need to assist relatives to become aware of the different stages of change in each other and to tolerate differences in progress (Fahrenwald & Walker, 2003).

Cognitive Interventions

Each family is unique in terms of its tolerance for change. Changes in the cognitive domain—the way a family perceives its situation—are the most profound and sustaining (Wright & Leahey, 2005). An example of a cognitive nursing intervention is teaching a family about postpartum depression and resources available to help manage it (Wright & Leahey, 2005). Nurses build on family strengths and assist family members to find tools and resources that improve their understanding of their situation and foster hopefulness.

Affective Interventions

The affective domain involves the emotions. Related nursing interventions focus on easing emotional pain to enable the family to focus on problem solving. For example, a nurse might connect a family who has just learned of a member's diagnosis of Alzheimer's disease to a support group. Another is referring parents of a child with bulimia to an advanced practice psychiatric nurse or other mental health care provider who can provide family therapy. Nurses can assist family members to communicate their thoughts and fears about their current health stress or crisis with one another. Often, relatives can lessen their fears by learning that others have similar concerns or that another family member has agreed to take on a new role or behavior.

Behavioral Interventions

Behavioral interventions assist family members to interact with one another differently. One example might be assisting members to be caregivers by teaching procedures and techniques needed for home care or by offering respite care for a member who needs rest and time alone. A mother can learn exercises to conduct with a child who has cognitive

NURSING SPOTLIGHT 15.1

NANDA, NOC, and NIC Labels in Psychiatric Family Care

NANDA

- Deficient Knowledge
- Risk for Impaired Parent/Infant/Child attachment
- Risk for Caregiver Role Strain
- Compromised Family Coping
- Disabled Family Coping
- Interrupted Family Processes
- Readiness for Enhanced Family Processes
- Impaired Parenting
- Ineffective Family Therapeutic Regimen Management
- Parental Role Conflict

NOC

- Abuse Cessation
- Abuse Protection
- Caregiver Home Care Readiness
- Caregiver Stressors
- Caregiver Well-Being
- Caregiver–Patient Relationship
- Family Coping
- Family Functioning
- Family Health Status
- Family Integrity
- Family Normalization
- Family Participation in Professional Care
- Family Physical Environment
- Family Resiliency
- Family Social Climate
- Family Support During Treatment
- Parenting Performance
- Role Performance

NIC

- Abuse Protection Support: Child
- Abuse Protection Support: Domestic Partner
- Abuse Protection Support: Elder
- Caregiver Role Strain
- Development Enhancement: Child
- Family Involvement Promotion
- Family Therapy
- Home Maintenance Assistance
- Parenting Promotion
- Respite Care
- Risk Identification
- Risk Identification: Childbearing Family
- Role Enhancement
- Sibling Support
- Support System Enhancement

Sources: Bulechek, G. M., Butcher, H. K., & McCloskey Dochterman, J. (2008). *Nursing interventions classification (NIC)* (5th ed.). St. Louis, MO: Mosby; Moorhead, S., Johnson, M., Maas, M. L., & Swanson, E. (2008). *Nursing outcomes classification (NOC)* (4th ed.). St. Louis, MO: Mosby; NANDA International. (2007). *Nursing International nursing diagnoses: Definitions and classification, 2009–2011.* Philadelphia, PA: Wiley-Blackwell.

dysfunction, and a husband may offer respite care so that she can spend time with other children in the family. This same family may also require visits from a home care nurse so that the parents and other children can spend time together or assume roles outside the family.

FAMILIES OF CLIENTS WITH MENTAL ILLNESS

And it's like you've got to constantly be on your toes, but you've got to, uh, make it all as normal as possible. It's like OK. Bad news, how do you do that? It seems like it's a matter of adjusting all the time, every day, hour to hour, you know minute to minute, you know (Wade, 2006).

Before state asylums were established in the mid-19th century, people with mental illness in the United States lived where vast numbers of them live now: on the streets, in homes for the poor or ailing, in jails, and *with their families.* During the past 150 years, Americans with **serious and persistent mental illness (SPMI)** have literally journeyed to the asylum and back. Today, most clients with SPMI live within the community. Associated stresses for their families can be tremendous (Saunders, 2003).

Family Burden

Researchers have conceptualized the stresses that families experience when a loved one has SPMI as **family burden**. Some families recall the exact moment they became aware that something was wrong with their relative. Others take years to identify the warning signs and try to normalize puzzling behaviors. This is commonly called *denial,* but it is more appropriate to call it *disbelief.* As the sister of a man with schizophrenia recalls, "When he quit Harvard to travel cross country, we thought he was 'finding himself.'" A father says, "When our daughter started to send hundred dollar bills to television evangelists, we didn't think 'manic'; we thought 'born again Christian.'"

When ill clients finally begin treatment, relatives learn the painful lesson that psychiatry is not an exact science. Many families expect a speedy recovery, only to find their loved ones never fully recover or that the process of healing is quite lengthy. Moreover, the first diagnosis is not always correct and can be one of many (Brady & McCain, 2004; Wade, 2006).

Objective Burden

Objective burden refers to the practical problems family members encounter while caring for ill relatives. Examples include housing, food and laundry, transportation, medication management, money management, companionship and recreation, crisis intervention, and mediation with the police (Figure 15.6) (Grandon et al., 2008). When hospitals discharge clients with mental illness, case managers employed by the mental health system are supposed to help navigate ongoing needs (see Chap. 20). However, because of high caseloads and a high rate of employee turnover, much responsibility falls to families.

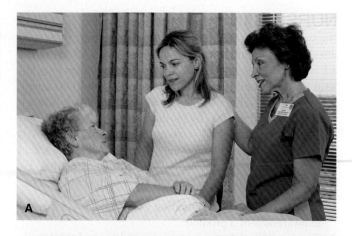

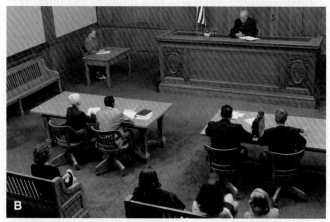

FIGURE 15.6 **(A)** Objective family burden in caring for loved ones with SPMI may involve dealing with crises related to illness relapse. **(B)** Families may also struggle with a loved one's ongoing legal problems as a consequence of actions taken while suffering from psychiatric symptoms.

Caregiving, even if construed as a labor of love, remains demanding. Families cope with behaviors that can be embarrassing, irresponsible, disturbing, bizarre, frustrating, and sometimes dangerous (Wynaden et al., 2006). Although violence is rare when clients are receiving treatment, relatives are the usual target when it does occur. Families are also painfully aware of the elevated suicide risk in clients with mental illness (Case Vignette 15.1).

One father recalled an incident with his daughter who had bipolar disorder, "She was picking out trees that she wanted to hang herself from. I talked to the maintenance people about cutting them down" (Wade, 2006).

Nurse researchers have described the seemingly endless effects of mental illness as a story with a beginning and middle—but no end (Tuck et al., 1997). Even when the relative's condition improves, a crisis can recall the caregiver to active duty. Parental concern about "what will happen when I am gone" is so widespread that more than 25 years ago, it acquired its own acronym, WIAG (Lefley, 1987). Siblings, the successor candidates, entertain mixed feelings about inheriting the caregiver role. In the words of a member of a sibling support group, "I am not looking forward to being in charge of my sister. I love her, but she is a very high maintenance person."

Case Vignette 15.1

I was in my office when I received a call informing me that the child of one of our members had committed suicide the night before. My first thought was "Oh, my God, how horrible!" Then came my next thought, "Thank God, it wasn't my son."

The next morning at the graveside, it was extremely hot and humid. Carrying my sport coat over my arm, I got under the canopy just to escape the direct sunlight. From that vantage point, I looked at the people who had assembled to pay their last respects.

A dozen or so immediate family members, including a twin sister, sat closest to the coffin. A group of about 15 people stood at the rear. They were from the community residential unit where Tommy lived and included several well-dressed professional staff members as well as the residents. The residents wore ill-fitting clothes and kept their eyes lowered toward the ground.

None of Tommy's friends from high school, college, or the Army was present. Many of us take for granted the ability to make and keep friends, but doing so is hard for people with psychiatric disorders. Their "inappropriate behavior," as we euphemistically call it, and their frequent "decompensations" often preclude lasting friendships.

The largest contingent was from our NAMI chapter, of which Tommy's mother is the secretary. Although the rest of us had never met Tommy, we could all empathize with the family's tragedy. Perhaps they have a sense of relief, knowing they no longer have to care for an adult who could not care for himself. Or they may be thinking, "If only we had visited him last weekend" or "If only we had him over to dinner more often." There will probably be no end to the "If onlys" the family thinks of. There is a definite limit, however, to the time and energy a family can devote to one member and still carry on somewhat normal lives.

Why Tommy took his life will never be fully known. Did he decide life was no longer worth living? Did a voice tell him to do it? What makes this tragedy even sadder is that only 2 days ago, I received a flyer from our state NAMI informing us that two new drugs for schizophrenia will soon be available. They might have improved Tommy's condition.

Since his discharge from the U.S. Army, Tommy had been a prisoner of a semi-functional mind that kept him from holding a job, maintaining friendships, managing his money, or even grocery shopping by himself. Tommy is now free of the mind that made him an outcast. He no longer has to grieve internally while watching his former friends do many things he could not. He no longer has to watch people self-righteously turning away from him or hear people whispering about him behind his back. In the words of an old Negro spiritual, He's free at last! Thank God Almighty, Tommy's free at last! All we can do now is extend our deepest sympathy to the family and continue to advocate for other people like Tommy.

Reflection and Critical Thinking

- Why do you think a 24-year-old college graduate and Army veteran with schizophrenia would commit suicide?
- What do you imagine Tommy's twin sister was thinking and feeling at the funeral?
- Would you predict that Tommy's family would continue to advocate for an improved mental health system?
- What kinds of thoughts were going through the minds of the residents of the mental health center?

Ron Schwarz, DVD, NAMI Georgia

Checkpoint Questions
8. What term is used to describe the stresses or effects of SPMI on a family?
9. In cases of violence involving a client receiving treatment for SPMI, who is the usual target?

Subjective Burden

Subjective burden refers to the grief, fear, guilt, anger, and other negative emotions that family members experience in response to a loved one's mental illness. Because the grief seems interminable, many relatives experience chronic sorrow. Several encounter health care professionals who misconstrue their signs of grief:

> In all the therapy we participated in and in all our communications with the professionals who worked with our son, it was never suggested to us that our responses (of fright, anxiety, guilt and self-doubt) were an expression of normal grief and indeed we as well as our son had lost something precious. Why is it that a discipline whose major focus is on feelings,

thoughts, and relationships has so little to say about grief and loss? (MacGregor, 1994)

Another common problem is *fear*. Many grieving relatives have experienced the same fear-like feeling: fluttering in the stomach and restlessness. But they also notice explicit fear, asking such questions as "Is this illness going to put us in the poor house?" and "It costs $10,000 per month to keep him in the hospital. How can we afford that?" Many family members feel as if they are walking along a precipice, afraid to make a wrong move. "I just panicked. I would cry, and I'd have to go to work, and I just spent all my energy trying to figure out what to do. I was so scared" (Mohr & Regan-Kubinski, 2001).

Guilt, a common response when a relative succumbs to any serious illness, is exaggerated in psychiatric illness because of unfounded beliefs related to parental causation. Siblings, too, often irrationally agonize over being well and living a "normal" life while their brothers or sisters must contend with mental problems.

Family members direct *anger* irrationally at themselves, one another, the ill relative, God, or treating professionals.

Kayla Bernheim and Anthony Lehman, co-authors of the first book on the subject of mental health professionals working with families, attributed family hostility to guilt and fear about the illness, resistance to acceptance of chronic disability and its implications for their lives, and previous, negative experiences with the treatment system. These authors urged families to use anger constructively to change the system and called advocacy sublimation of the healthiest, most adaptive kind (Bernheim & Lehman, 1985). See Case Vignette 15.2.

Iatrogenic Burden

Iatrogenic burden is attributable to a flawed mental health system and to the attitudes and behaviors of some professionals who cling to outmoded theories about families and mental illness. In addition to generalized system failure, families identify confidentiality laws, involuntary treatment laws, and discrimination in insurance, treatment, housing, and employment as specific sources of burden.

Confidentiality Issues

With respect to confidentiality, families have a legitimate need for information related to diagnosis, current treatment, medications, community resources, and effective strategies for managing the illness. When family caregivers are not involved, the client's progress is likely to be slower. In worst-case scenarios, the results can be tragic. In the

---

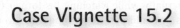

Case Vignette 15.2

My husband and I will celebrate 25 years of married life this April. Twenty-five years ago, I did not know how our marriage would go. He was diagnosed with schizophrenia, and I knew next to nothing about mental illness. I only knew that I loved him, and I had to try to make marriage work. He was a doctoral candidate then, and now is retired from 30 years in state service, working with the most seriously mentally ill as a clinical psychologist.

Initially I had hoped that the schizophrenia would go away, but I learned that mental illnesses are long-term, even lifetime conditions. When he would become symptomatic, I would get very anxious; torturing myself with all kinds of "what ifs...." Eventually, I learned the pattern: excitement leading to expansive thinking; a rush of activity and self-absorption (living in his head); increased medication followed by a period of crashing; and then back to normal. These episodes occurred every year to 18 months; and with each passing episode they became less worrisome to me.

I also had to learn what the illness meant on a daily basis. Some activities are more difficult for him than others, such as those requiring attention to details or high degrees of organization. Gradually, a division of labor evolved that worked for us. I picked up those responsibilities that were problematic for him, and he supported me in taking care of things that were hard for me to attend to while teaching at the university. He was very successful with his work and was always able to provide for us, and we were very fortunate that insurance always covered our mental health expenses.

Although these illnesses have a genetic component, we had hoped that our children would escape them. One by one, however, as they entered puberty, they began to exhibit symptoms. I later discovered that depression runs in my side of the family, so our children were getting genes from both sides. Because by this time we were active in the family movement, and Fred was a Board member of NAMI, we had a broad circle of friends who could support us with good advice. Getting help for our children was not easy, as childhood mental illnesses were only beginning to appear on the radar screen, and we had some scary times with children whose lives were rapidly deteriorating—but once again Providence carried us. We decided to be very open about mental illness in our family, treating it as one would any other medical disorder. Mental health providers and the children's school systems really worked with us to help bring them through the onset of their illnesses.

When the worst was over and our children's lives were stabilized, we all dedicated ourselves more diligently to increasing understanding of mental illness in the general public. We accepted speaking engagements as a family, and eventually produced a video on childhood depression. This advocacy work increased our children's self-esteem while educating them about their illness. As it turned out it also gave them wonderful resumes for college. Their advocacy was admired at school, and they were even called on to talk with other students who were experiencing difficulties.

With everyone in the family diagnosed with a mental illness and taking medication, except me, sensitivity and compassion among family members increased. We learned to recognize the heightened sensitivity that comes with these disorders and to soften our interactions with one another. It was OK to back off from tasks that were overwhelming and return to them later when we felt better equipped to deal with them. It was OK to sleep at just about anytime. In fact, in our house, you could probably find someone asleep and someone awake at almost any time of the day or night.

A zany, delightful sense of humor prevailed, the kind that happens with people who go through difficult times together. And in the dark times, faith saw us through. Today we are doing well, aware that there are still difficult times ahead, but having enough successes behind us to give us confidence that we will be able to meet the hard times when they come.

Reflection and Critical Thinking

- What signs did Penny Frese learn to recognize as signaling the return of her husband's symptoms?
- What accommodations in their daily routine did the couple make to cope with the illness?
- To what mission did the family members dedicate themselves after everyone's conditions were stabilized?
- Name three factors that contributed to this family's resiliency. (Hint: One of them is love.)

Penny Frese, PhD

well-publicized case of Andrea Yates, the Texas woman who murdered her five children while suffering from severe depression, her husband testified that her professional caregivers never told him that she had fantasies of violence and voiced fears of harming others (McLellan, 2006).

Despite this, nurses and other health care providers must work within strict laws that protect against the divulgence of confidential information without the explicit permission of clients themselves. In cases in which clients are struggling with mental illness, the difficulty for families in accessing information to help their loved ones can be challenging, frustrating, and time consuming.

Involuntary Treatment Statutes

Involuntary treatment statutes originally intended to protect citizens from being "put away" by unconcerned or conniving families now prevent *caring families* from getting loved ones into treatment before their symptoms escalate dangerously. Families point to people with psychiatric disorders eating out of garbage cans and cite media accounts of violent acts committed by untreated people. They contend that the *right to treatment* should outweigh the *right to refuse treatment* when a person does not recognize that he or she is ill simply because he or she is ill. In such cases, the illness blocks the ability to evaluate one's health objectively.

Discrimination

Discriminatory practices persist in insurance coverage despite advocacy for parity with nonpsychiatric disorders, and in housing and employment despite statutes that forbid it. Managed care companies discriminate by limiting access to rehabilitation strategies on the grounds that they are not a medical necessity.

Burden Attributable to Professionals

Burden attributable to professionals is decreasing as those schooled in theories that led to the misunderstanding of families experiencing SPMI retire from practice and academia or change their treatment approaches. Unfortunately, old attitudes—even as they fade away—leave a legacy in terms of disinterest in the needs of families and failure to provide family services. For example, mothers have been prevented from visiting their ill children in psychiatric hospitals because they were believed to have caused the illness (e.g., "schizophrenogenic mothers") (Johnson, 2001).

Family members and professionals from the National Alliance on Mental Illness (NAMI) have been advocating for change in the preservice training programs of psychiatric disciplines since 1980. One of NAMI's ongoing goals is to make the training of mental health professionals *more relevant to the needs of people with SPMI and their families.* The first objective in nursing education was to produce graduates prepared to respond to the needs of the most vulnerable populations. Echoing the distinguished nursing leader who questioned whether nursing would ever respond to the unmet needs of people who are chronically mentally ill (Aiken, 1987), NAMI advocated for nurses prepared to work "in the

trenches" with the community residents who in years past would have been in state hospitals. The second objective was to dispel the delusion that families caused mental illness and to cast them in new roles as treatment allies. That message is welcome. Families are allies to be consulted, not pathologized and excluded from treatment.

> ### Checkpoint Questions
> **10.** What four common subjective burdens do family members experience in response to a loved one's mental illness?
> **11.** How does iatrogenic burden affect the care of people with SPMI and their families?

Families as a Population at Risk

Although psychiatric nursing textbooks mention **secondary prevention** with respect to other types of trauma, they often fail to mention it in relation to mental illness. Caregiver burnout (which then puts clients at risk of homelessness); damaged interpersonal relationships, including broken marriages; developmental delay in younger family members; and stress-related health problems for all members are significant risks for families experiencing mental illness. There are also known genetic risks for mental illness that vary according to the family member's relationship to the ill person (Sadock & Sadock, 2007).

Risk attributable to living in proximity to mental illness has received less attention than genetic risk, and research examining correlates and outcomes of the effects of mental illness on family caregivers is lacking. Potential consequences of caregiver burden include depression, sleep deprivation, irritability, substance abuse, marital discord, and other stress-related health problems (e.g., stroke, cardiac conditions, asthma, smoking). Subjective family burden may also correlate with self-reports of poor health among family caregivers (Awad & Voruganti, 2008).

Family Consultation

Family consultation is a secondary prevention strategy based on the assumption that the model family dealing with SPMI is healthy and competent, but lacks sufficient knowledge and skills. In the role of family consultant, nurses *mentor* families to expand their experientially based knowledge and to help them access NAMI or other family organizations. They also *support* families with empathic understanding, help them set priorities and problem solve, and refer them to clinical services, including psychotherapy, grief counseling, marital counseling, or medications. Ultimately, it is up to the family members to select the interventions they want to receive, and the choice is likely to vary with their evolving needs and circumstances.

Components

Families consult with a mental health professional for advice about mental illness. In a typical situation, the family consultant makes a "secondary prevention scan" by asking how

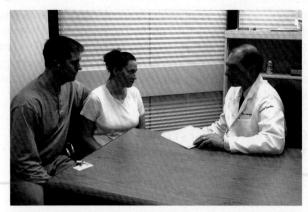

FIGURE 15.7 Health providers performing family consultation concentrate on what will be most helpful for the family in question based on their communicated interests, needs, desires, and requests.

family members are getting along and how he or she can help them (Figure 15.7). The format for family consultation is flexible; this discussion reviews the "Three F" approach: feeling, focus, and finding.

• In the *feeling stage,* the consultant acknowledges the feelings of all family members and tries to normalize them with statements such as "If that happened to me, I'd be angry, too."

• In the *focus stage,* the consultant helps relatives set priorities, a process that may depend on finding the common denominator in competing issues. If the mother of a daughter with bipolar disorder is concerned because the daughter is a messy housekeeper, the father worries because she runs up the telephone bill, and the sister is tired of lending her clothes, the common denominator is "setting limits."

• *Finding the solution* is the final stage. As the expert on mental illness, the consultant takes the lead in finding solutions, but the family also contributes their own experientially based expertise.

Nurses as Family Consultants

Family consultation can take place in family sessions called specifically for this purpose, on an impromptu basis whenever the nurse and family members happen to meet, and even by telephone. The knowledge base required by nurses functioning as family consultants includes thorough understanding of SPMI and treatment, empathy about family burden, caregiving skills, and awareness of government entitlement programs and community resources, including those offered by family advocacy organizations. Consultants also need teaching skills and the ability to communicate with clarity and respect.

The need for *clarity* is not based on the belief that family members experience *communication deviance,* as was once assumed. Rather, it is based on the recognition that families are under stress and likely to be preoccupied and anxious. Furthermore, some family members share (to a lesser degree) the same problems with concentration and memory that trouble their ill relatives. Consultants

try to compensate for possible cognitive problems by repeating information and writing down key points. Some consultants advise family members to use a tape recorder.

Respect is an indispensable component of effective communication. To be respectful means to recognize the expertise that family caregivers have acquired through experience and to assume until proved otherwise that they are doing the best they can and have the best interests of their relatives at heart. In family language, the concepts of *enabling* and *codependency* translate into *adding insult to injury.* Family members are especially affronted when these labels are used stereotypically, without taking time to get to know the people involved. In Therapeutic Communication 15.1, the nurse in the ineffective dialogue not only fails to respond to Mr. Silverman's distress when he enters the office, but she assumes that he and his wife had something to do with the son's explosive behavior. This assumption strikes the father as both irrelevant and disrespectful, and he turns defensive. The nurse actually intends no disrespect; she is simply pursuing a line of reasoning suggested to her by family systems theory (ie, the putative association between marital discord and the client's symptoms). Nevertheless, her comment angers the father and ends the session before the real reason for Eric's behavior becomes apparent.

In the effective dialogue, the nurse responds with empathy to Mr. Silverman before they even began to talk about Eric. With his feelings validated, the father relaxes and, with the nurse's prompting, relates the events that turned out to be the probable cause of Eric's behavior. The information can be useful in terms of Eric's vulnerability to relapse, but in the meantime, the nurse again empathizes with the father, who truly was "having a rough time."

Checkpoint Questions

12. What are the three stages of family consultation?

13. When the nurse is acting as a family consultant and communicating with the family, which two elements are crucial?

Family Empowerment

All communication, regardless of its specific purpose in terms of conveying information or teaching skills to family members, must support the family members' sense of self-worth. In the vocabulary of the community support program movement, this is called **family empowerment**, the companion piece to *client empowerment.*

Currently, family empowerment is more of a dream than a reality. Family support services for family caregivers are lacking despite the evidence of their value for clients and caregivers (Doornbos, 2002). Family advocacy organizations have tried to address this shortage by starting support groups for caregivers in all parts of the country. Peer support groups can be beneficial in terms of reducing family burden and increasing coping and adaptation. NAMI affiliates offer a wide range of support and educational services, with programs such as:

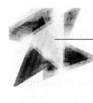

Therapeutic Communications 15.1

Family Consultation

Mr. Silverman, the father of a 30-year-old man with schizophrenia, enters the community mental health center office of the nurse who sees his son for weekly blood work to ensure that his treatment with Clozaril is not affecting his white cell count.

INEFFECTIVE DIALOGUE

NURSE: Is Eric with you?

Mr. S.: No, he refused to come.

NURSE: Mr. Silverman, it's very important that Eric gets his blood work done. What is wrong?

Mr. S.: Eric threw a chair through the living room wall. That's what's wrong!

NURSE: *(Thinking)* Hmmm. Mr. Silverman, what is going on at home?

Mr. S.: *(Baffled)* I just told you. Eric got mad and threw a chair through the wall.

NURSE: I heard what you said, Mr. Silverman. But, i mean, have you and Mrs. Silverman been having any problems lately? Arguments perhaps?

Mr. S.: *(Defensively)* What's that got to do with anything? It's Eric we're talking about!

EFFECTIVE DIALOGUE

NURSE: Good morning, Mr. Silverman. Is eric with you?

Mr. S.: No, he refused to come.

NURSE: Why? What's wrong?

Mr. S.: Eric threw a chair through the living room wall.

NURSE: You must be very upset.

Mr. S.: To tell the truth, i am. I just can't figure out what got into Eric.

NURSE: Maybe we can figure it out together. Tell me more about it.

Mr. S.: Well, for one thing, i suspect he hasn't been taking medicine the way he's supposed to. His mother keeps tabs on that, and she's been away since friday.

NURSE: Where did she go?

Mr. S.: She went to ohio to see her mother, and while she was there, her mother had a slight stroke.

NURSE: I am so sorry to hear that. Eric has mentioned his grandmother to me, and I know he's very fond of her. How did he take the news?

Mr. S.: You know that's a funny thing. Eric didn't seem bothered at all when his mother called about the stroke. He just went into his room for a real long time, and when he came out, that's when he threw the chair through the wall.

NURSE: Mr. Silverman, i can see you're having a rough time. What can i do to help?

Reflection and Critical Thinking

- How do you think Mr. Silverman was feeling when he entered the office? How did he feel as a result of the nurse's responses in the ineffective dialogue? The effective dialogue?
- What was the nurse's hypothesis about the cause of Eric's behavior in the ineffective dialogue? Was she on the right track or the wrong track?
- What did the nurse in the effective dialogue accomplish when she said, "Tell me more about it." What did she accomplish when she said, "What can I do to help?"

- Hand-to-Hand, an educational course of eight sessions for families with children or adolescents with mental illness or emotional disorders
- Family-to-Family, a 12-session, 36-hour course for families of adults with serious mental illness
- NAMI-CAN, a monthly support group for families of children and adolescents with mental illness
- NAMI Rap Session, a monthly group for families of adults with serious mental illness

- NAMI-CARE, support groups for adult clients
- Grief and Loss group, monthly support meetings with a nurse in attendance
- Depression and Manic/Depression group, a monthly support group (NAMI, 2011)

Family Education

Although family education has been part of the nurse's role since the days of Florence Nightingale, the families of people with medical illnesses (e.g., diabetes, heart disease) have been the primary beneficiaries. In contrast, the families of clients with psychiatric problems seldom receive educational services from any mental health professional. A 1998 report by the Schizophrenia Patient Outcomes Research Team (PORT) confirmed that only 10% of the family caregivers of people with schizophrenia received any kind of education (Lehman & Steinwachs, 1998). The 10% included caregivers who were merely handed a brochure or a package insert from a pharmaceutical company. More than 10 years later, the Schizophrenia PORT summarized effective evidence-based psychosocial interventions and recommended that key elements of family interventions include illness education, crisis intervention, emotional support, and training in how to cope with illness symptoms and related problems. The selection of a family intervention should be guided by collaborative decision making among the client, family, and clinician (Dixon et al., 2010).

Components

Agnes Hatfield, a professor of education at the University of Maryland and a founding member of NAMI, introduced **family education**. She asked NAMI families what they wanted from family therapists and found that they wanted education, not therapy (Hatfield, 1983). Using her training in the principles of adult education, her personal experience as a caregiver for an ill son, and extensive interviews with other caregivers, Hatfield wrote the manual *Coping With Mental Illness in the Family* for family use and to train providers in community mental health centers to offer family education. Hatfield since has written extensively on family education and acquired an international reputation as a specialist in this area.

The successful outcome measures for family education are reduced family burden and improvement in the family's quality of life. Client improvement often accompanies this outcome, but it is not a primary goal.

Nurses as Family Educators

Mary Moller and Jo Ann Wer (1989) pioneered family education by nurses but referred to it as *simultaneous family/patient education* because they taught families and clients in the same classes. Moller made a series of videos on preventing relapse and communicating with people who were hallucinating or delusional and made them available to both family and professional caregivers. Today family psychoeducational interventions are commonplace and used successfully with clients experiencing severe mental illness such as schizophrenia (Lukens & Thorning, 2010) and mood disorders (Miklowitz & Goldstein, 2010).

Peer-Taught Family Education

Social workers in collaboration with NAMI Kansas introduced peer-taught family education in 1987. The first program to reach families throughout the entire country was the NAMI Family-to-Family Education Program, a 12-session, 36-hour curriculum based on a trauma-recovery model. The course is taught by a team of trained family members, using a curriculum written by Joyce Burland, PhD, a NAMI family member psychologist. To qualify for training as teachers, applicants must have a relative with SPMI and be recommended by a local NAMI affiliate. Many course teachers are nurses.

NAMI's Family-to-Family Education Program reduces subjective family burden and increases the family's sense of empowerment with respect to the mental health system, the community, and the family (Dixon et al., 2004). The Family-to-Family course is one of several programs offered free of charge through NAMI state affiliates. In addition to the NAMI programs, other community-based, family-led programs, such as the Journey of Hope education course, seek to strengthen families' coping competencies. Curricula cover brain biology, medications, the mental health systems, problem-solving skills, and mechanisms of family support (Pickett-Schenk et al., 2008).

Psychotherapy and Medication

Although the nonclinical services described earlier in the chapter meet the needs of most families, an important minority chooses more extensive services. For example, some family members choose psychotherapy, medication, or both. Some couples want to receive counseling to help them work together constructively as caregivers.

In a study of siblings and offspring, 77% of participants reported using psychotherapy as adults; among those who were younger than 10 years when their relative became ill, the percentage rose to 90% (Marsh, 1998). Many of these siblings and offspring regretted that no one had offered them supportive or therapeutic services when they were children. Optimally, support services should be provided to pregnant women with mental illness to help them have the best start possible in child rearing (Mowbray et al., 2004).

Another factor creating the need for clinical services for caregivers is that in many families, more than one member has a psychiatric diagnosis. Instead of a "well spouse" caring for an "ill spouse," two ill spouses may serve as one another's caregivers. This situation is more common today because clients living in the community have opportunities to meet one another, date, and marry. It is also not unusual for mental illness to span two generations, as was reported by a client member of the NAMI Provider Course teaching team:

> Because my mother had schizophrenia, my father left us when we were small. My grandparents helped raise us, but they both died before I got through college. I took off on a trip around the world, but in Crete I thought I saw my grandparents rising from their graves. The authorities decided I had schizophrenia and sent me home. My mother and my brother—who by then were also diagnosed with schizophrenia—met me at the airport. I have now been taking Clozaril for 10 years. My mother and my brother and I try to help one another.

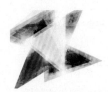

Reviewing and Applying Your Knowledge

Chapter Summary

- Nurses, working with the family unit, can promote family health and assist families to adapt to stressors such as psychiatric illness, divorce, or death.

- The family is a system that interacts with the subsystems of family members and larger systems, such as the community and health care. Families follow a path called the *family life cycle*. The family has the role of protecting those in the unit and socializing members with the values and culture of past generations. The family unit, when faced with a crisis, must make a second-order change that reorders the roles and interactions of family members.

- Nurses intervene to assist families in building on strengths and helping perceive crises with hope. By connecting families to resources within and without, nurses collaborate with them to improve their situation and bring them to a higher level of functioning.

- Nurses work with families of those with psychiatric disorders for two purposes: to help them cope with the traumatic effects of mental illness and caregiving and to involve them as allies in their ill relatives' treatments.

- The stress associated with caregiving is conceptualized as family burden, further divided into objective (the practical aspects of caregiving) and subjective (the emotional response).

- A large part of family burden is iatrogenic, meaning that it stems from a dysfunctional mental health system or from the attitudes and behaviors of mental health professionals who generalize about families on the basis of outdated theories. Stigma and discrimination in housing, employment, and insurance coverage, as well as confidentiality laws and involuntary commitment laws, are additional sources of burden.

- The family members of people with SPMI are a population at risk for genetically linked mental illnesses, stress-related medical disorders and social problems, or both.

- Family consultation designed to reduce family burden is a prime example of a needed secondary prevention strategy.

- Nurses functioning as family consultants mentor families, meaning they provide information and advice about mental illness and caregiving; support families with empathy, grief counseling, and conflict mediation; and provide access to psychotherapy, marriage counseling, and medication, as needed.

- Effective communication with families is clear and respectful and based on the assumption (unless proven otherwise) that families are doing their best and have the client's best interests at heart.

- Although most family members' needs are met by non-clinical services (support and education), a minority (including caregivers who are also clients) needs clinical services (psychotherapy, marriage counseling, and medication prescription).

- Family advocacy organizations, such as NAMI, are excellent resources for family and professional caregivers.

Study Questions

1. The nurse, using the family as the unit of care, approaches the illness of a family member by

   a. including the family as the context for the ill member.

   b. assessing how the family views the illness of the member.

   c. maintaining his or her role as the person in charge.

   d. partnering with the family.

2. When assessing a family, which of the following roles would lead the nurse to suspect that the family is healthy? Select all that apply.

   a. Socializing members with societal values

   b. Passively coping with stresses

   c. Maintaining rigid boundaries

   d. Promoting positive personal health practices

   e. Encouraging interaction with the community

   f. Distributing power equally to accomplish tasks

3. When developing a plan of care using the resiliency model for a family experiencing a crisis, which of the following would the nurse expect to include to achieve family adaptation?

   a. Maintaining usual family roles

   b. Making first-order changes

   c. Limiting connections to resources

   d. Building on family strengths

(continues on page 282)

4. The nurse is interviewing the 81-year-old mother of a 51-year-old client who has had schizophrenia since 16 years of age. Which of the mother's concerns is likely to dominate?

   a. Will my retirement funds outlast me?

   b. Who will handle my funeral arrangements?

   c. What will become of my son when I am gone?

   d. How can I get my son's doctor to talk to me?

5. Which of the following statements by family members would the nurse identify as an example of subjective burden?

   a. "Our daughter's illness has really drained our savings account."

   b. "If only we had been able to realize he was sick sooner."

   c. "We don't know how we're going manage the day-to-day things."

   d. "We've had to call the police several times when he got out of control."

Critical Thinking Questions

1. What aspects of family burden do siblings and offspring share? What option does a spouse have that other family members lack? What prevents this option from being a good one?

2. Which family member is likely to help out when one parent is ill and the other one has to earn a living?

3. What is likely to be an aging parent's primary concern about an ill child?

References

Aiken, H. L. (1987). Unmet needs of the chronically mentally ill: Will nursing respond? *Image: Journal of Nursing Scholarship, 19*(3), 121–125.

Awad, A. G., & Voruganti, L. N. (2008). The burden of schizophrenia on caregivers: A review. *Pharmacoeconomics, 26*(2), 149–162.

Bernheim, K. F., & Lehman, A. F. (1985). *Working with families of the mentally ill.* New York, NY: W. W. Norton.

Boss, P. (2006). *Loss, trauma, and resilience: Therapeutic work with ambiguous loss.* New York, NY: W. W. Norton.

Brady, N., & McCain, G. C. (2004). Living with schizophrenia: A family perspective. *Online Journal of Issues in Nursing, 10*(1), 7.

Dixon, L. B., Dickerson, F., Bellack, A. S., Bennett, M., Dickinson, D., Goldberg, R. W., ... Kreyenbuhl, J. (2010).The 2009 schizophrenia PORT psychosocial treatment recommendations and summary statements. *Schizophrenia Bulletin, 36,* 48–70.

Dixon, L., Lucksted, A., Stewart, B., Burland, J., Brown, C. H., Postrado, L., ... Hoffman, M. (2004). Outcomes of the peer-taught 12-week family-to-family education program for severe mental illness. *Acta Psychiatrica Scandinavia, 109*(3), 207–215.

Doornbos, M. M. (2002). Family caregivers and the mental health system: Reality and dreams. *Archives of Psychiatric Nursing, 16*(1), 39–46.

Duvall, E. (1977). *Marriage and family development* (6th ed.). New York, NY: Harper & Row.

Early, T., & GlenMaye, L. (2000). Valuing families: Social work practice with families from a strengths perspective. *Social Work, 45*(2), 118–130.

Fahrenwald, N., & Walker, S. N. (2003). Application of the transtheoretical model of behavior change to the physical activity behavior of WIC mothers. *Public Health Nursing, 20*(4), 307–317.

Grandon, P., Jenaro, C., & Lemos, S. (2008). Primary caregivers of schizophrenia outpatients: Burden and predictor variables. *Psychiatry Research, 158,* 335–343.

Greff, A. P., Vansteenwegen, A., & Ide, M. (2006). Resiliency in families with a member with a psychological disorder. *American Journal of Family Therapy, 34,* 285–300.

Hatfield, A. B. (1983). What families want from family therapists. In W. R. McFarlane (Ed.), *Family therapy of schizophrenia* (pp. 41–65). New York, NY: Guilford Press.

Hill, R. (1958). Generic features of families under stress. *Social Caseworker, 49,* 139–150.

Hill, R. (1970). *Family development in three generations.* Cambridge, MA: Schenkman.

Jackson, D. (1967). Play, paradox, and people: Power and education. *Medical Opinion and Review, 3,* 41–47.

Johnson, D. (2001, First Quarter). Psychoeducation or family education: What's it all about? *Newsletter of the World Fellowship for Schizophrenia and Allied Disorders, 12,* 3–4.

Lefley, H. P. (1987). Aging parents as caregivers of mentally ill adult children: An emerging social problem. *Hospital and Community Psychiatry, 38*(10), 1063–1070.

Lehman, A. F., & Steinwachs, D. M. (1998). At issue: Translating research into practice: The Schizophrenia Patient Outcomes Research Team (PORT) treatment recommendations. *Schizophrenia Bulletin, 24*(1), 10.

Lukens, E., & Thorning, H. (2010). Psychosocial family groups. In A. Ruben, D. W. Springer, & K. Trawver (Eds.), *Psychosocial treatment of schizophrenia* (pp. 89–144). Hoboken, NJ: John Wiley & Sons.

Lynch, E., & Hanson, M. (2004). *Developing cross-cultural competence: A guide for working with children and their families* (3rd ed.). Baltimore, MD: Paul H. Brookes.

MacGregor, P. (1994). Grief: The unrecognized parental response to mental illness in a child. *Social Work, 39*(2), 160–166.

Marsh, D. T. (1998). *Serious mental illness and the family: The practitioner's guide.* New York, NY: John Wiley & Sons.

Marsh, D. T. (2001). *A family-focused approach to serious mental illness: Empirically supported interventions.* Sarasota, FL: Professional Resource Press.

McCubbin, H. I., Thompson, E. A., Thompson, A. L., & Futrell, J. A. (1999). *The dynamics of resilient families.* Thousand Oaks, CA: Sage Publications.

McCubbin, M. (1995). The Typology Model of Adjustment and Adaptation: A family stress model. *Counseling and Guidance, 10*(4), 31–37.

McGoldrick, M., & Carter, B. (2007). The family life cycle. In F. Walsh (Ed.), *Normal family process: Growing diversity and complexity* (3rd ed.). Philadelphia, PA: Taylor & Francis.

McGoldrick, M., Carter, B., & Garcia-Preto, N. (2010). *The expanded family life cycle: Individual, family, and social perspectives* (4th ed.). New York, NY: Allyn & Bacon.

McLellan, G. (2006). Mental health and justice: The case of Andrea Yates. *The Lancet, 368,* 1951–1954.

Miklowitz, D. J., & Goldstein, T. R. (2010). Family-based approaches to treating bipolar disorder in adolescence: Family-focused therapy and dialectical behavior therapy. In D. J. Miklowitz & D. Cicchetti (Eds.), *Understanding bipolar disorder: A developmental psychopathology perspective* (pp. 466–493). New York, NY: Guilford Press.

Mohr, W. K., & Regan-Kubinski, M. J. (2001). Living in the fallout: Parents' experiences when their child becomes mentally ill. *Archives of Psychiatric Nursing, 15*(2), 69–77.

Moller, M. D., & Wer, J. (1989). Simultaneous patient/family education regarding schizophrenia: The Nebraska model. *Archives of Psychiatric Nursing, 3*(6), 332–337.

Moore, B. C. (2005). Empirically supported family and peer interventions for dual disorders. *Research on Social Work Practice, 15,* 231–245.

Mowbray, C. T., Bybee, D., Oyserman, D., MacFarlane, P., & Bowersox, N. (2004). Psychosocial outcomes for adult children of parents with severe mental illness: Demographics and clinical history predictors. *Health & Social Work, 31,* 99–108.

National Alliance on Mental Illness (NAMI). (2011). *About NAMI.* Retrieved from http://www.nami.org/template.cfm?section=About_NAMI

Nichols, M. P. (2010). *Family therapy. Concepts and methods* (9th ed.). Boston, MA: Allyn & Bacon.

Olson, D. H., & DeFrain, J. (2007). *Marriages and families: Intimacy, diversity, and strengths* (6th ed.). New York, NY: McGraw-Hill.

Pickett-Schenk, S. A., Lippincott, R. C., Bennett, C., & Steigman, P. J. (2008). Improving knowledge about mental illness through family-led education: The Journey of Hope. *Psychiatric Services, 59,* 49–56.

Prochaska, J. O., DiClemente, C., & Norcross, J. (1992). In search of how people change: Applications to addictive behavior. *American Psychologist, 47,* 1102–1114.

Sadock, B. J., & Sadock, V. A. (2007). *Kaplan & Sadock's synopsis of psychiatry* (10th ed.). Philadelphia, PA: Lippincott Williams & Wilkins.

Saunders, J. C. (2003). Families living with severe mental illness: A literature review. *Issues in Mental Health Nursing, 24,* 175–198.

Tuck, I., duMont, P., Evans, G., & Shupe, J. (1997). The experience of caring for an adult child with schizophrenia. *Archives of Psychiatric Nursing, 11*(3), 118–125.

Wade, J. (2006). "Crying alone with my child": Parenting a school age child diagnosed with bipolar disorder. *Issues in Mental Health Nursing, 27,* 885–903.

Walsh, F. (2007). *Normal family process: Growing diversity and complexity* (3rd ed.). Philadelphia, PA: Taylor & Francis.

Wright, L., & Leahey, M. (2005). *Nurses and families: A guide to family assessment and intervention* (4th ed.). Philadelphia, PA: F. A. Davis.

Wynaden, D., Ladzinski, U., Lapsley, J., Landsborough, I., Butt, J., & Hewitt, V. (2006). The caregiving experience: How much do health professionals understand? *Collegian, 13*(3), 6–10.

Web Resource

National Alliance on Mental Illness (NAMI): http://www.nami.org

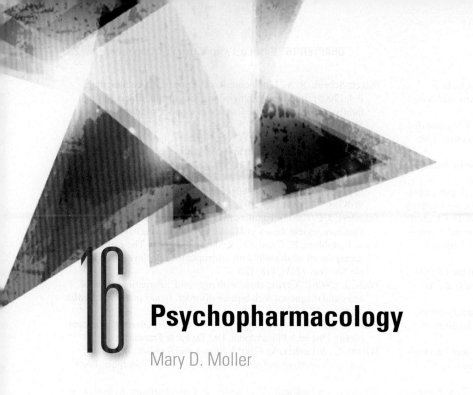

16

Psychopharmacology

Mary D. Moller

LEARNING OBJECTIVES

On completion of this chapter, you should be able to accomplish the following:

- Explain the FDA's process of approving new drugs and labeling restrictions in psychiatry.
- Review the relationship of neurons to the administration and effectiveness of psychotropic drugs.
- Describe pharmacokinetics and pharmacodynamics, including the P450 liver enzyme system and drug–drug and drug–food interactions.
- Discuss the pharmacologic principles of adherence, efficacy, response, and remission.
- Identify important classes and subclasses of psychotherapeutic drugs, including the neurotransmitters involved and the disorders for which they are used commonly.
- Discuss the therapeutic indication, mechanism of action, recommended dosage, routes of administration, side effects, potential adverse effects, contraindications, and nursing implications for major psychotropic medications.
- Apply the nursing process to the care of clients prescribed a psychotropic medication.

This chapter provides a comprehensive summary for nurses of the art and science of a **psychopharmacology** (the formal study of drugs specifically developed to treat psychiatric disorders). The field changes rapidly as new **psychotropic medications** (drugs used primarily for psychiatric conditions and approved for other conditions but also used in psychiatry) are continually developed and discovered. Psychopharmacology is exquisitely complex. It encompasses pharmacodynamics (the specific properties of drugs), pharmacokinetics (how drugs move through the body), and the requisite skills needed to prescribe, administer, and monitor clients using these agents. A single chapter can provide only an overview of the most basic and important concepts and topics. Nurses must be alert to new advances and changes in the field to best facilitate clients' therapeutic needs.

Before proceeding, it is important to emphasize that nurses, clients, and families must understand the inexactitude of current psychopharmacologic treatment, a topic that this chapter explores further in pertinent sections. In addition, health care providers must avoid judging clients who do not adhere to medication regimens. Many clients cannot tolerate the side effects (eg, weight gain, sexual dysfunction) caused by these drugs. In many ways, psychotropic medications serve as mixed blessings for the clients who must take them daily to function.

THE FOOD AND DRUG ADMINISTRATION DRUG-APPROVAL PROCESS

The purpose of the U.S. **Food and Drug Administration (FDA)** is to ensure public safety related to available foods and drugs. Its approval protocol for new medications is rigid and based on clinical trials (Table 16.1). For every 100 drugs that start the process, approximately 70 successfully complete phase 1 trials and move to phase 2. Approximately 33 of the original 100 complete phase 2, from 25 to 30 of the original 100 clear phase 3, and approximately 20 of the original 100 move forward for marketing. Before reaching phase 1, a drug has been in initial synthesis and animal-testing phases for at least 1 to 3 years. Thus, it takes a drug 2 to 10 years to go from phase 1 to phase 3. Only after phase 3 can a company submit a new drug application to the FDA. From submission to approval takes another 2 to 84 months (average 24 months). Finally, the FDA grants a *labeled indication* to a drug for use in a specific illness. After FDA approval, phase 4 begins with a postmarket surveillance process that includes adverse reaction reporting, surveys, sampling and testing, and inspections. Phase 4 typically lasts another 2 years. Each phase costs the pharmaceutical industry millions of dollars. Understanding the rigor of this process may help students better understand one reason why new drugs cost so much.

Clinical Trials

A **clinical trial** is a research study in which people volunteer to answer specific health questions related to new treatments. All clinical trials have guidelines and criteria for inclusion and exclusion based on such variables as age, sex, problem being treated, treatment history, and medical condition. For all clinical trials of psychotropic medications, criteria for inclusion are strict, with safety as the predominant goal. Participants must give informed consent and exhibit understanding of the study and its specific risks, as well as the overall potential risks and benefits of any clinical trial.

Clinical trials are essential to the research and development of new drugs. Health care providers are required ethically to screen and protect participants carefully before beginning. This is especially crucial with psychotropic drugs, which impose special vulnerabilities and have related potential consequences.

Clinical trials are considered the gold standard of research. Ideally, prescribed drugs are studied thoroughly through clinical trials. Nevertheless, many medications are used **off label** clinically. *Off label* means use of a drug for an indication other than that for which the FDA has given approval.

Special Considerations with Psychotropic Agents

FDA approval for psychotropic agents has a unique consideration. Typically, the FDA approves medications based on mechanism of action to counteract demonstrable pathology in a given organ or system. For example, beta blockers

TABLE 16.1 The FDA Drug Testing Protocol for Humans

Phase	Number of Participants	Length	Purpose	% of Drugs Successfully Tested
1	20–80	Several months	Mainly safety	70
2	50–300	Several months to 2 years	Some short-term safety, but mainly effectiveness	33
3	Up to 3,000	1–4 years	Safety, dosage, effectiveness	25–30
4	Several thousand in multiple testing sites	Up to 2 years	General safety and tolerability, as well as emergence of adverse events	90

are an approved treatment for hypertension. However, the FDA bases approval of psychotropic drugs on descriptive diagnoses from the *Diagnostic and Statistical Manual of Mental Disorders*, 4th edition, text revision (*DSM-IV-TR*) (American Psychiatric Association, 2000). While research is validating that psychiatric illnesses have neurochemical and neuroelectrical causes, the current diagnostic methodology for such illnesses remains poorly defined. Unlike hypertension, illnesses such as schizophrenia and borderline personality disorder cannot be confirmed through objective laboratory values or visual imaging (see Chap. 2).

Because of this dilemma, a cumbersome regulatory process requires pharmaceutical companies to repeat the entire FDA protocol for each new indication of an already approved psychotropic drug before providers can administer that same drug on label for the new condition. For example, in 1997 the FDA approved quetiapine, developed by Astra Zeneca, for acute schizophrenia. Because diagnostic overlap between schizophrenia and bipolar disorders is common, prescribers soon administered quetiapine off label to clients with various bipolar presentations. However, not until 2006 did the FDA grant approval for the use of quetiapine in the treatment of bipolar depression. Oftentimes, when a drug is already being widely used off label, pharmaceutical companies will not even pursue FDA approval for new diagnoses because of the cost associated with the approval process.

PHARMACODYNAMICS

Pharmacodynamics is the study of the mechanisms of action and biochemical and physiologic effects of drugs (essentially, what the drug does to the body). The following sections discuss principles of pharmacodynamics of clinical relevance to psychiatric–mental health nursing.

Neurons and Neurotransmission

A basic principle of psychopharmacology is that symptoms of mental illness result from a chemical imbalance within the nervous system. As described in Chapter 2, the *central nervous system* (CNS) consists of the brain and spinal cord. The *peripheral nervous system* includes the *autonomic nervous system* (ANS), which controls heart muscle, smooth muscle, and exocrine glands. The ANS contains the sympathetic (adrenergic) and parasympathetic (cholinergic) nerves that branch from cells located throughout the spinal cord. Generally, adrenergic impulses stimulate, whereas cholinergic impulses relax. Most medication side effects occur within the ANS (Figure 16.1).

Interactive neurochemical and neuroelectrical systems help the brain navigate myriad stimuli arising from within the body and from the environment. The system of navigation is called *neurotransmission*, which allows the brain to create conscious awareness of sensory perceptions. The brain then decides how to respond to stimuli and stores memories of its decisions. Subsequent responses are usually behavioral, with some accompanying emotions.

Errors in any part of neurotransmission can affect *cognition*, or the ability to accurately perceive incoming information. Students are directed to Chapter 2 for an in-depth discussion about neuroanatomy and neurophysiology.

Affinity

Receptors are specific protein-binding sites inside or on the cellular surface. They are the cellular components with which drugs are presumed to interact. Binding of drug chemicals to receptors either activates or inhibits various cellular functions. Cell bodies create receptors to accommodate the amount of neurotransmitter produced. Receptors upregulate (increase in number) or downregulate (decrease in number), depending on how much neurotransmitter is available. They also fully open (agonize) or fully close (reverse agonize), depending on the neurotransmitter and speed of transmission.

Drugs usually affect receptors by binding to them or changing their behavior toward the host cell (Brunton et al., 2011). The chemical property of **affinity** (degree of attraction between a drug and a specific receptor) influences binding. Affinity is the product of the mutual attraction between the molecular structures of a drug and a receptor. A drug with a high affinity for a given receptor possesses great complementarity with the binding site of that receptor. The more tightly bound a drug is to a receptor, the stronger the drug's action.

Axons and dendrites have their own receptors. Axon receptors are called *presynaptic*, whereas dendrite receptors are called *postsynaptic*. Both are sensitive to even small chemical fluctuations and have the ability to self-regulate. Other specialized receptors called *autoreceptors* act like light switches to help individual neurons downregulate, upregulate, or both.

Receptor–Pharmacology Spectrum

The intent of psychopharmacologic therapy is to "reset" receptor openings, adjust the number of available receptors by altering the amount of available neurotransmitter designated for a particular neuroreceptor, or both. Medications do so by stimulating chemical release, adjusting the enzymes required to destroy neurochemicals, and adjusting the storage/reuptake process. The receptor–pharmacology spectrum includes the following:

- **Agonist**. An agonist triggers an action from a cell or another drug. It is attracted to, binds with, and activates a given receptor, subsequently causing a change in cellular function (Aschenbrenner & Venable, 2009). An agonist medication opens a receptor to full capacity.
- **Partial agonist**. This substance exerts a similar but weaker effect than an agonist. For example, an agonist might open a certain ion channel fully, whereas a partial agonist opens it halfway.
- **Antagonist**. An antagonist blocks the actions of everything in the agonist spectrum. It binds to and blocks a receptor, producing no response and preventing agonists

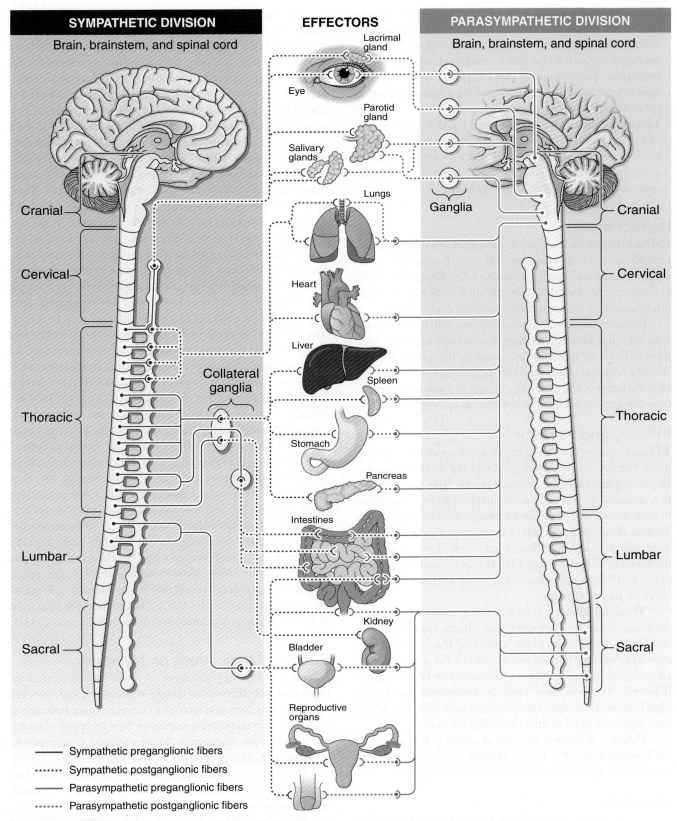

SYMPATHETIC DIVISION	EFFECTORS	PARASYMPATHETIC DIVISION
Brain, brainstem, and spinal cord		Brain, brainstem, and spinal cord

Lacrimal gland

Eye

Parotid gland

Salivary glands

Ganglia

Cranial

Cervical

Lungs

Heart

Liver

Spleen

Collateral ganglia

Stomach

Pancreas

Thoracic

Intestines

Lumbar

Kidney

Sacral

Bladder

Cranial

Cervical

Thoracic

Lumbar

Sacral

Reproductive organs

—— Sympathetic preganglionic fibers
······· Sympathetic postganglionic fibers
—— Parasympathetic preganglionic fibers
······· Parasympathetic postganglionic fibers

FIGURE 16.1 The autonomic nervous system, where many side effects of psychotropic medications occur.

from binding. An example of a drug antagonist is naltrexone, which blocks endogenous opioids at opiate receptors. Naltrexone is a treatment for narcotic and alcohol dependence because it also blocks exogenous opioids from binding to opiate receptors (see Chap. 30). Antagonists have inhibitory action and compete for agonist-binding sites. Alone, they have no activity.

- **Inverse agonist**. An inverse agonist has the *opposite effect of an agonist* (Stahl, 2006). An inverse agonist would neither open the ion channel nor block an agonist from doing so. Rather, it would bind the receptor to provoke an opposite response to that of the agonist.

Refractoriness

Refractoriness (also called *downregulation*) means the desensitization of cells to a drug over time. It usually happens when agonists continually stimulate cells. Repeated cellular exposure to the same drug concentration leads to diminished effectiveness of the medication (Brunton et al., 2011).

Refractoriness is common in clients with mental illness who take the same medication for months to years. Over time, effectiveness diminishes, leading the symptoms that initially required treatment to reemerge. Early identification of refractoriness and resulting changes in medication type or dose can prevent relapses of psychiatric disorders.

Efficacy and Potency

Efficacy means how well, under ideal conditions, a treatment, therapy, or procedure produces the desired outcome. In psychopharmacology, efficacy results from the information encoded in the drug's chemical structure; that information causes the receptor to change accordingly during binding (Brunton et al., 2011). Some psychoactive medications lose efficacy over time, even when clients have used them successfully for years. Clients may present with a complaint that "my medication just stopped working." This is a result of **loss of efficacy**.

Maximal efficacy refers to the greatest effect that a drug can produce. Undesired side effects may limit how much of a drug can be given, rendering true maximal efficacy unachievable (Brunton et al., 2011). For example, psychotic symptoms may improve in clients who take clozapine (Clozaril); however, they need to discontinue the drug if blood studies show agranulocytosis. In such cases, the health care team may need to limit or change the dosage.

Potency is another measure of efficacy. It is related to the concentration of a drug in plasma, transport across cell membranes, and influence of competitive antagonists.

Rule of 5s

Steady state means that a fairly constant level of medication is affecting neurons continuously. Only when steady state is reached do neurons really begin to pay attention to a drug. It then takes approximately 4 more weeks before the neurons adapt to new medications and can make consistent changes in electrical charge, release of neurotransmitters, and responses from autoreceptors and postsynaptic receptors.

An important rule of pharmacology is the "Rule of 5s," which states that it takes a drug *five half-lives* to build to steady state in the body. **Half-life** refers to how long it takes the body to eliminate half of a drug dose. The liver is responsible for making a drug more water soluble so that the kidneys can eliminate it. By the time five half-lives have occurred, the body has eliminated a single dose. *The Rule of 5s is only a guideline.* Few people eat and drink the exact same things each day, so each person's body chemistry is ever changing. Dietary fluctuations are one reason medications work better some days than others.

Some medications such as nefazodone (Serzone) and quetiapine (Seroquel) have half-lives of only a few hours. Thus, they reach steady state quickly, and clients must take them more than once a day because they are eliminated so quickly. Other medications such as fluoxetine (Prozac) have an extended half-life, taking several days to advance to steady state. For this reason, many clients do not seem to have a response to fluoxetine when they first start taking the drug. Their dosing schedule may be only once every other day because the drug takes so long to wash out of the body. Drugs with long half-lives (such as fluoxetine) often metabolize into more than one drug. After the first-pass metabolism, the liver processes the first compound (fluoxetine) into the second (norfluoxetine).

Some medications such as haloperidol (Haldol) have a 24-hour half-life but are *fat soluble*, which means they accumulate in body fat. Depending on how the body uses fat, a person can stop taking haloperidol, but the body may continue to release it into the bloodstream for several months.

Generally, clients need to take drugs with a half-life of 18 hours or more only once a day after reaching steady state. *The Rule of 5s is only a generalization.* Some people are rapid metabolizers and feel the effects of stopping medications only a few hours after missing a dose. Slow metabolizers do not notice any change for several days after stopping medications. The half-lives of major psychiatric medications are identified in charts throughout this chapter. The actual length of time a drug is available in the circulation is called the *area under the curve* (AUC). Peak plasma concentration is *T-Max*, whereas maximum serum concentration is *C-Max*.

Effect of Medications on Neurons

Scientific technology continues to reveal information about the individual differences among neurons. Researchers are tracking many human responses to the exact brain structure(s) responsible for stimulating responses. New receptors or receptor subtypes are discovered almost monthly. Consequently, pharmacology also progresses at warp speed.

Psychotropic medications are *not* "silver bullets." Unfortunately, psychotropic drugs used in an effort to target neurotransmitters thought to contribute to mental problems can also affect other neurotransmitters, leading to adverse effects or new problems. Because of the proximity of the 200 billion neurons in the brain, the effect of psychotropic drugs on target neurons is more like buckshot than an intravenous drip—medications affect a wide and indiscriminate target area (Stahl, 2006). They hit not only the intended receptors, but also everything around the target. One synaptic reaction can affect up to 25,000 surrounding neurons. Prescribed drugs may shut down neurotransmitter systems other than those intended. They may affect target receptors not only in the problematic region, but also in other healthy parts of the brain that control vital functions (Table 16.2). Although psychotherapeutic drugs may improve symptoms of mental illness, they may cause clients to experience entirely new dysfunctions and discomforts, called **side effects**.

Effects of Medications on Synapses

Upregulation and downregulation make it virtually impossible to alter only one type of receptor at a time. The body basically treats drugs as invading foreign chemicals and attempts to adjust in response. As a result, some clients have difficulty adjusting to psychiatric medications and the subsequent changes they trigger. The fundamental action of psychotropic medications is to alter either the transmission or the reception of nerve impulses. The result is increased or slowed nervous system function, depending on the targeted neurotransmitter and receptor. Medications usually work on one part of the neuron to regulate the level of neurotransmitter within the synapse and, it is hoped, keep the correct amount of chemical-stimulating receptors on both axon and dendrite.

Antipsychotics (chlorpromazine, haloperidol, risperidone, clozapine) antagonize selected postsynaptic receptor sites, causing the function of those nerve cells to "slow down." Most antidepressants block the reuptake of certain neurotransmitters, which keeps more of them in the synapse stimulating the receptors. The result is an eventual "return-to-normal" function once the neurotransmitter has been restored to a normal level in the synapse. Agonists such as some benzodiazepines, narcotics, and stimulants tend to fit

TABLE 16.2 Effects of Receptor Antagonism

Specific Receptor	Source Location	Effects of Blockade
Alpha adrenergic 1	Sympathetic/motor	Dizziness, postural hypotension, tachycardia
Alpha adrenergic 2	Sympathetic/motor	Anxiety, tachycardia, dilated pupils, tremor, sweating
Beta adrenergic 1	Sympathetic neurons	Orthostatic hypotension, sedation, sexual dysfunction
Muscarinic	Hippocampus and cortex; activates K^+ channels, postsynaptic parasympathetic sites	Constipation, blurred vision, dry mouth, memory dysfunction, urinary retention, tachycardia
Histaminic	Hypothalamus converts histamine	Weight gain, drowsiness, hypotension, sedation
Nicotinic	Spinal autonomic ganglia; preganglion	Muscle irritability, restlessness, insomnia
Dopaminergic 1/5	Substantia nigra, striatum, basal ganglia, nucleus accumbens, olfactory, amygdala	Extrapyramidal side effects (EPSE): dystonias, dyskinesia, akathisias
Dopaminergic 2	Striatum, olfactory, nucleus accumbens, substantia nigra	EPSE: dystonias, dyskinesia, akathisias
Dopaminergic 3	Pituitary, nucleus accumbens, olfactory, hypothalamus	Endocrine problems, weight gain, sexual dysfunction
Dopaminergic 4	Frontal cortex, midbrain, medulla	Psychosis
Serotonergic 1	Hippocampus, raphe, cortex	1_a: anxiety (buspirone is agonist) 1_d: cerebral artery dilation (sumatriptan is agonist)
Serotonergic 2a	Cortex, olfactory system; claustrum	Antipsychotic symptoms, antianxiety, sleep restoration
Serotonergic 2c	Frontal cortex	Antagonist action is antidepressant and helps regulate dopamine, also causes many SSRI side effects
Serotonergic 3	Area postrema, cortex, "leaky" blood–brain barrier around posterior pituitary and supra-ventricular areas, bowel wall	Antagonist is antinausea due to slowed bowel motility (ondansetron); questionable antianxiety effect;
Serotonergic 4	Gastrointestinal tract; limbic system	Agonist (used for weight loss in research)
Serotonergic 5	Central nervous system (mood, sleep, circadian rhythms	Agonists used to treat hypermotility and depression
Serotonergic 6	Involved in alcohol metabolism and depression	Antagonist is antidepressive and antipsychotic
Serotonergic 7	CNS, GI tract, blood vessels (anxiety, memory, mood, sleep)	Antagonist is antidepressive and antipsychotic

Nichols, D. E., & Nichols, C. D. (2008). Serotonin receptors. *Chemical Reviews*, 108 (5): 1614–41. doi:10.1021/cr078224o.

directly into certain receptors. This effect stops a "craving" for the substance because the brain receives feedback that the receptor is "coated." Unfortunately, this often sets up a process called *negative feedback*, in which the brain slows down production of an already deficient neurotransmitter or receptor site. That nerve eventually does not function normally without the outside chemical. This process is thought to be the basis of addiction (see Chap. 30).

Checkpoint Questions

1. What name is given to specific protein-binding sites inside or on the surface of the cell?
2. What chemical property influences binding?
3. What term refers to the specific symptoms a medication aims to alter?

PHARMACOKINETICS

Drugs interact with the whole person, leading to individual outcomes. Each medication can potentially alter multiple body functions. Thus, drugs used to treat a particular psychiatric illness can significantly affect other body functions.

Complex drug interactions involve biochemical and physiologic responses related to how the drugs move through the body. The process of such movement from ingestion to elimination is called **pharmacokinetics** (essentially, what the body does to the drug). The four basic stages are absorption, distribution, metabolism, and elimination. Drug interactions (effects on receptors between two or more drugs) can occur in each (Figure 16.2).

Absorption

Absorption means the ability of a drug to transfer from the stomach, intestine, or both into the bloodstream. It is expressed as amount per time (eg, grams per minute or milliliters per hour). Absorption indicates the speed and degree with which a drug leaves its site of administration and enters the circulation. The drug's physiochemical properties affect absorption, as do its size, shape, and charge. Most drugs move by passive diffusion (from areas of high concentration to areas of low concentration). However, some use carrier-mediated transporters for active transport and facilitated diffusion.

Other factors that influence absorption include the nature of the absorbing surface, blood flow to the site of absorption, drug concentration (ie, dose—the easiest way to increase a drug response is to increase the dose), dose form, and route of administration. Some drugs (eg, antacids) prevent absorption and thereby inhibit or decrease the effects of other drugs.

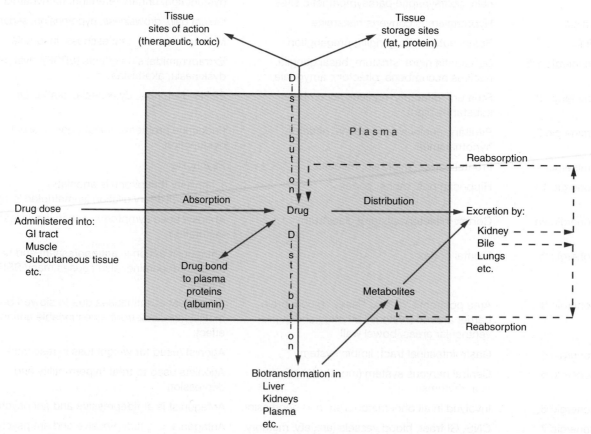

FIGURE 16.2 Drug interactions can occur in the absorptive, digestive, metabolic, or elimination phases of pharmacokinetics.

Acidity or alkalinity governs absorption. Most medications are designed to be broken down by gastric acid but not absorbed until they pass from the stomach to the intestine. Excess stomach acid can inactivate a drug, preventing it from reaching the brain. Conversely, an overly alkaline digestive environment never breaks down a drug enough for intestinal absorption. See also Table 16.3.

Distribution

Distribution refers to how the drug moves through the bloodstream to various body target sites. Factors that affect distribution include the drug's physiochemical properties, cardiac output and blood flow, the blood–brain barrier, and drug reservoirs.

The body perceives most drugs as foreign, toxic substances. Pharmaceutical companies know and have allowed

TABLE 16.3 Effects of Psychotropic Medications on Appetite, Gastrointestinal Function, Nutrient Absorption, and Metabolism

Drug	Effects
Antipsychotics in general	Dry mouth, constipation, weight gain (except molindone and loxapine), riboflavin (B_2) depletion (clinical significance not established)
fluphenazine, trifluoperazine	Peripheral edema; false $\uparrow$ urinary bilirubin; $\downarrow$ absorption of B_{12}; $\downarrow$ appetite
loxapine	Possible edema
thioridazine	Possible peripheral edema; false $+$ $\uparrow$ of urinary bilirubin (false)
thiothixene	$\uparrow$ appetite; peripheral edema; $\uparrow$ food intake; $\downarrow$ alkaline phosphatase, SGOT, SGPT; $\downarrow$ uric acid
chlorpromazine	$\downarrow$ Absorption of B_{12}; peripheral edema; $\uparrow$ cholesterol by altering lipid metabolism; $\uparrow$ bilirubin; possible increased salivation
clozapine	Hypersalivation; constipation; $\uparrow$ or $\downarrow$ blood pressure; weight gain
risperidone	Weight gain; hypersalivation; excessive sweating; dry mouth; nausea, vomiting, constipation
Cyclic antidepressants	Dry mouth; nausea and vomiting; constipation; epigastric distress (upset stomach, bloating); weight gain; stomatitis (mouth sores)
amitriptyline	Swollen parotid gland; $\uparrow$ appetite for carbohydrates; fluctuating blood glucose levels; take with food/milk
nortriptyline	Weight fluctuation; take with food
desipramine	$\uparrow$ Appetite for sweets; weight fluctuation; take with food
imipramine	Contains tartrazine; take with food; dilute liquid form with 4 oz (118.2 mL) water, milk
doxepin	Sour or metallic taste; $\uparrow$ appetite for sweets; alters blood glucose
Selective serotonin/ norepinephrine reuptake inhibitor venlafaxine	$\uparrow$ Liver enzymes, $\uparrow$ serum cholesterol; nausea and vomiting; dry mouth
SSRIs	Weight loss or weight gain; nausea and vomiting
Monoamine oxidase inhibitors	Dry mouth; constipation; B_6 deficiency; weight gain (especially phenelzine); $\downarrow$ blood glucose levels
Antianxiety agents	Taking with food increases the overall effect; jaundice (from $\uparrow$ bilirubin); nausea, constipation, hiccoughs; $\uparrow$ appetite, $\uparrow$ weight; salivary changes; $\uparrow$ SGOT, SGPT, alkaline phosphatase
Lithium	Nausea/vomiting/abdominal cramps/gas; loose stools/diarrhea; extreme thirst/excessive urination $\rightarrow$ inhibits the effects of ADH on the kidneys; weight gain (up to 20 pounds); impairs glucose tolerance and $\uparrow$ sensitivity to insulin; affects metabolism by decreasing efficiency of thyroid gland ($\downarrow T_4$); $\uparrow$ urinary CA, glucose, albumin; $\uparrow$ serum MG; $\downarrow$ calcium uptake by bone; anemia; metallic taste
Anticonvulsants, including diphenylhydantoin (Dilantin), mephenytoin (Mesantoin), trimethadione (Tridione), valproic acid (Depakene), and carbamazepine (Tegretol)	Decreased transport of folic acid into CNS Accelerated folic acid metabolism, altered pyridoxine metabolism (mechanism unknown), decreased transport of B_{12} into the cerebrospinal fluid, increased excretion of cholecalciferol and diminished calcium absorption, inhibited synthesis of vitamin K Nutritional complications related to the newer anticonvulsants, such as lamotrigine (Lamictal), gabapentin (Neurontin), tiagabine (Gabitril), and topiramate (Topamax), have not yet been determined.

for this factor in medication dosages. One or two plasma proteins circulating in the bloodstream (eg, albumin, globulin) "grab up" most drug molecules. Only the milligrams not attached to albumin are free for transport to the brain and other body tissues. For example, if a pill has 10 mg of medication in it, only 1 or 2 mg actually distribute to the brain (Figure 16.3).

A body with insufficient protein does not have enough albumin to bind the drug appropriately. Side effects can result.

A second highly protein-bound drug in the blood can intensify the activity of some strongly bound drugs by displacing their molecules from the plasma proteins. Consequently, more drug is free to leave the blood and diffuse into tissues. The pattern of initial distribution in body fluids depends on the nature of the drug, cardiac output, and regional blood flow.

Metabolism

Metabolism, or *biotransformation*, is how the body increases the electrical charge on drugs and targets them for excretion.

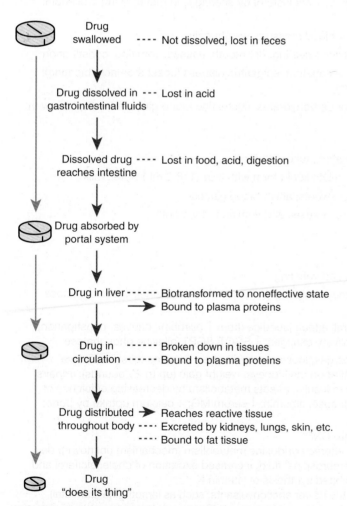

Drug swallowed - - - - Not dissolved, lost in feces

Drug dissolved in - - - Lost in acid
gastrointestinal fluids

Dissolved drug - - - - Lost in food, acid, digestion
reaches intestine

Drug absorbed by
portal system

Drug in liver - - - - - - Biotransformed to noneffective state
→ Bound to plasma proteins

Drug in - - - - - - Broken down in tissues
circulation - - - - - - Bound to plasma proteins

Drug distributed → Reaches reactive tissue
throughout body - - - - Excreted by kidneys, lungs, skin, etc.
- - - - Bound to fat tissue

Drug
"does its thing"

FIGURE 16.3 Very little of an oral dose of a medication actually reaches receptors. The discrepancy between the amount of drug swallowed and the amount that actually acts on target symptoms is shown.

Biotransformation reactions alter a medication's chemical structure. They occur primarily in the liver and involve enzymatic breakdown for excretion in urine and feces. Although biotransformation reactions convert active drugs to inactive metabolites, they also convert active drugs into active metabolites and inactive drugs into active metabolites. Thus, they do not necessarily inactivate drugs. An example is the increased solubility (biotransformation and elimination) of some drugs, such as gabapentin, in the urine.

Biotransformation is accomplished primarily by the cytochrome P450 liver enzyme systems, composed of hundreds of enzymes that metabolize many drugs. When two or more drugs use the same enzyme system, the presence of one drug can increase or inhibit the other's rate of metabolism. Related important definitions are substrate, inhibitor, and inducer.

- A **substrate** is the material or substance (drug) on which an enzyme acts. Enzymes are proteins characterized by two properties. First, they increase the rate of a chemical reaction without themselves being consumed or permanently altered. Second, they increase reaction rates without altering the chemical equilibrium between products and reactants. Products result when an enzyme acts on a substrate. Both enzymes and substrates are involved in the inhibition and binding of drug receptors and determine a drug's selectivity of action, relation between dose and effects, and therapeutic effectiveness.
- An **inhibitor** refers to a drug that blocks a specific P450 enzyme system.
- An **inducer** is a drug that increases the amount of P450 enzyme production.

For example, a client is taking clozapine, which uses the P450 1A2 system for metabolism. If the same client smokes 1 pack of cigarettes, which induces the 1A2 system, the effect of clozapine will be reduced greatly. Conversely, if a client is taking fluvoxamine, which inhibits the 1A2 system, and ingests caffeine, the caffeine will not be metabolized. As a result, the half-life of the caffeine will have a net increase of up to 32 hours. Fluvoxamine can also increase the effects of haloperidol and olanzapine by severalfold. Prescribing handbooks will identify specific P450 system interactions for all drugs.

Elimination

Elimination refers to how drugs are removed from the body. Most drugs are excreted via the kidneys. Like metabolism, elimination can be enhanced or inhibited. *Most drugs continue to exert their effects until they are excreted, either unchanged or as active metabolites.* The liver only changes the drugs to a water-soluble form so they can be eliminated by either the kidneys or the gastrointestinal tract. Elimination of drugs by the kidneys is pH dependent and closely related to the rate at which the drug is absorbed from the gastrointestinal tract.

TABLE 16.4 Foods That Contribute to Acid or Alkaline Urine

Foods	Acid	Alkaline
Meats	Fish, fowl, shell-fish, eggs, cheese, peanut butter	
Vegetables	Corn and lentils	All types
Fat	Bacon Nuts: Brazil, filberts, peanuts, walnuts	Almonds, chest-nuts, coconut
Fruit	Cranberries, plums, prunes	Citrus fruits
Breads	All types, crackers, pasta	
Desserts	Cakes, cookies	
Milk products		Milk, cream, buttermilk

All foods and beverages affect the acidity and alka-linity of urine. Simply put, what goes into the stomach as acid comes out in the urine as alkaline and vice versa. See Table 16.4.

Elimination of one drug can slow elimination of another based on pH preference by the kidney. A common drug–drug interaction occurs when clients have the flu and drink a lot of juice, which is acid. If such clients then take aspirin (also acid), they will not experience relief from the symptom of headache. People dependent on amphetamines have learned that they can increase the half-life of those drugs by alkalin-izing their urine with antacids or baking soda.

Psychotropic drugs can also have a deleterious effect on nutrition, including changes in taste, appetite, gastrointesti-nal function, nutrient absorption, and metabolism of foods. See Table 16.5 and Box 16.1.

Checkpoint Questions
4. What are the four components of pharmacokinetics?
5. What are two properties of enzymes?

TABLE 16.5 Effects of Food and Drug pH on Elimination

Drug pH	GI pH	Urine pH	Drug Elimination
Acid	Acid Ψ	Base	Increased
Acid	Base Ψ	Acid	Decreased
Base	Acid Ψ	Base	Decreased
Base	Base Ψ	Acid	Increased

BOX 16.1 Effects of Dietary Substances on Psychotropic Medications

Antipsychotics
- Use with alcohol results in sedation.
- Use with ascorbic acid decreases absorption of fluphenazine.
- Use with caffeine decreases effectiveness of the medication.

Heterocyclic Antidepressant
- Use with coffee or tea results in precipitation.
- Use with alcohol leads to sedation.
- Use with ascorbic acid increases elimination of antidepressant.

Selective Serotonin Reuptake Inhibitors
- Use with caffeine increases agitation and excitation.
- Use with alcohol increases sedation and somnolence.

Monoamine Oxidase Inhibitors
- Use with alcohol can result in neurotoxicity.
- Use with foods high in tryptophan and tyramine can lead to hypertensive crisis (fatally elevated blood pressure).

Lithium
- Increased caffeine intake can increase lithium elimination.
- Sudden decrease in caffeine intake may cause lithium toxicity from change in urination.
- Use with sodium increases lithium elimination, while a low-sodium diet may lead to lithium retention and toxicity.

Antianxiety Agents
- Use with alcohol causes sedation.
- Use with caffeine leads to decreased effectiveness of the medication.

MAJOR CLASSES OF PSYCHOTROPIC DRUGS

This section explores the most important psychotherapeu-tic drugs in current use: antidepressants, mood stabilizers, anxiolytics, antipsychotics (neuroleptics), stimulants, and memory/cognitive enhancers. Later chapters contain more discussions about these and other drugs as they relate to specific disorder groups and conditions. However, all nurses working in psychiatric–mental health care must be familiar with the particulars of the drugs discussed here.

Antidepressants

Antidepressants are used regularly to treat major depression, depressive phases of bipolar disorder, and depressive symp-toms not associated with major depression. Symptoms that indicate a possible need for antidepressants include dyspho-ria, change in appetite and energy, *anhedonia* (lack of interest in routine activities), difficulty concentrating, hopelessness, and suicidality (see Chap. 27). Antidepressants are also used to treat anxiety disorders (see Chap. 23).

Before clients begin taking antidepressants, they should undergo a thorough physical examination to determine cardiovascular irregularities and the potential for seizures, because antidepressants can lower the seizure threshold. A baseline electrocardiogram is usually recommended (Figure 16.4).

Ingestion of large amounts of certain antidepressants (tricyclic antidepressants) is potentially life-threatening; therefore, providers use caution when dispensing all categories of these drugs to clients at risk for self-harm. Outpatient providers frequently give only a few days' to 1 week's worth of medication, requiring clients to return for evaluation before dispensing more.

A classic landmark study comparing antidepressants is the *Sequenced Treatment Alternatives to Relieve Depression* (STAR*D) (Rush et al., 2004). Numerous publications have been mined from this study. Nurses are encouraged to read it for the latest data regarding antidepressant therapy.

See Understanding Psychopharmacology 16.1 for a summary of specific antidepressants.

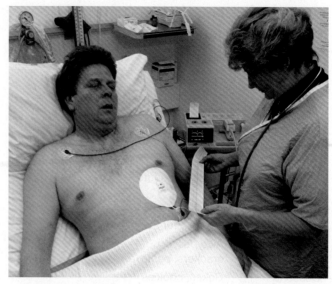

FIGURE 16.4 A baseline electrocardiogram is usually recommended for clients before they begin antidepressant therapy.

UNDERSTANDING PSYCHOPHARMACOLOGY 16.1

Antidepressants

GENERIC AND BRAND NAMES	USUAL DOSE	SEDATION LEVEL/ HALF-LIFE	SIDE EFFECTS	RELIEF OF SYMPTOMS
Tricyclic Antidepressants (TCAs)				
desipramine (Norpramin, Pertofrane)	100–350 mg/day	Less sedating than other TCAs	Dry mouth, tremors, blurred vision, bloating and weight gain, urinary retention	2–4 wk; side effects may be discouraging
imipramine (Tofranil)	100–150 mg/day PO in divided doses; gradually increase to 200 mg/day; if no response after 2 wk, may be increased to 250–300 mg/day	May be sedating, at least initially; half-life is 8–16 hr	Sedation, anticholinergic effects, confusion, disturbed concentration, dry mouth, constipation, orthostatic hypotension	Decreased anxiety immediately evident; antidepressant response may require 2–3 wk
nortriptyline (Pamelor)	25 mg TID-QID PO; doses > 150 mg/day not recommended	Sedating; half-life is 18–28 hr	Sedation and anticholinergic effects, confusion (especially in elderly), disturbed concentration; seizures, orthostatic hypotension, dry mouth, constipation, nausea; avoid abrupt withdrawal of medication	Gradual; 2–4 wk
doxepin (Sinequan)	25 mg PO TID for mild to moderate anxiety and depression; 50 mg PO TID (up to 300 mg/day) for more severe anxiety and depression	May be sedating; half-life is 8–25 hr	Sedation, anticholinergic effects, confusion, disturbed concentration, dry mouth, constipation, orthostatic hypotension	2–4 wk

amitriptyline (Elavil)	Initially, 75–100 mg/day PO in divided doses; gradually increase to 200–300 mg/day PO	May be sedating; half-life is 10–50 hr	Sedation, anticholinergic effects, confusion, disturbed concentration, dry mouth, constipation, orthostatic hypotension	Beginning relief of symptoms may take 2–4 wk
protriptyline (Vivactil)	5–40 mg/day PO in three to four divided doses with gradual increase to 60 mg/day; make increases in AM dose	Activating; half-life is 67–89 hr	Sedation and anticholinergic effects, confusion (especially in elderly), disturbed concentration, seizures, orthostatic hypotension, myocardial infarction, stroke, dry mouth, constipation	24–30 hr
amoxapine (Asendin)	50 mg PO BID-TID with gradual increase to 100 mg BID-TID by end of first week; increase above 300 mg/day only if this dosage ineffective for at least 2 wk	Sedating; half-life is 8–30 hr	Disturbed concentration, sedation and anticholinergic effects, confusion, orthostatic hypotension, dry mouth, constipation; avoid abrupt withdrawal of medication	Gradual; 2–4 wk
trimipramine (Surmontil)	Inpatient: 100 mg/day PO in divided doses with gradual increase to 200 mg/day; outpatients: initially 75 mg/day PO in divided doses with increase to 150 mg/day; maintenance dose is 50–150 mg/day given as single HS dose	Sedating; half-life is 7–30 hr	Sedation and anticholinergic effects, confusion (especially in elderly), disturbed concentration, orthostatic hypotension, myocardial infarction, precipitation of congestive heart failure, stroke, dry mouth, constipation; avoid abrupt withdrawal of medication	2 hr
clomipramine (Anafranil)	75–250 mg/day	Sedating	Cognitive impairment, memory loss, confusion, dry mouth, tremors, blurred vision, bloating and weight gain, urinary retention	Can be lethal in a suicide attempt; 2–4 wk; side effects may be discouraging

Tetracyclic Antidepressant

| maprotiline (Ludiomil) | Initially 75 mg/day PO with gradual increases in 25-mg increments; most clients respond to 150 mg/day, but some may require 225 mg/day; severe depression may require 100–150 mg/day PO with gradual increase to 300 mg/day; usual maintenance dose is 75–150 mg/day PO | Sedating; half-life is 27–58 hr | Sedation and anticholinergic effects, confusion (especially in elderly), disturbed concentration, seizures, orthostatic hypotension, dry mouth, constipation, nausea; avoid abrupt withdrawal of medication | Gradual; 2–4 wk |

(continues on page 296)

UNDERSTANDING PSYCHOPHARMACOLOGY 16.1

Antidepressants (continued)

GENERIC AND BRAND NAMES	USUAL DOSE	SEDATION LEVEL/ HALF-LIFE	SIDE EFFECTS	RELIEF OF SYMPTOMS
Monoamine Oxidase Inhibitors-A				
phenelzine sulfate (Nardil)	Initially, 15 mg PO TID; increase dose to at least 60 mg/day at rapid pace according to client tolerance; some may require 90 mg/day	Likely to energize; half-life is unknown	Dizziness, vertigo, headache, overactivity, hyperreflexia, tremors, muscle twitching, mania, hypomania, jitteriness, confusion, memory impairment, insomnia, weakness, fatigue, drowsiness, restlessness, overstimulation, increased anxiety, agitation, blurred vision, sweating, constipation, diarrhea, nausea, abdominal pain, edema, dry mouth, anorexia, weight changes, hypertensive crisis, orthostatic hypotension, disturbed cardiac rate and rhythm	Up to 4 wk for maximum response
tranylcypromine (Parnate)	Most effective dose is usually 30 mg/day PO in divided doses; if no improvement within 2 wk, increase dosage in 10 mg/day increments to a maximum of 60 mg/day	May be stimulating, especially to clients with agitation or schizophrenia; half-life is unknown	Dizziness, vertigo, headache, overactivity, hyperreflexia, tremors, muscle twitching, mania, hypomania, jitteriness, confusion, memory impairment, insomnia, weakness, fatigue, drowsiness, restlessness, overstimulation, increased anxiety, agitation, blurred vision, sweating, constipation, diarrhea, nausea, abdominal pain, edema, dry mouth, anorexia, weight changes, hypertensive crises, orthostatic hypotension, disturbed cardiac rate and rhythm	Improvement within 48 hr to 3 wk
isocarboxazid (Marplan)	30–60 mg/day	Half-life is unknown; energizing	Similar to Parnate and Nardil	Improvement seen within 3–6 wk

Monoamine Oxidase Inhibitors-B

selegiline transdermal (Emsam)	Transdermal patchs Initially apply a 6-mg patch that must be changed every 24 hr. The dose can be increased every 2 wk to a maximum of 9 mg.	Activating; half-life is 10 hr	Headache, increased blood pressure. Same dietary and OTC precautions as for MAOI-A.	Up to 7 days

Selective Reuptake Inhibitors (Serotonin-2 Antagonist/Reuptake Inhibitor) (SARIs)

nefazodone (Serzone)	200 mg/day PO in two divided doses; increase at 1-wk intervals to 100–200 mg/day; usual range is 300–600 mg/day	May cause nervousness or insomnia or be slightly sedating; half-life is 2–3 days	Headache, nervousness, insomnia, drowsiness, anxiety, tremor, dizziness, light-headedness, nausea, vomiting, diarrhea, dry mouth, anorexia, dyspepsia, constipation, taste changes, sweating, rash, pruritus	Beginning relief of symptoms may take 2–4 wk
trazodone (Desyrel)	Initially, 150 mg/day PO with increase of 50 mg/day every 3–4 days; maximum dose should not exceed 600 mg/day in divided doses for clients who are severely depressed	May cause drowsiness or agitation; half-life is 3–6 hr and then 5–9 hr	Anger, hostility, agitation, nightmares/vivid dreams, hallucinations, delusions, hypomania, confusion, disorientation, decreased concentration, impaired memory, impaired speech, dizziness, lack of coordination, drowsiness, fatigue, gastric disorder, decreased/increased appetite, dry mouth, bad taste in mouth, nausea, vomiting, diarrhea, flatulence, constipation, hypertension, hypotension, shortness of breath, syncope, tachycardia, palpitations, decreased libido, allergic skin conditions, edema	10–14 days and up to 2–4 wk

Selective NE/DA Reuptake Inhibitors

bupropion (Wellbutrin)	300–450 mg	Low; if anything, energizing; half-life is 8–24 hr	Weight loss, agitation, risk of seizures, relative absence of sexual dysfunction	10–14 days

Alpha 2 Reuptake Inhibitor

mirtazapine (Remeron)	Initial dose of 15 mg/day PO as a single evening dose; may be increased up to 45 mg/day PO as needed	May be sedating; half-life is 20–40 hr	Sedation and anticholinergic effects, confusion, disturbed concentration, dry mouth, constipation, nausea, agranulocytosis, neutropenia	Clinical response in 3–7 days or up to 2–3 wk

(continues on page 298)

UNDERSTANDING PSYCHOPHARMACOLOGY 16.1

Antidepressants (continued)

GENERIC AND BRAND NAMES	USUAL DOSE	SEDATION LEVEL/ HALF-LIFE	SIDE EFFECTS	RELIEF OF SYMPTOMS
Selective Serotonin Reuptake Inhibitors (SSRIs)				
fluoxetine (Prozac)	Initial dose of 20 mg/ day PO in AM; if no improvement after several weeks, increase dose on a BID schedule up to 80 mg/day PO	May be energizing; half-life is 2–9 days	Headache, nervousness, insomnia, drowsiness, anxiety, tremor, dizziness, light-headedness, nausea, vomiting, diarrhea, dry mouth, anorexia, dyspepsia, constipation, taste changes, upper respiratory infections, pharyngitis, painful menstruation, sexual dysfunction, frequency, sweating, rash, pruritus, weight loss, asthenia, fever	Up to 4 wk
paroxetine (Paxil)	20 mg/day PO as a single dose; may be increased up to 50 mg/day	May be energizing; half-life is 1 hr	Somnolence, dizziness, insomnia, tremor, nervousness, headache, nausea, dry mouth, constipation, diarrhea, ejaculatory disorders, male genital disorders, sweating, headache, asthenia	1–4 wk
sertraline (Zoloft)	Administer daily, AM or PM, 50 mg/ day PO; may be increased up to 200 mg/day; increases occur at 1-wk intervals	May be energizing; half-life is 26 hr	Headache, nervousness, drowsiness, anxiety, tremor, dizziness, insomnia, nausea, diarrhea, dry mouth, rhinitis, painful menstruation, sweating	Beginning relief of symptoms may take 2–4 wk
fluvoxamine maleate (Luvox)	Initially 50 mg PO HS with increase in 50-mg increments at 4- to 7-day intervals; usual range is 100–300 mg/day with divided doses and larger dose at HS	May be activating; half-life is 15 hr	Headache, nervousness, insomnia, drowsiness, anxiety, tremor, dizziness, light-headedness, sweating, rash, pruritus, nausea, vomiting, diarrhea, dry mouth, anorexia, dyspepsia, constipation, taste changes, sexual dysfunction, frequency, upper respiratory infection, pharyngitis; avoid abrupt withdrawal of medication	2–4 weeks
citalopram (Celexa)	Initially 20 mg PO/day as a single dose; may be increased to 40 mg/day if needed	May be energizing; half-life is 35 hr	Nausea, dry mouth, sweating, somnolence, dizziness, insomnia, ejaculatory disorders	4–6 wk

e-citalopram (Lexapro)	Initially 5 mg PO/day as a single dose; may be increased to 20 mg/day if needed	May be energizing; half-life is 35 hr	Nausea, dry mouth, sweating, somnolence, dizziness, insomnia, ejaculatory disorders	4–6 wk
vilazodone (Viibryd)	Initially 10 mg PO/day as a single dose; may be increased to 40 mg/day	Energizing; half-life is 20–24 hr	Diarrhea, nausea, vomiting, insomnia	2–4 wk

Selective Serotonin/Norepinephrine Reuptake Inhibitors (SNRIs)

venlafaxine (Effexor)	Initially 75 mg PO/day as a single dose may be increased to 375 mg/day	May be energizing; half-life is 3–7 hr, 9–13 hr, metabolite	Dry mouth, nausea, headache, sweating, dizziness, hypertension, sexual dysfunction, anxiety	Beginning relief of symptoms up to 2 wk
desvenlafaxine (Pristiq)	Initially 50–100 mg as a single dose	Energizing; half-life is 11 hr	Nausea, dizziness, sweating, constipation, decreased appetite	Beginning relief of symptoms up to 2 wk
duloxetine (Cymbalta)	Initially 30–60 mg as a single dose, may be increased to120 mg	Energizing; half-life is 8–19 hr	Nausea, dry mouth, headache, drowsiness, fatigue, dizziness, insomnia, constipation, diarrhea, loss of appetite, sweating, abdominal pain	Beginning relief of symptoms up to 2 wk

Dopamine Agonist

pramipexole (Mirapex)	Oral doses Week 1: 0.125 mg TID Week 2: 0.25 mg TID Week 3: 0.5 mg TID Week 4: 0.75 mg TID Week 5: 1 mg TID Week 6: 1.25 mg TID Week 7: 1.5 mg TID	May cause sleepiness; half-life is 8 hr	Headache, dizziness, insomnia, somnolence, nausea, constipation, asthenia	Relief of symptoms at therapeutic dose

Tricyclic Antidepressants (TCAs)

The orally administered TCAs were the first inhibitors of neuronal reuptake of serotonin and norepinephrine. They are anticholinergic at the CNS and peripheral receptors and act as sedatives. All TCAs have a three-ring molecular core and most share pharmacologic and clinical (antidepressant and anxiolytic) properties (Brunton et al., 2011).

Developed in the 1960s, the TCAs were the first drugs used to combat major depression. Currently, they are used for severe depression. The typical related symptom pattern of early morning wakening, feeling worse in the morning, anxiety, and weight loss is predictive of a good response to TCAs. These drugs also may be used for panic and obsessive-compulsive disorders (see Chap. 23).

Because TCAs have the "buckshot" properties discussed earlier, they block reuptake not only of norepinephrine and serotonin, but also of acetylcholine (ACh), which controls the cholinergic system and histamine. Blockage of both ACh and histamine leads to the predominant side effects of sedation, dry mouth, blurred vision, urinary retention, delayed micturition, dizziness, and fainting. Other side effects of confusion, disturbed concentration, weight gain, and constipation may lead to clients' reluctance to continue use. Abrupt withdrawal of TCAs may cause nausea, headache, and vertigo. Nurses monitor for orthostatic hypotension in clients beginning TCA therapy.

As a rule, the more sedating the TCA, the more anticholinergic properties it has. The tetracyclic antidepressant mirtazapine (Remeron) has been developed to reduce the discomfort of anticholinergic side effects. Other ways to control side effects include starting with low doses and increasing slowly, or changing to another antidepressant. Clients taking TCAs frequently do not experience improvement in symptoms for 2 to 6 weeks. They require support and encouragement during this time of adjustment.

The most drastic potential consequence of TCAs is lethality when taken in overdose. If a 10-day supply is taken at one time, the overdose can cause cardiac and cerebral toxicity. With clients beginning antidepressant therapy, practitioners should limit the amount of medication prescribed at any one time. Moreover, they should monitor clients starting these drugs carefully because risk for suicide increases when clients begin to "feel better" or energized.

Clients who take TCAs in conjunction with oral anticoagulants may be at risk for bleeding. Administration with clonidine may cause severe hypertension. Although monoamine oxidase inhibitors (MAOIs) and TCAs can be used together for refractory depression, adverse reactions (including hyperpyretic crises and hypertensive episodes) may be severe. Nurses observe and document adverse reactions to TCAs, especially if administration is in conjunction with other psychotropic agents (Karch, 2011).

> ### Think About It 16.1
> A client with major depression has been taking a TCA for several months. She comes to the clinic with decreased appetite and energy and lack of interest in daily activities. She states, "I feel like I did before I started taking the medicine." Explain what may be happening.

Monoamine Oxidase Inhibitors (MAOIs)

The MAOIs were first derived from hydrazone, a potent hepatotoxic substance (Anderson, 2005). These drugs inhibit monoamine oxidase-A (MAO), a gut enzyme that breaks down the amines hypothesized to be deficient in those with depression. Decreased MAO enables the previously deficient amines to accumulate in neuronal storage sites, alleviating depression (Karch, 2011). Drugs in this category include isocarboxazid (Marplan), phenelzine (Nardil), and trancyclopromine (Parnate).

MAOIs are administered orally. The MAOI-As are used with atypical depression and depression unresponsive to other drug regimens. They have been largely replaced by the selective serotonin reuptake inhibitors.

Side effects of MAOIs include dizziness, vertigo, headache, overactivity, manic behavior, constipation, diarrhea, and nausea. Clients should not take them with herbal remedies, particularly ginseng. The most serious risk of MAOI-As is hypertensive crisis. Clients taking them must avoid foods containing tyramine and over-the-counter medications containing amine derivatives such as phenylpropanolamine. Normally, MAO breaks down tyramine; however, because MAOIs inhibit MAO, tyramine can accumulate in the bodies of clients taking these drugs and eating tyramine-containing foods. Tyramine also releases norepinephrine from nerve endings. These metabolic actions can precipitate a hypertensive crisis. Examples of tyramine-containing foods include aged cheeses, processed meats, and dried, processed, or fermented fish. Beer, red wine, avocados, figs, raisins, and bananas also have significant amounts of tyramine. Regular assessment of blood pressure is necessary to detect signs of hypertensive crisis (Figure 16.5) (Karch, 2011). The nurse and client should carefully review every aspect of the client's diet to ensure the elimination of foods that could precipitate a hypertensive crisis. These drugs are contraindicated in any client unable or unwilling to give up eating such things.

Selective Serotonin Reuptake Inhibitors (SSRIs)

Developed in the 1980s to eliminate the cholinergic and histaminergic side effects caused by the TCAs, SSRIs are effective antidepressants with minimal toxic potential. Because SSRIs have a more tolerable side-effect profile than earlier antidepressants, pose no risk of lethal overdose, and are effective in 70% of cases, they are now the first choice for depression. SSRIs immediately block the neuronal transport of serotonin via the reuptake mechanism. This stimulates many postsynaptic receptor sites and probably contributes to the side effects, which include nausea, vomiting, weight changes, and delayed or impaired orgasm. The SSRIs also may cause agitation or restlessness. Unfortunately, many people who take them find that these drugs interfere with sexual performance, response, and arousal. This side effect may compromise adherence to the drug regimen.

Late and indirect actions of SSRIs are less well understood than are those of TCAs. Response to SSRIs may take anywhere from 3 weeks to 3 months (Stahl, 2006). Nurses must explain carefully the need for an adequate medication trial to people beginning this drug therapy.

Side effects are immediate; some experts believe that beginning with a subtherapeutic dose to improve initial

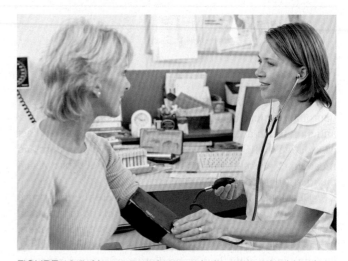

FIGURE 16.5 Nurses need to regularly assess the blood pressure of clients taking MAOIs to detect any signs of hypertensive crisis.

tolerance can minimize side effects. Others posit that the starting dose should be the same as the maintenance dose (Stahl, 2006). Taking the SSRIs with St. John's wort (*Hypericum perforatum*) increases the risk of a severe reaction. Clients should not take SSRIs with lithium; cigarette smoking decreases the effectiveness of SSRIs (Karch, 2011).

Use of SSRIs can cause *serotonin syndrome*, a potentially fatal condition that accompanies elevated blood levels of serotonin. Signs and symptoms include tachycardia, hypertension, fever, sweating, shivering, confusion, anxiety, restlessness, disorientation, tremors, muscular spasms, and rigidity. Risk factors for serotonin syndrome include the following:

* Concomitant use of antidepressants from different classes (eg, TCAs and SSRIs)
* Inadequate time between discontinuing use of one antidepressant and initiating use of another
* Combined use of serotonergic agonists with SSRIs
* Combined use of SSRIs with St. John's wort

If serotonin syndrome develops, temporary withdrawal of the SSRI is necessary and administration of a serotonin antagonist such as cyproheptadine occurs. Short-term use of an antianxiety drug, such as diazepam (Valium), may be helpful as an adjunct to control muscle spasms.

Nurses highlight several teaching points when educating clients about serotonergic agents. Many clients take medications with juice. Studies have shown that grapefruit juice can potentially alter the plasma concentrations of many oral medications, including SSRIs, through the P450 liver enzyme system. In some cases, the result may be undesirable clinical effects. Thus, nurses encourage clients not to take their medications with grapefruit juice. Another teaching point involves the discontinuation of SSRIs and serotonin/norepinephrine reuptake inhibitors. Each person responds differently to stopping the use of these drugs. Some people have only mild side effects; others have severe reactions from just lowering the dosage. In clients who react strongly to decreases, their neural serotonergic system has become dependent on the actions of the antidepressant. In such cases, stopping abruptly causes serotonergic activity to drop drastically. Thus, discontinuation "side effects" may appear, such as electrical surges/shocks in the head (brain shivers), body, or both; pins and needles on the skin; feelings of being on the verge of losing consciousness; blackouts; and short-term memory problems. Nurses advise clients never to stop taking these medications abruptly but to taper use very slowly, in conjunction with guidance from health care providers.

Other Selective Antidepressants
SELECTIVE SEROTONIN/NOREPINEPHRINE REUPTAKE INHIBITORS (SNRIS). Newer antidepressants affect both noradrenergic and serotonergic neurotransmission through dual presynaptic reuptake inhibition. SNRIs are more activating than SSRIs, causing more of an increase in energy. SNRIs include venlafaxine (Effexor, Effexor XR), desvenlafaxine (Pristiq), and duloxetine (Cymbalta) (Brunton et al., 2011).

* VENLAFAXINE. Venlafaxine (Effexor, Effexor XR) is approved for depression and hot flashes associated with perimenopausal symptoms. This drug's structure does not resemble any other currently used antidepressant. In doses under 125 mg, it is primarily an SSRI (Stahl, 2008). Doses over 150 mg cause reuptake inhibition on norepinephrine. Its action on both serotonin and norepinephrine means that venlafaxine may be a successful antidepressant for those who have not experienced response to SSRIs. Side effects that typically disappear in a week or two include drowsiness, weakness or tiredness, dizziness, headache, nightmares, nausea, vomiting, stomach pain, constipation, diarrhea, flatulence, heartburn, burping, dry mouth, change in ability to taste food, loss of appetite, weight loss, tremors, paresthesias, muscle tension, twitching, yawning, sweating, hot flashes or flushing, frequent urination, difficulty urinating, changes in libido, and dilated pupils. Venlafaxine should not be discontinued abruptly. Even missing one dose can cause withdrawal symptoms such as flashes in the peripheral vision, dizziness, headache, blurred vision, and nausea.
* DESVENLAFAXINE. Desvenlafaxine (Pristiq) is the active isomer (metabolite) of venlafaxine. It is a long-acting antidepressant and only needs to be taken once a day. Common side effects include constipation, loss of appetite, dry mouth, dizziness, extreme tiredness, unusual dreams, yawning, sweating, tremors, paresthesias, dilated pupils, blurred vision, difficulty urinating, and decreased libido.
* DULOXETINE. Duloxetine (Cymbalta) is approved for depression, generalized anxiety disorder, and pain associated with diabetic neuropathy, fibromyalgia, muscle aches, and osteoarthritis. A potent SNRI, duloxetine is available in a long-acting time-release capsule and only needs to be taken once a day. It can cause extreme nausea and dosage should be gradually increased. Nurses should encourage duloxetine to be taken with yogurt or ginger ale to decrease nausea. The side effects are similar to those of the other SNRIs.

SEROTONIN ANTAGONIST/REUPTAKE INHIBITORS (SARIS). In addition to blocking the reuptake of presynaptic serotonin, drugs in this category act as potent blockers of serotonin 2A and serotonin 2C. They also block alpha-1 norepinephrine receptors.

* TRAZODONE. Trazodone (Desyrel) is a psychoactive compound with sedative and antidepressant properties. Because of its sedative qualities, due to histamine-1 receptor antagonism, trazodone often is prescribed to augment other antidepressants and is to be taken at night to help treat insomnia. It has been associated with priapism (prolonged or inappropriate erections)

in men. Approximately 33% of reported cases required surgery; some of these clients experienced permanent erectile dysfunction. Men taking trazodone who experience priapism should discontinue the drug immediately and consult their physician. Clinical studies in clients with preexisting cardiac disease indicate that trazodone may contribute to dysrhythmias and should not be used (Schatzberg & Nemeroff, 2003).

• NEFAZODONE. Nefazodone (Serzone) is an excellent antidepressant, with particular efficacy in individuals with alcohol dependency; however, it can be hepatotoxic, and several deaths are directly attributable to the drug. As such, the brand-name drug was voluntarily removed from distribution in the United States in 2004. Because of demand due to efficacy, however, some generic formulations are still produced and distributed. The side effect profile is very similar to that of the SNRI category.

SELECTIVE DOPAMINE REUPTAKE INHIBITOR (SDRI).

• BUPROPION. Bupropion (Wellbutrin, Wellbutrin XL) is a weak blocker of serotonin and a potent blocker of norepinephrine reuptake, and partially inhibits reuptake of dopamine. It also is an antagonist to the nicotinic acetylcholine receptor and is an approved treatment for smoking cessation. Bupropion does not inhibit MAO, nor does it cause the sexual side effects that accompany many SSRIs. However, it does lower the seizure threshold, contraindicating its use in clients with seizure disorders. An additional contraindication is use in clients with a history of eating disorders because of a higher incidence of seizures noted in these clients (Schatzberg & Nemeroff, 2003).

ALPHA-2 REUPTAKE INHIBITOR (ARI).

• MIRTAZAPINE. Mirtazapine (Remeron) is a presynaptic alpha-2 antagonist with the dual action of increasing noradrenergic and serotonergic neurotransmission. Mirtazapine also has the unique ability to block two specific serotonin receptors, leading to minimal serotonergic side effects. Mirtazapine also causes fewer anticholinergic, cardiovascular, and cognitive disturbances than found with TCAs (Schatzberg & Nemeroff, 2003).

Drugs for Refractory Depression

Direct dopamine agonists used primarily for Parkinson disease, such as pramipexole (Mirapex) and the MAOI-B selegiline (Eldepryl), have been found effective for refractory depression (Aiken, 2007). Selegiline has been formulated in a transdermal patch (Emsam) approved for use in major depression (Morgan, 2007). It selectively blocks the MAO enzyme in the brain and, to a lesser extent, in the gut. The same dietary precautions associated with the MAOI-A drugs also apply to selegiline transdermal.

Checkpoint Questions

6. What are common categories of antidepressants?
7. What is the most serious risk associated with MAOIs?
8. What class of drugs is considered the first choice for treating depression?

Mood Stabilizers

Mood stabilizers are used primarily to treat bipolar and impulse-control disorders (Understanding Psychopharmacology 16.2; see Chaps. 28 and 32). For several decades, lithium carbonate (Eskalith) has been the predominant treatment for mania. Other major categories of mood stabilizers include anticonvulsants and medications for refractory mania.

Lithium Carbonate

Lithium carbonate is the first-line agent against bipolar disorders (Goodwin & Jamison, 2007). Its mechanism of action is unknown. Lithium alters sodium transport in nerve and muscle cells and inhibits the release of norepinephrine and dopamine. However, it does not inhibit the release of serotonin (Karch, 2011). It usually takes 2 to 3 weeks of gradually increasing doses to achieve a therapeutic level of lithium. More than half of clients with bipolar disorders are refractory to lithium, meaning that the drug does not work or they cannot tolerate its side effects. In other cases, lithium loses efficacy with time. Those for whom lithium succeeds must stay on it; stopping lithium is related directly to later loss of efficacy. When effective, lithium quells the frequency and severity of both mania and depression (Goodwin & Jamison, 2007).

In acute mania, lithium is usually prescribed as 600 to 900 mg three times a day. It is administered orally in slow-release form to produce therapeutic serum levels from 1 to 1.5 mEq/L (Karch, 2011). Maintenance doses range from 0.6 to 1.2 mEq/L. Regular serum levels must be drawn to ascertain correct dosage and to monitor for potential toxicity. In the early weeks of administration, blood should be drawn twice each week before clients take the morning dose. Maintenance therapy requires nurses to assess clients' blood levels of lithium at least every 2 months (Figure 16.6).

Lithium toxicity can occur when sodium levels are low and absorption is disrupted. Predisposing factors include excessive heat, diaphoresis, concurrent use of diuretics, and decreased sodium intake. Nurses evaluate blood levels immediately if clients show any symptoms of lithium toxicity. With levels below 1.5 mEq/L, toxicity symptoms include lethargy, slurred speech, muscle weakness, hand tremor, nausea, vomiting, and diarrhea. At a mild to moderate toxicity level (1.5 to 2 mEq/L), symptoms include coarse hand tremor, mental confusion, drowsiness, lack of coordination, gastrointestinal upset, and electrocardiographic changes. At levels of 2 to 2.5 mEq/L, symptoms of toxicity include ataxia, blurred vision, stupor, coma, and respiratory failure. Levels above 2.5 mEq/L are considered life-threatening (Karch, 2011).

UNDERSTANDING PSYCHOPHARMACOLOGY 16.2

Mood Stabilizers

GENERIC AND BRAND NAMES	USUAL DOSE	SEDATION LEVEL/ HALF-LIFE	SIDE EFFECTS	RELIEF OF SYMPTOMS
lithium carbonate (Lithobid, Lithonate, Lithotabs)	Acute mania: 600 mg PO TID or 900 mg in oral slow-release form BID to produce serum levels between 1 and 1.5 mEq/L; for longer use: 300 mg PO TID or QID for serum levels between 0.6 and 1.2 mEq/L	May initially cause lethargy; half-life is 17–36 hr	Adverse effects related to serum levels; in acute treatment, blood should be drawn twice a week, 8–12 hr after previous dose; in long-term management, blood should be drawn every 2 mo; lethargy, slurred speech, muscle weakness, fine hand tremor, nausea, vomiting, diarrhea, thirst, polyuria, moderate to severe toxicity (blood serum of 2.0–2.5 mEq/L), pulmonary complications; life-threatening toxicity (blood serum >2.5 mEq/L), death	Takes several weeks
carbamazepine (Tegretol)	Initial dose of 200 mg PO TID with gradual increase of 200 mg in divided doses, not to exceed 1,200 mg/ day PO	May cause drowsiness; half-life is initially 25–65 hr, followed by 12–17 hr	Dizziness, drowsiness, unsteadiness, nausea, vomiting, fatal hepatitis, fatal massive hepatic cellular necrosis with total loss of intact liver tissue, fatal cardiovascular complications	Relief of symptoms when on maintenance dose
divalproex sodium (Depakote)	For mania: 750 mg orally TID in divided doses; do not exceed 60 mg/kg per day	May cause sedation; half-life is 6–16 hr	Sedation, nausea, vomiting, indigestion, life-threatening pancreatitis, hepatic failure	Relief of symptoms when on maintenance dose
lamotrigine (Lamictal) APPROVED FOR BIPOLAR DEPRESSION ONLY	Initially, 25 mg/day PO for 2 wk, then 100 mg/day PO in two divided doses for 2 wk; may increase by 100 mg/day every week up to a maintenance dose of 300–500 mg/day in two divided doses	May cause insomnia; half-life is 29 hr	Dizziness, ataxia, nausea, potentially life-threatening Stevens-Johnson syndrome and toxic epidermal necrolysis with multiorgan failure	Relief of symptoms at therapeutic dose
tiagabine HCl (Gabitril) OFF LABEL	4 mg PO daily for 1 wk with increases of 4–8 mg/wk until desired response; maximum dose of 56 mg/ day in three to four divided doses	Activating half-life 7–9 hr	Dizziness, asthenia, somnolence, gastrointestinal upset, pain; avoid abrupt withdrawal of medication	30–60 min
oxcarbazepine (Trileptal)	300 mg PO BID with increases to 1,200 mg PO BID	May be activating; half-life 2 hr, then 9 hr	Dizziness, drowsiness, unsteadiness, hypotension, hypertension, bradycardia, tachycardia, nausea, vomiting, impaired fertility, hyponatremia; avoid abrupt withdrawal of medication	4–5 hr

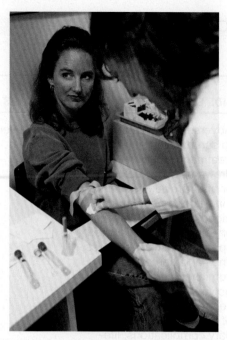

FIGURE 16.6 Clients starting lithium therapy must have their blood drawn twice each week before taking the morning dose. Once they are on maintenance therapy, their blood levels of lithium should be assessed at least every 2 months.

Before initial administration, clients undergo a thorough physical examination that includes electrolyte studies, complete blood count, and thyroid function tests. Identification of preexisting physical problems provides a baseline for the health care team to effectively monitor side effects, such as weight gain and thyroid dysfunction.

Clients often do not take their lithium as prescribed because of knowledge deficits and side effects, among other factors. They and their families also are often unaware of the care that is required for such clients to remain physically healthy. Client and family education is essential to prevent toxicity. Teaching points include avoiding the sun, potential overheating, and dehydration. See also Client-Centered Education 16.1.

Anticonvulsants

Several anticonvulsants have been used successfully as mood stabilizers. Some scientists theorize that they affect *kindling* (a neuroelectrical phenomenon in which the brain becomes increasingly sensitive to stress and eventually shows constant abnormal neuroelectrical activity). Results of kindling include increased frequency of relapse and longer duration of an episode of either mania or depression. It has been theorized that lithium blocks the early stages of kindling, carbamazepine and valproic acid act later, and lamotrigine works through the glutamate system.

- **VALPROIC ACID.** Valproic acid (Depakote) appears to act by increasing the activity of the inhibitory neurotransmitter gamma-amino-butyric acid (GABA). This action facilitates the entrance of chloride into the neuron to bind with calcium, thus stabilizing the nerve action potential and eventually decreasing mania. It is necessary to obtain periodic liver function tests as well as valproic acid levels to check for toxicity. It is common for hair

Client–Centered Education 16.1

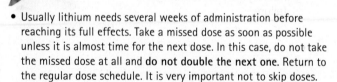

Teaching Points for Clients Taking Lithium

- Usually lithium needs several weeks of administration before reaching its full effects. Take a missed dose as soon as possible unless it is almost time for the next dose. In this case, do not take the missed dose at all and **do not double the next one**. Return to the regular dose schedule. It is very important not to skip doses.
- Because the kidneys cannot tell the difference between lithium and salt, anything that changes the amount of salt in the body automatically changes the level of lithium. Thus, consume a consistent amount of sodium every day.
- Drink at least 2 quarts of water each day.
- Do not increase or decrease the amount of salt and salty foods (cheese, hot dogs, potato chips, pizza) you normally eat. An increase in salt will cause lithium to decrease. A decrease in salt will cause lithium to increase.
- Use extra care in hot weather and during activities that cause heavy sweating, such as hot baths, saunas, or exercise. The loss of too much water and salt from your body may lead to serious side effects.

- Lithium may cause you to become drowsy or less alert. It is dangerous to take it with alcohol, sleeping pills, or pain medication.
- Weight increase is common with lithium. Be sure to eat balanced meals and avoid snacking on sweets.
- **Avoid all caffeine**: it greatly interferes with the effectiveness of lithium.
- Receive an annual physical to check the following:
  - Kidney function tests, including electrolytes, blood urea nitrogen, and creatine clearance to rule out possible kidney damage
  - Liver enzyme tests, including LDH, SGOT, and SGPT, to rule out possible liver damage
  - Thyroid function tests, including T_3, T_4, free T_3, free T_4, and TSH to rule out possible thyroid damage. Lithium sometimes alters thyroid function; clients may need thyroid medication.
  - Cardiac function tests, including periodic electrocardiograms (EKG) to rule out arrhythmias or other possible cardiac defects

loss to occur shortly after initiating therapy. Taking at least 100 to 200 mg of zinc at night has been found helpful in reducing and eliminating hair loss. Other common side effects include headache, talkativeness, sweating, severe nausea, vomiting, diarrhea, constipation, inflammation of the oral mucosa, and slurred speech. Valproic acid should be taken with yogurt or ginger ale to decrease nausea. Female clients of childbearing years should be closely monitored due to the potential of developing polycystic ovary syndrome.

- Carbamazepine. Carbamazepine (Tegretol) is chemically related to the TCAs and has complex pharmacokinetics. It is the third most common drug used for mania, following lithium and valproic acid. Carbamazepine is particularly effective against aggressive and hostile symptoms. Absorption after oral administration is slow, with peak plasma concentrations 4 to 8 hours after ingestion (Brunton et al., 2011). Acute toxicity can result in stupor or coma, hyperirritability, convulsions, and respiratory depression. Less dangerous side effects include drowsiness, vertigo, ataxia, diplopia, and blurred vision. Tolerance can develop; however, dose changes can control it (Brunton et al., 2011). Another side effect is feeling uncoordinated and less mentally "sharp." Carbamazepine can also make clients feel bloated or uncomfortable. Of concern with the use of carbamazepine are the numerous drug–drug interactions that can occur through the P450 liver enzyme system.
- Oxcarbazepine. Oxcarbazepine (Trileptal), an analogue of carbamazepine, is structurally similar but differs slightly in composition. The difference makes oxcarbazepine much less likely to cause aplastic anemia. Oxcarbazepine has been found to be useful in bipolar disorder (Pratoomsri et al., 2006).
- Lamotrigine. Lamotrigine (Lamictal) has been approved for bipolar depression with documented effectiveness as both monotherapy and adjunctive therapy (Stahl, 2006). Lamotrigine decreased manic symptoms in 74% of clients, but a severe and potentially fatal rash indicative of Stevens-Johnson syndrome developed in 15% of those studied. *Nurses advise any client taking anticonvulsants in whom a rash develops to go immediately to the local emergency department.* Coadministration with valproic acid and doses above those recommended appear to increase the risk of rash (Stahl, 2006).

Medications for Refractory Mania

Refractory mania is completely or marginally unresponsive to drug therapy with conventional mood-stabilizing agents. It is particularly debilitating. Associated behaviors include rapid cycling with dangerous, impulsive behaviors alternating with severe depression. Morbidity and mortality increase during depressed and mixed phases (Goodwin & Jamison, 2007).

For people with mania refractory to first-line treatment for bipolar disorder, several different medications can be used (Stahl, 2006). Several drugs that have been successful against refractory mania were not designed for this purpose. Clozapine (Clozaril), used to treat resistant schizophrenia (see Chap. 29), is an example. Green and colleagues (2000) found that a 12-week trial of clozapine was highly effective in clients with mania unresponsive to other agents. Most atypical antipsychotic agents are now used to stabilize both acute and refractory phases of bipolar disorder (Goodwin & Jamison, 2007). Approximately two-thirds of clients with refractory bipolar disorder experienced response to lamotrigine plus lithium (Ghaemi et al., 2006).

Anxiolytics

Anxiolytic (antianxiety) medications are used for generalized anxiety disorder, acute anxiety states, social phobia, performance anxiety, and simple phobias (see Chap. 23). They also are prescribed for short-term relief of insomnia. They include buspirone (BuSpar) and benzodiazepines (as well as SSRIs). Benzodiazepines are also used in alcohol withdrawal, agitation, and also may prevent seizures. Benzodiazepines also are used for mania and for acute psychoses when safe and rapid sedation with relatively few side effects is desired. The main difference between the various benzodiazepines involves half-life. See Understanding Psychopharmacology 16.3.

Buspirone

Buspirone (BuSpar) is a serotonin-1A partial agonist. It lacks anticonvulsant, sedative, and muscle relaxant properties (Karch, 2011). Due to the potential for headache, adults should begin with 5 mg twice a day for 3 days and then increase to 5 mg three times a day, with increases of 5 mg/day occurring every 2 to 3 days. The maximum dose should not exceed 60 mg/day.

Buspirone is contraindicated in clients with marked renal or liver impairment and lactating women. Adverse effects include dizziness, headache, nervousness, insomnia, light-headedness, nausea, dry mouth, and gastrointestinal distress. Buspirone must be used cautiously in clients who use alcohol or other CNS depressants; fluoxetine decreases the drug's effects. If taken with erythromycin, itraconazole, or nefazodone, serum levels of buspirone may increase and must be monitored (Karch, 2011).

Benzodiazepines

Benzodiazepines have the pharmacologic effects of anxiolysis, sedation, centrally mediated muscle relaxation, and elevation of the seizure threshold (Karch, 2011). They act directly on GABA-A receptors and are thought to increase GABA available to dampen neural overstimulation (Figure 16.7). They are classified according to half-life. Benzodiazepines are generally considered safe and effective for short-term use only. Adverse effects are extensions of their central actions. Benzodiazepines may be excessively sedating, and concurrent use with narcotics or alcohol can potentiate their effects. In addition to these effects and the side effects also found

UNDERSTANDING PSYCHOPHARMACOLOGY 16.3

Anxiolytics

GENERIC AND BRAND NAMES	USUAL DOSE	SEDATION LEVEL/ HALF-LIFE	SIDE EFFECTS	RELIEF OF SYMPTOMS
buspirone (BuSpar)	Initially 15 mg/day PO (5 mg TID); increase dose 5 mg/day at intervals of 2–3 days to achieve maximum therapeutic response; do not exceed 60 mg/day	Energizing; half-life of 3–11 hr	Dizziness, headache, nervousness, insomnia, light-headedness, nausea, dry mouth, vomiting, abdominal/gastric distress, diarrhea	Maximum benefit after reaching therapeutic dose
Benzodiazepines				
diazepam (Valium)	For anxiety disorder: 2–10 mg BID-QID	Transient, mild drowsiness; half-life of 20–50 hr	Transient, mild drowsiness initially, sedation, depression, lethargy, apathy, fatigue, light-headedness, disorientation, restlessness, confusion, possible mild paradoxical excitatory reactions during first 2 wk of treatment, constipation, diarrhea, bradycardia, tachycardia, incontinence, urinary retention, changes in libido, drug dependence with a withdrawal syndrome	Immediately effective at therapeutic dose
lorazepam (Ativan)	PO: 2–6 mg/day IM: 0.05 mg/kg	Transient, mild drowsiness; half-life 10–20 hr	Depression, lethargy, apathy, fatigue, light-headedness, disorientation, restlessness, constipation, dry mouth, nausea	Intermediate
alprazolam (Xanax)	PO: 0.25–1 mg TID	Transient, mild drowsiness; half-life 6–20 hr	Depression, lethargy, apathy, fatigue, light-headedness, disorientation, restlessness, constipation, dry mouth, nausea	Intermediate
chlordiazepoxide (Librium)	PO: 5–10 mg TID-QID IM/IV: 50–100 mg/day	Transient, mild drowsiness; half-life 30–100 hr	Depression, lethargy, apathy, fatigue, light-headedness, disorientation, restlessness, constipation, diarrhea, bradycardia, tachycardia, urinary retention, incontinence, changes in libido	Intermediate
flurazepam (Dalmane)	10–30 mg/day	Transient, mild drowsiness; half-life 50–160 hr	Depression, lethargy, apathy, fatigue, light-headedness, disorientation, restlessness, asthenia, constipation, diarrhea, dyspepsia, bradycardia, tachycardia, urinary retention, incontinence, changes in libido	Rapid
clonazepam (Klonopin)		Mild; half-life 19–60 hr	Depression, fatigue, drowsiness, short term memory impairment, decreased coordination, confusion, agitation, insomnia	Rapid

Anticonvulsant

| gabapentin (Neurontin) | 900–1,800 mg/day PO in three divided doses; maximum time between doses should not exceed 12 hr; up to 2,400–3,600 mg/day has been used | May cause insomnia; half-life is 5–7 hr | Dizziness, insomnia, somnolence, ataxia | Relief of symptoms at therapeutic dose |

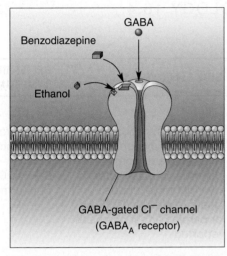

FIGURE 16.7 Benzodiazepines act directly on GABA receptors and increase GABA available. Effects include the decreased stimulation of the nervous system that accompanies anxiety. However, use with alcohol (ethanol) can be dangerous because a different side can bind with ethanol and further enhance responsiveness to GABA. The result can be oversedation.

with buspirone, benzodiazepines can stimulate a mild paradoxical excitatory reaction at the beginning of treatment.

Benzodiazepines have the potential to lose efficacy due to the development of tolerance. Clients may begin increasing doses to achieve previous response and discover that they are developing drug dependence. Dependence means that when clients stop taking the medication, they experience pathologic symptoms and signs. In the past, a distinction was made between *physical* and *psychological* dependence, with physical withdrawal syndromes being the key indicator of "addiction." Moreover, stigma was attached to the idea of being "physically dependent" to these drugs. However, as stressed in Chapter 2, there is no psychology without physiology. The concept of dependence (addiction) is a cluster of cognitive, behavioral, affective, and physiologic signs that indicate compulsive use of a substance. Thus, the distinction between psychological and physiologic dependence is not useful.

Use of benzodiazepines requires caution in older adults and debilitated clients because of the potential for falling and mental confusion. They should also not be used in depressed or suicidal clients and clients with a history of substance abuse. Withdrawal syndrome is possible on discontinuation and most common with high doses used for more than 4 months (Karch, 2011). Symptoms of withdrawal syndrome include anxiety, irritability, tremulousness, sweating, lethargy, diarrhea, insomnia, depression, abdominal and muscle cramps, vomiting, and convulsions. Discontinuation of benzodiazepines should be gradual with careful monitoring of symptoms. Onset of symptoms related to withdrawal or discontinuation usually reflects the half-life of the specific drug (1 to 2 days for short-acting drugs and 2 to 5 days for long-acting drugs). However, withdrawal symptoms have been known to develop 7 to 10 days after discontinuation. Symptoms usually peak several days after onset and disappear slowly during a period of 1 to 3 weeks (Rosenbaum et al., 2005; Stahl, 2006). Nurses need to caution clients not to abruptly discontinue use of these medications because of the certain risk of severe seizures.

Other Anxiolytics

In addition to buspirone and the benzodiazepines, other drug classes used to treat anxiety include the sedating antidepressants (eg, trazodone, TCAs) and the sedating antihistamines (eg, diphenhydramine [Benadryl]). Anticonvulsants such as gabapentin also have been found useful, as has low-dose olanzapine (Pollack et al., 2006). Most of the SSRIs have also received FDA approval for treatment of anxiety. Newer nonbenzodiazepine sedative-hypnotics are rapidly becoming first-line treatment for insomnia (Stahl, 2006). Examples are zaleplon (Sonata), zolpidem (Ambien), and eszopiclone (Lunesta), and also ramelteon (Rozerem), which is a melatonin-1 and -2 receptor agonist (see Chap. 22).

> ### Checkpoint Questions
> 9. Which neurotransmitter is not affected by lithium?
> 10. What manifestations develop when serum lithium levels range from 2 to 2.5 mEq/L?
> 11. How are benzodiazepines believed to achieve anxiolysis?

Antipsychotic (Neuroleptic) Agents

Antipsychotic (neuroleptic) medications are used to treat severe thought disorders such as schizophrenia (see Chap. 29). They also are used for acute and chronic confusion that commonly accompanies psychoses, extreme aggression, and dementia (see Chap. 31). Target symptoms include disorganized speech and behavior, flat or inappropriate affect, delusions, hallucinations, and catatonia. Antipsychotics are subdivided into typical (traditional) antipsychotics and atypical antipsychotics. See Understanding Psychopharmacology 16.4 for an overview of specific agents.

Typical or Traditional Antipsychotics

For many years, traditional antipsychotic agents were the only class of medications for the treatment of psychosis. They block dopamine receptors in the brain, thus altering the release and turnover of dopamine. Antipsychotics are lipophilic and metabolized by hepatic mechanisms (Brunton et al., 2011). All clients taking them require close monitoring for side effects. Unlike antidepressants, the risk of overdose is low, even with large amounts. Lethality also is low (Brunton et al., 2011). The greatest hazards involve extrapyramidal symptoms (EPSs) and tardive dyskinesia (TD).

UNDERSTANDING PSYCHOPHARMACOLOGY 16.4

Antipsychotics/Neuroleptics

GENERIC AND BRAND NAMES	USUAL DOSE	SEDATION LEVEL/ HALF-LIFE	SIDE EFFECTS	RELIEF OF SYMPTOMS
Typical (Traditional) Antipsychotics				
fluphenazine (Prolixin)	PO: 0.5–10.0 mg/day in divided doses every 6–8 hr; give doses of 20 mg/day with caution IM: initial dose of 12.5–25 mg; determine subsequent doses based on client response; dose not to exceed 100 mg	Initially causes drowsiness; half-life: PO, 4.5–15.3 hr; IM, 6.8–9.6 days	Drowsiness, pseudoparkinsonism, dystonia, akathisia, autonomic disturbances, refractory dysrhythmias; sudden death related to asphyxia or cardiac arrest has been reported	Full therapeutic effects may require 6 wk to 6 mo of treatment
chlorpromazine (Thorazine)	May be given IM, 25 mg, repeated in 1 hr; dose can be increased to 400 mg every 4–6 hr with move to oral administration; 25–50 mg PO TID up to 800 mg, increase oral dose by 20–50 mg semi-weekly until optimum dose achieved	Sedating; half-life is 2 hr, then 30 hr	Drowsiness, insomnia, vertigo, extrapyramidal syndromes, dry mouth, salivation, nausea, vomiting, anorexia, constipation, hypotension, orthostatic hypotension, anemia, urinary retention, photophobia, blurred vision, urticaria, photosensitivity	Immediate relief of agitation from psychiatric symptoms
thioridazine (Mellaril)	50–100 mg PO TID with gradual increase to maximum of 800 mg/day if needed to control symptoms	Sedating; half-life is 10–20 hr	Drowsiness, pseudoparkinsonism, dystonia, akathisia, neuroleptic malignant syndrome, refractory dysrhythmias, photophobia, blurred vision, dry mouth, salivation, nasal congestion, nausea, urine discolored pink to red-brown	Relief of symptoms at most effective dose
trifluoperazine (Stelazine)	PO: 2–5 mg BID with optimum response at 15–20 mg/day IM: for prompt relief of severe symptoms, 1–2 mg by deep IM injection every 4–6 hr (should not need to exceed 6 mg/day)	Sedating; half-life is 47–100 hr	Drowsiness, pseudoparkinsonism, dystonia, akathisia, refractory dysrhythmias, photophobia, blurred vision, dry mouth, salivation, nasal congestion, nausea, urine discolored pink to red-brown	Relief of symptoms at optimum dosage in 2–3 wk if orally administered

haloperidol (Haldol)	PO: 0.5–2.0 mg BID or TID; daily doses up to 100 mg have been used, but safety not demonstrated	Sedating; half-life is 21–34 hr for oral administration and 3 wk for decanoate	Drowsiness, pseudoparkinsonism, dystonia, akathisia, neuroleptic malignant syndrome, refractory dysrhythmias, suppression of cough reflex and potential for aspiration, anaphylactoid reactions	Relief of symptoms at optimum PO dose; immediate relief of acute symptoms with IM
	IM: 2–5 mg and up to 10–30 mg every 30–60 min or every 4–8 hr as necessary for relief of acute agitation and severe symptoms			
	Decanoate: initial dose is 10–15 times the daily oral dose; repeat at 4-wk intervals			
thiothixene (Navane)	PO: Initially 2 mg BID or TID or 5 mg BID; increase dose as needed to optimum dose of 20–30 mg/day; may increase to 60 mg/day but few benefits reported	Sedating; half-life is 34 hr	Drowsiness, pseudoparkinsonism, dystonia, akathisia, autonomic disturbances, refractory dysrhythmias, photophobia, blurred vision, dry mouth, salivation, nasal congestion, nausea, urine discolored pink to red-brown	Immediate relief, especially with IM administration
	IM: usual dose is 4 mg BID-QID with most clients controlled on 16–20 mg/day; maximum IM dose is 60 mg/day			

Atypical Antipsychotics

clozapine (Clozaril)	25 mg BID; gradually increase to a maximum of 900 mg	Initially sedating	Weight gain, sedation, salivation, seizures, danger of agranulocytosis, sexual dysfunction. Requires monthly testing of WBC.	Takes 6 mo or more to show effectiveness
risperidone (Risperdal; Consta, depot; Invega, long acting)	Initially 0.25–1 mg daily, increasing to a maximum of 9–12 mg/day. Available in 0.25, 0.5, 1, 2, 3, 4, and 6 mg, IM (Consta)	Low-may be energizing	Insomnia, agitation, anxiety, headache, nausea, vomiting, neuroleptic malignant syndrome	Some relief immediately; more at peak dose
	Invega in 3-6-9: Invega is dosed 3:2 compared with Risperdal.			
olanzapine (Zyprexa)	Initially 5–10 mg PO QID, increase to 10 mg PO QID within several days; may be increased by 5 mg/day at 1-wk intervals; do not exceed 20 mg/day. Also available in IM immediate action	May be sedating, at least initially; half-life is 30 hr	Excessive weight gain, somnolence, dizziness, neuroleptic malignant syndrome, constipation, postural hypotension, fever	Relief of symptoms when therapeutic dose achieved
quetiapine (dibenzothiazine, Seroquel, Seroquel XR)	Initial dose of 25–50 mg PO BID; increase in increments of 50–100 mg BID or TID to reach a therapeutic level. XR only needs to be taken once daily.	May be sedating, at least initially; half-life is 6 hr		Relief of symptoms when therapeutic dose achieved

(continues on page 310)

UNDERSTANDING PSYCHOPHARMACOLOGY 16.4

Antipsychotics/Neuroleptics (continued)

GENERIC AND BRAND NAMES	USUAL DOSE	SEDATION LEVEL/ HALF-LIFE	SIDE EFFECTS	RELIEF OF SYMPTOMS
ziprasidone (Geodon)	Initially 20 mg PO BID, then effective range of 20–80 mg PO BID	High sedation; half-life is 3 hr	Drowsiness, neuroleptic malignant syndrome, orthostatic hypotension, somnolence, sedation, headache, dysrhythmias, nausea, dyspepsia, constipation, fever. Must be taken with a gram of fat for maximum efficacy.	6–8 hr
aripiprazole (Abilify)	2–30 mg PO QD Available in 2, 5, 10, 15, 20 mg, and IM for immediate response.	Moderate sedation; half-life is 75–146 hr	Headache, anxiety, insomnia, light-headedness, tremor, asthenia, orthostatic hypotension, nausea, vomiting, constipation, diarrhea, rhinitis, cough, seizures, malignant neuroleptic syndrome	3–5 hr
iloperidone (Fanapt)	Initial dose is 1m g BID increasing to therapeutic range of 6–12 mg BID	Moderate sedation; half-life is 18 hr	Dizziness, dry mouth, sedation, stuffy nose, orthostatic hypotension, hypersomnolence, tachycardia, weight gain, hyperglycemia	Some effects may be felt within 2 wk; full benefit may take 6–12 wk to develop
asenapine (Saphris)	5–10 mg sublingual tablet BID	Moderate sedation; half-life is 24 hr	Slight weight gain, hyperglycemia, orthostatic hypotension, akathisia, tremors, muscle stiffness	Some effects may be felt within 2 wk; full benefit may take 6–12 wk to develop
Lurasidone (Latuda)	Initial dose of 40 mg daily. Therapeutic dose ranges from 40 to 120 mg daily.	Moderate sedation; half-life is 18 hr	Akathisia, tremors, muscle stiffness, agitation, nausea	Full benefit may take 6–12 wk to develop

Tremors, shufflegate, ↑ drooling

Risk of EPSs and other movement disorders is highest for clients who use older, high-potency neuroleptic agents, such as haloperidol or perphenazine, for long periods. They set up a powerful dopamine blockade to control psychosis, but they also block dopamine receptors in the part of the brain that controls finely coordinated movements. This "secondary blockade" leads to movement disorders. Table 16.6 summarizes the potential motor side effects of antipsychotic medications and suggested treatments. Complex monitoring for EPSs should involve client and family. Before initiating any neuroleptic drug, clients must understand its risks and hazards. If acute psychiatric symptoms are compromising a client's ability to learn, health care providers involve relatives and significant others. Early diagnosis of beginning symptoms may result in prompt withdrawal of or a change in

medication. Thoroughly understanding symptoms and their causes alleviates client and family anxiety if a movement disorder emerges. *snakemotion, rollingtongue*

Tardive dyskinesia, the most serious side effect of long-term use of neuroleptics, is often irreversible and severely disabling. Characteristics include involuntary choreoathetotic movements affecting the face, tongue, and perioral, buccal, and masticatory muscles. TD also may involve the neck, torso, and extremities. Risk of irreversible TD increases with cumulative dose and duration of neuroleptic treatment. Fine, wormlike movements of the tongue may be the first sign of TD; discontinuing the medication immediately may prevent the full-blown syndrome (Brunton et al., 2011). Whereas decreasing or discontinuing neuroleptic medication is the best treatment for TD, it also

TABLE 16.6 Extrapyramidal Motor Side Effects of Antipsychotic Medications

Side Effect	Definition	Description	Treatment
Acute dystonic reactions	Severe muscle spasms that can be life-threatening if not treated immediately	1. **Torticollis:** Severe twisting of the neck and back 2. **Opisthotonus:** Severe arching of the back 3. **Oculogyric crisis:** Severe rolling back of the eyes into the head 4. **Laryngospasm:** Spasm of the throat in which breathing and swallowing become severely impaired and emergency tracheotomy may be required 5. **Oral-facial-maxillary spasms:** Spasms of the face, lips, and tongue making it very difficult to talk, chew, and eat	IM administration of diphenhydramine, 25 mg, or benztropine, 0.5–1.0 mg EPSs are caused by an imbalance between acetylcholine and dopamine. The antiparkinsonian drugs antagonize the muscarinic receptors to ease the side effects.
Dyskinesias	Abnormal muscle movements, not as severe as spasms	1. Facial tics and twitches 2. Chewing movements 3. Lip smacking 4. Blinking 5. Aimless movements of the tongue 6. Shoulder shrugging 7. Pedaling movements of legs 8. Flailing arms	Decrease dose. Some clients require prophylactic treatment with antiparkinsonian agents such as benztropine 1–2 mg up to QID.
Tardive dyskinesia	Late onset of any of the dyskinesias. Usually does not occur until 4–6 mo after treatment with a neuroleptic has begun.	Tardive dyskinesia can become permanent and must be treated at the first symptom. Can also occur with antidepressants that affect dopamine neurons.	Prevention (ie, regular reevaluation of drug dose and assessment for beginning side effects) along with maintenance on lowest dose of medication
Parkinsonian reactions	Muscle movements that resemble symptoms of Parkinson's disease	1. Stiffness and slowness of voluntary movement 2. Masklike immobility of facial muscles 3. Stooped posture 4. Slow, monotonous speech 5. Shuffling gait speeds up on its own 6. Immobility	IM or IV administration of diphenhydramine or benztropine
Akathisia	Nearly continual muscle activity, less intense than dystonias or dyskinesias	1. Intolerance of inactivity 2. Continuous agitation and restlessness 3. Pacing 4. Constant leg and finger movements	Changing to a different neuroleptic or decreasing the dose

can precipitate withdrawal dyskinesia. These symptoms are the same as those of TD, but they tend to resolve within a few weeks. Clients need to understand that it may take time for symptoms to resolve, even if use of the medication is discontinued.

LOW-POTENCY TYPICAL ANTIPSYCHOTICS. These drugs include chlorpromazine (Thorazine) and thioridazine (Mellaril). Chlorpromazine decreases arousal (Brunton

et al., 2011). Thioridazine depresses the parts of the brain involved with wakefulness and emesis and is an anticholinergic, antihistaminic, and alpha-adrenergic blocking agent (Karch, 2011).

Chlorpromazine is available in tablets, sustained-release capsules, liquid concentrate, suppositories, and as an injection. As much as 2,000 mg/day can be given to inpatients; the usual dose is 200 to 800 mg/day. Adverse effects include drowsiness, insomnia, vertigo, dry mouth, salivation, nausea, vomiting, and constipation. Side effects include hypotension, anemia, urinary retention, blurred vision, and photosensitivity (Karch, 2011). The risk of tachycardia and hypotension increases if chlorpromazine is taken with epinephrine or norepinephrine. An additive effect is possible if chlorpromazine is taken with beta blockers. CNS depression and hypotension can occur if chlorpromazine is taken with barbiturate anesthetics, alcohol, or meperidine. Chlorpromazine is contraindicated in clients with bone marrow suppression, respiratory disorders, or liver disorders, severe depression, coma, bone marrow suppression, and cerebral or arterial arteriosclerosis (Karch, 2011).

When administering chlorpromazine, nurses caution clients to take the medication exactly as prescribed and to avoid getting the irritating oral concentrates on skin or clothes. Clients must avoid alcohol; they also should not operate machinery or drive because the drug may cause drowsiness. They should wear sunscreen because chlorpromazine precipitates photosensitivity (Karch, 2011). Low-potency neuroleptics have the same anticholinergic properties as TCAs, causing the same symptoms of dry mouth, constipation, blurred vision, and drowsiness.

HIGH-POTENCY TYPICAL ANTIPSYCHOTICS. Fluphenazine (Prolixin), trifluoperazine (Stelazine), haloperidol (Haldol), and thiothixene (Navane) are typical moderate- to high-potency antipsychotics. Like other drugs in this class, these dopaminergic-blocking agents pose an increased risk of side effects.

Movement disorders accompany treatment with low-dose, high-potency phenothiazine medications such as fluphenazine. The most serious and potentially fatal side effect is **neuroleptic malignant syndrome**, characterized by severe muscular rigidity, altered consciousness, disorientation, dysphagia, elevated creatine phosphokinase, stupor, catatonia, hyperpyrexia, and labile pulse and blood pressure. This life-threatening condition can occur after a single dose; however, it is more common in the first 2 weeks of administration or with an increased dose (Brunton et al., 2011). It can continue for as long as 2 weeks after discontinuation of the medication; treatment involves immediate cessation of the drug and hospitalization to stabilize acute symptoms.

Black box warnings alert and inform health professionals of potentially severe, life-threatening adverse events associated with a particular medication. The FDA has "black boxed" trifluoperazine because of life-threatening dysrhythmias that have accompanied its use. These problems are more likely with higher doses of trifluoperazine and are not correlated with duration of treatment. Clients who overdose on trifluoperazine remain vulnerable to ventricular tachycardia or fibrillation for as long as 10 days after discontinuing the drug. *Haldol — for severe aggitation*

Haloperidol continues to be widely used despite its negative effects on motivation and cognition in some clients and the availability of atypical antipsychotics, which are less prone to causing side effects. Haloperidol is a potent blocker of postsynaptic dopamine receptors in the brain. Haloperidol is administered in several forms, including orally as capsules and liquid concentrate and through intramuscular injection. The initial oral dose is 2 or 5 mg three times daily, with an optimal dose of 20 to 30 mg/day. Doses may be as high as 60 mg/day, but further increases rarely yield sufficient benefits (Karch, 2011). Side effects include drowsiness, pseudoparkinsonism, dystonia, akathisia, and more serious, albeit rare, autonomic disturbances. Others include refractory dysrhythmia, photophobia, dry mouth, salivation, nasal congestion, and nausea (Karch, 2011). Haloperidol is contraindicated in clients with severe CNS depression, blood dyscrasia, Parkinson's disease, liver disease, or compromised renal function. Nurses advise clients to take the medication exactly as prescribed and to avoid driving if CNS or vision changes result. Clients must maintain fluid intake and avoid situations that could precipitate heatstroke (Karch, 2011).

Atypical Antipsychotics *Extreme Weight Gain*

Although revolutionary in their time, typical or traditional antipsychotics had a serious drawback: they did not improve the negative symptoms of schizophrenia. Atypical antipsychotic drugs differ because they minimally block dopamine and potentially block serotonin receptors, which accounts for their decreased side effects. This simultaneous blocking may account for their increased efficacy in improving negative symptoms of schizophrenia with few EPSs (Brunton et al., 2011). Additionally, newer research is demonstrating that blocking dopamine may not be the most important in decreasing psychosis (Karch, 2011). Many health care providers choose atypical antipsychotics because of their markedly decreased risk of long-term, irreversible side effects, such as TD. When switching from a typical to an atypical antipsychotic, at least a 12-week crossover titration (slowly decreasing the dosage of the typical while slowly increasing the dosage of the atypical) is recommended for all drugs in the class (Stahl, 2008).

Although use of atypical agents has increased, many clients continue to take the traditional agents they have used for many years. Regardless of the specific antipsychotic agent, all clients require careful monitoring for side effects (Table 16.7). Whereas incidence of EPSs is decreased with atypical drugs, they are still possible (Conley & Kelly, 2007). Neuroleptic malignant syndrome remains a risk. Other side effects include orthostatic hypotension, dizziness, tachycardia, weight gain, sleep disturbance, constipation, and rhinitis. Despite reduced EPSs, atypical antipsychotics can also contribute to seizures, weight gain, diabetes, and hyperprolactinemia (Lieberman et al., 2005).

With the arrival of clozapine (Clozaril) in 1990, the treatment of schizophrenia improved dramatically. More than 30% of people with schizophrenia did not experience response to traditional neuroleptics. For many of them, atypical antipsychotics have enabled a degree of functioning they never would have thought possible (Table 16.8). Many

TABLE 16.7 Comparisons of Antipsychotic Side Effects Based on Receptor Blockade

Classification/Generic Name	Trade Name	EPSE	Sedation	Anticholinergic	∴B/P	Antiemetic
Phenothiazines						
Chlorpromazine	Thorazine	**	***	***	***	Strong
Promazine	Sparine	**	***	***	***	Moderate
Triflupromazine	Vesprin	**	**	***	**	Strong
Thioridazine	Mellaril	*	***	***	***	Weak
Mesoridazine	Serentil	*	***	**	**	Weak
Piperacetazine	Quide	**	**	*	**	Moderate
Perphenazine	Trilafon	***	*	**	*	Weak
Trifluoperazine	Stelazine	***	*	*	*	Weak
Fluphenazine	Prolixin	****	*	*	*	Weak
Acetophenazine	Tindal	**	**	*	*	Weak
Prochlorperazine	Compazine	***	**	*	*	Strong
Nonphenothiazine						
Thiothixene	Navane	***	*	**	**	0
Haloperidol	Haldol	****	*	*	*	0
Loxapine	Loxitane	***	**	*	**	0
Molindone	Moban	***	*	*	*	0
Atypicals						
Clozapine	Clozaril	0	***	***	***	0
Risperidone	Risperdal	*	**	*	**	0
Olanzapine	Zyprexa	0	**	**	**	0
Quetiapine	Seroquel	0	**	**	**	*
Ziprasidone	Geodon	0	*	*	*	Causes
Aripiprazole	Abilify	*/-	*	*	*	Nausea
Iloperidone	Fanapt	*/-	*	*/0	*/*	0
Asenapine	Saphris	**	**	*	*	0
Lurasidone	Latuda	***	**	*	**	0

EPSE: extrapyramidal side effects. The greater the number of asterisks, the more the characteristic is present; 0 = absent.

TABLE 16.8 Actions of Atypical Antipsychotic Medications by Receptor Blockade

Medication	D$_1$	D$_2$	D$_3$	D$_4$	5HT1$_a$	5HT1$_d$	5HT$_{2a}$	5HT$_{2c}$	A$_1$	A$_2$	H$_1$	M$_1$
Clozapine	85	126	473	35	875	980	16	16	7	50	6	1.9
Risperidone	430	4	10	9	210	100	0.5	25	0.7	0.81	20	>10.000
Olanzapine	31	11	49	27	>10,000	800	4	23	19	500	7	1.9
Quetiapine	−55	160	340	1,600	2,800	—	295	1,500	7	500	11	120
Ziprasidone	525	5	7	32	3	2	0.4	1	11	>1,000	50	0.1000
Aripiprazole	265	3PA	0.80	44	5.6	—	3.4	15	26	38	61	>10.000
Iloperidone	216	21.4	7.1	—	92.1	—	5.6	42.8	0.4	162	—	>1,000
Asenapine	9	9	9	9	9	—	10	10.5	9	9	9	5
Lurasidone	—	0.994	—	—	7PA	—	0.047	—	48	10.8	>1,000	>1,000
Haloperidol	210	0.7	2	3	1,1000	—	45	>10,000	6	20	440	>1,500

* The closer to 1.0, the tighter the drug binds to a given receptor.

Sources

Newman-Tancredi, A., & Kleven, M. S. (2011). Comparative pharmacology of antipsychotics possessing combined dopamine D(2) and serotonin 5-HT (1A) receptor properties. *Psychopharmacology* Mar 11; [Epub ahead of print]

Preskorn, S. H. (2010). CNS drug development: Part II: Advances from the 1960s to the 1990s. *Journal of Psychiatric Practice*, 16(6), 413–415.

Richelson , E. (210) New antipsychotic drugs: How do their receptor-binding profiles compare? *Journal of Clinical Psychiatry*, 71(9), 1243–1244.

experts in the treatment of schizophrenia recommend the use of atypical antipsychotics as first-line treatment.

- Clozapine. Clozapine (Clozaril) produces little to no TD and may decrease or eliminate existing TD (Lieberman et al., 2005). TD tends to return once clients stop taking clozapine. Before clozapine, the only option for treating TD was to stop the drug that was causing symptoms and attempt behavioral interventions. Clozapine suppresses development of white blood cells (WBCs) in a small minority of clients who take it. Use of clozapine requires weekly monitoring of WBC counts for the first 6 months of treatment, every 2 weeks for the next 6 months, and monthly thereafter, to assess for agranulocytosis. If WBC levels decrease significantly from baseline, immediate discontinuation of clozapine is recommended. Clients should never use the drug with other agents that suppress WBC production (eg, carbamazepine). Increased risk of potentially life-threatening blood disorders makes clozapine most appropriate for clients with severe schizophrenia who have not experienced response to other antipsychotics or who are at risk for worsened TD.

- Risperidone. Risperidone (Risperdal-oral, Consta-IM) has fewer side effects than traditional agents. Its mechanism of action is not fully understood, but it blocks dopamine and serotonin receptors in the brain and has anticholinergic, antihistaminic, and alpha-adrenergic blocking activity (Karch, 2011). It is administered in tablets or as an oral solution. Because of its short half-life, it must be taken twice a day. Initial adult dose is 1 mg twice a day with gradual increases to a target dose of 3 mg twice a day. Side effects include insomnia, anxiety, agitation, headache, nausea, vomiting, constipation, and rarely, neuroleptic malignant syndrome. The risk of therapeutic and toxic effects increases if risperidone is given with clozapine; clinical effects are diminished if risperidone is administered with carbamazepine (Karch, 2011). Risperidone is contraindicated during pregnancy; women should use contraception while taking it. Clients should not abruptly stop taking risperidone and should gradually decrease the dose to avoid side effects. Nurses monitor for underlying signs of infection (eg, fever) and observe carefully to rule out a drug reaction (Karch, 2011).

- Paliperidone. Paliperidone (Invega) is the active isomer of risperidone. It has the same side effect profile, but only needs to be taken once a day.

- Olanzapine. Olanzapine (Zyprexa) is anticholinergic and antihistaminic and produces fewer EPSs than do traditional antipsychotics. Olanzapine is prescribed in tablets of 2.5 to 20 mg. Initial doses are usually 2.5 to 5 mg two times a day, with increases to 10 mg two times a day within several days. Maximum dose is not to exceed 20 mg/day (Karch, 2011), but many clients require higher doses for maximum effect. Eventually, clients are able to take the entire dose at once at bedtime. Side effects include somnolence, dizziness, neuroleptic malignant syndrome (rare), constipation, fever, and postural hypotension. The risk of orthostatic hypotension increases when clients take olanzapine with antihypertensives, alcohol, or benzodiazepines; thus, clients should avoid such concomitant use. Olanzapine increases risk of seizures and may have decreased effectiveness with rifampin, omeprazole, carbamazepine, and smoking. The risk of toxicity increases with coadministration with fluvoxamine (Karch, 2011). Nurses monitor for orthostatic hypotension, instruct clients to take the medication exactly as prescribed, and observe for fever, lethargy, weakness, or sore throat (Figure 16.8). Olanzapine is not safe in pregnancy.

- Symbyax. Symbyax, a combination of olanzapine and fluoxetine, was approved as the first medication for bipolar depression. Symbyax is administered once daily at night, usually beginning with a 6-mg/25-mg capsule. Antidepressant efficacy was demonstrated with Symbyax in a dose range of olanzapine 6 to 12 mg and fluoxetine 25 to 50 mg.

- Quetiapine. Quetiapine (Seroquel, Seroquel XR) is a dibenzothiazine antipsychotic that blocks dopamine and serotonin receptors in the brain. It also is an antagonist at histaminergic and adrenergic receptor sites, which likely contributes to adverse effects that include somnolence and orthostatic hypotension (Karch, 2011). It is approved for schizophrenia, bipolar disorder (both depressed and manic phases), and for major depression. Quetiapine is administered in tablets of 25, 100, 200, 300, and 400 mg and is available in both immediate and extended-release formulations. Dosage is determined by symptoms. The initial adult dosage for mania is 100 mg at bedtime, increasing to 400 to 600 mg over 3 days. The dosage for depression is approved up to 300 mg and for psychosis up to 800 mg. The immediate-release formulation needs to be taken twice a day. The maximum dose is 800 mg/day (Karch, 2011). An extended-release formulation eliminates the twice-daily dosing that can contribute to lack of

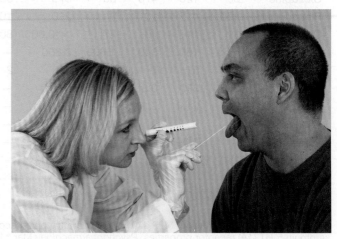

FIGURE 16.8 **The nurse is checking for signs of fever and sore throat in a client taking olanzapine.**

adherence. Alcohol and other CNS depressants potentiate quetiapine's CNS effects. Phenytoin, thioridazine, carbamazepine, phenobarbital, rifampin, levodopa, dopamine antagonists, and glucocorticoids decrease the effects of quetiapine; antihypertensives and lorazepam increase them. Nurses monitor carefully for side effects and teach clients to report unusual symptoms (Karch, 2011). Quetiapine should be given to suicidal clients in small quantities. Those exposed to extreme heat require careful monitoring; administration is not safe in pregnancy. Clients should monitor their own health for sore throat, fever, unusual bleeding or bruising, rash, weakness, and tremors, reporting any such findings to providers, because they may be indications of a serious side effect (Karch, 2011). Quetiapine has been found to lower free and total T_4 by as much as 90%. Thyroid function should be closely monitored.

- ZIPRASIDONE. Ziprasidone (Geodon) is chemically unrelated to phenothiazine or butyrophenone. It has low risk of EPSs, causes little to no elevation of prolactin levels, and does not seem to cause weight gain (Lieberman et al., 2005). Ziprasidone is used to treat schizophrenia and mania. Because it is a serotonin-1A agonist and a serotonin-1D antagonist, it may have additional antidepressant and anxiolytic effects. It is available in capsules of 20, 40, 60, and 80 mg and needs to be taken twice daily. The maximum effect is reached at a total daily dose of at least 120 mg. The current formulation requires taking ziprasidone with 1 g of fat (eg, peanut butter) for full absorption. When taken on an empty stomach, more than 40% of the absorption is lost.

- ARIPIPRAZOLE. Aripiprazole (Abilify) represents a departure from the usual mechanism of action of antipsychotics. Technically called a D_2 partial agonist, this drug can stimulate the D_2 receptor under certain circumstances and contribute to an activating, not sedating, response. When dopamine levels in the brain are too high, aripiprazole may switch its role and block dopamine from getting to the receptor. Because researchers now believe that some negative and cognitive symptoms of schizophrenia result from too little dopamine, whereas positive symptoms result from too much (see Chap. 2), a drug that could regulate dopamine activity accordingly is especially beneficial. Aripiprazole showed a relatively low rate of adverse side effects in clinical trials. The most common were headache, anxiety, and insomnia. Moreover, aripiprazole does not cause the distressing weight gain associated with many antipsychotics. Initially the activating response can cause akathisia-type symptoms; thus, starting with a low

dose is best. Aripiprazole comes in capsules of 2, 5, 10, and 20 mg. Daily dosage can range from 5 to 30 mg.

Stimulant and Nonstimulant Cognitive Enhancers

Stimulants (amphetamine and methylphenidate), both FDA Class II controlled substances, are commonly used to treat attention-deficit hyperactivity disorder (ADHD) in children (see Chap. 36). This same drug class was approved for treatments of adults with ADHD in 2004. Stimulants also have been used to augment treatment for refractory depression (Understanding Psychopharmacology 16.5). Use of stimulants requires careful diagnosis of the disorder, the lowest possible effective dosage, and careful monitoring of response.

Amphetamines have two major mechanisms of action. They stimulate the release of stored dopamine and norepinephrine and also prevent the reuptake of dopamine back into the synapse by reversing the dopamine transporter system. The net results are increased stimulation of dopamine to both presynaptic and postsynaptic dopamine receptors. The primary form of amphetamine is dextroamphetamine, the single dextro isomer. It is available in both short- and intermediate-acting formulations. Mixed amphetamine salts are also available in both short- and long-acting formulations and include a combination of both levo and dextro amphetamine isomers. Side effects include nervousness, insomnia, anorexia, nausea, increased or decreased pulse and blood pressure, and tachycardia.

Methylphenidate has actions and side effects similar to those of amphetamines. It blocks the dopamine transporter and releases dopamine from presynaptic dopamine terminals. It is contraindicated in clients with glaucoma, motor tics, and severe depression. It is used cautiously in clients with seizure disorders (Karch, 2011). Methylphenidate is available in tablets from 5 to 20 mg and in sustained-release tablets in 18- and 36-mg doses. It is usually given in divided doses two or three times daily, 30 minutes before meals. Oral doses range from 10 to 60 mg/day. Sustained-release tablets usually start at an oral dose of 18 mg in the morning; doses increase weekly from 18 mg/day to a maximum of 54 mg/day.

Effects and toxicity increase if methylphenidate is given with MAOIs; phenytoin, TCAs, oral anticoagulants, and SSRIs show increased serum levels if administered with methylphenidate. Coadministration decreases the effects of guanethidine.

Children on long-term methylphenidate therapy require careful monitoring of their growth. If insomnia occurs, the last dose should be given before 6 PM. Nurse emphasizes that clients must swallow whole, not chew, timed-release tablets. Clients must take methylphenidate exactly as prescribed (Karch, 2011). Adults should keep methylphenidate in a secure place because it has a high value as a street drug.

The FDA has approved atomoxetine HCl (Strattera) as the first nonstimulant for the treatment of ADHD in all age groups. Atomoxetine is a norepinephrine reuptake inhibitor that facilitates focus and attention. Dosages range from 10 to

---

Checkpoint Questions

12. When is neuroleptic malignant syndrome most common?

13. What follow-up is essential for clients taking clozapine?

14. What receptors does quetiapine affect?

UNDERSTANDING PSYCHOPHARMACOLOGY 16.5

Stimulants and Cognitive Enhancers

GENERIC AND BRAND NAMES	USUAL DOSE	SEDATION LEVEL/ HALF-LIFE	SIDE EFFECTS	RELIEF OF SYMPTOMS
methylphenidate (Ritalin, Ritalin-SR, Concerta, Metadate-ER)	Tablets: 5, 10, 20 mg SR tablets: 20 mg ER tablets: 18, 36 mg Doses range from 10 to 60 mg/day PO	None, may be energizing; half-life is 1–3 hr	Nervousness, insomnia, increased or decreased pulse or blood pressure, tachycardia	Immediate response if dosing is correct
dextroamphetamine sulfate (Dexedrine, Dexedrine Spansules, Dextrostat)	Tablets: 5, 10 mg SR capsules: 5, 10, 15 mg Usual dose: 5–60 mg/day PO	None, may be energizing; half-life is 10–30 hr	Overstimulation, restlessness, dizziness, insomnia, dry mouth, unpleasant taste, diarrhea, palpitations, tachycardia, hypertension	Immediate response if dosing is correct
Mixed amphetamine salts, D-amphetamine, L-amphetamine (Adderall)	Capsules: 5, 10, 15, 20, 30 mg take BID up to a maximum of 60 mg daily. Also available in XR.	Energizing; half-life is 2–4 hr	Overstimulation, restlessness, dizziness, insomnia, dry mouth, unpleasant taste, diarrhea, palpitations, tachycardia, hypertension	Immediate response if dosing is correct
Lisdexamfetamine dimesylate (D-amphetamine) (Vyvanse)	Capsules: Available 30, 50, and 70 mg that equate to Adderall 10, 20, and 30 mg	Energizing; half-life is 6 hr. Formulation of the drug is designed to decrease abuse potential.	Overstimulation, restlessness, dizziness, insomnia, dry mouth, unpleasant taste, diarrhea, palpitations, tachycardia, hypertension	Immediate response if dosing is correct
The first Pro-drug; does not release until after first-pass through liver modafinil (Provigil)	200 mg/day PO as single dose; up to 400 mg/day as single dose may be used	Activating; half-life is 8–10 hr	Insomnia, headache, nervousness, anxiety	2–3 hr

15 mg in children up to 100 mg in adults. Careful monitoring of blood pressure is required. Some clients discontinue the drug because of severe urinary retention. It has been found helpful in adult women with ADHD who also experience symptoms of depression. Because it is not a controlled substance, it does not carry the risk of abuse.

The wake-promoting agent modafinil (Provigil) has been approved for the treatment of narcolepsy and shift work-related sleep disorders (see Chap. 22). Its exact mechanism and sites of action are unknown, but modafinil may block reuptake of central histamine and other neurotransmitters active in the sleep–wake cycle. Modafinil was tested in ADHD, but higher doses caused a rash and the drug was not approved for treatment of ADHD.

Memory and Cognition Enhancers

Studies have shown three cholinesterase inhibitors—donepezil (Aricept), galantamine (Reminyl), and rivastigmine (Exelon)—to delay cognitive decline in people with Alzheimer's disease (Understanding Psychopharmacology 16.6). Cholinesterase breaks down ACh. With cholinesterase inhibitors, the goal is to inhibit cholinesterase so that ACh will break down more slowly, thereby making more ACh available for the brain (Leonard, 2004; Stahl, 2006). Cholinesterase inhibitors stabilize memory, language, and orientation. They also promote the client's ability to cope with daily life. They may not improve the ability to do things such as plan a meal or decide what to wear. However, they do slow the loss of these skills and can make people less apathetic or indifferent.

UNDERSTANDING PSYCHOPHARMACOLOGY 16.6

Cognitive and Memory Enhancers

GENERIC AND BRAND NAMES	USUAL DOSE	SEDATION LEVEL/ HALF-LIFE	SIDE EFFECTS	RELIEF OF SYMPTOMS
Nonstimulant Cognitive Enhancer				
atomoxetine HCl (Strattera)	Adults and children >70 kg: 40 mg/day PO with daily total target dose of 80 mg PO; maximum dose of 100 mg/day Pediatric clients <70 kg: 0.5 mg/kg per day PO with target dose of approximately 1.2 mg/kg per day PO as single daily dose in the morning; not to exceed 1.4 mg/kg or 100 mg/day, whichever is less	Activating; half-life is 5 hr	Headache, dry mouth, nausea, decreased appetite, constipation, upper abdominal pain, vomiting, cough	1–2 hr
Memory and Cognition Enhancers				
donepezil HCl (Aricept)	5 mg PO at HS with increases to 10 mg/day after 4–6 wk	Activating; half-life is 70 hr	Insomnia, fatigue, rash, nausea, vomiting, diarrhea, dyspepsia, anorexia, abdominal pain, muscle cramps, hepatotoxicity	2–4 hr
galantamine hydrobromide (Reminyl)	Initial 4 mg PO BID with increase to 8 mg PO BID after 4 wk; increase to 12 mg PO BID maximum dose	Activating; half-life is 7 hr	Insomnia, dizziness, nausea, vomiting, diarrhea, dyspepsia, anorexia, abdominal pain	8 hr
rivastigmine tartrate (Exelon)	Initial dose of 1.5 mg PO BID with food; usual dose range of 6–12 mg/day, should not exceed 12 mg/day	Activating; half-life is 1 hr	Insomnia, fatigue, rash, nausea, vomiting, diarrhea, dyspepsia, anorexia, abdominal pain	12 hr
memantine (Namenda)	Dose escalation over 1 mo: 5 mg/day for 7 days, 5 mg BID for 7 days, 10 mg AM and 5 mg PM for 7 days, 10 mg BID	Activating; half-life is 60–100 hr	Confusion, agitation, insomnia, mild to moderate dizziness, headaches	1–2 hr

The benefits of cholinesterase inhibitors are temporary (ie, they disappear if clients stop treatment for a few weeks). Improvements peak 3 months after initiating the drug, with a slow return to the starting point during a period of 9 to 12 months. After that, clients show a slower decline than those who have not taken the medication.

A second class of memory enhancers is the type that blocks the excitatory neurotransmitter glutamate. The glutamatergic neurotransmitter system plays a crucial role in memory formation and information processing. Disturbances in this system caused by Alzheimer' disease contribute to the symptoms of the disease. Memantine (Namenda) is approved for use in the later stages of Alzheimer's to delay the progression of the illness. Memantine has a mild side effect profile that consists primarily of dizziness, confusion, headache, and constipation. It can be administered with or without food. A suggested gradual dosing schedule over 1 month includes 1 to 5 mg/day for the first week, 5 mg twice a day for the second week, 5 to 10 mg a day for the third week, and 10 mg twice a day the fourth week. Memantine has also been used off label in the treatment of schizophrenia with some positive responses (Dedeurwaerdere et al., 2011).

Checkpoint Questions

15. What is the first nonstimulant approved for the treatment of ADHD?

16. What three cholinesterase inhibitors are used to treat Alzheimer's disease?

APPLYING THE NURSING PROCESS

Clients Using Psychopharmacologic Agents

Nurses across many treatment settings assume a valuable role in assisting clients and families to manage psychotropic medications. For example, nurses coordinate outpatient medication groups for clients with schizophrenia and monitor their symptoms, general functioning, and health needs throughout treatment. Home care nurses discuss issues related to medication during visits. Nurses in psychiatric hospitals teach about medicines while preparing clients for discharge to the community. All nurses consider multiple aspects of the client's life, monitor response to medications, and continually assess needs to maximize functioning. In most states, nurse practitioners have prescriptive authority, meaning that they prescribe and manage the administration and monitoring of medications.

Nurses are likely to encounter clients with psychiatric problems in all settings and situations. Many clients benefit from psychopharmacologic treatment. Nurses must understand the importance of brain-based psychiatric illness within the broader context of client-centered care. They need to focus on aspects of care that traditional medical models ignore: health education, case management, family issues, client management, and advocacy (see Chap. 13).

The proliferation of available medications to treat psychiatric disorders makes it imperative for nurses to understand the actions and side effects of specific drugs. Also essential to professional nursing care is a thorough appreciation for the client taking the prescribed medication. For many, medication is an adjunct therapy to other interventions that nurses coordinate, including family counseling or individual therapy. Medications can enhance the effectiveness of other nursing interventions by alleviating symptoms and making clients more emotionally open to change. They can help clients avoid hospitalization and allow them to remain at home. However, medications alone do not magically facilitate communication, help clients get jobs, or cause chronic, long-term problems to disappear.

▲ ASSESSMENT

Nursing assessment related to psychopharmacology focuses on reviewing clients' health history, experience with psychotropic medications, past side effects, and past efficacy. The care setting influences the type and extent of assessment. For example, is the client experiencing a psychiatric crisis requiring hospitalization? Is the request for services part of routine psychiatric care in an outpatient clinic? Is the need for medication part of a long-term treatment strategy that involves few changes? Clients with acute disorders usually take medication for a prescribed time, and the crisis may be traceable to a specific event. These clients also are more likely to experience brief psychiatric hospitalizations. In such cases, nurses tailor assessment questions to focus on the events leading to the episode and immediate problems. Clients with chronic difficulties may have longer and more frequent needs for inpatient care. A client's place along the continuum of care can change according to acuity of psychiatric symptoms and varying needs for services.

Regardless of setting, nurses assess the client's life history, including history of psychiatric illness, past hospitalizations, and past use of medication. They review the target symptoms requiring need for medication, client's perception of the problem, type and quality of any community and family supports, and need for adjunct care, such as group, individual, or family treatment.

Target Symptoms

Target symptoms are the specific problems that a medication aims to alter. The health care team must identify and understand the client's target symptoms before initiating a medication regimen. Certain drugs target particular symptoms, and symptoms, rather than illnesses, are the foci of psychiatric treatment.

Clients also must understand and participate in identifying and monitoring changes in target symptoms. Instruments such as the Brief Psychiatric Rating Scale (BPRS) help clients rate symptoms systematically before and after drug administration (Lachar et al., 2001) (Assessment Tool 16.1). Health care personnel should use results from the BPRS in conjunction with interdisciplinary observations.

ASSESSMENT TOOL 16.1

Brief Psychiatric Rating Scale

DIRECTIONS: Place an X in the appropriate box to represent level of severity of each symptom.

	Not Present	Very Mild	Mild	Moderate	Mod. Severe	Severe	Extremely Severe
SOMATIC CONCERN—preoccupation with physical health, fear of physical illness, hypochondriasis.	☐	☐	☐	☐	☐	☐	☐
ANXIETY—worry, fear, overconcern for present or future, uneasiness.	☐	☐	☐	☐	☐	☐	☐
EMOTIONAL WITHDRAWAL—lack of spontaneous interaction, isolation deficiency in relating to others.	☐	☐	☐	☐	☐	☐	☐
CONCEPTUAL DISORGANIZATION—thought processes confused, disconnected, disorganized, disrupted.	☐	☐	☐	☐	☐	☐	☐
GUILT FEELINGS—self-blame, shame, remorse for past behavior.	☐	☐	☐	☐	☐	☐	☐
TENSION—physical and motor manifestations of nervousness, over-activation.	☐	☐	☐	☐	☐	☐	☐
MANNERISMS AND POSTURING—peculiar, bizarre unnatural motor behavior (not including tic).	☐	☐	☐	☐	☐	☐	☐
GRANDIOSITY—exaggerated self-opinion, arrogance, conviction of unusual power or abilities.	☐	☐	☐	☐	☐	☐	☐
DEPRESSIVE MOOD—sorrow, sadness, despondency, pessimism.	☐	☐	☐	☐	☐	☐	☐
HOSTILITY—animosity, contempt, belligerence, disdain for others.	☐	☐	☐	☐	☐	☐	☐
SUSPICIOUSNESS—mistrust, belief others harbor malicious or discriminatory intent.	☐	☐	☐	☐	☐	☐	☐
HALLUCINATORY BEHAVIOR—perceptions without normal external stimulus correspondence.	☐	☐	☐	☐	☐	☐	☐
MOTOR RETARDATION—slowed weakened movements or speech, reduced body tone.	☐	☐	☐	☐	☐	☐	☐
UNCOOPERATIVENESS—resistance, guardedness, rejection of authority.	☐	☐	☐	☐	☐	☐	☐
UNUSUAL THOUGHT CONTENT—unusual, odd, strange, bizarre thought content.	☐	☐	☐	☐	☐	☐	☐
BLUNTED AFFECT—reduced emotional tone, reduction in formal intensity of feelings, flatness.	☐	☐	☐	☐	☐	☐	☐
EXCITEMENT—heightened emotional tone, agitation, increased reactivity.	☐	☐	☐	☐	☐	☐	☐
DISORIENTATION—confusion or lack of proper association for person, place, or time.	☐	☐	☐	☐	☐	☐	☐

Global Assessment Scale (Range 1-100)

Reprinted with permission from Overall, J. E. (1998). The Brief Psychiatric Rating Scale (BPRS). Recent developments in ascertainment and scaling. *Psychopharmacology Bulletin, 24,* 97–99.

Nurses encourage clients to carry a list of medications with dose, time of administration, and prescribing mental health professional for each. Clients then can show this list to other caregivers who provide emergency or routine medical care. Family members can also provide supplemental knowledge of medications if clients choose to use their support in obtaining medical care.

Understanding the psychosocial needs of clients who potentially benefit from psychotropic medications implies an awareness of their basic needs for food, shelter, family, and kinship. It also involves appreciating the personal meanings of their psychiatric disorders. Nurses must be willing to consider the prejudices and biases often leveled at people with chronic psychiatric problems; understand the role of gender, culture, and ethnicity in provision of psychiatric care; and consider whether psychotropic medication is in the client's best interests (Chee et al., 2008).

Caffeine Use

Of particular importance in the management of psychotropic medications is assessment of daily caffeine intake (DeLeon, 2004). Many people use toxic amounts of caffeine, which can dramatically affect the efficacy of psychotropic medications. Caffeine changes the pH of gastric acid, thus altering drug absorption. As a result, clients need higher doses of psychotherapeutic drugs, increasing their risk for side effects. Clients who eliminate or decrease caffeine to no more than 225 mg/day also may be able to decrease their required doses of psychotropics. This outcome has economic ramifications because decreasing the number of doses means less drug is needed.

Caffeine both agonizes and antagonizes selected neural receptors. Its antagonistic effect on tranquilizing adenosine receptors is the partial cause of caffeine-induced nervousness. Caffeine also stimulates the release of excitatory neurotransmitters (eg, norepinephrine) and actually increases norepinephrine synthesis. Caffeine is pharmacologically similar to amphetamines and cocaine in that it stimulates the frontal lobes of the brain, increasing energy and concentration. However, it does not yield the euphoria of street drugs. Some people believe caffeine helps them think better, but it can be addicting. Pharmacologically speaking, caffeine is singularly the most devastating, legally available stimulant that clients with unstable mood can ingest. More than 225 mg/day of caffeine is considered excessive because this amount affects the action of *all* psychotropic medications and can lead to a *DSM-IV-TR* diagnosis of caffeine intoxication. Thus, nurses should calculate each client's daily caffeine intake to identify any potential for interactions or tendency to worsen mood (Box 16.2). Most clients do not experience severe caffeine intoxication simply because of the substance's limited water solubility.

Nicotine Use

Nicotine has become one of the most closely scrutinized legal drugs. It has long been known to be extremely addictive, but only recently has research begun to uncover what effects it can have on prescription medications. Many people taking psychotropic drugs are addicted to nicotine. The ability of nicotine to increase the release of dopamine is thought to be one reason many clients with schizophrenia who smoke require such high doses of medications. In such cases, use of nicotine may actually counteract the effects of antipsychotics. Nicotine receptors have been found to be deficient in people with schizophrenia (Levin & Rezvani, 2007), which may be one reason people with schizophrenia become so easily addicted to smoking. Because nicotine is also a stimulant, it may reduce the drowsiness caused by neuroleptics and antianxiety agents. Nicotine also causes the release of stimulating neurotransmitters and begins a series of nervous system and endocrine (hormonal) functions, including the release of stored glycogen in the liver (which is

---

BOX 16.2 Assessing Caffeine Intake

The following formula can be used as a helpful guide for caffeine detoxification. Adhering to the following guidelines will guarantee a safe withdrawal with minimal discomfort. This protocol must be done in collaboration with the prescriber because the client will need medication dosage decreases during the withdrawal. Clients should not attempt to withdraw from benzodiazepines or nicotine until they have finished caffeine withdrawal.

Formula for Caffeine Withdrawal

1. Calculate daily caffeine intake (in milligrams).
2. Divide daily amount by 6.
3. Decrease by 1/6 each week for 5 weeks (eg, if total amount is 3,000 mg, eliminate 500 mg/day or 2 cups of regular coffee).
4. At week 5, decrease by 250 mg/day.
5. At week 6, the client will be at 250 mg day.
6. The ultimate goal is 0 mg of caffeine.

At week 2, the client will start to notice a greater sedative effect from most medications. At this time, begin a slow decrease in dose of prescribed medications **in collaboration with the prescriber**. Ultimately, the client will be at one half of the previous dose of antipsychotic medication and/or one-third to one half of the dose of the antidepressant.

---

what causes the nicotine kick). Nicotine can also go directly to the serotonin receptors in a manner similar to alcohol. *These functions become self-rewarding, and the brain begins to require it for the person to feel normal.*

Smoking creates another problem. When people smoke, they ingest compounds called arial carbons, of which carbon monoxide is one of the most deadly. These hydrocarbons induce the P450 liver enzyme systems. Smoking in general can create interactions with other drugs by affecting their metabolism as a result of the liver enzymes induced. The simple act of smoking can raise the dose required to create a therapeutic response from antipsychotic medications, causing unpleasant side effects. One study shows that 33% of all nicotine users become addicted, as compared with 25% of heroin users, 16% of cocaine users, 15% of alcohol users, 11% of amphetamine users, and 9% of marijuana users (Kapusta et al., 2007).

Polypharmacy

Polypharmacy is the use of two or more psychotropic drugs, two or more drugs of the same chemical class, or two or more drugs with the same or similar pharmacologic actions to treat different conditions (Stahl, 2006). The frequency of polypharmacy is high, especially in clients with serious psychiatric disorders (Essock et al., 2011). Although polypharmacy often is necessary, it can increase the chance of adverse effects, drug interactions, client nonadherence, and medication errors. However, polypharmacy can result in symptom amelioration in clients with severe psychosis, resistant schizophrenia, and depression (Essock et al., 2011).

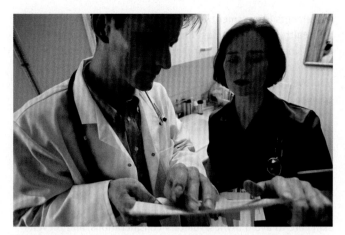

FIGURE 16.9 A nurse reviews a client's chart with a physician to pinpoint issues of polypharmacy and possible concerns.

Nurses must question the use of several agents to treat a disorder and understand the rationale for polypharmacy (Figure 16.9). They must explore specific target symptoms, drug interactions, and the client's understanding of medication management. Taking more than one agent can confuse a client, especially if dosing times for each drug differ. Health education can assist clients to understand the purpose, side effects, and efficacy of their medications. The goal of pharmacology management always is optimal treatment with the fewest medications possible. Nurses also must recognize that taking multiple agents increases the potential for side effects.

Nurses should understand the philosophy regarding polypharmacy held by the treatment setting where they practice. Although not appropriate for all clients, careful management of the practice can provide symptom relief to clients with refractory disorders.

▲ NURSING DIAGNOSIS

Nursing diagnoses for clients taking psychotherapeutic drugs are as varied and specific to the client's needs as the drugs themselves and the disorders being treated. A list of common nursing diagnoses related to the effects of pharmacotherapy is found in Nursing Spotlight 16.1. In addition, a few diagnoses are common for most clients requiring psychopharmacotherapy. For example, those just starting their medication regimens will meet the criteria for Deficient Knowledge. Clients who have problems following their drug regimens may qualify for Ineffective Therapeutic Regimen Management or Ineffective Coping. These are just a few examples; nurses should remember that all diagnoses must be individualized to meet particular assessment data and desired outcomes (Aschenbrenner & Venable, 2009).

▲ OUTCOME IDENTIFICATION AND PLANNING

Planning for care involves ascertaining the length of the medication trial, the client's need for follow-up, and monitoring of side effects. Ensuring safety is the most important aspect of planning medications.

NURSING SPOTLIGHT 16.1

Selected Nursing Diagnoses Pertaining to Drug Effects

- Constipation
- Diarrhea
- Acute Pain
- Chronic Pain
- Fatigue
- Risk for Infection
- Risk for Injury
- Disturbed Sensory Perception
- Ineffective Sexuality Patterns
- Disturbed Sleep Pattern
- Disturbed Thought Processes
- Interrupted Breast-Feeding
- Acute Confusion
- Deficient Fluid Volume
- Excess Fluid Volume
- Imbalanced Nutrition: More Than Body Requirements
- Imbalanced Nutrition: Less Than Body Requirements
- Impaired Urinary Elimination
- Urinary Retention

Prescribed and Maximum Dose

Nurses are responsible for knowing essential information about a prescribed drug before administering it. This information includes the class of drug, target symptoms for which it is prescribed, route of administration, dosing information, adverse effects, contraindications, and nursing implications. Nurses clearly communicate this information to clients and families (if appropriate) as part of education.

Nurses carefully monitor drug administration, noting if the correct drug is being given in the correct manner, prescribed dose, and time to the intended client (Karch, 2011). Nurses are aware of storage issues for particular medications (eg, refrigeration, protection from light). They consider interventions associated with drug administration, such as monitoring vital signs, giving the medication with food, and implementing other physical parameters.

If a prescribed dose of a drug appears outside normal dosing standards, nurses contact prescribers for clarification. They clarify all questions about a medication, whether these involve confusion about spelling, dosage, or administration. When nurses administer medication, they assume responsibility under their nursing license. For example, clonidine and clozapine are different psychotropic medications with similar-sounding names. Clarification of confusion is essential when administering medication.

Method of Administration

Determining the best mode of administration is important when tailoring a plan of care to suit a client's particular needs. For example, many clients with schizophrenia prefer oral tablets or capsules. Some who take neuroleptics for long periods find

BOX 16.3 Decanoate Injections

- Antipsychotics are the only medications currently available in decanoate form. Such injections are usually given every 4 to 6 weeks. Clients receiving them require close monitoring for side effects after the first few administrations of the drug.
- Research data supporting the use of decanoates are inconclusive. An increasing body of knowledge suggests that nursing approaches to drug therapy that empower clients might be as effective. Examples of this empowerment include encouraging the client to make an informed choice about medication and the effects on lifestyle and functioning. Further research is needed.

that decanoate injectables of fluphenazine or haloperidol are more convenient and eliminate the need to remember to take oral medications (Box 16.3). Some clients prefer liquid forms. Disadvantages to liquids include difficulties obtaining an accurate dose, risk of overdose, and the need for juice or other liquid for mixing. Many older clients in long-term care settings and nursing homes receive liquid forms of haloperidol or chlorpromazine in their juice for ease of administration. Most of these clients do not independently pour their medication; nurses perform this function for them. These examples illustrate ways in which nurses must consider method of administration when planning care.

Expected Drug Action

Before giving a drug, nurses must understand the client's physical and psychiatric functioning. They should understand the baseline from which to gauge the client's response after drug therapy begins. Such knowledge can assist clients and nurses to ascertain whether side effects come specifically from the psychotropic medication or another source. Influences on drug action include other drugs that the client takes, allergies, past health care patterns, and general physical health. Nurses are aware of the client's health history and current health strengths and weaknesses to manage the effects of psychotropic medication. They have the most direct and ongoing contact with clients, and thus the best opportunity to notice small changes that can determine the success or failure of drug therapy and client adherence to medication regimens (Karch, 2011).

Side Effects

As discussed, most psychotropic medications have side effects that range from common and well established to rare and idiosyncratic. Nurses instruct clients about side effects of their drugs, tailoring information to meet each person's specific learning abilities and needs. Clients have a right to know about all side effects and changes they might encounter when taking a particular medication.

Nurses use a combination of techniques to monitor side effects. For example, visual observation illuminates the overt presence of TD. Use of the Abnormal Involuntary Movement Scale is a definite and precise way to evaluate abnormal

movements (Assessment Tool 16.2) (National Institute of Mental Health, 1995). The most important monitoring comes from discussing with clients their perceptions of responses. Clients may share that they believe their psychiatric symptoms have improved (a positive response) but that they are experiencing adverse effects (negative). Careful discussion, monitoring, and follow-up may be necessary to ensure that clients continue with drug regimens. Thorough review of the consequences of discontinuing medications also is essential.

Nurses plan interventions to decrease anticipated side effects of particular drugs while promoting safety (Karch, 2011). Such planning might include education about sensitivity to light or heat, use of sunscreen, avoiding driving, maintaining skin care to avoid dryness, dietary considerations, and prevention of constipation. For example, dehydration can precipitate toxicity and severe illness in clients taking lithium carbonate. Thus, nurses advise such clients to take special care to hydrate regularly in hot weather. They might instruct clients to carry water bottles. Nurses plan to manage side effects according to the client's ability to understand, lifestyle needs, and psychiatric status.

Nurses must establish careful, thoughtful relationships with clients that foster discussion of adverse effects and planning for appropriate management. Clients need to understand that different drugs in the same class can have varying effects. If a client does not tolerate one medication, another may have fewer adverse effects and better treat symptoms. The nurse–client relationship is essential to assisting clients as they manage all effects of a drug. This is crucial in promoting adherence to a drug regimen aimed at amelioration of a symptom.

▲ IMPLEMENTATION

Often, clients receive medicine without understanding its purpose, risks, and benefits. Nurses absolutely must make client and family education an integral part of practice, particularly when administering psychotropic drugs. See Client-Centered Education 16.2.

Other aspects of intervention involve the following:

- Assessing where and how the client will receive medication
- Arranging follow-up appointments and prescription renewal
- Understanding the client's financial resources
- Educating about safe storage of medication if young children live in or visit the home frequently

Promoting Medication Adherence

One of the most difficult aspects of treatment with psychotropic medications involves **adherence,** or the client's ability to engage in recommended treatment for the duration of treatment as a caregiver prescribes. It involves the client's right to know and understand all aspects of the medication, including potential side effects, benefits, and dangers. In the landmark CATIE study (Clinical Antipsychotic Trials of Intervention Effectiveness; Lieberman et al., 2005), approximately 74% of all clients discontinued antipsychotic medication for a variety of reasons over the 18-month course of the study.

ASSESSMENT TOOL 16.2

Abnormal Involuntary Movement Scale

		None	Minimal	Mild	Moderate	Severe
Facial and Oral Movements						
	1: Muscles of facial expression (eg, movements of forehead, eyebrows, periorbital area, cheeks; include frowning, blinking, smiling, grimacing)	0	1	2	3	4
	2: Lips and perioral area (eg, puckering, pouting, smacking)	0	1	2	3	4
	3: Jaw (eg, biting, clenching, chewing, mouth opening, lateral movement)	0	1	2	3	4
	4: Tongue Rate only increase in movement both in and out of mouth, *not* inability to sustain movement	0	1	2	3	4
Extremity Movements						
	5: Upper (arms, wrists, hands, fingers) Include choreic movements (ie, rapid, objectively purposeless, irregular, spontaneous), athetoid movements (ie, slow, irregular, complex, serpentine). Do *not* include tremor (ie, repetitive, regular, rhythmic).	0	1	2	3	4
	6: Lower (legs, knees, ankles, toes) (eg, lateral knee movement, foot tapping, heel dropping, foot squirming, inversion and eversion of foot)	0	1	2	3	4
Trunk Movements						
	7: Neck, shoulders, hips (eg, rocking, twisting, squirming, pelvic gyrations)	0	1	2	3	4
	8: Severity of abnormal movements	0	1	2	3	4
Global Judgment						
	9: Incapacitation due to abnormal movements	0	1	2	3	4

10: Patient's awareness of abnormal movements Rate only patient's report	No awareness	0
	Aware, no distress	1
	Aware, mild distress	2
	Aware, moderate distress	3
	Aware, severe distress	4

(continues on page 324)

ASSESSMENT TOOL 16.2   Abnormal Involuntary Movement Scale (continued)

		None	Minimal	Mild	Moderate	Severe
Global Judgment						
	11: Current problems with teeth and/or dentures		No		0	
			Yes		1	
	12: Does patient usually wear dentures?		No		0	
			Yes		1	

Examination Procedures for AIMS

Either before or after completing the examination procedure, observe the patient unobtrusively, at rest (eg, in waiting room). The chair to be used in this examination should be a hard, firm one without arms.

1: Ask patient whether there is anything in his/her mouth (ie, gum, candy, etc.) and if there is, to remove it.

2: Ask patient about the *current* condition of his/her teeth. Ask patient if he/she wears dentures. Do teeth or dentures bother patient *now*?

3: Ask patient whether he/she notices any movements in mouth, face, hands, or feet. If yes, ask to describe and to what extent they *currently* bother patient or interfere with his/her activities.

4: Have patient sit in chair with hands on knees, legs slightly apart, and feet flat on floor. (Look at entire body for movements while in this position.)

5: Ask patient to sit with hands hanging unsupported. If male, between legs, if female and wearing a dress, hanging over knees. (Observe hands and other body areas.)

6: Ask patient to open mouth. (Observe tongue at rest within mouth.) Do this twice.

7: Ask patient to protrude tongue. (Observe tongue at rest within mouth.) Do this twice.

*8: Ask patient to tap thumb with each finger, as rapidly as possible for 10–15 seconds; separately with right hand, then with left hand. (Observe facial and leg movements.)

9: Flex and extend patient's left and right arms (one at a time). (Note any rigidity and rate on Notes.)

10: Ask patient to stand up. (Observe in profile. Observe all body areas again, hips included.)

*11: Ask patient to extend both arms outstretched in front with palms down. (Observe trunk, leg, and mouth.)

*12: Have patient walk a few paces, turn, and walk back to chair. (Observe hand and gait.) Do this twice.

---

*Activated movements.

Reprinted from Guy, W. (1976). *ECDEU: Assessment manual for psychopharmacology* (DHEW Publication No. 76–338). Washington, DC: Department of Health, Education, and Welfare, Psychopharmacology Research Branch.

Some providers believe that complete knowledge of a drug may cause a client to refuse to follow the regimen. For example, if a client knows that a likely side effect of a certain drug is significant weight gain, he may refuse to start the medication or stop taking it once weight gain begins (Case Vignette 16.1). Nevertheless, all clients have the right to refuse all treatments unless they are judged legally incompetent to make treatment decisions (see Chap. 5). Nurses are responsible for understanding specifics related to legal competence and adherence to treatment regimens within their geographic area of practice. Legalities differ among states.

Factors Contributing to Nonadherence

Clients may have many reasons for failing to adhere to medication regimens (Velligan et al., 2009). The most common are adverse effects, many of which are debilitating and difficult to manage, lack of social support, and lack of insight into illness. Some clients with chronic psychiatric disturbances believe that they have little control over their lives or environment and may refuse medication to exert more control over their situation.

Unfortunately, many clients experience social stigma associated with mental illness. For some, the need for psychotropic drugs means that they can no longer deny their symptoms or problems. Others perceive that taking psychotropic medications means that they agree with the label of "crazy" or "psychotic," regardless of whether they experience symptom relief and improved functioning as a result.

Other clients fear addiction, especially if they or relatives have a history of treatment for substance abuse. Some clients have memories of relatives receiving primitive forms

Client-Centered Education 16.2

Psychopharmacology Teaching Plan

Assess the information needs of the client and family.

- Are the client and family fully able to comprehend information?
- What do the client and family think about taking medication regularly?
- Do the client and family have any cultural or other biases about use of medication?
- Has the client had past problems with medication adherence? If so, were these issues resolved? How?
- Are the client and family willing to adhere to a medication schedule?

Plan education.

- Do handouts provide clear, useful information about medication, intended effects, side effects, treatment implications, and self-care?
- Is educational material appropriate to the language needs and developmental levels of client and family?

- Does the educational presentation meet the client and family's learning needs?

Implement medication teaching.

- Would individual or joint client–family teaching be more effective?
- Has the nurse carried out follow-up teaching several times to determine information gaps and the need for further education?
- What issues has the client or family expressed about adherence, especially regarding medication side effects and taking medication regularly?

Evaluate effectiveness of medication teaching.

- Is the nurse frequently monitoring the client and family to elicit their perceptions of medication, efficacy, and adherence?
- Do others who work with client and family have access to this medication information?

---

of psychiatric treatment. Others had difficult experiences with the mental health system as children and adolescents, when long stays in state psychiatric hospitals meant custodial care and high doses of medication often used as chemical restraints.

Baloush-Kleinman and colleagues (2011) recommended using a health belief model. In this model, health care providers determine adherence to treatment through assessment of the client's perceived benefits of treatment and risk of illness versus

cost of treatment, including adverse side effects. Clients who believed that the risks of treatment were worth the benefits were more likely to adhere to prescribed medication regimens.

Lack of awareness of illness (anosognosia) is a major cause of nonadherence in psychiatric illnesses (Pia & Tamietto, 2006). Nurses can assess the client's level of awareness of illness with the Beck Cognitive Insight Scale (Beck et al., 2004). Nurses need to consider the client's level of self-certainty and ability for self-reflection before judging a client as refusing to

---

Case Vignette 16.1

Michelle, 20 years old, presents to the community mental health clinic. She seems annoyed that she was kept waiting for a few minutes past her appointment time. Michelle reports feelings of depression. "My medicines aren't working anymore. I'm getting fat." She mentions that she recently spent 2 weeks at home during spring break from college. The nurse notes that Michelle is wearing a skirt and sandals with no coat or socks, although it is cold. During the interview Michelle alternately sits across from the nurse and paces in front of the window.

Michelle states that she started taking desipramine prescribed by a college physician last semester because she was feeling "sad." She has gained 30 lb (13.6 kg) in 6 months. Michelle angrily states that the physician did not listen when she complained during follow-up sessions about weight gain and asked to take "something else." She denies suicidality or homicidality but notes that, at times, she feels "hyper," with extreme depression following. At one point, Michelle stands

and says, "If you don't change these pills, I'll find someone who will." She responds to a firm, supportive request from the nurse to "work together to figure out the best plan of action" by crying and sitting huddled in her chair.

Reflection and Critical Thinking

- Although she denies suicidality or homicidality, Michelle's behavior suggests impulsivity that might increase her risk for self-harm. What should the nurse do? Should the nurse involve Michelle's parents or a supportive friend? Is it safe for Michelle to leave the clinic? Should the nurse consider psychiatric hospitalization?
- What information about Michelle's family history should the nurse gather?
- Should the nurse contact the college physician? Is a release of information necessary?

participate in treatment or accusing the client of denial (Cooke et al., 2010).

Nursing Responses

Nurses must treat clients who are having difficulty adhering to medication regimens with compassion and understanding. If clients are struggling with side effects to the point that they want to discontinue the medication, dosage adjustments are often helpful. It is important to understand that clients will stop medications if the symptoms go away, if they don't go away, and if they are simply tired of taking them. Continuing discussion with the client and family and regular monitoring of the client's treatment plan are useful interventions.

Families want medication to "cure" or "fix" their psychiatrically ill relative. When symptoms abate and clients no longer have problems, they may decide to stop taking the drug, believing that they have been "cured." However, many chronic disorders require long-term medication use. It is essential for clients and families to understand this aspect of illness management (Velligan et al., 2010). Nurses assist both client and family to realize that mental health conditions are no different from other chronic illnesses that require medication (eg, diabetes, hypertension).

Caregiver sensitivity to each client's specific issues can have a positive influence on adherence. Psychiatric nurses adopt objective approaches that combine psychoeducation and brief motivational interviewing to assist with adherence. Other methods include the following:

- Keep in close contact with the client, including performing careful follow-up.
- Respond immediately to client complaints and change dose, time of administration, and medication if it helps alleviate the difficulty (Figure 16.10).
- Develop a strong therapeutic alliance with the client.
- Understand community and family supports available to the client.

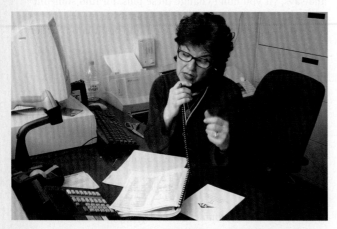

FIGURE 16.10 This nurse practitioner is discussing concerns related to a client's psychotropic medications and is ready to take necessary actions to make needed adjustments.

Working With the Family

Family members play essential roles in medication management. Many adults with psychiatric illness depend on parents and siblings for housing, monetary assistance, and emotional guidance. Lack of adequate housing has resulted in increased dependence of clients on families and community-based models of care (Piat et al., 2011). Furthermore, the families of clients with persistent mental illness are caring for the most disabled and underserved populations in society. Informal and formal networks of care available to the aging parents of adults who are chronically disturbed often are inadequate (see Chap. 15).

Medication management is usually a part of a care network and requires nurses to approach case management with client and family as a collaborative partnership (Hensley, 2011). Parents of adults who are chronically ill often feel that they are in conflict with caregivers, mostly involving their adult child's issues of autonomy and integrity in managing self-care. Nurses can help by viewing families as a resource and avoiding adversarial relationships. Families can assist with and support medication adherence and management of adverse side effects (Hensley, 2011).

"Family" can be defined broadly for clients with psychiatric illness and may include a significant other who is not a spouse, a caring neighbor, or a good friend. The client must identify a person as a support, and this person must agree to provide assistance in medication and illness management.

Families may positively influence adherence to medication regimens, act as the first line of assessment for adverse side effects, and supervise administration of medications and refilling of prescriptions. Nurses must help to resolve any conflicts between a client's confidentiality and the family's need for information (Wynaden & Orb, 2005). Family education about mental illness and the medications used to treat it should focus on family coping skills rather than family problems.

Although many adult clients prefer not to have relatives involved in medication management, parents may be available as support for their offspring with mental illness. Including them in decision making regarding medication management, especially when they are actively assisting a family member who is psychiatrically ill, can only enhance the benefits of psychotropic medication and the client's positive response to this treatment.

Lifespan Considerations
Pregnancy

Pregnant women who require psychotropic medications to stabilize their psychiatric symptoms present special problems. Whereas studies of the teratogenic effects of psychotropic medications have had mixed findings, maternal use of several drugs (eg, lithium, valproic acid, carbamazepine) during pregnancy can increase the risk of fetal congenital malformations (Brunton et al., 2011).

Unfortunately, the first trimester is when a woman is most likely to be unaware that she is pregnant. Nurses must thoroughly assess women of childbearing age starting drug therapy who may be pregnant or planning to conceive (Case

Case Vignette 16.2

Teresa, 24 years old, presents to an outpatient crisis center with complaints of hearing voices and "seeing things on television that aren't really there." Her husband Anthony accompanies her and reports that his wife's behavior has become increasingly odd and frightening. "She is not sleeping and believes that someone is poisoning her." He urged her to come to the clinic.

The couple has been married for 2 years. They have no children, although Anthony reports that they were going to start a family before Teresa's recent symptoms. They live in the urban neighborhood where they both grew up. Extended family on both sides lives nearby.

Teresa reports a history of psychiatric problems that began at age 18 during her first semester living at college. She had her "first breakdown," came home, was hospitalized, and did not return to school. She believes that she recovered from what she calls "my psychosis," but was intermittently plagued with auditory and visual hallucinations.

After the first breakdown, Teresa began working with a private psychiatrist (her parents paid for the treatment). During the 6 years of care, the psychiatrist attempted several drugs for the hallucinations. Teresa reports that she was taking clozapine (Clozaril) approximately 1 year ago and was "much

better," even taking college courses again. However, she adds that her psychiatrist retired 2 months ago. This development, coupled with a 45-lb (20.4 kg) weight gain, caused her to stop taking the drug.

Health care team members note Teresa's increasing paranoia and vague threats toward Anthony. They recommend a brief hospitalization. Teresa reluctantly agrees. During admission, the hospital psychiatrist prescribes clozapine for Teresa. At discharge 7 days later, the client agrees to visit the clinic nurse for help in managing her medication. Teresa also begins to attend a therapy group for women and resumes college classes.

Reflection and Critical Thinking

- What teaching will the nurse need to address with Anthony or other family members?
- What steps should the nurse take to develop an ongoing relationship that allows Teresa to discuss her concerns about medication, rather than abruptly discontinuing it in the future?
- What teaching points should a nurse consider for this client, a woman of childbearing age with severe psychiatric problems?

Vignette 16.2). However, doing so can be especially difficult if a client is in an acute psychotic state and cannot give an adequate or reliable sexual history.

At any time during pregnancy, the major concern involves the transfer of medications across the placenta, given that the placenta is not an absolute barrier to drugs taken by the mother. The fetus cannot safely metabolize the medication or its by-products. After delivery, the placenta is no longer available to assist with secretion, and drug toxicity may result (Brunton et al., 2011).

When it is imperative for a pregnant woman to receive psychotropic medication, the prescriber should use the lowest possible dose (Hendrick, 2010). Careful fetal monitoring should be part of the nursing care plan. Hypervigilance to potential pregnancy also assists in planning and managing medications.

Because psychotropic drugs are improving quality of life in clients with psychiatric disabilities, more women with psychiatric disorders are choosing to become pregnant. The deleterious effect of untreated depression and mania on the fetus makes it imperative for nurses to discuss the benefits of continuing to use existing psychotropic medications during pregnancy. Recent improvements in techniques to determine concentrations of psychotropic medications in both the fetus and in breast milk assist nurses to provide state-of-the-art information to clients (Fortinguerra et al., 2009).

Lactation

The benefits of breast-feeding for both mother and baby are well documented; however, the postpartum period is a time of

increased onset and relapse of mental illness (Banti et al., 2011). Breast-feeding also poses dilemmas when nursing mothers take psychotropic medications because all major classes of them pass into maternal breast milk, transferring undetermined amounts of medication to the infant (Fortinguerra et al., 2009). The goal of treatment should be to minimize infant exposure while maintaining maternal emotional health.

Children and Adolescents

Psychotropic medications have been administered to children for several decades. Whereas the standard of care for most practitioners makes such use acceptable, questions and controversy surround the need for these medications in the pediatric population. Researchers have identified issues related to efficacy, side effects, and long-term developmental consequences. Nurses must clarify their personal attitudes about use of psychotropic medications for children and teens.

The same principles of medication administration and management with adults apply to children and adolescents with psychiatric disturbances. In addition, nurses must be aware of the legal, physical, and emotional dependence that children younger than the age of consent have on their parents or guardians. Nurses must explain the principles of informed consent and health education to youthful clients and their family members. They must ensure that health teaching is developmentally based and gear it to the level of the client's understanding.

Medication management becomes more complicated with the involvement of school personnel, pediatric care providers, and after-school or day care providers. Supervision of medication administration, assessment of efficacy through parent and school reports, and careful monitoring of family response to the pediatric client's difficulties are greater issues than they are with adult clients.

Psychotropic medications commonly used to treat psychiatric disorders in pediatric populations include TCAs, SSRIs, lithium, and clozapine (see Chap. 36) (Zuddas et al., 2011). Most psychotropic medications have not been FDA approved for the pediatric population. Nevertheless, the clinical usefulness of such drugs in children and adolescents must be approached rationally and in a balanced way that considers the clinical needs of pediatric clients.

The effect of the 2005 FDA black box warning on the risk of suicidality in pediatric clients has severely limited the use of antidepressants. See Chapter 36 for discussion of this issue.

Issues particular to psychotropic treatment of children and adolescents include diagnosis and assessment, measurement of change, education, and the role of the family in supporting and managing treatment (Chrisman et al., 2007). An understanding that medication management in youthful populations is more complicated than with adults is essential and requires a developmental perspective for maximum clinical effectiveness (see Chap. 36).

Older Adults

The pharmacologic actions of psychotropic medications change dramatically for people older than 60 years. These changes may result from differences in drug absorption secondary to diminished gastrointestinal motility, decreased plasma proteins, decreased kidney function, or congestive heart failure. Other explanations include normal age-related changes in body composition, lean body mass, muscle mass, and fatty tissue (Hutchison & Sleeper-Irons, 2010).

Regardless of the reasons, nurses must be aware that older adults may respond differently than younger people to psychotropic medications. Because many older clients take several drugs simultaneously for various ailments, the need for hypervigilance concerning side effects from polypharmacy is increased. Coordination among medical and psychiatric providers is essential (Anderson & Bjorklund , 2010).

Psychiatric syndromes in older adults produce suffering, disability, and loss of independence (Hutchison & Sleeper-Irons, 2010). These problems also increase burdens for caregivers. Nevertheless, psychotropic medications can dramatically improve functioning in older clients when drugs are administered cautiously. Atypical antipsychotic medications have increased safety and efficacy. Older clients still present particular challenges to caregivers because of their propensity for chronic medical conditions. See Chapter 37 for more discussion of older adults.

Pharmacogenetics

Pharmacogenetics is the study of how the actions of and reactions to drugs vary with a person's genes. Since the unraveling of the human genome, pharmacogenetic research has exploded (Relling & Giocomini, 2011). In the not so distant future, pharmacogenetics will be able to predict side effects for individual clients (Zandi & Judy, 2010). People of African, Native American, Hispanic, Asian, Caucasian, and European descent often respond differently to the same doses of medication used to treat psychiatric illness (Chaudrey et al, 2008). The three predominant aspects of pharmacogenetics are (1) the biologic response that varies by ethnicity; (2) the client's cultural belief system and culturally based expectations about psychotropic medication management; and (3) the ways that caregiver perception of ethnicity influences care decisions. Recognizing the client's culture, belief system, and racial background and their influence on response to medication is essential for nurses managing care.

Since the 1920s, research has suggested that ethnicity affects response to medication (Camilleri, 2007; Nnadi & Malhotra, 2007). Several research studies suggest that African Americans tend to be misdiagnosed and overmedicated compared with other ethnic groups. They may have an increased risk of neuroleptic toxicity (Fijal et al., 2009) and have a higher incidence of side effects when given lithium (Chee et al., 2008). They are also less likely to experience response to fluoxetine. Similarly, it has been found that Korean American clients achieved significantly lower clozapine concentrations than did Caucasians. Asians tend to metabolize TCAs more slowly than do Caucasian populations (Chee et al., 2008). Hispanic populations have different responses to antidepressants than other ethnicities (Dong et al., 2009). Cultural factors affecting response to medication can include attitudes toward disease and cure, beliefs about psychiatric illness, and spiritual beliefs in relation to illness (Relling & Giocomini, 2011). Although research has suggested that genetic factors influence differences in drug response, belief systems can influence drug response, as well as drug adherence. Believing the medication is helpful is likely to influence the client's willingness to take it and the response to treatment.

A basic tenet of nursing care involves awareness of clients' belief systems, their culture, and their willingness to accept treatment. Although many of the exact cultural influences on biologic response to medication have not been researched, there is a significant focus on nursing care that attempts to understand a client's culture and belief system and to plan care based on this understanding.

Complementary and Alternative Modalities (CAM)

In 1991, Congress established the Office of Alternative Medicine at the National Institutes of Health. The status, mandate, and authority of this office were expanded in 1998 to create the National Center for Complementary and Alternative Medicine (NCCAM), which now supports a robust research department (http://nccam.nih.gov). The task of the NCCAM is to conduct and support basic and applied research regarding the identification, investigation, and validation of CAM treatments; diagnostic and prevention modalities; disciplines; and systems. Types of CAM include herbal medicine, massage, megavitamins, acupuncture, chiropractic manipulation, fields of mind–body medicine, and self-help groups (Ravven et al., 2011). CAM is discussed in detail in Chapter 17.

The most common alternative agent used in psychiatry is St. John's wort for depression (Dwyer et al., 2011; Monti & Beitman, 2010). Its chemical composition has been well studied, and pharmacologic benefits include antidepressant, antiviral, and antibacterial effects (Sarris et al., 2011). Several studies using meta-analysis confirm the benefit of St. John's wort in treating mild to moderately severe depression (Sarris et al., 2011). Nevertheless, several difficulties accompany the use of St. John's wort for this problem. For example, clients who take both St. John's wort and an antidepressant drug are at risk for serotonin syndrome (discussed earlier). Because agents such as St. John's wort are available in health food stores and over the counter, they are unregulated in terms of content and manufacturing. If clients choose to self-medicate without consulting a health care provider, there is no opportunity to evaluate their complete health status or to identify other metabolic or health-related causes for depression. Providers would also be unable to evaluate other substances that these clients use or factors that may contraindicate the use of St. John's wort or other alternative remedies.

Omega-3 polyunsaturated fatty acids found in fish, fish oil, and flaxseed have been found to ameliorate the symptoms of bipolar disorders and schizophrenia (Mischoulon & Rosenbaum, 2008). Several studies show that fish oil might possess elements that assist in stabilizing mood. The omega-3 polyunsaturated fatty acids are recommended as an adjunct therapy, rather than a first-line monotherapy for any psychiatric illness (Freeman & Rapaport, 2011). The predominant adverse effect of taking omega-3 polyunsaturated fatty acids is mild gastrointestinal distress.

For nurses, the most important consideration in treating clients with mental illness taking psychotherapeutic drugs is to assess carefully what other agents they may be using to alleviate symptoms. Nurses should contact a pharmacist or homeopathic physician familiar with alternative therapies if they have any doubt about a vitamin or other substance clients are taking concurrently with a psychotropic medication.

Performing Self-Clarification

Nurses must clarify their own values about the benefit of psychotropic medication to treat psychiatric disorders. This clarification will influence the care they provide to clients who may refuse medication. Should nurses support a client's decision to refuse medication, even if refusal lowers quality of life or increases the risk of psychiatric hospitalization or incarceration? Nurses must understand the multiple factors influencing their attitudes, including legal rights, institutional values of their working environment, and personal value system about client care.

Checkpoint Questions

17. What are two potentially lethal dysrhythmias that may be associated with psychopharmacologic agents?

18. What is meant by the term *adherence*, and what does it involve?

▲ EVALUATION

Evaluation of a client's medication regimen involves the following:

- Review the efficacy of the drug in improving functioning.
- Discuss the client's subjective perception of response to medication.
- Regularly monitor perceived response, feelings about the medication, and potential difficulties.

Clients may spontaneously discontinue medication without consulting caregivers. When this happens, the best treatment strategy is to avoid criticism, rejection, or ultimatums. Nevertheless, the treatment team, including the nurse, needs to decide, after carefully considering all factors, whether care can continue should the individual choose not to take psychiatric medication.

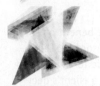

Reviewing and Applying Your Knowledge

Chapter Summary

- The development of psychopharmacology has paralleled the increasingly important role of the nurse in medication management.

- The administration of psychotropic medication involves specific nursing responsibilities.

- Principles of medication management are applicable to psychiatric clients.

- Particular psychotropic medications are characterized by side effects and administration guidelines. Medications should be used to treat psychiatric target symptoms for a specified period.

- Specific client populations who may require psychotropic medication include pregnant and lactating women, older adults, and children and adolescents.

- Families provide essential support to clients receiving psychotropic medication.

- Nurses must be aware of the specific management issues inherent in polypharmacy in client use of alternative substances to treat mental health disorders.

- Nurses can blend an understanding of psychosocial needs with specific symptoms to provide optimal nursing care.

- Nurses must engage in a research process that evaluates multiple effects of medication on a client's life and functioning.

Study Questions

1. After a nurse teaches a client and family about the use of psychoactive medications, which of the following statements from family members indicates successful teaching?

   a. "The drugs act primarily on specific target sites."

   b. "The drugs help the symptom but may lead to other problems."

   c. "The effects of drugs on other body systems are usually minimal."

   d. "Drug therapy is highly effective in treating psychiatric problems."

2. Which of the following would be most important for the nurse to do for a client who is beginning therapy with a TCA?

   a. Have the client change positions slowly.

   b. Assess for prompt elevation in mood.

   c. Monitor for hypertensive crisis.

   d. Anticipate the need for an antidiarrheal agent.

3. After teaching a client who is prescribed phenelzine sulfate (Nardil) about dietary restrictions, which of the following client statements indicates the need for additional teaching?

   a. "I'll have to stop using blue cheese salad dressing."

   b. "I'll have a turkey sandwich instead of a salami sandwich for lunch."

   c. "I'm going to have tacos with sour cream and guacamole tonight."

   d. "I'll switch to drinking orange juice in the mornings with breakfast."

4. Which of the following instructions would the nurse include in a teaching plan for a client who is receiving lithium?

   a. "Avoid getting overheated when you're outside."

   b. "Have your blood levels checked every 6 months."

   c. "Limit your water intake to two to three glasses per day."

   d. "Expect some weight loss with this drug."

5. Which of the following would be most important for the nurse to monitor for in a client receiving clozapine (Clozaril)?

   a. Signs of TD

   b. Refractory dysrhythmia

   c. Decreased WBC count

   d. Orthostatic hypotension

Critical Thinking Questions

1. What aspects of a biopsychosocial evaluation must the nurse consider before the client begins psychotropic medication?

2. What are some possible legal, ethical, and social issues involved when a client who has a chronic psychiatric illness refuses to adhere to a medication regimen?

3. How can a nurse's personal attitudes about psychiatric medications influence (positively or negatively) the care that he or she provides to clients?

References

Aiken, C. B. (2007). Pramipexole in psychiatry: A systematic review of the literature. *Journal of Clinical Psychiatry, 68,* 1230–1236.

American Psychiatric Association. (2000). *Diagnostic and statistical manual of mental disorders* (4th ed., text rev.). Washington, DC: Author.

Anderson, K. S., & Bjorklund, P. (2010). Demystifying federal nursing home regulations to improve the effectiveness of psychopharmacological care. *Perspectives in Psychiatric Care, 46*(2), 152–162.

Anderson, S. (2005). Making medicines: A brief history of pharmacy. London, UK: Pharmaceutical Press.

Aschenbrenner, D. S., & Venable, S. J. (2009). *Drug therapy in nursing* (3rd ed.). Philadelphia, PA: Lippincott Williams & Wilkins.

Baloush-Kleinman, V., Levine, S. Z., Roe, D., Shnitt, D., Weizman, A., & Poyurovsky, M. (2011). Adherence to antipsychotic drug treatment in early-episode schizophrenia: A six-month naturalistic follow-up study. *Schizophrenia Research*, May 31; [Epub ahead of print] PMID: 21636254

Banti, S., Mauri, M., Oppo, A., Borri, C., Rambelli, C., Ramacciotti, D., et al. (2011). From the third month of pregnancy to 1 year postpartum. Prevalence, incidence, recurrence, and new onset of depression. Results from the Perinatal Depression-Research & Screening Unit study. *Comprehensive Psychiatry, 52*(4), 343–351.

Beck, A. T., Baruch, E., Balter, J. M., Steer, R. A., & Warman, D. M. (2004). A new instrument for measuring insight: The Beck Cognitive Insight Scale. *Schizophrenia Research, 68,* 319–329.

Brunton, L., Chabner, B., & Knollman, B. (2010). *Goodman and Gilman's: The pharmacological basis of therapeutics* (12th ed.). New York, NY: McGraw Hill.

Camilleri, M. (2007). Pharmacogenomics and serotonergic agents: Research observations and potential clinical practice implications. *Neurogastroenterology Motility, 19*(S2), 40–45.

Chaudhry, I., Neelam, K., Duddu, V., & Husain, N. (2008). Ethnicity and psychopharmacology. *Journal of Psychopharmacology, 22*(6), 673–680.

Chee, H. N., Lin, K. L., Singh, B. S, & Chiu, E. Y. K. (2008). *Ethnopsychopharmacology: Advances in current practice.* New York, NY: Cambridge Medicine.

Chrisman, A. K., Enderlin, H. T., Landry, K. L., Colvin, J. S., & De-John, M. R. (2007). Teaching evidence-based medicine pediatric psychopharmacology: Integrating psychopharmacologic treatment into the broad spectrum of care. *Child and Adolescent Psychiatric Clinics of North America, 16,* 165–181.

Conley, R., & Kelly, D. L. (2007). Clinical pharmacology and medication-associated side effects: A review of second-generation antipsychotics for schizophrenia. *Clinical Schizophrenia and Related Psychoses, 1,* 135–146.

Cooke, M. A., Peters, E. R., Fannon, D., Aasen, I., Kuipers, E., & Kumari, V. (2010). Cognitive insight in psychosis: the relationship between self-certainty and self-reflection dimensions and neuropsychological measures. *Psychiatry Research*, 178(2), 284–289.

Dedeurwaerdere, S., Wintmolders, C., Straetemans, R., Pemberton, D., & Langlois, X. (2011). Memantine-induced brain activation as a model for the rapid screening of potential novel antipsychotic compounds: Exemplified by activity of an mGlu2/3 receptor agonist. *Psychopharmacology, 214*(2), 505–514.

DeLeon, J. (2004). Atypical antipsychotic dosing: The effect of smoking and caffeine. *Psychiatric Services, 55,* 491–493.

Dong, C., Wong, M. L., & Licinio, J. (2009). Sequence variations of ABCB1, SLC6A2, SLC6A3, SLC6A4, CREB1, CRHR1 and NTRK2: Association with major depression and antidepressant response in Mexican-Americans. *Molecular Psychiatry, 14*(12), 1105–1118.

Dwyer, A. V., Whitten, D. L., & Hawrelak, J. A. (2011). Herbal medicines, other than St. John's Wort, in the treatment of depression: A systematic review. *Alternative Medicine Reviews, 16*(1), 40–49.

Essock, S. M., Schooler, N. R., Stroup, T. S., McEvoy, J. P., Rojas, I., Jackson, C., et al. (2011). The Schizophrenia Trials Network: Effectiveness of switching from antipsychotic polypharmacy to monotherapy. *American Journal of Psychiatry*, May 2; [Epub ahead of print] PMID: 21536693.

Fijal, B. A., Kinon, B. J., Kapur, S., Stauffer, V. L., Conley, R. R., Jamal, H. H., et al. (2009). Candidate-gene association analysis of response to risperidone in African-American and white patients with schizophrenia. *Pharmacogenomics Journal, 9*(5), 311–318.

Fortinguerra, F., Clavenna, A., & Bonati, M. (2009). Psychotropic drug use during breastfeeding: A review of the evidence. *Pediatrics, 124*(4), e547–e556.

Freeman, M. P., & Rapaport, M. H. (2011). Omega-3 fatty acids and depression: from cellular mechanisms to clinical care. *Journal of Clinical Psychiatry, 72*(2), 258–259.

Ghaemi, S., Schrauwen, E., Lugman, J., Berv, D., Shirzadi, A. A., Pardo, T. B., et al. (2006). Long-term lamotrigine plus lithium for bipolar disorder: One-year outcome. *Journal of Psychiatric Practice, 12,* 300–305.

Goodwin, F. J., & Jamison, K. R. (2007). *Manic-depressive illness: Bipolar disorders and recurrent depression* (2nd ed.). New York, NY: Oxford University Press.

Green, A. I., Tohen, M., Patel, J. K., Banov, J., DuRand, C., Berman, I., et al. (2000). Clozapine in the treatment of refractory psychotic mania. *American Journal of Psychiatry, 157,* 982–986.

Hendrick, V. (2010). *Psychiatric disorders in pregnancy and the postpartum.* Totowa, NJ: Humana Press.

Hensley, M. A. (2011). Roles of community helpers in using the Medicare Part D benefit. *Journal of Health Care for the Poor and Underserved, 22*(1), 258–270.

Hutchison, L. C., & Sleeper-Irons, R. (2010). *Fundamentals of geriatric pharmacotherapy: An evidenced approach.* Bethesda, MD: American Society of Health System Pharmacists.

Kapusta, N. D., Plener, P. L., Schmid, R., Thau, K., Walter, H., & Lesch, O. M. (2007). Multiple substance use among young males. *Pharmacology, Biochemistry, and Behavior, 86,* 306–311.

Karch, A. M. (2011). *2011 Lippincott's nursing drug guide.* Philadelphia, PA: Lippincott Williams & Wilkins.

Lachar, D., Bailley, S. E., Rhoades, H. M., Espadas, A., Aponte, M., Cowan, K. A., et al. (2001). New subscales for an anchored version of the Brief Psychiatric Rating Scale: Construction, reliability, and validity in acute psychiatric admission. *Psychological Assessment, 13,* 384–395.

Leonard, B. E. (2004). Pharmacotherapy in the treatment of Alzheimer's disease: An update. *World Psychiatry, 3,* 84–88.

Levin, E. D., & Rezvani, A. H. (2007, July). Nicotinic interactions with antipsychotic drugs, models of schizophrenia and impacts on cognitive function. *Biochemical Pharmacology*. Retrieved from http://www.ncbi.nlm.nih.gov/sites/entrez?Db=pubmed& Cmd= ShowDetailView&TermToSearch=17714691&ordinalpos=1& itool=EntrezSystem2. PEntrez.Pubmed.Pubmed_ResultsPanel. Pubmed_RVDocSum.

Lieberman, J. A., Stroup, T. S., McEvoy, J. P., Swartz, M. S., Rosenheck, R. A., Perkins, D. O., et al. (2005). Effectiveness of antipsychotic drugs in patients with chronic schizophrenia. *New England Journal of Medicine, 353,* 1209–1223.

Mischoulon, D., & Rosenbaum, J. F. (2008). *Natural medications for psychiatric disorders.* Philadelphia, PA: Lippincott Williams & Wilkins.

Monti, D. A., & Beitman, B. D. (2010). *Integrative psychiatry* (Weil Integrative Medicine Series). New York, NY: Oxford University Press.

Morgan, P. (2007). Treatment-resistant depression: Response to low-dose transdermal but not oral selegiline. *Journal of Clinical Psychopharmacology, 27,* 313–314.

National Institute of Mental Health. (1995). Abnormal involuntary movement scale (AIMS). Retrieved from http://www.NIMH.nih.gov

Nnadi, C. U., & Malhotra, A. K. (2007). Individualizing antipsychotic drug therapy in schizophrenia: The promise of pharmacogenetics. *Current Psychiatry Reports, 9,* 313–318.

Pia, L., & Tamietto, M. (2006). Unawareness in schizophrenia: Neuropsychological and neuroanatomical findings. *Psychiatry and Clinical Neuroscience, 60*(5), 531–537.

Piat, M., Sabetti, J., Fleury, M. J., Boyer, R., & Lesage, A. (2011). "Who believes most in me and in my recovery": The importance of families for persons with serious mental illness living in structured community housing. *Journal of Social Work and Disability Rehabilitation, 10*(1), 49–65.

Pollack, M. H., Simon, N. M., Zalta, A. K., Worthington, J. J., Hoge, E. A., Mick, E., et al. (2006). Olanzapine augmentation of fluoxetine for refractory generalized anxiety disorder: A placebo controlled study. *Biological Psychiatry, 59,* 211–215.

Pratoomsri, W., Yatham, L., Bond, D., Lam, R., & Sohn, C. H. (2006). Oxcarbazepine in the treatment of bipolar disorder: A review. *Canadian Journal of Psychiatry, 51,* 540–545.

Ravven, S. E., Zimmerman, M. B., Schultz, S. K., & Wallace, R. B. (2011). 12-month herbal medicine use for mental health from the national Comorbidity Survey Replication (NCS-R). *Annals of Clinical Psychiatry, 23*(2), 83–94.

Relling, M. V., & Giocomini, K. M. (2011). Pharmacogenetics. In L. L. Brunton, J. S. Lazo, & K. Parker (Eds.), *Goodman & Gilman's the pharmacological basis of therapeutics* (12th ed., pp. 145–168). New York, NY: McGraw-Hill.

Rosenbaum, J. F., Arana, G. W., Hymen, S. E., Labbate, L. A., & Fava, M. (2005). *Handbook of psychiatric drug therapy* (5th ed.). Philadelphia, PA: Lippincott Williams & Wilkins.

Rush, A. J., Fava, M., Wisniewski, S. R., Lavori, P. W., Trivedi, M. H., Sackeim, H. A., et al. (2004). Sequenced treatment alternatives to relieve depression (STAR*D): Rationale and design. *Controlled Clinical Trials, 25,* 119–142.

Sarris, J., Panossian, A., Schweitzer, I., Stough, C., & Scholey A. (2011). Herbal medicine for depression, anxiety and insomnia: A review of psychopharmacology and clinical evidence. *European Neuropsychopharmacology,* May 20; [Epub ahead of print] PMID: 21601431

Schatzberg, A. F., & Nemeroff, C. B. (2003). *Textbook of psychopharmacology.* Washington, DC: American Psychiatric Publishing.

Stahl, S. M. (2006). *Essential psychopharmacology: The prescriber's guide: Revised and updated edition. (Essential Psychopharmacology Series).* New York, NY: Cambridge University Press.

Stahl, S. M. (2008). *Stahl's essential psychopharmacology: Neuroscientific basis and practical applications.* New York , NY: Cambridge University Press.

Velligan, D. I., Weiden, P. J., Sajatovic, M., Scott, J., Carpenter, D., Ross, R., & Docherty, J. P. (2010). Strategies for addressing adherence problems in patients with serious and persistent mental illness: Recommendations from the expert consensus guidelines. *Journal of Psychiatric Practice, 16*(5), 306–324.

Velligan, D. I., Weiden, P. J., Sajatovic, M., Scott, J., Carpenter, D., Ross, R., et al. (2009). Expert Consensus Panel on Adherence Problems in Serious and Persistent Mental Illness. The expert consensus guideline series: Adherence problems in patients with serious and persistent mental illness. *Journal of Clinical Psychiatry, 70*(Suppl 4), 1–46.

Wynaden, D., & Orb, A. (2005). Impact of patient confidentiality on careers of people who have a mental disorder. *International Journal of Mental Health Nursing, 14*(3), 166–171.

Zandi, P. P., & Judy, J. T. (2010). The promise and reality of pharmacogenetics in psychiatry. *Clinical Laboratory Medicine.* 30(4), 931–974.

Zuddas, A., Zanni, R., & Usala, T. (2011). Second generation antipsychotics (SGAs). for non-psychotic disorders in children and adolescents: A review of the randomized controlled studies. *European Neuropsychopharmacology,* May 5; [Epub ahead of print] PMID: 21550212

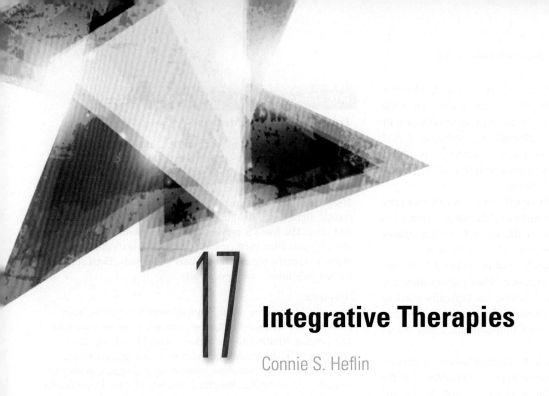

17

Integrative Therapies

Connie S. Heflin

KEY TERMS

allopathic
alternative therapy
complementary therapy
energy medicine
holism
integrative therapy
manipulative and body-based
    practices
mind–body medicine
whole medical systems

LEARNING OBJECTIVES

On completion of this chapter, you should be able to accomplish the following:

- Differentiate between the terms "complementary therapy" and "alternative therapy."
- Explain what is meant by "integrative therapy."
- Identify the categories of complementary and alternative therapies as classified by the National Center for Complementary and Alternative Medicine (NCCAM).
- Construct a list of complementary and alternative therapies used to treat specific psychiatric–mental health conditions.
- Incorporate complementary and alternative therapies into evidence-based psychiatric–mental health nursing practice.

Complementary and alternative medicine (CAM) has become a mainstream part of U.S. health care. One reason for this development is the general dissatisfaction of many clients with Western (**allopathic**) medicine. CAM therapies, many of which are based on Eastern philosophies, incorporate a holistic, integrative approach in unifying physical, mental, and spiritual well-being.

The terms **alternative therapy** and **complementary therapy** have different meanings. Alternative therapies are those used *in place of* Western therapies. Complementary therapies are used *in conjunction* with Western therapies. CAM generally refers to practices not considered "conventional" in Western medical practice. That means they are not taught widely in medical schools, not typically used in hospitals, and not usually reimbursed by medical insurance companies (National Center for Complementary and Alternative Medicine [NCCAM], 2010).

CAM practices may not readily integrate into the dominant Western health care model because they pose challenges to diverse societal beliefs and practices. However, attitudes toward CAM have evolved as health care professionals have become more culturally competent and responsive to clients' needs and requests for practices instead of or in addition to those that mainstream medicine offers. The more comprehensive term **integrative therapy** may be used, instead of complementary or alternative, implying the use of practices in conjunction with traditional health care modalities in the care of clients.

NCCAM'S CATEGORIES OF PRACTICE

In 1998, Congress established the National Center for Complementary and Alternative Medicine as an institute under the auspices of the National Institutes of Health (NIH). The NIH operates under the Public Health Service in the U.S. Department of Health and Human Services. The mission of NCCAM is to support research and dissemination of information on CAM in an effort to integrate evidence-based CAM therapies into Western medicine (NCCAM, 2010).

One area that the NCCAM studies involves **whole medical systems**. Several of these methods have existed for centuries. Examples include traditional Chinese medicine, Ayurveda, homeopathic medicine, and naturopathic medicine. Box 17.1 lists the major whole medical systems with underlying beliefs and common treatments for each.

The NCCAM groups individual integrative therapies into broad categories that often overlap:

- **Mind–body medicine**. These approaches use mindful stress-reduction techniques to restore bodily functions. Primary examples include meditation, yoga, and acupuncture. Other mind–body practices are deep breathing exercises, guided imagery, hypnotherapy, progressive relaxation, *qi gong*, and *tai chi*. As the name indicates, the mind and body working as one are thought to be integral to the healing process. This

---

BOX 17.1 Whole Systems of Medical Practice

Traditional Chinese Medicine

Common practices include acupuncture, moxibustion (application of heat from burning the herb moxa at the acupuncture point), Chinese Materia Medica (catalog of natural products), and massage/manipulation. *Qi* is the vital life force in the body. *Yin/yang* is the interaction of opposing forces (hot/cold, male/female, light/dark). Health results from a balance of *qi* and *yin* and *yang*. The focus is prevention of illness with a balance of five elements (fire, earth, metal, water, and wood) that correspond to specific organs and systems in the body. Each client is treated individually and specifically.

Ayurveda

Literally "the science of life," practitioners believe that inner harmony and balance (body, mind, and spirit) are necessary for self-healing. Methodologies include lifestyle analysis, determination of dosha (body type), change in healing processes, special diets, herbs, vitamins, meditation, massage, exposure to sunlight, and controlled breathing. It comprises the major health care system in India.

Homeopathic Medicine

Practitioners give minerals, plant extracts, chemicals, and disease-producing germs in minute doses to effect a cure, when these same substances can cause illness in larger doses. For example, they may give arsenicum (arsenic) in minute doses for digestive problems. Practitioners select therapies based on how closely symptoms produced by a remedy match the symptoms of the client's disease (principle of similars). The method originated in Germany.

Naturopathic Medicine

Literally "nature disease," this method posits that nature and each person possess inherent healing power. The healing power of nature underscores the concept of "first do no harm," treatment of the whole person, and prevention. Practitioners advocate changes in lifestyle and prevention techniques to promote health. It originated in Europe.

Adapted from National Center for Complementary and Alternative Medicine (NCCAM). (2010). *What is CAM?* Retrieved from http://nccam.nih.gov.

---

concept is part of traditional Chinese medicine and Ayurvedic medicine.

- **Natural products**. These methods rely on substances such as herbs and diet and nutrition supplements, including probiotics (live microorganisms such as bacteria found in yogurt). Natural products are the most widely used category of CAM in the United States. According to a 2007 National Health Interview Survey, adults reported using fish oil/omega-3s most often (reported by 37.4% of all adults who said they used natural products). The most widely reported products for children included echinacea (37.2%) and fish oil/omega-3s (30.5%) (NCCAM, 2010).
- **Manipulative and body-based practices**. Modalities in this classification focus on the manipulation or movement of one or more body parts. Two common examples are spinal manipulation and massage therapy. Spinal

manipulation was used by the ancient Greeks. Interestingly, Hippocrates claimed that medicine was the "art of rubbing" (NCCAM, 2010).

There are a variety of other CAM practices that do not fit into the above categories. Movement therapies such as Pilates are purported to promote physical, mental, emotional, and spiritual health. **Energy therapies** such as magnet therapy, *qi gong*, Reiki, or therapeutic touch focus on energy fields that originate from inside (biofields) or outside (electromagnetic fields) the body. There is no research-based evidence of these energy fields. Other CAM therapies include light therapy, aromatherapy, and practices of traditional healers such as Native American shamans.

Many therapies belong to more than one category. For example, yoga and tai chi can be considered mind–body and movement therapies. In addition, clients and practitioners may use modalities in combination. For example, some people use aromatherapy concurrently with massage or meditation in conjunction with guided imagery.

See Table 17.1 for an illustrated review of various common integrative therapies within the various NCCAM categories.

TABLE 17.1 Illustrated Review of Common Integrative Modalities

Mind–body medicine: Approaches use mindful stress-reduction techniques to restore physiologic functions. Additional approaches to those covered include art therapy, dance therapy, guided imagery, humor, hypnotherapy, prayer and spirituality (see Chap. 7), and support groups.

Acupuncture 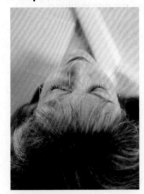	Acupuncture involves the placement of needles on specific points of the body to treat specific illnesses. Needle placement helps correct and rebalance energy flow and consequently relieve pain and restore health. It redirects energy to organs with health deficiencies.
Meditation 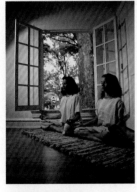	Clients try to achieve awareness without thought and positively alter physiology. Moment-to-moment attention leads to perceptual and cognitive changes. Focus on breathing diverts concentration from stressors. Meditation is done at prescribed frequencies and durations.
Music therapy 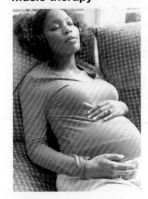	Use of music can alter behavior, emotions, or physiology. Musical vibrations and artistic expressions can help restore or enhance regulatory function. Such modalities may help clients develop self-awareness and creativity, improve learning, clarify values, and cope with various illnesses.

(continues on page 336)

TABLE 17.1 **Illustrated Review of Common Integrative Modalities** (continued)

Pet therapy

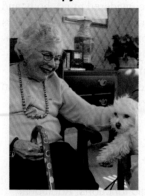

Pet therapy programs are found nationwide. Studies support the benefits of interaction with pets, which include decreased blood pressure, enhanced mood and socialization, and improved cardiovascular symptoms. Pets can be helpful companions for depressed clients, as well as those with cognitive challenges.

Yoga

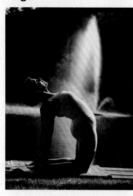

Yoga is used to relieve anxiety, stress, and pain; treat addictions and migraines; enhance spatial memory; and increase auditory and visual perceptions. There are many styles of yoga; each is a unique combination of physical postures and exercises (*asanas*), breathing techniques (*pranayamas*), relaxation, diet, and proper thinking.

Natural products: These methods use natural substances to restore health and healing. Additional approaches to those covered include apitherapy, probiotics, macrobiotics, nutritional supplements, and vitamin therapy.

Herbal therapy

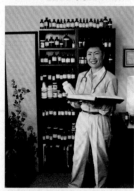

Herbal therapy uses plants or their parts to manage illness. Most herbs act by correcting underlying causes of disease. Each herb has a complex mixture of active ingredients, often making it difficult to identify the effective agent. Use of herbs requires knowledgeable practitioners and reliable products because the strength and purity of preparations vary.

Aromatherapy

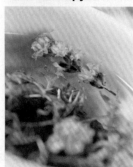

Aromatherapy uses essential oils for health benefits. It is not known if aromatherapy achieves its efficacy from placebo response, effects of touch and smell on the nervous system, learned memory of aromas, pharmacokinetic potentiation of drugs by essential oils, or pharmacologically active ingredients that have analgesic effects.

Manipulative and body-based practices: These modalities involve the manipulation or movement of one or more body parts. Additional approaches to those covered include chiropractic, massage (more than 80 forms), osteopathy, and reflexology.

Reflexology

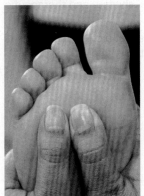

Reflexology involves massaging specific areas of the hands or feet to relieve stress or pain in corresponding related body areas. Use of reflexology is reported to improve pain, digestion, insomnia, premenstrual syndrome, menopausal symptoms, fertility, respiratory conditions, asthma, and cardiovascular problems.

Spinal manipulation

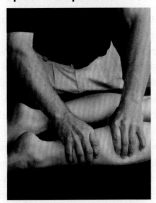

Spinal manipulation involves using the hands to apply force to a joint of the spine, moving it beyond its passive range of motion. It is most commonly used for chronic back pain.

Massage therapy

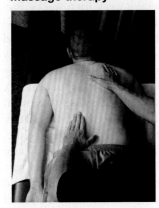

Massage therapy encompasses manipulating soft tissue and muscle by pressing and rubbing them with the hands. Massage is used to reduce anxiety and stress and to assist with sports injuries.

Tai chi

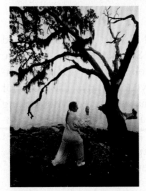

Tai chi consists of a series of choreographed, continuous slow movements performed with mental concentration and coordinated breathing. Clients learn to connect with energies, balance energies within the body, and maintain equilibrium with the opposing forces of nature (*yin* and *yang*). This powerful centering activity may precede meditation, prayer, or other exercises.

(continues on page 338)

TABLE 17.1 **Illustrated Review of Common Integrative Modalities** (continued)

Other CAM therapies: Energy therapies focus on energy fields that originate from inside (biofields) or outside (electromagnetic fields) of the body. Additional approaches to those covered include acupressure, Reiki, shiatsu, and therapeutic touch.

Bioelectromagnetic therapy

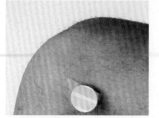

Clients use magnetic fields to prevent and treat disease and as first aid. Natural mineral magnets are used for insomnia, chronic pain, broken bones, stress, and musculoskeletal disorders.

Each category includes a sampling of common methods only.

Checkpoint Questions

1. According to traditional Chinese medicine, what five basic elements make up the body?
2. What are the underlying beliefs of Ayurveda?
3. What are three examples of mind–body practices thought to affect mental health?

PSYCHIATRIC CONDITIONS AND INTEGRATIVE THERAPIES

Nursing students should be familiar with the major integrative modalities from their fundamentals and other courses. The following sections discuss the status of various integrative therapies in relationship to common psychiatric conditions and disorders. Nurses should be familiar with these modalities, so they can answer questions from clients and families seeking methods of mental health promotion or options for the management of psychiatric challenges. Many clients and families are increasingly aware that alternatives exist, but they may desire advice or need guidance from nurses to separate unsubstantiated claims from facts (see Chap. 4).

Anxiety Disorders

Many people with anxiety disorders, especially those with panic attacks, use CAM therapies to manage stress and their conditions, largely because many CAM therapies involve methods to reduce stress levels in general. Mind–body techniques such as relaxation and breathing, guided imagery, meditation, hypnosis, and biofeedback are frequently used approaches to anxiety management.

Herbal remedies such as passion flower, valerian root, chamomile, skullcap, and lemon balm have soothing effects on the nervous system. Nurses should be aware that use of the herb kava (*Piper methysticum*) is associated with liver damage and should not be recommended to clients. The U.S. Food and Drug Administration (FDA) Center for Food Safety and Applied Nutrition posted an advisory regarding kava in 2002 (FDA, 2011), and this was reiterated by an NCCAM Consumer Advisory in 2010 (NCCAM, 2010).

Furthermore, herbal remedies may potentiate or otherwise alter the effect of prescription antianxiety medications. Nurses should carefully assess current medication and herbal uses in clients with anxiety. See Table 17.2.

Music therapy may foster a sense of inner peace and feelings of relaxation. Some studies have shown that music therapy contributes to hypometabolic alterations in the autonomic, immune, and endocrine systems, resulting in decreased tension and anxiety. Participants in an experimental group received a 30-minute music listening intervention based on personal preferences. This was delivered by trained nursing staff in midafternoon twice a week for 6 weeks. Participants in a control group received the standard care with no music. Results indicated that the older adults who received the preferred music listening intervention had significantly lower anxiety at 6 weeks as compared with the control group (Sung et al., 2010) (Evidence-Based Practice Spotlight 17.1).

Aromatherapy with essential oils, especially lavender, vanilla, and chamomile, can have calming effects. Other therapies for anxiety include massage, yoga, acupuncture, energy healing, and humor therapy. Engineers in Japan have incorporated "aroma systems" into the construction of new buildings. Lavender and rosemary scents are pumped into customer areas to help keep customers calm while they wait (Holistic-Online.com, 2007b).

Mood Disorders

Clients employ a wide variety of CAM therapies for mood disorders, especially depression. Some clients with chronic depression do not experience relief from prescribed antidepressants and short-term psychotherapy. The costs of conventional medicine and stigma associated with seeking treatment for mood alterations are likely contributors toward the use of CAM therapies in these clients. The most common CAM modalities for depression are light therapy, meditation, and herbal/dietary therapy.

TABLE 17.2 Selected Herbs, Minerals, and Vitamins for Mental Health Use

Herbs, Minerals, and Vitamins	Uses	Actions and Precautions	Dose
California poppy, yellow and orange	Relieves pain Acts as sedative Relieves mild anxiety	Poppy contains mild alkaloids similar to codeine and morphine. Do not use with monoamine oxidase inhibitors (MAOIs).	1 tsp/cup tea 2–3 times a day
Ginkgo biloba *Memory* (handwritten)	Reduces senility Reduces short-term memory loss in normal older adults Improves peripheral circulation	Use as a circulatory aid and antioxidant. Fruit or seed should not be handled or eaten. May enhance papaverine. Possible side effects include gastrointestinal (GI) distress, headache, and allergic reaction. Cautious use is recommended if taking aspirin or other blood-thinning drugs.	60 mg BID Alzheimer's—240 mg divided 2–3 times a day
Ginseng (Asian and American) *Energy* (handwritten)	Reduces stress and fatigue Improves physical and mental function, especially with elderly clients Assists smoking cessation efforts	Use the root. Use may raise blood pressure and serum glucose levels and can increase the growth of estrogen-dependent cancer.	American—0.03% ginsenoside, 1–2 g fresh root Asian—1.5% ginseng, 1–2 g fresh root For both, 200–600 mg liquid extract daily
Guarana	Enhances cognition Reduces combat fatigue Acts as a "cerebral stimulant"	It is a food additive/dietary supplement. It contains an extremely high caffeine level: 2.6%–7%, compared to coffee beans with 1%–2% and dried tea leaves with 1%–4%.	Not recommended for use Range for use: 250–1,200 mg/day
Hops	Has a sedative effect Reduces anxiety	Forms include tea, extract, or capsule. The active ingredient is in glandular hairs on its scaly, conelike fruits.	1 tsp/cup tea 2–3 times a day or 30–40 drops tincture
Passion flower	Causes mild hypnosis Reduces insomnia Reduces nervousness, restlessness, and agitation	Depresses the central nervous system (CNS) for mild sedative effect. Forms include tea, capsules, and extracts.	Infusion of 2–5 g (1 tsp) dried herb TID
Rosemary and other mints	Normalizes nerve impulses Acts as an antioxidant Relieves headache Acts as a sedative Helps improve memory and prevent dementia	Slows/inhibits action of acetylcholinesterase to acetylcholine, which stays in synapse longer. Antioxidant is carnosic acid that is concentrated in young growing leaves, peaks in the summer, lessens in older leaves, and is hardly present in old wood stems. Forms include whole essential oils for external use (see Aromatherapy section in text).	Tincture (1:5) 2–4 mL TID

(continues on page 340)

TABLE 17.2 Selected Herbs, Minerals, and Vitamins for Mental Health Use (continued)

Herbs, Minerals, and Vitamins	Uses	Actions and Precautions	Dose
St. John's wort	Treats mild to moderate depression, loss of interest, anorexia, fatigue, chronic fatigue immune dysfunction syndrome, and anxiety	Leaves or flowering tips can be used; hypericin is the active ingredient. May interfere with HIV drugs. Use may cause light sensitivity. Use with other drugs can be dangerous; do not take with other psychoactive medications (ie, selective serotonin reuptake inhibitors [SSRIs], tricyclics, and MAOIs). Has fewer side effects compared with antidepressants. May lower activity of nonsedating antihistamines, oral contraceptives, antiepileptics, calcium channel blockers, cyclosporins, macrolides, and some antifungals.	300–500 mg TID with meals for 4–6 wk 0.5 mg hypericin per capsule
SAM-e (S-adenosylmethionine)	Treats mild to moderate depression and arthritis, protects the liver, eases fibromyalgia	SAM-e is a naturally occurring compound that regulates action of serotonin and dopamine. Approved as prescription drug in Italy, Germany, Spain, and Russia. Takes effect in 10 days, faster than prescription drugs. Use enteric-coated tablets with 96% pure product. Do not use for bipolar disorder. Must take 800 µg folic acid and 1,000 µg vitamin B_{12} daily; the herb will not work if these vitamin levels are low.	200–800 or 1,600 mg BID 1 hr before breakfast and lunch For arthritis 400–800 mg a day For fibromyalgia, 800 mg a day
Valerian	Relieves anxiety and insomnia	Forms include a tea (2–3 g dried root several times a day) or capsules. Herb is nonaddictive. Do not take with tranquilizers, sedatives, or alcohol. Possible side effects include blurred vision, excitability, and changes in heartbeat if taken in large doses or for more than 2 weeks.	300–400 mg 1–2 times a day
5-Hydroxytryptophan (5-HTP)	Treats bipolar disorder in conjunction with lithium Reduces depression Relieves insomnia	This amino acid is a precursor of serotonin. Taken from *Griffonia simplicifolia* seed.	Bipolar disorder—200 mg, depression—150–300 mg, insomnia—200–600 mg

Preferred Music Listening Intervention to Lower Anxiety in Older Adults With Dementia

The level of anxiety in older adults with dementia is often misdiagnosed or undiagnosed. A study was conducted by Sung and colleagues (2010) using a preferred music intervention to lower anxiety levels in older adults with dementia in a nursing home. The experimental group consisted of 29 participants who received a 30-minute music listening intervention based on personal preferences delivered by trained nursing staff in midafternoon, twice a week for 6 weeks. The control group of 23 participants received the usual standard care, but with no music. Anxiety levels were measured by use of the Rating Anxiety in Dementia scale at baseline and again at 6 weeks.

The experimental group showed a significant decrease in anxiety at 6 weeks as compared with the control group. Implications from this study are that nurses can add the preferred music listening intervention to individualize the plan of care and contribute to the mental health of their clients with dementia.

Reference

Sung, H. C., Chang, A., & Lee, W. L. (2010), A preferred music listening intervention to reduce anxiety in older adults with dementia in nursing homes. *Journal of Clinical Nursing, 19*(7/8), 1056.

Light Therapy

Light therapy primarily serves as a treatment for seasonal affective disorder (SAD) (see Chaps. 18 and 27). This modality exposes clients during the fall and winter months (when natural light is in short supply) to artificial light approximately 200 times stronger than normal indoor lighting. Clients sit in front of a light box or lamp for several hours each week to improve mood and functioning. Another light therapy is *dawn simulation*. Clients time a special bedside light to gradually become brighter upon awakening. The light suppresses nocturnal melatonin secretion and normalizes melatonin levels, which affect mood balance (Holistic-Online.com, 2007a).

Meditation

Meditation for depression can take several forms (Cultural Spotlight 17.1). Two basic types are *concentrative meditation* and *mindfulness meditation.*

Concentrative meditation involves focusing on one point of attention such as a mantra or sound. Transcendental Meditation, associated with the principles of the Maharishi Mahesh Yogi, is a form of concentrative meditation in which clients repeat a sound or phrase. Another method is to use a phrase or question, called a *koan,* to occupy the mind (Essortment, 2010). Meditation can also involve focus on a single object, such as a candle flame.

Mindfulness meditation (vipassana or insight meditation) focuses more on breathing techniques to facilitate concentration and to develop a higher state of present awareness (Client-Centered Education 17.1). Mindfulness meditation originated in Buddhist philosophy, but it is not considered a religious practice. All types of clients use it, regardless of religious belief.

Herbal and Dietary Supplements

The top-selling herbal product for depression in the United States is St. John's wort (*Hypericum perforatum*). The FDA classifies St. John's wort as a dietary supplement. Because it classifies herbs as foods, there is no FDA approval for herbs as medicines (phytomedicinals). The Dietary Supplement Health and Education Act (DSHEA) of 1994 established "good manufacturing practices" to aid in identity, cleanliness, and quality control of herbal products. As with other phytomedicinals, St. John's wort is available in capsule, dried, and tincture forms, but with varying degrees of potency. It is not a proven treatment for depression, but it is thought to increase serotonin levels. Therefore, taking St. John's wort along with a prescription antidepressant may cause central serotonin syndrome (see Chap. 16) (Figure 17.1). In addition, St. John's wort interferes with the action of other medications such as indinavir (Crixivan) for HIV infection, anticancer drugs such as irinotecan (Camptosar), and antirejection medications such as cyclosporine (Sandimmune). The *Cochrane Database of Systematic Reviews* lists a review abstract of a study by Berner and Kriston (2008) that compared treatment with extracts of St. John's wort with placebo treatment or standard antidepressants. They reviewed studies that included over 5,000 clients with mild to moderately severe symptoms of depression from

Cultural *Spotlight* 17.1

Drumming and Chanting

Some Native Americans use drumming and chanting as forms of meditation. Drumming brings clients in balance with the "heartbeat of the Earth." Symbolically, the drum represents all life in some Native cultures. The wood was once a tree, and the skin covering the drum was once life. Chanting is a form of prayer through music. Clients use different chants to attract good, cure illness, or remove evil. The rhythm of drumming alters the level of consciousness, while the sounds made by chanting and singing provide noise to interfere with the evil spirits of disease (Spector, 2009).

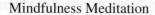

Client–Centered Education 17.1

Mindfulness Meditation

Centering is a term for relaxing and achieving mental, physical, and emotional quiet. It is accomplished by deep breathing, visualization, and focusing. Nurses may recommend the following centering exercise for clients with stress, anxiety, or depression.

1. Sit or lay comfortably on the floor or outside on the ground. Close your eyes.
2. Breathe in slowly and deeply from the abdomen. Feel your abdominal muscles slowly move upward and outward on inspiration, holding the breath for several seconds.
3. Breathe out, your abdomen falling with slow, measured expiration. Visualize breathing in peace, while breathing tension out.

4. Imagine a clearing in the woods. Feel the softness of the leaves on the trees overhead, and the warm, gentle breeze. Feel the sun shining down on you, the light filtering through the canopy of the trees. The warmth travels down through your body and out your legs. You are at peace. This is your special place.

Adapted from Fontaine, K. L., & Kaszubski, B. (2004). *Absolute beginner's guide to alternative medicine.* Indianapolis, IN: Que Publishing.

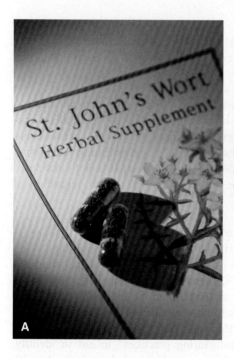
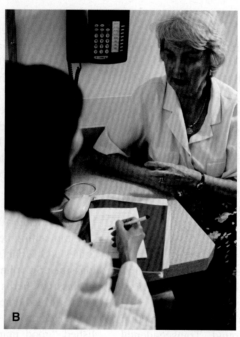

FIGURE 17.1 **(A)** Nurses and other health care providers must carefully assess and document use of St. John's wort. **(B)** The herb has many interactions and can result in life-threatening serotonin syndrome if used concomitantly with antidepressants and other substances.

a variety of countries. The results indicated that St. John's wort was superior to placebo for clients with major depression and was similarly as effective as standard antidepressants. They also found that St. John's wort had fewer side effects than standard antidepressants.

Another herbal preparation touted for depression that has gained popularity in the United States is the dietary supplement S-adenosylmethionine, known as SAM-e. SAM-e is found naturally in every human cell. The National Institute of Mental Health funded a 6-week, single-site trial in which 73 clients received either SAM-e or a placebo added to their prior stable medication (most commonly escitalopram, duloxetine, or fluoxetine). Results showed that there were significantly better responses with SAM-e than with placebo. No instances of serotonin syndrome were observed

with the SAM-e and serotonin reuptake inhibitor combination (Papakostas et al., 2010).

Yet another dietary supplement for depression is the fatty acid omega-3. Research has demonstrated that consumption of omega-3 polyunsaturated fatty acids (found in fish, fish oil, and flaxseed oil) can lower rates of depression by its effect on the brain's endocannabinoid system (Fundazoia, 2011).

Other Modalities for Depression

Spirituality/prayer, yoga, tai chi chuan, art therapy, dance therapy, music therapy, pet therapy, and humor therapy are used for depression (see Table 17.1). In addition, transcranial magnetic stimulation (TMS) has also shown success in alleviating symptoms, especially with refractory depression.

In a sham-controlled randomized trial by George and colleagues (2010), antidepressant drug-free clients with unipolar nonpsychotic major depressive disorder were treated with daily left prefrontal TMS. (See Chap. 18.) The group receiving daily TMS experienced a significant improvement in depression symptoms over the control group.

Schizophrenia and Other Thought Disorders

Clients with schizophrenia and other thought disorders generally do not use many CAM therapies, which may be a direct result of their fluctuating patterns of disordered thinking and ability to maintain routines and consistently manage their own health (see Chap. 29). Many modalities simply are too challenging to implement because of client symptoms. For example, energy therapies involving touch or application of devices would not be appropriate for clients with paranoia, who may misinterpret the activities of practitioners as attempts at harm.

Traditional Chinese herbal medicines have been used for thousands of years to treat people with mental illness. In a Cochrane systematic review of randomized controlled trials, Rathbone and colleagues (2007) found that combining Chinese herbs with traditional antipsychotics improves depression. Another CAM treatment thought to be beneficial for people with schizophrenia is music therapy. A benchmark Cochrane review by Gold and associates (2005) showed that music therapy was effective for clients with thought disorders when used in conjunction with antipsychotic drugs. Results showed improved global state of functioning and enhanced communication and expression.

Addictive Disorders

Validating studies of CAM in relationship to addictions is challenging because of the variations in the frequency and quantity of individual drug use, as well as polydrug abuse. Many smoking cessation programs employ hypnosis as a mind–body therapy (Figure 17.2). A major difficulty in assessing research findings for results is that hypnotic procedures are not standardized.

Mind–body interventions such as biofeedback, prayer, and meditation (particularly Transcendental Meditation) may be helpful for alcohol or drug abuse. *Eye movement desensitization and reprocessing* (EMDR) has been used with some success in clients with dual diagnoses. In this method, rapid lateral eye movements are combined with guided imagery recall of a traumatic event to decrease negative thoughts and emotions. Products such as botanicals and special diets with amino acids and vitamins are also used. Some clients view spirituality as an alternative approach; it is an inherent component of many 12-step programs, including Alcoholics Anonymous (see Chap. 30). Research has shown that spirituality may be underestimated in its positive effects toward assisting with long-term sobriety (Galanter et al., 2007).

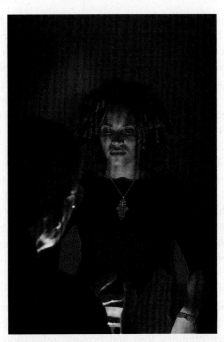

FIGURE 17.2 Some clients elect to use hypnotherapy as a way to conquer addictive problems, such as smoking, gambling, and overeating.

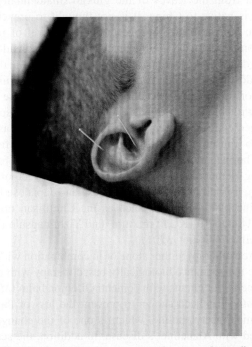

FIGURE 17.3 Auricular acupuncture is a growing adjunct treatment for chemical dependency. Practitioners place small needles under the skin of the outer ear to deliver an electrical impulse to the brain. Resulting relaxation may foster adherence to other substance abuse treatments and manage stress so that clients do not feel the need to engage in drinking or use of drugs.

Auricular acupuncture is a specialized modality touted as an adjunct treatment in traditional chemical dependency treatment programs (Figure 17.3). In this technique, practitioners place eight small needles under the skin of the client's outer ear for 45 minutes. (The outer ear has more than 200 acupuncture points, with each point corresponding to certain areas of the body.) When stimulated, each acupoint delivers an electrical impulse to the brain, and then to the specific area of the body being treated. Clients report feeling more relaxed and better able to focus on treatment after the procedure, resulting in lower program attrition rates and decreased rates of relapse (National Acupuncture Detoxification Association, 2010).

The U.S. Department of Health and Human Services has identified obesity as a priority area for action. The NCCAM is supporting studies on popular diets such as Atkins, the Zone, and Ornish. Other studies focus on maintaining weight loss primarily through yoga, but also with meditation, acupuncture, massage, and Eastern martial arts (Sharpe et al., 2007).

Cognitive Disorders

Most types of dementia have common symptoms such as memory loss and anxiety. The aim of CAM therapies is to improve memory loss and provide relaxation. *Ginkgo biloba* has been found to be the most useful herbal therapy in treating memory loss (see Chap. 31). Ginkgo extract is derived from the leaves of the ginkgo (maidenhair) tree, which is native to China. It is not thought to prevent dementia, but rather to improve the current level of mental functioning. Nurses should teach clients to consult with health care professionals or herbalists regarding the correct dose; dosing is not standardized, and there are significant variations in quality. In addition, ginkgo may cause problems with blood clotting if clients are taking anticoagulant medications such as warfarin (Coumadin) or aspirin. Ginkgo causes antagonism of platelet-activating factors. Other herbal preparations that have been studied for improving dementia include Silymarin (an extract of milk thistle), as well as traditional Chinese and Japanese herbal medicine plant mixtures, such as the Choto-san mixture, Kami-Umtan-To (KUT) mixture, and Yizhi capsule (YZC) (Alzheimer's Society, 2011).

Aromatherapy, either alone or in combination with therapeutic massage, is a biologically based therapy with potential benefits for clients with dementia. Lemon balm (*Melissa officinalis*) has been shown to prevent the loss of the neurochemical acetylcholine, which is one of the changes associated with Alzheimer's disease. In addition, the scent of lavender oil has been linked to reduced agitated behavior. The combination of aromatherapy and massage may reduce excessive wandering (Alzheimer's Society, 2011).

> **Think About It 17.1**
> The daughter of an older adult client with Alzheimer's disease comes to the clinic with her father. During the interview, the daughter states, "I've been reading about *ginkgo biloba*. Maybe we should try this with Dad?" Describe the necessary topics that need to be addressed when responding to the client's daughter.

INTEGRATIVE CARE: INCORPORATING CAM INTO EVIDENCE-BASED NURSING PRACTICE

Holism focuses on treating the person, rather than the illness. Holistic nursing involves integrating principles of the mind, body, and spirit into clinical practice. The current U.S. health care system, based on a Western disease-based model, approaches illness management with the use of medications and surgery, rather than the body's natural healing abilities. Integrative approaches are rooted in a "whole system" philosophy that clients are more than their physical bodies. It is incumbent upon the nurse to be aware of cultural differences in clients when planning care. A European American asking to take shark cartilage for cancer treatment is seeking an alternative therapy. A Chinese American asking to use acupuncture for chronic pain may be using a traditional treatment (Spector, 2009).

Individual state nursing laws outline the scope of practice for registered nurses. Psychiatric nurses need to know and understand the parameters of their state nurse practice acts before practicing CAM treatments. Nurses should seek credentialing in specific treatments through professional specialty organizations. In addition, nurses who work for CAM therapists should be aware of appropriate levels and principles of delegation (Cherry & Jacobs, 2008). These measures help ensure that nurses are practicing within legal guidelines and also offer protection against professional liability.

> **Checkpoint Questions**
> **4.** How do thoughts and feelings influence health?
> **5.** How is healing related to the mind?

Importance of Assessment

For all clients, nurses must carefully assess for use of CAM and integrative therapies. For example, many herbs may interact negatively with other compounds. A thorough nursing assessment is essential before clients use any herbal supplements. Most importantly, this includes asking clients about all medications they take, including over-the-counter drugs, herbal preparations, and nutritional supplements. Direct questions about caffeine and alcohol intake, as well as use of any street drugs, are also important (Case Vignette 17.1).

Ethical, Legal, and Research-Oriented Obligations

Ethically, nurses have an obligation to explain the philosophical foundations underlying various CAM therapies. This is necessary for clients to be fully informed about the treatment. The philosophical underpinnings of the treatment should be compatible with the client's own spiritual beliefs. The American Holistic Nurses' Association provides standards of care as guidelines for practice (http://www.ahna.org).

Case Vignette 17.1

Emmett, 31 years old, presents at the clinic stating that he has been depressed "off and on" for 2 years. He sleeps 5 to 6 hours per night and has a low energy level. In addition, he has progressively isolated himself from others, not attending church or weekly bowling matches that he used to enjoy. He has recently started a new job and is anxious about the travel that it requires of him.

The psychiatric nurse practitioner performs a complete physical examination, with no unusual findings. During the health history, Emmett states that he is not currently taking any medications. The nurse practitioner completes a mental status examination, in which Emmett denies suicidal ideation. The nurse practitioner prescribes venlafaxine (Effexor XR) 75 mg/day and refers Emmett to a counselor.

Three weeks later, Emmett once again presents at the clinic with a temperature of 101°F, blood pressure of 180/100 mm Hg, and pulse of 115 bpm. His lungs are clear, but he has nasal congestion. This time the nurse practitioner asks Emmett if he is using any dietary supplements or any type of street drugs. Emmett denies use of street drugs; he states that the only unusual thing he has been taking is St. John's wort capsules three times a day. He has been using this preparation for several months in hopes that he would "feel better." This past week, he also has been taking over-the-counter cold medications for his nasal congestion.

The nurse practitioner correctly diagnoses Emmett with central serotonin syndrome and explains that St. John's wort interacts adversely with cold medications and also with venlafaxine. Emmett verbalizes his understanding of the medication side effects and agrees to stop taking St. John's wort while taking the venlafaxine.

Reflection and Critical Thinking
- What measures are necessary to ensure that practitioners find out pertinent information from clients to protect and optimize their health?
- Describe the relevance of a client's cultural beliefs on the use of CAM therapies.
- How do current trends and attitudes in U.S. health care impose barriers to holistic treatment, comprehensive assessment, and safe care for clients? Do CAM approaches negate or compound these problems? Explain your rationale.

▲

The growth and demand for CAM therapies in the current health care system are undeniable. Nurses must be knowledgeable about basic CAM treatments and resources to assist clients in selecting the most effective care. They should incorporate client education about CAM into the planning of nursing care. Nurses serve as the client's advocate in supporting decisions to use complementary and alternative treatments. Nurses may also want to pursue further instruction and education about holistic and CAM practices. Opportunities for doing so are growing, especially online offerings.

As always, nurses should respect clients' beliefs and wishes in terms of their pursuing any therapies. In addition, nurses are obligated to provide empirical and high-quality information on both CAM and conventional therapies. Some sources and agencies that nurses can use for their own and clients' education include the following:

- The *Agency for Healthcare Research and Quality (AHRQ),* a component of the U.S. Public Health Service, was established in 1989 to enhance the quality, appropriateness, and effectiveness of health services. Formerly called the Agency for Health Care Policy and Research, it has published many clinical practice guidelines in separate versions for clinicians and consumers.
- The *American Medical Association's (AMA's) Council on Scientific Affairs* studies many medical issues and reports to the AMA's House of Delegates. Once accepted, these reports help shape AMA public policies and may be published in the *Journal of the American Medical Association.*
- The *Cochrane Database of Systematic Reviews* is an electronic journal produced by the *Cochrane Collaboration,* an international network of individuals and institutions, established in 1993, that hopes to cover the entire spectrum of medical interventions.
- The *National Academy of Sciences* issues the Dietary Reference Intakes and many other reports by expert committees.
- The *National Guidelines Clearinghouse (NGC)* is an Internet-based public resource sponsored by the AHRQ, in partnership with the AMA and the American Association of Health Plans. The NGC Web site summarizes more than 1,000 clinical practice guidelines that have met its criteria.
- The *National Institutes of Health Consensus Development Program,* begun in 1977, has held about 100 consensus conferences in which experts meet for several days to discuss a topic and issue a report.
- The *U.S. Preventive Services Task Force* publishes recommendations for preventive services that prudent health professionals should offer their clients in the course of routine clinical care. These recommendations represent the pooled judgment of many experts.

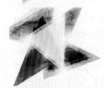

Reviewing and Applying Your Knowledge

Chapter Summary

• CAM refers to practices not considered "conventional" in Western medical practice. They are used instead of (alternative) or in addition to (complementary) mainstream modalities. This chapter suggests that these practices may be integrated into the client's current care plan.

• The National Center for Complementary and Alternative Medicine (NCCAM) supports research and dissemination of information on CAM therapies.

• The three categories of CAM are (1) mind–body medicine, (2) natural products, (3) and manipulative and body-based practices. Whole systems of practice include traditional Chinese medicine, Ayurveda, homeopathy, and naturopathy.

• CAM research focusing on psychiatric and mental health is limited. New research studies on St. John's wort for depression and *ginkgo biloba* for dementia are completed or in progress. Additional funding for research using herbals and other indigenous therapies to treat schizophrenia and bipolar disorder has been approved.

• The cost of conventional medicine and the stigma associated with seeking psychiatric–mental health treatment are likely factors in turning clients toward CAM therapies.

• CAM therapies used with anxious clients focus on reducing stress levels through use of herbal medications such valerian root and chamomile, music therapy, and aromatherapy with lavender or vanilla essential oils.

• Clients with depression have been shown to benefit from light therapy (SAD), concentrative or mindfulness meditation, and herbal products, particularly St. John's wort and SAM-e.

• Clients with schizophrenia or other psychotic disorders do not generally use CAM therapies.

• EMDR and auricular acupuncture have been used as adjunct treatments in traditional chemical dependency treatment programs.

• CAM therapies in clients with dementia focus on improving memory loss and providing relaxation through the use of herbal therapy with ginkgo extract, aromatherapy, and therapeutic massage.

• Holistic nursing embraces an integrative approach through the "whole system" belief that clients are more than their physical bodies.

• The psychiatric nurse practicing CAM therapies should follow legal and ethical guidelines, including consulting state nursing laws for scope of practice, obtaining certification through specialty organizations, and fully informing clients of the philosophical underpinnings of treatments.

• Nurses have the opportunity to obtain data from clients, relate information to them, and facilitate the blending of CAM and traditional healing modalities.

Study Questions

1. Alternative therapies differ from complementary therapies in that they are used

   a. instead of Western (allopathic) therapies.

   b. only for refractory disorders.

   c. in addition to Western (allopathic) therapies.

   d. only for psychiatric disorders.

2. The National Center for Complementary and Alternative Medicine (NCCAM) studies practices of whole medical systems. Which of the following are whole medical systems? Select all that apply.

   a. Homeopathic medicine

   b. Feng shui

   c. Naturopathic medicine

   d. Ayurveda

   e. Biomagnetic medicine

   f. Traditional Chinese medicine

3. Client teaching regarding the use of the herb kava should include that it may be toxic to the

   a. brain.   c. liver.

   b. kidneys.   d. eyes.

4. The top-selling herbal product for depression in the United States is

   a. St. John's wort.   c. chamomile.

   b. calendula.   d. echinacea.

5. The nurse should teach the client taking *ginkgo biloba* that certain medications may cause which type of problem?

   a. Urinary retention

   b. Bone marrow suppression

   c. Loss of visual acuity

   d. Blood clotting

Critical Thinking Questions

1. What is the most effective way to obtain information about CAM practices from the psychiatric client?

2. How can nurses best evaluate a client's feelings and concerns about both conventional and CAM practices?

3. How could you incorporate a client's routine CAM practices (eg, meditation twice a day) into care given in a hospital, the client's home, or a group home?

References

Alzheimer's Society (2011). *Complementary and alternative medicine and dementia*. Retrieved from http://www.alzheimers.org.uk/site/scripts/documents_info.php?documentID=134

Berner, L. K., & Kriston, L. (2008). St. John's wort for major depression. *Cochrane Database of Systematic Reviews, 2008*(4). doi:10.1002/14651858.CD000448.pub3

Cherry, B., & Jacobs, S. R. (2008). *Contemporary nursing: Issues, trends, & management* (4th ed.). St. Louis, MO: Elsevier.

Essortment (2010). *Understanding the meaning of Zen koans*. Retrieved from http://www.essortment.com/understanding-meaning-zen-koans-42451.html

Fontaine, K. L., & Kaszubski, B. (2004). *Absolute beginner's guide to alternative medicine*. Indianapolis, IN: Que Publishing.

Fundazoia, E. (2011, February 4). Scientific research reveals brain alterations linking omega 3 deficit with depression. *e! Science News*. Retrieved from http://esciencenews.com/articles/2011/02/04/scientific.research.reveals.brain.alterations.linking.omega.3.deficit.with.depression

Galanter, M., Dermatis, H., Bunt, G., Williams, C., Trujillo, M., & Steinke, P. (2007). Assessment of spirituality and its relevance to addiction treatment. *Journal of Substance Abuse Treatment, 33*(3), 257–264.

George, M. S., Lisanby, S. H., Avery, D., McDonald, W. M., Durkalski, V., Pavlicova, M., ... Sackeim, H. A. (2010). Daily left prefrontal transcranial magnetic stimulation therapy for major depressive disorder. *Archives of General Psychiatry, 67*(5), 507. Retrieved from http://archpsyc.ama-assn.org/cgi/content/abstract/67/5/507

Gold, C., Heldal, T. O., Dahle, T., & Wigram, T. (2005, April). Music therapy for schizophrenia or schizophrenia-like illnesses. *Cochrane Database of Systematic Reviews, 2005*(2). CD004025.

Holistic-Online.com. (2007a). *Light therapy for seasonal affective disorders*. Retrieved from http://www.holisticonline.com/Light_Therapy/hol_LightTherapy.htm

Holistic-Online.com. (2007b). *What is aromatherapy?* Retrieved from http://www.holistic-online.com/Aromatherapy/aroma_what_is_htm

National Acupuncture Detoxification Association. (2010). *Welcome to NADA*. Retrieved from http://www.acudetox.com

National Center for Complementary and Alternative Medicine (NCCAM). (2010). *What is CAM?* Retrieved from http://nccam.nih.gov

Papakostas, G. I., Mischoulon, D., Shyu, I., Alpert, J. E., & Fava M. (2010). *S*-adenosyl methionine (SAM-e) augmentation of serotonin reuptake inhibitors for antidepressant nonresponders with major depressive disorder: A double-blind, randomized clinical trial. *American Journal of Psychiatry, 167*, 942–948.

Rathbone, J., Zhang, L., Zhang, M., Xia, J., Liu, X., Yang, Y., & Adams, C. (2007). Chinese herbal medicine for schizophrenia. *British Journal of Psychiatry, 190*, 379–384.

Sharpe, P. A., Blanck, H. M., Williams, J. E., Ainsworth, B. E., & Conway, J. M. (2007). Use of complementary and alternative medicine for weight control in the United States. *Journal of Alternative and Complementary Medicine, 13*(2), 217–222

Spector, R. E. (2009). *Cultural diversity in health and illness* (7th ed.). Upper Saddle River, NJ: Pearson Prentice Hall.

Sung, H. C., Chang, A., & Lee, W. L. (2010), A preferred music listening intervention to reduce anxiety in older adults with dementia in nursing homes. *Journal of Clinical Nursing, 19*(7/8), 1056.

U.S. Food and Drug Administration (FDA). (2011). *Kava* (Piper methysticum). Retrieved from http://www.fda.gov/Safety/MedWatch/SafetyInformation/SafetyAlertsforHumanMedicalProducts/ucm154577.htm

Web Resources

American Holistic Nurses' Association (AHNA): http://www.ahna.org

CAM on PubMed: http://www.nlm.nih.gov/nccam/camonpubmed.html

National Institutes of Health, National Center for Complementary and Alternative Medicine (NCCAM): http://nccam.nih.gov

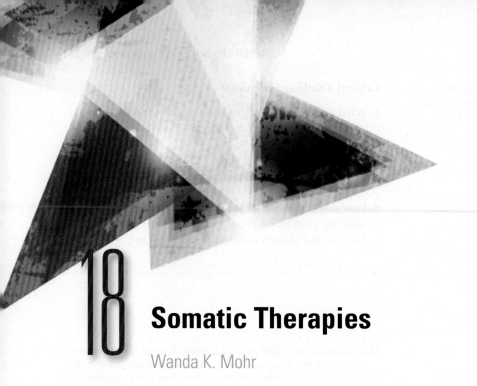

18

Somatic Therapies

Wanda K. Mohr

KEY TERMS

deep brain stimulation (DBS)
electroconvulsive therapy (ECT)
magnetic seizure therapy (MST)
phototherapy
psychosurgery
somatic therapies
transcranial direct current
   stimulation (tDCS)
transcranial magnetic
   stimulation (TMS)
vagus nerve stimulation (VNS)

LEARNING OBJECTIVES

On completion of this chapter, you should be able to accomplish the following:

- Explain what is meant by somatic therapies and the types of modalities this classification includes.
- Describe the procedure for electroconvulsive therapy (ECT), its indications, and its potential side effects.
- Identify the nurse's role in caring for people undergoing ECT and their families.
- Discuss phototherapy for seasonal affective disorder, including teaching points for clients using this modality.
- Explain the current status and general approaches of transcranial magnetic stimulation, vagus nerve stimulation, and deep brain stimulation.
- Describe promising, but unapproved, treatments such as transcranial direct current stimulation (tDCS) and magnetic seizure therapy (MST).
- Describe indications for psychosurgery and why its use is so rare.

Unit IV discusses several treatment modalities that assist people with varying psychiatric disorders. In addition to psychotherapies, which rely on clients working with professionals to change dysfunctional thinking and behaviors, **somatic** (biologic) **therapies** represent another arsenal of available psychiatric tools. Also sometimes referred to as *neuromodulation* and *brain-stimulation techniques*, somatic therapies include psychopharmacotherapeutics (medications) and nonpharmacologic, body-based modalities.

To some extent, differentiating psychotherapies from somatic or biologic therapies is incorrect. All therapies in mental health involve biology, in that all human experiences result in physical changes, even if only at the molecular level. As mentioned in Chapter 2, cognitive–behavioral therapy has been shown to result in brain changes, related to the remarkable capacity of *neuroplasticity*. Nevertheless, most texts categorize psychotherapies and somatic therapies in different sections for simplicity and to make content more approachable and containable.

Chapter 16 describes psychopharmacology, one type of somatic therapy, in extensive detail. In addition, because of the importance and prevalence of medications as first-line treatment for most psychiatric disorders, specific medications and related issues are covered throughout many portions of this book. The content in this chapter describes nonpharmacologic somatic therapies, their purposes, and their current standing in terms of efficacy and approval.

ELECTROCONVULSIVE THERAPY

Electroconvulsive therapy (ECT) involves the administration of anesthesia, the application of electricity, and the induction of a seizure. ECT is performed under anesthesia in order to avoid the motor convulsion that would otherwise occur in the absence of a muscle relaxant, and in order to ensure adequate oxygenation throughout the procedure (Rowny & Lisanby, 2008).

Inducing seizures as a means of therapy for mental illnesses dates to the early 1700s, when camphor was used for this purpose. Modern ECT was introduced to psychiatric practice in the 1930s in Italy. By 1940, ECT had made its way to psychiatry in the United States.

From the 1940s to the early 1960s, people with various psychiatric disorders were subjected to seizure therapies by way of insulin-induced hypoglycemia and ECT. With the advent of modern psychotropic medications, ECT fell into disfavor and its use started to wane. The therapy began to be viewed as barbaric. Reports of fractures and amnestic effects from ECT were grossly exaggerated, although its use was unregulated and sometimes inappropriate, as documented in Ken Kesey's classic *One Flew Over the Cuckoo's Nest*. In the 1960s, several state hospital systems banned ECT (Dukakis & Tye, 2006).

Over time, ECT overcame its tarnished image and has been reintroduced as an important treatment in the therapeutic tool kit. Approximately 100,000 U.S. citizens receive ECT annually (Abrams, 2002). It is the most effective treatment available for refractory major depression (i.e, depression that recurs and does not respond to other modalities). Some psychiatric researchers consider ECT the standard against which other somatic therapies, including medications, should be compared (Abrams, 2002).

Pretreatment Evaluation

Assessment of clients for whom ECT is a consideration should happen as close to the first treatment with ECT as possible. From a medical standpoint, clients should undergo a complete health history and physical examination. Laboratory and diagnostic tests should include a blood count, evaluation of electrolyte levels, complete metabolic panel, electrocardiography (ECG), and chest x-ray. Clients should be evaluated as to their ability to tolerate anesthesia. From a psychiatric standpoint, a baseline of symptoms should be recorded against which clinicians can monitor progress and symptom alleviation (American Psychiatric Association [APA], 2001). Clients are generally asked to fast after midnight the day of the procedure.

Procedure

Prior to the procedure, clients undergo brief general anesthesia with succinylcholine to prevent severe muscle contractions that might result in muscle or bone injuries. Some clients receive anticholinergic medications to lessen secretions that might interfere with respiration. Ultra-brief anesthetic agents are used to induce unconsciousness. ECT itself involves placing an electrode on the temple and inducing a grand mal seizure (Figure 18.1). Bilateral (both

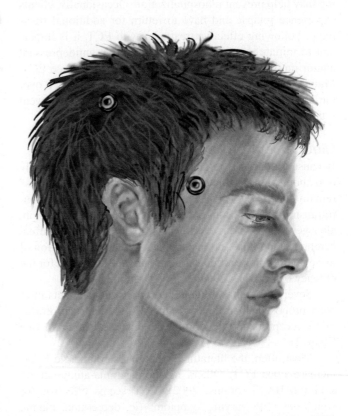

FIGURE 18.1 **Placement of unilateral electrodes during ECT.**

temples) placement of electrodes has happened in the past and sometimes is used now; however, such placement leads to an increase in cognitive adverse effects, such as memory loss. An electric current is passed through the electrode for 0.10 to 1.0 second. Clients experience a convulsion that lasts approximately 1 minute. During this entire time, clients receive oxygen, and clinicians monitor oxygen saturation and cardiac functioning (Folk et al., 2000). Typically, ECT is given twice weekly on nonconsecutive days; treatments may range from a few to 15 sessions, depending on a client's response. The entire procedure lasts less than 1 hour, although each client's recovery time varies.

Indications

Generally, ECT is used in clients for whom all other therapeutic interventions have failed and whose lives are at risk. Approximately 85% of clients receiving ECT have major depression as the indication for use, with the remainder having schizoaffective disorders, mania, schizophrenia, and occasionally Parkinson's disease (Abrams, 2002). ECT will typically relieve the most profound symptoms of depression within 2 to 3 weeks, with treatments usually given 2 to 3 times per week during the acute course of the treatment (Rowny & Lisanby, 2008). When repeated episodes of depression or other serious life-threatening symptoms occur after a series of treatments with ECT, the physician may opt to taper ECT over several weeks to months. Typically, a tapering schedule is once a week for 1 month, once every 2 weeks for 2 months, once every 3 weeks for 2 months, and once every month for 2 to 4 months. This kind of tapering may help prevent rehospitalization. Occasionally, clients experience relapse and have to return for additional treatment. Following effective treatment with ECT, it is important to initiate maintenance therapy with an antidepressant and/or mood stabilizer or in some cases maintenance ECT. Maintenance ECT refers to the continued use of ECT over the months following a successful ECT course to prevent relapse (Rowny & Lisanby, 2008).

Mechanism of Action

Because the brain is relatively inaccessible for direct study of pathophysiology, the mechanisms by which ECT "works" remain speculative. It is known that seizures release neurotransmitters, alter neurotransmitter receptor expression, alter gene expression, exert neurotrophic effects, and affect cerebral blood flow and metabolism. Which constellation of these neurobiologic effects is necessary and sufficient for the efficacy of ECT is still under investigation.

Several hypotheses about neurotransmitter effects have been proposed. One theory is that ECT alters neurotransmitter receptors and thereby the chemistry of the brain (see Chap. 2).

Most often, the literature posits that serotonergic levels increase after ECT. Others mention gamma-aminobutyric acid (GABA) (Abrams, 2002). ECT seems effective for conditions with varying symptoms (ie, depression, mania,

schizophrenia), and much remains unknown; more research is needed. Recent work in this area is exploring ECT's effect on neuropeptides and growth factors. Other research includes investigating the effects of the large increases in cerebral blood flow that happen during a grand mal seizure. Other scientists are exploring the possible structural changes associated with neuronal plasticity and promotion of neurogenesis (Erraji-Benchekroun et al., 2007). All of these studies are at the level of basic science with human and animal brains.

Side Effects

Following ECT, clients may have a headache, muscle aches, or nausea. Approximately 50% of clients report throbbing headaches. These side effects can be treated with medications before or after ECT. In addition, some people may exhibit postictal confusion, which typically lasts for 30 to 60 minutes (Abrams, 2002).

Memory loss is one of the important and legitimate concerns that people have about ECT. The first type is a short-term memory loss limited to the period involving the course of treatment. An example of this kind of memory loss might be the client forgetting what he or she had for a meal. This situation generally corrects itself, with the client returning to pretreatment levels of functioning within a few weeks to several months. The second type of memory loss is of past events, with recent past events being more sensitive to ECT. This retrograde amnesia may persevere for several months after treatment. In some instances, it may be permanent. This memory loss is more common with bilateral electrode placement.

ECT is generally considered a low-risk procedure and is one of the safest procedures performed under anesthesia. Nevertheless, any medical condition involving anesthesia carries some danger. Potential risks include cardiac dysrhythmias and respiratory arrest. Deaths resulting from respiratory or cardiac arrest following ECT are fewer than 1 in 10,000 cases (Folk et al., 2000).

Nursing Role and Care

In addition to carefully assessing clients about to undergo ECT, nurses can tell them and their families what to expect immediately before and after the procedure. They should reassure clients and families that the procedure is safe and that most side effects are transitory.

Immediately after the procedure, nurses should closely observe the client's cardiovascular status and airway patency. Likewise, they should closely watch for postictal confusion and record the duration and severity of any disorientation. Nurses should provide gentle but firm direction to clients, so that they remain in bed during disorientation. Because clients have been fasting and may have received anticholinergic medications during anesthesia, nurses can provide for their comfort by giving small sips of water, ice chips, or juice.

Nurses also have a supportive and educative role relative to ECT. Much information on the Internet is helpful, but some sites supply untrue and dangerous material. Web sites that seem to make a specialty of fear-mongering abound, and clients and families may be exposed to such content. Some discussions are difficult to distinguish from legitimate research or best-practice information. Nurses can help families and clients to "sift the wheat from the chaff." In general, the National Institutes of Mental Health and APA provide the most up-to-date research and information on ECT and other somatic therapies. They also have hyperlinks to other well-regarded sites that have undergone scientific scrutiny.

Checkpoint Questions

1. ECT is the most effective treatment for which condition?
2. What drug is used to provide brief general anesthesia prior to ECT?
3. How often is ECT usually given?
4. Which type of memory loss is more common with bilateral electrode placement?

MAGNETIC SEIZURE THERAPY

A new convulsive technique, **magnetic seizure therapy (MST)**, is under development. MST uses alternating magnetic fields to cross the scalp and the calvarium and induce a more localized electric current in targeted regions of the cerebral cortex than is possible with ECT. The aim is to produce a seizure whose focus and patterns of spread can be controlled. Like ECT, MST is performed under general anesthesia and using muscle relaxants. The seizure is induced using a modified transcranial stimulation device that can administer higher output than conventional transcranial stimulation devices (Lisanby et al., 2003). Research is needed to establish its efficacy and safety. MST is not U.S. Food and Drug Administration (FDA) approved as of this writing.

PHOTOTHERAPY

Phototherapy (light therapy) was introduced during the 1980s as a treatment for seasonal affective disorder (SAD), a mood disorder with a seasonal pattern (see Chap. 27). Typically, symptoms of SAD begin in the fall or early winter and resolve in the spring. Clients with SAD experience the symptoms of general depression during this time, such as sleep disturbance, sadness, loss of energy, and irritability. They may also develop cravings for sugar and starch, resulting in significant weight gain. Women seem to be more susceptible, and there seems to be a familial tendency for the disorder (Avery et al., 2001).

Although competing theories of the etiology of SAD exist, it is generally accepted that SAD develops in predisposed people as a result of insufficient exposure to sunlight. Thus, the most common treatment for SAD is phototherapy. In this procedure, the person exposes his or her eyes to bright

artificial light for approximately 2 hours per day. See Understanding Biologic Foundations 18.1.

Several phototherapy devices are on the market, but the fluorescent light box with a filter to screen out ultraviolet rays is the gold standard. Recommended treatment is exposure in the morning to mimic the natural circadian rhythm. Relief of symptoms generally occurs within 4 days of beginning the treatment, with 50% of clients experiencing relief of symptoms after 1 week (Avery et al., 2001). Treatment continues throughout the winter months because symptoms are likely to return if light exposure stops.

In addition to being an effective treatment for SAD, light therapy can be a useful and safe alternative or adjunct to treatment of other types of depression during pregnancy, when concerns about medications can prompt women to seek psychiatric consultation about safety to the fetus (Epperson et al., 2004). Moreover, for clients suffering from nonseasonal depression, bright light therapy offers modest though promising antidepressive efficacy, especially when administered during the first week of treatment (Tuunainen et al., 2004).

Recent research has suggested that light has a modest benefit in improving some cognitive and noncognitive symptoms of dementia (Riemersma-van der Lek et al., 2008). However, the results of a rigorous meta-analysis in the Cochrane databases indicated that more research on this population is needed. Scholars conducting the review opined that there was insufficient evidence to assess the value of light therapy for people with dementia and that most available studies examined were not of high methodological quality (Forbes et al., 2009).

Phototherapy tends to be well tolerated. Some people complain of headaches, eyestrain, nausea, sweating, visual disturbances, and sedation. Ophthalmic damage was reported from the use of earlier, less sophisticated boxes, but newer boxes screen out harmful rays that may damage the eyes. Clients should be instructed to consult an ophthalmologist prior to commencing treatment and not to look directly into the light. As with any other treatment for depression, there is a rare chance that a person may develop mania or hypomania (Avery et al., 2001). Clients should be made aware of this possibility. See Client-Centered Education 18.1.

Think About It 18.1

A woman with SAD is to receive phototherapy as treatment. She says, "What good would light do? Can't I just take a pill?" How should the nurse respond?

TRANSCRANIAL MAGNETIC STIMULATION

Transcranial magnetic stimulation (TMS) is a technique in which rapidly changing magnetic fields induce electrical current to the superficial cerebral cortex of the brain (George & Belmaker, 2006). The magnetic pulses are roughly the

UNDERSTANDING BIOLOGIC FOUNDATIONS 18.1

Light Therapy for Seasonal Affective Disorder

Levels of melatonin and serotonin depend on the exposure of the pineal gland to sunlight. The decreased amount of such exposure that occurs in the fall and winter months is thought to be the cause of seasonal affective disorder (SAD). Clients with SAD have symptoms similar to those of depression (see Chap. 27). Symptoms tend to disappear once the days become longer in the springtime.

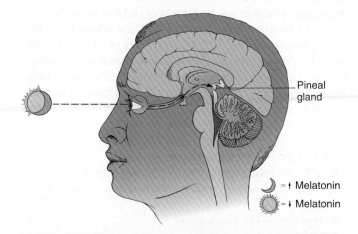

Pineal gland

= ↑ Melatonin

= ↓ Melatonin

To treat symptoms of SAD, health care providers may recommend that clients expose themselves to light therapy devices. The photograph shows a light box that emits powerful light that mimics the amount and intensity emitted by the sun. A common prescription is to sit by the box from 30 to 120 minutes per day, preferably in the morning. (Courtesy of Light Therapy Products.)

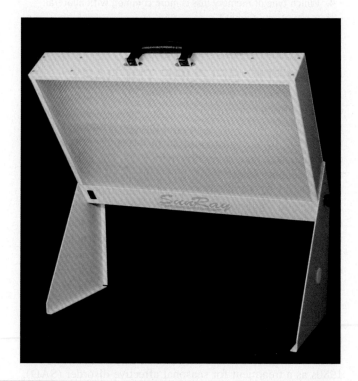

Client–Centered Education 18.1

Seasonal Affective Disorder

The nurse must teach the client who experiences SAD and his or her family the following:

- Avoid the use of eyeglasses or contact lenses that are coated to shield ultraviolet radiation because the coating interferes with light transmission to the pineal gland.
- Add more lamps and bright fixtures at home and work.
- Install skylights.

- Trim shrubs and trees from around windows.
- Use translucent curtains or shades rather than heavy drapes.
- Sleep and work in an east-facing room.
- Take brief walks outside around noon without sunglasses.
- Jog after sunup and before sundown.
- Take up an outdoor winter sport.

strength of the magnetic scanner used in magnetic resonance imaging (MRI), but are considerably more focused. They pass easily through the skull, just as the MRI scanner fields do. However, because they are short pulses and not a static field, they can stimulate the underlying cerebral cortex (brain).

TMS was developed in the 1980s, but it has only piqued researchers' interest in the last decade or so. It is currently being investigated as a potential treatment for major depression, schizophrenia marked by auditory hallucinations, acute and chronic pain, and various other psychiatric and neurologic disorders (George et al., 2007). TMS is considered the safest and least invasive of the new stimulating techniques now under research. Its advantage is that it has no side effects (Figure 18.2).

The mechanism of action of TMS involves the use of magnetic fields to indirectly induce focal electrical currents in the brain, which in turn trigger the firing of functional neuronal circuits. This leads to observable behavioral effects.

As of this writing, numerous people have participated in studies involving TMS (O'Reardon et al., 2007). TMS appears to achieve clinical improvement in clients with depression, but the body of evidence is by no means conclusive and the results are modest compared with those achieved with ECT (Rowny & Lisanby, 2008). As technology has advanced and stronger stimulation has been employed, the results seem to have improved.

Relative to people who have schizophrenia and auditory hallucinations, the research on TMS is limited. Some studies show it might reduce this distressing symptom, but currently TMS treatment of schizophrenia is not approved. Additional study is needed.

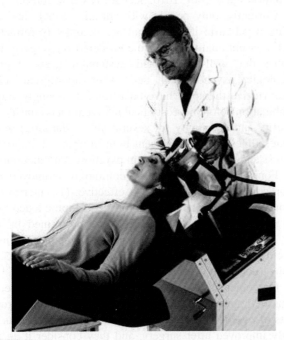

FIGURE 18.2 A practitioner observes as a client undergoes therapy with transcranial magnetic stimulation. (Courtesy of Neuronetics, Malvern, PA.)

Researchers are also exploring TMS for the treatment of pain, hypothesizing that if mood-regulating centers overlap so significantly with neural pathways involved in pain regulation, TMS might be effective. Although results appear promising, additional research is needed.

TMS has been approved in Canada and Israel for refractory depression. In 2008, the FDA approved TMS in the United States for the treatment of depression (DeNoon, 2008).

VAGUS NERVE STIMULATION

Vagus nerve stimulation (VNS) is an FDA-approved treatment that involves implantation of a device under the client's skin. The action of VNS is on the phrenic nerve, which feeds back to the brain's limbic system. The device emits a steady pulse, like a pacemaker. Studies have demonstrated the effectiveness of VNS for medically refractory partial-onset seizures; VNS has been used successfully and safely for years in clients with seizures (Benbadis et al., 2000). VNS also seems to help clients with treatment-refractory depression (Rush et al., 2005b).

The implantation of the VNS device is done under general anesthesia on an outpatient basis. Side effects include coughing, hoarseness, voice changes, dyspnea, neck pain, and irritation at the site of the implant. These results are usually transient. VNS does not appear to cause any cognitive side effects; in fact, neurocognitive performance seems to slightly improve with VNS, probably due to its efficacy in improving depression (Rowny & Lisanby, 2008).

Studies on VNS for refractory depression seem to be promising, with depression being relieved and relief sustained, in some studies, for as much as 24 months (George et al., 2007). Other studies find no difference in adjunctive VNS versus sham treatment in the overall improvement of depression (Rush et al., 2005a).

The mechanism of action of VNS is as well (or as poorly) understood as that of many procedures discussed in this chapter. Moreover, the available long-term studies are open label, raising some doubts about their accuracy. An open-label study is one in which both health providers and clients are aware of the drug or treatment being given.

TRANSCRANIAL DIRECT CURRENT STIMULATION

Transcranial direct current stimulation (tDCS) is an investigatory treatment for depression that appears to be effective in some clinical trials (Boggio et al., 2008). It involves the application of weak electrical currents to the scalp (1 to 2 mA) to modulate the activity of neurons in the brain. The fields are applied using direct current rather than the alternating current used in ECT, VNS, and deep brain stimulation. Work with this technology is at very early stages and little is known about its mechanism of action. Research suggests that tDCS may enhance certain brain functions. It is not FDA approved and is considered experimental.

DEEP BRAIN STIMULATION AND OTHER PSYCHOSURGERIES

The most invasive form of brain stimulation involves implanting an electrode directly into the brain. The technique, **deep brain stimulation (DBS),** is used in end-stage Parkinson's disease for relief of distressing tremors (Figure 18.3). Studies on DBS for refractory depression are scant and highly experimental. Most of them have been done in Europe over a long span of years between the 1970s and the 1990s with a subset of people reporting relief (Riddle & Roberts, 1978; Starr et al., 1998).

Because of the invasiveness of the procedure, lack of data, and availability of less invasive techniques, DBS is mainly of research interest at this point, with very early U.S. studies being conducted at Brown University and the Cleveland Clinic. Given past misuses of psychosurgery, guidelines to protect clients have been issued for the use of these invasive procedures (OCD-DBS Collaborative Group, 2002).

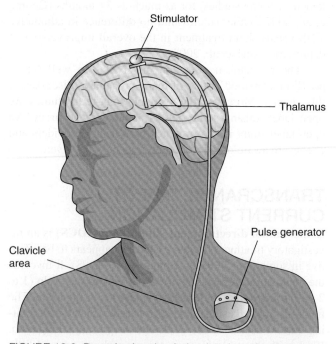

FIGURE 18.3 Deep brain stimulation involves the implantation of a neurostimulator that sends electrical impulses to block abnormal nerve signals that cause the tremors that accompany Parkinson's disease.

Psychosurgery refers to brain surgery on humans intended to relieve severe and otherwise intractable mental or behavioral problems. It is not a new phenomenon. In the recent history of psychiatry, it was recommended for curing or ameliorating schizophrenia, depression, homosexuality, childhood behavior disorders, criminal behavior, and uncontrolled violence. Estimates are that more than 50,000 psychosurgery procedures were performed in the United States alone from the 1930s to the 1950s (Greenberg et al., 2003; Greenberg, 2005). Much of the controversy surrounding psychiatric neurosurgery may relate to its overzealous and sometimes indiscriminate application during this period. Although the number of psychosurgical procedures for the purpose of psychiatric intervention performed internationally today is unknown, estimates are that fewer than 25 clients are operated on annually in the United States and Great Britain (Greenberg, 2005).

Psychiatric neurosurgery involves the disconnection of brain tissue (referred to as ablation) with the intent of altering affective and behavioral states caused by mental illnesses. The goal is to restore clients to a better level of functioning. Several of these procedures have differing targets, such as the cerebral cortex, nuclei, or other pathways that display abnormal physiologic activity. The temporal lobe may be the target in intractable epilepsy. Surgical treatment of Parkinson's disease may involve making lesions in the basal ganglia (Greenberg, 2005).

Unfortunately, as other chapters in this text have discussed, the biologic basis of most psychiatric illnesses is poorly understood and defined. Consequently, surgical results may vary. Thus, psychosurgery remains exceedingly controversial in psychiatry, with traditional forms of surgery (ablation) being supplanted with deep brain stimulation (Kahane & Depaulis, 2010; Rodriguez-Oroz, 2010; Sachdev & Chen, 2009).

Currently, only people with chronic, severe, and disabling psychiatric illnesses that are completely refractory to all conventional therapy are considered for surgery. This implies that well-documented, systematic trials of pharmacologic, psychological, and, when appropriate, electroconvulsive therapies have been tried both singly and in combination before neurosurgical intervention is considered. Severity and chronicity (of several years' duration) of the client's illness must be present both in terms of subjective distress and a severe alteration in psychosocial functioning.

Four procedures are most commonly employed and regarded as the safest and most effective: (1) anterior cingulotomy, (2) subcaudate tractotomy, (3) limbic leucotomy, and (4) anterior capsulotomy. All are performed bilaterally, and all involve creating lesions of limbic or paralimbic structures and interruptions of their connections with deeper brain structures (Greenberg, 2005).

Outcomes of surgery are an important parameter in terms of improved postoperative functional status. Proponents of psychosurgery have observed that some clients are vastly improved after surgery, and they consider it an important therapeutic option when other treatments have failed (Greenberg et al., 2003; Price et al., 2001).

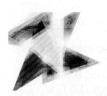

Reviewing and Applying Your Knowledge

Chapter Summary

- Somatic therapies are biologically based therapies and generally include psychopharmacotherapeutics and non-pharmacologic, bodily oriented modalities.

- Electroconvulsive therapy (ECT) involves placement of an electrode on the temple or temples of a client under general anesthesia to induce a grand mal seizure. ECT is indicated for clients with psychiatric illnesses in whom all other treatment modalities have failed and whose lives are subsequently at risk. Potential side effects include short- and long-term memory loss and the dangers associated with all procedures conducted under anesthesia.

- Nurses caring for people undergoing ECT and their families are responsible for initial and ongoing assessment, teaching about the procedure, and instruction regarding myths and facts relative to ECT, other somatic therapies, and all psychiatric care.

- Phototherapy involves exposure of the eyes to artificial light during the fall and winter to prevent or treat seasonal affective disorder.

- Transcranial magnetic stimulation, vagus nerve stimulation, transcranial direct current, stimulation, magnetic seizure therapy and deep brain stimulation are modalities in various stages of international acceptance, approval, and use for varying psychiatric conditions. More research on these modalities and their outcomes is needed.

- Psychosurgery is indicated only when clients have psychiatric illnesses that are chronic, severe, disabling, and completely refractory to all conventional treatments. Because surgical results are so uncertain, the risks involved are high, and less invasive and controversial modalities are available, neurosurgery for psychiatric conditions remains rare.

Study Questions

1. Which instruction would the nurse include when preparing a client scheduled for ECT?

   a. "You'll be awake, but you won't remember anything about the treatment."

   b. "Don't eat or drink anything after midnight of the day of the treatment."

   c. "One treatment session is usually all that you'll need for treatment."

   d. "Avoid looking directly into the light when the doctor shines it at you."

2. Which assessment would be the priority for a client immediately after ECT?

   a. Airway patency   c. Hydration

   b. Neurologic status   d. Skin integrity

3. When describing various somatic therapies to a group of students, which therapy would the nursing instructor identify as having no side effects?

   a. ECT   c. Vagus nerve stimulation

   b. Deep brain stimulation   d. Transcranial magnetic stimulation

4. Which of the following responses from a group of nursing students indicates that the instructor's teaching about psychosurgery has been successful?

   a. Psychosurgery is used as treatment for seasonal affective disorder.

   b. Magnetic fields are changed to electrical current to stimulate the brain.

   c. It involves ablation of brain tissue to alter affective and behavioral states.

   d. A pacemaker-like device acts on the phrenic nerve to affect the limbic system.

5. The nurse is assisting a client in scheduling his first four ECT treatments. Which schedule would be most appropriate?

   a. Monday, Tuesday, then Thursday, Friday

   b. Tuesday, Friday, then Monday, Thursday

   c. Tuesday, Wednesday, then Thursday, Friday

   d. Wednesday, Thursday, Monday, Tuesday

Critical Thinking Questions

1. A client and his wife visit the mental health clinic. The client has a history of major depression. He was receiving antidepressants, which were initially effective. However, during the past 2 years, recurrent episodes have not responded to treatment. After discussing various options with the health care provider, the client has decided to try ECT, with the support of his wife. Develop a client teaching sheet that addresses ECT and could be given to this couple.

2. Compare and contrast transcranial magnetic stimulation, vagus nerve stimulation, and deep brain stimulation.

References

Abrams, R. (2002). *Electroconvulsive therapy.* New York, NY: Oxford University Press.

American Psychiatric Association. (2001). *A task force report on the practice of electroconvulsive therapy.* Washington, DC: Author.

Avery, D. H., Eder, D. N., Bolte, M. A., Hellekson, C. J., Dunner, D. L., Vitiello, M. V., & Prinz, P. N. (2001). Dawn stimulation and bright light in the treatment of SAD: A controlled study. *Biological Psychiatry, 50,* 205–216.

Benbadis, S. R., Tatum, W. O., & Vale, F. L. (2000). When drugs don't work: An algorithmic approach to medically intractable epilepsy. *Neurology, 55*(12), 1780–1784.

Boggio, P. S., Rigonatti, S. P., Ribeiro, R. B., Myczkowski, M. L., Nitsche, M. A., ... Fregni, F. (2008). A randomized, double-blind clinical trial on the efficacy of cortical direct current stimulation for the treatment of major depression. *International Journal of Neuropsychopharmacology, 11,* 249–254.

DeNoon, D. J. (2008, October 9). FDA approves first transcranial magnetic stimulation device for depression. *Medscape Today.* Retrieved from http://www.medscape.com/viewarticle/581830

Dukakis, K., & Tye, L. (2006). *Shock: The healing power of electroconvulsive therapy.* New York, NY: Avery.

Epperson, C. N., Terman, M., Terman, J. S., Hanusa, B. H., Oren, D. A., Peindl, K. S., & Wisner, K. L. (2004). Randomized clinical trial of bright light therapy for antepartum depression: Preliminary findings. *Journal of Clinical Psychiatry, 65,* 421–425.

Erraji-Benchekroun, L., Lisanby, S. H., Arango, V., Galfalvy, H., Pavlidis, P., & Underwood, M. D. (2007). Effect of electroconvulsive shock and magnetic seizure on gene expression profiles in the prefrontal cortex of the rhesus monkey. *Biological Psychiatry, 61,* 173–187.

Folk, J. W., Kellner, C. H., Beale, M. D., Conroy, J. M., & Duc, T. A. (2000). Anesthesia for electroconvulsive therapy: A review. *Journal of ECT, 16,* 187.

Forbes, D., Culum, I., Lischka, A. R., Morgan, D. G., Peacock, S., Forbes, J., & Forbes, S. (2009). Light therapy for managing cognitive, sleep, functional, behavioural, or psychiatric disturbances in dementia. *Cochrane Database of Systematic Reviews, 2009*(4). CD003946.

George, M. S., & Belmaker, R. H. (2006). *TMS in clinical psychiatry.* Washington, DC: American Psychiatric Press.

George, M. S., Nahas, Z., Borckardt, J. J., Anderson, B., Foust, M. J., Burns, C., ... Short, E. B. (2007). Brain stimulation for the treatment of psychiatric disorders. *Current Opinion in Psychiatry, 20*(3), 250–254.

Greenberg, B. D., Price, L. H., Rauch, S. L., Friehs, G., Noren, G., Malone, D., ... Rasmussen, S. A. (2003). Neurosurgery for intractable obsessive-compulsive disorder and depression: Critical issues. *Neurosurgery Clinics of North America, 14*(2), 199–212.

Greenberg, M. S. (2005). *Handbook of neurosurgery.* New York, NY: Thieme Medical Publishing.

Kahane, P., & Depaulis, A. (2010). Deep brain stimulation in epilepsy: What is next? *Current Opinion in Neurology, 23*(2), 177–182.

Lisanby, S. H., Luber, B. Schlaepfe, T. E., & Sackeim, H. A. (2003). Safety and feasibility of magnetic seizure therapy (MST) in major depression: Randomized within-subject comparison with electroconvulsive therapy. *Neuropsychopharmacology, 28,* 1852–1865.

OCD-DBS Collaborative Group. (2002). Deep brain stimulation for psychiatric disorders. *Neurosurgery, 51,* 519.

O'Reardon, J. P., Solvason, H. B., Janicak, P. G., Sampson, S., Isenberg, K. E., Nahas, Z., ... Sackeim, H. A. (2007). Efficacy and safety of transcranial magnetic stimulation in the acute treatment of major depression: A multisite randomized controlled trial. *Biological Psychiatry, 62*(11), 1208–1216.

Price, B. H., Baral, I., Cosgrove, G. R., Rauch, S. L., Nierenberg, A. A., Jenike, M. A., & Cassem, E. H. (2001). Improvement in severe self-mutilation following limbic leucotomy: A series of 5 consecutive cases. *Journal of Clinical Psychiatry, 62*(12), 925–932.

Riddle, M., & Roberts, A. H. (1978). Psychosurgery and the Porteus maze tests: Review and reanalysis of data. *Archives of General Psychiatry, 35*(4), 493–497.

Riemersma-van der Lek, R. F., Swaab, D. F., Twisk, J., Hol, E. M., Hoogendijk, W. J., & Van Someren, E. J. (2008). Effect of bright light and melatonin on cognitive and noncognitive function in elderly residents of group care facilities: a randomized controlled trial. *Journal of the American Medical Association, 299*(22), 2642–2655.

Rodriguez-Oroz, M. C. (2010). Deep brain stimulation for advanced Parkinson's disease. *Lancet Neurology, 9*(6), 558–559.

Rowny, S., & Lisanby, S. II. (2008). Brain stimulation in psychiatry. In A. Tasman, J. Kay, J. A. Lieberman, M. B. First, and M. Maj (Eds.), *Psychiatry* (3rd ed., Vol. 2, pp. 2354–2368). West Sussex, UK: John Wiley & Sons.

Rush, A. J., Marangell, L. B., Sackeim, H. A., George, M. S., Brannan, S. K., Davis, S. M., ... Cooke, R. G. (2005a). Vagus nerve stimulation for treatment-resistant depression: A randomized, controlled acute phase trial. *Biological Psychiatry, 58*(5), 347–354.

Rush, A. J., Sackeim, H. A., & Marangell, L. B. (2005b). Effects of 12 months of vagus nerve stimulation in treatment-resistant depression: A naturalistic study. *Biological Psychiatry, 58,* 355–363.

Sachdev, P. S., & Chen, X. (2009). Neurosurgical treatment of mood disorders: traditional psychosurgery and the advent of deep brain stimulation. *Current Opinion in Psychiatry, 22*(1), 25–31.

Starr, P. A., Vitek, J. L., & Bakay, R. A. (1998). Deep brain stimulation. *Neurosurgery Clinics of North America, 9,* 381–402.

Tuunainen, A., Kripke, D. F., & Endo, T. (2004). Light therapy for non-seasonal depression. *Cochrane Database of Systematic Reviews, 2004*(2). CD004050.

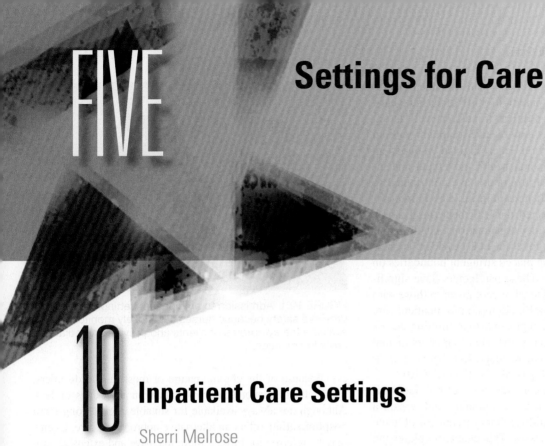

FIVE

Settings for Care

19

Inpatient Care Settings

Sherri Melrose

LEARNING OBJECTIVES

On completion of this chapter, you should be able to accomplish the following:

- Define the various levels of care within inpatient treatment settings.
- Describe variations of psychiatric settings.
- Explain the role of psychiatric nurses in inpatient settings.
- Explain elements and methods of fostering a therapeutic milieu.
- Explain transfer and discharge in relation to inpatient psychiatric care.

Treatment settings for clients with mental illnesses have undergone a paradigm shift in recent years. Because of economic and political trends, as well as advances in care, many clients now receive treatment without institutional-based intervention or care given in inpatient settings. The community mental health movement and intensive community outreach programs have contributed to this trend (see Chap. 20). Changes in health care reimbursement also have greatly affected the U.S. behavioral health care system. Preferred provider organizations, health maintenance organizations, and governmental providers such as Medicare and Medicaid have placed stringent boundaries on treatment length and focus. These parameters have significantly affected the type and level of care given to those with mental health needs. Criteria for admission to inpatient care settings have become more regulated, thus limiting access to services for many. Nationally, the rate of inpatient mental health beds per 100,000 people declined 45% between 1990 and 2004 (National Center for Health Statistics, 2010).

Nevertheless, inpatient care settings still provide critical services to the mental health community and remain a vital component of the multidisciplinary treatment of acute exacerbations of mental illnesses. This chapter explores the current role of inpatient facilities in the continuum of psychiatric care. It reviews key nursing activities and foci from admission through discharge, particularly elements that contribute to a safe and optimal therapeutic milieu.

INPATIENT CARE CRITERIA AND VARIATIONS

For clients to receive **inpatient care** (also called **hospital-based treatment**), they must meet specific criteria, which insurance providers generally set forth. Candidates most likely to receive inpatient treatment are those who pose a risk of harm to self (Doerfler et al., 2011) or those who pose a risk of harm to others (Kynoch et al., 2009). The safety of clients, their families, and the community remains of paramount concern throughout care. Clients who qualify for admission may need short-term (acute) or long-term hospitalization, depending on their unique circumstances (Bowers, 2005).

Levels of Care

Acute care hospitals provide a highly structured setting (the **milieu**) that optimizes safety. The milieu is also conducive to decreasing anxiety. Clients experiencing suicidal or homicidal ideation, acute psychoses, confusion, or disorientation and those in need of acute detoxification are all candidates for acute care admission. Clients admitted to psychiatric units typically have an Axis I or Axis II disorder, are experiencing a clinical crisis that renders them unable to function or care for themselves, and are unable to access other less restrictive treatments (Sharfstein & Dickerson, 2009). Workers in inpatient settings can closely monitor and evaluate such clients, as well as provide immediate crisis intervention (see Chap. 35) (Figure 19.1). The average length of stay for acute care psychiatric admissions is 3 to 7 days.

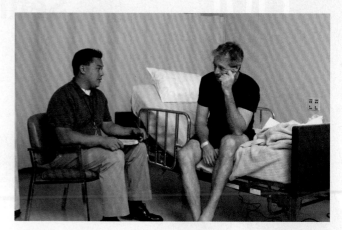

FIGURE 19.1 Admission to an inpatient setting helps to preserve safety because nurses can closely monitor and evaluate the symptoms of clients and provide immediate crisis intervention.

Because of the chronic nature of most mental disorders, many clients cannot achieve stabilization in 7 days or less. Although not always available for suitable clients, **long-term hospitalization** offers an alternative approach to care. Clients may be referred for further, more intensive and extensive support to safely manage both their psychiatric and comorbid medical conditions. Long-term psychiatric facilities often provide certain areas where high-security measures, such as close staff supervision, locked doors, and security cameras, are implemented. These institutions may also provide short-term therapy for specific client groups, outpatient therapy groups, and community wellness programs. Many long-term psychiatric hospitals are state-supervised facilities. Conditions in such settings have improved dramatically during the past 50 years.

During the past several decades, many hospitals have begun step-therapy settings known as **partial (day) hospitalization** (PHPs), which are ideal alternatives for those who continue to need some supervision but are not appropriate clients for long-term admission. PHPs are best suited for clients whose symptoms are not severe enough to warrant inpatient treatment (Priebe et al., 2011). PHPs provide opportunities for clients to attend group therapy sessions, life skills workshops, and individual psychotherapy and counseling for 6 to 8 hours per day. Clients then return to their primary residence or workplace. PHPs may be in the daytime or evening hours and can mainstream clients back into the workplace and their homes effectively. Family therapy may also be available. PHPs provide socialization and social support, medication administration and education, and opportunities for ongoing assessment and therapies.

Types of Settings

Inpatient psychiatric treatment is not delivered exclusively in general hospitals. A wide range of treatment settings includes psychiatric units within general hospitals, psychiatric specialty units, nonpsychiatric units, and scatter beds.

Although only a small percentage of nurses specialize in psychiatric nursing, all nurses care for clients with psychiatric challenges. Therefore, it is imperative for all nurses, regardless of discipline, to incorporate concepts of psychiatric nursing into their repertoire of care. Whether clients are receiving treatment in nonpsychiatric units, specialty psychiatric units, or some other variation, nurses need to provide the most competent, up-to-date, comprehensive, and compassionate care possible.

Psychiatric Units

Many large general hospitals offer psychiatric services. They often use a triage system through their emergency departments (EDs), where an attending physician may order psychiatric consultations for clients who need them. Once health care providers evaluate and determine that a client is in need of psychiatric hospitalization, they transfer him or her to the in-house psychiatric unit. Such units are usually a single entity within the matrix of the hospital but have divisions based on client age. The general-hospital psychiatric setting is primarily for acute treatment, with the main goal of stabilization.

Psychiatric Specialty Units

Psychiatric specialty units treat clients with specific circumstances, symptoms, or diagnoses. Examples include older adults, pediatric populations, dementia care, substance abuse/dependency, eating disorders, and intensive care for adults. Specialization enables units to be better equipped and employ more personnel who are fully prepared to manage the unique needs of the population in question. Personnel tailor and focus interventions to meet the needs of clients with specific symptoms.

Nonpsychiatric Units

Some clients receive initial treatment within nonpsychiatric units. Often, such clients need physiologic stabilization before psychological treatment can ensue. Examples include drug or alcohol detoxification, overdose, eating disorders, and older adults with multiple medical diagnoses. Once health care providers have stabilized the medical conditions of these clients, the clients are transferred to psychiatric units within the hospital or at another facility.

Scatter Beds

When clients in crisis need the safety and support of an inpatient admission, but beds are not available on designated psychiatric units, they can be admitted to medical–surgical units. Beds for psychiatric clients on units that have not been organized and staffed specifically to treat psychiatric disorders are "scattered" through the hospital and are known as "scatter beds" (Mark et al., 2010).

Checkpoint Questions

1. What is the average length of stay in an acute care psychiatric institution?

2. What is the main goal of the general hospital psychiatric setting?

NURSING ROLES IN INPATIENT CARE MANAGEMENT

The role of psychiatric nurses who care for clients in inpatient environments is complex and includes multiple responsibilities. Many interventions discussed throughout this book apply and require slight or no modifications for correct implementation within inpatient facilities. The following sections review important issues and areas needing adjustments when nurses give care to clients admitted to health care facilities for psychiatric problems.

Admission

When clients are admitted to inpatient psychiatric settings, nurses often are the first health care providers they meet. Beginning with admission, nurses begin to form rapport with clients and initiate the assessment phase of care. Establishing a trusting relationship is paramount at this time (see Chaps. 10 and 11). Depending on the diagnosis and associated symptoms, establishing rapport may be difficult. It is critical for psychiatric nurses to be patient and reassuring. Clients may be frightened, angry, defensive, paranoid, anxious, or despondent (Figure 19.2). Through the eyes of our clients, inpatient units can be seen as unsafe places where they are subject to aggression, bullying, theft of their personal property, and widespread use of drugs and alcohol (Jones et al., 2010). Giving reminders to clients that they are safe is a nursing priority.

Another priority is ensuring the safety of other clients, staff, and visitors. For this reason, admission may take place in a separate area of the facility until providers have completed a thorough assessment of the client's safety needs. Nurses respectfully but thoroughly check clients' personal belongings for items that could be used to harm themselves or others. Sharp objects including knives and glass, smoking supplies including lighters and matches, and corded items including electrical equipment and belts are usually confiscated (Cardell et al., 2009). Psychiatric symptoms are likely to be most pronounced soon after admission (Allen et al., 2009). During the first 24-hour period after admission,

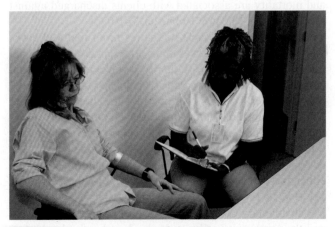

FIGURE 19.2 Nurses need to be prepared to address the difficult emotions clients experience while hospitalized, especially during the admission phase.

nurses must observe clients frequently, document behaviors carefully, review and evaluate medication orders, assess the environment for risks, listen carefully to client and family concerns, and ask in-depth questions that go well beyond the checklists available for charting convenience. Nurses working on such units with clients who are acutely ill must be able to assess in multiple domains and in different ways. For example, clients may deny that they are suicidal, but when probed may tell the nurse that they have experienced a significant loss and that they feel hopeless. These kinds of statements, although not addressing suicide directly, should cue the nurse to further assessment of self-harm potential.

Types

Clients may be admitted to hospitals on a voluntary or involuntary basis (see Chap. 5). With *voluntary admission,* clients make an autonomous decision to seek inpatient treatment by submitting a formal, written request. They may also give a parent or mental health or legal guardian the authority to request inpatient treatment for them. Many such clients have tried outpatient strategies without achieving optimal results. Informal voluntary admissions based on verbal requests from clients occur more often in private, freestanding facilities and general psychiatric units, whereas voluntary admissions by written request are more common in state psychiatric hospitals.

Because clients voluntarily participate in treatment, they may also willingly suspend it. However, although clients request discharge, the physician and interdisciplinary treatment team ultimately decide whether discharge is appropriate. A client's status may change from voluntary to involuntary if the treatment team decides the person is a threat to self or others. Many facilities have clearly designated guidelines for when clients can request discharge. There may be a grace period of 24 hours to several days from when a client requests discharge against medical advice and the treatment team completes its assessment. This grace period gives the staff sufficient time to evaluate the client and, if necessary, attempt to convince him or her to maintain inpatient status. Increased rates of rehospitalization, morbidity, and mortality are associated with clients discharged against medical advice (Sclar & Robinson, 2010).

Involuntary commitment requires proof that a client is mentally ill, a danger to self or to others, and unable to care for self. States have the authority to involuntarily commit people for psychiatric treatment by police power or *parens patriae* power. Police power provides for committing those who are deemed dangerous to others. *Parens patriae* allows the state to take responsibility for those who cannot care for and are considered a danger to themselves. Each state designates guidelines for involuntary commitment, which either the court system or a group of physicians initiates. See Box 19.1.

Involuntary commitment is useful in protecting clients and the community at large. It also has drawbacks. Unfortunately, the power to commit people against their will is

---

BOX 19.1 Types of Involuntary Commitment

Emergency

- Duration is temporary.
- The client is at risk for distinct harm to self or others.
- Time frame is limited to 24 to 72 hours, by which time a hearing must occur to decide the next phase of treatment.

Observational

- Duration varies widely, from a few days to several months.
- Goal is to allow time for an appropriate diagnosis.
- After adequate diagnosis is made, the client may be discharged, stay voluntarily for continued treatment, or continue hospitalization under an extended commitment order.

Extended

- The court system or physicians decide to commit a client for an undetermined duration.
- The judicial system often remits the client to a state psychiatric setting until further notice.
- The client can participate in the hearing, although often clients choose not to.

Outpatient

- Client is remanded to attend regularly scheduled outpatient appointments with a psychiatrist; this decision usually occurs following an involuntary hospitalization.
- Client is stable enough for discharge; however, he or she still needs close supervision and frequent monitoring.
- Many times, a clause states that noncompliance with outpatient treatment will result in involuntary rehospitalization. Clients with mental illnesses who are also judicial offenders may also be remanded for outpatient commitment after release from prison.

---

sometimes used inappropriately. Clients must be proven to exhibit behaviors deemed dangerous and unpredictable. Critics of involuntary commitments have voiced concern that the label of "dangerous" adds to the stigma already associated with mental illness and perpetuates society's fear of psychiatric illness (see Chap. 8).

Assessment

Nurses must frequently monitor the mental health status of clients throughout inpatient treatment. They are responsible for assessing physiologic, psychological, and mental status, and all other holistic dimensions of the clients for whom they care.

When a client is being admitted to inpatient settings, the nurse first obtains the client's psychiatric history. The nurse gathers data about the client's immediate status, reason for coming to hospital, risk of harm to self or others, comorbid medical conditions, current medications, and past diagnoses and treatments. The nurse also documents the client's family history of mental illness and previous psychiatric treatments and interventions. Clients may be able to supply much of the data for the psychiatric history; however, health care providers may also need to obtain information from family, court officials, and documentation of treatment from other mental health practitioners. See Chapter 10 for more details.

Therapeutic Strategies

Inpatient treatment settings allow psychiatric nurses to manage the therapeutic environment and implement strategies that contribute to the overall community. An environment is deemed as therapeutic when it meets several criteria (Box 19.2). In general, the main elements of such environments are that they facilitate safety, optimal daily functioning, appropriate interpersonal interactions, and movement toward independent living.

Scheduled client observations are critical in establishing a safe inpatient environment. During client care conferences, psychiatric workers establish observation levels, or how frequently they will check each client. While staff may not interact with clients during each observation, they record the observation times and the client's behavior. Formal, routine, or general observation usually involves hourly checks, frequent observation usually involves 30- to 15- minute checks,

---

BOX 19.2 Criteria for Establishing a Therapeutic Milieu

The therapeutic milieu should:

- Be purposeful and planned to provide safety from physical danger and emotional trauma. It should have furniture to facilitate a homelike atmosphere. Provisions for privacy and physical needs are necessary.
- Promote interaction and communication among clients and personnel and provide safety from emotional trauma.
- Provide a testing ground for new patterns of behavior while clients take responsibility for their actions. Behavioral expectations—including the existing rules, regulations, and policies—should be explained to clients.
- Provide for consistent limit-setting. This criterion reflects aspects of a democratic society. All clients are treated as equally as possible with respect to restrictions, rules, and policies.
- Encourage participation in group activities and free-flowing communication in which clients are free to express themselves in a socially acceptable manner.
- Provide for client respect and dignity. Adult–adult interactions should prevail when appropriate, promoting equal status among the parties involved, exchange of interpersonal information, and avoidance of any "power plays." Clients should be encouraged to use personal resources to resolve problems or conflicts.
- Convey an attitude of overall acceptance and optimism. Conflict among staff members must be handled and resolved in some manner to maintain a therapeutic milieu. Clients are perceptive of such reactions and may feel that they are the cause of conflicts among personnel.
- Allow for continual assessment and evaluation of clients' progress, with modifications in treatment and nursing interventions as needed.

---

and constant observation usually involves a staff member remaining with the client at all times (Manna, 2010).

Similarly, scheduled environmental tours (Joint Commission Resources, 2007) or "walk-arounds" of the unit also establish a safe inpatient environment. Nurses continually assess all unit spaces for objects clients might use to harm themselves or others (Cardell et al., 2009). Psychiatric inpatient units are designed with attention to environmental safeguards and nurses must remain aware of dangers that seemingly ordinary objects might pose. Everyday medical supplies and self-care items readily available on other hospital units must be considered thoughtfully when left in client areas and are generally kept at the nursing station rather than at the bedside. Visitors may inadvertently bring in items than can be harmful and psychiatric staff maintain discreet but vigilant observations of people who come to the unit.

Psychiatric nurses play a pivotal part in inpatient settings and can implement strategies that assist in maintaining a therapeutic atmosphere. Most inpatient settings are for acute exacerbations of mental illness. Therefore, it is not the intent or desire of facilities to maintain inpatient status for clients any longer than necessary. Treatment goals should be realistic and achievable. Unrealistic goals lead to feelings of hopelessness and despair. Clients also should actively participate in treatment planning (if they are able). Those who actively contribute to their own treatment plan are more likely to feel empowered and in control. These elements eventually contribute to increased accountability for maintaining adherence to the treatment regimen for their illness.

Professional Relationships

Professionalism within all workplaces is important; however, it is a heightened concern in inpatient psychiatric settings. Because of the continual interactions between nurses and clients, as well as the personal nature of psychiatric care, nurses must be cautious about protecting personal boundaries. To maintain professionalism, nurses must examine their own feelings and biases regarding clients and settings. Self-awareness can assist nurses to provide unbiased treatment for all clients. A therapeutic and professional nurse–client relationship depends on the nurse's ability to maintain appropriate communication, understand client behaviors, and recognize the contributions that they can bring to the nurse–client relationship.

Many clients are concerned about their right to privacy during hospitalization. Stigma associated with mental illness leads to concerns regarding confidentiality (see Chaps. 6 and 8). Nurses learn information of a highly personal nature. Maintaining discretion and respect for the client's personal information is a major nursing responsibility. Clients may also feel as if they are continually under the watchful eye of staff. By respecting a client's privacy while he or she bathes, showers, and dresses, nurses can alleviate some anxiety that clients experience as a result of continual supervision. The task of balancing clients' needs for privacy while maintaining needed scheduled observation times is not straightforward. The physical environment contributes significantly to the cause of inpatient suicides. Suicide attempts are likely to occur in quiet areas such as bathrooms, closets, and client sleeping spaces—86% of inpatient suicide attempts involved hanging from bathroom doors (Joint Commission Resources, 2007). To ensure safety, nurses must unobtrusively remain aware of the activities their clients are engaged in at all times. Nurses also should work to protect vulnerable clients, such as those receiving psychiatric care, from inappropriate disclosures of the nurse's own personal information.

Nurse–Client Contracts

Inpatient settings often use contracts to facilitate communication of expected behaviors. The most widely used nurse–client contract is known as a *no self-harm contract*, in which clients agree not to harm themselves but rather to seek out staff for direction on alternatives to self-harm. Many inpatient settings include this contract as a component of initial documentation and paperwork that clients complete at admission. The goal is for clients to seek other ways of dealing with their distress, especially by calling on nurses and the nurse–client relationship.

Other contracts may focus on maladaptive behaviors such as acting out or inappropriate behaviors that staff are attempting to modify. Clients help develop contracts so that their stipulations are meaningful. Contracts frequently outline predetermined consequences for specific behaviors. All participants agree on the guidelines and sign the document prior to implementation. The goal is to achieve a sense of accountability for the client and nurse within the boundaries of the working relationship.

> ### Checkpoint Questions
> **3.** What two methods do states use to involuntarily commit people for psychiatric treatment?
> **4.** What are the general elements of a therapeutic environment?
> **5.** What three levels of client observation do nurses usually establish on psychiatric inpatient units?
> **6.** What assessments do nurses implement during environmental tours of the unit?

Milieu Management

Milieu therapy is also known as the maintenance of the therapeutic environment. The provision of such a setting helps to stabilize clients with mental illness—specifically in terms of improving their thought processes and fostering more appropriate behaviors. Therapeutic relationships between staff and clients improve social functioning. To achieve and maintain a therapeutic environment, it is paramount for staff members to display professional attitudes. Clients learn and assimilate appropriate group dynamics through milieu therapy (Yalom & Leszcz, 2005). Nurses play an important role in the management of symptoms.

Although care within the mental health community has evolved and changed, the concepts within traditional milieu therapy remain applicable (Mahoney et al., 2009; Thibeaut et al., 2010). Traditional milieu therapy consists of containment, support, validation, structure, and involvement (Gunderson, 1978).

- *Containment* involves the provision of basic needs: food, shelter, safety, and security. Inpatient settings can be locked units to ensure that clients are not at risk for harm to self or others. Current environmental strategies involve the use of the least restrictive methods possible for controlling dangerous behaviors, such as time-out, therapeutic holds, verbal de-escalation, and chemical restraints. Health care providers still sometimes use restraints and seclusion with out-of-control or aggressive clients (see Chap. 32). Nurses contribute integrally to containment by observing clients continuously and vigilantly for their psychological and physical needs. Maintenance of safety for both clients and staff is the crux of containment (Moylan & Cullinan, 2011).
- Providing *support* is essential to a positive nurse–client relationship. Nurses offer clients encouragement, praise, and positive feedback. A supportive environment helps clients to achieve autonomy and improve their coping mechanisms. Supportive interventions include education, management of symptoms, and facilitation of social and interpersonal skills.
- *Validation* begins with the first interaction between nurse and client. By providing for and respecting each client's sense of privacy, cultural needs, and feelings, nurses can contribute to the client's holistic health. Doing so ultimately improves the client's independence and overall sense of self-worth.
- *Structure* within inpatient settings assists in the control and limitation of maladaptive behaviors, such as yelling, screaming, and cursing, that may accompany aggressive outbursts. Nurses must use skills in verbal de-escalation to lead to the cessation of such negative actions (see Chap. 32). Setting limits is another important skill in maintaining structure. Nurses examine and determine trends in behaviors and develop preventive interventions that diminish self-destructive and high-risk behaviors. Examples of methods for fostering structure include written guidelines for acceptable behavior and behavioral contracts.
- The concept of *involvement* has evolved over time. Involvement currently refers to promoting the self-efficacy of the client. The client's involvement in treatment is critical to his or her improvement. Nurses help engage clients to become more self-efficacious by promoting self-care, assessing education needs, facilitating stress-management strategies, and assisting with the development of social skills. Through the promotion of self-care activities, nurses assist clients to become independent.

Think About It 19.1

A client is hospitalized in an inpatient facility for an acute exacerbation of bipolar mania. He is very talkative with grandiose delusions, uses flamboyant gestures, and is extremely active. He often enters the rooms of other clients and touches items that belong to them. The client cannot sit for any period of time, even to eat a meal. How would the nurse apply the elements of containment and structure in the milieu of this client?

INTERDISCIPLINARY MANAGEMENT. Professionals from several disciplines collaborate to promote a therapeutic milieu. Examples include psychiatric–mental health nurses; psychiatric nurse assistants; psychiatrists; psychologists; social workers; occupational, educational, art, music, recreational, play, pet, and speech therapists; chaplains; and dietitians. Frequently, psychiatric–mental health nurses are responsible for managing and coordinating milieu activities. Treatment teams meet regularly and as scheduled to discuss the progress of clients and to review individualized plans of care. See Chapter 12 for more information.

FOSTERING SELF-CARE. Some clients receiving inpatient care cannot manage hygiene, grooming, feeding, or other activities because of their illnesses, adjustments to medications, or other challenges. One benefit of hospitalization is that nurses and other personnel can assist clients with such practices until they are stable enough to resume self-care (Figure 19.3). Nurses also encourage client participation in bathing, dressing, and eating and encourage clients to independently assume such activities as soon as they are able.

CLIENT EDUCATION. Client education promotes involvement, prevents complications, and reduces hospital readmissions. In today's health care environments, nurses often must face challenges from inside and outside the institution.

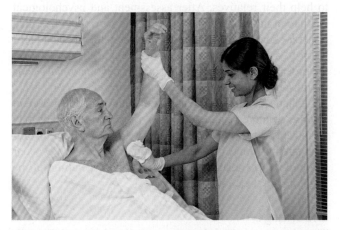

FIGURE 19.3 Nurses help hospitalized clients with self-care whose conditions limit their ability to attend to hygiene, eating, and other activities of daily living. When performing personal care and maintaining frequent observation, nurses strive to maintain as much privacy and dignity for clients as possible.

Examples include insufficient resources, limited time to spend with each client, and language or cultural barriers with clients.

Before beginning teaching, nurses must determine the knowledge base and knowledge deficits of clients (Burlingame et al., 2006). They also must work to determine whether clients are open to education before beginning to provide information. Teaching sessions should follow these basic guidelines:

1. Prioritize needs in a hierarchy from basic to complex.
2. Give specific information.
3. Use the simplest terminology and language possible to avoid confusion.
4. Tailor approaches to best meet each client's particular learning style.
5. Reinforce previously taught information while providing care.

LIVING SKILLS GROUPS. Nurses can greatly affect the lives of their clients through the seemingly simple task of teaching basic living skills. The lack of performing these basic life skills can contribute to the inability of clients to maintain stability once they return to the community. Clients with acute mental illnesses, especially altered perceptions of reality, have difficulty performing even the simplest of daily living skills. As clients achieve a more reality-based thought process, the nurse can assist in the development of these necessary living skills.

MEDICATION ADMINISTRATION. Psychiatric nurses are responsible for administering medications and monitoring effectiveness, associated side effects, and potential health concerns. Because mental disorders are often chronic, the process of pharmacologic management is often tedious and lengthy. To stay stable, many psychiatric clients must remain on medication regimens for the rest of their lives. Because pharmacologic intervention is an important aspect of treatment, psychiatric nurses must not only administer medications, but also provide education to clients and families regarding the effects of medication, side effects, and need for adherence. Nurses must also become proficient at documenting client responses to psychopharmacology and any potential issues that may warrant further evaluation of the current medications.

When giving medication within inpatient settings, psychiatric nurses must be aware of potential associated safety issues. It is always important to verify each client prior to administration by checking the "five rights" (right client, right drug, right dose, right time, and right route). Some clients may be disoriented or confused; they may be experiencing altered thought processes that affect their ability to identify themselves. Nurses should be able to definitively identify each client prior to administering medications (Figure 19.4).

Other clients may attempt to manipulate staff by "cheeking" medications. Cheeking medication is done by hiding oral medications within the cheek and gum or under

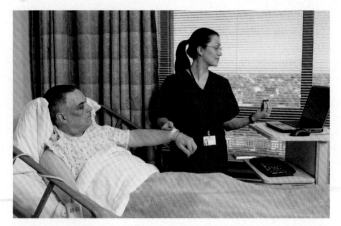

FIGURE 19.4 The nurse is checking to make sure she has the right medication for the right client before administering the drug.

the tongue. It may appear as if the client has swallowed the medications, when, in fact, he or she has not. Clients at risk for suicide, those who have a history of medication nonadherence, and those who display other manipulative behaviors require careful assessment for medication adherence. Clients who have "cheeked" medications may hoard medications for several days prior to overdosing. Nursing staff should ask clients to open their mouths and lift up their tongues to be certain that they swallowed medication.

Although clients within inpatient psychiatric settings may experience thought distortions, they still have a sense of and a right to autonomy. Clients have the right to refuse medication unless otherwise decided by the court system. Nurses should make every effort to administer medication safely, observe for adverse effects, and behave ethically.

WORKING WITH SUPPORT SYSTEMS/FAMILIES.
An important aspect of any client's treatment plan is involvement of a support system. Clients who have a support system have a better chance of adhering to medications and other intervention plans. The National Alliance for the Mentally Ill has placed a premium on the addition of family-focused support groups to help those with mental illness and their loved ones. It is important for psychiatric nurses to remain supportive of families, yet nonjudgmental. Many relatives have a difficult time coping with the illness of their loved one. When family members are considered a viable component of the treatment plan, clients can receive more comprehensive care.

Checkpoint Questions

7. What are the five elements of traditional milieu therapy?

8. What is meant by "cheeking" medications?

Documentation and Reporting

A primary responsibility of nurses is to observe, assess, and thoroughly document behaviors, actions, and responses of clients. Documentation is done for the welfare of the client

and for the legal welfare of the nurse and the institution. Complete documentation can ensure that the events of today are remembered in the future. The client's medical record should directly reflect what occurred at any given time during a client's hospitalization.

The medical record should include a comprehensive history of presenting illness, chief complaint, previous treatment approaches, diagnoses, safety risks because of specific behaviors, levels of observations maintained, and direct explanation of all behaviors during hospitalization. Particular concern occurs when clients are at risk for violence toward self or others. If a client has expressed thoughts of self-harm or an intention to harm others, it is critical that the nursing staff document the plan, as stated by the client, and the level of intent and lethality. Self-harm documentation must include assessment of impulsive behaviors, access to means, family adversity or social loss, recent clinical condition, past suicide history, evidence of poor coping, medication noncompliance, living environment, and substance abuse (Joint Commission Resources, 2007). If a client has expressed an intention to harm others, documentation must include past levels of risk, previous dangerous behavior, severity of mental illness, degree of impulsivity, level of insight, nonadherence to treatment, missed contact with clinicians, access to weapons, and substance abuse (Ignelzi et al., 2007). The existence of any contracts (eg, no self-harm) also need to be recorded. Behaviors may change rapidly in clients with mental illness, so detailed, accurate, and ongoing documentation is a necessity.

Transfers

Many clients are transferred either into or out of inpatient treatment settings. Clients may first present to EDs, either verbally expressing psychological distress or showing signs of overdose or intoxication. Or they may arrive through emergency first responders. Often, family members bring their loved ones to the ED because they are unsure of how to help their relatives. After assessment and psychological evaluation have been completed, health care providers may transfer clients to a psychiatric unit within the medical facility or to a freestanding psychiatric hospital. In some cases, the order of a judge (either from a court hearing or jail) leads to transfer of clients to an inpatient setting.

Clients can also be transferred from inpatient treatment settings to more secure settings. For example, a client may be moved from an acute care facility to a long-term institution, nursing home, jail, or group home. Transfers may occur to more or less restrictive environments, depending on the level of care the client needs.

Discharge

The ultimate goal of the treatment plan is to stabilize clients and prepare them for discharge. Discharge planning begins at the moment of admission. Inpatient interventions are intended to help individuals learn strategies that are transferable to their lives outside of the hospital (Nolan, 2011).

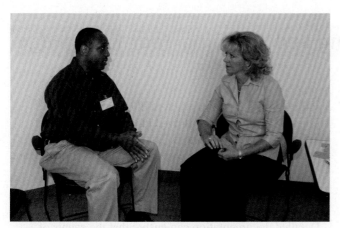

FIGURE 19.5 The nurse is discussing important components of follow-up care with the spouse of a client about to be discharged from an acute care psychiatric facility.

A lient's optimal level of functioning is the primary goal. Therefore, if a client has lived independently prior to admission to an inpatient setting, the goal is to return the client back home. However, doing so may not always be realistic or feasible. In such cases, the goal is to stabilize and discharge the client to the least restrictive environment possible.

Discharge planning also involves family members who assume care and responsibility for clients (Figure 19.5). The plan for discharge should be appropriate for all parties involved: the client, the family, and the institution. Many discharge plans are time consuming and require more intensive medical and psychological testing. A client may need to be medically cleared, or the team may need to prove that the client is, in fact, in need of further placement. This process can take days or weeks to complete, and the whole team's expertise is utilized. A client's insurance carrier also affects the direction of discharge planning. One's insurance may dictate where an individual can go after discharge. Discharge planning is especially difficult when clients are in need of additional services that are not covered by their insurance, or perhaps they do not have insurance benefits. In such cases, the case manager and social worker become a critical component of the treatment plan.

Once a client is discharged from the inpatient treatment setting, continued treatment and follow-up are imperative for continued progress. Assertive Community Treatment (ACT) teams have become more of a mainstay of the community mental health center. ACT teams are comprised of multiple disciplines, including nurses, physicians, and social workers who provide intensive support for clients who may be at risk for decompensation after discharge. This approach is client centered and provides holistic care that allows for reintegration into the community environment (see Chap. 20).

Checkpoint Questions

9. When does discharge planning begin?

10. If a client cannot reach his or her optimal level of function, what would be the most realistic goal of treatment?

Reviewing and Applying Your Knowledge

Chapter Summary

• Inpatient care, also referred to as hospital-based treatment, requires fulfillment of specific criteria that insurance providers generally set forth. Candidates most likely to receive inpatient treatment are those who pose a risk of harm to self or others or those who are unable to function or care for themselves.

• Acute care hospitals are highly structured to optimize safety. Clients with psychiatric diagnoses admitted to hospitals generally remain there for 3 to 7 days. Long-term hospitalization occurs for clients whose conditions require more than 7 days for stabilization. Partial (day) hospitalization programs are for clients who continue to need supervision but not long-term admission.

• Inpatient psychiatric treatment does not occur exclusively in general hospitals. A wide range of treatment settings includes psychiatric units within general hospitals, psychiatric specialty units, nonpsychiatric units, and scatter beds.

• The role of psychiatric nurses caring for clients in inpatient environments is complex and includes multiple responsibilities.

• Clients may be admitted on a voluntary or involuntary basis. With *voluntary admission*, clients (or parents or mental health or legal guardians with authority) make an autonomous decision to seek inpatient psychiatric treatment by submitting a formal, written request. *Involuntary commitment* requires proof that a client is (1) mentally ill, (2) a danger to self or to others, and (3) unable to care for self. States have the authority to involuntarily commit people for psychiatric treatment by either police power or *parens patriae* power.

• Psychiatric nurses manage the therapeutic environment and implement strategies that contribute to the overall community. A therapeutic community facilitates safety, optimal daily functioning, appropriate interpersonal interactions, and movement toward independent living.

• Observation levels are scheduled as formal, routine, or general (hourly checks); frequent (30- to 15-minute checks); or constant (staff member remains with the client at all times).

• Psychiatric workers conduct frequent environmental tours to ensure that no spaces, objects, or people on the unit will pose a danger to clients, staff, and visitors.

• Milieu therapy is also known as the maintenance of the therapeutic environment. The provision of such a setting assists in stabilization of clients with mental illness—specifically, improved thought processes and more appropriate behaviors. Traditional milieu therapy consists of containment, support, validation, structure, and involvement.

• Documentation is done for the welfare of the client and for the legal welfare of the nurse and the institution. Detailed documentation can ensure that the events of today are remembered in the future. The client's medical record should directly reflect what occurred at any given time during a client's hospitalization.

• Discharge planning begins at the time of admission and aims to promote client achievement of his or her optimal level of functioning. Discharge planning involves family members who assume care and responsibility for clients and should be appropriate for all parties involved.

Study Questions

1. Within the inpatient milieu, which of the following freedoms does the client retain?

   a. Expressing feelings in a socially acceptable manner that is not verbally or physically abusive to others.

   b. Collaborating with psychiatric professionals on a care plan addressing presenting complaint, inpatient treatment, and discharge planning.

   c. Recovering from crisis in a structured environment where safeguards disallow objects that can be used to harm self or others.

   d. Participating in the least restrictive containment measures of restraint and seclusion when needed to ensure the safety of self and/or others.

2. A nurse is preparing to orient a group of new staff members at an acute care psychiatric hospital. When describing the therapeutic milieu, which of the following would the nurse review? Select all that apply.

   a. Multidisciplinary care

   b. Participation from family and support people of clients

   c. Limit setting

   d. Behavioral interventions

   e. Client and family education

3. Which of the following reflects most accurately the direct effects of managed care on inpatient treatment?

   a. Psychiatric care must occur in a short period of time.

   b. Family members need to be involved in planning care.

   c. Clients require follow-up or provision for continuum of care.

   d. All treatment team members should be involved with planning.

References

Allen, D., Nesnera, A., & Souther, J. (2009). Executive-level reviews of seclusion and restraint promote interdisciplinary collaboration an innovation. *Journal of the American Psychiatric Nurses Association, 15*(4), 260–264.

Bowers, L. (2005). Reasons for admission and their implications for the nature of acute inpatient psychiatric nursing. *Journal of Psychiatric Mental Health Nursing, 12*(2), 231–236.

Burlingame, G. M., Ridge, N., Matsuno, J., Hwang, A. D., & Earnshaw, D. (2006). Educational needs of inpatients with severe & persistent mental illness: A partial replication. *Journal of Psychosocial Nursing and Mental Health Services, 44*(5), 38–43.

Cardell, R., Bratcher, K., & Quinnett, P. (2009). Revisiting "suicide proofing" an inpatient unit through environmental safeguards: A review. *Perspectives in Psychiatric Care, 45*(1), 36–44.

Doerfler, L., Moran, P., & Hannigan, K. (2011). Situations associated with admission to an acute care inpatient psychiatric unit. *Psychological Services, 7*(4), 254–265.

Gunderson, J. (1978). Defining the therapeutic processes in psychiatric milieus. *Psychiatry, 41,* 327–335.

Ignelzi, J., Stinson, B., Raia, J., Osinowo, T., Ostrowski, L., & Schwirian, J. (2007). Utilizing risk-of-violence findings for continuity of care. *Psychiatric Services, 58*(4), 452–454.

Joint Commission Resources. (2007). *Suicide prevention: Toolkit for implementing national patient safety goal 15A.* Oakbrook Terrace, IL: Author.

Jones, J., Bowers, L., Whittington, R., & Bhui, K. (2010). Psychiatric wards: Places of safety? *Journal of Psychiatric and Mental Health Nursing, 17,* 124–130.

Kynoch, K., Wu, C., & Chang, A. (2009). The effectiveness of interventions in the prevention and management of aggressive behaviours in patients admitted to an acute hospital setting: A systematic review. *Joanna Briggs Institute Library of Systematic Reviews, 7*(6), 175–223.

Mahoney, J., Palyo, N., Napier, G., & Giordano, J. (2009). The therapeutic milieu reconceptualised for the 21st century. *Archives of Psychiatric Nursing, 23*(6), 423–429.

Manna, M. (2010). Effectiveness of formal observation in inpatient psychiatry in preventing adverse outcomes: The state of the science. *Journal of Psychiatric and Mental Health Nursing, 17,* 268–273.

Mark, T. L., Vandivort-Warren, R., Owens, P. L., Buck, J. A., Levit, K. R., Coffey, R. M., & Stocks, C. (2010). Psychiatric discharges in community hospitals with and without psychiatric units: How many and for whom? *Psychiatric Services, 61*(6), 562–568.

Moylan, L. B., & Cullinan, M. (2011). Frequency of assault and severity of injury of psychiatric nurses in relation to the nurses' decision to restrain. *Journal of Psychiatric and Mental Health Nursing, 18,* 526–534.

National Center for Health Statistics. (2010). *Health, United States, 2010: With special feature on death and dying.* Hyattsville, MD: Author. Retrieved from http://www.cdc.gov/nchs/data/hus/hus10.pdf

Nolan, P. (2011). Disengaging from acute inpatient psychiatric care: A description of service users' experiences and views. *Journal of Psychiatric and Mental Health Nursing, 18,* 359–367.

Priebe, S., McCabe, R., Schutzwohl, M., Kiejna, A., Nawka, P., Raboch, J., ... Kallert, T. (2011). Patient characteristics predicting better treatment outcomes in day hospitals compared with inpatient wards. *Psychiatric Services, 62*(3), 278–284.

Sclar, D., & Robinson, L. (2010). Hospital admission for schizophrenia and discharge against medical advice in the United States. *The Primary Care Companion to the Journal of Clinical Psychiatry, 12*(2). Retrieved from http://www.ncbi.nlm.nih.gov/pmc/articles/PMC2911003

Sharfstein, S., & Dickerson, F. (2009). Hospital psychiatry for the twenty-first century. *Health Affairs, 28*(3), 685–688.

Thibeaut, C., Trudeau, K., d'Entremont, M., & Brown, T. (2010). Understanding the milieu experiences of patients on an acute inpatient psychiatric unit. *Archives of Psychiatric Nursing, 24*(4), 216–226.

Yalom, I., & Leszcz, M. (2005). *Theory and practice of group psychotherapy* (4th ed.). New York, NY: Basic Books.

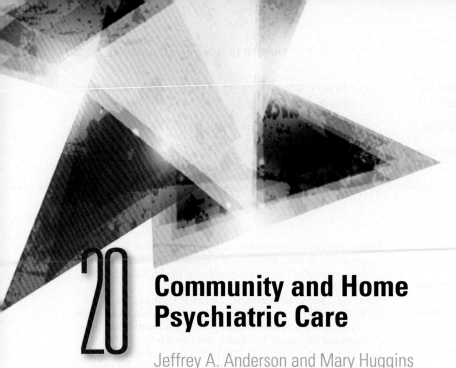

20 Community and Home Psychiatric Care

Jeffrey A. Anderson and Mary Huggins

LEARNING OBJECTIVES

On completion of this chapter, you should be able to accomplish the following:

- Identify the levels of prevention of mental illness.
- Describe potential interventions for primary, secondary, and tertiary prevention of mental health problems.
- Define the term *community support system.*
- Describe the philosophical context of the community support initiative.
- Identify essential components of a community support system.
- Compare models of community support programs.
- Outline the purpose of systems of care for children with multisystem needs and their families.
- Explain the importance of service coordination to the effectiveness of a community support system.
- Identify trends that affect social policy regarding the care of people with severe mental illnesses.
- Explain essential features of psychiatric home care.
- Analyze factors that influence psychiatric home care nursing, including policy, economics, client populations, and the structure of interdisciplinary collaboration.

This chapter gives an overview of the promotion and protection of mental health in communities. It explains levels of prevention, which help shape a community's health and determine systems and programs that it needs. The chapter also describes the importance of community support systems and rehabilitation to prevent the development, recurrence, or exacerbation of psychiatric disorders. It explores the effects of the community support movement on delivery systems and projects trends that will affect the continued provision of appropriate and effective community-based care.

An important component of community health involves the delivery of **psychiatric home care nursing**. Nurses who work in this specialty provide holistic psychiatric nursing care on a visiting basis to people needing and qualifying for assistance. They conduct psychiatric and physical assessment and direct interventions such as behavioral management, crisis intervention, psychoeducation, in-home detoxification, medication management, case management, consultation with colleagues, and others. This chapter reviews dynamics and special considerations related to this unique setting for practice.

COMMUNITY MENTAL HEALTH

Nurses focus on *holistic health,* or all aspects of physical, emotional, and spiritual well-being. They encourage individuals, families, and communities to engage in and support various practices to avoid health problems or to prevent their recurrence. Such practices involve both physical health and mental health.

Each person functions not in isolation but within a larger society. Additionally, family and group systems interact, communicating with one another to produce accepted societal norms. As a result, a network forms through which individuals, families, and groups influence entire societies. In turn, the larger society shapes and influences individuals, families, and groups. This network system has required the field of nursing to expand its understanding of *client* to mean not only one person but an entire community. In this way, the community becomes the client (Nies & McEwan, 2007).

The concept of *community mental health* addresses the collective mental health of all people within a particular community. To evaluate and address a community's mental health needs, nurses first must assess internal aggregate groups. An **aggregate group** is a group of people that has at least one commonality among its members. Examples related to psychiatric nursing may include people who are homeless (see Chap. 38), adolescents with mood disorders (see Chap. 36), and victims of abuse (see Chap. 33). **Aggregate mental health** refers to the way in which families and groups within a given environment contribute to or enhance interactions among people along the mental health–illness continuum (Nies & McEwan, 2007).

Evolution

Historical, political, cultural, and economic factors have contributed to the current understanding of and circumstances surrounding community mental health. In 1955, Congress passed the Mental Health Study Act to examine the needs of people with mental illness. The findings of this effort led to recommendations for community-based residential and educational programs, as well as early and intensive treatment of acute mental illness. They also suggested a need for fewer and smaller mental institutions, with a shift of care for mental illness from long-term government-run hospitals to community health clinics.

The provisions of the Community Mental Health Center Act of 1963 included prevention, early intervention, and quality clinical mental health centers. The deinstitutionalization of clients began (ie, moving clients from more restrictive hospital-type settings to less restrictive community-based settings), saving many dollars (see Chaps. 1, 15, and 38). The U.S. government was supposed to make funding available to develop community mental health clinics. Unfortunately, the needs of people with mental illness exceeded the services offered. As a result, many people who were deinstitutionalized became homeless, resorted to crime to survive, or both (see Chaps. 21 and 38).

In the 1970s, the first community support program introduced the concept of the **case manager**, a person who would coordinate the many functions required to address the various needs of clients with mental illness living in the community. One case manager would be responsible for several clients within a community. The intended goal was to reduce inpatient hospitalizations.

In 1980, Congress passed the Mental Health Systems Act to address the needs of people with chronic mental illness, including older adults, minorities, and children. At the time, the government failed to implement its provisions. However, subsequent policies and programs incorporated several of its key concepts, among them increasing the role of the states in developing mental health services and focusing on high-risk, high-need target populations.

The 1990 Americans With Disabilities Act helped to address the needs of people with mental and physical disabilities. Its major provisions mandated the inclusion of people with disabilities in employment, public service programs and activities, and public accommodations (Perlin, 1994). At the same time, many advocacy groups were beginning to form and emerge. These included the National Alliance on Mental Illness (NAMI) and the National Alliance for Mental Patients, two organizations that involve consumers and families (see Chaps. 1 and 15). These are just two examples of many groups that offer valuable services to the community by representing mental health issues and participating in discussions on national health care reform.

The current focus on **psychosocial rehabilitation (PSR)** represents a paradigm shift in how services are provided. The traditional medical model of doctors directing care and focusing efforts on curing illnesses is being replaced by an interdisciplinary model in which professionals collaborate with the client and his or her family to improve and maximize function within the client's normal daily environment. Models of PSR focus on strengths, skills, and community supports, rather than diseases and illnesses. Programs purposely are informal and age and culturally appropriate. Their focus is empowerment so that people with serious and persistent mental illness (SPMI) become contributing members of the community within a supportive setting. Many programs developed by the federal community support program are PSR programs (Corrigan et al., 2007).

Legislatures currently need to address the continued needs of people with mental illness in community settings. Areas of concern include access to and reimbursement for rendered health care services. The power of change lies within each local community. Nurses can help to address these needs.

Levels of Prevention

As noted, health care delivery traditionally focused on treating ill people, rather than preventing illness. With the emergence of the *Healthy People* initiative (U.S. Department of Health and Human Services [USDHHS], 2007), both society and the health care industry have shifted focus, emphasizing health promotion and health maintenance. These ideas include levels of prevention: primary, secondary, and tertiary (Table 20.1). For individuals and communities, nurses use the levels of prevention to identify and implement strategies to maintain and attain optimal mental health.

Primary Prevention

The goals of **primary prevention** are to *stop* mental disorders from occurring and to *reduce* identified cases of psychiatric disorders and disabilities within a population. Primary prevention consists of two concepts: health promotion and disease prevention. *Health promotion* aims to ensure the continued well-being of people and communities already considered healthy. *Disease prevention* focuses on protecting against any potentially harmful threat. Its goal is to protect as many people as possible from any harmful consequences of a specific health threat.

Nurses design primary prevention interventions not only to address general health concerns but also to target populations known to be at high risk for mental health problems. Although the focus of mental health promotion is prevention, these efforts also help prevent relapse in consumers who already experience mental distress. For example, children who live in poverty or experience undue mental distress comprise a high-risk group (Dashiff et al., 2009). If these children do not receive appropriate and effective interventions, poor mental health and social outcomes are likely when they become adults. Schools throughout the country also are pursuing primary prevention efforts in mental health (Adelman & Taylor, 2000).

Certain adults also are at high risk for mental health problems, including those experiencing adverse life situations such as unemployment, divorce, or loss of a loved one. Mental health interventions enable these individuals to deal with and grow from a current crisis. Such interventions also can prevent further deterioration and associated problems. Research has shown that employment is the single most important factor in assisting people with mental illness to recover and to avoid relapse (Resnick et al., 2003). Thus, research can function as a form of primary prevention. In the field of mental health recovery, former "mental patients" have begun to advocate and work together to form highly effective prevention strategies. Efforts also are under way to implement evidence-based practices (EBPs) in community mental health settings. EBPs are well-defined clinical interventions that have *demonstrated effectiveness* and *can be replicated* across settings (Salyers & Tsemberis, 2007).

Community mental health nurses try to incorporate health promotion and primary prevention by interacting with healthy people and attempting to maintain and enhance their well-being. Nurses include family members and caregivers in developing strategies to promote mental health because caregivers who also become incapacitated are less apt to continue caring for the person with mental illness (see Chap. 15). Examples of mental health promotion include promoting parent–infant bonding, developing age-appropriate social skills, and creating environments that favor positive adaptation. Other examples are reviewed in Box 20.1.

Findings from many studies have shown that most adults with SPMI experience comorbid symptoms such as panic, anxiety, depression, phobias, and substance abuse (Sokal et al., 2004). For this reason, children and adolescents require appropriate efforts to prevent problems from accumulating. Interventions at onset as well as a smooth

TABLE 20.1 Interventions According to Levels of Prevention

Level of Prevention	Definition	Examples
Primary	Prevent problem from occurring	Nurse promotes self-esteem, teaches alternatives to violence, and encourages political involvement for clients.
Secondary	Early diagnosis and treatment	Nurse holds conflict management classes, teaches gun safety, conducts mental health screenings, and makes necessary referrals.
Tertiary	Continued support and rehabilitation	Nurse leads support groups, holds refresher courses on conflict management, and supports and reinforces nonviolent behavior.

BOX 20.1 Mental Health Promotion Interventions

For Adults

- Home visits to provide social support to pregnant women from disadvantaged communities
- Cognitive–behavioral therapy
- Job-searching skills
- Problem-solving skills
- Communication techniques
- Stress management
- Respite care or some type of psychological support for long-term caregivers
- Coping skills (job loss, birth, caregiving, separation, divorce, bereavement, poverty)
- Parent–child interaction training
- Exercise programs

For Children

- Early intervention education for preschoolers from disadvantaged communities
- Social skills training to deal with behavioral problems, improve peer relationships, enhance positive attitudes
- Cognitive–behavioral skills training
- Wraparound supports
- Functional Family Therapy
- Emotional support for children experiencing death of a loved one or divorce or separation of parents
- Social support visits for parents (to target available community resources or ways to achieve educational and occupational goals)
- Support groups for children with divorced parents
- Bereavement groups

transition from the child to the adult mental health systems can interrupt the downward spiral many people experience. Such strategies, along with recognition of the genetic components of several psychiatric disorders, assist nurses in better identifying familial and environmental factors to focus their early intervention efforts.

Secondary Prevention

Secondary prevention focuses on interventions that identify mental health problems early and reduce the duration and prevalence of mental illness. It includes early diagnosis and prompt treatment of any disabilities. Examples for community mental health nurses include conducting screening surveys that focus on identifying mental illness in people within schools or the community, referring clients for mental health treatment, and providing crisis intervention to a community that has encountered a natural or man-made disaster (see Chap. 35). Another example is the provision of depression screenings in conjunction with Mental Health month in May (see Chap. 27). For school-aged individuals, secondary prevention can include having a mental health therapist who sees student-clients during the school day or a social worker who provides social skills training to targeted students in need of such training.

Tertiary Prevention

Tertiary prevention is the final level of prevention. Its focus is rehabilitation and ways to minimize residual effects and ongoing challenges for people who have encountered mental health problems. Examples include Assertive Community Treatment, vocational rehabilitation, self-help groups, systems of care and wraparound for children and families, and sufficient residential and independent living services.

Checkpoint Questions

1. What is the focus of psychosocial rehabilitation?
2. What two concepts are associated with primary prevention?

COMMUNITY SUPPORT SYSTEMS

A **community support system** is a network of people committed to helping a vulnerable population meet its needs and reach its potentials without unnecessary isolation or exclusion. This basic philosophy of care is meant to address, humanely, the needs of adults whose SPMI limits their ability to function in the primary areas of daily living.

The Center for Mental Health Services (CMHS) is the U.S. agency that leads national efforts to improve prevention and treatment of mental illness for all Americans. "CMHS pursues its mission by helping states improve and increase the quality and range of their treatment, rehabilitation, and support services for people with mental illness, their families, and communities. Further, it encourages a range of programs—such as systems of care—to respond to the increasing number of mental, emotional, and behavioral problems among America's children" (Substance Abuse & Mental Health Services Administration, 2012). Community support is a primary focus of CMHS. The agency influences the delivery of broadranged services and support needed for people with SPMI to live in the least-restrictive environment possible. It also recognizes the importance of quality of life and focuses on moving service provision from restrictive settings (eg, residential placements) to home and community settings.

To help improve documented poor outcomes for children with serious emotional disturbances and related mental health problems, the Child and Adolescent Service System Program (CASSP) was established in 1984. Its ongoing goal is to ensure that all children considered emotionally disturbed or at risk for psychiatric illnesses receive needed mental health services (New York State Office of Mental Health, 2006).

Components of a Community Support System

A community support system creates and delivers community-based care to a specific population who traditionally required long-term hospitalization. It includes a range of services: health care, mental health care, rehabilitation, social networks, housing arrangements, and educational and employment opportunities. In addition, it provides several different program models (discussed later). The goal is to move clients from restrictive settings into the community.

Typically, a single agency coordinates the community support system and negotiates among the various agencies that form the network of services (ie, the provider network). This agency is responsible for articulating the philosophical and operational basis for the network and promoting the active participation of all those invested (eg, clients, family members, government officials, and health care providers). The community support system will incorporate many programs in an effort to provide comprehensive services needed to meet the diverse needs of individuals with SPMI. To achieve the comprehensiveness required, the system needs to both maintain flexibility and incorporate the positive elements of several generic models, while at the same time, promoting seamless service delivery.

Essential components of a community support system are listed in Box 20.2.

Community Support Programs

Within community support systems, community support programs (CSPs) address the specific needs of individuals. Since 1977, all 50 states, the District of Columbia, and several U.S. territories have developed CSPs. These CSPs need visibility and continuing support from all levels of government to effect services at the systems level (eg, police,

housing authorities, local planning boards). CSPs are based on values implemented at three levels: individual, agency, and network. These values focus on the person; the consumer is central to the system. As such, the person stays involved in decisions that affect the needed services. The central theme is empowerment, recognizing the following three tenets:

1. All people are valuable and should be afforded dignity, respect, and the opportunity to take full advantage of their human, legal, and social rights.
2. Every human being is capable of growth, development, and learning.
3. Services should be provided in a normative and socially valued way.

This approach requires a holistic understanding that each person is an individual with hope for a wide range of outcomes, including considerable improvement and recovery. SPMI, although devastating, is no longer associated with hopelessness. Hope is essential, not only for the person, but for those helping him or her (Stein & Santos, 1998).

Guiding Principles

The overriding principles of CSPs are respect for each person's dignity and specific needs and the fostering of empowerment, rather than dependency. The goal is to enable those with SPMI to remain in the community and

---

BOX 20.2 Essential Components of a Community Support System

- Identification and assertive outreach to the at-risk population to inform clients of and ensure their access to needed services
- Adequate mental health care, including diagnostic evaluations, management of prescribed psychotropic medications, periodic examinations, community-based psychiatric or psychological services, and specialized counseling or treatment (eg, for substance abuse)
- Links with medical and dental services, including help in applying for medical assistance benefits
- Twenty-four-hour quick-response assistance to enable both family and client to cope effectively with crises while maintaining the client's status as a functioning community member; this element requires all-day crisis services provided by trained professionals at various sites, including at home, in the criminal justice system, and on the job (see Chap. 21)
- Psychosocial and vocational services through various rehabilitative options for an indefinite duration, focusing primarily on improving the client's ability to function in normal social roles (ie, training in daily living and community living skills, social skills, interests, and leisure activities) and assisting him or her to find and use appropriate employment services
- A range of rehabilitative and supportive housing options based on choice and offering necessary support, incentives, and encouragement for the client to accept increasing responsibility for his or her own life
- Backup support, assistance, consultation, and education for families, friends, landlords, employers, and community

agencies as well as referrals to family self-help or advocacy programs (eg, NAMI, Reach) to maximize the benefits of and minimize the problems associated with the client living in the community
- Recognition and involvement of concerned community members and endorsement of the natural support system, including consumer and family self-help groups, churches, community organizations, commerce, and industry in the development and implementation of community support systems
- Assistance with application for entitlements (financial, medical, housing, and other benefits) that are crucial to meeting basic human needs, including food, clothing, shelter, general medical and dental care, and personal safety
- Protection of the client's rights, provision of information regarding basic civil rights and available resources, and access to advocacy and grievance procedures to ensure that appropriate mechanisms are in place to protect these rights
- Case management (a single person or team) responsible for helping the person make informed choices, ensuring timely access to needed assistance, providing opportunities and encouragement for self-help, and coordinating all services to meet the client's needs
- Provision of these components through an integrated system that responds to the person's needs, including those individualized to specific circumstances (eg, older adult, child, homelessness, parole, developmental disability, hearing impairment)

function as independently as possible. People facing psychiatric challenges are a diverse group. Each person has unique concerns, abilities, motivations, and problems. Therefore, CSPs must include services that provide for self-determination, individuation, normalization of settings and treatment offerings, least restrictive settings, and maximization of mutual assistance and self-help. In addition, they must be culturally competent and accountable to their clients (see Chap. 6).

Models of Community Support Programs
A major influence in the development of various models has been the increased voice of consumers in recovery. People recovering from mental illness have influenced legislation and policies, services, and assessments (both at individual and system levels). Their efforts have contributed to substantial gains in integrating the social service system.

Although all CSPs share similarities, they differ in comprehensiveness and the degree to which they provide or broker services. The preferred model for people with SPMI embraces psychosocial rehabilitation, although the configuration of offerings may be distinct because of factors relating to local policies, demographics, or funding. However, all models embrace the principles of psychiatric rehabilitation and focus on individually tailored programs, with realistic goals based on assessment of the client's strengths and weaknesses.

Principles basic to psychiatric rehabilitation, and thus to all CSPs, include the following:

- The primary focus is to improve the capabilities and competence of the person with mental illness. Alleviation of symptoms is secondary.
- Insight is not a primary goal. The focus is on the person's ability to function.
- Provision of services is eclectic and uses various therapeutic constructs.
- Improvement of vocational outcomes is a central focus.
- Positive expectations and hope are essential to the process.
- A deliberate increase in dependency, as in sheltered settings, may or may not be a first step.
- The program seeks the active participation and involvement of the person in rehabilitation, the operation of programs, and the delivery of services so that rehabilitation occurs *with,* rather than *to,* the person.
- Development of individual skills and environmental resources is a fundamental intervention.

The services in CSPs are delivered mostly in real-life communities (in vivo) to promote the transfer of learning through modeling and immediate reinforcement. These sites include, but are not limited to, home, school, and work.

Assertive Community Treatment
Assertive Community Treatment (ACT) is a service delivery model that provides comprehensive, locally based treatment to people with SPMI (eg, see Salyers & Tsemberis, 2007). Unlike other community-based programs, ACT is not a linkage or brokerage case-management program, but a direct provider of highly individualized consumer services. Recipients have access to multidisciplinary, around-the-clock staffing from a psychiatric unit in the comfort of their own homes. To have the competencies and skills to meet multiple treatment, rehabilitation, and support needs, ACT team members are trained in psychiatry, social work, nursing, substance abuse treatment, and vocational rehabilitation.

The elements of ACT include the provision of psychopharmacology, individual supportive therapy, mobile crisis intervention, hospitalization (if necessary), and substance abuse treatment, including group therapy (for clients with a dual diagnosis). They also include rehabilitation services such as behaviorally oriented skill teaching (supportive and cognitive–behavioral therapy) and employment and education training and opportunities. Finally, ACT provides support services such as education and skill teaching to family members, assistance with legal and advocacy services, financial support, supported housing, money management services, and transportation (Allness, 2003).

Clients who receive ACT spend significantly less time in hospitals, have higher rates of employment, earn more income, experience more positive social relationships, express greater satisfaction with life, and are less symptomatic than are those in non-ACT treatment groups. They spend more time in the community, resulting in decreased family burden (see Chap. 15). In addition, the ACT model has shown a small economic advantage over institutional care. Despite ACT's documented treatment success, only a fraction of those with the greatest needs have access to this uniquely effective program.

Examples of Programs
Nurses must recognize that no one program fits the needs of all people with mental illness. A system based on a single model is not inclusive and when promoting programs, health care providers must avoid falling into a one-size-fits-all mentality (the "model trap"). Effective service systems provide various program types so that people requiring treatment can obtain services that best meet their specific needs. All the programs identified as examples in the next section share the core elements necessary for effective psychosocial programming. They are based on the principles of psychiatric rehabilitation and focus on individually tailored program plans with realistic goals.

All psychiatric rehabilitation programs follow the same basic principles; however, implementation of these principles varies. A movement is burgeoning to ensure the implementation of evidence-based strategies and approaches (Evidence-Based Practice Spotlight 20.1). The following sections discuss some models.

CLUBHOUSE MODEL. The clubhouse model evolved from Fountain House, founded in New York City in 1948. Its members fully participate in the program's operation. Services

---

EVIDENCE-BASED PRACTICE SPOTLIGHT 20.1

Psychiatric Rehabilitation

Recently, the Substance and Mental Health Services Administration and its Center for Mental Health Services announced the development of the first six Evidence-Based Practice Implementation Resource Kits, which were created to encourage mental health programs to use evidence-based practices and science-to-service strategies. The six identified areas are as follows:

1. *Illness Management and Recovery*, which strongly emphasizes helping people set, pursue, and implement personal goals through teaching about mental illnesses and recovery strategies
2. *Medication Management Approaches in Psychiatry* as an overall treatment for severe mental illness

3. *Assertive Community Treatment* to assist people to stay out of the hospital
4. *Family Psychoeducation* involving partnerships
5. *Supported Employment* focusing on competitive employment with supports
6. *Co-occurring Disorder* to assist people in recovering from both mental health and substance abuse at the same time

Although many PSR programs have not yet been included specifically, they have demonstrated in practice their effectiveness with clients.

---

usually are divided into four major areas: (1) social-recreational, (2) vocational, (3) residential, and (4) educational.

Members can participate in various activities (eg, meal preparation, newsletter publication, janitorial services), as well as in decisions regarding program operation. Evaluation indicates that this model is effective in reducing hospitalizations and improving community functioning, particularly in vocation and independent living for long-term members (Mowbray et al., 2006; Schonebaum et al., 2006).

FAIRWEATHER LODGE. Fairweather Lodge began in 1960. It uses the hospital as a training center for clients who subsequently move into the community to live in a lodge and operate a small business. Group norms and peer support form the foundation for this model. All members participate fully in the lodge and the workplace, using appropriate roles and habits. Evaluation indicates reduced recidivism and increased community employment activities (Fairweather Lodge, 2007).

CONSUMER-RUN ALTERNATIVES. These self-help programs are based on the idea that planning, administering, delivering, and evaluating services should be done *for* consumers *by* consumers. Their core elements are voluntary participation, consumer control, and empowerment. Several such alternatives have been developed. Social, recreational, and educational services frequently are added, and also may include community and public education and advocacy at both the individual and public policy levels. Consumer alternatives also have been started in residential, crisis, and vocational services.

Several states have developed offices devoted to consumer programming and advocacy within their offices of mental health. The focus on outcomes and satisfaction with this model have led to several grants to states to assess the effects of these programs.

COMMUNITY WORKER PROGRAMS. Community worker programs rely on ordinary citizens, called community workers, to provide a range of services, including companionship, emotional support, teaching, and assistance in accessing appropriate services. The community worker complements professional mental health services by modeling appropriate behaviors and monitoring the consumer's level of functioning. In the community supportive care variation (Rhinelander model), which originated in rural Wisconsin, the county pays lay citizens to provide community support. This model emphasizes one-to-one relationships. The Compeer variation uses volunteers to provide caring, supportive relationships. It originated in Rochester, New York, as an adjunct to therapy and fills gaps when clients lack natural supports.

Checkpoint Questions

3. What four areas of service does the Clubhouse Model provide?
4. Who provides services in community worker programs?

Systems of Care

As a group, children with serious emotional and behavioral challenges have the poorest long-term outcomes of any group with a disability (Blanchard et al., 2006). These children have serious problems in several domains, including social behavior, emotional and behavioral functioning, educational performance, and overall functioning. Reform efforts have focused on alternative ways to provide services in which solutions to problems are based on the social contexts of children with serious emotional and behavioral challenges (Adelman & Taylor, 2000). Contemporary approaches indicate that interventions should be individualized, coordinated, and informed by the best available research (Hernandez & Hodges, 2003). Although different practice disciplines (eg, education, nursing, child welfare) continue to focus on different outcomes, improving cross-system collaboration among them is critical in the children's social services arena (Hodges et al., 2003). Entire systems and the networks that make up those systems must be considered to maintain organizational changes.

Although system-level change in children's social services might be initiated in various ways, the focus of this discussion turns to systems of care as an emerging mechanism for reform.

Beginning with the CASSP in 1984, a new philosophy of service provision for children with serious emotional disturbances evolved that emphasized several important principles (New York State Office of Mental Health, 2006):

• Services should be community based and provided in the least-restrictive setting possible.
• Services, assessments, and values should be strength based, instead of deficit oriented.
• Parents or caregivers should be partners in providing services, by both identifying needed services and designing individual service plans for their children.
• Service systems and providers should be culturally competent and provide all services within each family's unique cultural and ethnic perspectives.

Since enactment of the CASSP, other essential values have been added: service coordination, individualization of services, local- and state-level leadership, focus on natural and informal supports, and flexible funding.

Service systems that adopt and use these principles often are referred to as **systems of care** (Stroul & Friedman, 1986). These comprehensive spectrums of mental health and other necessary services are organized into coordinated networks. In that way, providers can address more appropriately the various and changing needs of children and adolescents with serious emotional disturbances and their families. All systems of care use methods to connect the various systems, agencies, and people (including family) that participate in the child's care. The goal is to ensure effective, ongoing communication among everyone involved so that services and interventions are consistent and directed toward common goals. In operationalizing systems of care, team-based **wraparound** approaches appear to be growing in popularity (Walker & Schutte, 2004). While both concepts often are used interchangeably, a wraparound approach focuses on what happens at the team level, while systems of care focus on creating and sustaining the structures and partnerships needed to bring various agencies and systems together.

Wraparound teams typically include one or more family members, individuals who support the family (eg, extended family members, family friends, a neighbor, a religious practitioner), a *care coordinator*, the young person her- or himself, and representatives from the various agencies involved with the family. The role of the care coordinator overseeing this process is to convene and guide a multiagency team (a.k.a. child and family team) responsible for organizing and managing all services a child receives (Dosser et al., 2002). The goal is to bring the resources, strengths, and concerns of all the systems and professionals involved with the family to bear on common objectives (Walker & Schutte, 2004). On "wrap-teams," family members and providers develop comprehensive plans, sharing ideas across agencies and systems. For example, a team might help a young person develop appropriate peer and adult relationships by implementing an intervention simultaneously in the home, community, and school. Then the team monitors cross-system goals and adjusts them as needed to ensure progress (Walker & Schutte, 2004). Teams typically meet once a month, but more often when necessary. Teams are both flexible in responding to individual situations and also standardized such that they adhere to the core system of care values described earlier. Systems of care challenge nurses, teachers, social workers, and others to move past professional barriers and create partnerships with families and one another.

The Dawn Project, located in Indianapolis, Indiana, is an example of a system of care (Choices, 2012). Founded in 1997, the Dawn Project is funded jointly by county and state governments and administered through a contract with a private, nonprofit care management organization. At its core, the Dawn Project provides a coordinated, community-based network of services for children, youth, and their families who are involved with multiple systems (Anderson et al., 2002). Its *provider network* includes more than 100 child-serving organizations and agencies. The impetus for the Dawn Project system of care was the recognition that increasing numbers of children with serious emotional and behavioral problems were being sent away from home, including costly placements out of the county or state. To date, the Dawn Project has provided services and support for Indiana children and youth with the most serious psychiatric challenges. Findings from a longitudinal evaluation suggested that clinical improvements in functioning, strengths, and symptoms over time are significant, use of more restrictive settings is reduced, and rates of recidivism are lower for those who successfully complete the program (Anderson et al., 2003, 2008).

Public Policy and Trends

Community support systems have focused on public policy issues. Certain areas have become obstacles at worst and challenges at best to the delivery of community-based care for people with severe mental illness.

Chronicity of SPMI

A growing body of knowledge continues to identify mental illness as a disease of the brain (see Chap. 2). SPMI can be chronic and debilitating, similar to multiple sclerosis or chronic heart disease. Recognition of this fact counters the myth of a "quick cure" and diminishes the belief that people with SPMI can live without supportive treatment such as medication and counseling.

Gross confusion persists about the relationship between diseases and their symptoms. Misunderstandings perpetuate the myth that SPMI precludes opportunities for rehabilitation. However, for most people mental illness is treatable. Services that focus on problem solving and the development of coping skills, in conjunction with administration of antipsychotic medications, can be effective ways to assist clients with SPMI. Health care providers must maintain and promote a vision of recovery within communities. They must facilitate processes that provide hope and optimism while

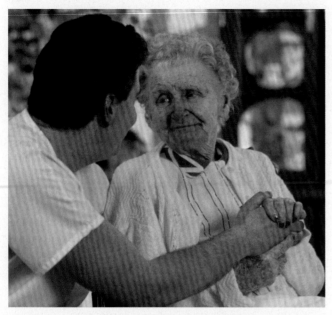

FIGURE 20.1 Nurses can help clients receiving ongoing psychiatric care in the community by coordinating services effectively and by instilling a sense of hope and optimism.

maintaining realistic expectations based on a client's specific coping abilities (Figure 20.1).

Stalled Resources

Conflicting federal, state, and local mandates have prevented resources, including funds and staff, from reaching communities. This can be best documented by reviewing the dramatic shift in funding responsibility during the past 50 years. In the late 1960s, most costs for those with mental illnesses rested with state governments (primarily in state hospitals). Recently, responsibility for community-based care has rested at the local level, with federal payments and reimbursements to support the individual. However, responsibility for overall planning and policy making has remained at the state level. Funding bases not intended to support people with mental illness have become the core for community-based treatment. Moreover, mental illness has been underreported systematically for several reasons, including stigma, lack of access, sensitivity of interviews, embarrassment, and reluctance to admit symptoms. This underreporting exacerbates the current system's inability to document accurately the need for services. The result is a system fragmented and characterized by multiple providers and inadequate funds (Stroul & Friedman, 1986). A consequence has been movement toward managed care.

Medicaid funding, although limited in noninstitutional settings, remains the primary source for poor people, including most people with SPMI. One result has been inappropriate admissions to nursing facilities and other institutions so that clients can receive appropriate care. In some states, commitment laws have become stringent to stem inappropriate admissions to state hospitals. Families and advocates of people with SPMI are trying actively to change these laws.

This activity is the result of both the difficulty they have experienced in admitting their friends and loved ones for treatment and their sense that hospitalization is necessary to address the client's needs appropriately. Although Medicaid is now paying for some community-based services for people with serious mental illness who need long-term support and maintenance, the fundamental policy question is how to fund those services known to be effective with a funding source developed primarily for medical services.

Poverty

Poverty is an overwhelming reality for many people with SPMI. Reliance on Supplemental Security Income (SSI) as the major source of financial support allows little opportunity for choices. Many people live in unlicensed facilities with little or no follow-up care. Their average monthly stipend barely meets their rent payments. Opportunities to improve finances are limited or nonexistent because these people lack funds for education, clothing, and transportation. In addition, limited stipends can buy only a level of housing found mostly in the poorest areas of cities.

When people in such circumstances find a job, the position usually is low paying and at entry level. Working clients with mental illness also risk losing the limited benefits available when they relied solely on SSI (eg, access to health care). Mental illness and stress further complicate this situation. Clients who are rehospitalized or cannot work on a long-term basis lose both benefits and medical insurance.

Reinstitutionalization

The fundamental lack of public policy and the potential dissolution of the current infrastructure have contributed to problems of "reinstitutionalization." Unlike the early institutions that housed those with mental illness in hospitals and asylums, current reinstitutionalization occurs in both hospitals and jails (see Chap. 21). As responsibility for people with SPMI remains in limbo, the large numbers of people who are inadequately housed or homeless can overwhelm local governments.

State hospitals that have not closed have downsized significantly. The result has been a second generation of people who have been deinstitutionalized and who have more serious disabilities than those in the past. Many of these individuals may have special behavioral problems that make living in the community difficult. The policy question becomes: What mix of services should replace the former state hospital system? Several community interventions have been developed to increase tenure and quality of life for people with SPMI. See Box 20.3.

Education

Another institution that experiences substantial challenges is education. Although the movement toward inclusion of children with disabilities into general education classrooms tends to require placement in the least-restrictive environment,

BOX 20.3 Community Alternatives to Rehospitalization for Clients With SPMI

- Community-based acute psychiatric intervention teams, treatment centers, or both to provide a positive environment either by moving the person to a homelike setting for short periods or by de-escalating and providing support in the person's own home
- Acute day care treatment or residential beds for people needing more support through an acute crisis
- Supported housing for people needing support while living in their own apartments or homes
- Cognitive–behavioral therapy for affective and anxiety disorders
- Consumer-focused outcomes such as quality of life, recovery, hope, and empowerment
- Employment as an expectation, including vocational coaches and peer-support programs that include self-help

schools have had a difficult time fully including children with serious emotional and behavioral challenges. Lack of funding, paucity of appropriate teacher training and supports, and issues related to stigma all present barriers to full and successful access to inclusive settings.

Psychopharmacology

People respond to medications differently. To provide accurate doses, providers need to understand how factors such as race, ethnicity, age, sex, and family history influence responses to drugs. Studies have shown variations in drug metabolism based on such factors. Improved availability and access to state-of-the-art medications will go far in reducing treatment disparities. However, effective interventions for minority subpopulations need further development to improve overall quality of care (USDHHS, 2001).

Stigma

Stigma toward those with psychiatric disorders may involve employment, housing, restrictive zoning, and segregated schooling. At the forefront of the antistigma campaigns are consumer and family movements. These groups demand involvement in the development of treatment alternatives. They provide advocacy, support, and knowledge regarding the disease—including realistic expectations—to other consumers, family members, and the general public. In many parts of the country, clients and families are involved in antistigma media watches and public education and advocacy. For more discussion on stigma, see Chapter 1.

Checkpoint Questions

5. What are the ongoing problems faced by providers of community support services?

6. What is a consequence of fragmentation of care versus implementing a system of care?

COMMUNITY PSYCHIATRIC NURSING

Nurses are in a unique position to assess the availability of individual and community supports. Furthermore, nurses can focus on a specific situation while retaining a holistic approach by blending the client's physical, mental, and social needs with community environmental norms. Nurses can serve to bridge the gaps among the medical model, hospital and rehabilitation model, and community; the psychiatrist and community caregiver; and the public and other health care providers. Nursing education emphasizes teamwork and shared responsibility to an extent rarely seen in other professions (Figure 20.2). When included in community teams, nurses enhance understanding of treatment alternatives, medications and side effects, and the importance of client education and teaching to reduce stress and thus alleviate episodes. This unique background is underscored as clients in the community are treated with new antipsychotic and other drugs requiring assertive outreach and monitoring to assist with compliance. Nurses understand the importance of physical movement to decrease muscle atrophy and other long-term effects resulting from lack of full range-of-motion exercise frequently associated with mental illness. They also work in many schools and participate on school committees responsible for designing and implementing individual education programs for children and youth with emotional disturbances, in addition to other disabilities.

As services shift from focusing on removal of disease to strengthening the ability of the individual to function in the community, nurses bring an understanding of the essential parts of treatment (medications, health care, and education) to the rehabilitative process. Thus, nurses can facilitate the shift from psychiatrically disabled to psychiatrically able.

The combination of inpatient, public health, and psychiatric nursing knowledge and physical assessment skills is imperative in community-based programs. Understanding the role of stress affords the nurse the ability to provide the integrative link among community resources, housing,

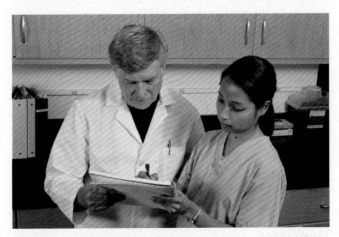

FIGURE 20.2 Collaboration and coordination are foundations of nursing education, making nurses eminently suitable to participating in community service teams for psychiatric clients.

vocation, social relationships, and psychiatric episodes. Nurses must be able to separate the disease from the social disability. Nursing education prepares nurses to teach consumers, professionals, and the public about psychiatric disability, medication effects and side effects, effects of stress on mental disorder, and interventions to diminish harm.

Nurses traditionally have worked with natural support systems in developing care plans. In many parts of the country, nurses have initiated contact with tribal healers, *curanderas,* midwives, or other healers. Thus, the integration of the nursing care process into the community support system is a logical extension of the nurse's role.

> ### Think About It 20.1
>
> At a community forum, several participants voice concern over a growing incidence of teenage drug use in the area. A task force is established to study the problem. You are selected as a member. Using the nursing process, explore steps that the task force might take to combat this problem.

PSYCHIATRIC HOME CARE

Home care provides an array of health-related services to clients and families in their places of residence, which include residential care facilities, group homes, and private homes, and is one part of a comprehensive continuous health care system. Home health care is one aspect of community health nursing, *not* an alternative to institutional care (Stanhope & Lancaster, 2008).

Psychiatric home health care services are appropriate for different age groups, clients with acute psychoses, clients with SPMI, and clients with AIDS. The psychiatric home care team customizes services for each client, depending on specific needs and problems, available services, and issues related to reimbursement (Case Vignette 20.1).

Services

Unlike hospital care, in which various services are delivered directly in the facility, home care agencies must outsource work and collaborate with mobile health care services to deliver comprehensive care in the homes of clients. The most commonly used services in psychiatric home care are medical care, social work, psychological services, pharmacy services, and various therapies such as physical, occupational, vocational, recreational, speech, and respiratory.

In addition, **home health aides** play a critical role. They often implement aspects of psychiatric home care in addition to providing transportation for clients to attend selected social functions necessary to regain psychological well-being. They also may deliver durable medical supplies and equipment when necessary.

Principles

Most home care agencies share the following principles:

- The home and community environments help clients sustain social, family, and self-care functions. Keeping

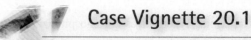
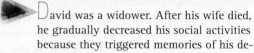

Case Vignette 20.1

David was a widower. After his wife died, he gradually decreased his social activities because they triggered memories of his deceased wife. This was emotionally overwhelming to him. David developed a depressive disorder as the first anniversary of his wife's death drew near. His condition became so acute that he required brief psychiatric hospitalization.

Once his depressive symptoms subsided, David was discharged to his home. His daughter and her family moved in with him. David acknowledged the importance of going out to meet friends and family, yet he could not make himself do so.

David's discharge plan included psychiatric home care nursing services to help him continue his recovery. The psychiatric home care nurse visited David weekly to provide brief psychotherapy. Also, she evaluated David's overall physical health and psychoneurologic status during each visit and monitored his medical and psychotropic medications. Occasionally, the psychiatric home care nurse called David's primary care physician to discuss David's proper medication adjustments. She also taught David's daughter to observe any change in her father's mood, behavior, and cognition.

The nurse visited David for 6 weeks. Gradually David began to go for walks in his neighborhood. He also began to visit his psychiatrist monthly accompanied by his daughter.

Reflection and Critical Thinking

- What advantages does psychiatric home care nursing afford clients? What about the health care industry overall?
- What follow-up issues are likely to require attention for this client? Would any other services be useful for him and his family?

▲

clients in their usual environments is preferred, as long as it is medically, socially, and economically feasible to do so.
- A health problem is a manifestation of several related problems and issues, residual or ongoing, in various aspects of life. A holistic approach is necessary.
- Cost effectiveness can be achieved only through well-coordinated and integrated services. Close monitoring of the balance between the costs of providing services and adequate reimbursement is critical.
- Home health care is delivered in a client's place of residence. When entering a client's home, health care professionals are in that person's cultural surroundings and must respect them, as well as integrate cultural preferences and expectations into services.
- High-quality client care is an indisputable goal, regardless of changes in policy and regulation of home care services.

Psychiatric home care nursing is integrated in a continuous and comprehensive system of general home care. Services of this specialty complement other types of psychiatric care, such as inpatient, outpatient, and long-term services, to maximize positive outcomes. Psychiatric home care nursing can be provided as a series of scheduled home visits or as single visits for crisis intervention (see Chap. 35). In addition to the principles of general home care listed previously, the following are specific principles of psychiatric home care nursing practice:

• Each person has a unique psychological makeup. Nurses must tailor an individualized care plan to the person's particular circumstances and consider his or her home and community surroundings. Goals for improving health status and developing personal resources must be realistic based on the client's condition.
• A consumer's or family's reaction to an alteration in mental health status, mental disability, or mental illness often is influenced by whether the condition is permanent, temporary, degenerative, or unknown. Empathy for emotional reactions from clients and families to various mental illnesses can help establish a positive therapeutic relationship.
• Nurses base client care on the therapeutic relationship (see Chap. 11). Therapeutic rapport is the foundation for providing appropriate psychiatric home care nursing services.

Goals

The goals of these efforts are to help clients regain, maintain, or improve psychological well-being to enhance their overall health status. Indicators of achieving these goals include decreased incidences of psychiatric hospitalization and maintenance of a stable state at home. General interventions directed toward achieving the goals of psychiatric home care nursing are as follows:

• Helping consumers and family members, including caregivers, understand mental illness and how to monitor signs of relapse, medication effects, and medication side effects (Figure 20.3)
• Providing respite and community resources to family members and caregivers
• Helping clients and family members and caregivers learn skills of problem solving, stress reduction, coping, and proper interpersonal communication
• Coordinating and integrating clients' medical, social, spiritual, vocational, and other community-based services, as well as teaching clients and families to do this independently

Funding and Eligibility

Home care services are reimbursed through many funding mechanisms. Medicare is currently the largest single source of reimbursement. Other funding sources include Medicaid, state and local government funding, private insurance, and out-of-pocket payments. As such, the Centers for Medicare and Medicaid Services publish many regulations of home care services. Most private insurance and managed care companies adopt Medicare rules, including criteria for eligibility of receiving home care, providers' certification of

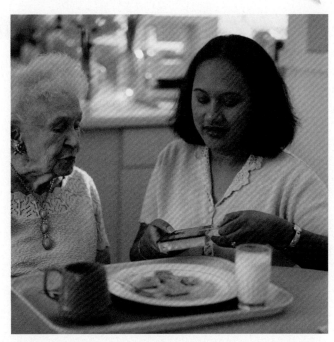

FIGURE 20.3 This home care nurse is reviewing medication issues during a visit with a client.

delivery of services, and mechanisms of reimbursement. This is true for psychiatric home care services as well.

According to Medicare regulations, to receive psychiatric home care services, a client must (1) be certified by a physician or psychiatrist as homebound, (2) have a psychiatric diagnosis and be under the care of a physician, (3) demonstrate intermittent needs for skilled psychiatric nursing care, and (4) receive services under a plan of care established and approved by a physician.

Criteria for homebound status include an inability to leave home alone because of physical, psychosocial, or medical problems; a need for assistance and taxing effort to leave home; and infrequent short absences from home only for medical or certain types of personal needs. Local Medicare intermediate offices review and interpret claims for service reimbursement. Their determinations of clients' eligibility and health conditions directly affect payment to psychiatric home care nursing services.

Medicare is a health insurance plan for older adults; therefore, most of the home care population consists of people 65 years of age or older. Most clients in psychiatric home care are referred from inpatient institutions. Other referral sources include social workers, family and friends, community agencies, and clergy. See Box 20.4.

Checkpoint Questions

7. What is the foundation for providing appropriate psychiatric home care nursing services?
8. Which two indicators determine achievement of the goals of psychiatric home care nursing?
9. What is the largest single source of reimbursement for psychiatric home care nursing services?

BOX 20.4 Common Indications for and Sources of Referral in Psychiatric Home Care

Indications

- Depression with or without previous inpatient treatment
- Increased anxiety, agitation, and manic behaviors
- Social isolation or refusal to leave a room or bed because of psychotic features
- Mismanagement, noncompliance, or misunderstanding of medication regimen
- Impaired or potentially dangerous self-care and activities of daily living
- Suicide risks, including potential or actual suicide attempts
- Mismanagement and exacerbation of a physical disease process
- Frequent falls secondary to impaired health status and functioning level
- Increased environmental or safety hazards secondary to impaired health status or disease process
- Preoccupation with somatic complaints, resulting in decreased personal functioning
- Panic attacks
- Anorexia with weight loss of more than 10 pounds per month

Referral Sources

- Case managers and hospital discharge planners
- Nurses, physicians, and social workers at outpatient clinics
- Clients and former clients
- Family members and caregivers
- Landlords and neighbors
- Health departments
- Police and fire departments and postal services
- Community agencies and clergy
- Interdisciplinary staff members at various health care settings
- Insurance companies, including health maintenance organizations, preferred provider organizations, and managed care organizations
- Employee assistance programs, senior care services, and attorneys
- Skilled nursing and other intermediate care facilities

Psychiatric Home Care Nurses

To be eligible to provide services to clients receiving Medicare coverage, psychiatric home care nurses must be certified by Medicare. Requirements include the following:

- A registered nurse (RN) with a master's degree in psychiatric or community mental health nursing
- An RN with a bachelor's degree in nursing and 1 year of related work experience in an active treatment program for adults or geriatric clients in psychiatric health care settings
- An RN with a diploma or associate degree and 2 years of related work experience in an active treatment program for adults or geriatric clients in psychiatric health care settings
- American Nurses Association certification in psychiatric or community health nursing
- Other qualifications (considered on an individual basis)

Advanced practice registered nurses in psychiatric–mental health (APRN-PMH), which include nurse practitioners and clinical nurse specialists (CNSs), are master's degree-prepared RNs with advanced training in psychiatric nursing. Most managed care organizations require that home care agencies utilize APRN-PMHs to deliver psychiatric home health nursing care. The APRN-PMH can provide nursing services with explicit theory-based psychiatric nursing interventions and therapies and, in some states, have certain levels of prescribing authority.

Psychiatric home care nurses work with clients and families in their immediate daily living environment. Those working in this specialty must remember that:

- Home is part of a larger community and social system heavily influenced by cultural considerations that the nurse should respect when planning and delivering care.
- Provision of home care services involves many different disciplines and services that must be well integrated to prevent fragmentation and confusion.
- Mental health problems often have high comorbidity with physical problems. These interwoven problems affect the client's overall health.

Psychiatric home care nurses use and adapt their fundamental knowledge and skills of psychiatric nursing to implement interventions appropriately in a client's home. They also address each client's unique cultural and societal norms. Indeed, home care requires a constant negotiating process between professional practice and the home environment. To provide high-quality care, psychiatric home care nurses first must attain excellence in the practice of psychiatric nursing, regardless of setting. Additional requirements for success include flexibility and willingness to modify practice according to conditions and available resources.

Think About It 20.2

An 80-year-old client with dementia and depression is referred for psychiatric home nursing services. The client also has a history of degenerative joint disease. He lives alone with his 77-year-old wife who had hip surgery approximately 1 year ago and uses a cane to ambulate. The couple has two children: a son who lives 30 miles away and visits once a month, and a daughter who lives 300 miles away, calls every week, and visits once or twice a year. Based on this situation, propose services that would be appropriate for this client along with the focus of each.

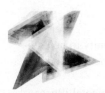

Reviewing and Applying Your Knowledge

Chapter Summary

- Community support is crucial to quality of life for those with SPMI residing in the community. The goal of community support systems is to enable those with severe mental illnesses to remain in the community while functioning at optimal levels of independence.

- A community support system encourages participation from all people in it: clients, family members, government officials, and providers. The objective is to deliver a full range of life-supportive care. Services are based on guiding principles that promote self-determination and individuation.

- Essential components of a community support system include active outreach efforts, help in ensuring access to services, psychosocial and vocational opportunities, rehabilitative and supportive housing options, crisis intervention services, case management, and family and community education programs.

- Reform efforts in children's social services have led to the establishment of systems of care, which create mechanisms for coordinating social services. They are designed to facilitate collaboration among parents, teachers, and other service providers so that they can gear services for students with multisystem needs toward common and agreed-on goals.

- Services must be developed with active participation from the consumer and family.

- Consumer and family movements are very active in promoting destigmatization of mental illness, developing treatment alternatives, and helping to shape policy at all levels of government.

- Nurses are an important link between hospital and community and bring essential knowledge and skills to a community-based treatment team or a school individual education plan team.

- Nurses have a leadership role in the development of comprehensive systems committed to the holistic approach of intervening at both client and community levels.

- Psychiatric home care nursing is a critical component in the continuum of psychiatric health care. This nursing service is an important resource to clients with psychiatric disorders and their family members to assist clients living independently or interdependently in communities.

- The goals of psychiatric home care are to assist clients with mental illness to gain, regain, maintain, or restore an optimal state of health and independence and to prevent institutionalization.

Study Questions

1. To be effective, which factors would be most important to include for a community support system? Select all that apply.

   a. The needs and functioning level of people with serious mental illness

   b. A care philosophy based on values and guiding principles

   c. Adoption of a specific program model

   d. Coordination of network by multiple agencies

   e. Assertive outreach programs for at-risk populations

   f. Vocational services for a specified period

2. The nurse is coordinating all of the various services needed to address the needs for housing, health care, mental health treatment, social contacts, and workups of a consumer with mental illness. The nurse is functioning as which of the following?

   a. Case manager

   b. Social worker

   c. Client advocate

   d. Home care nurse

3. The nurse assesses a group and determines that it has at least one commonality among its members. The nurse identifies this as a(n):

   a. Support group

   b. Self-help group

   c. Advocate group

   d. Aggregate group

4. When describing the characteristics of clients eligible to receive Medicare-reimbursed psychiatric home care services, which of the following would the nurse be least likely to include?

   a. Plan of care for services that are established and approved by a physician

   b. Demonstration of needs requiring continuous skilled psychiatric nursing care

   c. A psychiatric diagnosis for which a physician is providing care

   d. Certification by a psychiatrist that client is confined to the home

(continues on page 382)

5. The nurse is developing a presentation about home care nursing, including psychiatric home care nursing, for an older adult community group. Which of the following would the nurse include in the presentation?

   a. The services provided address a single problem or issue at one time.

   b. The costs of services are easily reimbursed through Medicare.

   c. The nurse acts as the controller in the client's home.

   d. The nurse tailors care to the client's particular circumstances.

Critical Thinking Questions

1. How can nurses work within the community to help ensure positive outcomes for clients with mental illness?

2. How do the issues faced by adults with mental illness differ from those faced by children and adolescents with mental illness?

3. How and why has psychiatric home care nursing developed and transformed to become a nursing specialty?

References

Adelman, H. S., & Taylor, L. (2000). Moving prevention from the fringes into the fabric of school improvement. *Journal of Emotional and Psychological Consultation, 11*(1), 7–37.

Allness, D. (2003). The ACT Standards (revised). In *A manual for ACT start-up: Based on the PACT model of community treatment for persons with severe and persistent mental illnesses.* Washington, DC: National Alliance for the Mentally Ill.

Anderson, J. A., McIntyre, J. S., Rotto, K., & Robertson, D. C. (2002). Developing and maintaining collaboration in systems of care for children and youth with emotional and behavioral disabilities and their families. *American Journal of Orthopsychiatry, 72*(4), 514–525.

Anderson, J. A., Wright, E. R., Kelly, K., & Kooreman, H. E. (2008). Clinical functioning over time for young people served in a system of care. *Journal of Emotional and Behavioral Disorders, 16*(2), 90–104.

Anderson, J. A., Wright, E. R., Kooreman, H. E., Mohr, W. K., & Russell, L. (2003). The Dawn project: A model for responding to the needs of young people with emotional and behavioral disabilities and their families. *Community Mental Health Journal, 39*(1), 63–74.

Blanchard, L. T., Gurka, M. J., & Blackman, J. A. (2006). Emotional, developmental, and behavioral health of American children and their families: A report from the 2003 National Survey of Children's Health. *Pediatrics, 117*(6), 1202–1212.

Choices. (2012). *Indiana choices—Cross system care coordination.* Retrieved from http://www.choicesteam.org/cscc

Corrigan, P. W., Mueser, K. T., Bond, G. R., Drake, R. E., & Solomon, P. (2007). *Principles and practice of psychiatric rehabilitation: An empirical approach.* New York, NY: Guilford Press.

Dashiff, C., DiMicco, W., Myers, B., & Sheppard, K. (2009). Poverty and adolescent mental health. *Journal of Child and Adolescent Psychiatric Nursing, 22*(1), 23–32.

Dosser, D. A., Handron, D., McCammon, S., & Powell, J. Y. (2002). *Child mental health: Exploring systems of care in the new millennium.* New York, NY: Haworth Press.

Fairweather Lodge. (2007). *Frequently asked questions.* Retrieved from http://theccl.org/Fairweather.htm

Hernandez, M., & Hodges, S. (2003). Building upon the theory of change for systems of care. *Journal of Emotional and Behavioral Disorders, 11*(1), 19–26.

Hodges, S., Hernandez, M., & Nesman, T. (2003). A developmental framework for collaboration in child-serving agencies. *Journal of Child and Family Studies, 12,* 291–305.

Mowbray, C. T., Lewandowski, L., Holter, M., & Bybee, D. (2006). The clubhouse as an empowering setting. *Health and Social Work, 31*(3), 167–179.

New York State Office of Mental Health. (2006). Child and Adolescent Service System Program (CASSP). Retrieved from http://www.omh.state.ny.us/omhweb/ebp/cassp.htm

Nies, M. A., & McEwan, M. (2007). *Community/public health nursing: Promoting the health of populations* (4th ed.). Philadelphia, PA: Elsevier.

Perlin, M. L. (1994). Law and the delivery of mental health services in the community. *American Journal of Orthopsychiatry, 64*(2), 194–208.

Resnick, S. G., Neale, M. S., & Rosenheck, R. A. (2003). Impact of public support payments, intensive psychiatric community care, and program fidelity on employment outcomes for people with severe mental illness. *Journal of Nervous and Mental Disease, 191*(3), 139–144.

Salyers, M. P., & Tsemberis, S. (2007). ACT and recovery: Integrating evidence-based practices and recovery orientation on Assertive Community Treatment teams. *Community Mental Health Journal, 43*(6), 619–641.

Schonebaum, A. D., Boyd, J. K., & Dudek, K. J. (2006). A comparison of competitive employment outcomes for the clubhouse and PACT models. *Psychiatric Services, 57*(10), 1416–1420.

Sokal, J., Messias, E., Dickerson, F. B., Kreyenbuhl, J., Brown, C. H., Goldberg, R. W., & Dixon, L. B. (2004). Comorbidity of medical illnesses among adults with serious mental illness who are receiving community psychiatric services. *Journal of Nervous and Mental Disease, 192*(6), 421–427.

Stanhope, M., & Lancaster, J. (2008). *Community health nursing: Process and practice for promoting health* (7th ed.). St. Louis, MO: Mosby.

Stein, L. I., & Santos, A. B. (1998). *Assertive community treatment of persons with severe mental illness.* New York, NY: W. W. Norton.

Stroul, B. A., & Friedman, R. M. (1986). *A system of care for children and youth with severe emotional disturbances* (rev. ed.). Washington, DC: Georgetown University Child Development Center, National Technical Assistance Center for Children's Mental Health.

Substance Abuse & Mental Health Services Administration. (2012). *Center for Mental Health Services.* Retrieved from http://www.samhsa.gov/about/cmhs.aspx

U.S. Department of Health and Human Services (USDHHS). (2001). *Mental health: Culture, race, and ethnicity. A supplement to Mental Health: A Report of the Surgeon General.* Rockville, MD: U.S. Department of Health and Human Services, Public Health Services, Office of the Surgeon General.

U.S. Department of Health and Human Services (USDHHS). (2007). *Healthy people 2010.* Retrieved from http://www.healthypeople.gov

Walker, J. S., & Schutte, K. M. (2004). Practice and process in wraparound teamwork. *Journal of Emotional and Behavioral Disorders, 12*(3), 182–192.

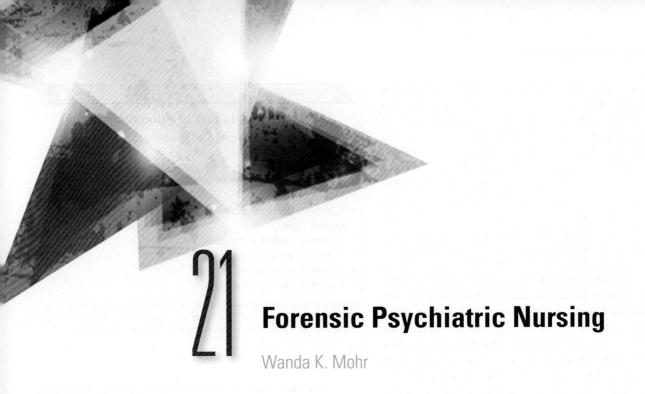

21

Forensic Psychiatric Nursing

Wanda K. Mohr

KEY TERMS

crime
custody and caring
expressive violence
gang violence
instrumental violence
interpersonal violence

LEARNING OBJECTIVES

On completion of this chapter, you should be able to accomplish the following:

- Describe the psychiatric nurse's role in the forensic milieu.
- Describe characteristics of psychiatric and mental health concerns specific to forensic populations, addressing implications for nursing care.
- Describe the steps of the nursing process as related to the care of clients in forensic settings and their families.

Forensic psychiatric nursing is a rapidly expanding specialty and has gained wider visibility in the contemporary health care era. With increased attention from nursing specialty professional organizations such as the International Association of Forensic Nurses (2012) and the American Psychiatric Nurses Association (2012), there is a greater awareness of the number of forensic roles and career choices for psychiatric nurses. Specifically, forensic psychiatric nurses work with clients and their families who seek mental health care through the criminal justice system.

Forensic clients share distinct legal, ethical, political, administrative, and professional concerns. Their issues and the associated response from professional nurses have strengthened the designation of forensic nursing as an emergent specialty (Lynch & Duval, 2010). Another contributing factor to its growth is the public's developing understanding of the overlap between the criminal justice and mental health systems. To truly legitimize this discipline, some researchers have argued for the need to create a curriculum in and establish a national certification process for forensic nursing. Although many leading nursing organizations, including the American Nurses Credentialing Center, American Nurses Association (ANA), and the International Association of Forensic Nurses (IAFN), are working toward these goals, they have not been met to date.

The terminology used to describe nursing with forensic populations has varied over the years and frequently is linked to a specific client group or care setting. Broadly, forensic nursing represents a diverse area of practice. To clarify its scope, the IAFN, in its combined efforts with the ANA (1997), established the *Scope and Standards of Forensic Nursing Practice,* which defines the role of forensic nurses globally to include those working with victims and perpetrators of crimes, as well as their families. Clarification of this role depends not only on what a nurse does (role expectations) but also on where he or she works (role setting); this would apply to psychiatric forensic nurses who may work in a wide variety of settings including correctional facilities and locked psychiatric facilities, and as psychiatric mental health liaisons in the hospital setting. Nursing Spotlight 21.1 lists the IAFN subspecialties.

This chapter views forensic psychiatric nurses as integrating psychiatric mental health nursing philosophy and practice within a sociocultural context that includes the criminal justice system to provide comprehensive care to clients, families, and communities. How different settings or jurisdictions define the role of nurses may restrict or enlarge their image and potential influence in forensic settings and communities at large. *Forensic nursing, jail nursing, prison nursing, correctional nursing,* and *forensic psychiatric nursing* are terms used in the literature, sometimes interchangeably, to refer to this specialty area. Other positions that continue to expand also include *clinical legal nurse consultant, nurse attorney, forensic nurse examiner, death investigator, forensic consultant,* and *expert witness.*

NURSING SPOTLIGHT 21.1

IAFN Subspecialties of Forensic Nursing

- Forensic nursing educators/consultants
- Nurse coroners
- Death investigators
- Legal nurse consultants
- Nurse attorneys
- Clinical nursing specialists in trauma, transplant, and critical care
- Forensic pediatric nurses
- Forensic gerontologic nurses
- Forensic psychiatric nurses
- Forensic correctional nurses

From the International Association of Forensic Nurses & American Nurses Association. (1997). *Scope and standards of forensic nursing practice.* Washington, DC: American Nurses Association.

As **crime** and violence continue to escalate, all nurses, regardless of setting, need forensic knowledge and skills. Nurses must view crime as a societal problem that transcends individual, family, and community boundaries and culminates in profound community health consequences (see Chaps. 32 and 33). Nurses are uniquely positioned to respond because the principles of psychiatric nursing apply to any setting in which criminal behavior and mental health problems occur (Lynch & Duval, 2010).

FORENSIC SETTINGS

The care and management of people with mental illness who come into conflict with the law challenge the collective wisdom of criminal justice and mental health systems. Enduring contradictions about how best to meet client needs prevail. Forensic psychiatric nursing occurs in various secure environments, which may belong to the mental health system or criminal justice system, and in the contemporary setting, in the community to serve those who are under "house arrest" or "home monitoring." The continuum of controlled environments includes community-based outpatient clinics, secure units in general hospitals, state psychiatric hospitals, forensic psychiatric hospitals, and custodial-type settings (eg, juvenile detention centers, jails, prisons). As such, nurses in different jurisdictions commonly have different roles, expectations, physical resources, and clinical and professional boundaries.

In his seminal work, Osborne (1995) declared "in these times of radical capitalism and individualism, there is a blurring of the mission of corrections and mental health facilities" (p. 5). Sadly, not much has changed since. Society continues to view correctional facilities, by default, as "primary mental health facilities" (Human Rights Watch [HRW], 2003). For example, Gondles (2005) notably declared that the two largest U.S. providers of mental health services are the Los Angeles County Jail and Riker's Island in New York.

FACTORS CONTRIBUTING TO INCARCERATION

Currently, the United States has the highest incarceration rate in the Western world. In 2006, 2,245,189 men, women, and juveniles were in federal, state, or local custody—the largest increase since 2000 (Sabol et al., 2007). Many factors contribute to the growing forensic population, including more drug-related activities (Williams, 2007), rising **interpersonal** and urban violence, anticrime and antidrug legislation, poor economic conditions and associated homelessness (see Chap. 38), and, perhaps most tragically, the pervasive issue of the "criminalization of the mentally ill" (Harrison & Beck, 2003; HRW, 2003). This criminalization directly results from the deinstitutionalization movement that began in the 1960s, peaked in the 1970s, and continues today (see Chap. 1). Sadly, the persistent lack of community-based services and appropriate mental health policies for clients with chronic mental illness has fragmented the mental health system. Many people cannot access appropriate and timely treatment and ultimately experience a "revolving door syndrome" that includes courts, jails, and prisons. Even those treated and released from hospitals or prisons are at increased risk for psychiatric problems (Wilson & Draine, 2006; World Health Organization [WHO], 2007). Correctional facilities have become the country's front-line mental health providers representing the mental health institutions of the 21st century (Adams & Ferrandino, 2012; White & Whiteford, 2006, p. 302) (Figure 21.1).

ALTERNATIVES TO INCARCERATION

Some jurisdictions divert offenders with mental disorders, particularly those who did not have criminal intent, from the court process and refer them directly for treatment, to mental health courts, or both. Effectiveness depends greatly on both availability and type (eg, with police, upon arrival to court, upon initial detention) (Statistics Canada, 2003; Steadman et al., 2001; Trupin & Richards, 2003; Watson et al., 2001). Although relatively new, diversion schemes are humane treatment, may be cost effective, and appear to contribute to reduced recidivism among people with mental illness (HRW, 2003; Munetz & Griffin, 2006).

Forensic assertive community treatment is another emerging approach. Its aim is to prevent the arrest and incarceration of people with severe mental illness by integrating assertive community treatment and community justice initiatives (see Chap. 20). Sadly, limited funding resources compromise refinements to programs and further research (Lamberti et al., 2004).

More recently, Munetz and Griffin (2006) have advocated for a *sequential intercept model.* It envisions five points of interception, from law enforcement to community corrections and support, to prevent people from entering or further penetrating into the criminal justice system.

The role of forensic nurses in alternatives to incarceration for offenders with mental illness varies according to the program. Thus, ongoing research and development are necessary.

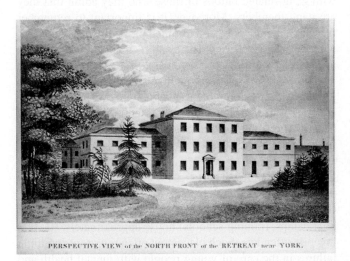

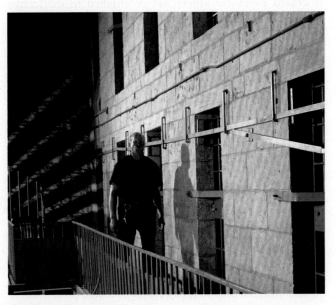

FIGURE 21.1 In some ways, treatment for many people with mental illness has moved from one type of institution to another, which is an unfortunate outcome of the deinstitutionalization movement and the "criminalization of the mentally ill." The image on the *left* depicts the York Retreat, founded in 1792 for those with mental disorders (U.S. National Library of Medicine, *Images from the History of Medicine.* National Institutes of Health, Department of Health and Human Services). The image on the right is a photo of a modern prison.

CHARACTERISTICS OF THE FORENSIC POPULATION

Forensic clients present with complex and multifaceted issues further complicated by the unique environmental and social factors of their milieu (Cultural Spotlight 21.1). In their seminal and poignant work, Love and Hunter (1999), assert that "The commingling of severe and persistent mental illness with criminality poses vexing clinical challenges and complex moral dilemmas not faced in either general psychiatric or correctional environments" (p. 35). Important considerations include the prevalence of mental disorders, cultural and demographic variations, and the needs of special at-risk groups.

Historically, forensic clients demonstrate poor judgment, limited reasoning, and a history of not learning from mistakes. They also report an exceptionally high level of substance abuse at the time of arrest (Freudenberg et al., 2005). In Canada, 80% of those housed in correctional facilities enter with substance abuse problems; more than 50% report that they were under the influence of drugs, alcohol, or both when they committed their crimes (Public Safety Canada, 2007). People with substance use disorders are also at increased risk for mental illness (see Chap. 30). However, the inaccurate caricature of offenders who have a mental illness as crazed psychotic killers has contributed to ineffective planning and treatment. Depending on the treatment setting, jurisdiction, location, and facilities available, populations may include both suspects or convicts, those sentenced or unsentenced, those not guilty by reason of insanity or incompetent to stand trial, and those not criminally responsible because of mental disorders. With such variation, psychiatric nurses must be aware of the laws and provisions governing their particular jurisdictions. See Case Vignette 21.1.

Offenders With Mental Illness

In forensic psychiatric nursing, the predominant client group is those with psychiatric disorders. As many as 15% of prison or jail inmates have a mental disorder; as many as 20% require psychiatric intervention while incarcerated (HRW, 2003; Quanbeck et al., 2003). The U.S. Department of Justice reports that 64% of local inmates, 56% of state prisoners, and 45% of federal prisoners have symptoms of serious mental illness (James & Glaze, 2006). Chronic severe schizophrenia, mood disorders, and organic syndromes with psychotic features are also common.

In addition, many forensic clients present with mental health problems associated with a criminal lifestyle. The coexistence of personality disorders, substance abuse, and violence and aggression often complicates psychotic presentations; many clients self-medicate with drugs and alcohol (Quanbeck et al., 2003; Woods et al., 2006) (see also Chaps. 25, 30, and 32).

Violent Offenders

Studies of violence among prison populations reveal two major types. **Expressive violence** involves interpersonal altercations, usually with people known to the assailant and of similar age, ethnicity, and cultural background. **Instrumental violence** usually involves premeditated, motive-driven acts (frequently for economic gain). Perpetrators and victims of instrumental violence usually are unknown to one another. A significantly emerging third type is **gang violence**, which is associated with group alliances and is committed for retaliation or revenge. Typical victims of gang violence within forensic settings include sex offenders, those who have hurt children, and those with mental illness or physical and mental handicaps. From a psychiatric nursing standpoint, it is important to be able to identify those clients who have gang affiliations; for example, individuals wearing gang colors or with gang-related tattoos or those who may admit that they are gang members. Moreover, it is important to remember that gang members have a troubled past, which typically includes a history of psychiatric and mental health challenges and issues (Clements & Akiyama, 2011).

Forensic nurses work with many clients who have a proven capacity for violence. Although staff injuries generally are rare, violence and its potential are occupational hazards. Personal, institutional, and community safety is a frequent topic of discussion.

Special Populations
Juvenile Offenders

On any day, U.S. custodial facilities (eg, detention centers, boot camps, training schools) house approximately 100,000 juvenile offenders. Such placement often represents multiple failures in the care of young people with mental health and criminal problems (Trulson, 2007). Juveniles presenting to the justice system often come from disadvantaged backgrounds and frequently experience developmental, mental health, and community risk factors (Bonham, 2006; Cashin, 2006). Although mental health treatment is legally mandated for them, juvenile offenders are a vastly underserved at-risk population who require special services to meet their growth and development, education, and special health needs

Cultural *Spotlight* 21.1

Minority Offenders

Clients from ethnic minorities are disproportionately represented in most North American forensic facilities. Specific ethnic groups may dominate, and traditional psychiatric practices often are incompatible with their cultural beliefs. Providers must consider cultural implications when providing mental health care. Failure by client and staff to recognize and respond appropriately to differences creates tension, with the potential to disrupt therapeutic relationships, cultivate stressful environments, and instigate violence (Hufft, 2006; Hufft & Kite, 2003).

Case Vignette 21.1

Robert, 42 years old, has a long history of antisocial behavior and difficulty getting along with others. His verbally and physically abusive father was an alcoholic. Robert had many problems in school and had to repeat fourth grade. When he was 11 years old, the courts ordered Robert to spend time in a closed-custody facility for juveniles because his parents could not provide required supervision. Anger and hatred quickly replaced initial feelings of loss. Reports indicate that Robert had a "short fuse" and responded to others with physical aggression.

On release from the juvenile facility, Robert stopped all communication with relatives and felt satisfied that he was inflicting his pain and loss on them. He moved among foster homes, primarily because of his acting-out behavior. School problems continued; eventually, he ran away to a large city far from home. With no education or job skills, he quickly became involved in robbery, drugs, and prostitution. He blamed the world for his problems, lashing out at those who tried to get close to him. He experienced great sadness but could not cry.

In his late teens, Robert was part of an experimental treatment group after an involuntary admission to a psychiatric facility. The material presented was beyond his level of comprehension. A controlling coping style soon replaced his feelings of powerlessness. After treatment, Robert further isolated himself. He began heavy use of alcohol and drugs to self-medicate depressive symptoms. His thoughts became increasingly irrational, and he believed that the only way to deal with his feelings was to hurt others before they could hurt him.

By 20 years of age, Robert's interpersonal difficulties, coupled with serious substance abuse, culminated in an indefinite sentence for a murder of which he had no recollection. Initially, he had no feelings about serving time. Two years passed before he began to question his future and despise his situation. He made numerous suicide and self-mutilation attempts. He lived one day at a time; his formula for success was morphine and opiates. He sold drugs to make money in prison. He usually was "high" on something, which gave him a temporary sense of control over his emotions and environment. Robert began to realize that he had feelings of depression and turned to the health care center for prescribed antidepressants. When medication failed to "solve all his problems," he turned to illicit substances for a temporary fix. He was in a vicious cycle of drugs, depression, and detoxification.

After 20 years in prison, Robert states he has matured and is ready to lead a prosocial lifestyle. He has entered a specialized treatment program designed to deal with dual diagnoses and is beginning to deal with some of the feelings he has ignored for most of his life. He states that he will never be able to forgive himself for what he has done to himself and those around him, particularly the victim of his crime.

Reflection and Critical Thinking

- What do you think is Robert's most immediate problem?
- In counseling Robert, what issues or problems might the therapist encounter?
- What factors make the care of this client different from that of other clients with depression?

—*Tracy Edmonds, RN, BN, Nurse Coordinator, Bow Unit, Regional Psychiatric Centre, Correctional Service of Canada, Saskatoon, Saskatchewan.*

(Shelton, 2005; Teplin et al., 2005). Unfortunately, the behavioral problems associated with their criminal activities often divert attention. Advanced clinical knowledge and skill and approaches that coordinate justice, law, social services, education, and health care are necessary (Bohnam, 2006; Shelton, 2005).

Female Offenders

Although women commit fewer crimes than men, one of the most dramatic trends of the past decade is the increased number of incarcerated women (Blanchette & Brown, 2006) (Figure 21.2). Although women comprise approximately 5% of global incarcerated populations, the percent increase in female offenders under the jurisdiction of U.S. state and federal prisons between 2005 and 2006 was almost twice the rate of males.

Incarcerated women often experience overlapping health challenges, including significant substance abuse, blood-borne infections, serious mental health concerns (including post-traumatic stress and personality disorders), diabetes, and hypertension. Many female offenders have histories of physical, emotional, and sexual abuse (Maeve, 2003; Peternelj-Taylor, 2005b; Roth & Pressé, 2003). Many of them struggle

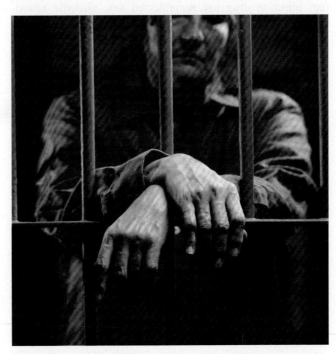

FIGURE 21.2 The number of incarcerated women is growing in the United States.

with the ever-present fear of losing custody of their children (Blanchard, 2004; Harner, 2004; Maeve, 2003). Development of appropriate relationships with peers, family members, and volunteers can assist them to cope with forced separation from loved ones, influence their adaptation to incarceration, and also positively influence their health (Harner, 2004).

Older Adult Offenders

The health care needs of an ever-increasing "graying population" clearly challenge traditional correctional resources, resulting in the need for special adaptations. Aging forensic clients are unique in terms of criminal patterns, health care needs, problems in adjustment to institutional life, and family issues. These factors pose special difficulties to the prison system, particularly in relation to custody, rehabilitation, and reintegration. In many ways, the health challenges that older clients in forensic settings experience are no different than those of the general population, although they are complicated by conditions of the milieu (see Chap. 37).

In addition to problems with mental health, older forensic clients have more debilitating effects from chronic illness and often require more services for physical illness. Increased knowledge and skill in gerontologic, geriatric, and forensic nursing are required to provide a standard of care that enhances their health outcomes (Rikard & Rosenberg, 2007). Community placement for elderly forensic clients with dementia is particularly challenging, given their criminal histories (Encinares, 2007).

Offenders With HIV/AIDS or Hepatitis

Issues related to HIV and AIDS represent challenges to clinical and administrative management. Rates of HIV, AIDS, and hepatitis B and C are higher in forensic clients than in the general population, primarily because of high-risk behaviors (eg, injection drug use, unprotected sex, unsterile tattooing, and body piercing) (Vlahov & Putnam, 2006). Health concerns extend beyond institutional walls because most forensic clients eventually reenter the community. Harm-reduction strategies in some facilities include available condoms, bleach kits, methadone maintenance, and needle exchange programs; these measures also serve as long-term prevention for outside communities (Thomas, 2005; Vlahov & Putnam, 2006). Nevertheless, these strategies are controversial; implementation varies greatly, and adoption is not the norm.

Offenders With Terminal Illness

"Dying in prison does not have to be seen as the 'ultimate failure' or feared, if it can be afforded dignity, sensitivity, care and understanding" (Bolger, 2005, p. 620). Palliative care for terminally ill forensic clients is a growing reality, particularly in areas that prohibit early release for compassionate reasons (Buckley, 2010). Forensic nurses need to address the adaptation and implementation of standard protocols, particularly in terms of training and development for pain and symptom management; availability and use of controlled substances; and palliative care teams, including community volunteers (Anno et al., 2004).

> **Checkpoint Questions**
>
> 3. Which type of violence usually involves premeditated and motive-driven acts with people unknown to one another?
> 4. What is the most common reason that the health care needs of juvenile offenders is overlooked?

EFFECTS OF INCARCERATION ON MENTAL HEALTH

Forensic psychiatric nurses provide care not only for offenders who enter correctional systems with mental disorders but also for people who become mentally ill while incarcerated. Daily living conditions affect all forensic clients. Creating a healing therapeutic environment in a forensic setting is a challenge. The physical conditions, client population, and authoritarian interpersonal atmosphere contribute to society's most extreme and stressful living environment (Peternelj-Taylor, 2005a) (Box 21.1).

BOX 21.1 Common Stressors to Mental Health in Secure Environments

Stressors That Affect the Client

- Loss of freedom
- Overcrowding
- Double stigmatization
- Grief, isolation, loneliness
- Gang violence
- Institutional violence: stabbing, beating, sexual assault
- Deteriorating living conditions
- Lack of privacy
- Protective custody
- Segregation
- Fear of the unknown
- Separation from loved ones
- Cumulative effects of losses

Stressors That Affect the Nurse

- Actual or implied threats of violence/personal safety
- Constant barrage of swearing
- Need to be constantly on guard against manipulation
- Dual responsibility of providing custody and caring
- Role confusion and ambiguity
- Professional isolation
- Stigma of "second-class nurse"
- Institutionalization
- Antagonistic relationships with correctional staff
- Fear of the unknown
- Ethical dilemmas
- Secondary trauma
- Understaffing

Some offenders cruelly abuse others through torment, beatings, and sexual assaults. Many victims have chronic mental illnesses, mental retardation, brain injuries, decreased social skills, or limited physical strength (especially among men). Their safety poses ongoing dilemmas for administrators, who often must confine them to protective custody units. Unfortunately, this measure can be counterproductive by further exacerbating mental illness (Aufderheide & Brown, 2005; Cloyes, 2007).

CHARACTERISTICS OF FORENSIC PSYCHIATRIC NURSES

Regardless of setting, forensic psychiatric nurses have dual obligations: (1) social necessity (custody) and (2) social good (caring). The "**custody and caring**" debate is framed by doing what is beneficial for the community while advocating for what is most therapeutic for clients. Nurses must comprehend and confront this paradox to provide competent care. Ramifications are at best perplexing, if not disconcerting, and nurses often feel torn between the needs of society and the needs of clients (Blair, 2002; Dumpel, 2006; Maroney, 2005; Smith, 2005).

Considerable anecdotal evidence suggests that forensic psychiatric nurses frequently experience role ambiguity and confusion, often because of overlapping and conflicting expectations. They must maintain security standards to provide safe working environments. Thus, they spend much time attending to issues related to the safety of the therapeutic milieu. Nurses who master the inherent dilemmas between the philosophies of custody and caring and achieve professional resolution and personal understanding can enjoy increased self-esteem and a sense of accomplishment. More commonly, however, nurses perceive the conflict as a source of stress (Blair, 2000; Dumpel, 2006; Smith, 2005). Rather than viewing these elements as competing interests, Maroney (2005) concludes that they can coexist, particularly when supported by focused educational interventions and research in correctional nursing practice.

The American Nurses Association's (2007) foundational document *Corrections Nursing: Scope and Standards of Practice* reflects the current state of knowledge within forensic nursing practice. It also provides direction for professional nursing practice within the criminal justice system (Nursing Spotlight 21.2). Perhaps the greatest challenge that forensic nurses experience is to remain true to their nursing roots and to avoid being co-opted into a custodial role that may define expectations and responsibilities more clearly (Blair, 2000; Maroney, 2005).

Attitudes

Forensic psychiatric nurses care for a frequently stigmatized and marginalized population. The mental health background and criminal history of clients may intensify and influence responses from nurses. How forensic nurses refer to the recipients of their care is informative. For example, what words do nurses use? What effects do labels such as "inmate," "psychopath," "con," "perp," and "psycho" have on nursing care (Hufft, 2006; Peternelj-Taylor, 2004)? (See Chap. 8.) Negative attitudes toward offenders can inhibit the entire nurse–client relationship and promote underinvolvement in client care.

Psychiatric nurses traditionally have based their practice on caring. This commitment does not change when those receiving care are in correctional settings. "Care is care no matter where. There is no reduced standard of care dependent on the clinical setting" (Klein, 2003, p. 45). An attitude that conveys an enduring conviction that caring for these vulnerable groups is appropriate and decent is a desirable approach (Peternelj-Taylor, 2003). Assessing and exploring common preconceptions, beliefs, and stereotypes help forensic nurses to decrease potential fears, anxieties, and negative attitudes. Participating in a tour, interacting with clients, or observing experienced nurses in practice are ways to confront thoughts and feelings, verify reality, and overcome natural apprehension to working with incarcerated clients.

The competing demands of custody and caring shape the moral climate of forensic settings (Austin, 2001). Exposure to the frequently profound associated issues provides numerous opportunities for moral and personal growth. Nurses who are most successful in mastering the complexities of the forensic role view clients as people who deserve respect and professionalism, believe that people can be rehabilitated, and see their role as caregiving (Hufft, 2006; Peternelj-Taylor, 2003). Being able to adopt a therapeutic role and "transcend judgmental and prejudicial attitudes toward those who have committed crimes" (Hufft & Fawkes, 1994) requires ongoing self-reflection and self-awareness. Nurses should reflect on the following questions:

- What has motivated my decision to work in forensic psychiatric nursing?
- What are my feelings about heinous violent crimes such as murder and sexual assault? Can I put them aside, see beyond the crime, and care for one who has done these things?
- How would I respond to questions like "How can you care for them?" "Why don't you just lock the door and throw away the key?"
- Can I work in an area where professional roles and responsibilities are not defined clearly, particularly in terms of balancing the custodial and caring roles?

Skills

Not all nurses are suited for forensic environments, nor is it appropriate to place all students in such settings. Those working in forensic institutions must be good communicators, have a wide range of physical and psychosocial assessment skills, and display solid critical thinking and decision making (ANA, 2007). Social maturity, adaptability,

NURSING SPOTLIGHT 21.2

ANA Standards for Forensic Nursing

Standards of Practice for Corrections Nursing

The corrections nurse is a registered nurse working in a corrections environment or with confined or detained individuals.

Standard 1. Assessment

The corrections nurse collects comprehensive data pertinent to the patient's health and condition or the situation.

Standard 2. Diagnosis

The corrections nurse analyzes the assessment data to determine the diagnoses or issues.

Standard 3. Outcomes Identification

The corrections nurse identifies expected outcomes for a plan individualized to the patient or the situation.

Standard 4. Planning

The corrections nurse develops a plan that prescribes strategies and alternatives to attain expected outcomes.

Standard 5. Implementation

The corrections nurse coordinates care delivery.

Standard 5A: Coordination of Services

The corrections nurse coordinates care delivery.

Standard 5B: Health Education and Health Promotion

The corrections nurse employs strategies to promote health and a safe environment.

Standard 5C: Consultation

The advanced practice registered nurse and the nursing role specialist provide consultation to influence the identified plan, enhance the abilities of others, and effect change.

Standard 5D: Regulatory Activities

The advance practice registered nurse uses prescriptive authority, procedure, referrals, treatments, and therapies in accordance with state and federal laws and regulations.

Standard 6. Evaluation

The corrections nurse evaluates progress toward attainment of outcomes.

Standards of Corrections Nursing Professional Performance

Standard 7. Quality of Practice

The corrections nurse systematically enhances the quality and effectiveness of nursing practice.

Standard 8. Education

The corrections nurse attains knowledge and competency that reflects current nursing practice.

Standard 9. Professional Practice Evaluation

The corrections nurse evaluates one's own nursing practice in relation to professional practice standards and guidelines, relevant statutes, rules, and regulations.

Standard 10. Collegiality

The corrections nurse interacts with and contributes to the professional development of peers and colleagues.

Standard 11. Collaboration

The corrections nurse collaborates with patient, family, and others in the conduct of nursing practice.

Standard 12. Ethics

The corrections nurse integrates ethical provisions in all areas of practice.

Standard 13. Research

The corrections nurse integrates research findings into practice.

Standard 14. Resource Utilization

The corrections nurse considers factors related to safety, effectiveness, cost, benefits, and impact on practice in the planning and delivery of nursing services.

Standard 15. Leadership

The corrections nurse provides leadership in the professional practice setting and the profession.

professionalism, and analytical skills are critical, as are confidence, nonjudgmental attitudes, ability to work independently and within teams, decisiveness, and ability to work in a secure environment while applying nursing knowledge to care decisions. Educational facilities and forensic agencies favorably view personal characteristics such as stability, integrity, assertiveness, maturity, and friendliness (Blair, 2000; Hufft, 2006; Reimer, 2007). Primary, secondary, and tertiary roles of forensic psychiatric nurses are highlighted in Box 21.2.

Levels of Prevention in Forensic Settings

Primary Prevention

- Illness prevention
- Mental health promotion
- Classification of stressors
- Political involvement
- Appropriate referrals
- Provision of education and information
- Advocacy

Secondary Prevention

- Assessment, evaluation, diagnosis
- Community consultation
- Crisis intervention
- Program planning and implementation
- Substance abuse treatment
- Sex offender treatment
- Aggressive behavior control
- Life and social skills training
- Acute inpatient psychiatric nursing
- Suicide prevention and management
- Creation and maintenance of a therapeutic milieu
- Short-term therapy
- Counseling, psychotherapy
- Medication administration and management
- Emergency care

Tertiary Intervention

- Case management
- After-care services/community reintegration
- Rehabilitation
- Vocational training
- Relapse prevention
- End-of-life/palliative care
- Compassionate release
- Spiritual care

Checkpoint Questions

5. What two obligations do nurses specializing in forensic psychiatric nursing face?
6. What three attitudes are necessary for nurses to master the complexities of the forensic psychiatric nursing role?

APPLYING THE NURSING PROCESS

Forensic Clients

In forensic settings, the effects of the distinctive environment modify the essence of nursing. Special adaptations are necessary to achieve professional standards and personal goals.

◢ ASSESSMENT

Regardless of setting, all forensic psychiatric nurses have a significant role to play in the observation and assessment of clients. Context of care, number of clients, and lengths of stay can facilitate or hamper the nurse's ability to provide comprehensive mental health services as per the community standard. Assessing clients in isolation from their support systems, homes, and daily routines can be problematic. Forensic clients are supervised closely, and institutional policies restrict and mandate their behaviors. The physical environment and lack of privacy further complicate assessment and diagnosis. Security concerns affect every aspect of forensic nursing practice and can interfere with the establishment of therapeutic relationships. Access to clients can be difficult, particularly in correctional (as opposed to mental health) facilities. Nurses often must rely on correctional staff to make appropriate referrals for offenders in need of assessment.

Interview rooms are designed to allow for maximum observation of nurses conducting assessments. These rooms are soundproof, but all can see inside, violating rights to privacy and confidentiality common to psychiatric nurse–client relationships (yet vital to security) (Figure 21.3). At times, correctional personnel are required, which further complicates the assessment process, because clients are reluctant to disclose information to nonmental health care staff. More importantly, however, many clients are reluctant to be identified with forensic psychiatric nurses because of the stigma associated with mental illness. In many prison environments, it is "better to be bad than mad" (Peternelj-Taylor & Johnson, 1995). "A control unit inmate has a much greater sense of legitimacy in prison discourse, while the other, mentally ill, is devalued and frequently disdained" (Cloyes, 2007, p. 207).

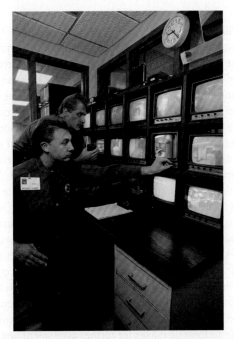

FIGURE 21.3 Frequently, forensic psychiatric nurses must conduct assessments and interventions for clients while being supervised by security and law enforcement staff. Such conditions can hamper the trust and sense of confidentiality that are hallmarks of the therapeutic relationship.

Content

Correctional facilities include mental health questions as part of receiving, screening, and conducting follow-up for every offender. Comprehensive assessments help identify the client's needs, particularly those requiring immediate attention. In addition, a separate mental health screening and evaluation process is performed on all admissions to mental health facilities or treatment centers to identify level of functioning and uncover less obvious mental conditions (Smith & Smith, 2006). Ford and colleagues (2007) released two particular screening tools for use in correctional facilities: the Correctional Mental Health Screen and the Brief Jail Mental Health Screen, which contribute to the overall mental health triage. As part of an effective triage system, nurses may be involved with training correctional staff regarding initial screening, conducting more in-depth psychiatric evaluations, or referring clients for a full-scale psychiatric evaluation.

Critical information needed to plan nursing care often includes police reports, correctional files, and previous mental health records. Crime histories and history of aggression also are essential (Schafer & Peternelj-Taylor, 2000). Assessments should include a history of psychiatric illness, hospitalization and outpatient treatment, current psychotropic medication, suicidal ideation, self-mutilating behavior, risk assessment, and drug and alcohol use. Nurses need to be alert to assessing substance use because many clients continue to abuse drugs and alcohol while hospitalized or incarcerated. Focused, in-depth assessments are conducted on clients admitted for fitness-to-stand-trial assessments and for special programming, such as sexual offenders (Scheela, 2001), parasuicidal clients (Roth & Pressé, 2003), and those with anger management or intermittent explosive disorders (Schafer & Peternelj-Taylor, 2000).

Risk of Suicide

Suicide rates among forensic clients have declined significantly during the past two decades (Mumola, 2005). Nevertheless, incidence of self-violence and suicide is much higher than in the general population, and suicide risk assessment remains a critical area of practice. Unrestricted access to psychiatric care must be available for any offender presenting with suicidal ideation or at-risk behavior. Youth who present with histories of suicidal behavior are at increased risk for suicide during incarceration and require vigilant monitoring throughout (Penn et al., 2003).

Factors contributing to the significantly higher rate of suicide in forensic clients include history of psychiatric illness, previous suicide attempts, substance abuse and associated withdrawal, psychological effects of arrest and imprisonment, difficulties facing the crime and length of sentence, actual or perceived victimization by other offenders, inability to cope in a confined environment, and lack of communication with family (WHO & International Association for Suicide Prevention, 2007). Correctional officers have a critical role to play in referring at-risk people to forensic nurses for further assessment and intervention (Blair, 2000; HRW, 2003). See Evidence-Based Practice Spotlight 21.1.

A full debriefing must follow suicide (or attempted suicide) in forensic settings. Forensic psychiatric nurses have a role to play as facilitators and can provide leadership for group processing of the event. They use critical incident stress management to minimize adverse effects of stressful or traumatic events such as inmate disorders, riots, and suicide by teaming mental health professionals and trained laypersons to debrief and manage incidents. The National Commission on Correctional Health Care (2003) has added this successful process to its accreditation standards for postsuicide care. (See also Chap. 34.)

▲ NURSING DIAGNOSIS

As in all settings, nurses use assessment data to formulate nursing diagnoses and care plans that meet each client's particular needs. Common relevant diagnoses for forensic populations include Ineffective Coping, Fear, Dysfunctional Grieving, Noncompliance, Chronic Low Self-Esteem, Risk for Self-Mutilation, Disturbed Sleep Pattern, Impaired Social Interaction, Social Isolation, and Risk for Violence: Self-Directed or Other-Directed (NANDA International, 2007).

▲ OUTCOME IDENTIFICATION AND PLANNING

In planning any treatment program with forensic clients, nurses consider the realities and limitations of the setting, which differs in terms of populations served and context of care (ie, within the health care or criminal justice/correctional system). Working knowledge of the operation and culture of secure or controlled environments is essential (Blair, 2000; Hufft, 2006).

Planning short-term goals, which frequently involve completion of tasks and practice of selected communication or self-care skills, must revolve around the mandatory regimens set up for clients. In many settings, therapy conflicts with the realities of structured environments, which include work details, lock-ups, formal countings, and endless security procedures. Nevertheless, manageable, feasible goals are necessary to achieve outcomes that maintain or improve client functioning, regardless of the environment. The challenge for forensic nurses is to be sensitive to scheduled assignments that can be changed and those that cannot. Planning also requires attention to the processes that allow for continuity. It is typical for clients to be transferred from facility to facility, often without health records. When possible, planning should include the client's active participation in the identification of realistic and attainable goals.

Long-term goals must be consistent with the reality of the client's circumstances. Although it may seem unrealistic to plan for reentry to the community for a client at the beginning of a long sentence, Marchese (2007) argues that successful reentry needs to begin when a client commences treatment (or incarceration), and not be left for the time of discharge. Often, it is important to acknowledge that long-term goals, such as developing trusting relationships with peers and staff, may be unrealistic.

> ### Think About It 21.1
> Review Case Vignette 21.1. Examine the scenario for problem areas. Formulate a list of issues that the nurse would need to address in the client's plan of care.

EVIDENCE-BASED PRACTICE SPOTLIGHT 21.1

Interventions for Suicide Prevention in Incarcerated Populations

Overview of Effective Treatment: Comprehensive suicide prevention programs have contributed to reduced rates of attempted and completed suicide among incarcerated populations. Not all suicides can be prevented; however, comprehensive programs provide for mechanisms to identify, assess, and treat potentially suicidal clients. Key components of a suicide prevention program based on contemporary evidence include training, intake screening, post-intake observation, management following screening, monitoring, communication, social intervention, attention to the physical environment and architecture, and mental health treatment. Screening tools such as the Suicide Risk Assessment Scale, a nine-item suicide checklist, can be particularly useful in practice; they provide standard or structured questions, they can facilitate communication between staff members, and they provide legal documentation. Moreover, checklists are not confined for use upon admission and can be used at any time during a client's confinement.

What Has Not Been Shown Effective: Suicide is a very private act and almost always occurs when a person is alone. There is a strong association between suicide and type of housing assignment. Placing at-risk individuals in single cells or in isolation should be avoided whenever possible. If isolation must be used, then constant observation and companionship should be provided. Ideally, dormitory or double bunking housing assignments should be implemented. Placement of juvenile offenders in adult facilities contributes to increased risk and should also be avoided whenever possible.

Implications for Practice: All staff who work with incarcerated clients should receive suicide prevention training as part of their orientation and ongoing professional development. Forensic nurses are in an ideal position to update staff regarding new developments regarding suicide prevention based on outcome studies. Peer monitoring programs that use "inmate buddies" or "listeners" can provide emotional support to at-risk clients but should not take the place of professional nurses. Forensic nurses must carefully assess the use of peers and also ensure that they are adequately screened, trained, and supervised. They should also continue to advocate for policies and resources to support best practices in suicide prevention.

References

Daigle, M. S., Labelle, R., & Cote, G. (2006). Further evidence for the validity of the Suicide Risk Assessment Scale for prisoners. *International Journal of Law and Psychiatry, 29,* 343–354.

Mumola, C. J. (2005). Suicide and homicide in state prisons and local jails. *Bureau of Justice Statistics Special Report* (NCJ 210036, pp. 1–12). Retrieved from http://www.ojp.usdoj.gov/bjs/pub/pdf/shsplj.pdf.

Way, B. B., Sawyer, D. A., Barboza, S., & Nash, R. (2007). Inmate suicide and time spent in special disciplinary housing in New York State Prison. *Psychiatric Services, 58*(4), 558–560.

World Health Organization & International Association for Suicide Prevention. (2007). *Preventing suicide in jails and prisons* (pp. 1–28). Retrieved from http://www.who.int/mental_health/prevention/suicide/resource_jails_prisons.pdf

▲ IMPLEMENTATION

The ability to establish therapeutic relationships with forensic clients is one of the most important competencies that forensic nurses need. Therapy issues can be stressful and complicated, and the effects of the forensic milieu on both nurses and clients cannot be ignored. Cultural and ideologic variations among correctional personnel, forensic clients, and helping professionals must be considered when navigating the counseling role (Peternelj-Taylor, 2002; Schafer & Peternelj-Taylor, 2003).

Recurring themes of power and control, negotiation, and trust building dominate therapeutic interventions in this setting; clients have, in varying degrees, learned to adapt to an environment that rewards distrust, manipulation, and deceit (Peternelj-Taylor, 2002) (Challenging Behaviors 21.1). Criminal histories, frequent diagnoses of antisocial and borderline personality disorder, and aggressive interpersonal styles can evoke strong emotional responses from nurses; countertransference and splitting reactions are common. Most would agree that diverse opinions make for a resource-rich team; however, when emotional reactions mix with sound clinical judgment, team members may become polarized, which negatively affects the overall integrity of therapeutic interventions (Roth & Pressé, 2003; Woods et al., 2006).

Establishing and maintaining therapeutic nurse–client relationships in forensic settings are trying and difficult tasks. Issues surrounding treatment boundaries frequently prevail (Box 21.3). The familiarity and trust that develop over time, coupled with the seductive pull of helping, can contribute to nurses becoming overly involved in their work, which also may erode boundaries. Nurses have been known to become intimately involved with forensic clients, a phenomenon that Peternelj-Taylor (1998) refers to as "forbidden love." The intensity of the forensic environment contributes to this immediate risk because institutions are considered "hotbeds" for problems. However, failing to engage a client and attend to his or her treatment needs is equally problematic, yet underinvolvement rarely is understood in relation to treatment boundaries (Peternelj-Taylor, 2002). Sexual dilemmas and other boundary violations should be considered occupational hazards, not just

Challenging Behaviors 21.1

The Client Who Requests Personal Information

Situation: A client with whom you work frequently asks personal questions or attempts to discuss your personal life (eg, "Do you have a boyfriend?" "Are you married?" "Do you have children?"). Likewise, she attempts to challenge your credibility by saying things like "How would you know how to deal with this problem, you had such a good life growing up?" "You know everything about me, but I know nothing about you," or "How can you help me with this problem? You don't know what it is like."

Your Potential Feelings: Uncertainty, awkwardness, unease.

What Is Going On? The client may be asking questions purely out of curiosity or may be engaging in social chitchat. Such requests, however, are more likely a form of manipulation and a way to control the situation (and information), as well as avoid talking about herself or her problem.

Strategy: The intent of self-disclosure is to be empathic and to let clients know that they are understood (see Chap. 11). Often nurses can share general rather than specific information. Self-disclosure requires thoughtful consideration and clinical judgment; the goal is always therapeutic. The nurse stays client focused and redirects the interview back to the client after the disclosure (eg, "Is that how you felt?"). Nurses avoid sharing personal problems with clients because this may lead to role reversal and transgression of the treatment boundaries.

Nurse Action/Communication: Refer to the policies and procedures specific to your employer (or your clinical placement). If the problem is ongoing, the treatment team should determine and apply consistently a course of action.

---

social and professional taboos (Peternelj-Taylor, 1998, 2002; Peternelj-Taylor & Yonge, 2003; Schafer & Peternelj-Taylor, 2003). See Challenging Behaviors 21.2.

Promoting Health

Forensic nursing includes health promotion. Unfortunately, because of fiscal constraints, mandates of the particular forensic facility, and a general preoccupation with acute care, it can be easily dismissed (Peternelj-Taylor, 2005a). Female offenders, in particular, are interested in their own health, and a discussion about contraception and birth control can be an opportunity to

express feelings related to abuse, powerlessness, or social awkwardness (Maeve, 2003; Sowers et al., 1999).

Nurses in forensic settings also are responsible for mental health and wellness promotion (Peternelj-Taylor, 2005a). Stress management is not just a health promotion strategy in this milieu, it is a real-life skill. Programs that promote adaptation and coping in selected situations may translate into life skills that promote more effective rehabilitation. Nevertheless, nurses must be aware that improving opportunities to achieve the highest level of physical, psychosocial, and social functioning puts clients in a catch-22 position. The skills to survive in prison are

---

BOX 21.3 Boundary Maintenance Strategies

- **Be aware of red flags of caution such as:**
  - "You are such a good nurse."
  - "You are the only one who understands me."
  - "I would never have gotten into trouble if I had someone like you in my life."
- **Do not become dependent on your clients to meet your social needs.** Have a good, intact, and separate social life.
- **Avoid inappropriate self-disclosure.** Self-disclosure that meets the needs of the nurse, not the client, can lead to role reversal.
- **Engage in boundary violation "spot checks."** Ask yourself the following questions:
  - "What do I do when I am attracted to a client, or when a client is attracted to me? How do I set the boundaries?"
  - "Am I having my intimacy needs met through my relationship with my clients?"

- "Would I say or do this in front of my other clients? My colleagues? My supervisor?"
- "Am I doing this for the client's benefit or to meet a need of my own? And if I think I am doing this for the client's benefit, am I fooling myself?"
- **Talk to trusted colleagues.** Be honest with yourself regarding your feelings about clients. Talking to trusted colleagues and supervisors will assist in effective boundary maintenance.
- **Seek clinical supervision.** This is an effective risk management strategy that can assist with the management of feelings related to the nurse–client relationship and prevent the gradual erosion of boundaries.
- **Contribute to meaningful practice guidelines.** Realistically, guidelines for every situation are unlikely. Hypothetical scenarios, however, can be used to educate team members and invite differing views and recommendations for practice.

For further information, see Peternelj-Taylor, C., & Yonge, O. (2003). Exploring boundaries in the nurse–client relationship: Professional roles and responsibilities. *Perspectives in Psychiatric Care, 39*(2), 55–66.

Challenging Behaviors 21.2

The Client Who Gives Compliments and Makes Sexually Explicit Remarks

Situation: Your assigned client frequently compliments you on your looks and has begun to act out seductively.

Your Potential Feelings: Embarrassment, anxiety, fear.

What Is Going On? Most forensic clients have poor interpersonal skills. The compliments might be genuine, but more often than not the client is "testing" you to see how you might respond. Furthermore, the client may be attempting to split you from the rest of the treatment team, hoping that you will regard the relationship as special or unique.

Strategy: Students and novice nurses often have a hard time dealing with compliments and sexually explicit remarks made

by forensic clients. Instead of confronting this inappropriate behavior, they often withdraw. A direct verbal approach is required. For example, "Thank you for the compliment (if appropriate), but I would appreciate that from this point on you keep your comments to yourself." Or "I'm not here to discuss my eyes, hair, or my body." And "Your remarks are irrelevant to my purpose in working with you." Avoid engaging in flirtatious and sexual banter with all clients.

Nurse Action/Communication: Discuss this situation with the treatment team and document your actions and the client's response. If the behavior continues and becomes more brazen and threatening, the client may need reassignment to another nurse, unit in the facility, or both.

---

not the same as those required to survive on the street (Hufft & Fawkes, 1994).

Maintaining an Interdisciplinary Approach

Teamwork is essential to working in forensic environments. Communication among nurses, other health care professionals, and correctional personnel is vital to safe and professional practice. The cross-training required for an interdisciplinary approach to forensic health requires sharing knowledge of therapeutic modalities while incorporating professional standards of practice (Aufderheide & Brown, 2005; Dumpel, 2006).

Many different health care providers are involved in forensic mental health services, and all need to work collaboratively to deliver high-quality care consistent with the community standard. In correctional settings, nurses work in partnership with correctional personnel to ensure appropriate health care to those who are confined (ANA, 2007). Correctional personnel need to be informed when suicidal, homicidal, or out-of-control behavior is suspected or is of concern (Peternelj-Taylor & Johnson, 1995). The most successful client outcomes are achieved when team members share a common philosophy: professionalism in providing security and quality health care to those in custody (Hufft, 2006; Maeve, 2003).

Focusing on the Family

Williams (2007) observes that "men and women confined to prisons and jail are not held in a vacuum. Even under lock and key, they remain parents, husbands, wives, daughters, sons and neighbors who will return to their homes once released. As such their health is inextricably linked to the health or our society" (p. 82). Unfortunately, family members comprise a hidden forensic population. They are seldom accounted for or discussed, yet they are linked to the total health profile of the forensic population and represent a significant portion of at-risk society. Too often, clinical practice with forensic clients occurs apart from family and the community. Families frequently experience guilt

and blame themselves for the crimes of their relatives (Encinares & Lorbergs, 2001). Support, guidance, and psychoeducational programs are important strategies to adopt when working with family members (Figure 21.4). Such approaches not only have the potential to contribute to the overall management and rehabilitation of forensic clients, but also can contribute to the well-being of the whole family, thereby preventing further involvement of other relatives with the criminal justice system (Freudenberg et al., 2005).

Current trends in health care are calling for increased access to mental health services, more emphasis on prevention, and community partnerships. Examples of effective, collaborative community-based partnerships include (1) early intervention programs that address the psychological risk factors in pregnancy for female forensic clients (Fogel & Belyea, 2001; Williams & Schulte-Day, 2006); (2) a home care program for

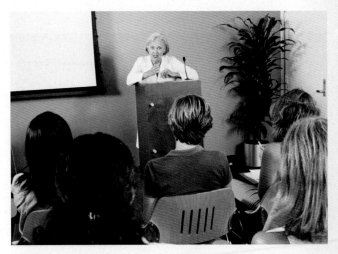

FIGURE 21.4 This forensic nurse practitioner is conducting a seminar and support group for wives and partners of incarcerated clients.

children, adolescents, and their families involved in the juvenile justice system (Shelton & Pearson, 2005); (3) working with the families of incarcerated women, as in the Girl Scouts Beyond Bars programs (Hufft, 1999); (4) a statewide implementation of a crisis intervention team program (Munetz et al., 2006); and (5) community-based reentry programming (Freudenberg et al., 2005). These questions are appropriate for forensic nurses to contemplate because they form the foundation for future forensic nursing practice.

Ensuring Continuity of Care

Continuity of care is virtually nonexistent for offenders who leave correctional or treatment settings. Offenders with mental illness in particular experience high rates of recidivism, high symptom levels, and poor quality of life. Little opportunity exists for long-term case management or discharge planning. Evaluating the progress of clients with a view of returning to the community is difficult if they have no opportunities to interact with that community (Kerns & Pinney, 2006; McCoy et al., 2004).

Dvoskin and Broaddus (1993) have proposed a mental health care model for the efficient and systematic treatment of offenders with mental illness. This approach advocates a seamless continuum of services that includes prisons and satellite services within the community, linking correctional and parole staff with community mental health care providers. The underlying premise is that forensic settings are communities in which people live and work together under various stressors. This model, designed to address stressors as challenges to community living, provides a framework that bridges the forensic and nonforensic settings. Components include screening and referral, crisis beds, intermediate care (residential care), outpatient services, predischarge planning services, and postrelease services, including mental health, probation, and parole. Although such a system may seem idealistic, the underlying assumptions are increasingly being actualized in practice (Smith & Smith, 2006), and nurses are ideally situated to embrace expanded roles in this regard (Figure 21.5).

Encinares and Lorbergs (2001) describe nursing practice in a comprehensive forensic outpatient clinic that emphasizes therapeutic alliance, vocational rehabilitation, employment and recreational activities, family involvement, community involvement, housing and financial support, knowledge of the legal system, and cultural and spiritual needs of clients. Likewise, Maeve (2003) describes an innovative Nursing Care Partnership Program designed to partner women with nurses before their release from jail, as a way to promote their health while attempting to break the cycle of repeated incarcerations. Finally, McCoy et al. (2004) describe a successful assertive community treatment program for people with mental illness who are released from jail. It demonstrates reductions in both psychiatric hospital use and jail recidivism, while contributing to the overall quality of life for participants.

Acting as Advocate

Traditional principles of advocacy involve informing clients of their choices and rights and then supporting their decisions. In any psychiatric setting, this standard is controversial; in forensic settings, it is inflammatory. Client actions and communications are not privileged information. Advocacy standards demand that nurses be honest with clients, informing them that disclosure of medical records is a reality and that court proceedings against clients may require testimony from nurses (Figure 21.6).

Frequently, conflicting priorities compromise the ability of forensic nurses to advocate for clients. Confinement, isolation, and security goals generally override the health care needs of many prisoners (Dumpel, 2006). The advocacy role differs in forensic psychiatric nursing from the role in other settings or specialties because nurses embrace the destigmatization and decriminalization of the client group. Rehabilitation into the public arena is difficult, particularly because of public and political antipathy toward offenders.

From a public health perspective, the state of health of the correctional population reflects that of the community at large.

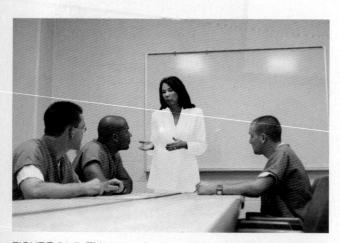

FIGURE 21.5 This nurse is discussing community supports and intervention programs for a group of forensic clients about to be released from prison.

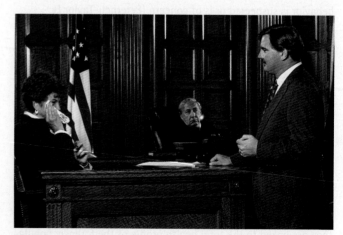

FIGURE 21.6 Nurses must make clear to clients the limits of disclosure in forensic settings. Clients need to understand that nurses may need to share information divulged in court proceedings against clients.

Nurses need to acquaint themselves with policies that affect the forensic population and overall society. Multisectoral collaboration is one avenue to meet the complex needs of forensic clients and includes not only health and justice, but also social and economic sectors (Freudenberg et al., 2005; Peternelj-Taylor, 2003). In addition, supporting the implementation of policies based on well-designed research and questioning those based on convenience or "conventional wisdom" are appropriate political roles.

▲ EVALUATION

To assess the effectiveness of the nursing process in forensic settings, nurses measure client behaviors that indicate resolution or change in diagnostic criteria, specifically the signs and symptoms that indicated a psychiatric problem. Depending on diagnosis and prognosis, nurses evaluate outcomes in terms of small successes, which many clients consider "giant steps."

Change that leads clients to solve problems, to demonstrate the ability to reason and show good judgment, or to comply with institutional rules is a form of success (Schafer & Peternelj-Taylor, 2000).

When measuring the effectiveness of treatment outcomes in forensic settings, health care professionals must be cognizant of the definition of the forensic mental health treatment being used (Greenwood, 1995). The goal is to address a mental disorder, whereas the goal of correctional treatment is to decrease recidivism. These terms are not mutually exclusive and do not always work in tandem. A person may deal well with a mental health problem but continue to break the law. Finally, researchers and practitioners alike need to continue to work together to learn more about treatment effectiveness: "for *whom* does it work, *when* does it work, and *how* does it work" (Wormith et al., 2007, p. 888).

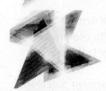

Reviewing and Applying Your Knowledge

Chapter Summary

- Forensic psychiatric nursing helps bridge the gap between the criminal justice and mental health care systems.

- Deinstitutionalization, homelessness, increased drug incarcerations, interpersonal and domestic violence, and anticrime legislation are contributors to the soaring forensic psychiatric population.

- Forensic clients are young and old, male and female, and victims and perpetrators of crime.

- Forensic settings include forensic psychiatric facilities, locked units of general hospitals, and state hospitals. However, common practice sites are jails and prisons.

- Legal and ethical issues related to forensic clients are pertinent to forensic psychiatric nursing, and nurses need to be familiar with relevant legislation governing the settings in which they are employed.

Study Questions

1. When reviewing trends in forensic nursing, the nurse notes that one of the largest changes in the composition of the forensic population requiring special adaptations is associated with

   a. an increased number of elderly offenders.

   b. the number of juvenile offenders.

   c. a decreased number of female offenders.

   d. an increased number of offenders charged with drug offenses.

2. A nurse is caring for a verbally aggressive forensic client who reminds her of her ex-boyfriend. At the end of the interview, she seeks out an experienced nurse colleague to explore her feelings about this client. The nurse's actions indicate

   a. inability to cope with the forensic milieu.

   b. the need for psychotherapy.

   c. boundary exploitation.

   d. appropriate self-awareness.

3. A nurse is preparing a teaching plan for a group of psychiatric nursing students about the three levels of prevention. Which of the following would the nurse include

   as an example of the forensic psychiatric nurse's role in primary prevention?

   a. Conducting a relapse prevention program for sexual offenders

   b. Applying principles of crisis management after a suicide attempt

   c. Developing a medication management program for an offender with schizophrenia

   d. Participating in a multidisciplinary committee focusing on domestic violence

4. Which of the following would the nurse identify as increasing a forensic client's risk for suicide?

   a. History of psychiatric illness, difficulties facing the crime, perceived victimization by other offenders

   b. Actual victimization by other offenders, dormitory-type housing, ability to cope with a confined environment

   c. Substance abuse, difficulties facing the length of the sentence, open communication with family and friends

   d. Age older than 45 years, previous suicide attempts, acceptance of the crime

5. When acting as an advocate for a forensic client, which of the following actions is crucial?

   a. Ensuring that the client's actions and behaviors remain privileged

   b. Supporting the client in decisions about choices made

   c. Informing the client that medical records are subject to disclosure

   d. Telling the client that nurse–client conversations will not be used against him or her

Critical-Thinking Questions

1. Correctional institutions are among the most extreme living environments. Can such an environment lead to healing and personal growth? Does it reinforce clients as criminals or inmates? How can psychiatric nurses create therapeutic environments in forensic milieus?

2. If you could rewrite history, would you change the deinstitutionalization movement? How and why?

3. How might a forensic nurse deal with ethical issues that emerge in practice?

References

Adams, K., & Ferrandino, J. (2012). Managing mentally ill inmates in prisons. *Criminal Justice and Behavior, 39*, 125–143.

American Nurses Association (ANA). (2007). *Corrections nursing: Scope and standards of practice.* Silver Spring, MD: Author.

American Psychiatric Nurses Association. (2012). *Forensic Psychiatric Nurses Council.* Retrieved from http://www.apna.org/i4a/pages/index.cfm?pageid=3737

Anno, B. J., Graham, C., Lawrence, J. E., & Shanksy, R. (2004). *Correctional health care: Addressing the needs of elderly, chronically ill, and terminally ill inmates* (Accession No. 018735). Washington, DC: National Institute of Corrections.

Aufderheide, D. H., & Brown, P. H. (2005, February). Crisis in corrections: The mentally ill in America's prisons. *Corrections Today,* 30–33.

Austin, W. (2001). Relational ethics in forensic psychiatric settings. *Journal of Psychosocial Nursing, 39*(9), 12–17.

Blair, P. (2000). Improving nursing practice in correctional settings. *Journal of Nursing Law, 7*(2), 19–30.

Blair, P. (2002). Correctional nursing: What's wrong with this picture? *CorrectCare, 16*(4), 8.

Blanchard, B. (2004). Incarcerated mothers and their children: A complex issue. *Forum on Correctional Research, 16*(1), 45–46.

Blanchette, K., & Brown, S. L. (2006). *The assessment and treatment of women offenders: An integrative perspective.* Chichester, UK: John Wiley & Sons.

Bolger, M. (2005). Dying in prison: Providing palliative care in challenging environments. *International Journal of Palliative Care, 11*(12), 619–620.

Bonham, E. (2006). Adolescent mental health and the juvenile justice system. *Pediatric Nursing, 32*(6), 591–595.

Buckley, C. (2010, January 29). Law has little effect on early release for inmates. *The New York Times.* Available from http://www.nytimes.com/2010/01/30/nyregion/30parole.html

Cashin, A. (2006). Extreme nursing: Forensic adolescent mental health nursing in Australia. *Journal of Child and Adolescent Psychiatric Nursing, 19*(3), 99–102.

Clements, P. T., & Akiyama, C. (2011). Youth gangs: Reason for concern. *Journal of Forensic Nursing, 7*(3), 105–107.

Cloyes, K. (2007). Prisoners signify: A political discourse analysis of mental illness in a prison control unit. *Nursing Inquiry, 14*(3), 202–211.

Dumpel, H. (2006, March). Critical patient advocacy issues facing correctional RNs in California, Part II. *California Nurse,* 22–26.

Dvoskin, J. A., & Broaddus, R. (1993). Creating a mental health care model. *Corrections Today, 55*(7), 114–115.

Encinares, M. (2007). Community care of elderly offenders with dementia. *Journal of Chinese Clinical Medicine, 21*(1), 34–41.

Encinares, M., & Lorbergs, K. A. (2001). Framing nursing practice within a forensic outpatient service. *Journal of Psychosocial Nursing, 39*(9), 35–41.

Fogel, C. I., & Belyea, M. (2001). Psychological risk factors in pregnant inmates: A challenge for nursing. *Maternal Child Nursing, 26*(1), 10–16.

Ford, J., Trestman, R. L., Osher, F., Scott, J. E., Steadman, H. J., & Robbins, P. C. (2007). Mental health screens for corrections. *National Institute of Justice Research for Practice* (NCJ216152, pp.1–18). Retrieved from http://www.ncjrs.gov/pdffiles1/nij/216152.pdf

Freudenberg, N., Daniels, J., Crum, M., Perkins, T., & Richie, B. E. (2005). Coming home from jail: The social and health consequences of community reentry for women, male adolescents, and their families. *American Journal of Public Health, 95*(10), 1725–1736.

Gondles, J. A. (2005, February). The mentally ill don't belong in jail. *Corrections Today,* 1.

Greenwood, A. (1995). Forensic mental health treatment: Do we really know what we are talking about? *Forum on Correctional Research, 7*(3), 27–29.

Harner, H. M. (2004). Relationships between incarcerated women: Moving beyond stereotypes. *Journal of Psychosocial Nursing, 42*(1), 38–46.

Harrison, P. M., & Beck, A. J. (2003, July). Prisoners in 2002. *Bureau of Justice Statistics Bulletin* (NCJ 200248, pp.1–14). Retrieved from http://www.ojp.usdoj.gov/bjs/ pub/pdf/p02.pdf

Hufft, A. G. (1999). Girl Scouts Beyond Bars: A unique opportunity for forensic psychiatric nursing. *Journal of Psychosocial Nursing, 37*(9), 45–51.

Hufft, A. G. (2006). Correctional nursing. In R. M. Hammer, G. Moynihan, & E. M. Pagliaro (Eds.), *Forensic nursing: A handbook for practice* (pp. 633–665). Sudbury, MA: Jones & Bartlett.

Hufft, A. G., & Fawkes, L. S. (1994). Federal inmates: A unique psychiatric nursing challenge. *Nursing Clinics of North America, 29*(1), 35–42.

Hufft, A., & Kite, M. M. (2003). Vulnerable and cultural perspectives for nursing care in correctional systems. *Journal of Multicultural Nursing & Health, 9*(1), 18–26.

Human Rights Watch (HRW). (2003). *Ill equipped: U.S. prisons and offenders with mental illness.* New York, NY: Author.

International Association of Forensic Nurses. (2012). What is forensic nursing? Retrieved from http://www.iafn.org/displaycommon.cfm?an=1&subarticlenbr=137

International Association of Forensic Nurses (IAFN) & American Nurses Association (ANA). (1997). *Scope and standards of forensic nursing practice.* Washington, DC: American Nurses Association.

James, D. J., & Glaze, L. E. (2006, September). Mental health problems of prison and jail inmates. *Bureau of Justice Statistics Special Report* (NCJ 213600, pp. 1–12). Retrieved from http://www.ojp.usdoj.gov/bjs/pub/pdf/mhppji.pdf

Kerns, J., & Pinney, B. (2006). Promoting systems for continuity of care. In M. Puisis (Ed.), *Clinical practice in correctional medicine* (2nd ed., pp. 472–488). Philadelphia, PA: Elsevier.

Klein, A. A. (2003). Care is care no matter where. *The Nurse Practitioner, 28*(7), 45.

Lamberti, J. S., Weisman, R., & Faden, D. I. (2004). Forensic assertive community treatment. Preventing incarceration of adults with severe mental illness. *Psychiatric Services, 55*(11), 1295–1298.

Love, C. C., & Hunter, M. (1999). The Atascadero State Hospital experience: Engaging patients in violence prevention. *Journal of Psychosocial Nursing, 37*(9), 32–36.

Lynch, V. A., & Duval, J. B. (2010). *Forensic nursing science* (2nd ed.). St. Louis, MO: Mosby.

Maeve, M. K. (2003). Nursing care partnerships with women leaving jail: Effects on health and crime. *Journal of Psychosocial Nursing, 41*(9), 30–40.

Marchese, J. T. (2007, October). Starting the reentry process in the beginning. *Corrections Today,* 20–21.

Maroney, M. K. (2005). Caring and custody: Two faces of the same reality. *Journal of Correctional Health Care, 11*(2), 157–169.

McCoy, M. L., Roberts, D. L., Hanrahan, P., Clay, R., & Luchins, D. J. (2004). Jail linkage assertive community treatment services for individuals with mental illnesses. *Psychiatric Rehabilitation Journal, 27*(3), 243–250.

Mumola, C. J. (2005). Suicide and homicide in state prisons and local jails. *Bureau of Justice Statistics Special Report* (NCJ 210036, pp. 1–12). Retrieved from http://www.ojp.usdoj.gov/bjs/pub/pdf/shsplj.pdf

Munetz, M. R., & Griffin, P. A. (2006). Use of sequential intercept model as an approach to decriminalization of people with serious mental illness. *Psychiatric Services, 57*(4), 544–549.

Munetz, M. R., Morrison, A., Krake, J., Young, B., & Woody, M. (2006). Statewide implementation of the crisis intervention team program: The Ohio model. *Psychiatric Services, 57*(11), 1569–1571.

NANDA International. (2007). *NANDA International nursing diagnoses: Definitions and classification, 2007–2008.* Philadelphia, PA: Wiley-Blackwell.

National Commission on Correctional Health Care. (2003). *Standards for health services in jails.* Chicago, IL: Author.

Osborne, O. (1995). Public sector psychosocial nursing. *Journal of Psychosocial Nursing, 33*(8), 4–6.

Penn, J. V., Esposito, C. L., Schaeffer, L. E., Fritz, G. K., & Spirito, A. (2003). Suicide attempts and self-mutilative behavior in a juvenile correctional facility. *American Academy of Child and Adolescent Psychiatry, 42*(7), 762–769.

Peternelj-Taylor, C. (1998). Forbidden love: Sexual exploitation in the forensic milieu. *Journal of Psychosocial Nursing and Mental Health Services, 36*(6), 17–23.

Peternelj-Taylor, C. (2002). Professional boundaries: A matter of professional integrity. *Journal of Psychosocial Nursing and Mental Health Services, 40*(4), 22–29.

Peternelj-Taylor, C. (2003). Guest editorial: Incarceration of the vulnerable. *Journal of Psychosocial Nursing and Mental Health Services, 41*(9), 6–7.

Peternelj-Taylor, C. (2004). An exploration of mothering in forensic psychiatric and correctional nursing. *Canadian Journal of Nursing Research, 36*(4), 130–146.

Peternelj-Taylor, C. (2005a). Mental health promotion in forensic and correctional environments. *Journal of Psychosocial Nursing and Mental Health Services, 43*(9), 8–9.

Peternelj-Taylor, C. (2005b). "Ordinary" women, extraordinary life circumstances. *Journal of Forensic Nursing, 1*(2), 84–85.

Peternelj-Taylor, C. A., & Johnson, R. L. (1995). Serving time: Psychiatric mental health nursing in corrections. *Journal of Psychosocial Nursing, 33*(8), 12–19.

Peternelj-Taylor, C., & Yonge, O. (2003). Exploring boundaries in the nurse–client relationship: Professional roles and responsibilities. *Perspectives in Psychiatric Care, 39*(2), 55–66.

Public Safety Canada. (2007). *Substance abuse.* Retrieved from http://www.publicsafety.gc.ca/prg/cor/acc/suba-eng.aspx

Quanbeck, C., Frye, M., & Altshuler, L. (2003). Mania and the law in California: Understanding the criminalization of the mentally ill. *American Journal of Psychiatry, 160*(7), 1245–1250.

Reimer, G. R. (2007). Transforming correctional health care through advanced correctional nursing education. *Journal of Correctional Health Care, 13,* 163–169.

Rikard, R. V., & Rosenberg, E. (2007). Aging inmates: A convergence of trends in the American criminal justice system. *Journal of Correctional Health Care, 13,* 150–162.

Roth, B., & Pressé, L. (2003). Nursing interventions for parasuicidal behaviors in female offenders. *Journal of Psychosocial Nursing, 41*(9), 20–29.

Sabol, W. J., Minton, T. D., & Harrison, P. M. (2007). Prison and jail inmates at midyear 2006. *Bureau of Justice Statistics Bulletin* (NCJ 217675, pp. 1–22). Retrieved from http://www.ojp.usdoj.gov/bjs/pub/pdf/pjim06.pdf

Schafer, P., & Peternelj-Taylor, C. (2000). Anger management. In D. Mercer, T. Mason, M. McKeown, & G. McCann (Eds.), *Forensic mental health care: A case study approach* (pp. 129–137). Edinburgh, UK: Churchill Livingstone.

Schafer, P., & Peternelj-Taylor, C. (2003). Therapeutic relationships and boundary maintenance: The perspective of forensic patients enrolled in a treatment program for violent offenders. *Issues in Mental Health Nursing, 24,* 605–625.

Scheela, R. A. (2001). Sex offender treatment: Therapists' experiences and perceptions. *Issues in Mental Health Nursing, 22*(8), 749–767.

Shelton, D. (2005). Patterns of treatment services and costs for young offenders with mental disorders. *Journal of Child and Adolescent Psychiatric Nursing, 18*(3), 103–112.

Shelton, D., & Pearson, G. (2005). ADHA in juvenile offenders: Treatment issues nurses need to know. *Journal of Psychosocial Nursing and Mental Health Services, 43*(9), 38–46.

Smith, H., & Smith, L. D. (2006). Correctional based mental health services: Designing a system that works. In M. Puisis (Ed.), *Clinical practice in correctional medicine* (2nd ed., pp. 292–305). Philadelphia, PA: Elsevier.

Smith, S. (2005). Stepping through the looking glass: Professional autonomy in correctional nursing. *Corrections Today,* 54–56, 70.

Sowers, W., Thompson, K., & Mullins, S. (1999). *Mental health in corrections: An overview for correctional staff.* Lanham, MD: American Correctional Association.

Statistics Canada. (2003). *Canadian Centre for Justice Statistics: Special study on mentally disordered in the criminal justice system.* Ottawa, Canada: Minister of Industry.

Steadman, H. J., Stainbrook, K. A., Griffin, P., Draine, J., Dupont, R., & Horey, C. (2001). A specialized crisis response site as a core element of police-based diversion programs. *Psychiatric Services, 52*(2), 219–222.

Teplin, L. A., Abram, K. M., McClelland, G. M., Washburn, J. J., & Pikus, A. K. (2005). Detecting mental disorder in juvenile detainees: Who receives services? *American Journal of Public Health, 95*(10), 1773–1780.

Thomas, G. (2005). *Harm reduction policies and programs for persons involved in the criminal justice system. Harm reduction for special populations in Canada.* Retrieved from http://www.ccsa.ca/NR/rdonlyres/B092A5D6-C627-4503-8F21-8A1AB8923B3A/0/ccsa0039002005.pdf

Trulson, C. R. (2007). Institutional corrections for juveniles: Special issue introduction. *Youth Violence and Juvenile Justice, 5*(1), 4–6.

Trupin, E., & Richards, H. (2003). Seattle's mental health courts: Early indicators of effectiveness. *International Journal of Law and Psychiatry, 26,* 33–53.

Vlahov, D., & Putnam, S. (2006). From corrections to communities as an HIV priority. *Journal of Urban Health: Bulletin of the New York Academy of Medicine, 83*(3), 339–348.

Watson, A., Hanrahan, P., Luchins, D., & Lurigio, A. (2001). Mental health courts and the complex issue of mentally ill offenders. *Psychiatric Services, 52*(4), 477–481.

White, P., & Whiteford, H. (2006). Prisons: Mental health institutions of the 21st century? *The Medical Journal of Australia, 185*(6), 302–303.

Williams, N. H. (2007). Prison health and the health of the public: Ties that bind. *Journal of Correctional Health Care, 13*(2), 80–92.

Williams, L., & Schulte-Day, S. (2006). Pregnant in prison—The incarcerated woman's experience: A preliminary descriptive study. *Journal of Correctional Health Care, 12*(2), 78–88.

Wilson, A. B., & Draine, J. (2006). Collaborations between criminal justice and mental health systems for prisoner reentry. *Psychiatric Services, 57*(6), 875–878.

Woods, P., Kettles, A., & Byrt, R. (2006). *Forensic mental health nursing: Interventions with people with "personality disorder."* London, UK: Quay Books.

World Health Organization (WHO). (2007). *Mental health in prisons.* Retrieved from http://www/who.iny/mental_health/policy/services/en/index.html

World Health Organization (WHO) & International Association for Suicide Prevention (IASP). (2007). *Preventing suicide in jails and prisons.* Retrieved from http://www.who.int/mental_health/prevention/suicide/resource_jails_prisons.pdf

Wormith, J. S., Althouse, R., Simpson, M., Reitzel, L. R., Fagan, T. J., & Morgan, R. D. (2007). The rehabilitation and reintegration of offenders: The current landscape and some future directions for correctional psychology. *Criminal Justice and Behavior, 4*(7), 879–892.

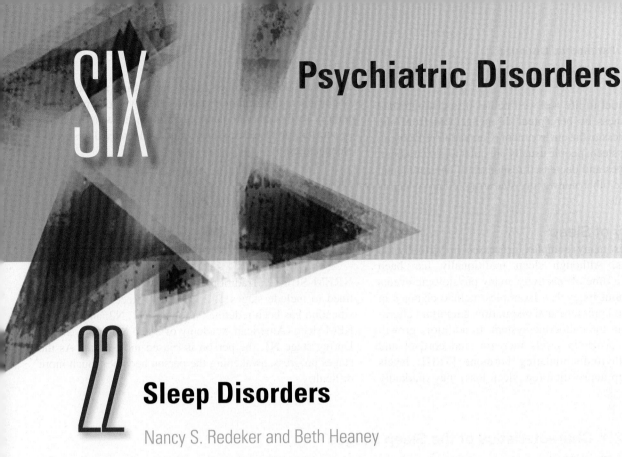

SIX

Psychiatric Disorders

22

Sleep Disorders

Nancy S. Redeker and Beth Heaney

KEY TERMS

circadian rhythm
homeostasis
hypersomnia
insomnia
multiple sleep latency testing
narcolepsy
nocturnal polysomnography
obstructive sleep apnea–hypopnea
  syndrome
parasomnias
periodic limb movement disorder
restless legs syndrome
sleep hygiene

LEARNING OBJECTIVES

On completion of this chapter, you should be able to accomplish the following:

- Define sleep.
- Explain normal changes in sleep across the human lifespan.
- Identify environmental, psychological, psychiatric, physiologic, and medical factors that can affect sleep.
- Discuss the significance of sleep disorders.
- Discuss methods used to diagnose sleep disorders.
- Explain interdisciplinary treatments and nursing interventions for clients with sleep disorders.
- Discuss the specific implications of sleep disorders for psychiatric clients.
- Apply the steps of the nursing process to clients with sleep disorders.

SLEEP

Sleep is essential to life and well-being. It is distinguished from wakefulness by perceptual disengagement from and unresponsiveness to the environment (Carskadon & Dement, 2005). During sleep, people usually are quiet and recumbent, with closed eyes and decreased responses to environmental stimuli. Unlike other nonwaking states (eg, coma), sleep is easily reversible.

Physiology of Sleep

Sleep involves many complex processes in virtually all body systems. Although sleep traditionally has been thought of as a time of inactivity, many physiologic events occur throughout its cycles. Examples include changes in heart rate, blood pressure, and respiration. Important alterations happen in the endocrine system. In addition, growth hormone and prolactin levels increase, and cortisol and thyrotropin (thyroid-stimulating hormone [TSH]) levels decrease. Sleep deprivation (eg, sleep loss) may markedly alter these normal events. Sleep deprivation may be acute or chronic and partial or complete. However, the most common is chronic partial sleep deprivation, in which sleep is of shorter duration than normal and/or decreased in specific sleep stages.

Sleep Stages

The two primary states of sleep are *non-rapid eye movement (NREM) sleep* and *rapid eye movement (REM) sleep*. In adult humans, NREM and REM states alternate throughout the night in approximately 90-minute cycles (Table 22.1).

NREM SLEEP. Traditionally, NREM sleep has been defined to include stages 1, 2, 3, and 4. Recently, this classification has been redefined as stages N1, N2, and NR and REM sleep (American Academy of Sleep Medicine, 2007). During stage N1, the person is roused most easily. As the stages progress, awakening the person becomes much more difficult.

TABLE 22.1 Characteristics of the Sleep Stages

Stage	Physiologic and Biochemical Correlates	Electroencephalogram	Dreaming and Subjective Awareness	Rebound
N1—Light	Muscles are relaxed; eyes display rolling movements; respirations are even; pulse rate is decreased.	Gradual loss of alpha waves	Person may feel a sense of floating or see idle images; if person is awakened, may say he or she was not asleep.	No
N2	Eyes may appear to roll.	Bursts of sleep spindles; sharp, slow waves	Person awakens easily and may report that he or she was thinking or daydreaming.	No
N3—Deep, slow wave	Muscles are very relaxed but tone is maintained; respirations are even; growth hormone and serotonin are released.	Delta (slow wave); person may respond to outside stimuli but is unaware; spindles are present.	Dreams are less dramatic, more realistic, and may lack plot; person requires stronger stimuli to awaken.	No
	Blood pressure, temperature, pulse rate, urine secretion, and oxygen consumption of muscle are decreased; snoring may occur.			Yes, priority
REM sleep	Muscles are at lowest tone; blood pressure, pulse, vaginal secretions, cerebral blood flow, and oxygen consumption are increased; respirations fluctuate; episodic cortisol and adrenocorticotropic hormone (ACTH) and catecholamine are released.	Desynchronized; extremely active; similar to wakefulness	Dreams have vivid content, full color, sounds, implausible settings, and may involve a sense of paralysis; person is difficult to awaken except with significant stimuli.	Yes

During NREM sleep the brain is relatively inactive, actively regulated in a movable body (Carskadon & Dement, 2005). During NREM sleep, heart rate, blood pressure, and respiratory rate generally decrease. Each stage is associated with characteristic patterns of brain wave activity. For example, stage N3 is called slow-wave sleep because of the high-voltage, slow-frequency brain waves that occur (Figure 22.1).

REM SLEEP. Rapid eye movements and vivid dreams occur during REM sleep, which also is associated with great

Awake:
low-voltage, fast

Awake, eyes closed:
alpha-waves, 8–12 cps

Stage 1:
theta-waves, 3–7 cps

Stage 2:
sleep spindles, 12–14 cps;
K-complex

sleep spindle

K-complex

Stages 3 and 4:
delta-waves, 0.5–2 cps

REM:
low-voltage mixed frequency
sawtoothed waves

sawtooth

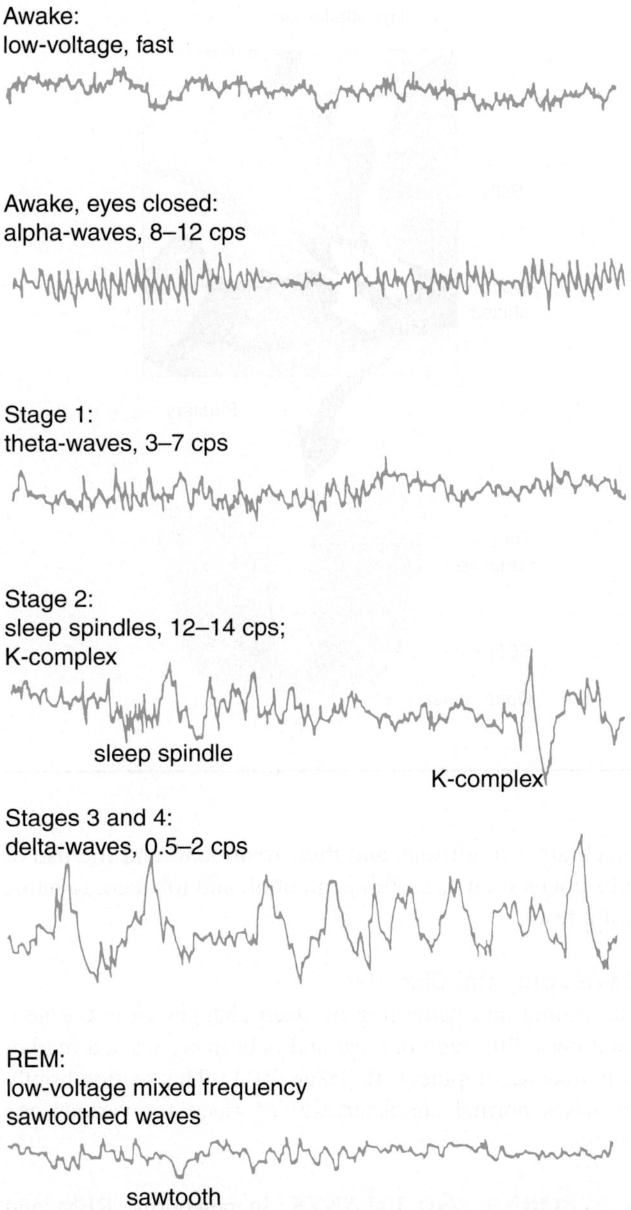

FIGURE 22.1 Each stage of sleep has characteristic patterns of brain wave activity. High-voltage, slow-frequency brain waves mark stages 3 and 4, whereas low-voltage, mixed-frequency waves are indicative of REM sleep. (Courtesy of the University of Washington School of Nursing, Sleep Laboratory, Seattle, WA.)

electrical brain activation and loss of muscle tension, or *atonia*. Heart rate and blood pressure are more variable and may increase during this stage.

Sleep-Regulating Processes

The two primary physiologic processes that regulate sleep cycles are the circadian rhythm and the homeostatic process. These processes work in tandem and the interaction of these two processes is described as the two-process model of sleep (Borbely & Acherman, 2005).

CIRCADIAN RHYTHM. The **circadian rhythm** is regulated by a pacemaker or biologic clock that balances the daily patterning of sleep. In mammals, this structure is the suprachiasmatic nucleus located in the hypothalamus (Understanding Biologic Foundations 22.1). The term *circadian* means "about a day," or a period of 24 hours. The circadian pacemaker stimulates changes in the daily patterns of sleep and wake that are endogenous (stimulated internally) to the organism. The changes occur in an approximately 24-hour rhythm. These circadian characteristics cause sleep and awakening to occur at predictable times of the day and night. For example, most adult humans are diurnal, meaning that they are awake during the day and asleep at night. The tendency to sleep is greatest in the midafternoon and early morning. Genetic predispositions and exogenous (external) factors, such as environmental changes (eg, light/dark exposure), drugs, and behavioral factors (eg, shift work), also influence the timing of the sleep–wake patterns (Czeisler et al., 2005).

Exogenous factors, such as night work or changes in time zones associated with airplane travel may result in changes in patterning of sleep across the 24-hour day. Western society, in which people work and play throughout the evening and night, also affects patterning of sleep–wake cycles. The outcome of these changes is displacement of sleep periods to times of the day that are not part of the person's typical sleep pattern.

HOMEOSTASIS. **Homeostasis** is the result of the coordinated physiologic processes that maintain most steady states in an organism (Cannon, 1939). In humans, the need for sleep increases with the time spent awake. Prolonged periods of wakefulness result in decreased alertness, increased sleepiness, and more slow-wave (stage N3) sleep once the person gets to sleep. Once sleep begins, homeostasis, or the steady state, is achieved, and the accumulated "sleep debt" is replenished. The client awakens feeling rested. This cycle continues over the next period of wakefulness.

Purposes of Sleep

Although experience suggests that sleep is a restorative process that results in the person feeling rested, researchers have not been able to establish the physiologic reasons

UNDERSTANDING BIOLOGIC FOUNDATIONS 22.1

The Suprachiasmatic Nuclei

The hypothalamus within the diencephalon serves as the control center for endocrine, somatic, and autonomic functioning (see Chap. 2). Two suprachiasmatic nuclei (SCN) within the hypothalamus are positioned just above the optic chiasm (where the optic nerves cross) and are next to the brain's third ventricle. The SCN contribute to human circadian rhythms.

Light that reaches the photoreceptors in the retina creates signals that travel along the optic nerve to the SCN. The 20,000 neurons of the SCN then send signals throughout the brain, including to the pineal gland, which responds by stopping production of melatonin. Levels of melatonin in the body normally increase with darkness, making people feel sleepy. Levels fall once the retina and in turn the SCN are again exposed to light, thus decreasing the need for (and the body's production of) melatonin.

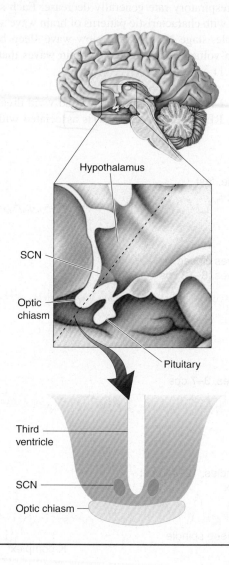

for this, despite many years of investigation. Scientists have proposed various theories about the purpose of sleep, but the function of sleep remains unknown. Yet there is very strong evidence that complete or even partial sleep deprivation contributes to decreases in human performance, such as problems with memory, learning, decision making, poor work performance, injuries, and other negative consequences. Recent evidence suggests that sleep deprivation can also contribute to the development of diabetes and cardiovascular disorders.

Influences on Sleep

Many factors contribute to sleep deprivation and the development of sleep disorders. These may include the person's developmental stage, voluntary patterns of work or leisure, the demands of work and family life, the environment (eg, noise, lighting, and temperature), medical and

psychiatric conditions and their treatment, and the use of substances such as caffeine, alcohol, and tobacco, to name just a few.

Developmental Changes

The timing and patterning of sleep changes from the neonatal period through old age and is in many ways a marker of human development (Redeker, 2011). This section briefly discusses normal characteristics of sleep for various age groups.

NEWBORNS AND INFANTS. In newborns, REM and NREM sleep alterations occur approximately every 50 to 60 minutes. Normal full-term newborns sleep 16 to 18 hours per day, in 3- to 4-hour cycles throughout the day and night. As infants develop during the first few months, more total daily sleep occurs at night. By the end of the first year, infants

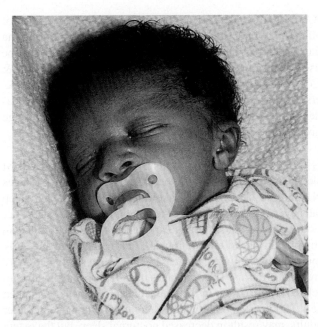

FIGURE 22.2 Infants normally spend more time each day asleep than awake. Their 14 to 15 hours of daily sleep usually consists of one or two naps and 10 to 12 hours of nighttime sleep.

spend approximately half of the day asleep, with most sleep at night with one or two daytime naps (Crabtree & Williams, 2009) (Figure 22.2).

CHILDREN AND ADOLESCENTS. Young children have large amounts of slow-wave and REM sleep relative to adults. Bedtimes and sleep times are earliest for children 12 months old and become later throughout the preschool years. Children 1 to 5 years old sleep approximately 9 hours each night. Napping is virtually universal until the second year of life, and then decreases. Children between the ages of 3 and 5 years who were in daycare slept about 76 minutes per day and usually stopped napping by the age of 4 or 5 (Ward et al., 2008). There are also important cultural behaviors that may have an impact on sleep. For example, sharing of a bedroom or parent–child co-sleeping, as well as nocturnal feedings, may decrease sleep duration and continuity (Jenni & O'Connor, 2005).

Lower socioeconomic status is associated with more variable bedtimes and sleep periods, as well as later rising times, longer times in bed, and more time awake at night (Acebo et al., 2005). As children move into adolescence, total daily sleep gradually declines to approximately 7 to 8 hours per night (Fredriksen et al., 2004). For children 3 to 17 years old, weekday times awake change little, but bedtimes become later. On weekends, bedtimes and wake times become later. The decline in sleep time is most dramatic from ages 8 to 9 years (Snell et al., 2007).

Experts estimate that although adolescents need approximately 9 hours of sleep, they typically get approximately 7 to 8 hours (Wolfson et al., 2007), especially by the end of

adolescence (Fredriksen et al., 2004; Knutson & Lauderdale, 2009). However, total sleep time is not decreased relative to younger children when only weekends are considered (Fredriksen et al., 2004; Knutson & Lauderdale, 2009; Ohayon et al., 2004). REM sleep increases relative to that experienced earlier in childhood (Ohayon et al., 2004).

Circadian changes in sleep timing, particularly later bedtimes, may be normal in adolescence (Carskadon et al., 1999). Teens may be difficult to rouse early in the morning and may experience excessive daytime sleepiness. Sleep deprivation may be a consequence of the mismatch between the adolescent's circadian tendency (stay up late, get up late) and school and work schedules, such as early school start times. Social activities and the use of computers and social media are also important factors that contribute to sleep loss. Sleep deprivation is a growing health concern for children, with estimates of prevalence ranging from 20% to 41% (Archbold et al., 2002; Mindell et al., 1999; Owens et al., 2000). Approximately 15 million U.S. children experience inadequate sleep (Smaldone et al., 2007) (Figure 22.3). This has serious implications for learning and for work and school performance. Sleep deprivation may be associated with obesity and the development of diabetes—important public health concerns.

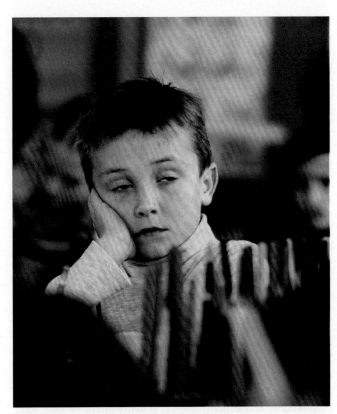

FIGURE 22.3 Inadequate sleep and sleep deprivation are chronic health concerns for pediatric populations. Nurses who work with children and teens must carefully question families about sleep habits and provide education to solve any problems or deficits related to sleep that children may have.

Environmental, behavioral, and social factors related to children's sleep include parenting behaviors, family stress, and family functioning. Children's sleep, in turn, appears to have an important influence on behavior and functioning in school (Bates et al., 2002; Smaldone et al., 2007). Sleep deprivation leads to poorer cognitive functioning, conduct problems, and depression, as well as poor performance in school.

Many environmental and behavioral factors that contribute to sleep problems are correctable, and nurses have many opportunities to teach children and their families about the importance of sleep, the characteristics of normal sleep across developmental stages, and the consequences of poor sleep. Promoting regular bedtimes even for very young children can assist in the development of lifelong patterns of healthy sleep. School-aged children and adolescents and their families often need guidance about managing demands related to schoolwork, sports, work, and social activities. It is also important to raise awareness among teachers and others who work with children and adolescents about these issues. Some school districts have rescheduled the school day to have later start and end times to accommodate the circadian patterns of adolescents. At the community level, nurses can play an important role in advocating for public policy and health education to promote healthy sleep patterns.

Sleep Disorders in Children. As many as 40% to 45% of children may experience sleep disorders sometime before the end of adolescence (Meltzer et al., 2009). Although many types of sleep disorders occur in children, the most common are sleep-onset insomnia, parasomnias, sleep disordered breathing (sleep apnea), and movement disorders (eg, restless legs syndrome) (Archbold, 2011a). As many as 3% of the pediatric population may have sleep apnea, a condition that may contribute to diabetes and cardiovascular disorders and seems to be growing in prevalence. An important factor that contributes to this disorder is obesity, a problem that is of epidemic proportions.

Although much is known about normal sleep and sleep disorders in pediatric settings, and effective treatments are available, sleep disorders are often underdiagnosed and undertreated. Evaluation of sleep and sleep disorders should be an essential part of nursing care for children in all settings, including schools (Archbold, 2011a, 2011b; Lee, 2011).

YOUNG AND MIDDLE ADULTS. Young adults typically report sleeping approximately 7.5 hours per night on weekdays and 8.5 hours or more per night on weekends. However, the amount of sleep varies greatly and is influenced by factors such as genetics, preferences, lifestyle, and environment (Carskadon & Dement, 2005). Usually there is one long sleep period and little or no daytime napping. REM stages account for 20% to 25% of the sleep period, with NREM stages occupying 75% to 80%. Slow-wave (NREM stages 3 and 4) sleep occurs mostly in the first third of the night, whereas REM sleep predominates near the end of the night

(Carskadon & Dement, 2005). Approximately one third of adults may intentionally sleep for a short period during the day (National Sleep Foundation, 2005). Napping may be used in response to sleep loss or for enjoyment (Milner & Cote, 2009), but may be especially beneficial for shift workers. Family stress, positive and negative life events, and academic pressure may contribute to sleep problems in this age group (Bernert et al., 2007).

OLDER ADULTS. As adults age, slow-wave and REM sleep, sleep efficiency, and total sleep time decrease. Stages N1 and N2 sleep, time awake after sleep onset, and sleep latency (time from bedtime to beginning of the sleep period) increase. Older adults experience a flattened circadian rhythm, advanced circadian phase (earlier bedtime and early morning awakenings), decreased slow-wave sleep, and more frequent arousals. These changes may be associated with age-related deterioration in the suprachiasmic nucleus (Cajochen et al., 2006). Napping, which is common among some older adults, may result in decreased nocturnal sleep, but the extent to which napping is associated with positive or negative health outcomes is not known (Ancoli-Israel & Martin, 2006).

Older adults may experience *advanced sleep phase syndrome,* which involves falling asleep early in the evening and awakening early in the morning. Although many sleep experts believe this finding to be a normal developmental pattern, advanced sleep phase syndrome becomes problematic when it interferes with preferred work and leisure activities.

Insomnia, a problem of initiating (prolonged time to fall asleep) and maintaining (staying asleep, frequent awakenings, or awakening too early) sleep is common among people older than 65 years; it also is more common in older women than in older men (Bliwise, 2005). As many as 44% of older adults have sleep-disordered breathing (sleep apnea) (Bliwise, 2005). Daytime sleepiness may be a sign of poor nocturnal sleep, sleep apnea, depression, or use of sedatives, hypnotics, or diuretics. Although many people believe that sleep disturbances and sleepiness among older adults are a normal part of aging, most sleep disturbances among older adults actually are associated with treatable sleep disorders or medical or psychiatric illnesses (Asplund, 2004; Foley et al., 2004). Nocturia and pain are common causes. The belief that sleep disturbance is part of normal aging may be a barrier to seeking help for genuine problems. Therefore, health care providers must be vigilant about sleep assessment and treatment. Changes in sleep patterns may be signs of treatable sleep disorders or other medical conditions, such as heart disease, pain, or mental health problems.

Sex and Gender

Although there are few gender differences in sleep in young children, gender differences in sleep begin during adolescence, and women often report more difficulty initiating and maintaining sleep across the adult lifespan. Sleep is closely tied to hormonal levels (Lee et al., 2008), with about one third of women reporting sleep disturbance during the premenstrual period (Lee et al., 2008). Disrupted sleep is also common during pregnancy and the postpartum period. These changes are associated with hormonal fluctuations, discomforts, emotions, and adoption of new roles. Sleep disruption is often associated with menopause, and may be associated with vasomotor symptoms, such as hot flashes, although some researchers have found that factors such as life stress play an equally important role (Minarik, 2011). Among men, gradual declines in testosterone levels associated with aging may also have a negative impact on sleep efficiency (Anderson & Tufik, 2008). Gender-related roles, such as motherhood, may also contribute to sleep disorders. Sleep-disordered breathing is more common among men (Minarik, 2011).

Race and Ethnicity

There are many cultural differences in sleep-related perceptions and behaviors, including perceptions about normal and abnormal sleep, although this is an understudied area. Nevertheless, there is growing recognition of health disparities related to the prevalence of sleep disorders. For example, Latino, African, and Asian Americans may be at greater risk for certain sleep disorders, such as sleep apnea, than their Caucasian counterparts. The reasons for this are not completely known, but disparities in access to health care and socioeconomic status may play an important role (Baldwin & Ornelas, 2011).

Medical Disorders and Treatments

Many problems related to physical illness can affect sleep. Sleep disturbances may be secondary to symptoms of a disease, related to an illness's underlying pathophysiology, or result from use of medications or side effects of treatments. For example, clients with asthma may report that their symptoms increase during the early morning hours. Angina, nocturia, diabetes, congestive heart failure, gastroesophageal reflux disease, hyperthyroidism, fibromyalgia, chronic obstructive pulmonary disease, Parkinson's disease, and HIV/AIDS are examples of other conditions associated with disrupted sleep (Parker, 2011).

Symptoms, treatments, and environmental conditions in hospitals and long-term care facilities almost universally have a negative impact on quality and quantity of sleep. Sleep disturbance due to acute illness or hospitalization may also improve with recovery. For example, sleep improves throughout recovery for clients who have undergone cardiac surgery (Redeker et al., 2004, 2011).

Drugs and Chemical Substances

Many prescribed and over-the-counter (OTC) drugs, herbal remedies, and illegal substances affect the central nervous system (CNS) and influence sleep. Examples of prescription and OTC drugs that can adversely affect sleep are listed in Box 22.1.

Caffeine, a stimulant, can delay sleep onset, decrease total sleep time, increase wakefulness after sleep onset, and decrease REM and slow-wave sleep (Obermeyer &

BOX 22.1	Drugs That Contribute to Disturbed Sleep
Alcohol	Diuretics
Alpha-hydroxybutyrate	Lithium
Alpha-methyldopa	Methylphenidate
Amphetamines	Methysergide
Antidepressants	Narcotics
Aspirin	Nicotine
Barbiturates	Phenothiazine
Benzodiazepines	Reserpine
Caffeine	Selective serotonin reuptake
Chloral hydrate	inhibitors
Cimetidine	Steroids
Clonidine	Trazodone
Cocaine	

Benca, 1996). Caffeine-containing beverages include coffee, tea, cola, chocolate, and some noncola soft drinks. OTC cold preparations also contain caffeine. Although people differ in the intensity and duration of their response to caffeine-containing products, effects may last as long as 14 hours. Therefore, afternoon or evening consumption of caffeine may have negative consequences relative to nocturnal sleep. Evaluation of caffeine consumption is an especially important component of nursing assessment of clients who present with difficulty falling asleep or staying asleep.

Nicotine also powerfully influences sleep, with higher doses producing more arousal. Withdrawal from nicotine can result in irritability and frequent waking from sleep. Pharmacologic treatments for smoking cessation, such as nicotine replacement therapy and bupropion, also may disrupt sleep, especially in women. Therefore, sleep disturbance and the resulting irritability and fatigue may be barriers to effective treatment for clients with tobacco addiction (Colrain et al., 2004).

Use of alcohol often is associated with sleep disorders (Teplin et al., 2006). Many people use alcohol to self-treat insomnia. Although its acute sedative effects lead to drowsiness and shorten sleep latency (time to fall asleep), long-term effects include arousal and wakefulness. Once alcohol is metabolized (4 to 5 hours), withdrawal results in shallow and disturbed sleep, sympathetic nervous system stimulation, increased REM, enhanced dream recall, and increased wakefulness. Sleep disturbance is a common problem for clients with alcoholism, who may report either insomnia or hypersomnia. Sleep problems appear to persist for months or even years in clients recovering from alcoholism, and sleep disturbance may be a predictor of alcoholic relapse (Gillin et al., 2005). Alcohol use also increases snoring and apnea in clients with obstructive sleep apnea. Therefore, people with this disorder should avoid alcohol consumption near bedtime.

Stimulants, such as methylphenidate, amphetamine, modafinil, and the newer drug armodafinil, are used to treat excessive daytime sleepiness in clients with sleep disorders such as narcolepsy. However, excessive use results in restlessness, anxiety, and sleep disturbance. Cocaine, an illegal stimulant, produces irritability and sleep disturbance. Clients withdrawing from cocaine may experience hypersomnolence.

Opiates, such as morphine, result in drowsiness and analgesia. They also may lead to decreased REM sleep, especially in those taking such drugs for the first time. Withdrawal from opiates may result in severe sleep disturbance, and poor sleep may predict relapse. However, the use of opiates may improve sleep in people for whom these drugs are prescribed for pain (Gillin et al., 2005).

SLEEP DISORDERS

As many as 50 to 70 million people in the United States have a sleep disorder (Centers for Disease Control and Prevention, 2008). Unfortunately, many of these are undiagnosed and untreated. This finding emphasizes the critical role of assessment and intervention by nurses and other health care professionals in every possible encounter with clients. See Therapeutic Communication 22.1.

Signs and Symptoms/Diagnostic Criteria

The *International Classification of Sleep Disorders* coding manual (American Academy of Sleep Medicine, 2005) lists the following categories of sleep disorders:

- Insomnia
- Sleep-related breathing disorders
- Hypersomnias
- Circadian rhythm sleep disorders
- Parasomnias
- Sleep-related movement disorders
- Isolated symptoms
- Other sleep disorders

The American Psychiatric Association (APA, 2007) updated the *Diagnostic and Statistical Manual of Mental Disorders,* 4th edition, text revision (*DSM-IV-TR*), to reflect these changes. Therefore, these two diagnostic classification systems are now consistent relative to sleep (DSM-IV-TR Box 22.1).

Insomnia

Insomnia, a perception of insufficient sleep or not feeling rested after habitual sleep, is the most common sleep disorder in adults. Approximately 30% to 35% of the adult population exhibits symptoms that include difficulty falling asleep, staying asleep, or both, or not feeling rested on awakening at least 3 nights per week (Mai & Buysse, 2008). Insomnia can range from a few days to many months or years. Clients with insomnia often report distress in social, occupational, or other areas of functioning.

Primary insomnia occurs when no cause of a sleep disturbance (eg, a psychiatric or medical diagnosis) can be identified. Primary insomnia occurs infrequently.

Psychophysiologic insomnia is chronic insomnia in which clients worry about sleep, are cognitively and physiologically overaroused at bedtime, and have poor daytime functioning. This leads to further worry about sleep. This, in turn, may lead to a vicious cycle in which insomnia leads to more insomnia (Figure 22.4). Most often, insomnia is comorbid with other psychiatric or medical disorders. Although treating the comorbid condition is important, it usually does not eliminate chronic comorbid insomnia.

A useful model for guiding evaluation and treatment of insomnia is the "3 P" model (Spielman, 1986; Spielman et al., 1987). This model posits that there are predisposing, precipitating, and perpetuating factors for insomnia. Predisposing characteristics may include genetics, personality, and coping style. Precipitating factors may include psychiatric or medical disorders, acute stressful events (eg, hospitalization, bereavement), or developmental events, such as pregnancy. Many clients have difficulty initiating or maintaining sleep in unfamiliar environments, such as hospitals or hotels. In health care settings, noise, lighting, and frequent care activities may contribute to disturbed sleep (Lorenz et al., 2011; Redeker, 2011). Factors that perpetuate insomnia are thoughts, perceptions, and behaviors. For example, some people may develop ineffective behaviors, such as lying in bed for extended periods of time in an attempt to obtain more sleep or engaging in activities during bedtime, such as watching TV, that may only worsen sleep. Clients with insomnia develop inaccurate beliefs about the causes and consequences of sleep, such as the belief that sleep loss will lead to catastrophic consequences (Jungquist, 2011). Although precipitating factors often resolve (eg, treatment of acute illness), insomnia becomes chronic because of dysfunctional behaviors and beliefs (perpetuating factors) (Espie, 2009).

A diagnosis of insomnia is made primarily through an interview with the client regarding the characteristics of the sleep complaint, related factors, and consequences. Polysomnography (see the sleep disorders Assessment section) may be used to rule out other sleep disorders.

The mainstays of treatment for insomnia are pharmacologic and behavioral. A combination of approaches may be helpful. Hypnotic medications are especially beneficial for acute (short-term) insomnia, but are not recommended for long-term use.

Cognitive–behavioral therapy for insomnia (CBT-I) addresses the factors that perpetuate insomnia. It is a structured approach that includes stimulus control (a set of instructions to reassociate the bedroom with sleep and to reestablish a consistent sleep–wake schedule), sleep restriction (designed to curtail time in bed to improve sleep efficiency), relaxation training (focuses on physical and physiologic relaxation), cognitive therapy (challenging and changing clients' misconceptions and faulty beliefs about sleep), and sleep hygiene (guidelines about health practices, such as exercise and caffeine intake and environmental factors that may affect sleep) (Morin et al., 2006). CBT-I can be provided in both individual and group formats of various durations.

Therapeutic Communication 22.1

Assessing Sleep Patterns

Joanna and Paco Estevez are parents of two small children: Enrique, who is 3 weeks old, and Theresa, who is 3 years old. Paco works nights, and Joanna has recently returned to work at her day job as a nurse's aide in a large nursing home. Emily Arana, a community health nurse, is at their home for a follow-up visit.

INEFFECTIVE DIALOGUE	EFFECTIVE DIALOGUE
CLIENT: I'm glad you came early, Ms. Arana. The kids are both asleep and so is Paco. We can talk in peace for a little while. *(Sits on sofa and motions Emily to sit down.)*	CLIENT: I'm glad you came early, Ms. Arana. The kids are both asleep and so is Paco. We can talk in peace for a little while. *(Sits on sofa and motions Emily to sit down.)*
NURSE: Sounds like it's been busy around here lately. *(Settles onto sofa and sits attentively.)*	NURSE: Sounds like it's been busy around here lately. *(Settles onto sofa and sits attentively.)*
CLIENT: You got that right! Enrique isn't sleeping through the night yet, and Theresa wakes up, too. Plus she has a cold so she isn't feeling too good. And Paco isn't around to help much since he's working nights. It gets pretty hairy around here at 2 AM. *(Smiles tightly.)*	CLIENT: You got that right! Enrique isn't sleeping through the night yet, and Theresa wakes up, too. Plus she has a cold so she isn't feeling too good. And Paco isn't around to help much since he's working nights. It gets pretty hairy around here at 2 AM. *(Smiles tightly.)*
NURSE: And I understand you're working, too. Day shift?	NURSE: How about you? *(Good eye contact.)*
CLIENT: Yes. *(Wearily.)* I had to go back or lose the job. I leave the kids with my mother all day until I get off at 3 PM. She lives close by. *(Yawns.)* Sorry! I didn't mean to yawn in your face!	CLIENT: I do what I can. *(Shrugs wearily.)* I had to return to work after the baby came home or lose my job. I get up at 5:00 to get the kids ready to take to my mother's while I work. So I don't get much rest. Or much time with Paco. I really hate this night shift he's on. But it's extra money and it won't be forever. *(Yawns.)* Sorry! I didn't mean to yawn in your face!
NURSE: No problem. And is your husband able to help or is he too tired? *(Begins to open bag and take out assessment equipment.)*	NURSE: No problem. You have reason to be tired. What are you doing to try and get more rest? *(Looks concerned, asking an open-ended question.)*
CLIENT: He helps on his days off. He's really good with both of them. *(Sounds a little defensive.)*	CLIENT: I try to nap here and there. Paco takes the night feedings on his nights off so I can sleep through at least 2 nights a week. Other than that, I wait for the baby to grow so he'll sleep through and for Theresa's cold to get better.
NURSE: I'm sure he is, having had three brothers and sisters of his own to take care of. Maybe I could see the baby now and see how he's doing. Do you think Theresa will be up soon? I can look at her, too, and see what we can do for her cold. What do you think?	NURSE: Would you be willing to discuss things that might help both kids move along faster?
CLIENT: Sure, you start on the baby, and I'll see if Theresa's about to wake up. *(Pauses to get a clean towel for the baby to lie on and goes in to the bedroom. Yawns again.)*	CLIENT: *(Looks surprised.)* Sure! I didn't know there was anything else I could do for them.

Reflection and Critical Thinking

- Determine the factors affecting this family's sleep and rest patterns.
- Explain how the nurse in the second dialogue elicited additional information from the client.
- Explain what information the nurse in the first dialogue missed.
- Formulate your ideas of what consequences further sleep deprivation may have for this family.

Adapted from Craven, R. C., Hirnle, C. J. (2009). *Fundamentals of nursing: Human health and function* (6th ed.). Philadelphia, PA: Lippincott Williams & Wilkins.

Many studies have documented its efficacy when provided by trained therapists, including nurses (Table 22.2.)

Many self-help resources are available for insomnia. These include books (bibliotherapy) and, increasingly, Internet-based treatments. Although there is beginning to be evidence of the efficacy of these nonprescribed treatments (Jungquist, 2011), little is known about their efficacy compared with treatment by a therapist (Jungquist, 2011).

Sleep-Related Breathing Disorders

Obstructive sleep apnea–hypopnea syndrome (OSAHS) is associated with repetitive episodes of reduced airflow

DSM-IV-TR BOX 22.1

Sleep Disorders

Insomnia

A. The predominant complaint is difficulty initiating or maintaining sleep, or nonrestorative sleep, for at least 1 month.

B. The sleep disturbance (or associated daytime fatigue) causes clinically significant distress or impairment in social, occupational, or other important areas of functioning.

C. The sleep disturbance does not occur exclusively during the course of Narcolepsy, Breathing-Related Sleep Disorder, Circadian Rhythm Sleep Disorder, or a Parasomnia.

D. The disturbance does not occur exclusively during the course of another mental disorder (eg, Major Depressive Disorder, Generalized Anxiety Disorder, Delirium).

E. The disturbance is not due to the direct physiologic effects of a substance (eg, a drug of abuse, a medication) or a general medical condition.

Sleep-Related Breathing Disorder

A. Sleep disruption, leading to excessive sleepiness or insomnia that is judged to be due to a sleep-related breathing condition (eg, obstructive or central sleep apnea syndrome or central alveolar hypoventilation syndrome).

B. The disturbance is not better accounted for by another mental disorder and is not due to the direct physiologic effects of a substance (eg, a drug of abuse, a medication) or another general medical condition (other than a breathing-related disorder).

Hypersomnia

A. The predominant complaint is excessive sleepiness for at least 1 month (or less if recurrent) as evidenced by either prolonged sleep episodes or daytime sleep episodes that occur almost daily.

B. The excessive sleepiness causes clinically significant distress or impairment in social, occupational, or other important areas of functioning.

C. The excessive sleepiness is not better accounted for by Insomnia and does not occur exclusively during the course of another Sleep Disorder and cannot be accounted for by an inadequate amount of sleep.

D. The disturbance does not occur exclusively during the course of another mental disorder.

E. The disturbance is not due to the direct physiologic effects of a substance (eg, a drug of abuse, a medication) or a general medical condition.

Circadian Rhythm Sleep Disorder

A. A persistent or recurrent pattern of sleep disruption leading to excessive sleepiness or insomnia that is due to a mismatch between the sleep–wake schedule required by a person's environment and his or her circadian sleep–wake pattern.

B. The sleep disturbance causes clinically significant distress or impairment in social, occupational, or other important areas of functioning.

C. The disturbance does not occur exclusively during the course of another Sleep Disorder or other mental disorder.

D. The disturbance is not due to the direct physiologic effects of a substance (eg, a drug of abuse, a medication) or a general medical condition.

Reprinted with permission from the *Diagnostic and Statistical Manual of Mental Disorders, Fourth Edition, Text Revision* (Copyright © 2000). American Psychiatric Association.

(*hypopnea*) or cessation of airflow (*apnea*) resulting from collapse of the upper airway (Figure 22.5). Clients with OSAHS experience sleep disruption and excessive daytime sleepiness. They typically snore loudly and may gasp or choke during sleep. Some clients have more severe OSAHS when they lie on their backs to sleep; thus, the side-lying or prone position for these clients may be recommended. Clients with OSAHS may be unaware of their episodes of apnea, hypopnea, or snoring during sleep. Therefore, reports from witnesses of these events help establish the diagnosis.

OSAHS occurs in 4% of men and 2% of women in the United States when the criterion of excessive daytime sleepiness is used, in addition to frequency of episodes of apnea and hypopnea. When only episodes of apnea and hypopnea are considered, prevalence is 24% in men and 9% in women (Young et al., 1993). Prevalence in women appears to increase during menopause (Anttalainen et al., 2006). General risk factors include age, gender, and obesity (Patil et al., 2007).

Clients with OSAHS are at risk for lapses in memory, slowed reaction time, and falling asleep while working, operating machinery, or driving a motor vehicle. Therefore, evaluation of excessive daytime sleepiness and the client's history for accidents or problems with performance are critical to ensuring safety and protecting the public. People at risk should be discouraged from operating machinery or driving motor vehicles until their OSAHS is treated. OSAHS is associated with hypertension, heart failure, stroke, metabolic syndrome, and type 2 diabetes (Nieto et al., 2000; Taub & Redeker, 2008; Van Cauter et al., 2008; Yaggi et al., 2005, 2006).

A diagnosis of OSAHS is made by history, physical examination, and a polysomnographic study. Risk factors that may suggest OSAHS in adults include overweight or obesity, large neck size, snoring, and witnessed apneas (cessations in breathing during sleep). Additional physical findings may include excess pharyngeal tissue, large tongue and/or

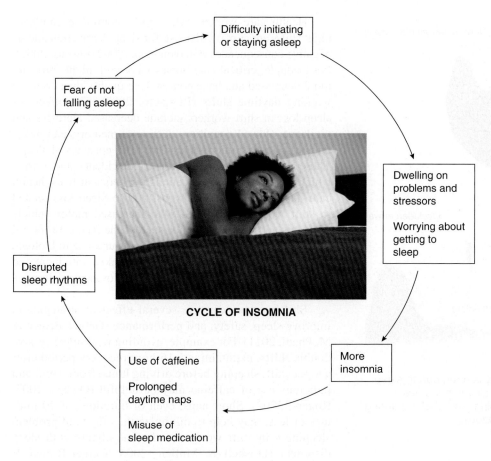

CYCLE OF INSOMNIA

FIGURE 22.4 Insomnia can be part of a vicious cycle in which worry about sleep and poor daytime habits to compensate for missed sleep lead to more sleep problems. In such cases, insomnia begets insomnia.

TABLE 22.2 Components of Cognitive–Behavioral Therapy for Insomnia

Strategy	Goal	Explanation
Stimulus control	To reduce maladaptive conditioning in which the client associates the bed with insomnia	The client is taught to limit activities in bed to sleep and sex and to get out of bed when sleep does not occur.
Sleep restriction	To restrict time in bed to the average sleep time, thus reducing time awake in bed and making sleep as efficient as possible	The client gradually increases time in bed as his or her sleep improves.
Relaxation training	To reduce physiologic arousal	Strategies may include progressive muscle relaxation, biofeedback, yoga, and other techniques.
Cognitive Therapy		
Paradoxical intention	To reduce anxiety associated with trying to fall asleep so that the client will fall asleep more quickly	Clients are instructed to try to stay awake when they go to bed.
Cognitive restructuring	To change irrational beliefs about sleep	The health care provider provides accurate information and assists the client to develop new beliefs about sleep.

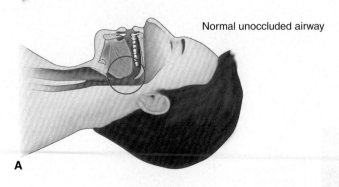

Normal unoccluded airway

A

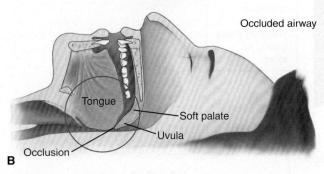

Occluded airway

Tongue

Soft palate

Uvula

Occlusion

B

FIGURE 22.5 **(A)** The normal airway is open during sleep. **(B)** In obstructive sleep apnea, the airway becomes occluded, leading to snoring, gasping, and choking during sleep and many potential complications.

tonsils, and a large uvula, although OSAHS may occur in the absence of these findings. In addition to obesity, large tonsils are a major risk factor in children. Effective treatments for OSAHS include weight loss, nightly nasal continuous positive airway pressure (CPAP), and oral appliances designed to maintain patency of the upper airway during sleep (Sawyer & Weaver, 2011). Surgical or laser procedures that reduce the volume of the soft palate and pharyngeal tissue also may be helpful. For the many clients whose OSAHS is a result of obesity, weight loss is also an important treatment. Although these treatments are highly effective, adherence (especially with CPAP) is a major problem for many clients. Assisting clients with adherence to these treatments is an important nursing intervention.

Other Sleep Disorders

HYPERSOMNIAS. Hypersomnias are disorders of excessive sleep, including significant daytime sleepiness, almost on a daily basis.

CIRCADIAN RHYTHM SLEEP DISORDERS. Sleep deprivation is the consequence of total or partial reduction in time spent asleep. Partial sleep deprivation, the most common form, is one consequence of the very busy lives many people lead today. At least 20% of the U.S. population works during times outside the 9:00 AM to 5:00 PM "typical" day, and about 30% of shift workers have clinically significant sleep disturbance or daytime sleepiness (Drake et al., 2004).

Health care workers who work rotating, evening, or night shifts are at particular risk for sleep deprivation and its negative consequences (Ohayon et al., 2002; Owens, 2007). For example, critical care nurses who work night shifts are more depressed and have poorer sleep quality than do those working daytime shifts (Ruggiero, 2003). The effects of sleep loss in shift workers include decreased alertness and vigilance, slowed cognition, decreased memory, and involuntary periods of microsleep (very brief episodes of sleep). These effects increase the risk of accidents and errors, which has important implications for personal lives, health care quality, and safety (Owens, 2007). Sleep loss related to shift work is associated with increased motor vehicle accidents and major accidents, such as the *Exxon Valdez* oil spill. Shift work and the subsequent disturbance in biologic rhythms and sleep loss also have been linked with increased gastrointestinal, psychiatric, and cardiovascular diseases (Dowling & Mastick, 2011).

Shift workers can use several effective strategies to improve sleep, safety, and performance (Geiger-Brown & McPhaul, 2011). For example, avoiding working excessive double shifts, maintaining a 16-hour recovery period after a night shift, sleeping before driving home from work, and judicious use of caffeine may be helpful (Owens, 2007; Rogers, 2002). Short naps, even of durations of 20 minutes or less, may help to minimize the effects of problem sleepiness in shift workers and some clients with sleep disorders (Driskell & Mullen, 2005; Geiger-Brown & McPhaul, 2011).

Problem sleepiness (sleepiness at inappropriate times) may be a symptom of many sleep disorders and is a major risk factor for injury to self and others. For example, researchers have shown that short sleep duration contributes to sleepiness and the potential for crashes in commercial truck drivers (Pack et al., 2006). Alcohol magnifies the consequences of problem sleepiness. Health care providers need to educate clients and families about these risks and advise them to avoid driving or operating equipment or motor vehicles when there is potential for sleepiness.

PARASOMNIAS. Parasomnias are primary sleep disorders characterized by unusual or undesirable behaviors during sleep. They interfere with sleep or happen during the threshold between sleep and wakefulness. Examples include nightmares, sleepwalking, and sleep terrors.

SLEEP-RELATED MOVEMENT DISORDERS. Periodic limb movement disorder (PLMD) is a condition in which the legs move repetitively during the night (periodic limb movements during sleep—PLMS) usually in approximately 90-second repetitive patterns. The movements result from contractions of the leg muscles during sleep. This condition causes frequent nighttime arousals, nonrestorative sleep, and excessive daytime sleepiness. **Restless legs syndrome** (RLS) is associated with disagreeable leg sensations, such as pain, cramping, and itching, which often interfere with the onset of sleep when they occur at bedtime (Cuellar & Redeker, 2011).

PLMD occurs in both adults and children. More than 6% of the population has periodic limb movements during sleep (Cuellar et al., 2007). Both RLS and PLMS have been associated with musculoskeletal disorders, heart disease, OSAHS, cataplexy, mental health problems, and physical activity near bedtime (Ohayon & Roth, 2002). Recent studies have shown that PLMD may have a negative impact on cardiovascular health (Allena et al., 2009; Siddiqui et al., 2007).

NARCOLEPSY. **Narcolepsy** is a disorder associated with loss of neurons in the hypothalamus that produce hypocretin, a neurotransmitter that influences wakefulness. Characteristics of narcolepsy include excessive daytime sleepiness, cataplexy (sudden bilateral loss of postural muscle tone), and other REM sleep phenomena. It occurs in 0.02% of the population. The disorder often begins in adolescence and young adulthood. Narcolepsy seems to have a genetic component, but its development also may be associated with environmental factors, the nature of which has not been completely determined (Dauvilliers et al., 2007).

In addition to excessive daytime sleepiness and cataplexy, clients also may have sleep paralysis, *hypnagogic hallucinations* (dreamlike images, sounds, or sometimes smells before falling asleep or waking up), automatic behaviors, or disruptions of nocturnal sleep episodes. Narcolepsy affects almost every aspect of daily life, including professional performance, ability to drive and operate machinery, and social interactions. Accompanying depression is common.

Treatment for narcolepsy focuses on managing excessive daytime sleepiness and cataplexy. Commonly used drugs include stimulants, hypnotics, selective serotonin reuptake inhibitors (SSRIs), tricyclic antidepressants (TCAs), and sodium oxybate (Rogers, 2011). Modafinil (Provigil) is the stimulant of choice because of its long half-life and low potential for abuse, although armodafinil (Nuvigil) may be preferred by some clients because of its longer-acting effects (Rogers, 2011). Stimulants, such as methylphenidate (Ritalin), also have been used to decrease daytime sleepiness, and are the safest for children (Rogers, 2011). Sodium oxybate is the only approved treatment for cataplexy. Tricyclic medications (clomipramine, desipramine, and protriptyline) and serotonin-specific reuptake inhibitors (fluoxetine) are also used but are associated with many side effects (Dauvilliers et al., 2003). Scheduled naps appear useful in assisting clients with severe sleepiness not addressed by stimulant medications (Rogers, 2001).

> ### Think About It 22.1
> A 24-year-old man is diagnosed with narcolepsy. The physician orders modafinil 200 mg PO daily. The client appears anxious about taking this drug. Develop a teaching plan to address the client's concerns about the medication.

Psychiatric Comorbidity and Sleep

Sleep disorders and psychiatric problems often coexist. Sleep problems are often symptomatic of underlying mental health issues, and many clients present initially for treatment because of sleep complaints (McEnany, 2011a). In fact, the *DSM-IV-TR* (APA, 2000) includes disordered sleep in the diagnostic criteria for many psychiatric disorders. Insomnia or hypersomnia are the most commonly reported sleep symptoms found in clients with psychiatric diagnoses. According to the National Comorbidity Survey Replication, approximately half of people with sleep problems also had a comorbid *DSM-IV-TR* diagnosis (Roth et al., 2006). Up to 90% of people with depression have demonstrated alterations in sleep architecture in polysomnographic studies, and over 80% of clients with schizophrenia complain of sleep symptoms (DeMartinis & Winokur, 2007; Wulff et al., 2010).

Medications prescribed to treat psychiatric disorders affect the central nervous system and may heighten arousal and lead to increased wakefulness at night. Some have sedating effects and may lead to excessive sleepiness. When educating clients regarding medications and symptoms, the nurse should remember to include information regarding sleep. The clinician should also consider the client's sleep patterns when prescribing or evaluating the effects of psychiatric medications. Effective treatment of the sleep disturbance may contribute to overall improvement of the psychiatric disorder, and untreated sleep disturbances may result in a relapse in psychiatric symptoms (Sateia, 2009).

Mood Disorders

Insomnia and depressive disorders often coincide. In fact, disturbed sleep and depression share common underlying pathophysiology (Sateia, 2009). Insomnia and hypersomnia are part of the diagnostic criteria for major depression (APA, 2000). Up to 90% of clients with depression report sleep difficulties, most commonly difficulty falling asleep and staying sleep, waking early in the morning and being unable to fall back asleep, distressing dreams, as well as nonrestorative sleep with daytime fatigue and sedation (Krystal et al., 2008; Szklo-Coxe et al., 2010). Clients with major depressive disorder (MDD) have decreased slow-wave sleep, with a shorter time to REM latency (Benca & Peterson, 2008). For many clients, insomnia symptoms, such as frequent awakenings or short sleep duration, are precursors to depression (Krystal et al., 2008; Szklo-Coxe et al., 2010). Clients with insomnia have a 10-fold increase in likelihood of developing depression (Benca & Peterson, 2008).These findings suggest that insomnia is both a risk factor for and an indicator of depression. Current research indicates that treating insomnia may prevent depression (Szklo-Coxe et al., 2010). Researchers continue to seek to understand the role of age and gender in relationships among sleep disorders, circadian rhythms, and depression (Armitage, 2007).

Medications for major depression may cause either sedation or insomnia (see Chap. 27). Sedating antidepressants, such as amitriptyline (Elavil) and doxepin (Sinequan), tend to

TABLE 22.3 Antidepressants and Sleep

Class	Sedating	Activating
TCA	Amitriptyline (Elavil) Doxepin (Sinequan)	Desipramine (Norpramin) Protriptyline (Vivactil)
SSRI	Paroxetine (Paxil)	Fluoxetine (Prozac) Sertraline (Zoloft)
Other	Trazodone (Desyrel) Nefazodone (Serzone) Mirtazapine (Remeron)	Venlafaxine (Effexor) Bupropion (Wellbutrin)

(Stahl, 2008.)

shorten sleep latency, increase total sleep time, increase short-wave sleep, and suppress REM sleep (DeMartinis & Winokur, 2007). Clients who take monoamine oxidase inhibitors may experience insomnia. SSRIs have significant effects on sleep architecture and may cause either arousal or sedation (DeMartinis & Winokur, 2007). Psychotropic medications can also affect REM sleep and increase nighttime wakefulness in both adults and older adults (DeMartinis & Winokur, 2007; Ensrud et al., 2006; Peterson & Benca, 2006). Remember to consider symptoms of insomnia or sleepiness when evaluating drug effects (Table 22.3).

Mania is closely associated with disturbed sleep. Decreased sleep predicts manic episodes in clients with bipolar disorder (Fiedorowicz et al., 2011; Harvey, 2008). Clients may have dramatically reduced sleep without reporting insomnia or fatigue, and often report increased energy. Sleep loss and disruption of the 24-hour sleep–wake cycle may contribute to both manic symptoms and the development of bipolar disorder (Benca et al., 2009; Wulff et al., 2010). During depressed phases of bipolar disorder, clients may have either insomnia or hypersomnia. Clients with bipolar disorder have more variable circadian rhythms of activity and rest, even when symptoms are not in the acute phase (Harvey, 2008). This suggests the importance of encouraging clients to obtain adequate sleep and maintain consistent sleep schedules.

Anxiety Disorders

Insomnia is the most reported sleep disturbance by clients with anxiety disorders (Kyung Lee & Douglass, 2010) (see Chap. 23); conversely, anxiety is prevalent in clients with insomnia (Roth et al., 2006). People with anxiety disorders frequently cannot relax or sleep, not only because they are worrying and thinking about their problems, but also because anxiety is a heightened physiologic state. People suffering from anxiety report prolonged sleep latency and frequent nighttime awakenings. A diagnosis of anxiety increased the risk of insomnia 3.5 times in one community-based survey of adolescents, but insomnia did not predict anxiety (Johnson et al., 2006). These findings suggest that anxiety may cause insomnia. Other studies have had similar results (Mellman, 2006).

Specific anxiety disorders may be associated with varied aspects of disturbed sleep. For example, generalized anxiety disorder and panic disorder are associated with decreased short-wave sleep and difficulty initiating and maintaining sleep. Between 44% and 71% of clients with panic disorder also may have sleep panic attacks (Kyung Lee & Douglass, 2010). Clients with obsessive compulsive disorder report problems with the initiation and maintenance of sleep, delayed onset of sleep, and multiple awakenings from obsessive-compulsive behaviors (Papadimitriou & Linkowski, 2005).

Clients with post-traumatic stress disorder (PTSD) chronically "relive" or reexperience previous traumatic events; they also have symptoms of arousal and avoidance (APA, 2000). They have intrusive thoughts, crying, and anxiety, and often are hypervigilant. Problems with initiating and staying asleep and frequent nightmares about the traumatic event are common symptoms (Kyung Lee & Douglass, 2010). Disrupted sleep is an almost universal finding in people with PTSD; conversely, 7.5% of clients with a sleep disorder had PTSD. The nature of the trauma, prior exposure, and other characteristics may influence the type and characteristics of the sleep disturbance. Common manifestations include insomnia, nightmares, recurrent awakenings, and more body movement during sleep (Mellman, 2006). Insomnia is the most common symptom reported in military personnel with PTSD (McLay et al., 2010). Sleep symptoms are positively correlated with PTSD symptoms (Waldrop et al., 2008). Given that core symptoms of PTSD are sleep related, a thorough sleep assessment and appropriate interventions related to sleep are important in caring for people with PTSD.

Attention Deficit/Hyperactivity Disorder

Children with attention deficit/hyperactivity disorder (ADHD) have more daytime sleepiness, movement during sleep, total sleep time, and sleep-disordered breathing problems than do healthy controls (Cortese et al., 2006; Kirov et al., 2007). Approximately 55% of children with ADHD report sleep disturbances, and many clients referred for ADHD actually have a primary sleep disorder (Konofal et al., 2010). Various manifestations of ADHD appear to be associated with characteristic sleep pattern disturbances. For example, attention problems are associated with shorter sleep onset latency, while hyperactivity is associated with more frequent sleep cycles (Kirov et al., 2007). One theory is that the hyperactivity present in ADHD develops as a coping mechanism for chronic daytime fatigue (Ming & Walters, 2009). ADHD is also associated with RLS and periodic limb movements. Studies in adults suggest that greater nocturnal motor activity and arousals from periodic leg movement may account for some ADHD symptoms (Gau et al., 2007; Ivanenko & Johnson, 2008; Philipsen et al., 2006). The potential contributions of sleep disorders, such as sleep apnea, periodic limb movements, and RLS suggest the importance of taking a careful sleep history, carefully evaluating differential diagnoses, and ruling out other comorbid sleep disorders in clients with ADHD.

Schizophrenia

Clients with schizophrenia (see Chap. 29) often have poor sleep efficiency and prolonged sleep latency. They may stay awake at night and sleep during the day; nightmares are also common (Benson & Zarcone, 1994, 2000; Krystal et al., 2008; Zarcone & Benson, 1997). Prolonged sleep latency, increased time awake at night, reduced REM sleep, and reduced slow-wave sleep appear to be associated with exacerbation of schizophrenia (Benson & Zarcone, 2000; Krystal et al., 2008; Yang & Winkelman, 2006; Zarcone & Benson, 1997). Clients with schizophrenia who stay awake at night have poorer sleep quality, more symptoms, and more cognitive deficits (Benson, 2006). Severe insomnia may be predictive of an acute psychotic episode (Krystal et al., 2008). During acute psychosis, clients with schizophrenia may have complete sleep loss.

Although much research is still needed regarding sleep disturbance in schizophrenia, sleep problems may be related to overactivity of dopamine or other neurotransmitters. Treatment of schizophrenia involves antipsychotic drugs, which exert effects on dopamine systems. First-generation antipsychotics and clozapine (Clozaril) cause sedation and increased total sleep time (Benson, 2006). Risperidone (Risperdal) and olanzapine (Zyprexa) cause less sedation. Giving antipsychotic medications at bedtime maximizes their sedative effects and improves sleep (Stahl, 2008). Discontinuation of antipsychotic medications may result in severe insomnia, an early sign of relapse (Benson, 2006; Stahl, 2008) (Table 22.4).

Cognitive Disorders

Disturbed sleep is highly prevalent in clients with dementia, including Alzheimer's disease (AD). Current studies estimate that 25% to 50% of clients with AD experience sleep disruptions, with up to 80% of AD clients experiencing obstructive sleep apnea (Rose & Lorenz, 2010). Disrupted sleep is more common in dementia with Lewy bodies than in AD, although with AD, disrupted sleep is associated with further disease progression (Bliwise et al., 2011). Reversal of day–night sleep patterns with increased daytime sleep, difficulty maintaining sleep, and decreased slow-wave and REM sleep are common in clients with AD (Rose & Lorenz, 2010). Studies found significant associations between sleep disturbances and aggressiveness (verbal outbursts, physical threats, and agitation) and the degree to which behavioral symptoms were troubling to caregivers. The duration of time in bed is associated with functional impairment; daytime sleepiness, sleep-disordered breathing, and primary arousal disorders were more common in clients with dementia (Tractenberg et al., 2006). Several studies indicate that REM behavior disorders may appear years prior to the diagnosis of Parkinson's disease or dementia, perhaps as a prodrome (Arnulf & Oudiette, 2008). Nursing care for AD clients should include education about sleep hygiene and exercise as options to help manage sleep symptoms.

Sleep–wake disturbances among people with dementia are also a significant cause of sleep loss among family caregivers (D. Lee et al., 2007; McCurry et al., 2007) and may lead to long-term placement for the AD client. Respite care has been found to improve the sleep of caregivers, while worsening the sleep of clients with dementia (J. H. Lee et al., 2007).

Treatment of Sleep Disorders in Clients with Comorbid Psychiatric Disorders

Treatment of sleep disorders in clients with psychiatric disorders often focuses on managing the environmental influences on sleep and may include adjusting drugs used to treat the psychiatric disorder for their somnolent or arousing effects. Hypnotic medications may also be useful for clients with insomnia. Light therapy, the application of bright light to pattern or "entrain" circadian rhythms, is helpful in treating seasonal affective disorder and improving sleep (McEnany, 2011a).

Sleep disturbance is an issue for acutely ill hospitalized clients who must deal with the acute effects of the illness as well as the illness itself. Acute psychiatric illness is often a life-threatening experience, and the focus of nursing care is on safety, providing a structured environment, and medication treatment. Unfortunately, sleep is an often overlooked but important symptom that should be addressed during hospitalization (McEnany, 2011b).

In the outpatient psychiatric setting, treatment may be episodic or continuous in the case of a chronic disorder. In these settings, individual or group-based treatments may be used. Behavioral approaches to insomnia, such as cognitive–behavioral therapy for insomnia (CBT-I), as well as hypnotic medications, may be particularly helpful (McEnany, 2011b). Clients also benefit from learning sleep hygiene strategies focused on managing environmental influences on sleep and regular sleep habits.

Interdisciplinary Goals and Treatment

The need for sleep is universal. Sleep disorders are found in clients across the lifespan in all states of health and illness and across the continuum of health care settings. Promoting sleep and assessing and treating sleep problems is the responsibility of a wide range of health professionals, including nurses, physicians, psychologists, and others who practice across specialty areas and health care settings.

TABLE 22.4 Antipsychotics and Sleep

	Sedating	Nonsedating
Atypical Antipsychotics	Clozapine (Clozaril) Olanzapine (Zyprexa) Quetiapine (Seroquel)	Aripiprazole (Abilify) Ziprasidone (Geodon)

(Stahl, 2008.)

When clients are suspected of having primary sleep disorders, such as narcolepsy, periodic limb movements during sleep, and obstructive sleep apnea, they need referral to specialized sleep centers for evaluation. These centers, usually staffed by interdisciplinary teams of sleep specialists, administer thorough sleep evaluations and specialized testing for sleep disorders, including **nocturnal polysomnography** (NPSG). NPSG uses continuous monitoring of at least one channel of electroencephalography (EEG) to monitor brain waves, electro oculography (EOG) to monitor eye movements, and chin electromyography (EMG) (Figure 22.6). Depending on the purposes of the study, the examiner may obtain other physiologic measurements. These commonly include cardiorespiratory (oximetry, airflow, and respiratory effort, electrocardiography) and neurologic measures (EMG of the anterior tibialis muscle). Sleep specialists can determine quantity and stages of sleep and evaluate for cardiorespiratory disorders, such as obstructive sleep apnea, periodic limb movements during sleep, and some parasomnias.

Multiple sleep latency testing (MSLT) is a procedure that determines the extent of daytime sleepiness by evaluating how long it takes clients to fall asleep during a series of daytime naps. MSLT is essential to the diagnosis of narcolepsy.

Checkpoint Questions

1. What specialized test is necessary to diagnose a primary sleep disorder?
2. What test is essential for diagnosing narcolepsy?

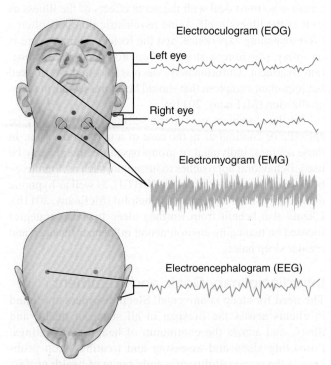

Electrooculogram (EOG)

Left eye

Right eye

Electromyogram (EMG)

Electroencephalogram (EEG)

FIGURE 22.6 Nocturnal polysomnography involves continuous monitoring of brain waves through electroencephalography, eye movements through electro oculography, and muscle activity through chin electromyography.

Sleep Hygiene

Sleep hygiene includes strategies to manipulate environmental conditions and personal behaviors to support effective sleep. Just as human beings need a balanced diet to promote and maintain health, they need habits and a structure to promote effective sleep. The general principles of sleep hygiene include environmental modifications, avoiding behaviors that contribute to poor sleep (eg, exercise or use of a computer near bedtime), and avoiding substances that contribute to poor sleep (eg, caffeine).

Clients should be taught to obtain sufficient sleep to meet developmental sleep needs, maintain a regular sleep schedule on weekdays and weekends, modify the sleeping environment to reduce noise and light, maintain a comfortable environmental temperature, and sleep in a comfortable bed. Health care providers discourage clients from eating a large meal or spicy foods near bedtime; conversely, they instruct clients to avoid going to bed on an empty stomach. Many sleep specialists recommend that clients consume a light snack of carbohydrate-containing foods or warm milk before bedtime and avoid caffeine within 6 hours of bedtime. Although sleep hygiene is the first step in promoting adequate sleep, it may be ineffective alone as a treatment for chronic insomnia.

Hypnotic Drugs

Hypnotic drugs, used primarily to treat insomnia, are among the most frequently prescribed medications in the United States today. Hypnotics are most appropriate for treatment of transient or intermittent insomnia; however, they can be used for treatment of chronic insomnia if the client's condition and response to medication are monitored carefully. Usually, the most effective approach is to combine treatment with hypnotic drugs with behavioral strategies, such as sleep hygiene.

Since the 1960s, benzodiazepines have been prescribed commonly to promote sleep. They work by promoting the effects of gamma-aminobutyric acid (GABA) receptors. Understanding Psychopharmacology Box 22.1 provides examples. They reduce anxiety and are highly effective in promoting sleep. Nevertheless, they reduce REM and stages 3 and 4 sleep, and tolerance may develop in clients. The effects of some benzodiazepines may last into the next day and produce "hangover" effects, particularly in older adults. Rebound insomnia may develop if the drugs are withdrawn quickly.

A newer classification of drugs, the nonbenzodiazepine benzodiazepine agonists, includes zolpidem (Ambien), zaleplon (Sonata), and eszopiclone (Lunesta). These drugs act more selectively on GABA receptors than the benzodiazepines to promote sleep. They are less likely to produce tolerance or hangover effects than the benzodiazepines (see Understanding Psychopharmacology Box 22.1). Ramelteon (Rozerem), a melatonin receptor agonist, appears to be effective in reducing transient insomnia in healthy adults and has been studied in chronic insomnia. However, there is a need for long-term clinical trials.

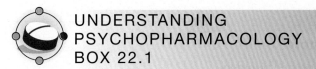

UNDERSTANDING PSYCHOPHARMACOLOGY BOX 22.1

Drugs Used to Treat Insomnia

Benzodiazepine Sedative-Hypnotics

Quazepam (Doral)	Temazepam (Restoril)
Triazolam (Halcion)	Triazolam (Halcion)
Estazolam (ProSom)	Flurazepam (Dalmane)

Nonbarbiturate Hypnotics

Zolpidem (Ambien)

Zaleplon (Sonata)

Eszopiclone

Chloral hydrate

Ramelteon

Sedating Antidepressants

Amitriptyline (Elavil)

Mirtazapine

Nortriptyline

Trazodone (Desyrel)

Doxepin (Sinequan)

Most OTC medications used for sleep contain the antihistamine diphenhydramine, which causes sedation, drowsiness, and tolerance. Daytime sleepiness is commonly associated with use of diphenhydramine. Antihistamines may have adverse effects when used with anticholinergic drugs and CNS depressants. Little research supports their use as hypnotic drugs and they are not recommended for use in older adults, who may experience daytime dysfunction, impaired memory, and possibly falls or other injuries as a result of their use (Jungquist, 2011).

Complementary and Alternative Modalities

Melatonin, an endogenous hormone responsible for regulating the circadian rhythm, may be useful in sleep disorders associated with circadian rhythms, such as jet lag and shift work. It has some sleep-promoting properties, especially when used outside of the biologic sleep period (daytime for people who typically sleep during the night). However, it has a short half-life and is associated with vasoconstriction. Medicinal plants and herbs, such as kava-kava, valerian, and plants used for aromatherapy, such as lavender, chamomile, and ylang-ylang, appear to have some hypnotic and anxiolytic effects and many people use these substances alone or in combination with prescribed medications. Scientific evidence supporting the effects and safety of these products is limited and some (eg, kava-kava) have toxic effects. In addition, available products may be inconsistent in dose and quality. Therefore, clients should be discouraged from using them until further evidence supporting their beneficial effects is available. Nevertheless, nursing care should include assessment for the use of these products, particularly because they may block or augment the effects of prescribed medications. Client teaching regarding these effects is also very important.

Tricyclic antidepressants that have sedating effects also may be prescribed to promote sleep. However, there are few data supporting their efficacy in insomnia, and the U.S. Food and Drug Administration has not approved them for this indication. These drugs increase the duration of NREM sleep, decrease awakenings, and decrease REM sleep. They may be especially useful for treating insomnia in clients with depression.

Checkpoint Questions

3. What are three areas addressed by sleep hygiene?

4. How do benzodiazepines act to promote sleep?

5. What are the daytime effects of hypnotic medications?

6. What are important elements of client teaching regarding the use of hypnotic medications?

APPLYING THE NURSING PROCESS

Sleep Disorders

▲ ASSESSMENT

Careful assessment of sleep is an important component of nursing care for clients of all ages and in virtually all health care situations (Assessment Tool 22.1) Sleep assessment should be an integral part of the health history. The nurse assesses the characteristics of sleep, including the client's perceptions of the need for sleep. The nurse asks about environmental, medical, psychiatric, situational, and treatment-related factors that may influence sleep patterns. A careful review of medications, including prescribed, OTC, and herbal substances, helps determine the contribution of these substances to the sleep complaint.

Assessment of the client's lifestyle and functioning in work, family roles, exercise, and leisure activities is useful in understanding the context for the sleep complaint. Some behaviors may be modifiable to improve sleep. For example, increasing exercise late in the afternoon (not in the evening) may improve nocturnal sleep quality. Late afternoon exercise has been associated with improved quality of sleep, whereas evening exercise is energizing.

The nurse considers the effects of the client's sleep disturbance on his or her functioning. Fatigue, problem sleepiness, disturbed mood, and difficulty with memory and cognitive functioning may be consequences. The nurse evaluates problem sleepiness by asking the client about inappropriate situations in

ASSESSMENT TOOL 22.1

Sleep Inventory

Typical Sleep Pattern

Bedtime
Wakeup time
Duration of sleep
Frequency of nighttime awakenings
Duration of time from lights out to sleep onset
Daytime napping
Perceived causes of nighttime awakenings
Differences in sleep patterns between weekdays and
  weekends
Events occurring during sleep: pain, parasomnias,
  snoring
Limb movements or limb discomfort during sleep
Recent changes in sleep pattern; perception of cause

Factors That May Influence Sleep

Environment: noise, lighting
Medical disorders

Psychiatric disorders
Stressors
Medications

Consequences of Sleep

Satisfaction with sleep
Daytime sleepiness
Cognitive function
Memory
Work performance
Social relationships
History of accidents/injury
Mood
Quality of life
Unusual events occurring during sleep
Snoring
Parasomnias
Sleep environment

---

which he or she has fallen asleep. The Epworth Sleepiness Scale may be useful (Johns, 1991; see Assessment Tool 22.2).

The nurse may recommend that the client keep a sleep log or diary to record details of sleep patterns, including bedtime, arising time, number of times awake, napping, overall quality of sleep, and sleeping aids. Recording these characteristics for several weeks can assist the nurse and client to evaluate the characteristics of the sleep experience (Figure 22.7).

Physical assessment is also useful in identifying clients at risk for sleep disorders, especially sleep-disordered breathing. Adult clients who are overweight or obese and have large necks are at particular risk for these disorders. Assessment of

---

ASSESSMENT TOOL 22.2

The Epworth Sleepiness Scale

How likely are you to doze off or fall asleep in the following situations, in contrast to feeling just tired? This refers to your usual way of life in recent times. Even if you have not done some of these things recently, try to work out how they would have affected you. Use the following scale to choose the most appropriate number for each situation:

- 0 = **no chance of dozing**
- 1 = **slight chance of dozing**
- 2 = **moderate chance of dozing**
- 3 = **high chance of dozing**

Situation	Chance of Dozing
Sitting and reading	
Watching television	
Sitting inactive in a public place (eg, a theater or a meeting)	
As a passenger in a car for an hour without a break	
Lying down to rest in the afternoon when circumstances permit	

Situation	Chance of Dozing
Sitting and talking to someone	
Sitting quietly after a lunch without alcohol	
In a car, while stopped for a few minutes in traffic	

To check your sleepiness score, total the points. Check your total score to see how sleepy you are.

1–6	Congratulations, you are getting enough sleep!
7–8	Your score is average
9 and up	Seek the advice of a sleep specialist without delay

Source: Johns, M. W. (1991). A new method for measuring daytime sleepiness. The Epworth Sleepiness Scale. *Sleep, 14,* 540–545.

Date		9:00 PM	10:00 PM	11:00 PM	12:00 AM	1:00 AM	2:00 AM	3:00 AM	4:00 AM	5:00 AM	6:00 AM	7:00 AM	8:00 AM	9:00 AM	Rate your quality of sleep* (1–3)	Rate your level of daytime alertness (1–3)	I took a nap (If yes, indicate time of nap and length. If no, leave blank.) Time	Length	Rate your mood today (1–3)

1. Answer the questions in the shaded areas.
2. Draw a line through the times you were asleep.
3. Put down (↓) arrows at the times you went to bed and up (↑) arrows at the times you got up.

(Each tick mark represents 1 hour)

Row	Sleep quality	Alertness	Nap Time	Nap Length	Mood
EXAMPLE	1	2	4:00 PM	45 min	2
NIGHT 1					
NIGHT 2					
NIGHT 3					
NIGHT 4					
NIGHT 5					
NIGHT 6					
NIGHT 7					
NIGHT 8					
NIGHT 9					
NIGHT 10					
NIGHT 11					
NIGHT 12					
NIGHT 13					
NIGHT 14					

*1=poor; 2=fair; 3=good

FIGURE 22.7 Clients can use a sleep log or diary to monitor the amount and quantity of sleep they have had, as well as effects on subsequent daytime functions. Nurses can review the information with clients to determine patterns, characteristics, and other factors in an effort to enhance sleep.

the pharynx for excessive pharyngeal tissue and large tongue or uvula may reveal the potential for nocturnal airway obstruction. Morphologic deviations, such as deviated nasal septa, small chin, and other abnormalities may also contribute to sleep-disordered breathing. Large tonsils and obesity in children are important risk factors.

▲ NURSING DIAGNOSIS

The primary nursing diagnosis of the client who has a sleep disorder is Disturbed Sleep Patterns. The following diagnoses also may be relevant, depending on the circumstances of the sleep disorder:

- Ineffective Coping
- Risk for Noncompliance
- Risk for Injury related to excessive daytime sleepiness
- Deficient Knowledge
- Fatigue

▲ OUTCOME IDENTIFICATION AND PLANNING

The overall goal of care for the client with Disturbed Sleep Patterns is to improve sleep. More specific goals for clients with this diagnosis include the following:

- The client will identify problematic sleep patterns and sleep-related behaviors.
- The client will adhere to recommended sleep promotion strategies.
- The client will verbalize knowledge relative to the importance of sleep and sleep promotion strategies.
- The client will avoid behaviors that may lead to injury.
- The client will seek specialized treatment for sleep disorders as appropriate.

Understanding Nursing Care 22.1 lists common interventions and outcomes appropriate in managing sleep problems. Case in Point 22.1 explores appropriate management of care for an actual client.

▲ IMPLEMENTATION

Sleep pattern disturbance occurs in many contexts. Therefore, nursing strategies to promote sleep vary depending on the client's developmental and health state. For clients with sleep disorders and comorbid medical or psychiatric illness, stressful situations, or environmental stimuli, it is important to address these conditions and their symptoms, but treating sleep itself may also improve the conditions. For clients with comorbid insomnia, the insomnia may not resolve simply by treating the underlying condition.

Education and counseling are essential nursing interventions for clients with a sleep disorder. Clients and significant others often need information about the nature of sleep and

UNDERSTANDING NURSING CARE 22.1

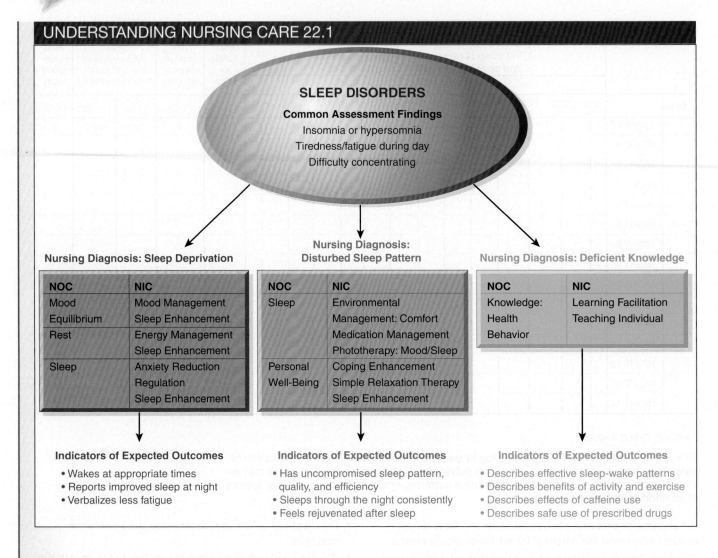

SLEEP DISORDERS

Common Assessment Findings

Insomnia or hypersomnia
Tiredness/fatigue during day
Difficulty concentrating

Nursing Diagnosis: Sleep Deprivation

NOC	NIC
Mood Equilibrium	Mood Management Sleep Enhancement
Rest	Energy Management Sleep Enhancement
Sleep	Anxiety Reduction Regulation Sleep Enhancement

Nursing Diagnosis: Disturbed Sleep Pattern

NOC	NIC
Sleep	Environmental Management: Comfort Medication Management Phototherapy: Mood/Sleep
Personal Well-Being	Coping Enhancement Simple Relaxation Therapy Sleep Enhancement

Nursing Diagnosis: Deficient Knowledge

NOC	NIC
Knowledge: Health Behavior	Learning Facilitation Teaching Individual

Indicators of Expected Outcomes

- Wakes at appropriate times
- Reports improved sleep at night
- Verbalizes less fatigue

Indicators of Expected Outcomes

- Has uncompromised sleep pattern, quality, and efficiency
- Sleeps through the night consistently
- Feels rejuvenated after sleep

Indicators of Expected Outcomes

- Describes effective sleep-wake patterns
- Describes benefits of activity and exercise
- Describes effects of caffeine use
- Describes safe use of prescribed drugs

Case in Point 22.1

Agatha's Story

Agatha, 28 years old, feels tired. She goes to bed at 10:30 PM every night. It takes her approximately 45 minutes to fall asleep, and she awakens often. She does not take any naps.

Agatha has always been a restless sleeper, but her problems have worsened since her mother died 3 months ago. She awakens at 6:00 AM, 1 hour before the alarm clock buzzes. She stays in bed, awake, because of her poor sleep at night. She has a prescription for zolpidem at bedtime; however, she does not take it for fear of becoming dependent on medications. Two cats stay in her bedroom at night; she reports that she can hear traffic in the street.

Agatha has no other medical problems and takes no prescribed or OTC medications. She has no history of psychiatric disorders. Agatha drinks two cups of coffee at breakfast and an additional cup after dinner. She occasionally has wine. She is happily employed full time as a teacher and sees friends, siblings, and their children regularly. Agatha walks approximately 2 miles for exercise three times per week in the early morning.

Key Assessment Findings

- Complaints of feeling tired during day
- Onset of problems with death of parent
- Recurrent pattern of sleep disruption for more than 1 month, with difficulty falling asleep, frequent night awakenings, early rising, and no naps
- Pets in room at night; environmental noise; ingestion of coffee with dinner
- Concern about dependency with use of zolpidem

Nursing DX: Disturbed Sleep **Pattern** related to inadequate sleep hygiene, grief, life change, and excessive stimulation as evidenced by frequent awakenings, difficulty falling asleep, and complaints of daytime fatigue

NOC: Sleep and Rest: The client will verbalize an improvement in sleep patterns.

NIC: Sleep Enhancement

- Record the client's sleep patterns and number of hours of sleep; encourage her to monitor sleep patterns (Fig. A). *Information about current sleep patterns provides a baseline for planning appropriate interventions.*
- Encourage the client to establish a bedtime routine. *It facilitates the transition from wakefulness to sleep.*
- Instruct the client to avoid bedtime foods and beverages that can interfere with sleep; for example, drinking coffee in the evening may contribute to problems; discourage caffeine intake after the late afternoon. *Caffeine, a stimulant, has a half-life of 8 to 14 hours. Its effects vary. People with sleep difficulties should avoid caffeine after the late afternoon.*
- Encourage the use of sleep medications as ordered. Explain the action and effect of zolpidem; reinforce that the drug is not habit forming. Adjust medication administration to support the client's sleep–wake cycle. *Short-term use of hypnotic drugs, particularly when combined with behavioral interventions, may help. Medications such as zolpidem are highly effective in promoting sleep. The timing of drug administration should be individualized to meet the client's needs, increasing the chances for effectiveness.*
- Encourage the client to talk about the loss of her parent and how this has affected her sleep. Suggest participation in a bereavement support group (Fig. B). *Understanding the relationship between the client's loss and sleep problems can aid in developing adaptive strategies, thus improving sleep. Participation in a support group promotes sharing of feelings and concerns.*

NIC: Environmental Management

- Explain the need for a clean, comfortable bed and environment; encourage the client to avoid unnecessary exposure, drafts,

overheating, or chilling. *Cleanliness and comfort promote relaxation, thereby facilitating the transition to sleep.*

- Encourage the client to participate in relaxing and enjoyable activities before bedtime. Monitor participation in fatigue-producing activities during wakefulness. *Enjoyable and relaxing activities prepare the body for sleep. Overactivity can lead to being overtired.*
- Urge the client to make the bedroom as quiet and dark as possible and to use the bed only for sleeping or sex; assist her to control or prevent undesirable or excessive noise when possible; encourage her to wear earplugs to decrease perceptions of noise from the street and to consider moving the cats to another room. *A sleep-promoting environment helps reduce stimuli that contribute to nocturnal arousal. Even low levels of movement or noise (eg, from pets) may disturb sleep.*

> 4/22/13: The client states that sleeping patterns have improved. She reports sleeping better through the night, with feelings of being rested and less fatigued during the day.
> Lorraine Allen, RN

Nursing DX: Deficient Knowledge related to factors that may influence sleep as evidenced by use of caffeine after dinner, avoidance of zolpidem, and presence of environmental stimuli.

NOC: Knowledge: Health Behavior: The client will identify factors contributing to sleep pattern disturbance that require modification.

NIC: Learning Facilitation

- Assess the client's readiness to learn; develop mutual goals with her. *Readiness to learn and mutual goal setting help facilitate effectiveness of teaching.*
- Adjust instruction to the client's level of knowledge and understanding. Provide information in terms she can understand. Review the use of medications to facilitate sleep. Reinforce the action of zolpidem and its non–habit-forming

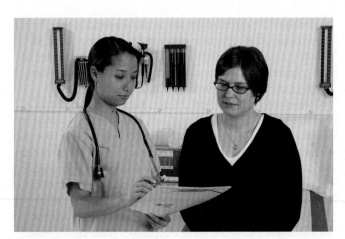

FIGURE A The nurse discusses the benefits of recording sleep patterns with the client.

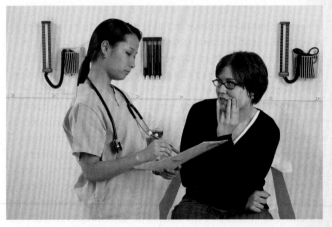

FIGURE B The nurse assists the client to discuss her feelings of loss after the death of her parent and introduces the idea of attending a bereavement support group.

(continues on page 422)

Case in Point 22.1 (continued)

Agatha's Story

nature. Discourage the use of caffeine late in the day. *Information provided at the client's level promotes better understanding and learning.*

- Provide memory aids as appropriate; use demonstration and return demonstration as appropriate. *Memory aids and demonstration encourage client participation in learning and help to provide mastery of the information.*

NIC: Teaching: Individual

- Teach the client about how the environment can influence sleep; encourage use of sleep hygiene strategies. *Environmental stimuli can interfere with an individual's sleep–wake cycle.*
- Explain the effects of the prescribed hypnotic. *Knowledge of the effects of the prescribed drug can help alleviate any anxiety or fears the client may have about using the medication.*
- Reinforce behavior, as appropriate (Fig. C). Work with the client to determine the most appropriate strategies for her. *Reinforcement provides positive feedback toward goal achievement and time for modifications if necessary. Collaboration with the client fosters empowerment.*
- Urge the client to continue exercise and activity early in the day, encouraging her to avoid exercise within 3 hours of bedtime. *Exercise is important; however, it acts as a stimulant and if done too late in the day, can interfere with sleep.*

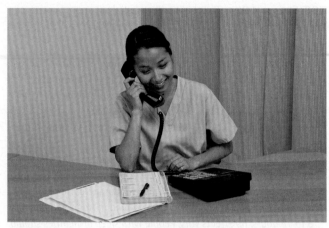

FIGURE C. The nurse is following up by phone to see how the client's treatment plan is working.

4/22/13: *The client reports improved sleep with use of appropriate sleep hygiene strategies. She demonstrates moderate to substantial understanding of sleep–wake patterns, strategies to promote efficient sleep, benefits of activity and exercise, safe use of prescription drugs, and effects of caffeine use.*

Lorraine Allen, RN

EPILOGUE

Two months have passed since Agatha's last visit. She reports that she continues to feel sad and tearful at times, but her grief is improving since she started going to a bereavement support group. She has dinner with friends at least once a week. "My nieces and nephews have been keeping me busy with all sorts of things lately." When asked about her difficulty sleeping, Agatha says, "I'm using the medicine. It helps. I've been sleeping better. I've also cut out that cup of coffee after dinner. I've started reading before going to bed; sometimes, I fall asleep while I'm reading." She also reports that her two cats now stay in the living room at night.

---

behaviors that may improve it that is appropriate to their developmental level, cultural beliefs, and health status. Many resources are available to supplement client teaching on this topic. See Client-Centered Education 22.1 for more information.

Clients suspected of having OSAHS, narcolepsy, parasomnias associated with violence, periodic limb movements during sleep, or chronic insomnia require referral to a sleep disorders center for evaluation by a sleep specialist. Once treatment begins in the sleep center, the nurse assists the client to adhere with the recommended treatment. Because treatment of sleep disorders often involves long-term behavioral change, some clients have difficulty maintaining their programs. The nurse helps the client to understand the treatment, solve problems that arise, and provide supportive feedback.

Nursing interventions for hospitalized clients include structuring the environment to promote sleep. Examples include reducing lighting and excessive noise, particularly at night, and

clustering client care interactions to allow adequate time for sleep (Figure 22.8). This time preferably should be at least 90 minutes to permit complete sleep cycles. For clients sleeping at home, adhering to the principles of sleep hygiene assists them to structure their home environment for sleep.

Administration of opioid and anesthetic medications may lead to respiratory depression in clients who have sleep-disordered breathing. Therefore, it is essential to identify clients who have this disorder prior to surgery or to administering these types of medications. Airway support, including positive airway pressure, and careful monitoring are essential. Clients may continue to be at risk in the postoperative period after anesthesia (Redeker et al., 2011).

Clients with problem sleepiness are at particular risk for accidents and injury. The nurse discourages these clients from engaging in activities that place them at risk, such as driving motor vehicles or operating machinery, until effective treatment has been instituted and the problem sleepiness has resolved.

Client-Centered Education 22.1

Recommended Sleep Hygiene Strategies

The nurse instructs the client and family as follows:

- Maintain a consistent bedtime and wakeup time every day, including weekends.
- Do something relaxing and enjoyable before bedtime.
- Avoid intellectually stimulating or stressful activity before bedtime. Try not to dwell on the troubles of the day when going to sleep.
- Avoid going to bed with a full stomach or hungry. Eat a light snack before bed if hungry.
- Make the bedroom as quiet and dark as possible.
- Use the bed only for sleeping and sexual activity.

- Avoid alcohol or caffeine within 6 hours of bedtime.
- Avoid taking naps during the day and early evening.
- Exercise as early in the day as possible. Be careful not to exercise within 3 hours of bedtime.
- Do not watch the clock.
- Avoid medications that are stimulants.
- Ban pets from the bedroom.
- Do not keep the television on at night.
- Avoid turning on bright lights if getting out of bed at night.
- Maintain a comfortable temperature in the bedroom.

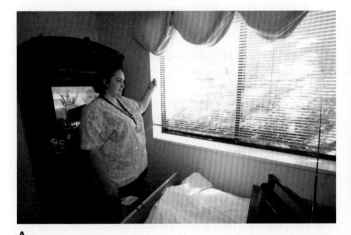
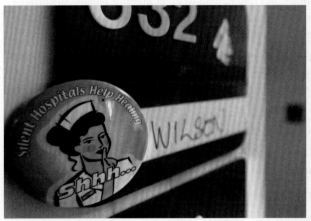

A **B**

FIGURE 22.8 **(A)** Nurses can make environmental modifications, such as closing blinds and using room-darkening devices to help enhance rest and sleep for clients as appropriate. **(B)** Some facilities use special mnemonics and devices to maintain quiet environments for their clients. An example is the "Shhh" sign, which stands for "Silent Hospitals Help Healing." (Frank Franklin II/AP.)

▲ EVALUATION

Indicators that the plan of care for the client with sleep disorders has been successful include the following:

- The client reports improvements in sleep.
- The client reports improvements in functioning, mood, and quality of life.

- The client reports reduced fatigue and daytime sleepiness.
- The client is at reduced risk of injury.
- The client reports minimal side effects of treatment.
- The client verbalizes satisfaction with care and quality of sleep.

Reviewing and Applying Your Knowledge

Chapter Summary

- Sleep disorders occur in clients across the lifespan and across a variety of health states.

- Sleep disorders are very common in clients with psychiatric mental health disorders; sleep disorders may contribute to the development of psychiatric–mental health disorders; conversely, psychiatric–mental health disorders may contribute to sleep disorders.

- Excessive daytime sleepiness or problem sleepiness is a major risk factor for accidents and injuries.

- Nurses and others who work at night or engage in shift work are at particular risk for excessive daytime sleepiness, accidents, and errors.

- Sleep disturbance is common in hospitalized clients. The nurse plays a critical role in promoting sleep in these environments.

Review Questions

1. The nurse expects that it would be most difficult to arouse a client during which stage of NREM sleep?

    a. Stage N1

    b. Stage N2

    c. Stage N3

2. When assessing a client's medication history, the nurse notes that the client is using a drug from a class that both contributes to disturbed sleep and is used for treating insomnia. Which drug class did the nurse identify?

    a. Amphetamines

    b. Benzodiazepines

    c. Selective serotonin reuptake inhibitors (SSRIs)

    d. Opiates

3. Which of the following strategies would the nurse include when teaching a client about appropriate sleep hygiene measures? Select all that apply.

    a. Eat a high-protein snack before bedtime.

    b. Take a short nap in the early evening.

    c. Avoid alcohol within 6 hours of bedtime.

    d. Exercise early in the day.

    e. Refrain from keeping the television on at night.

    f. Keep the bedroom at a comfortable temperature.

4. A client with insomnia is receiving cognitive–behavioral treatment. He asks, "Why am I supposed to stay in bed for a shorter period of time?" The nurse responds based on the understanding that this action accomplishes which of the following?

    a. Reduces anxiety associated with trying to fall asleep

    b. Reduces physiologic arousal

    c. Changes irrational beliefs about sleep

    d. Restricts time in bed to reduce awake time and promote efficient sleep

5. When planning the care for a hospitalized client who also has a sleep disorder, which of the following interventions would be least effective?

    a. Having a small night-light on in the room at night

    b. Providing the client with a glass of warm milk before bed

    c. Keeping the client's door open to the hallway

    d. Offering the client a back rub before bed

Critical Thinking Questions

Consider Case in Point 22.1 and answer the following questions:

1. List the symptoms that led you to think that Agatha had insomnia.

2. What are the factors that contributed to the development of insomnia?

3. What are some additional NANDA International diagnoses that may be appropriate for Agatha at this time?

4. What symptoms would lead the nurse to refer Agatha to a sleep disorders center?

5. If her sadness over the loss of her mother persists or worsens, what additional interventions might be needed?

References

Acebo, C., Sadeh, A., Seifer, R., Tzischinsky, O., Hafer, A., & Carskadon, M. A. (2005). Sleep/wake patterns derived from activity monitoring and maternal report for healthy 1- to 5-year-old children. *Sleep, 28*(12), 1568–1577.

Allena, M., Campus, C., Morrone, E., De Carli, F., Garbarino, S., Manfredi, C., et al. (2009). Periodic limb movements both in non-REM and REM sleep: Relationships between cerebral and autonomic activities. *Clinical Neurophysiology, 120*, 1282–1290.

American Academy of Sleep Medicine. (2005). *International classification of sleep disorders.* Westchester, IL: Author.

American Academy of Sleep Medicine. (2007). *Manual for the scoring of sleep and associated events: Rules, terminology, and technical specifications.* Westchester, IL: Author.

American Psychiatric Association (APA). (2000). *Diagnostic and statistical manual of mental disorders* (4th ed., text rev.). Washington, DC: Author.

American Psychiatric Association (APA). (2007). *DSM-IV-TR coding alert.* Retrieved from http://www.dsmivtr.org/codingalert.cfm

Ancoli-Israel, S., & Martin, J. L. (2006). Insomnia and daytime napping in older adults. *Journal of Clinical Sleep Medicine, 2*(3), 333–342.

Anderson, M. L., & Tufik, S. (2008). The effects of testosterone on sleep and sleep disordered breathing in men: Its bidirectional interaction with erectile function. *Sleep Medicine Reviews, 12*, 363–379.

Anttalainen, U., Saaresranta, T., Aittokallio, J., Kalleinen, N., Vahlberg, T., Virtanen, I., et al. (2006). Impact of menopause on the manifestations and severity of sleep-disordered breathing. *Acta Obstetrics and Gynecology Scandinavia, 85*(11), 1381–1388.

Archbold, K. H. (2011a). Pediatric sleep disorders. In N. S. Redeker & G. P. McEnany (Eds.), *Sleep disorders and sleep promotion in nursing practice* (pp. 219–223). New York, NY: Springer.

Archbold, K. H. (2011b). Sleep promotion in child health settings. In N. S. Redeker & G. P. McEnany (Eds.), *Sleep disorders and sleep promotion in nursing practice* (pp. 277–290). New York , NY: Springer.

Archbold, K. H., Pituch, K. J., Panahi, P., & Chervin, R. D. (2002). Symptoms of sleep disturbances among children at two general pediatric clinics. *Journal of Pediatrics, 140*(1), 97–102.

Armitage, R. (2007). Sleep and circadian rhythms in mood disorders. *Acta Psychiatry Scandinavia, Suppl* (433), 104–115.

Arnulf, I., Leu, S., & Oudiette, D. (2008). Abnormal sleep and sleepiness in Parkinson's disease. *Current Opinion in Neurology, 21*, 472–477.

Asplund, R. (2004). Nocturia, nocturnal polyuria, and sleep quality in the elderly. *Journal of Psychosomatic Research, 56*(5), 517–525.

Baldwin, C. M., & Ornelas, L. R. (2011). Racial/ethnic health disparities and sleep disorders. In N. S. Redeker & G. P. McEnany (Eds.), *Sleep disorders and sleep promotion in nursing practice* (pp. 243–260). New York, NY: Springer.

Bates, J. E., Viken, R. J., Alexander, D. B., Beyers, J., & Stockton, L. (2002). Sleep and adjustment in preschool children: Sleep diary reports by mothers relate to behavior reports by teachers. *Child Development, 73*(1), 62–74.

Benca, R., Duncan, M. J., Frank, E., McClung, C., Nelson, R. J., & Vicentic, A. (2009). Biological rhythms, higher brain function, and behavior: Gaps, opportunities, and challenges. *Brain Research Reviews, 62*, 57–70.

Benca, R., & Peterson, M. (2008). Insomnia and depression. *Sleep Medicine, 9*(1), S3–S9.

Benson, K. L. (2006). Sleep in schizophrenia: Impairments, correlates, and treatment. *Psychiatric Clinics of North America, 29*(4), 1033–1045.

Benson, K. L., & Zarcone, V. P. (1994). Sleep abnormalities in schizophrenia and other psychotic disorders. In J. M. Oldham & M. B. Riba (Eds.), *Review of psychiatry* (Vol. 13, pp. 677–705). Washington, DC: American Psychiatric Press.

Benson, K. L., & Zarcone, V. P. (2000). Schizophrenia. In M. H. Kryger, A. J. Roth, & W. C. Dement (Eds.), *Principles and practice of sleep medicine* (3rd ed., pp. 1159–1167). Philadelphia, PA: W. B. Saunders.

Bernert, R. A., Merrill, K. A., Braithwaite, S. R., Van Orden, K. A., & Joiner, T. E., Jr. (2007). Family life stress and insomnia symptoms in a prospective evaluation of young adults. *Journal of Family Psychology, 21*(1), 58–66.

Bliwise, D. (2005). Normal aging. In M. Kryger, T. Roth, & W. C. Dement (Eds.), *Principles and practice of sleep medicine* (4th ed., pp. 24–38). Philadelphia, PA: Elsevier.

Bliwise, D., L., Mercaldo, N., D., Avidan, A., Y., Boeve, B., F., Greer, S., A., & Kukull, W., A. (2011). Sleep disturbance in dementia with Lowy bodies and Alzheimer's disease: A multicenter analysis. *Dementia & Geriatric Cognitive Disorders, 31*, 239–246.

Borbely, A., & Acherman, P. (2005). Sleep homeostasis and models of sleep regulation. In M. Kryger & T. Roth (Eds.), *Principles and practice of sleep medicine* (4th ed., pp. 405–417). Philadelphia, PA: Elsevier.

Cajochen, C., Munch, M., Knoblauch, V., Blatter, K., & Wirz-Justice, A. (2006). Age-related changes in the circadian and homeostatic regulation of human sleep. *Chronobiology International, 23*(1–2), 461–474.

Cannon, W. B. (1939). *The wisdom of the body.* New York, NY: W. W. Norton.

Carskadon, M. A., & Dement, W. C. (2005). Normal human sleep: An overview. In M. H. Kryger, T. C. Roth, & W. C. Dement (Eds.), *Principles and practice of sleep medicine* (4th ed.). Philadelphia, PA: W. B. Saunders.

Carskadon, M. A., Labyak, S. E., Acebo, C., & Seifer, R. (1999). Intrinsic circadian period of adolescent humans measured in conditions of forced desynchrony. *Neuroscience Letters, 260*, 129–132.

Centers for Disease Control and Prevention. (2008). Percentage of adults who reported an average of ≤6 hours of sleep per 24-hour period by sex and age group—United States, 1985 and 2004. *Morbidity and Mortality Weekly Report, 54*, 933.

Colrain, I. M., Trinder, J., & Swan, G. E. (2004). The impact of smoking cessation on objective and subjective markers of sleep: review, synthesis, and recommendations. *Nicotine & Tobacco Research, 6*(6), 913–925.

Cortese, S., Konofal, E., Yateman, N., Mouren, M. C., & Lecendreux, M. (2006). Sleep and alertness in children with attention-deficit/hyperactivity disorder: A systematic review of the literature. *Sleep, 29*(4), 504–511.

Crabtree, V. M., & Williams, N. A. (2009). Normal sleep in children and adolescents. *Child and Adolescent Psychiatric Clinics of North America, 18*, 799–811.

Cuellar, N., & Redeker, N. S. (2011). Sleep-related movement disorders and parasomnias. In N. S. Redeker & G. P. McEnany (Eds.), *Sleep disorders and sleep promotion in nursing practice* (pp. 121–141). New York, NY: Springer.

Cuellar, N., Strumpf, N., & Ratcliffe, S. (2007). Symptoms of restless legs syndrome in older adults: Outcomes on sleep quality, sleepiness, fatigue, depression, and quality of life. *Journal of the American Geriatrics Society, 55*, 1387–1392.

Czeisler, C. A., Buxton, O. M., & Khalsa, S. B. S. (2005). The human circadian timing system and sleep–wake regulation. In M. H. Kryger, T. C. Roth, & W. C. Dement (Eds.), *Principles and practice of sleep medicine* (4th ed., pp. 375–394). Philadelphia, PA: Elsevier.

Dauvilliers, Y., Arnulf, I., & Mignot, E. (2007). Narcolepsy with cataplexy. *Lancet, 369*(9560), 499–511.

Dauvilliers, Y., Billiard, M., & Montplaisir, J. (2003). Clinical aspects and pathophysiology of narcolepsy. *Clinical Neurophysiology, 114*(11), 2000–2017.

DeMartinis, N. A., & Winokur, A. (2007). Effects of psychiatric medications on sleep and sleep disorders. *CNS & Neurological Disorders Drug Targets, 6,* 17–29.

Dowling, G., & Mastick, J. (2011). Circadian rhythm disorders. In N. S. Redeker & G. P. McEnany (Eds.), *Sleep disorders and sleep promotion in nursing practice* (pp. 159–176). New York, NY: Springer.

Drake, C. L., Roehrs, T., Richardson, G., Walsh, J. K., & Roth, T. (2004). Shift work sleep disorder: Prevalence and consequences beyond that of symptomatic day workers. *Sleep, 27,* 1453–1462.

Driskell, J. E., & Mullen, B. (2005). The efficacy of naps as a fatigue countermeasure: A meta-analytic integration. *Human Factors, 47,* 360–377.

Ensrud, K. E., Blackwell, T. L., Ancoli-Israel, S., Redline, S., Yaffe, K., Diem, S., et al. (2006). Use of selective serotonin reuptake inhibitors and sleep disturbances in community-dwelling older women. *Journal of the American Geriatrics Society, 54*(10), 1508–1515.

Espie, C. A. (2009). "Stepped Care:" A health technology solution for delivering cognitive behavioral therapy as a first line insomnia treatment. *Sleep, 32,* 1549–1558.

Fiedorowicz, J., Endicott, J., Leon, A., Solomon, D., Keller, M., & Coryell, W. (2011). Subthreshold hypomanic symptoms in progression form unipolar major depression to bipolar disorder. *American Journal of Psychiatry, 168*(1), 40–48.

Foley, D., Ancoli-Israel, S., Britz, P., & Walsh, J. (2004). Sleep disturbances and chronic disease in older adults: Results of the 2003 National Sleep Foundation Sleep in America Survey. *Journal of Psychosomatic Research, 56*(5), 497–502.

Fredriksen, K., Rhodes, J., Reddy, R., & Way, N. (2004). Sleepless in Chicago: Tracking the effects of adolescent sleep loss during the middle school years. *Child Development, 75*(1), 84–95.

Gau, S. S., Kessler, R. C., Tseng, W. L., Wu, Y. Y., Chiu, Y. N., Yeh, C. B., et al. (2007). Association between sleep problems and symptoms of attention-deficit/hyperactivity disorder in young adults. *Sleep, 30*(2), 195–201.

Geiger-Brown, J., & McPhaul, K. M. (2011). Sleep promotion in occupational health settings. In N. S. Redeker & G. P. McEnany (Eds.), *Sleep disorders and sleep promotion in nursing practice* (pp. 355–370). New York, NY: Springer.

Gillin, J. C., Drummond, S. P. A., & Moore, P. (2005). Medication and substance abuse. In M. Kryger, T. Roth, & W. C. Dement (Eds.), *Principles and practice of sleep medicine* (4th ed., pp. 1345–1358). Philadelphia, PA: Elsevier.

Harvey, A. (2008). Sleep and circadian rhythms in bipolar disorder: Seeking synchrony, harmony, and regulation. *American Journal of Psychiatry, 168,* 820–829.

Ivanenko, A., & Johnson, K. (2008). Sleep disturbances in children with psychiatric disorders. *Seminars in Pediatric Neurology, 15,* 70–78.

Jenni, O. G., & O'Connor, B. B. (2005). Children's sleep: An interplay between culture and biology. *Pediatrics, 115*(Suppl 1), 204–216.

Johns, M. W. (1991). A new method for measuring daytime sleepiness: The Epworth Sleepiness Scale. *Sleep, 14,* 540–545.

Johnson, E. O., Roth, T., & Breslau, N. (2006). The association of insomnia with anxiety disorders and depression: Exploration of the direction of risk. *Journal of Psychiatric Research, 40*(8), 700–708.

Jungquist, C. (2011). Insomnia. In N. S. Redeker & G. P. McEnany (Eds.), *Sleep disorders and sleep promotion in nursing practice* (pp. 71–94). New York, NY: Springer.

Kirov, R., Kinkelbur, J., Banaschewski, T., & Rothenberger, A. (2007). Sleep patterns in children with attention-deficit/hyperactivity disorder, tic disorder, and comorbidity. *Journal of Child Psychology and Psychiatry, 48*(6), 561–570.

Knutson, K. L., & Lauderdale, D. S. (2009). Sociodemographic and behavioral predictors of bed time and wake time among U.S. adolescents aged 15–17 years. *The Journal of Pediatrics, 154,* 426–430.

Konofal, E., Lecendreux, M., & Cortese, S. (2010). Sleep and ADHD. *Sleep Medicine, 11,* 652–658.

Krystal, A. D., Thakur, M., & Roth, T. (2008). Sleep disturbance in psychiatric disorders: Effects on function and quality of life in mood disorders, alcoholism, and schizophrenia. *Annals of Clinical Psychiatry, 20,* 39–46.

Kyung Lee, E., & Douglass, A. B. (2010). Sleep in psychiatric disorders: Where are we now? *Canadian Journal of Psychiatry, 55,* 403–412.

Lee, D., Morgan, K., & Lindesay, J. (2007). Effect of institutional respite care on the sleep of people with dementia and their primary caregivers. *Journal of the American Geriatric Society, 55*(2), 252–258.

Lee, J. H., Bliwise, D. L., Ansari, F. P., et al. (2007). Daytime sleepiness and functional impairment in Alzheimer disease. *American Journal of Geriatric Psychiatry, 15*(7), 620–626.

Lee, K. A. (2011). Sleep promotion and the child-bearing family. In N. S. Redeker & G. P. McEnany (Eds.), *Sleep disorders and sleep promotion in nursing practice* (pp. 261–276). New York, NY: Springer.

Lee, K. A., Baker, F. C., Newton, K. M., & Ancoli-Israel, S. (2008). The influence of reproductive status and age on women's sleep. *Journal of Women's Health, 17,* 1209–1214.

Lorenz, R. A., Harris, M., & Richards, K. C. (2011). Sleep in adult long-term care. In N. S. Redeker & G. P. McEnany (Eds.), *Sleep disorders and sleep promotion in nursing practice* (pp. 339–354). New York, NY: Springer.

Mai, E. & Buysse, D. J. (2008). Insomnia: Prevalence, impact, pathogenesis, differential diagnosis, and evaluation. *Sleep Medicine Clinics, 3,* 167–174.

McCurry, S. M., Logsdon, R. G., Teri, L., & Vitiello, M. V. (2007). Sleep disturbances in caregivers of persons with dementia: Contributing factors and treatment implications. *Sleep Medicine Review, 11*(2), 143–153.

McEnany, G. P. (2011a). Sleep and psychiatric disorders. In N. S. Redeker & G. P. McEnany (Eds.), *Sleep disorders and sleep promotion in nursing practice.* New York, NY: Springer.

McEnany, G. P. (2011b). Sleep in psychiatric-mental health settings. In N. S. Redeker & G. P. McEnany (Eds.), *Sleep disorders and sleep promotion in nursing practice* (pp. 309–320). New York, NY: Springer.

McLay, R. N., Klam, W. P., & Volkert, S. L. (2010). Insomnia is the most commonly reported symptom and predicts other symptoms of post-traumatic stress disorder in U.S. service members returning from military deployments. *Military Medicine, 175,* 759–762.

Mellman, T. A. (2006). Sleep and anxiety disorders. *Psychiatric Clinics of North America, 29,* 1047–1058.

Meltzer, L. J., Johnson, C. Crossette, J., Ramos, M. & Mindell, J. A. (2009). Prevalence of sleep disorders in pediatric primary care practice. *Sleep, 32,* A66–A67.

Milner, C. E., & Cote, K. A. (2009). Benefits of napping in healthy adults: Impact of nap length, time of day, age, and experience with napping. *Journal of Sleep Research, 18,* 272–281.

Minarik, P. (2011). Gender and sleep. In N. S. Redeker & G. P. McEnany (Eds.), *Sleep disorders and sleep promotion in nursing practice* (pp. 33–42). New York, NY: Springer.

Mindell, J. A., Owens, J. A., & Carskadon, M. A. (1999). Developmental features of sleep. *Child & Adolescent Psychiatric Clinics of North America, 8*(4), 695–725.

Ming, X., & Walters, A. S. (2009). Autism spectrum disorders, attention deficit/hyperactivity disorder, and sleep disorders. *Current Opinion in Pulmonary Medicine, 15,* 578–584.

Morin, C.M., Bootzin, R. R., Buysse, D. J., Edinger, J.D., Espie, C. A., & Lichstein, K. L., (2006). Psychological and behavioral treatment of insomnia: Update of the recent evidence (1996–2004). *Sleep, 29,* 1398–1414.

NANDA International. (2007). *Nursing diagnoses: Definitions and classification (2007–2008).* Philadelphia, PA: Author.

National Sleep Foundation. (2005). Retrieved from http://www .sleepfoundation.org/article/sleep-america-polls/2009-health-and-safety

Nieto, F. J., Young, T. B., Lind, B. K., Shahar, E., Samet, J. M., Redline, S., et al. (2000). Association of sleep-disordered breathing, sleep apnea, and hypertension in a large community-based study: Sleep heart health study. *Journal of the American Medical Association, 283,* 1829–1836.

Obermeyer, W. H., & Benca, R. M. (1996). Effects of drugs on sleep. *Neurologic Clinics, 14,* 828–840.

Ohayon, M. M., Carskadon, M. A., Guilleminault, C., & Vitiello, M. V. (2004). Meta-analysis of quantitative sleep parameters from childhood to old age in healthy individuals: developing normative sleep values across the human lifespan. *Sleep, 27*(7), 1255–1273.

Ohayon, M., Lemoine, P., Arnaud-Briant, V., & Dreyfus, M. (2002). Prevalence and consequences of sleep disorders in a shift worker population. *Journal of Psychosomatic Research, 53,* 577–583.

Ohayon, M., & Roth, T. (2002). Prevalence of restless legs syndrome and periodic limb movement disorder in the general population. *Journal of Psychosomatic Research, 53,* 547–554.

Owens, J. A. (2007). Sleep loss and fatigue in healthcare professionals. *Journal of Perinatal and Neonatal Nursing, 21*(2), 92–100; quiz 101–102.

Owens, J. A., Spirito, A., McGuinn, M., & Nobile, C. (2000). Sleep habits and sleep disturbance in elementary school-aged children. *Journal of Developmental & Behavioral Pediatrics, 21*(1), 27–36.

Pack, A. I., Maislin, G., Staley, B., Pack, F. M., Rogers, W. C., George, C. F., et al. (2006). Impaired performance in commercial drivers: Role of sleep apnea and short sleep duration. *American Journal of Respiratory and Critical Care Medicine, 174*(4), 446–454.

Papadimitriou, G. N., & Linkowski, P. (2005). Sleep disturbance in anxiety disorders. *International Review of Psychiatry, 17*(4), 229–236.

Parker, K. P. (2011). Sleep in medical disorders. In N. S. Redeker & G. P. McEnany (Eds.), *Sleep disorders and sleep promotion in nursing practice* (pp. 177–194). New York, NY: Springer.

Patil, S. P., Schneider, H., Schwartz, A. R., & Smith, P. L. (2007). Adult obstructive sleep apnea: Pathophysiology and diagnosis. *Chest, 132*(1), 325–337.

Peterson, M. J., & Benca, R. M. (2006). Sleep in mood disorders. *Psychiatric Clinics of North America, 29*(4), 1009–1032; abstract ix.

Philipsen, A., Hornyak, M., & Riemann, D. (2006). Sleep and sleep disorders in adults with attention deficit/hyperactivity disorder. *Sleep Medicine Review, 10*(6), 399–405.

Redeker, N. S. (2011). Developmental aspects of normal sleep. In N. S. Redeker & G. P. McEnany (Eds.), *Sleep disorders and sleep promotion in nursing practice* (pp. 19–32). New York, NY: Springer.

Redeker, N. S., Hedges, C., & Booker, K. (2011). Sleep in adult acute and critical care settings. In N. S. Redeker & G. P. McEnany (Eds.), *Sleep disorders and sleep promotion in nursing practice* (pp. 321–338). New York, NY: Springer.

Redeker, N. S., Ruggiero, J., & Hedges, C. (2004). Patterns and predictors of sleep disturbance after cardiac surgery. *Research in Nursing and Health.*

Rogers, A. E. (2001). A comparison of three different sleep schedules for reducing daytime sleepiness in narcolepsy. *Sleep, 24,* 385–391.

Rogers, A. E. (2002). Sleep deprivation and the ED night shift. *Journal of Emergency Nursing, 28,* 469–470.

Rogers, A. E. (2011). Narcolepsy. In N. S. Redeker & G. P. McEnany (Eds.), *Sleep disorders and sleep promotion in nursing practice* (pp. 141–158). New York, NY: Springer.

Rose, K. M., & Lorenz, R. (2010). Sleep disturbances in dementia: What they are and what to do. *Journal of Gerontological Nursing, 36,* 9–14.

Roth, T., Jaeger, S., Jin, R., Kalsekar, A., Stang, P. E., & Kessler, R. C. (2006). Sleep problems, comorbid mental disorders, and role functioning in the national comorbidity survey replication. *Biologic Psychiatry, 60*(12), 1364–1371.

Ruggiero, J. (2003). Correlates of fatigue in critical care nurses. *Research in Nursing and Health, 26,* 434–444.

Sateia, M. J. (2009). Update on sleep and psychiatric disorders. *Chest, 135,* 1370–1379.

Sawyer, A., & Weaver, T. (2011). Sleep-related breathing disorders. In N. S. Redeker & G. P. McEnany (Eds.), *Sleep disorders and sleep promotion in nursing practice* (pp. 95–120). New York, NY: Springer.

Siddiqui, F., Strus, J, Ming, X., Lee, I. a., Chokroverty, S., & Walters, A. S. (2007). Rise of blood pressure with periodic limb movements in sleep and wakefulness. *Clinical Neurophysiology 118,* 1923–1930.

Smaldone, A., Honig, J. C., & Byrne, M. W. (2007). Sleepless in America: Inadequate sleep and relationships to health and well-being of our nation's children. *Pediatrics, 119*(Suppl 1), S29–S37.

Snell, E. K., Adam, E. K., & Duncan, G. J. (2007). Sleep and the body mass index and overweight status of children and adolescents. *Child Development, 78*(1), 309–323.

Spielman, A. (1986). Assessment of insomnia. *Clinical Psychology Review, 6,* 11–25.

Spielman, A. J., Caruso, L. S., & Glovinsky, P. B. (1987). A behavioral perspective on insomnia treatment. *The Psychiatric Clinics of North America, 10,* 541–553.

Stahl, S. (2008). *Stahl's essential psychopharmacology neuroscientific basis and practical applications* (3rd ed.). Cambridge, UK: Cambridge University Press.

Szklo-Coxe, M., Young, T., Peppard, P., Finn, L., & Benca, R. (2010). Prospective associations of insomnia markers and symptoms with depression. *American Journal of Epidemiology, 171*(6), 709–720.

Taub, L. F., & Redeker, N. S. (2008). Sleep disorders, glucose regulation, and type 2 diabetes. *Biological Research for Nursing, 9,* 231–243.

Teplin, D., Raz, B., Daiter, J., Varenbut, M., & Tyrrell, M. (2006). Screening for substance use patterns among patients referred for a variety of sleep complaints. *American Journal of Drug and Alcohol Abuse, 32*(1), 111–120.

Tractenberg, R. E., Singer, C. M., & Kaye, J. A. (2006). Characterizing sleep problems in persons with Alzheimer's disease and normal elderly. *Journal of Sleep Research, 15*(1), 97–103.

Van Cauter, E., Spiegel, K., Tasali, E., & Leproult, R. (2008). Metabolic consequences of sleep and sleep loss. *Sleep Medicine, 9*(Suppl 1), S23–S28.

Waldrop, A. E., Back, S. E., Sensenig, A., & Brady, K. T. (2008). Sleep disturbances associated with posttraumatic stress disorder and alcohol dependence. *Addictive Behaviors, 33,* 328–335.

Ward, T. M., Gay, C., Anders, T. F., Alkon, A., & Lee, K. A. (2008). Sleep and napping patterns in 3- to 5- year old children attending full-day childcare centers. *Journal of Pediatric Psychology, 33,* 66–672.

Wolfson, A. R., Spaulding, N. L, Dandrow, C., & Baroni, E. M. (2007). Middle school start times: The importance of a good night's sleep for young adolescents. *Behavioral Sleep medicine, 5,* 194–209.

Wulff, K., Gatti, S., Wettstein, J. G., & Foster, R. G. (2010). Sleep and circadian rhythm disruption in psychiatric and neurodegenerative disease. *Nature Reviews Neuroscience, 11*, 589–599.

Yaggi, H. K., Araujo, A. B., & McKinlay, J. B. (2006). Sleep duration as a risk factor for the development of type 2 diabetes. *Diabetes Care, 29*(3), 657–661.

Yaggi, H. K., Concato, J., Kernan, W. N., Lichtman, J., Barass, L. M., & Mohesenin, V. (2005). Obstructive sleep apnea as a risk factor for stroke and death. *New England Journal of Medicine, 358*, 2034–2041.

Yang, C., & Winkelman, J. W. (2006). Clinical significance of sleep EEG abnormalities in chronic schizophrenia. *Schizophrenia Research, 82*(2–3), 251–260.

Young, T., Palta, M., Dempsey, J., Skatrud, J., Weber, S., & Badr, S. (1993). The occurrence of sleep-disordered breathing among middle-aged adults. *New England Journal of Medicine, 328*(17), 1230–1235.

Zarcone, V. P., & Benson, K. L. (1997). BPRS symptom factors and sleep variables in schizophrenia. *Psychiatry Research, 66*, 111–120.

Web Resources

American Academy of Sleep Medicine MEDSleep Educational Resources: http://www.aasmnet.org/MEDSleepprogram.htm

American Sleep Apnea Association: www.sleepapnea.org

American Sleep Disorders Association: www.aasmnet.org

National Center for Sleep Disorders Research: www.nhlbi.nih.gov/about/ncsdr

National Sleep Foundation: www.sleepfoundation.org

Sleep Research Society: www.sleepresearchsociety.org/education/sleepnet.com

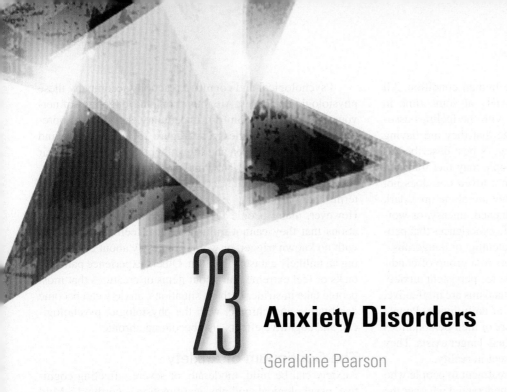

23

Anxiety Disorders

Geraldine Pearson

KEY TERMS

acute stress disorder
agoraphobia
anxiety
anxiety disorder
compulsions
generalized anxiety disorder
obsessions
obsessive-compulsive disorder
panic attack
panic disorder
phobia
post-traumatic stress disorder
(PTSD)
social phobia

LEARNING OBJECTIVES

On completion of this chapter, you should be able to accomplish the following:

Define the term *anxiety.*
Explain what is meant by *anxiety disorder.*
Describe the incidence and prevalence of anxiety disorders.
Discuss proposed etiologies for anxiety disorders.
Identify symptoms of anxiety disorders.
Explain the different types of anxiety disorders.
Discuss treatments for anxiety disorders.
Apply the nursing process to the care of clients with anxiety disorders.

Feeling anxious is part of the human condition. All people experience some anxiety at some time in their lives. Most people are familiar with the feelings associated with anxiety and can verbalize that they are having them. **Anxiety**, largely rooted in fear, is best described as a sense of psychological distress. People may feel transient anxiety before a job interview, when a loved one does not arrive home as expected, or when they are alone on a dark street at night. Feeling anxious, frightened, uneasy, or worried is a normal response to various life experiences that people could perceive as disruptive, threatening, or dangerous.

The term **anxiety disorder** refers to a group of conditions in which affected clients experience persistent anxiety that they cannot dismiss. Coping mechanisms are ineffective, and anxiety interferes with activities of daily living. People with anxiety disorders feel that the core of their personalities is being threatened, even when no actual danger exists. They perceive a threat, even if it is not present in reality.

To effectively plan and provide treatment to people who are anxious, nurses need to carefully understand whether the anxiety is a transient, normative response to stress or a long-term response to a real or perceived threat that is negatively influencing the person's ability to function in daily activities. This chapter explains anxiety as an appropriate response and its associated manifestations. It then explores in detail anxiety disorders, reviewing causes, symptoms and diagnostic criteria, interdisciplinary care, and nursing strategies.

ANXIETY

Anxiety should be differentiated from stress. Stress is not a disorder. It is a normal part of everyday life and does not have good or bad connotations. The perception of stress is individually based; an event that one person views as threatening may be tolerated easily or enjoyed by others. Therefore, the feeling of stress as a negative emotional state is based substantially on the person's appraisal of the stressor and assessment of his or her ability to respond to it. Still, stressors frequently are cited as causes of anxiety, and when the mind interprets events as threatening, it responds accordingly, with symptoms of anxiety.

To help people cope effectively with stressful, anxiety-provoking situations, the brain initiates physiologic mechanisms that protect against injury and allow them to either fight or flee. The widespread effects of the *fight-or-flight response,* mediated by the sympathetic nervous system, include the following:

- Heart rate and blood pressure increase.
- Blood flows to the muscles.
- Breathing rate increases.
- Perspiration increases.
- Blood clotting ability increases.
- Saliva production decreases.
- Digestion decreases.
- Immune response decreases.
- Energy-producing stored glycogen is released.

Psychological and cognitive reactions accompany these physiologic responses. Anxious people have feelings of nervousness, vague discomfort, uncertainty, self-doubt, apprehension, dread, or restlessness (Figure 23.1). They may find it hard to concentrate on anything other than the threat. Their senses are heightened. They may appear upset.

The fight-or-flight reaction is protective in the short term and particularly effective against physical threats. However, many people feel anxious about long-term situations that they cannot influence, have feelings of anxiety with no known trigger, or worry helplessly about events taking an unlikely catastrophic turn. Others experience panic attacks or feel extreme fear about items or creatures that most people take in stride. In these situations, anxiety can become debilitating and chronic, with the physiologic, psychological, and cognitive effects also becoming chronic.

The Continuum of Anxiety

Anxiety can be mild, moderate, or severe, affecting cognitive, psychological, and physical function accordingly. Mild anxiety results in improved functioning; however, as anxiety increases, people become less and less able to function. Cognitive functioning becomes distorted, and bodies must endure extended periods of high physical alert.

Effects on Sensation

Anxiety affects the ways people perceive and process sensory input. Mild anxiety actually heightens sensory awareness (ie, sight, hearing, taste, smell, and touch). Moderate anxiety dulls perception; however, people can attend to greater sensory input if directed to do so. In severe anxiety, perception becomes increasingly distorted, sensory input diminishes, and processing of sensory stimuli becomes

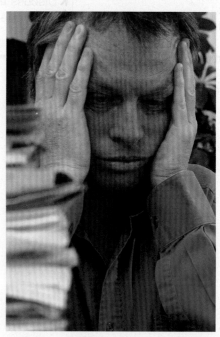

FIGURE 23.1 Increasing uncontrolled anxiety limits the ability to cope and function.

scattered and disorganized. In panic, perception becomes grossly distorted. At the level of panic, people cannot differentiate real from imaginary stimuli.

Effects on Cognition

Anxiety greatly influences *cognition,* the ability to concentrate, learn, and solve problems. Mild and moderate levels of anxiety are still conducive to concentration, learning, and problem solving. People of average intelligence who are mildly to moderately anxious discern relationships between and among concepts with relative ease and can concentrate and solve problems without much difficulty. In contrast, severe anxiety hinders cognitive function. Severely anxious people (such as those with anxiety disorders) have difficulty concentrating and may fail to discern even obvious conceptual relationships. Panic-stricken people have even greater cognitive impairment; concentration, learning, and problem solving are virtually impossible during panic.

Effects on Verbal Ability

In mild anxiety, speech content and form reflect heightened sensory awareness and cognitive function. Thoughts are verbalized logically; speech rate and volume are appropriate to the context of the content and communication. Mildly anxious people typically appear alert, confident, and relatively secure.

The verbal behavior of those with moderate anxiety is commonly marked by frequent changes of topic, repetitive questioning, joking, and wordiness. *Blocking,* or loss of train of thought, also may occur. Speech rate often accelerates, and speech volume often increases. Moderately anxious people may change body position frequently, use excessive hand gestures, and assume aggressive body postures toward others. Furthermore, because moderately anxious people do not perceive and process sensory input as efficiently as mildly anxious people, they tend to hesitate and procrastinate in meeting routine social and vocational expectations. Such behaviors often present an overall picture of restlessness and discontent that may provoke feelings of irritation in others.

Those with severe anxiety display verbal behavior that indicates highly disordered perceptual and cognitive function. They may verbalize emotional pain through such assertions as "I can't stand this" or "I can't think" or by vociferously demanding help and relief. Nonverbal behavior typically involves fine and gross motor tremors, grimaces, and other forms of purposeless activity, such as pacing and hand-wringing. Severely anxious people present an overall picture of extreme emotional discomfort and behavioral disorganization.

Panic-level anxiety results in even greater emotional pain and behavioral disorganization. Verbal and nonverbal behaviors suggest a psychotic-like state, rendering people virtually helpless and unable to negotiate simple demands (Figure 23.2). People may scream, run wildly, or cling tenaciously to something or someone they perceive as a source of safety and security. Others must initiate protective and calming measures promptly because prolonged panic is incompatible with life.

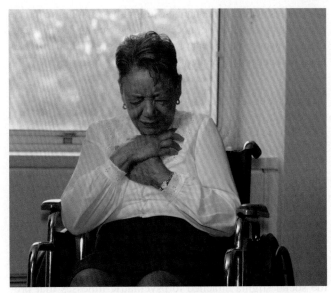

FIGURE 23.2 Clients in a state of panic may be unable to communicate at all. They may feel like they are choking, being smothered, or having a heart attack.

Normal Versus Abnormal Anxiety

All the behaviors described previously are normal in certain situations. Even panic may be a normal response to terrifying, life-threatening situations. So when does anxiety become a psychiatric disorder?

Pathologic anxiety is suspected when people are anxious despite no real threat, when a threat has passed long ago but continues to impair functioning, or when people substitute adaptive coping mechanisms with maladaptive ones. Other indicators of a need for intervention or treatment include anxiety with the following characteristics:

- Is of greater-than-expected intensity based on the context
- Prevents fulfillment of professional, personal, or social roles
- Is accompanied by flashbacks, obsessions, or compulsions
- Curtails daily or social activities
- Lasts longer than expected given the precipitating stress

Unrelieved anxiety causes physical and emotional problems, and people may use various adaptive or maladaptive coping mechanisms to try to manage it (Box 23.1). Short-term

---

BOX 23.1 Adaptive and Maladaptive Coping Mechanisms for Anxiety

- Withdrawal: Retreat from anxiety-provoking experiences
- Acting out: Discharge of anxiety through aggressive behavior
- Psychosomatization: Visceral or physiologic expression of anxiety
- Avoidance: Management of anxiety-laden experiences through evasive behaviors
- Problem solving: Systematic method for addressing difficult situations

use of these coping mechanisms might be a natural response to a stressor and does not necessarily indicate a need for treatment. However, persistent or recurrent anxiety requires evaluation to determine if a client has an anxiety disorder.

Checkpoint Questions
1. What is the effect of mild anxiety on sensation?
2. When do the symptoms of anxiety warrant further assessment and treatment?

ANXIETY DISORDERS

Currently, two major barriers exist to treating clients with anxiety disorders. One is lack of general knowledge about the nature and prevalence of anxiety disorders and about their positive response to effective treatment. The other is the social stigma attached to psychiatric illnesses that prevents many people from obtaining prompt treatment before complications arise (Roy-Byrne et al., 2010). Despite these barriers, early identification of anxiety disorders and evidence-based care for those with them is essential to preventing comorbidity and complications arising from misdiagnosis and inadequate treatment (Biederman et al., 2007).

Incidence and Prevalence

Anxiety disorders affect approximately 40 million Americans 18 years or older in any given year (Kessler et al., 2008). They are the most common psychiatric disorders for adults and children. Pediatric prevalence rates vary greatly, but approximately 20% of youth experience an anxiety disorder (Merikangas, 2005). See Chapter 36 for more discussion of anxiety disorders in children and adolescents.

Anxiety disorders pose a human and economic burden affecting quality of life and workplace productivity (Hoffman et al., 2008). They appear to affect females more often than males in both adult and pediatric populations. Anxiety disorders are often misdiagnosed and undertreated, thus leading to complications. Medical illness can increase the prevalence of anxiety disorders (Fava et al., 2010).

Etiology

According to current research, anxiety disorders have several possible causes. It is likely that most anxiety disorders result from a combination of neurobiologic vulnerabilities, developmental stage, and psychosocial stress.

Neurobiologic Theories

Hereditary predisposition contributes to the development of anxiety disorders. Martin and colleagues (2010) note that "each anxiety disorder, as well as major depressive disorder (MDD), has both genetic and environmental contributions to vulnerability" (p. 869). It is now thought that there is a developmental dynamic operative upon the development of depressive and anxious symptoms. In other words, risk factors for development of the disorder may vary by age and development (Kendler et al., 2008).

Biologic vulnerability to certain anxiety disorders varies. With clients who have a family history of panic disorder, evidence suggests that their heritable neuronal state may generate a lower threshold for their response to incidents that might generate anxiety. In other words, they are predisposed to a more intense response to emergencies and thus are more likely to experience anxiety. However, this vulnerability may never be stressed, and people with the same family history may not have the disorder.

All anxiety disorders have some commonalities. These include hyperactivity in limbic regions of the brain, particularly the amygdala. Higher cortical executive areas are unable to normalize the limbic response to stimuli (Martin et al., 2010). "Repeated, prolonged, or particularly severe stress could increase the magnitude and duration of CRF, glucocorticoid, and catecholaminergic signaling, and these three signaling classes can explain the psychiatric, circulatory, metabolic, and immune manifestations of stress-related illness" (Martin et al., 2010, p. 883). Severe stress can influence the brain's ability to regulate and avoid anxiety.

Several interacting brain structures influence and mediate fear and anxiety. The amygdala serves as a communications center for parts of the brain that intercept and process sensory input (Figure 23.3). It can identify incoming sensory

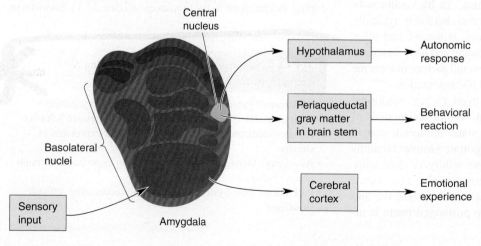

FIGURE 23.3 In the amygdala, sensory information is processed and sent out to other components of the nervous system. If it interprets input as threatening, responses in other regions lead to autonomic, behavioral, and emotional manifestations of fear and anxiety.

information as threatening and then instigate feelings of anxiety or fear. In addition, researchers theorize that emotional memories stored in the central part of the amygdala play a role in phobic disorders, whereas other parts of the amygdala are involved in other forms of anxiety. The amygdala also coordinates fear, memory, and emotion with heart rate, blood pressure, and other physical responses to stressful events.

Etkin and Wager (2007) conducted a meta-analysis of neuroimaging studies involving emotional processing in post-traumatic stress disorder, social anxiety disorder, and specific phobia. They concluded that "patients with all three disorders demonstrated hyperactivity in the amygdala and insula" (p. 1485). They also noted the same pattern of activation in healthy subjects experiencing anticipatory anxiety as part of the research. These findings suggest that all people experience the same neurobiology of a fear response and subsequent anxiety symptoms. Stein and colleagues (2007) similarly found increased amygdala and insula reactivity to certain types of emotional processing in young adults who were prone to anxiety-related temperamental traits.

It is thought that the symptoms of anxiety disorders occur as the result of an imbalance in the emotional centers of the brain. These cognitive centers are in the frontal lobe and include the prefrontal frontal cortex (PFC), which is responsible for executive functions of the brain such as decision making and planning, moderating, and understanding social behavior. The orbitofrontal cortex (OFC) is responsible for coding information, controlling impulses, and regulating mood (Martin et al., 2010). The *hippocampus* is responsible for processing threatening stimuli and is thought to play a role in anxiety disorders by encoding this information into memories. The research suggests that individuals exposed to traumatic events may use their dorsal executive network to process emotional/affective issues and, as a result, diminish their executive control (Martin et al., 2010). Additional biologic factors that may contribute to the onset of anxiety disorders include physical illness; exposure to substances such as cocaine, amphetamines, cannabis, and caffeine; and exposure to physical or psychological danger, trauma, or both. Research examining the link between brain chemistry and specific environmental or psychosocial stresses regarding anxiety disorders is ongoing.

Psychological Theories

Empirical research has shown that many clients with anxiety disorder share certain features, including low self-esteem, a shy or timid nature in childhood, parents whom they perceived as critical or angry, and discomfort with aggression. Long-term exposure to abuse, violence, or poverty may affect a person's susceptibility to anxiety disorders. Gal and colleagues (2011) found that abuse occurring in childhood and adolescence predisposed adults to anxiety and mood disorders. Anxiety disorders also can commonly co-occur with depressive disorders.

According to learning theory, anxiety results from conditioning, by which people develop an anxious response by linking a dangerous or fear-inducing event (eg, a house fire) with a neutral event (eg, watching someone light a match; see Chap. 3). In cases of general anxiety, people may learn the anxiety response when they begin to liken any anxious symptoms with a full-fledged anxiety attack, perpetuating a vicious anxiety cycle.

Cognitive theorists see anxiety as a manifestation of distorted thinking. They suggest that such disorders are the result of perceptions or attitudes that overestimate the danger. According to these theorists, many people with anxiety have an exaggerated need for approval and tend to view even the most minor mistakes as catastrophes.

> ### Checkpoint Questions
> 3. What are the two major barriers to the care of clients with anxiety disorders?
> 4. What four brain structures are believed to influence fear and anxiety?
> 5. How do cognitive theorists view anxiety?

Signs and Symptoms/Diagnostic Criteria

Anxiety disorders include generalized anxiety disorder, phobic disorders, panic attacks and panic disorder, obsessive-compulsive disorder, and stress disorders. Individual conditions are discussed in the following paragraphs.

Generalized Anxiety Disorder

Generalized anxiety disorder (GAD) is characterized by chronic and excessive worry and anxiety more days than not for at least 6 months, encompassing many aspects of the person's life (American Psychiatric Association [APA], 2000). The worry and anxiety of GAD cause so much discomfort that they interfere with daily life and relationships. Clients tend to exhibit persistent and chronic signs of severe anxiety, such as motor tension, autonomic hyperactivity, and apprehensive expectation. Some also may exhibit chronic hypervigilance for potential threats. Generalized anxiety disorder is the most commonly occurring anxiety disorder in primary care clients and may present with associated physical pain symptoms (Romera et al., 2011).

Because of this tense hyperarousal, clients may be unable to concentrate, suffer chronic fatigue, and experience sleep pattern disturbances. In addition, they may exhibit tenseness and distractibility in social situations. Anxiety has been linked to depression; approximately 50% of outpatients with major depression also suffer from anxiety disorders (Fava et al., 2008). See Case Vignette 23.1.

Phobic Disorders

A **phobia** is a persistent, irrational fear attached to an object or situation that objectively does not pose a significant danger. Affected clients experience anticipatory anxiety followed by a compelling desire to avoid the dreaded object or situation, even though they usually recognize that the fear is unreasonable or excessive in proportion to the actual threat

Case Vignette 23.1

For most of her life, Marcia, 34 years old, has been a "worrywart." She still has frequent nightmares about dropping out of college, even though she graduated with honors 10 years ago. Recently, she has been even more anxious, feeling like she is "falling off a precipice."

Marcia was promoted 9 months ago to assistant buyer at a large upscale department store. "I thought this position was a great opportunity to further my career," she tells the nurse. "I had no idea I would feel so uptight, afraid of getting in over my head. It's hard for me to concentrate. My boss has no patience and wants everything done yesterday."

Marcia was taking prescribed diazepam (Valium) initially, but felt too drowsy and stopped. She has never had a panic attack, but she reports considerable irritation with her husband and children. Marcia also complains of insomnia. She denies depression. She reports enjoying her ceramics class. She says that she is not having any sexual difficulties with her husband.

Marcia tried relaxation exercises and meditation but found herself dwelling on job worries during them. Her husband encouraged her to drink a glass or two of wine before or during dinner. She found that this initially helped but soon became fearful of becoming an alcoholic.

Marcia complains of a nagging uneasiness and sense of dread. She denies obsessions, compulsions, phobias, delusions, and hallucinations. She scores a 30 (of a possible 30) on the Mini-Mental State Examination. Her speech is clear, coherent, relevant, and spontaneous. She looks apprehensive, although she is well dressed and somewhat fidgety.

Reflection and Critical Thinking

- What additional data would you consider exploring with Marcia? Explain your answer.
- How can nurses help clients separate valid concerns from things that are causing them unnecessary anxiety?

(APA, 2000). Unlike panic attacks (discussed later in this chapter), phobias are always anticipated and never unexpected. They may be simple and specific to certain situations, events, or objects. They also may be globally incapacitating, as with severe agoraphobia. When phobias accompany panic attacks, the condition is diagnosed as panic disorder (APA, 2000). The degree to which phobias are disabling depends largely on how central the phobia is in the person's life. See DSM-IV-TR Box 23.1.

AGORAPHOBIA. Agoraphobia is a marked fear of being alone or in a public place from which escape would be difficult or help would be unavailable in the event of becoming disabled (APA, 2000). As such, it is the most severe and persistent phobic disorder. People with agoraphobia often fear such scenarios as being outside the house alone, using public or mass transportation, and being in a crowd. As a response, many of them avoid such situations or endure them with so much agony that they rearrange their lives to minimize these occurrences (eg, restrict travel, stop leaving the house). Eventually, the limitations of agoraphobia may diminish enjoyment of life and lead to depression (National Institute of Mental Health [NIMH], 2010).

SPECIFIC PHOBIA. A specific phobia is a persistent, irrational fear of and compelling desire to avoid a circumstance or thing other than those specific to agoraphobia or social phobia. Common specific phobias include acrophobia (fear of heights), claustrophobia (fear of closed spaces), blood phobia (fear of the sight of blood or injury), and fears of birds, cats or other furry animals, house dust, microbes, snakes, or insects (APA, 2000).

SOCIAL PHOBIA. Social phobia represents a persistent, irrational fear of and compelling desire to avoid situations in which people may be exposed to strangers or to scrutiny from others. In addition, clients fear behaving in a way that may prove humiliating or embarrassing. They experience marked anticipatory anxiety if confronted with such a situation and attempt to avoid it. Examples of social phobias include fear of speaking in public, eating or taking a test in the presence of others, or using public restrooms (NIMH, 2011).

Panic Attacks

Panic attacks typically are characterized by a discrete period of intense apprehension or terror without any real accompanying danger, accompanied by at least 4 of 13 somatic or cognitive symptoms (APA, 2000) (DSM-IV-TR BOX 23.2). The clinical picture involves a physiologic and psychological overresponse to stressors. Clients experiencing a panic attack incorrectly perceive their circumstances to be life threatening; therefore, they have physiologic reactions such as chest pain, choking or smothering sensations, dizziness, dyspnea, fainting, hot and cold flashes, palpitations, paresthesias, sweating, and vertigo. They also may report feelings of depersonalization or derealization, fears of dying or going crazy, or uncontrollable behaviors.

Panic attacks are exceedingly frightening and uncomfortable. While they are happening, clients may make extreme efforts to escape from what they believe to be causing the reaction. They may develop anticipatory anxiety about when the next panic attack will happen. The disorder is closely linked with generalized anxiety disorders but occurs in addition to this. Although panic attacks are unpredictable, they may occur in specific situations, such as driving

DSM-IV-TR BOX 23.1

Phobic Disorders

Agoraphobia

A. Anxiety about being in places or situations from which escape might be difficult (or embarrassing) or in which help may not be available in the event of having an unexpected or situationally predisposed Panic Attack or panic-like symptoms. Agoraphobic fears typically involve characteristic clusters of situations that include being outside the home alone; being in a crowd, or standing in a line; being on a bridge; and traveling in a bus, train, or automobile.

B. The situations are avoided (eg, travel is restricted) or else are endured with marked distress or with anxiety about having a Panic Attack or panic-like symptoms, or require the presence of a companion.

C. The anxiety or phobic avoidance is not better accounted for by another mental disorder.

Specific Phobia

A. Marked and persistent fear that is excessive or unreasonable, cued by the presence or anticipation of a specific object or situation (eg, flying, heights, animals, receiving an injection, seeing blood).

B. Exposure to the phobic stimulus almost invariably provokes an immediate anxiety response, which may take the form of a situationally bound or situationally predisposed Panic Attack. **Note**: In children, the anxiety may be expressed by crying, tantrums, freezing, or clinging.

C. The person recognizes that the fear is excessive or unreasonable. **Note**: In children, this feature may be absent.

D. The phobic situation(s) is avoided or else is endured with intense anxiety or distress.

E. The avoidance, anxious anticipation, or distress in the feared situation(s) interferes significantly with the person's normal routine, occupational (or academic) functioning, or social activities or relationships, or there is marked distress about having the phobia.

F. In individuals under age 18 years, the duration is at least 6 months.

G. The anxiety, Panic Attacks, or phobic avoidance associated with the specific object or situation are not better accounted for by another mental disorder.

Social Phobia

A. A marked and persistent fear of one or more social or performance situations in which the person is exposed to unfamiliar people or to possible scrutiny by others. The individual fears that he or she will act in a way (or show anxiety symptoms) that will be humiliating or embarrassing. **Note**: In children, there must be evidence of the capacity for age-appropriate social relationships with familiar people and the anxiety must occur in peer settings, not just in interactions with adults.

B. Exposure to the feared social situation almost invariably provokes anxiety, which may take the form of a situationally bound or situationally predisposed Panic Attack. **Note**: In children, the anxiety may be expressed by crying, tantrums, freezing, or shrinking from social situations with unfamiliar people.

C. The person recognizes that the fear is excessive or unreasonable. **Note**: In children, this feature may be absent.

D. The feared social or performance situations are avoided or else are endured with intense anxiety or distress.

E. The avoidance, anxious anticipation, or distress in the feared social or performance situation(s) interferes significantly with the person's normal routine, occupational (academic) functioning, or social activities or relationships, or there is marked distress about having the phobia.

F. In individuals under age 18 years, the duration is at least 6 months.

G. The fear or avoidance is not due to the direct physiologic effects of a substance (eg, a drug of abuse, a medication) or a general medical condition and is not better accounted for by another mental disorder.

H. If a general medical condition or another mental disorder is present, the fear in Criterion A is unrelated to it.

Reprinted with permission from the *Diagnostic and Statistical Manual of Mental Disorders, Fourth Edition, Text Revision* (Copyright © 2000). American Psychiatric Association.

an automobile. Attacks do not necessarily occur every time a person confronts the situation. Moreover, panic attacks may occur in other circumstances.

Panic Disorder

The essential features of **panic disorder** are recurrent, unexpected panic attacks that cause affected clients to worry persistently about recurrences or complications or to undergo behavioral changes in response to the attacks for at least 1 month. Panic disorder may be with or without agoraphobia.

Obsessive-Compulsive Disorder

In **obsessive-compulsive disorder** (OCD) clients experience recurrent obsessions or compulsions that are time consuming (ie, taking more than 1 hour per day), cause significant impairment or distress, or both (APA, 2000). M**O**VIE viewing **GUIDES** The term **obsessions** used in this diagnosis refers to recurrent, intrusive, and persistent ideas, thoughts, images, or impulses. People with OCD do not voluntarily produce obsessions but feel cognitively invaded by them, usually finding them repugnant or meaningless.

DSM-IV-TR BOX 23.2

Panic Disorders

Panic Attack

A discrete period of intense fear or discomfort, in which four (or more) of the following symptoms developed abruptly and reached a peak within 10 minutes:

1. Palpitations, pounding heart, or accelerated heart rate
2. Sweating
3. Trembling or shaking
4. Sensations of shortness of breath or smothering
5. Feeling of choking
6. Chest pain or discomfort
7. Nausea or abdominal distress
8. Feeling dizzy, unsteady, light-headed, or faint
9. Derealization (feelings of unreality) or depersonalization (being detached from oneself)
10. Fear of losing control or going crazy
11. Fear of dying
12. Paresthesias (numbness or tingling sensations)
13. Chills or hot flushes

Panic Disorder

A. Both (1) and (2):
1. Recurrent unexpected Panic Attacks

2. At least one of the attacks has been followed by 1 month (or more) of one (or more) of the following:
a. persistent concern about having additional attacks
b. worry about the implications of the attack or its consequences (eg, losing control, having a heart attack, "going crazy")
c. a significant change in behavior related to the attacks
B. The absence [or presence] of Agoraphobia*
C. The Panic Attacks are not due to the direct physiologic effects of a substance (eg, a drug of abuse, a medication) or a general medical condition (eg, hyperthyroidism).
D. The Panic Attacks are not better accounted for by another mental disorder, such as Social Phobia (eg, occurring on exposure to feared social situations), Specific Phobia (eg, on exposure to a specific phobic situation), Obsessive-Compulsive Disorder (eg, on exposure to dirt in someone with an obsession about contamination), Posttraumatic Stress Disorder (eg, in response to stimuli associated with a severe stressor), or Separation Anxiety Disorder (eg, in response to being away from home or close relatives).

*The two types of Panic Attack are **without agoraphobia** and **with agoraphobia** (see DSM-IV-TR BOX 23.1 for diagnostic characteristics of agoraphobia).

Reprinted with permission from the *Diagnostic and Statistical Manual of Mental Disorders, Fourth Edition, Text Revision* (Copyright © 2000). American Psychiatric Association.

Despite efforts to ignore or dismiss them, clients remain preoccupied with these obsessive ideations.

Compulsions are ritualistic behaviors that people feel compelled to perform either in accord with a specific set of rules or in a routine manner. Clients engage in such rituals to prevent or reduce anxiety, not to increase pleasure or satisfaction. In fact, they can resist the compulsion for a short period, but the delay creates a tremendous, anxious tension that is relieved only by performing the compulsive act. Usually, the compulsion is linked with an obsession, in that people engage in compulsive behavior to decrease the anxiety from the obsession (APA, 2000). For example, a person who is obsessed with fear of dirt or germs may engage in repetitive, excessive handwashing or housecleaning (Figure 23.4). At the same time, clients invest compulsive acts with symbolic significance by unrealistically believing that they will magically solve problems or atone for past misdeeds. If affected clients or others intervene to stop the compulsive act, anxiety results.

At one time, there was speculation that OCD, an anxiety disorder, was closely related to obsessive-compulsive personality disorder (see Chap. 25). However, more recent evidence suggests no real connection between them. To illustrate, clients with obsessive-compulsive personality disorder

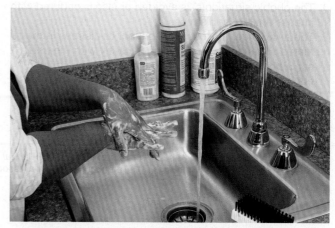

FIGURE 23.4 People with obsessive-compulsive disorder may engage in repeated behaviors, such as excessive handwashing, as a mechanism for managing anxiety.

do not experience symptoms as uncomfortable, distressful, or bothersome. Moreover, they do not have actual obsessions or compulsions. Clients with OCD, the anxiety disorder, experience their symptoms as alien to themselves and intrusive (APA, 2000).

Case Vignette 23.2

Graham, a 28-year-old registered nurse, is referred for assessment and treatment by the employee assistance program (EAP) at his hospital because he washes his hands to the point that he cannot perform clinically. He says to the nurse therapist, "I know my hands are clean and that I'm following the necessary precautions to prevent exposure to germs. I just feel this pressure that compels me to wash my hands. I can't help myself, much less anyone else." The nurse notices that Graham's hands are severely chapped and appear painful. As he talks, Graham occasionally wrings his hands; during pauses, he straightens the paperweight and files on the nurse's desk.

Graham agrees to cognitive–behavioral therapy and treatment with psychoactive medications. The initial prescription is 20 mg of fluoxetine (Prozac) every day for 7 days and then increased 20 mg each week until symptoms subside or a maximum dose of 80 mg is achieved.

Reflection and Critical Thinking

* What disorder does Graham seem to be exhibiting?
* Would you expect Graham's problems to increase or decrease after a stressful encounter with a client? Explain your response.

▲

Symptoms of OCD may be mild to severe. Whatever the degree of impairment, symptoms that interfere with occupational pursuits and quality of life usually lead affected clients to seek assistance. If people do not seek treatment or treatment is unsuccessful, they may become so uncomfortable that they become depressed or even suicidal. See Case Vignette 23.2.

Stress Disorders

Stress disorders consist of acute stress disorder, acute PTSD, chronic PTSD, and delayed PTSD. They are all similar in that they result from exposure to a severe or extraordinary stressor (DSM-IV-TR BOX 23.3). They differ in terms of timing, duration, and degree of impairment. The acknowledgment of stress disorder by the psychiatric community occurred primarily in response to the psychological problems experienced by veterans returning from Vietnam. These people experience various psychiatric symptoms and difficulties directly associated with their traumatic combat experiences. It is now generally accepted that traumatic experiences across the life span can profoundly and permanently change psychiatric health and functioning (Lanius, 2007).

Examples of traumatic events include natural disasters, accidents resulting from human error, and intentional harm. Common natural disasters include earthquakes, floods, hurricanes, tornadoes, and volcanic eruptions. Accidents may include train derailments and crashes, automobile or airplane crashes, or work-related accidents. Intentional human harm may result from murder, military combat, rape, assault, armed robbery, terrorism, muggings, stalking, hazing, and all forms of abuse (see Chap. 33).

ACUTE STRESS DISORDER. **Acute stress disorder (ASD)** occurs within the first month of exposure to extreme trauma: combat, rape, physical assault, near-death experience, or witnessing a murder. Symptoms begin during or shortly after the event. The symptom of *dissociation,* a state of detachment in which people experience the world as dreamlike and unreal, is a primary feature (see Chap. 24). Poor memory of specific events surrounding the trauma also may accompany the dissociative state, a condition referred to as *dissociative amnesia.* Usually, ASD resolves within 2 to 28 days after exposure to the trauma (APA, 2000; U.S. Department of Veterans Affairs, 2010).

POST-TRAUMATIC STRESS DISORDER. When symptoms of ASD continue for more than 1 month and are accompanied by functional impairment or stress, the diagnosis changes to acute **post-traumatic stress disorder (PTSD).** Symptoms include generalized anxiety, intrusive thoughts or images of the trauma, flashbacks, nightmares, and other sleep disturbances. In addition, clients feel a need to avoid situations or stimuli that elicit recollections of the trauma. When symptoms of acute PTSD persist beyond 3 months, the disorder at that point is referred to as *chronic PTSD.* Another variant is *delayed PTSD,* a diagnosis applied when clients develop symptoms of PTSD at least 6 months after exposure to the trauma. Bryant (2011) found, in a systematic review of research, that diagnosed ASD had positive predictive power for eventual development of PTSD. In contrast, the proportion of people who developed PTSD without a prior diagnosis of ASD was high. This suggests that the ASD diagnosis may not predict future development of PTSD.

Because PTSD is a sustained disorder compared with ASD, people with PTSD often experience decreased self-esteem, loss of positive and trusting attitudes toward people and society, a sense of being damaged, and difficulty establishing relationships. In addition, such clients are at increased risk for substance abuse or dependence, especially with alcohol, cannabis, and sedative-hypnotics. Danielson and associates (2009) found a link between substance-abusing adolescents and PTSD resulting from sexual or physical abuse. They noted that PTSD has lifetime implications for substance abuse or dependence and urged that trauma assessment be conducted when dealing with substance issues.

Checkpoint Questions

6. How commonly do people with GAD experience acute anxiety?

7. What term describes a marked fear of being alone or in a public place from which escape would be difficult or help would be unavailable in the event of becoming disabled?

8. What are compulsions?

DSM-IV-TR BOX 23.3

Stress Disorders

Acute Stress Disorder

A. The person has been exposed to a traumatic event in which both of the following were present:
  1. The person experienced, witnessed, or was confronted with an event or events that involved actual or threatened death or serious injury, or a threat to the physical integrity of self or others
  2. The person's response involved intense fear, helplessness, or horror
B. Either while experiencing or after experiencing the distressing event, the individual has three (or more) of the following dissociative symptoms:
  1. A subjective sense of numbing, detachment, or absence of emotional responsiveness
  2. A reduction in awareness of his or her surroundings (eg, "being in a daze")
  3. Serialization
  4. Depersonalization
  5. Dissociative amnesia (ie, inability to recall an important aspect of the trauma)
C. The traumatic event is persistently reexperienced in at least one of the following ways: recurrent images, thoughts, dreams, illusions, flashback episodes, or a sense of reliving the experience; or distress on exposure to reminders of the traumatic event.
D. Marked avoidance of stimuli that arouse recollections of the trauma (eg, thoughts, feelings, conversations, activities, places, people).
E. Marked symptoms of anxiety or increased arousal (eg, difficulty sleeping, irritability, poor concentration, hypervigilance, exaggerated startle response, motor restlessness).
F. The disturbance causes clinically significant distress or impairment in social, occupational, or other important areas of functioning or impairs the individual's ability to pursue some necessary task, such as obtaining necessary assistance or mobilizing personal resources by telling family members about the traumatic experience.
G. The disturbance lasts for a minimum of 2 days and a maximum of 4 weeks and occurs within 4 weeks of the traumatic event.
H. The disturbance is not due to the direct physiologic effects of a substance (eg, a drug of abuse, a medication) or a general medical condition, is not better accounted for by Brief Psychotic Disorder, and is not merely an exacerbation of a preexisting Axis I or Axis II disorder.

Post-Traumatic Stress Disorder

A. The person has been exposed to a traumatic event in which both of the following were present:
  1. The person experienced, witnessed, or was confronted with an event or events that involved actual or threatened death or serious injury, or a threat to the physical integrity of self or others

  2. The person's response involved intense fear, helplessness, or horror. **Note:** In children, this may be expressed instead by disorganized or agitated behavior.
B. The traumatic event is persistently reexperienced in one (or more) of the following ways:
  1. Recurrent and intrusive distressing recollections of the event, including images, thoughts, or perceptions. **Note:** In young children, repetitive play may occur in which themes or aspects of the trauma are expressed.
  2. Recurrent distressing dreams of the event. **Note:** In children, there may be frightening dreams without recognizable content.
  3. Acting or feeling as if the traumatic event were recurring (includes a sense of reliving the experience, illusions, hallucinations, and dissociative flashback episodes, including those that occur on awakening or when intoxicated). **Note:** In young children, trauma-specific reenactment may occur.
  4. Intense psychological distress at exposure to internal or external cues that symbolize or resemble an aspect of the traumatic event
  5. Physiologic reactivity on exposure to internal or external cues that symbolize or resemble an aspect of the traumatic event
C. Persistent avoidance of stimuli associated with the trauma and numbing of general responsiveness (not present before the trauma), as indicated by three (or more) of the following:
  1. Efforts to avoid thoughts, feelings, or conversations associated with the trauma
  2. Efforts to avoid activities, places, or people that arouse recollections of the trauma
  3. Inability to recall an important aspect of the trauma
  4. Markedly diminished interest or participation in significant activities
  5. Feeling of detachment or estrangement from others
  6. Restricted range of affect (eg, unable to have loving feelings)
  7. Sense of a foreshortened future (eg, does not expect to have a career, marriage, children, or a normal life span)
D. Persistent symptoms of increased arousal (not present before the trauma), as indicated by two (or more) of the following:
  1. Difficulty falling or staying asleep
  2. Irritability or outbursts of anger
  3. Difficulty concentrating
  4. Hypervigilance
  5. Exaggerated startle response
E. Duration of the disturbance (symptoms in Criteria B, C, and D) is more than 1 month.
F. The disturbance causes clinically significant distress or impairment in social, occupational, or other important areas of functioning.

Comorbidities and Dual Diagnoses

Anxiety disorders often accompany other serious psychiatric conditions, which can impede accurate diagnosis and treatment of either condition, causing needless suffering and further psychiatric complications, including increased risk for suicidality (Nepon et al., 2010). In particular, anxiety often co-occurs with depression, substance abuse, eating disorders, personality disorders, and schizophrenia. Practitioners should suspect and actively assess clients presenting with an anxiety disorder for other psychiatric conditions, including other types of anxiety disorders. Some clues to look for are as follows:

- High intake of alcohol or use of prescribed or illicit mood-altering drugs
- History of barbiturate or benzodiazepine dependence
- Chronic difficulties in interpersonal relationships or occupation
- History of frequent use of health care services for somatic complaints
- Negative outlook on self, others, and society
- Distorted thinking
- Obsessive or compulsive behavior
- History of an eating disorder

Differential Diagnosis

Because anxiety disorders have multiple differential diagnoses, health care personnel must recognize the importance of conducting diagnostic tests to rule out problems with the central nervous and endocrine systems. A complete blood count (CBC), chemistry profile, thyroid function test, urinalysis, and urine drug screen as part of a complete physical examination are basic tests to rule out other problems that may account for presenting complaints and symptoms of anxiety. Clients with physical abnormalities require more detailed and extensive testing. For example, they may need diagnostic testing to identify unrecognized medical problems, such as acute respiratory distress syndrome, asthma, atrial fibrillation, atrial tachycardia, encephalopathy, thyroid dysfunction, diabetic ketoacidosis, acute or chronic gastritis, or meningitis. See also Box 23.2.

Implications and Prognoses

Concurrence of an anxiety disorder with other psychiatric diagnoses complicates the clinical implications and prognoses. Fava and others (2008) found that people with anxious depression treated with antidepressants had poorer outcomes than did those with nonanxious depression. Chronic stress also may contribute to poorer physical health as a result of immunosuppression, increased blood pressure, and increased corticosteroid release. Even without comorbid psychiatric diagnoses or physical illnesses, the unitary effects of an anxiety disorder can be debilitating, diminishing quality of life and relationships.

BOX 23.2 Differential Diagnoses for Anxiety Disorders

Medical Disorders

Asthma
Cancer
Cardiac dysrhythmias
Chronic obstructive pulmonary disease
Collagen-vascular disease
Congestive heart failure
Coronary insufficiency
Cushing's syndrome
Epilepsy
Hypertension
Hyperthyroidism
Hyperventilation syndrome
Hypoglycemia
Hypothyroidism
Menopause
Mitral valve prolapse
Multiple sclerosis
Organic brain syndrome
Pheochromocytoma
Premenstrual syndrome
Vestibular dysfunction
Wilson's disease

Substances

Anticholinergics
Caffeine
Cannabis
Cocaine
Hallucinogens
Steroids
Sympathomimetics

Think About It 23.1
Review Case Vignette 23.1. Analyze this situation for indicators that would place Marcia at risk for possible complications, and predict possible complications.

Interdisciplinary Goals and Treatment

The first step in identifying treatment strategies for an anxiety disorder is to ascertain whether any physical condition could be precipitating anxiety. Identification and treatment of any physical precipitant may help differentiate medical illness from an anxiety disorder, which underscores the importance of holistic assessment in client care (see Chaps. 10 and 39).

Once a diagnosis of an anxiety disorder is established, the goal is to improve symptoms of anxiety and decrease the chance of recurrence. Treatments for symptoms fall into two categories: pharmacologic and cognitive–behavioral. Individualized plans for clients may include one or both categories, depending on the severity of symptoms, client motivation and preference, recommendations of health care professionals, and costs. Desired outcomes include fewer or no anxious symptoms; resumption or enhancement of productive professional, social, and family roles; replacement of maladaptive coping strategies with adaptive ones; and improved quality of life.

Cognitive–Behavioral Therapy

Cognitive–behavioral therapy (CBT) includes both cognitive and behavioral interventions (Evidence-Based Practice Spotlight 23.1). It is based on the theory that people can recognize the thoughts that produce and maintain anxiety and use various techniques to alter those thoughts. Cognitive interventions include problem-solving strategies, education, and help in identifying irrational thinking. Behavioral interventions rely on reinforcement and exposure to change aberrant behaviors and abnormal responses to anxiety-provoking situations.

Health care providers use various methods of CBT to treat different anxiety disorders. Several CBT approaches treat both general symptoms of anxiety and problems related to specific disorders. See Table 23.1.

⚠ EVIDENCE-BASED PRACTICE SPOTLIGHT 23.1 ⚠

Interventions for Anxiety Disorders

Overview of Effective Treatment: Studies have consistently found that cognitive–behavioral therapy (CBT), also called cognitive therapy, is the most effective behavioral intervention for anxiety disorders. Cognitive therapy is a system of psychotherapy, empirically supported, that is useful for a wide range of psychiatric and medical problems (Beck & Dozois, 2011). The essential principal is that information processing is vital to human adaptation and survival. "The cognitive (or information processing) system is intricately tied to other affective, motivational, and behavioral repertoires" (Beck & Dozois, 2011, p. 398).

Extensive empirical testing of efficacy has illustrated that CBT is an accepted, well-researched, evidence-based modality against anxiety disorders and depression. One of the most used treatments with the highest rate of symptom reduction, CBT assists people across the life span with various anxiety disorders. Butler and colleagues (2006) conducted a meta-analysis that showed that CBT ameliorated symptoms of anxiety, depression, and trauma. CBT is useful for nurses in many types of settings, with many different clients.

What is not effective? Medication can provide short-term relief for anxiety but is not indicated for long-term management of the disorder. It is essential that comorbid conditions be considered when providing treatment. If a client is depressed, this must also be treated; anxiety symptoms might improve with resolution of depression. Trauma-based anxiety requires careful assessment and treatment by a trauma-trained clinician; medication may be useful with this client.

Implications for Practice: Nurses are ideally suited to provide CBT in a variety of settings to clients with anxiety. CBT can be effective in late-life generalized anxiety disorder. Stanley and others (2009) identified primary care as an ideal setting in which to provide this treatment. Many older adults seek care from a primary care setting. In this study, treatment included education and awareness, motivational interviewing, relaxation training, cognitive therapy, exposure, problem-solving skills training, and behavioral sleep management. CBT significantly improved worry severity, depressive symptoms, and general mental health when compared with care as usual.

CBT is useful with older adults with anxiety and depression (Ayers et al., 2007), and adults with chronic nightmares after exposure to trauma (Davis & Wright, 2007). Trauma-focused CBT (TF-CBT) is an evidence-based treatment for traumatized individuals (Lang et al., 2010).

References

Ayers, C. R., Sorrell, J. T., Thorp, S. R., & Wetherell, J. L. (2007). Evidence-based psychological treatment for late-life anxiety. *Psychology and Aging, 22,* 8–17.

Beck, A. T., & Dozois, D. J. A. (2011). Cognitive therapy: Current status and future directions. *Annual Review in Medicine, 62,* 397–409. doi:10.1146/annurev-med-052209-100032

Butler, A. C., Chapman, J. E., Forman, E. M., & Beck, A. T. (2006). The empirical status of cognitive–behavioral therapy: A review of meta-analyses. *Clinical Psychology Review, 26,* 17–31.

Davis, J. L., & Wright, D. C. (2007). Randomized clinical trial for treatment of chronic nightmares in trauma-exposed adults. *Journal of Traumatic Stress, 20,* 123–133.

Lang, J. M., Ford, J. D., & Fitzgerald, M. M. (2010). An algorithm for determining use of trauma-focused cognitive-behavioral therapy. *Psychotherapy (Chic), 47*(4), 554–569.

Stanley, M. A., Wilson, N. L., Novy, D. M., Rhoades, H. M., Wagener, P. D., Greisinger, A. J., & Kunik, M. E. (2009). Cognitive behavior therapy for generalized anxiety disorder among older adults in primary care. *Journal of the American Medical Association, 301*(14), 1460–1467. doi:10.1001/jama.2009.458

TABLE 23.1 Selected Cognitive–Behavioral Treatment Strategies for Clients With Anxiety Disorders

Disorder	Cognitive–Behavioral Treatment
Panic attacks	Use cognitive restructuring to reframe catastrophic thinking. Desensitize client to feared situations. Educate about the disorder. Teach breathing techniques.
Generalized anxiety disorder	Teach relaxation techniques, stress management, and biofeedback. Use cognitive interventions to reframe catastrophic thinking. Assist the client with problem solving.
Obsessive-compulsive disorder	Desensitize client to feared situations. Educate about the disorder. Teach relaxation techniques.
Acute stress disorder	Assist the client to find a support group. Engage in therapeutic dialogues with the client. Teach problem solving. Teach relaxation techniques.
Specific phobias	Desensitize client to feared situations.
Social phobia	Challenge negative beliefs. Teach realistic appraisal of social situations.
Post-traumatic stress disorder	Encourage client to attend group therapy.

BASIC COGNITIVE THERAPY FOR ANXIETY. The goal of basic cognitive therapy is to gain insight into situations that provoke anxiety and then to learn new responses to those situations. It includes education and problem-solving strategies but primarily focuses on learning to identify and change faulty thinking that can lead to emotional distress. Treatment may last 12 to 20 weeks.

Initially, practitioners may ask clients to keep a diary of anxious feelings and any accompanying thoughts or events (Figure 23.5). In this way, clients can begin to recognize patterns in their anxious responses, which will increase awareness of anxious thoughts as they occur. Practitioners may then challenge these deep-rooted and habitual reactions to help clients gain insight. Clients receive homework so that they have a concrete plan for developing new behaviors. The following week, clients share with a group or therapist how effective the new approaches have been. As implementation continues, clients, through self-observation and coaching, gain insight into the faulty assumptions that trigger anxiety and begin substituting new ways of managing stressful situations.

Some common cognitive strategies include the following:

- Covert rehearsal: Practitioners help clients imagine themselves successfully confronting an anxiety-provoking situation.
- Positive coping statements: Clients make positive self-statements to prevent anxiety from escalating when facing

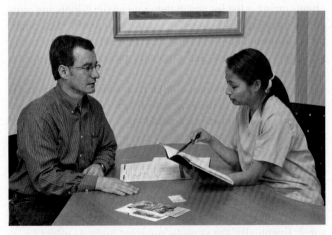

FIGURE 23.5 This client with OCD is keeping a diary to monitor his patterns of ritualistic behavior and to better understand triggers of and responses to anxiety.

emotionally difficult situations. For example, clients face a stressor and tell themselves, "I can handle this. I've done it before."

- Cognitive reframing: Practitioners help clients change their interpretation of anxiety-provoking situations from catastrophic to realistic. For example, a client states, "I will not lose everything if I do not do well on my evaluation. If my boss has criticisms, I will work with management on a plan to address those weak points."

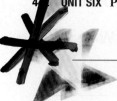

Client-Centered Education 23.1

Progressive Relaxation

Practicing relaxation techniques will help reduce muscle tension, anxiety, fears, and worry. Clients can and should use them when feeling anxious, but they should also use them regularly to help prevent anxiety. Teach the client and the family the following steps:

1. Sit in a comfortable chair or lie down in a quiet place away from phones or distractions.
2. Clear your mind by focusing on your breathing. Do not try to influence your breathing; just notice how the breath feels as it flows in and out. You can focus on your chest moving up and down or on the way the air feels as it moves in and out of your nose.
3. As thoughts come up, do not respond to them; rather imagine them just floating away and return to focusing on your breath.

Picture a calm, peaceful place to help stop the interruption of thoughts or worries or imagine a perfectly still lake or ocean.
4. Take several controlled breaths (breathe in through the nose for 3 seconds, hold the breath for 1 second, breathe out through the mouth for 3 seconds).
5. Beginning with your hands, tense each area of your body for 8 to 10 seconds (count slowly to yourself) and then release the tension and relax for 8 to 10 seconds. Proceed up your arms to your shoulders, neck, forehead, eyes, and jaws. Then proceed to the stomach, buttocks, thighs, calves, feet, and toes.
6. After all areas have been tensed and relaxed, focus again on your breathing for a few minutes. Sit quietly for a minute or two before opening your eyes.

SYSTEMATIC DESENSITIZATION AND EXPOSURE TREATMENT. *Systematic desensitization* is a classical conditioning technique by which clients learn to replace gradually a panic response with a relaxation response. It is a behavior therapy for specific phobias, social phobias, agoraphobia, and PTSD. Clients progressively confront an object of fear in very small, controlled steps while in a deeply relaxed state. In another type of systematic desensitization, clients create a list by which they rate anxiety-inducing situations by degree of fear, using a scale of 0 to 10. They begin by confronting situations that they rate as 1 or 2, practicing relaxation techniques and gradually progressing to higher-rated situations.

Exposure treatment is similar to desensitization in that it involves exposure to the feared object or situation, but it does not involve relaxation or a gradual approach to the source of anxiety. It does allow clients to have some control over how long they are exposed to the fear-causing object, if desired, and is therefore known as either *flooding* or *graduated exposure*. In flooding, clients are exposed to the anxiety-producing stimulus for as long as 1 to 2 hours; graduated exposure allows clients to control the length and frequency of exposures. Eventually, the stimulating event loses its effect.

RELAXATION TECHNIQUES AND BREATHING RETRAINING. One recurrent, effective component of any cognitive–behavioral strategy for reducing anxiety is teaching clients how to reduce the physical effects of anxiety through controlled breathing and relaxation exercises. For example, hyperventilation is one of the prime features of panic attacks and, in itself, results in uncomfortable physical feelings that panic-stricken people may interpret as life threatening. People who hyperventilate may experience chest pain, dizziness, tingling of the mouth and fingers, muscle cramps, and fainting. By practicing controlled breathing techniques in the early stages of a panic attack, clients may

be able to minimize the attack. Specific steps to follow for breath control are described in the Applying the Nursing Process section of this chapter.

Relaxation methods are extremely helpful in managing anxiety and stress. The *relaxation response,* a term coined by mind–body medicine pioneer Herbert Benson, is a physical state of deep rest that counters the fight-or-flight response (ie, it results in a feeling of peacefulness and decreased heart rate, blood pressure, and muscle tension). To gain the full benefit of the relaxation response, clients should practice relaxation techniques daily. See Client-Centered Education 23.1 for tips.

Psychopharmacology

Many medications to treat anxiety disorders are available, although medication is not necessarily recommended for every anxiety disorder and should not be considered the sole treatment. Each client's specific circumstances will suggest whether medication is indicated. Prior to initiating medication therapy, providers should thoroughly assess clients for attitudes about medication management, biases, values, cultural belief systems, and willingness to adhere to a prescribed regimen. All clients should have a thorough physical examination prior to beginning medication treatment to rule out medical causes for anxiety.

Drug classes commonly used for anxiety disorders include selective serotonin reuptake inhibitors (SSRIs), benzodiazepines (BZDs), buspirone, beta blockers, and tricyclic antidepressants (TCAs). See Chapter 16 for general information; the discussions below review details pertinent for drug therapy within the context of management of anxiety disorders.

SELECTIVE SEROTONIN REUPTAKE INHIBITORS. SSRIs and serotonin-norepinephrine reuptake inhibitors (SNRIs) have been established as effective in the management of anxiety disorders and are now considered first-line alternatives. Doses for anxiety are similar to those for depression. To prevent side effects, clinicians initially should prescribe smaller loading doses followed by gradual increases. Commonly used SSRIs include fluoxetine (Prozac), sertraline (Zoloft), paroxetine (Paxil), escitalopram (Lexapro), citalopram (Celexa), and fluvoxamine (Luvox). SNRIs include venlafaxine (Effexor), duloxetine (Cymbalta), and desvenlafaxine (Pristiq). Some are available in extended-release form and are designated with the letters CR or XR.

Unlike the TCAs, SSRIs and SNRIs are relatively free of anticholinergic, orthostatic, and sedative effects. Common side effects include sexual dysfunction, nervousness, nausea, insomnia, and anxiety. Like the TCAs, these medications should not be given with other antidepressants or other serotonergic agents to avoid the risk of life-threatening serotonin syndrome. This toxic hyperserotonergic state is characterized by restlessness, confusion, agitation, hyperreflexia, diaphoresis, shivering, tremors, muscle rigidity, hyperthermia, and autonomic instability. It typically develops within hours or days of the addition of a new medication or an increase in dosage. Herbal products and food supplements also may contribute to this syndrome. Thus, health care providers must question clients carefully about what natural products they use and advise clients about over-the-counter products that influence serotonin metabolism. Herbals can include St. John's wort, melatonin, ginkgo, flaxseed, and echinacea.

Given that SSRIs may require as long as 4 to 6 weeks to reach their maximum therapeutic effects, a benzodiazepine may be used in the initial phase of treatment to control anxiety.

BENZODIAZEPINES. BZDs have long been the drugs of choice for treatment of anxiety disorders, although they have not been shown to have more long-term effectiveness than antidepressants. Their advantages include rapid onset and high tolerability. Disadvantages are the risk of physical dependence and high potential for abuse. Abrupt discontinuation can trigger severe withdrawal symptoms and intense rebound anxiety. These medications potentiate the effects of alcohol and other sedative-hypnotics, are commonly abused, and have several significant side effects. The most common are sedation, ataxia, impaired coordination, slurred speech, memory impairment, paradoxical agitation, and dizziness.

They also cause psychomotor impairment; clients should not drive or operate machinery while taking them. Also, the cognitive disturbances induced by BZD therapy, especially in the early phase of treatment, can delay clients' positive engagement and response to CBT (Helms & Quan, 2007).

BZDs always require caution but are indicated for certain clients, such as those with panic disorder, those who have not experienced response to other medications or therapies, or those who need to reduce anxiety while waiting for other medications, such as antidepressants, to have a therapeutic effect. They also can be useful to decrease early anxiety associated with initiation of antidepressants and to treat residual anxiety of antidepressant treatment. See Understanding Psychopharmacology Box 23.1. Commonly prescribed BZDs include alprazolam (Xanax and Xanax CR), diazepam (Valium), lorazepam (Ativan), clorazepate (Tranxene), and oxazepam (Serax).

BUSPIRONE. Buspirone (BuSpar) is approved for the treatment and management of anxiety. Unlike the BZDs, buspirone lacks anticonvulsant, muscle relaxant, and hypnotic properties. It has been shown effective for generalized anxiety disorder. The most common side effects include nausea, dizziness, headache, insomnia, agitation, drowsiness, and dysphoria. Buspirone does not produce tolerance and is not addictive. Unlike the BZDs, buspirone requires 1 to 2 weeks before it produces antianxiety effects, and maximal effects may not appear until 6 weeks of therapy. Often, BZDs are given during the first few weeks of treatment with buspirone to control anxiety; they are then gradually reduced and discontinued.

BETA BLOCKERS. Propranolol is considered less effective in treating anxiety disorders than other medications because it affects only the physical ramifications of anxiety. However, in clients with prominent cardiovascular symptoms of anxiety, this drug may be the most effective. Like the BZDs, beta blockers should not be discontinued abruptly but should be reduced gradually to avoid rebound anxiety symptoms. In addition, beta blockers can cause side effects in the central nervous system, such as depression and nightmares. Common side effects such as bradycardia and hypotension necessitate careful monitoring of vital signs.

UNDERSTANDING PSYCHOPHARMACOLOGY BOX 23.1

Guidelines for Use of Benzodiazepines

- Use the lowest dose necessary to obtain symptom relief.
- Monitor sedative effects and the client's risk for injury.
- Use for short periods.
- Use cautiously in clients with a history of substance abuse.
- Use cautiously in clients with family members who have a history of substance abuse.
- Do not discontinue abruptly.

TRICYCLIC ANTIDEPRESSANTS. Clinical evidence shows that TCAs are effective against generalized anxiety disorder in clients without comorbid major depression. TCAs also have been shown to be highly effective for PTSD. Commonly used TCAs include imipramine (Tofranil), clomipramine (Anafranil), amitriptyline (Elavil), desipramine (Norpramin), and nortriptyline (Pamelor). These medications are relatively easy to dose and often can be conveniently administered once daily at bedtime to take advantage of the sedative effect. Common side effects include sedation, orthostatic hypotension, and anticholinergic effects. Concurrent use of these drugs with other medications such as monoamine oxidase inhibitors (MAOIs) and SSRIs is contraindicated. TCAs are contraindicated in clients with cardiac disorders.

Checkpoint Questions

9. Which type of cognitive strategy involves helping clients to imagine themselves successfully confronting an anxiety-provoking situation?
10. How does exposure treatment differ from desensitization?
11. Why would a BZD be given initially to a client receiving an SSRI for anxiety?
12. Which drug may be most effective for clients with prominent cardiovascular symptoms of anxiety?

APPLYING THE NURSING PROCESS

Clients With Anxiety Disorders

All nurses are likely to encounter many clients experiencing anxiety. Not all anxious clients have an anxiety disorder. The goals of nursing care are to identify clients with anxiety, identify its etiology, plan interventions, and assist with their implementation. These goals are true whether anxiety is a component of a client's long-term psychiatric illness or a transient response to a stressor.

▲ ASSESSMENT

Because anxiety and anxiety disorders are so prevalent in the general population, nurses carefully assess all clients for signs and symptoms of anxiety. Although several formal assessment tools exist (eg, State-Trait Anxiety Inventory, the Hamilton Anxiety Rating Scale, the Beck Anxiety Inventory), nurses begin by simply asking clients if they are currently feeling anxious or worried or have experienced such feelings recently. The client's response focuses the depth of the remaining assessment. For clients who answer positively, nurses assess them through observation and interview for psychological, physiologic, and cognitive indicators of anxiety.

An anxiety disorder is likely when clients report that they are experiencing persistent anxiety that they cannot dismiss,

that is interfering with activities of daily living, or both. Nurses also might observe signs and symptoms of anxiety during the interview or while providing other care. They must remember that many physical disorders and reactions to medications could potentially result in signs and symptoms that mimic or induce anxiety. The health care team must rule out such problems before establishing a diagnosis of an anxiety disorder. Some of the more common signs and symptoms to assess for include those reviewed in Assessment Tool 23.1.

Nurses also ask clients about obsessive thinking patterns, worrying, compulsions, repetitive activities, specific phobias, and exposure to traumatic events. Traumatic events could include indirect exposure to community or domestic violence, natural disasters (eg, floods, hurricanes), or automobile accidents. If clients answer positively to any of these questions, nurses follow up with additional questions aimed at eliciting specific details about the behavior or response to the feared object or trauma. Once nurses have established the presence of signs and symptoms of anxiety, they assess the possible underlying causes and inquire about family history, recent life events, current stress level, personal history of anxiety, medical and medication history, history of substance abuse, and other possible causes of the anxiety.

▲ NURSING DIAGNOSIS

Many nursing diagnoses may apply to clients with anxiety disorders, depending on their specific disorder and symptoms. Major diagnoses that can be applied to most clients with different anxiety disorders are as follows (NANDA, 2007):

- **Anxiety** related to perceived threat or stress
- **Ineffective Coping** related to inadequate individual resources
- **Ineffective Breathing Pattern** related to hyperventilation related to severe anxiety

▲ OUTCOME IDENTIFICATION AND PLANNING

Despite the differences among clients with anxiety or panic disorders, several common goals for nursing care apply. Some identified desired outcomes, organized according to the Nursing Outcomes Classification (NOC), might include the following (Moorhead et al., 2008):

- **Aggression Control:** The client will report a decreased intensity of anxiety.
- **Coping:** The client will use effective coping strategies to deal with symptoms of anxiety.
- **Anxiety Control:** The client will use breathing techniques to control anxiety and hyperventilation.

▲ IMPLEMENTATION

To help clients accomplish the established goals, nurses must first establish a supportive therapeutic relationship, which is characterized by trust, empathy, respect, and calmness on the nurse's part (see Chap. 11). Displaying these behaviors consistently lays the groundwork for a successful therapeutic

▲ ASSESSMENT TOOL 23.1 ▲

Common Findings Associated With Anxiety Disorders

Cognitive

- Fear of dying, going "crazy," or another unspecified fear
- Diminished problem-solving capability
- Preoccupation with worrisome thoughts
- Decreased ability to concentrate

Affective

- Irritable, worried, tense, or fearful affect
- Feelings of helplessness or inadequacy
- Overly excited, wary, or anguished affect

Physiologic

- Palpitations, chest pain, or tachycardia
- Hyperventilation or shortness of breath
- Dizziness, headache, paresthesia, or shakiness
- Choking sensation, dry mouth, nausea, vomiting, or diarrhea
- Muscle aches and tension, restlessness

Behavioral

- Pacing or fidgeting
- Appearance of overvigilance
- Restlessness

---

relationship and enhances the effectiveness of interventions. Common strategies for clients with anxiety disorders, organized by the Nursing Interventions Classification (NIC), include but are not limited to **Anticipatory Guidance, Anxiety Reduction, Behavior Modification: Social Skills, Calming Technique, Cognitive Restructuring, Complex Relationship Building, Coping Enhancement, Decision–Making Support, Emotional Support, Impulse Control Training, Security Enhancement, Self–Awareness Enhancement, Simple Guided Imagery,** and **Simple Relaxation Therapy** (Bulechek et al., 2008).

Case in Point 23.1 reviews the steps of the nursing process applied to a client dealing with PTSD.

Alleviating Anxiety

Successful management of an anxiety disorder involves helping clients identify thoughts and behaviors as anxiety induced and finding effective coping strategies. Some steps can be taken immediately, regardless of whether nurses care for clients at home, in a clinic, or in an acute care setting.

Initiating a Therapeutic Dialogue

Simply listening and gently counseling anxious clients can be beneficial. Nurses must start the process of therapeutic dialogue by asking what clients would find helpful. This information, followed by the use of therapeutic questioning techniques that elicit responses and reflective listening, can help clients feel valued, understood, and supported. Nurses avoid comments that block communication, such as statements that minimize or challenge a client's feelings (eg, "Things could be worse" or "Why do you think you'll die if you go outside?"). Likewise, false, nonchalant reassurances ("Don't worry, you're fine") or superficial pep talks ("You can get a grip on yourself") undermine trust. Clients dealing with anxiety do not feel "fine" at the moment, nor can they will themselves to "get a grip." Instead, nurses can help anxious clients by making factual observations and offering concrete interventions ("You're hyperventilating, which is causing you to feel worse physically. Let me coach you into breathing more slowly and deeply."), by providing realistic reassurance, by listening, and by just being present with the client

until uncomfortable, panicky feelings subside. See Therapeutic Communication 23.1.

Nurses provide a quiet environment, display calmness, listen carefully, make clear, simple statements, repeat statements calmly and quietly as often as necessary, help clients identify events leading up to the anxiety attack, and assist clients to identify and use past successful coping techniques.

Countering Faulty Thinking

Nurses also can help clients by providing facts that can counter anxiety-provoking misconceptions that often underpin anxiety and panic attacks. Clients can then learn to substitute objective appraisals of circumstances for unrealistically threatening appraisals. The ability to restructure anxiety-producing events as less threatening enables clients to gain control and make situations more predictable. For example, clients experiencing anxiety attacks may interpret physical feelings as serious symptoms of an impending health problem (ie, heart attack or stroke). Nurses can inform clients about the very common physical feelings associated with anxiety and teach clients objectively to assess symptoms when they occur again. Clients can then say, "This is how I feel when I have an anxiety attack. This is not a heart attack. These feelings will subside soon, as they have when I have had them before."

Managing Hyperventilation

Hyperventilation is a sign of anxiety as well as a symptom that can trigger panic. To decrease hyperventilation, it is necessary to increase the carbon dioxide level in the blood. Breathing into a paper bag is effective but not always practical or acceptable in certain (social, professional) situations. Also, it does not prevent a panic attack. Slow or controlled breathing exercises treat and help prevent panic attacks by correcting habitual faulty breathing patterns.

Nurses first help clients identify their own patterns of hyperventilating. They can teach clients to self-monitor respiratory rate and to begin breathing exercises if the rate is more than 12

(continues on page 446)

Case in Point 23.1

Ruth's Story

Ruth, 42 years old, is married with three children. Six months ago, she was in a fast-food restaurant when a man entered and began shooting with an automatic rifle. Several people were killed before the gunman turned his weapon on himself and died.

Ruth was doing "OK" until recently. She describes her current anxiety level as "very high" most days and states that life no longer seems real to her. She has nightmares about the incident and wakens from them sweating and with her heart pounding. When she drives by fast-food restaurants, something she avoids at all costs, she feels panicky and confused. Sometimes, she imagines that she hears screaming. She states she has had headaches, fatigue, and irritability.

The nurse at the mental health clinic asks about other findings associated with PTSD. Ruth admits that she feels tremendous guilt and wonders why she wasn't killed when others were. She relates that she has lost interest in most things, except her children, whom she now watches "like a hawk." Ruth states: "I don't let them go out with friends anymore because I'm afraid of what will happen to them." Ruth denies using any drugs but says she has begun drinking wine each night to help her sleep. She says she feels powerless to help herself. She states her husband has been impatient with her to "get over it" and to be thankful she was spared.

Key Assessment Findings

- Exposure to a traumatic event
- Intense fear experienced during event
- Reexperience and disturbing dreams of event
- Physiologic distress: diaphoresis, heart pounding
- Avoidance of fast-food restaurants; experience of panic and confusion when near one
- Headaches, fatigue, and irritability
- Reports of high anxiety level and feelings of detachment
- Feelings of guilt, extreme fear for children
- Sleep disturbances, including use of alcohol
- Distress in the home

Nursing Dx: Post–Trauma Syndrome related to being a victim of violent crime as evidenced by reexperiencing the trauma, psychic numbing, and hypervigilance

NOC: Coping and **Fear Control:** The client will recover from the intense emotional trauma and her symptoms will resolve.

NIC: Coping Enhancement

- Encourage the client to discuss her feelings of guilt. To help her adopt a more realistic appraisal, help her to identify evidence for and against her feelings. Assist her to develop an objective appraisal of the event. Discuss the consequences of not dealing with guilt. *The client's emotional response is understandable but ultimately irrational and self-defeating. Rational examination of her feelings can help her to restructure faulty thought patterns.*

- Discuss the event with the client. Listen to her verbalizations of feelings, perceptions, and fears. Provide an accepting, calm, and reassuring atmosphere (Figure A). *Avoidance behaviors are attempts to reduce stress. Fear levels will remain high, however, until the client confronts the fear often enough for it to dissipate. Discussing the event is a form of exposure therapy.*

- Encourage and assist the client gradually to expose herself to the environment in which the event occurred. *Avoiding driving by fast-food restaurants is impractical and an ineffective response to stress. Gradual, controlled exposure eventually will desensitize her to that trigger.*

NIC: Counseling

- Provide facts as necessary and appropriate; assist the client to identify the problem causing distress. Point out discrepancies between her feelings and behaviors. *Facts are necessary to help dispel irrational and self-defeating responses.*

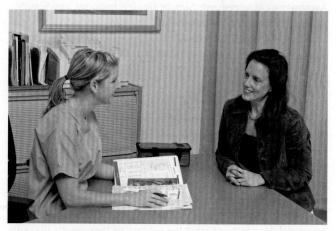

FIGURE A. A calm atmosphere that allows the client to emote is necessary.

3/2/13: The client is confronting emotional triggers that remind her of the event. She is learning and using behaviors to reduce stress. She also reports fewer physical symptoms and negative feelings, as well as more psychological comfort and interest in her everyday life and routines.

G. Bailey, RN, MSN

- Assist the client to identify strengths; encourage new skill development; reinforce new skills. *Development of new strategies enhances her ability to deal with stress; drawing on strengths promotes feelings of control.*

Case in Point 23.1 (continued)

Ruth's Story

Nursing Dx: Anxiety related to post-traumatic stress response as evidenced by poor sleep, irritability, and cognitive impairment

NOC: Anxiety Control: The client will verbalize a decreased anxiety level and improved mood, sleep, and thinking abilities.

NIC: Anxiety Reduction
- Help the client identify situations that precipitate anxiety and when her anxiety level changes. *Knowledge of anxiety-producing situations and indicators of increasing anxiety can assist her to exert control over the feelings.*
- Support the use of appropriate defense mechanisms. *They can assist in reducing anxiety.*
- Assist the client to appraise situations objectively. *Objective appraisals enable the client to gain control over and make the situation more predictable.*

NIC: Anticipatory Guidance
- Determine the client's usual methods of problem solving. Help her identify maladaptive strategies; provide suggestions for replacing them with appropriate ones. Encourage the client to refrain from using alcohol and to engage in regular exercise. *These interventions help the client determine the most beneficial strategies and substitute them for those that are maladaptive. Lifestyle changes can help make the client more resilient to stress.*
- Rehearse with the client various strategies to cope with anxiety. *Rehearsing enhances the chances for success when the client uses these techniques.*
- Refer the client to appropriate community agencies. Suggest that she consider joining a support group (Figure B). *Community agencies and support groups are tremendous resources for people who feel alone with their disorder.*

NIC: Simple Relaxation Therapy
- Teach controlled breathing methods. Describe relaxation interventions. Individualize content according to the client's preferences and demonstrate appealing techniques. *Controlled breathing and relaxation techniques decrease the sympathetic arousal that accompanies high anxiety. They also help to improve sleep.*
- Assist the client to identify situations when use of relaxation techniques would help. *Appropriate use of techniques enhances the chances for a successful outcome.*
- Encourage frequent repetition and practice of techniques. *Practice increases the chances that the client will use the technique correctly when needed.*

NIC: Therapy Group
- Encourage self-disclosure and discussion of the past only as related to the function and goals of the group. Encourage the

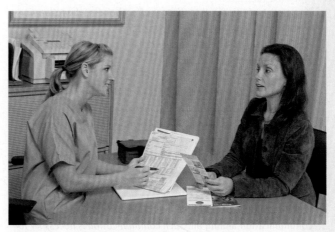

FIGURE B. The nurse gives the client referral information for a support group for people with PTSD.

client to share with the group such commonalities as anger, sadness, humor, mistrust, and other feelings. *Self-disclosure and discussion in conjunction with sharing promotes group cohesiveness and effectiveness.*
- Provide social reinforcement, structured group exercises, role playing, and problem solving as appropriate. *Specific therapeutic activities within a group promote group function and help clients gain insight into their behaviors and responses.*

> 4/5/13: The client regularly uses relaxation exercises. She reports improvements in her concentration, physical manifestations of anxiety, and sense of well-being. She has attended two group therapy sessions, which she describes as "helpful" to normalizing her responses and assisting her to work through them.
>
> J Bailey, RN, MSN

Nursing Dx: Compromised Family Coping related to temporary family disorganization as evidenced by husband's comments about "getting over it" and client's statement about watching her children "like a hawk"

NOC: Family Coping and Family Normalization: Family will provide more emotional support to the client.

NIC: Family Involvement Promotion
- Identify family expectations for the client, family structure, and family roles. Meet with the family to educate them about PTSD.

(continues on page 448)

Case in Point 23.1 (continued)

Ruth's Story

Knowledge of this family enhances effectiveness when planning specific interventions. Increasing the family's understanding of PTSD will help them view the client's behavior differently, thereby fostering support for the client.

- Listen to the family's concerns; accept coping styles without judgment. *Hearing family members without judgment promotes a feeling of being understood and valued as well.*
- Engage husband and family in treatment plan. Teach them how to listen reflectively (Figure C). *Partnering with family members and encouraging family decision making increases the likelihood of successful treatment.*

NIC: Family Support

- Listen to family concerns, feelings, and questions; facilitate communication among all. *Such communication is necessary to facilitate trust and promote a positive outcome.*
- Respect and support adaptive coping mechanisms; provide feedback regarding the family's coping. *Supporting adaptive coping and providing feedback promote the use of the most effective methods for the situation.*
- Refer to family therapy as appropriate.

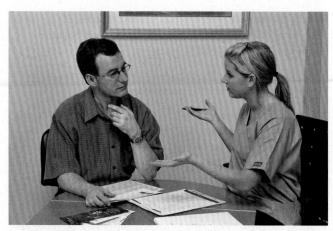

FIGURE C. The client's husband is learning to listen reflectively to better understand his wife's experience with anxiety.

5/14/13: The client reports more consistent demonstrations of support from her family. She also reports less anxiety and worry over the safety and well-being of her husband and children.

G. Bailey, RN, MSN

EPILOGUE

It has been 4 months since Ruth came to the mental health clinic. She is exercising three times a week and has stopped drinking alcohol before bedtime. She reports that although she still occasionally has upsetting dreams, their frequency has decreased. When she does have nightmares, she uses deep breathing and relaxation techniques that she has learned. Her family has participated in support groups. She says, "I can drive by a fast-food restaurant now. I still get a little nervous, but breathing helps. And I still worry when my children go out, but I realize that it is impossible to watch them all the time." Ruth also says her husband has been kind, concerned, and supportive.

to 16 breaths per minute (average at-rest respiratory rate is 10 to 12 breaths per minute). Nurses then demonstrate and teach clients how to perform a slow breathing exercise (Figure 23.6). Although such exercises vary, a common approach to use is to:

1. Hold the breath and count to 5.
2. On 5, breathe out, slowly and calmly saying the word "relax."
3. Then breathe in for 3 seconds and out for 3 seconds, saying the word "relax" with each exhalation.
4. After 1 minute, hold the breath for 5 seconds again and then continue breathing using the 6-second cycle (3-second inhalation, 3-second exhalation).
5. Continue until hyperventilation is under control and all symptoms have subsided.

Sometimes clients report increased anxiety when they first start to use the breathing exercise. Nurses inform clients that this occasionally happens but to continue with the breathing

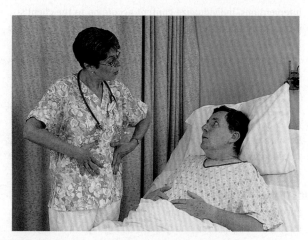

FIGURE 23.6 This nurse is teaching an anxious hospitalized client how to perform a slow breathing exercise.

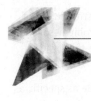

Therapeutic Communication 23.1

The Client With Generalized Anxiety Disorder

In working with Marcia, the client discussed in Case Vignette 23.1, the nurse tries to discuss the job-related anxiety she is experiencing.

INEFFECTIVE DIALOGUE

CLIENT: What will I do if I lose my job?

NURSE: Why do you think that you will lose your job?

CLIENT: I just feel that I might.

NURSE: Well, you seem to be worrying over nothing. I'm sure you're doing fine.

CLIENT: I still feel like I'm going to explode under the pressure.

NURSE: Well, maybe you should look for an easier job or not work at all.

CLIENT: *(Looks defeated and about to cry.)*

EFFECTIVE DIALOGUE

CLIENT: What will I do if I lose my job?

NURSE: What has happened to make you think that you will lose your job?

CLIENT: I just feel that I might.

NURSE: Has anything in particular happened that is worrying you?

CLIENT: I don't know. I guess not.

NURSE: What does your boss say about your work performance?

CLIENT: She says I do a good job as a buyer. I got a raise about 6 months ago.

NURSE: Then what is there for you to worry about?

CLIENT: I don't know. I've always been a worrier.

NURSE: What's different now?

CLIENT: I guess it's the promotion, more responsibility, maybe believing that I can't take the pressure.

Reflection and Critical Thinking

- Compare the approaches the nurse used in both dialogues. What techniques did the nurse in the Effective Dialogue use to improve communication with the client?
- What assumptions did the nurse in the Ineffective Dialogue make that served to shut down communication with the client?
- How would you recommend that the nurse in the second scenario proceed to continue the dialogue?
- How can nurses remember what it is like to be on the receiving end of health care when working with clients?

exercises and the anxiety will eventually subside. They tell clients to practice the exercise four times a day and whenever they notice sensations of anxiety.

Suggesting Lifestyle Changes

Nurses can suggest lifestyle changes that help reduce stress. Such changes can minimize the severity and frequency of anxiety or panic attacks and other anxiety symptoms and may help reduce the risk for anxiety disorders. Some changes to suggest include the following:

- Maintain a regular aerobic exercise program.
- Eat a well-balanced diet.
- Establish good sleep habits.
- Eliminate or minimize alcohol or recreational drug use.
- Reduce sources of stress (eg, cut back on commitments).
- Eliminate caffeine and nicotine.

Teaching Adaptive Coping Strategies

Clients learn to reduce their anxiety in either functional or dysfunctional ways. Functional responses lead to healthier, more productive lives. They tend to be voluntary, conscious behaviors that address and acknowledge the stressful situation and help clients to find solutions. Dysfunctional responses tend to be involuntary, inflexible, avoidance-type solutions that impair productivity.

Nurses first explore with clients techniques they have used in the past, and then help clients identify and enhance those strategies that are most beneficial. Together, they identify maladaptive coping strategies such as social withdrawal or alcohol use and replace them with adaptive strategies that suit personal, cultural, and spiritual values. This process can be difficult

(continues on page 450)

because clients may be afraid or unwilling to abandon "successful" coping strategies, as in the case of those with addictions to drugs or alcohol.

Nurses should not ask clients to give up coping mechanisms, even maladaptive ones, without offering other replacement alternatives. In other words, it is not appropriate to expect clients to just stop worrying, compulsively checking doors, or otherwise trying to cope with anxiety. Nurses should be prepared to suggest and teach new coping strategies and to support currently used adaptive defense mechanisms. Two possible strategies that are easy to teach are relaxation exercises and problem-solving strategies. Although these strategies are easily taught and learned, clients must practice them regularly to gain the full benefits.

Teaching Relaxation

Many people find relaxation techniques to be effective coping tools for managing anxiety. Regularly inducing the relaxation response reduces the general level of autonomic arousal in anxious clients. It lowers blood pressure, heart rate, metabolic rate, and oxygen demands. This physiologic effect may result from effects on the production of cortisol, a hormone the body releases in response to stress. Cortisol is helpful during the fight-or-flight response, but its prolonged release in chronically anxious or stressed clients can inhibit the immune system and have other deleterious physical effects.

Many methods can elicit the relaxation response, including meditation, yoga, progressive muscle relaxation, visualization, and hypnosis. Nurses discuss with clients the method that is most culturally acceptable to them and then teach that technique or refer clients to appropriate professionals or resources. See Client-Centered Education 23.1, which describes a common technique for inducing relaxation through progressive muscle relaxation.

Visualization is another technique some people use to manage stress and anxiety. Those who practice visualization begin with some relaxation techniques such as focused breathing or progressive muscle relaxation. Clients may then be guided, by a health care practitioner, audiotape, or independent means, to visualize a peaceful, calming environment in which they work through a stressful situation. Often clients are encouraged to include a mentor, spiritual presence, or loved one in the image as a source of wisdom and guidance. Whatever method clients choose to relax and reduce stress, nurses encourage them to practice it daily to receive the most benefit.

Teaching Problem-Solving Skills

Helping clients develop a method for problem solving is another intervention for teaching adaptive coping strategies. Instead of avoiding, worrying endlessly, or making a catastrophe out of anxiety-producing situations, clients can use a problem-solving technique for making decisions. Nurses can teach the basic steps of problem solving:

1. Answer the question: "*What is the problem?*" Be as specific as possible. Determine a goal.
2. *List all possible solutions,* including those you think may not work. Come up with as many as possible. Even though a solution may at first seem ridiculous, the idea may help to generate better solutions than those that are more obvious.
3. Briefly *discuss the advantages and disadvantages of each solution.* No solution is ideal, given that every good idea has some faults and most bad ideas also have some merit.
4. *Choose the solution or combination of solutions that will solve the problem or achieve the goal.* It may be best to choose a solution that clients can implement quickly and easily, even though it may not be "ideal." Getting started quickly and avoiding a solution that is too difficult to implement (even though "ideal") will make a difference in the problem.
5. *Plan how to implement the solution.* A detailed practical plan of action is critical to the successful resolution of the problem.
6. *Review the results.* The effectiveness of the solution is determined during the review process. If the problem was not solved, point out to clients that difficulties usually result from inadequate planning, not personal failure. Identify any attempt as a partial success, consider it a learning experience, and encourage clients to try again.

▲ EVALUATION

Nurses base evaluation of the effectiveness of their care on client reports about their feelings and observed behavior changes. Fewer cardinal symptoms associated with anxiety disorders also signify improvement, as does increased self-awareness and the ability to cope effectively with anxiety-provoking situations. Outcomes that indicate improvement include the following:

• The client identifies and uses adaptive coping strategies that are congruent with personal values.
• The client demonstrates one or more relaxation techniques.
• The client reports decreased incidence or intensity of anxiety or panic attacks.
• The client uses deep-breathing exercises to prevent and manage anxiety and panic attacks.
• The client uses problem-solving techniques to help manage difficult situations.

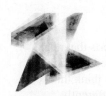

Reviewing and Applying Your Knowledge

Chapter Summary

• Anxiety can be a normal response to a threatening situation.

• Levels of anxiety include mild, moderate, severe, and panic. Anxious people may report feelings of dread, apprehension, restlessness, and jitteriness. Physiologic signs of anxiety may include increased heart rate, blood pressure, depth and rate of respirations, and perspiration.

• Anxiety disorders occur when a state of anxiety is exaggerated or prolonged without any threat, or when anxiety impairs functioning. These most common of all psychiatric syndromes affect children, adolescents, adults, and older adults. They are often misdiagnosed and undertreated, compounding the problems they cause. They occur more frequently in females than in males.

• Anxiety disorders frequently co-occur with depression.

• Common phobic disorders include agoraphobia, specific phobia, and social phobia.

• A panic disorder is characterized by recurrent, unpredictable panic attacks.

• Generalized anxiety disorder is characterized by chronic anxiety that is so uncomfortable that it interferes with daily life.

• A person with OCD experiences recurrent obsessions (persistent thoughts, images, or impulses) and compulsions (ritualistic behaviors performed routinely).

• Post-traumatic stress disorder is the development of certain characteristic symptoms after exposure to a severe, extraordinary, traumatic life experience.

• Nonpharmacologic methods used to treat anxiety disorders include relaxation techniques, such as deep breathing and progressive muscle relaxation; covert rehearsal; positive coping statements; cognitive reframing; systematic desensitization; and problem-solving strategies.

• Commonly prescribed antianxiety medications include SSRIs, BZDs, buspirone, beta blockers, and TCAs.

• Assessment reference points for nurses include knowing the definition of anxiety and being able to recognize the signs and symptoms of different anxiety levels.

• Important interventions nurses perform for clients with anxiety disorders include assisting them through anxiety attacks, helping them identify sources of anxiety, reinforcing use of adaptive coping mechanisms, and teaching new coping mechanisms.

• Nurses base evaluation of the effectiveness of nursing care for anxiety disorders on the client's report of feelings and observed behavior changes.

Study Questions

1. Which of the following topic areas would the nurse include in the teaching plan for a client with a panic disorder who is prescribed alprazolam?

   a. Serotonin syndrome

   b. Interactions with MAOIs

   c. Tardive dyskinesia

   d. Potentiation of alcohol effects

2. A client comes to the mental health clinic saying she has been "on edge" lately. She states she has been preoccupied with work, is making mistakes because she can't concentrate, and is forgetting important meetings. She says she thinks she's "going crazy." The nurse categorizes these assessment findings as which of the following?

   a. Affective

   b. Cognitive

   c. Physiologic

   d. Behavioral

3. A client with generalized anxiety disorder states, "I'm worried about my finances. I have substantial savings, and although my financial company is reputable, I'm afraid that the company will go bankrupt and I'll lose all my money." Which response would be most therapeutic?

   a. "It sounds like you have managed your money responsibly."

   b. "Your money is insured; there is no need to worry."

   c. "Has something changed that is causing you to worry?"

   d. "Why do you think the company will go bankrupt?"

(continues on page 452)

4. A 42-year-old man with a history of panic attacks complains that they are occurring more frequently. He is in good health and exercises regularly. He states he occasionally drinks wine with dinner. When planning care for this client, which of the following interventions would the nurse expect to discuss with the client?

a. Desensitization

b. Lifestyle changes

c. Problem-solving strategies

d. Controlled breathing techniques

5. A 22-year-old woman who arrived in the United States 1 week earlier from a country in Central America has complained to her family that she cannot stop crying and has been having nightmares and flashbacks. A few days before she left her home country, armed men had kidnapped her and returned her unharmed when her family paid the ransom. Analysis of this information would lead the nurse to suspect which of the following?

a. Acute stress disorder

b. PTSD

c. Normal anxiety after a traumatic event

d. Generalized anxiety disorder

Critical Thinking Questions

1. Refer to Case Vignette 23.1. Marcia reports that relaxation exercises and meditation only caused her to dwell on her problems more. Analyze why you think this occurred. Explain what Marcia could do differently.

2. Refer to Case vignette 23.2. What is Graham's fear about? What function does washing his hands have in dealing with the fear? Consider the various CBTs described in the chapter and explain which one might be most effective for Graham.

3. Consider the problem-solving method outlined in the text. Compare and contrast it with the nursing process. Use it to make a decision about a current event in your life. Discuss how (or if) going through the process changed your thinking about the event.

References

American Psychiatric Association (APA). (2000). *Diagnostic and statistical manual of mental disorders* (4th ed., text rev.). Washington, DC: Author.

Biederman, J., Petty, C. R., Hirshfeld-Becker, D. R., Henlin, A., Faragone, S. V., Fraire, M., et al. (2007). Developmental trajectories of anxiety disorders in offspring at high risk for panic disorder and major depression. *Psychiatry Research, 153*, 245–252.

Bryant, R. A. (2011). Acute stress disorder as a predictor of post-traumatic stress disorder: A systematic review. *Journal of Clinical Psychiatry, 72*, 233–239.

Bulechek, G. M., Butcher, H. K., & McCloskey Dochterman, J. (2008). *Nursing interventions classification (NIC)* (5th ed.). St. Louis, MO: Mosby.

Danielson, C. K., Amstadter, A. B., Dangelmaier, R. E., Resnick, H. S., Saunders, B. E., & Kilpatrick, D. G. (2009). Does typography of substance abuse and dependence differ as a function of exposure to child maltreatment? *Journal of Child & Adolescent Substance Abuse, 18*, 323–342.

Etkin, A., & Wager, T. D. (2007). Functional neuroimaging of anxiety: A meta-analysis of emotional processing in PTSD, social anxiety disorder, and specific phobia. *American Journal of Psychiatry, 164*, 1476–1488.

Fava, G. A., Porcelli, P., Rafanelli, C., Mangelli, L., & Grandi, S. (2010). The spectrum of anxiety disorders in the medically ill. *Journal of Clinical Psychiatry, 71*, 910–914.

Fava, M., Rush, J., Alpert, J. E., Balasubramani, G. K., Wisniewski, R. S., Carmin, C. N., et al. (2008). Difference in treatment outcome in outpatients with anxious versus nonanxious depression:

A STAR*D report. *American Journal of Psychiatry, 165*(3), 342–351.

Gal, G., Levav, I., & Gross, R. (2011). Psychopathology among adults abused during childhood or adolescence: Results from the Israel-based world mental health survey. *Journal of Nervous and Mental Disorders, 199*, 222–229.

Helms, R. A., & Quan, D. J. (2007). *Textbook of therapeutics: Drugs and disease management* (8th ed.). Philadelphia, PA: Lippincott Williams & Wilkins.

Hoffman, D. L., Dukes, E. M., & Wittchen, H-U. (2008). Human and economic burden of generalized anxiety disorder. *Depression and Anxiety, 25*, 72–90.

Kendler, K. S., Gardner, C. O. & Lichtenstein, P. (2008). A developmental twin study of symptoms of anxiety and depression: Evidence for genetic innovation and attenuation. *Psychological Medicine, 38*, 1567–1575.

Kessler, R. C., Gruber, M., Hettema, J. M., Hwang, I., Sampson, N., & Yonkers, K. A. (2008). Co-morbid major depression and generalized anxiety disorders in the National Comorbidity Survey follow-up. *Psychological Medicine, 38*(3), 365–374.

Lanius, R. (2007). Complex adaptations to traumatic stress: From neurobiological to social and cultural. *American Journal of Psychiatry, 164*, 1628–1630.

Martin, E. I., Ressler, K. J., Binder, E., & Nemeroff, C. B. (2010). The neurobiology of anxiety disorders: Brain imaging, genetics, and psychoneuroendocrinology. *Clinical Laboratory Medicine, 30*, 865–891.

Merikangas, K. R. (2005). Anxiety disorders: Epidemiology. In B. Sadock & V. Sadock (Eds.), *Kaplan & Sadock's comprehensive textbook of psychiatry* (8th ed., pp. 1720–1727). Philadelphia, PA: Lippincott Williams and Wilkins.

Moorhead, S., Johnson, M., Maas, M. L., & Swanson, E. (2008). *Nursing outcomes classification (NOC)* (4th ed.). St. Louis, MO: Mosby.

NANDA International. (2007). *Nursing diagnoses: Definitions and classification (2007–2008)*. Philadelphia, PA: Author.

National Institute of Mental Health (NIMH). (2010, July 29). *Agoraphobia among adults*. Washington, DC: Author. Retrieved from http://www.nimh.nih.gov/statistics/1AGOR_ADULT.shtml

National Institute of Mental Health (NIMH). (2011, January 21). *Social phobia (social anxiety disorder): Always embarrassed*. Retrieved from http://www.nimh.nih.gov/health/publications/social-phobia-social-anxiety-disorder-always-embarrassed/social-phobia-social-anxiety-disorder-always-embarrassed.shtml

Nepon, J., Belik, S-L., Bolton, J., & Sareen, J. (2010). The relationship between anxiety disorders and suicide attempts: findings from the National Epidemiologic Survey on Alcohol and Related conditions. *Depression and Anxiety, 27*, 791–798.

Romera, I., Montejo, A. L., Caballero, F., Caballero, L., Arbesu, J., Polavieja, P., et al. (2011). Functional impairment related to painful physical symptoms in patients with generalized anxiety disorder with or without comorbid major depressive disorder: post hoc analysis of a cross-sectional study. *BMC Psychiatry, 11*, 69 (epub ahead of print; PMID: 21510887

Roy-Byrne, P., Craske, M. G., Sullivan, G., Rose, R. D., Edlund, M. J., Lang, A. J., et al. (2010). Delivery of evidence-based treatment for multiple anxiety disorders in primary care. *Journal of the American Medical Association, 303*, 1921–1928.

Stein, M. B., Simmons, A. N., Feinstein J. S., & Paulus, M. P. (2007). Increased amygdala and insula activation during emotion processing in anxiety-prone subjects. *American Journal of Psychiatry, 164*, 318–327.

U.S. Department of Veterans Affairs. (2010). *Acute stress disorder*. Retrieved from http://www.ptsd.va.gov/public/pages/acute-stress-disorder.asp

Web Resources

Anxiety Disorders Association of America: http://www.adaa.org

Association for the Advancement of Behavior Therapy: http://www.aabt.org

Freedom from Fear: http://www.freedomfromfear.com

National Anxiety Foundation: http://lexington-on-line.com/naf.html

National Institute of Mental Health Public Inquiries: http://www.nimh.nih.gov

Obsessive-Compulsive Foundation, Inc.: http://www.ocfoundation.org

Obsessive Compulsive Information Center: http://www.miminc.org

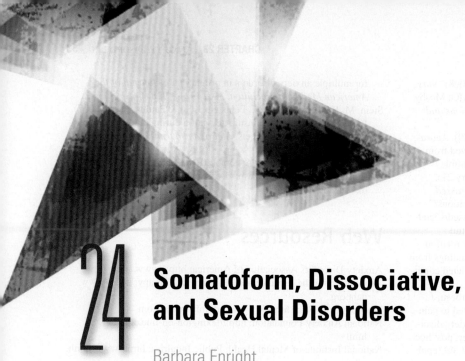

24

Somatoform, Dissociative, and Sexual Disorders

Barbara Enright

Abraham, E., Friedman, R. A., & Brenner, R. (1996). Verapamil for the treatment of agitated... Hillsdale, NJ: Erlbaum Mosby.

Psychiatric Association. (2007). American Journal of Psychiatry (Online source). Retrieved

Barondes, S. (2003). Better than Prozac (pp. 1-20). Boston:

New technology...

...American Journal of Psychiatry (Online source). Retrieved

KEY TERMS

alter
body dysmorphic disorder
conversion disorder
depersonalization disorder
dissociation
dissociative amnesia
dissociative disorders
dissociative fugue
dissociative identity disorder
dissociative trance
dyspareunia
factitious disorder
hypervigilance
hypochondriasis
malingering
pain disorder
paraphilias
premature ejaculation
primary gain
secondary gain
sexual dysfunction
somatization disorder
somatoform disorders
transsexual
transvestite
vaginismus

LEARNING OBJECTIVES

On completion of this chapter, you should be able to accomplish the following:

- Describe possible etiologies for somatoform disorders.
- Explain the features of various somatoform disorders.
- Identify the most common interdisciplinary goals and treatments for clients with somatoform disorders.
- Apply the steps of the nursing process to clients with somatoform disorders.
- Differentiate the types of dissociative disorders.
- Describe other psychiatric problems commonly associated with dissociative disorders.
- Identify the most common interdisciplinary goals and treatments, as well as nursing interventions for clients with dissociative disorders.
- Compare and contrast common sexual disorders.
- Outline interdisciplinary and nursing strategies for the management of sexual dysfunction.

This chapter discusses conditions that pose challenges to personal identity and self-concept: somatoform, dissociative, and sexual/gender disorders. In general, basic-level psychiatric nurses work with clients having these problems less frequently than they do clients with other disorders described in this unit. However, nurses may encounter such clients across many health care settings and need to understand how these problems affect clients and families. They also need to know appropriate interdisciplinary and nursing approaches for them.

SOMATOFORM DISORDERS

Clients with **somatoform disorders** experience physical symptoms despite no underlying medical explanation for them. They report severe symptoms with no organic or physical basis. Although the symptoms are physical, somatoform disorders are classified as mental disorders because physical examination and laboratory tests reveal no demonstrable organic pathology.

Somatoform disorders vary in severity, from mild and self-limited to chronic and disabling. Clients usually seek treatment not only in outpatient settings, such as primary care, but also in medical specialty practices such as dermatology and neurology.

Incidence and Prevalence

In general, somatoform disorders are diagnosed more commonly in women than in men (Holloway & Zerbe, 2000). Women in medical and community samples report more frequent, numerous, and intense physical symptoms than do men (Barsky et al., 2001; Leiknes et al., 2007; Silverstein, 1999). Estimated prevalence of unexplained medical symptoms ranges from 2% to 5% of inpatient neurology admissions (Allet & Allet, 2006). The first symptoms of

somatoform disorders usually appear in adolescence; clients may meet full diagnostic criteria by 30 years (Ford, 1995).

Etiology

Why do some people express emotional and psychological distress through somatic symptoms? The basis for somatoform disorders is often unclear and complicated. Most clinicians advocate for a multidimensional causal model encompassing a complex interplay of neurobiologic, psychological, and familial factors.

A careful review of the history of a client's physical complaints is essential to rule out any existing medical illness. Data about lifestyle, emotional status, and relationships are also critical because psychological distress and interpersonal problems often are common in these clients. For example, childhood abuse is associated with somatoform disorders, and providers should consider severe environmental stress in all cases of somatoform illness in children and adolescents (Bowman, 2000; Brown et al., 2005; Didie et al., 2006; Katon et al., 2001).

In the past decade, studies (Spence, 2000; Ward et al., 2003) utilizing neuroimaging techniques have revealed that complex brain mechanisms are involved in preventing normal cortical activity in specific somatoform disorders. The work in neuroimaging is incomplete and has not provided full understanding or effective treatment models. However, the identification of physiologic mechanisms and structures reduces derogatory labeling, helps relieve client stress, and may ultimately improve provider attitudes about care of this population.

Signs and Symptoms/Diagnostic Criteria

The major finding in all types of somatoform disorders is symptoms with no demonstrable pathology on testing or examination (*DSM-IV-TR* Box 24.1). Roots of symptoms

---

DSM-IV-TR BOX 24.1

Somatoform Disorders

Somatization Disorder

A. A history of many physical complaints beginning before age 30 years that occur over a period of several years and result in treatment being sought or significant impairment in social, occupational, or other important areas of functioning.

B. Each of the following criteria must have been met, with individual symptoms occurring at any time during the course of the disturbance:

 1. *Four pain symptoms:* a history of pain related to at least four different sites or functions (eg, head, abdomen, back, joints, extremities, chest, rectum, during menstruation, during sexual intercourse, or during urination)

 2. *Two gastrointestinal symptoms:* a history of at least two gastrointestinal symptoms other than pain (eg, nausea,

bloating, vomiting other than during pregnancy, diarrhea, or intolerance of several different foods)

 3. *One sexual symptom:* a history of at least one sexual or reproductive symptom other than pain (eg, sexual indifference, erectile or ejaculatory dysfunction, irregular menses, excessive menstrual bleeding, vomiting throughout pregnancy)

 4. *One pseudoneurologic symptom:* a history of at least one symptom or deficit suggesting a neurologic condition not limited to pain (conversion symptoms such as impaired coordination or balance, paralysis or localized weakness, difficulty swallowing or lump in throat, aphonia, urinary retention, hallucinations, loss of touch or pain sensation, double vision, blindness, deafness, seizures; dissociative symptoms such as amnesia; or loss of consciousness other than fainting)

(continues on page 456)

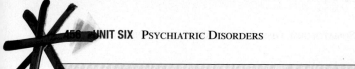

DSM-IV-TR BOX 24.1 Somatoform Disorders (continued)

C. Either (1) or (2):
   1. After appropriate investigation, each of the symptoms in Criterion B cannot be fully explained by a known general medical condition or the direct effects of a substance (eg, a drug of abuse, a medication)
   2. When there is a related general medical condition, the physical complaints or resulting social or occupational impairment are in excess of what would be expected from the history, physical examination, or laboratory findings
D. The symptoms are not intentionally feigned or produced (as in Factitious Disorder or Malingering).

Undifferentiated Somatoform Disorder

A. One or more physical complaints (eg, fatigue, loss of appetite, gastrointestinal or urinary complaints).
B. Either (1) or (2):
   1. After appropriate investigation, the symptoms cannot be fully explained by a known general medical condition or the direct effects of a substance (eg, a drug of abuse, a medication)
   2. When there is a related general medical condition, the physical complaints or resulting social or occupational impairment is in excess of what would be expected from the history, physical examination, or laboratory findings
C. The symptoms cause clinically significant distress or impairment in social, occupational, or other important areas of functioning.
D. The duration of the disturbance is at least 6 months.
E. The disturbance is not better accounted for by another mental disorder
F. The symptom is not intentionally produced or feigned (as in Factitious Disorder or Malingering).

Conversion Disorder

A. One or more symptoms or deficits affecting voluntary motor or sensory function that suggest a neurologic or other general medical condition.
B. Psychological factors are judged to be associated with the symptom or deficit because the initiation or exacerbation of the symptom or deficit is preceded by conflicts or other stressors.

C. The symptom or deficit is not intentionally produced or feigned (as in Factitious Disorder or Malingering).
D. The symptom or deficit cannot, after appropriate investigation, be fully explained by a general medical condition, or by the direct effects of a substance, or as a culturally sanctioned behavior or experience.
E. The symptom or deficit causes clinically significant distress or impairment in social, occupational, or other important areas of functioning or warrants medical evaluation.
F. The symptom or deficit is not limited to pain or sexual dysfunction, does not occur exclusively during the course of Somatization Disorder, and is not better accounted for by another mental disorder.

Hypochondriasis

A. Preoccupation with fears of having, or the idea that one has, a serious disease based on the person's misinterpretation of bodily symptoms.
B. The preoccupation persists despite appropriate medical evaluation and reassurance.
C. The belief in Criterion A is not of delusional intensity and is not restricted to a circumscribed concern about appearance.
D. The preoccupation causes clinically significant distress or impairment in social, occupational, or other important areas of functioning.
E. The duration of the disturbance is at least 6 months.
F. The preoccupation is not better accounted for by Generalized Anxiety Disorder, Obsessive-Compulsive Disorder, Panic Disorder, a Major Depressive Episode, Separation Anxiety, or another Somatoform Disorder.

Body Dysmorphic Disorder

A. Preoccupation with an imagined defect in appearance. If a slight physical anomaly is present, the person's concern is markedly excessive.
B. The preoccupation causes clinically significant distress or impairment in social, occupational, or other important areas of functioning.
C. The preoccupation is not better accounted for by another mental disorder (eg, dissatisfaction with body shape and size in Anorexia Nervosa).

Reprinted with permission from the *Diagnostic and Statistical Manual of Mental Disorders, Fourth Edition, Text Revision* (Copyright © 2000). American Psychiatric Association.

are linked to psychology, rather than physiology (American Psychiatric Association [APA], 2000).

People may negatively and pejoratively label clients with somatoform disorders as "doctor shopping" or "attention seeking." Affected clients do not intentionally cause and have no conscious or voluntary control over their symptoms. Lack of voluntary control is in contrast to *factitious disorder* and *malingering*. In **factitious disorder,** clients

deliberately make up or inflict symptoms. An example is *Munchausen syndrome by proxy*. In this condition, an adult (usually a parent) continuously brings a child to the attention of health care personnel for inexplicable and sudden illnesses. In reality, the parent induces or fabricates the sickness to gain attention. With **malingering**, clients consciously create or exaggerate false symptoms to avoid work or other responsibilities.

Some researchers argue that the current *Diagnostic and Statistical Manual of Mental Disorders,* 4th edition, text revision (*DSM-IV-TR*) (APA, 2000) classifications of somatoform disorders need revision (Creed, 2006; Kroenke, 2006; Sharpe & Carson, 2001; Sykes, 2006). Hypochondriasis might be an anxiety disorder, body dysmorphic disorder might be an obsessive-compulsive disorder, and conversion disorder might be a dissociative disorder (Mayou et al., 2005). Other somatoform disorders might be coded on Axis III as general medical conditions with a corresponding Axis I designation of "psychological factors affecting a medical condition" (see Chap. 39). Such debate about current classifications is important because the somatoform disorders encompass a broad spectrum of problems (Kroenke, 2006).

Some clinicians think somatoform disorders provide clients with **primary gain,** meaning that symptoms block psychological conflict or anxiety from conscious awareness. They also offer **secondary gain** by relieving clients from expected responsibilities and increasing the attention they receive. Such gains may positively reinforce and help to perpetuate somatic symptoms.

Checkpoint Questions

1. How do somatoform disorders differ from factitious disorder or malingering?
2. How do the symptoms associated with many somatoform disorders provide clients with primary and secondary gain?

Somatization Disorder

Clients with **somatization disorder** (*hysteria* or *Briquet's syndrome*) usually present exaggerated, inconsistent, yet complicated medical histories. They often seek treatment from multiple health care providers when their physical complaints are not addressed to their satisfaction. Medically unexplained and unintentionally expressed physical symptoms and their relationship to psychological well-being are dramatic.

Undifferentiated Somatoform Disorder

The persistent, unexplained physical symptoms of *undifferentiated somatoform disorder* last for at least 6 months and do not fully meet the criteria for somatization disorder or any other somatoform disorder. Common complaints include fatigue, loss of appetite, and gastrointestinal or urinary symptoms. Clients do not feign their symptoms, and they experience negative interpersonal, occupational, or other repercussions. History, physical examination, and laboratory tests do not explain or verify the physical symptoms or disruptions to life (APA, 2000).

Conversion Disorder

The predominant feature of **conversion disorder** is loss of voluntary motor or sensory functioning that appears to represent physiologic pathology but, instead, relates to psychological conflict or need. Symptoms follow a greatly distressing event or experience. One study showed a correlation between childhood traumatization and pseudoepileptic seizures in clients with conversion disorder (Roelofs et al., 2002). Symptoms provide a way for clients to defend against intrapsychic anxiety. Conversion symptoms are defined as "pseudoneurologic" because medical tests or laboratory findings cannot fully explain them. Examples include paralysis or localized weakness, impaired balance, aphonia, urinary retention, and difficulty swallowing. The illness occurs in approximately 2% to 4% of clients seen by neurologists (Allet & Allet, 2006). Although the term *la belle indifference*— clients' lack of anxiety or concern with their symptoms and disabilities—historically has been used to discriminate conversion disorders from organic neurologic disorders, Aybek and colleagues (2008) question its validity. In a systematic review of 11 published studies, Stone and associates (2006) found that the median frequency of "la belle indifference" in clients with conversion disorder was 21%, whereas it was 29% in clients with organic disease.

Hypochondriasis

Clients with **hypochondriasis** fear or believe that they have a serious disease despite no significant pathology or other reason for thinking so (APA, 2000). **Hypervigilance** of the body and its sensations leads clients to misinterpret and overreact to physical signs and symptoms, which are usually prolonged and chronic. Much energy may be bound up in unrealistic fears that health care providers are missing diagnoses, such as cancer, cardiac disease, or sexually transmitted infections. Some researchers suggest that health care providers inadvertently may reinforce this hypervigilance by instructing clients to "monitor their symptoms" (Abramowitz & Braddock, 2006). Clients may then notice and misinterpret normal body sensations and changes as serious illness.

People with hypochondriasis often seek medical care from numerous sources. When they do not obtain satisfaction from one provider, they go to others in an attempt to find an answer. Preoccupation with bodily distress and the accompanying expectation that others should also focus on their well-being may disrupt social relationships and work. In contrast to the lack of anxiety seen in clients with conversion disorder, clients with hypochondriasis often appear anxious. They sometimes can acknowledge that their fear of a dreaded disease is unfounded; however, they are unaware of their anxiety or depression.

Pain Disorder

The classic symptom in **pain disorder** is the inexplicable presence of physical pain, which is the major focus in clients' lives. Clients frequently access health care services and commonly take medications for the symptoms. Pain disorders are expressed in various areas (eg, abdomen, back, bone, breast), each of which is coded individually in the *DSM-IV-TR* (APA, 2000).

Body Dysmorphic Disorder

The primary feature of **body dysmorphic disorder (BDD)** is preoccupation with an imagined defect in appearance. Clients obsess about minor or nonexistent facial abnormalities, such as wrinkles, spots on the skin, facial asymmetry, or facial hair (Cunningham et al., 2000). Other body parts, such as the genitals, breasts, buttocks, hands, or feet, may be the focus of distress and embarrassment. Thinking that others notice the imagined flaw is an associated feature. BDD is underrecognized and underdiagnosed. Clients are reluctant to talk about their perceived defects with friends or health providers, fearing that they will be seen as silly or vain. If questioned, they are often relieved to be invited to talk about their concerns with body image.

One study found gender differences in BDD presentations (Figure 24.1). Men were more likely to be older, live alone, and obsess about thinning hair and body building, whereas women were more likely to have concerns about many body areas, camouflage imagined flaws, and perform obsessive actions such as mirror checking and skin picking (Phillips et al., 2006). Because of extreme self-consciousness about the imagined defect, clients may retreat from usual activities, become socially isolated, and display decreased academic and occupational functioning. Some clients even become housebound (Phillips & Dufresne, 2002). Those with severe forms of BDD are at increased risk of suicide (Phillips et al., 2005).

Compulsive skin picking is an underrecognized form of BDD. Clients with this condition spend hours a day picking at their skin, which can result in serious damage (Grant et al., 2001; Phillips & Dufresne, 2002).

Comorbidities and Dual Diagnoses

Many somatoform disorders coexist with other psychiatric disorders, such as major depression, anxiety disorders, and personality disorders. Community studies have shown that psychological distress, stressful events, depression, and anxiety often are associated with medical symptoms with no identifiable physiologic etiology, increased use of health care services, and increased costs (Katon et al., 2001; Lieb et al., 2007). In addition, clients with medical diagnoses characterized by an ill-defined pathology (eg, irritable bowel syndrome, fibromyalgia) have significantly higher rates of anxiety and depressive disorders than do clients with comparable, well-defined diseases and similar symptoms (Katon et al., 2001). Approximately 22% to 49% of clients with BDD have comorbid substance abuse (Grant et al., 2005). Other psychiatric comorbidities include major depression, social phobia, and OCD (Gunstad & Phillips, 2003). With hypochondriasis, the literature frequently describes comorbid mood disorders (Abramowitz & Braddock, 2006).

Implications and Prognosis

Somatoform disorders are usually difficult to treat and require long-term management. In 1997, 30% of people retiring

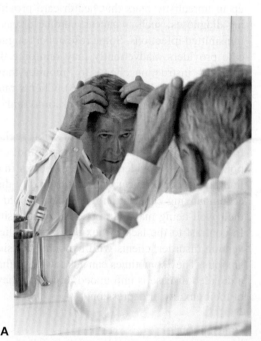
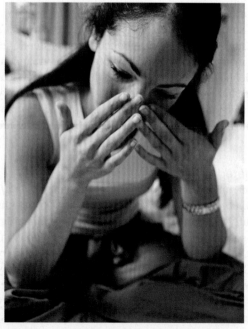

FIGURE 24.1 Presentations of body dysmorphic disorder may have patterns related to the client's gender. **(A)** Men with BDD may be preoccupied with body building or with concerns over losing their hair. **(B)** Women may have more pervasive body concerns or focus on and try to cover up imagined flaws, such as their noses or complexions.

early because of occupational disability had psychosomatic illness (Huber, 2000). For most somatoform disorders, more severe symptoms, longer durations, and psychiatric co-morbidities predict a more unremitting course and poorer prognosis. Research suggests that antidepressants may be efficacious in treating functional somatic disorders such as fibromyalgia, irritable bowel syndrome, chronic back pain, and noncardiac chest pain (Stahl, 2003).

Without an informed, experienced health care provider who can work with a client regarding underlying dependency needs, prognosis is not good. Often, clients go from provider to provider seeking a remedy for their ailments; this process may continue for many years. It is imperative that health care providers recognize the somatoform syndromes and either treat them accordingly or refer clients to psychiatric care providers.

Interdisciplinary Goals and Treatment

Multidimensional treatment requires interdisciplinary strategies for maximum effectiveness. Many authors have advocated a clinical approach that encompasses several overarching interventions (Box 24.1). Nevertheless, management may be fragmented and uncoordinated because these disorders often are unrecognized. Many clients with them receive treatment through primary care. Early detection and diagnosis are critical in primary care and psychiatric settings.

BOX 24.1 Selected Multidisciplinary Interventions for Clients With Somatoform Disorders

- Early screening and diagnosis
- Multidisciplinary care coordination
- Finding meaningful language with which to name the illness that is acceptable to the care provider and client
- Regular, brief office visits that minimize the client's need unconsciously to develop additional symptoms to meet dependency needs
- Management by nursing clinical specialists that includes frequent, supportive contacts, reassurance, and monitoring of physical status
- Regular health maintenance screenings and appropriate physical examinations to avoid missing symptoms that may have a medical basis
- Normalization of and empathy for the client's distress
- Exploration of predisposing factors that create vulnerability to development of a disabling condition, precipitating factors that trigger illness episodes, and perpetuating factors that serve to make maladaptive illness behaviors stable over time
- Safe environment for the client to express feelings
- Chronic disease and rehabilitative models that focus primarily on client functioning
- Appropriate control of access to medical services

Ideally, clients benefit most from early diagnosis coupled with a coordinated, comprehensive, long-term treatment plan. Effective management is based primarily on an established and strong therapeutic relationship with a team of providers who coordinate their efforts. Therapeutic relationships must be built on trust, coupled with gradual understanding by health care personnel about the client's ongoing struggles. In addition, empathy regarding the client's difficulty in expressing and meeting emotional needs is a critical prerequisite (Johns, 1999; Margo & Margo, 2000).

Kroenke's (2007) review of randomized trial studies of treatment efficacy for somatoform disorders found that five of seven randomized trials with CBT were effective, as were three of four trials with antidepressant medication, and three of four trials with psychiatric consultation with the primary care provider (PCP). Providing specialized training to PCPs and aerobic exercise were not found to be effective. Hypochondriasis and body dysmorphic disorder were treated most effectively, conversion disorder treatment has not been studied, and pain disorder has not been responsive to either cognitive–behavioral therapy (CBT) or antidepressants.

Experts advocate rehabilitative or chronic-disease approaches, with the long-term goal of maintaining optimal functioning (Becker, 1998; Epstein et al., 1999). Clients with mild somatic symptoms that are recognized early may respond to reassurance and support. Unrecognized and untreated early symptoms often progress to more debilitating disorders and unnecessarily dangerous, costly, and frustrating diagnostic procedures and treatments (Servan-Schreiber et al., 2000).

Individual and Group Psychotherapies

Individual and group psychotherapies have been advocated as the treatments of choice for somatoform disorders. Cognitive–behavioral psychotherapy has been shown effective in relieving symptoms of hypochondriasis and BDD (Kroenke, 2007; Phillips et al., 2002; Sumathipala, 2007; Taylor et al., 2005). Clients with other somatoform disorders also may benefit from CBT (Slaughter & Sun, 1999). See Evidence-Based Practice Spotlight 24.1.

Psychopharmacology and Somatic Therapies

Although psychopharmacologic agents have been of limited use in reducing symptoms of selective somatoform disorders, their appropriate use can sometimes help. Selective serotonin reuptake inhibitors (SSRIs), given in sequential trials of one or more medications, are the cost-effective and helpful drugs of choice for the reduction of symptoms of undifferentiated somatoform disorder, hypochondriasis, and BDD (Han et al., 2008; Holloway & Zerbe, 2000; Kroenke, 2007). Alternative somatic therapies are often useful, including biofeedback, meditation, and relaxation.

EVIDENCE-BASED PRACTICE SPOTLIGHT 24.1

Interventions for Hypochondriasis

Overview of Effective Treatment: Cognitive–behavioral interventions are effective in the treatment of hypochondriasis. Methods include psychoeducation, behavioral stress management, cognitive and cognitive–behavioral therapy (CBT), and exposure and response prevention. Psychoeducation helps clients adopt rational responses to normal physiologic sensations and is effective in treating mild cases of hypochondriasis. Group psychoeducational sessions have the additional benefit of exposing clients to a support group. The client and therapist collaborate on techniques to incorporate into the treatment. Exposure and response prevention techniques are beneficial in reducing the health anxiety symptoms and have been maintained at follow-up intervals. CBT and a trial of paroxetine were found to be similarly effective in reducing health anxiety in these clients.

What Has Not Been Shown Effective: Psychodynamic psychotherapy has not been shown to be an effective

treatment for hypochondriasis. Clients may reject this long-term therapy in favor of continued doctor-shopping. Reassurance from the therapist that there is no evidence of disease is not helpful to the hypochondriac because this perpetuates the initial health anxiety.

Implications for Practice: The most important intervention is to demonstrate empathy toward the client and to build a therapeutic alliance with the client. It is important to empower the client to take control of his or her anxieties and to become an active participant in the course of therapy. CBT fosters a collaborative partnership and allows the client to have maximum input in the direction of the therapy. Because medications and a short course of CBT have been shown to be equally effective for hypochondriasis, the client should be encouraged to decide which is the best course to take.

References

Abramowitz, J. S., & Braddock, A. E. (2006). Hypochondriasis: Conceptualization, treatment, and relationship to obsessive-compulsive disorder. *Psychiatric Clinics of North America, 29,* 503–519.

Barsky, A., & Ahern, D. (2004). Cognitive–behavior therapy for hypochondriasis: A randomized controlled trial. *Journal of the American Medical Association, 291,* 1464–1470.

Bouman, T. K., & van Duijn, M. A. (2006). Psychoeducation for hypochondriasis: A comparison of a cognitive-behavioral approach and a problem-solving approach. *Behaviour Research and Therapy, 45,* 887–899.

Buwalda, F. M., Bouman, T. K., & van Duijn, M. A. (2006). Psychoeducation for hypochondriasis: A comparison of a cognitive–behavioral approach and a problem-solving approach. *Behaviour Research and Therapy, 45,* 887–899.

Greeven, A., van Balkom A. J., Visser, S., Merkelbach, J., van Rood, Y. R., van Dyck, R., et al. (2007). Cognitive behavior therapy and paroxetine in the treatment of hypochondriasis: A randomized controlled trial. *American Journal of Psychiatry, 164*(1), 91–99.

Taylor, S., Asmundson, G. J. G., & Coons, M. J. (2005). Current directions in the treatment of hypochondriasis. *Journal of Cognitive Psychotherapy, 19*(3), 285–304.

Thomson, A. (2009). Psychotherapies for hypochondriasis. *Cochrane Database of Systematic Reviews, 2009*(3). Retrieved from EBSCO*host.*

Visser, S., & Bouman, T. K. (2001). The treatment of hypochondriasis: Exposure plus response prevention vs cognitive therapy. *Behaviour Research and Therapy, 39,* 423–442.

Warwick, H. M., Clark, D. M., Cobb, A. M., & Salkovskis, P. (1996). A controlled trial of cognitive–behavioral treatment of hypochondriasis. *British Journal of Psychiatry, 169*(2), 189–195.

APPLYING THE NURSING PROCESS

Somatoform Disorders

Although specific somatoform disorders may respond to different interventions, nurses work with all clients using an approach with similar general outcomes and interventions designed to address basic shared components of care. They assist clients with the overarching goal of developing and maintaining functional patterns of adaptation. They direct activities toward:

- Developing trust and establishing a therapeutic relationship
- Demonstrating genuine concern and caring with supportive interactions
- Assisting clients to improve physical health and adapt to stress
- Enhancing self-knowledge

- Helping clients examine ways to express and meet needs directly and to consider alternatives for coping other than through physical symptoms and illness

Ideally, one clinical care provider assumes responsibility for clients and coordinates treatment with others. Psychiatric–mental health clinical nurse specialists are in an ideal position to work with clients over long periods and to coordinate care closely with physicians (Figure 24.2).

▲ ASSESSMENT

Nurses in all settings must provide astute assessment of clients with somatic symptoms. A holistic approach is especially critical for clients with somatoform disorders. Viewing clients as a system greater than the sum of its parts assists nurses to assess the whole person, rather than focusing only on the obvious physical body. Knowledge and understanding of multidimensional causes

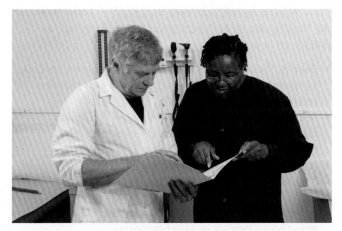

FIGURE 24.2 Collaboration with the physicians involved in the care of a client with somatoform disorders is crucial to preserving the client's holistic health and to ensuring appropriate use of health care resources.

of illness facilitate a comprehensive assessment that includes psychological, physiologic, and social influences.

Analysis of assessment data focuses on a thorough examination of the possible interrelationships of all systems. During assessment, nurses simultaneously practice therapeutic use of self and convey understanding and genuine concern, thus developing a strong, trusting, and therapeutic relationship with clients from the start (see Chap. 11).

Mental Status

Nurses obtain information about behavior within interpersonal relationships (including expressing needs and feelings) and intrapersonal experiences that focus on emotional life. Because depression and anxiety may be at the root of the physical symptoms, nurses are especially sensitive to those areas. Assessment is critical to determining the coexistence of other psychiatric disorders, such as depression, anxiety, or personality disorders. See Assessment Tool 24.1 for a review of the components of mental status and common findings seen with somatoform disorders.

Physical Examination

A complete review of systems, including vital signs and laboratory work, is indicated. Nurses must elicit information about current and past medical history. In particular, a complete history of help-seeking behaviors through the medical care system is essential, including any diagnostic testing, workups, hospitalizations, and outpatient surgeries. Critical areas of assessment include sleep, appetite, weight gain or loss, and bowel function. Evaluating these can help to rule out psychiatric comorbidities, such as sleep, eating, mood, or anxiety disorders.

These clients often present with complaints of low to no energy. Nurses examine such findings and determine how they affect daily functioning. Have clients felt "slowed down?" Do they complain of having to rest frequently or remain in bed during the day? If so, what are the family members', employers', or friends' responses? Have clients experienced increased daily activity or spurts of energy? What tasks has illness kept clients from performing?

One important consideration for clients with BDD involves gender differences in presentation. For example, females are more likely to camouflage skin excoriations or imagined defects with makeup and apparel, whereas males may deny hours spent "bulking up" on obvious body building. Nurses should take note of any evidence of skin damage, attempts to camouflage spots or pimples, or changes in a client's appearance that might indicate evidence of a problem.

Social Assessment

Comprehensive social assessment includes family functioning, social support, and cultural and ethnic ties. Families at high risk for communicating psychological distress through physical symptoms are those in which one or both parents express needs and feelings in this way. Thorough nursing assessment and analysis may reveal information about the family functioning. Nurses also assess social network, occupation, and education.

▲ NURSING DIAGNOSIS

Nursing diagnoses for clients with somatoform disorders focus on identifying the causes of dysfunctional coping and issues

---

▲ ASSESSMENT TOOL 24.1 ▲
Common Mental Status Findings in Somatoform Disorders

Behavior

• An alarming, crisis-oriented symptom presentation, focusing on particular physical concerns
• Excessive fear, dread, worry, apprehension, or rigid or obsessional thinking
• Restlessness, diaphoresis, palpitations, shortness of breath, muscle tension

Mood and Affect

• Reports of difficulty concentrating, thinking clearly, completing tasks, or enjoying usual activities

• Unemotional affect while describing anguishing symptoms
• In conversion disorders, description of situation without any affective display at all (*la belle indifference*)

Thought Process and Content

• Thorough knowledge of illnesses or illnesses associated with specific symptoms
• Expressed concerns about a specific aspect of physical appearance

related to the family and psychosocial interaction. Selected potential diagnoses include the following (NANDA, 2007):

- Ineffective Coping related to unresolved psychological issues as evidenced by somatization
- Anxiety related to perceived threat and excessive concern over physical symptoms or physical illness
- Powerlessness related to lifestyle of helplessness and perceived inability to effect a change in physical health as evidenced by excessive dependency
- Chronic Low Self-Esteem related to perceived inability to participate in daily functional activities
- Social Isolation related to inability to leave home and participate with others in social events
- Interrupted Family Processes related to client's ongoing, severe physical disability and assumption of the sick role

△ OUTCOME IDENTIFICATION AND PLANNING

Nurses collaborate with clients and family to create plans of care that include appropriate goals and ways to meet

them. Possible desired outcomes, incorporating labels from the Nursing Outcomes Classification (NOC), are as follows (Moorhead et al., 2008):

- **Coping:** The client will spend less time focusing on physical symptoms and make fewer visits to health care providers, the emergency department, or both.
- **Decision Making:** The client will become increasingly independent and will verbalize decreased feelings of powerlessness.
- **Anxiety Control:** The client will report increased feelings of relaxation and decreased anxiety.
- **Self-Esteem:** The client will demonstrate increased self-esteem by verbalizing positive elements of self and by reporting an increase in daily functioning.

△ IMPLEMENTATION

Implementation often begins in inpatient settings (if clients are hospitalized) and continues on an outpatient basis. This section focuses on outpatient care. See also Case in Point 24.1,

Case in Point 24.1

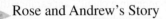

Rose and Andrew's Story

Rose, 62 years old, has been married to Andrew for 39 years. They have three grown children. Rose's internist of 5 years has referred Rose to psychotherapy. During those 5 years, Rose has complained of persistent, unrelenting pain in her head, back, arms, and joints, with occasional difficulty urinating. Just before her last visit, a kidney specialist had been treating her. Two courses of antibiotics were unsuccessful in relieving her complaints of severe pain on urination. While taking the antibiotics, Rose began to complain of increasing difficulty with coordination and balance, often "holding onto the walls" as she walks through her home. The internist has told Rose and Andrew that he believes the problems are stemming from somatoform illness.

Andrew accompanies his wife to the therapy session. On arrival, Rose produces a 10-page typewritten paper of her entire medical history since she was 18. She asks the nurse to read it, saying, "It's too detailed for me to really tell you about in 1 hour." Rose had two exploratory abdominal surgeries at 22 and 25 years for "extensive pain, diarrhea, and abdominal distention"; a history of irregular menses followed by a total hysterectomy at 32 years; and many multiple, unusual symptoms that have been tested individually, usually by different physicians, and resulted in negative apparent physiologic etiology. Rose angrily states, "The doctor acts like my problems are all in my head. But he has no idea of the pain I'm in!" Later, Rose says, "I can't do anything from day to day. Andrew helps me with everything. It's been this way a long time. I'm so tired of hurting, but I know there is no help for me."

Additional questioning reveals that the couple's typical day revolves around Andrew assisting Rose with multiple, complicated, and time-consuming activities designed to help her feel better and to function at home. He states, "I get her food, supplies, and anything else that she needs. I feel exhausted and burned out." Rose and Andrew also say that they "used to have a good social life, with our old high school friends, but that has stopped in the past year because Rose has been feeling so bad."

Key Assessment Findings

- **Numerous physical symptoms and complaints spanning years**
- **Persistent and unrelenting pain**
- **Difficulty urinating; severe pain on urination**
- **Problems with coordination and balance**
- **History of exploratory surgeries for intense pain, diarrhea, and distention; irregular menses; hysterectomy at 32 years**
- **Multiple unusual symptoms with no apparent physiologic etiology**
- **Social isolation**
- **Decreased level of client functioning**
- **Statements of hopelessness about condition**
- **Feelings of exhaustion by husband as primary caregiver**

Case in Point 24.1 (continued)

Rose and Andrew's Story

Nursing Diagnosis: Ineffective Coping related to unresolved psychological issues as evidenced by history of frequent bodily complaints unsupported by diagnostic testing, excessive use of medical resources, restricted lifestyle, persistent focus on physical symptoms, and inability verbally to express emotional content

NOC: Coping and Role Performance: The client will verbalize feelings about her life, stressors, and physical symptoms with less time spent focusing on physical symptoms.

NIC: Coping Enhancement

- Establish a therapeutic relationship. Provide calm reassurance and an accepting atmosphere. Show empathy for the client's distress but focus on feelings rather than physical complaints. Encourage verbalization of feelings, perceptions, and fears. Refocus client to express feelings rather than to describe physical complaints. *Clients with possible or diagnosed somatoform disorders often have little or no trust in the health care system and its providers. Therapeutic intervention is possible only when the client's trust has been gained. Focusing on feelings rather than physical complaints conveys interest in the client as a person and reduces her need to garner attention through physical complaints. Refocusing provides a model for gaining insight into the behavior.*

- Collaborate with the primary physician to coordinate physical care and appropriate use of medical services. Provide the client with realistic choices about certain aspects of care. *Care coordination is an important aspect of treatment. It helps ensure appropriate use of resources, medical screening, and care. It conveys to the client that health care providers are working together to protect her health.*

- Recommend insight-oriented therapy to explore psychological motivation for somatization. Assist the client to objectively appraise events. Discuss triggering factors to help the client gain insight into patterns associated with increased somatization. *Fewer symptoms and increased functioning may result as the client gains insight into behavior patterns. Recognizing triggering events will help her manage her behavior.*

- Encourage the client to identify strengths and abilities. Assist her to identify maladaptive strategies; provide suggestions for replacing them with appropriate ones. Support the use of appropriate defense mechanisms. Develop techniques that do not encourage focusing on bodily sensations (eg, developing an absorbing hobby, volunteering). *Clients cannot relinquish a coping strategy, no matter how dysfunctional, until they can replace it with another.*

NIC: Role Enhancement

- Review with the couple tasks that need to be done. Assist the client to identify tasks in which she can participate. Encourage her to start out with small ones and to participate in one task each week. *Identifying tasks and level of participation help*

the client visualize what she can do. Keeping activities and tasks small and manageable reduces the pressure on the client to perform, allows her to achieve success, and minimizes anxiety associated with expectations of independence.

- Assist the client to identify her usual role in the family and specific role changes from her current problems. *These measures aid in developing appropriate care strategies.*

- Facilitate discussion of role adaptations of client's husband to compensate for the client's role changes. *Discussion of his role helps improve the client's understanding of the situation.*

- Serve as a role model for learning new behaviors; facilitate opportunities for the client to role play new adaptive behaviors. Provide positive reinforcement for use of new behaviors. *Role modeling and role playing promote increased client participation in care and positive coping responses. Positive reinforcement enhances the continued use of adaptive behaviors.*

> *1/7/13: The client discusses feelings and demonstrates a beginning ability to use adaptive behaviors with a decreasing emphasis on physical complaints. She verbalizes fewer urinary symptoms and balance problems. She mentions being able to fold clothes, sort mail, and make grocery lists.*
>
> *K. Benes, RN*

Nursing Diagnosis: Caregiver Role Strain (husband) related to client's increased dependency needs and inability of client to provide self-care independently as evidenced by husband's statements of being exhausted and burned out and cessation of social activities.

NOC: Caregiver Physical/Emotional Health and Caregiver–Patient Relationship: Client will demonstrate participation in care activities.

NIC: Caregiver Support

- Acknowledge the difficulties of the caregiving role and of the client's dependency on her husband. Encourage the caregiver to give attention to the client in ways unrelated to her physical complaints. *Doing so will minimize the client's need to gain attention through a "sick role." It also will help reestablish husband-wife roles.*

- Encourage the client to participate in one activity outside the home per week. Offer positive reinforcement for any activity performed. Encourage the caregiver to slowly resume social activities with the client. *Engaging in an activity outside the home in conjunction with positive reinforcement provides an opportunity for the client to experience success at leaving the home and expanding her circle of experience. Social activities will help reverse the social isolation, promote a feeling of togetherness as a couple, provide an outlet for the caregiver, and help the client regain a more balanced sense of self as a friend and companion of others.*

(continues on page 464)

Case in Point 24.1 (continued)

Rose and Andrew's Story

- Monitor caregiver for indicators of stress; teach caregiver stress management techniques; encourage caregiver participation in support groups. *Stress management techniques and support groups are positive coping strategies to deal with the demands of caregiving.*
- Provide encouragement to the caregiver during times of client setback; support him in setting limits and taking care of himself. *Encouragement provides positive feedback to the caregiver and helps to decrease feelings of powerlessness. Limit setting and self-care are important in maintaining the caregiver's health and ability to function.*

NIC: Respite Care
- Monitor the endurance of the caregiver. Help the couple identify other family members who can assist; arrange for a substitute caregiver as necessary. *Assistance from others reduces the stress associated with the role of a constant caregiver.*

NIC: Presence
- Demonstrate acceptance; verbally communicate empathy or understanding of the client's experience. *An accepting attitude and demonstration of empathy are key to establishing a trusting*

relationship; the client needs to feel that others hear her complaints and understand her.
- Limit time spent discussing physical complaints; help the client realize that help is available but do not reinforce dependent behaviors. Stay with the client and provide assurance of safety and security during periods of anxiety; be available for the caregiver. *Limit setting helps the client to focus on feelings rather than the physical manifestations and aids in reducing dependency issues. This in turn helps alleviate some of the stress of the caregiver. Being available conveys understanding of the client's problems and caregiver's needs and helps to reduce anxiety for both.*

> 4/9/13: The couple reports that the client has increased her level of participation in activities and exhibited less reliance on the husband for care. The couple have engaged their children to help different days of the week so that the father can get some rest and relief from caregiving. The client also has been going to church once a week and eating dinner at her daughter's house on Friday nights.
>
> K. Benes, RN

EPILOGUE

Rose and Andrew have been meeting with a therapist for the past 8 months. Rose has not developed any new physical complaints. She reports that she still has pain but "it's not as bad." She has begun to help around the house with laundry, setting the table, and "some cooking." Andrew mentions that he still helps Rose but is feeling less exhausted. "Over the last few weeks, Rose had been getting up in the morning and making us coffee." When asked about their activities, Rose smilingly says, "I went to the grocery store with my neighbor for the first time last week. And next week, Andrew and I are going out to dinner with our son." Rose and Andrew plan to continue with therapy.

which outlines nursing care for a client who has somatization disorder.

The primary care coordinator and multidisciplinary team members collaborate. Coordinating care is vital to preventing clients from seeking multiple appointments with different team members. Possible nursing interventions, derived from the Nursing Interventions Classification, include **Anxiety Reduction, Body Image Enhancement, Calming Technique, Cognitive Restructuring, Coping Enhancement, Emotional Support, Security Enhancement, Self-Awareness Enhancement,** and **Self-Esteem Enhancement** (Bulechek et al., 2008).

Establishing a Trusting Relationship
The gold standard in caring for these clients is to establish a trusting relationship with them. This includes making and keeping periodic appointments spaced at appropriate intervals—weekly at first. Regular and planned appointments prevent clients from changing, canceling, or otherwise manipulating

times. Care coordinators, in consultation with medical care providers, work with clients to communicate the terms and goals of the care plan.

A crucial component is empathy. Clients need to feel that others hear their complaints and understand what they are experiencing. Therapeutic interventions might include responses such as "I hear that it has been a very difficult time for you. I can't imagine how trying it has been to get through all of this." Empathy serves several purposes. One is to establish a connection between care provider and client so that the provider conveys an understanding of the client's difficulties. The second is that empathy highlights the "feeling" or "emotional" aspect of the experience, which is what clients have difficulty verbalizing. Empathic statements serve as a powerful method for establishing trust while modeling the expression of emotional feelings and encouraging clients to engage in emotional, rather than physical, expressions of discomfort (Evidence-Based Practice Spotlight 24.2).

EVIDENCE-BASED PRACTICE SPOTLIGHT 24.2

Interventions for Body Dysmorphic Disorder

Overview of Effective Treatment: Clinical trials have shown that SRIs are effective for BDD. Trials of fluvoxamine, sertraline, and fluoxetine reduce the symptoms of obsession-compulsion often present in BDD. SSRIs also have been found effective to help control skin picking. Clomipramine (SRI) was more effective than desipramine, a tricyclic antidepressant.

These clients also benefit from a course of therapy combined with cognitive–behavioral techniques. Exposure and response prevention techniques encourage clients to expose themselves to situations where their perceived bodily flaw or defect is open to others. Clients are not allowed to hide or camouflage the defect. Response prevention techniques prohibit clients from performing activities that reduce the anxiety created by the perceived flaw. So, for example, clients are not allowed to check mirrors or ask others for reassurance about their appearance. Psychoeducation about BDD is helpful, as is follow-up with assertiveness training and behavioral modeling of socially appropriate skills.

What Has Not Been Shown Effective: Clinical assessment in which practitioners attempt to ensure clients with BDD that their symptoms do not exist (ie, that they are attractive) does not work. Nonpsychiatric treatment such as surgery or cosmetic procedures to correct the perceived defect is not likely to be effective. Some clients may even fixate on new appearance preoccupations following surgical procedures. Long-term psychodynamic psychotherapy has not been shown effective with these clients.

Implications for Practice: An empathic relationship is important because it is the foundation for any course of therapy that clients undergo. Attempts at reassurance that perceived deficits are imaginary are likely to backfire and may undermine the therapeutic alliance. Psychoeducation and cognitive–behavioral techniques enable clients to examine dysfunctional beliefs about their appearance and empower them to actively participate in therapy. Encouragement is most beneficial.

References

Allen, A., & Hollander, E. (2000). Body dysmorphic disorder. *Psychiatric Clinics of North America, 23*(3), 617–628.

Carroll, D. H., Scahill, L., & Phillips, K. A. (2002). Current concepts in body dysmorphic disorder. *Archives of Psychiatric Nursing, 16*(2), 72–79.

Cororve, M. B., & Gleaves, D. H. (2001). Body dysmorphic disorder: A review of conceptualizations, assessment, and treatment strategies. *Clinical Psychology Review, 21*(6), 949–970.

Grant, J. E., Menard, W., & Phillips, K. A. (2006). Pathological skin picking in individuals with body dysmorphic disorder. *General Hospital Psychiatry, 28,* 487–493.

Hollander, E., Allen, A., Kwon, J., Aronowitz, B., Schmeidler, J., Wong, C., & Simeon, D. (1999). Clomipramine vs desipramine crossover trial in body dysmorphic disorder: Selective efficacy of a serotonin reuptake inhibitor in imagined ugliness. *Archives of General Psychiatry, 56*(11), 1033–1039.

Ipser, J. (2008). Pharmacotherapy and psychotherapy for body dysmorphic disorder. *Cochrane Database of Systematic Reviews, 2008*(1). Retrieved from EBSCO*host.*

Neziroglu, F., & Khemlani-Patel, S. (2003). Therapeutic approaches to body dysmorphic disorder. *Brief Treatment and Crisis Intervention, 3,* 307–322.

Phillips, K. A., Albertini, R. S., & Rasmussen, S. A. (2002). A randomized placebo-controlled trial of fluoxetine in body dysmorphic disorder. *Archives of General Psychiatry, 59,* 381–388.

Rabinowitz, D., Neziroglu, F., & Roberts, M. (2007). Clinical application of a behavioral model for the treatment of body dysmorphic disorder. *Cognitive and Behavioral Practice, 14,* 231–237.

Wilhelm, S., Phillips, K. A., Fama, J. M., Greenberg, J. L., & Steketee, G. (2011). Modular cognitive–behavioral therapy for body dysmorphic disorder. *Behavior Therapy,* doi:10.1016/j.beth.2011.02.002

Williams, J., Hadjistavropoulos, T., & Sharpe, D. (2006). A meta-analysis of psychological and pharmacological treatments for body dysmorphic disorder. *Behaviour Research and Therapy, 44,* 99–111.

Managing Ineffective Coping

One primary manifestation of somatoform disorders is excessive use of health care services. Nurses encourage discussion about frequent visits to physicians, focusing on how clients feel when scheduling and going to visits. For example, "Can you talk about Dr. Jones and how it has been for you to go to him?" Nurses do not explore symptoms. For example, they avoid statements such as "Why did you go to see Dr. Jones?" or "What did you tell the doctor was wrong with you?"

Nurses use the opportunity to learn about the client's perception of physicians and to assess the dynamics of health-seeking behaviors. Clients frequently express angry, negative feelings about their health care providers, focusing on how others have been unable to find a physiologic cause for their complaints. Nurses inquire about how this feels, helping clients

to express anger and frustration. Verbalization of such feelings can be powerful.

It usually takes time before clients can begin to express feelings. Many clients with somatoform disorders have a strong tendency to revert to talking about physical problems (eg, low back pain, headaches). Gently refocusing them provides a model for moving toward expressing feelings, rather than describing physical states. Over time, this modeling can help clients become more familiar with how it feels to discuss emotions instead of physical problems. Nurses provide positive reinforcement when clients discuss feelings (Therapeutic Communication 24.1).

Care coordinators also can collaborate with primary physicians to facilitate periodic, appropriately timed appointments. Such planning fosters trust between clients and physicians and helps establish productive long-term relationships. At the same

Therapeutic Communication 24.1

Addressing Somatization Disorder

The dialogues are between Rose from Case in Point 24.1 and her nurse, with whom she has established a therapeutic relationship. They have been working together for 2 weeks, meeting biweekly in the psychiatric outpatient unit.

Ineffective Dialogue

NURSE: Good morning, Rose. I noticed you arrived early today and had a chance to get some coffee already. Are you ready to start? *(Tries to begin without making any references to Rose's body and focusing on the day's events)*

ROSE: Yes, I got up really early today. *(Sounds and appears exhausted, and her speech lacks energy)* My back and hip pain and my dizziness bothered me all night. I could hardly sleep; I was up and down the entire night. I'm so exhausted!

NURSE: Really? I'm sorry. Where was the pain? *(Note: Rose has undergone a thorough physical examination, which revealed no arthritis, joint problems, inflammatory processes, or other medical conditions. Pain and dizziness have been long-standing complaints.)*

ROSE: Well, it started at first at the bottom of my spine, then it went up my back and then down into my right hip. At the same time, I start to get real dizzy. From my hip, it goes to my legs, usually, and sometimes even my ankles. I've had trouble with that hip before, too. Last year, I ended up on bed rest when it got so sore.

NURSE: But it's great that you could get up this morning. *(Tries to refocus and give positive reinforcement about Rose's activity)*

ROSE: Well, if you want to call it "great," yeah. It's pathetic that "great" is a word that describes just getting out of bed. Most people do that without even thinking, so I wouldn't call it "great." This whole problem is causing me a lot of pain, and I know it is going to go around my body, joint by joint.

NURSE: How do you know that?

ROSE: Because that's what it always does.

NURSE: When has it done this before?

ROSE: Well, last winter, I had a really bad bout of dizziness and joint pain that circulated through all my joints—my hips, back, shoulders, knees, and then ankles. I was a mess! It was the worst thing I've ever been through! *(Continues a lively discussion of her history and the pain and comfortably avoids the work of talking about her feelings)*

Effective Dialogue

NURSE: Good morning, Rose. I noticed you arrived early today and had a chance to get some coffee already. Are you ready to start?

ROSE: Yes, I got up really early today. *(Sounds and appears exhausted, and her speech lacks energy)* My back and hip pain bothered me all night. I could hardly sleep; I'm so exhausted!

NURSE: When you got here was the coffee made already? I know you like your coffee.

ROSE: Yeah, it was. Your office manager is so nice. He offers me coffee as soon as I arrive. But, I have to tell you, it was very hard to pick up the cup because I was still dizzy, and my hands and fingers were so stiff. *(Returns to bodily sensations)*

NURSE: Rose, I notice that you mentioned how nice Tom is, but you quickly began to talk about your pain again. *(Observes and reflects the pattern of communication to reinforce that Rose has difficulty staying away from the topic of her body)*

ROSE: Well, I guess so. But I thought about it because I was talking about the coffee. I can't help it. *(Sounds irritated but acknowledges her behavior)*

NURSE: Rose, we've discussed how your focus on your body is unconscious, so I realize that sometimes you can't help it. You're working so hard to become better able to observe yourself and to notice when you do this. *(Uses positive reinforcement carefully)*

ROSE: I think so, but it is such hard work. Sometimes I feel like I'm being criticized.

NURSE: I noticed that you sounded a bit irritated with me, like you needed to defend yourself. How do you feel when I raise the topic of your focusing on your body? *(Realizes that Rose is progressing with self-observation. Takes the opportunity to ask how Rose feels about confrontation.)*

ROSE: Well, I don't know. I wasn't mad. I just felt criticized.

NURSE: Sometimes when we work on the issues of your body and talk about feelings, it may seem like criticism. A very normal emotional response is anger. *(Continues to focus on one emotional or feeling aspect of the exchange. She is trying to [1] point out that anger is normal, and [2] help Rose to understand that her emotions are normal responses to events.)*

Reflection and Critical Thinking

- In addition to the responses of the nurse in the effective dialogue, give two other examples of potentially therapeutic responses.
- How do you feel about giving positive and negative reinforcement? Can you link these behaviors to the concepts of "sick role" and "healthy role?" Give another example of how providing positive reinforcement can prematurely push a client with somatization disorder into the "healthy role."
- Carry on a conversation with another student and attempt to focus only on physical symptoms (with no references to feelings or emotions) throughout the conversation. Try to understand what it would feel like if you had somatization disorder. Ask your partner how it feels to have someone dwell on physical sensations.

time, it is imperative for care coordinators to maintain frequent contact with primary physicians. Physicians should be aware of all treatment goals and ideally should participate in planning. Calling at least once every 1 to 2 months and sending copies of a client's care plan and progress notes will maintain contact and provide physicians with an overview of the therapeutic goals and interventions.

When speaking with physicians, nurses ascertain that they are continuing to monitor the client's physical health. Frequently, because clients somatize so much, physicians become "immune" to their complaints and can miss critical changes in health. Nurses explore when physical examinations and routine diagnostic tests have been scheduled. They convey to clients that health care providers are making a team effort to protect health.

Depending on how much care-seeking behavior clients display, it may be advantageous to contract with clients not to obtain health care from any unknown provider without speaking with their primary provider first. Often, referrals are necessary for insurance purposes. If not, it is helpful for clients to understand that their primary providers are working closely to determine the best plan of care and should be included collaboratively in decisions for further medical intervention. Clients who know this can feel "taken care of" and reassured that the team is concerned about their welfare.

Addressing Powerlessness and Dependency

Care coordinators work with clients over time to establish and maintain a regular schedule of therapy sessions. Doing so helps prevent clients from developing more physical symptoms to ensure that their needs are met.

Therapists encourage clients to speak to their feelings rather than focusing on physical complaints. They do so by limiting time during the session spent reviewing symptoms (eg, "Can you take the first 15 minutes to update me as to how you are feeling physically, and then we will spend the rest of the time talking about how things are going in your life at home?"), or indirectly, by guiding the discussion away from symptoms toward emotional feelings and reactions to events.

Enhancing Self-Esteem

Encouraging clients to complete small activities between visits enhances independence and self-esteem. Keeping activities small and manageable avoids pressuring clients to divest themselves of the "sick role" too soon. Activities such as gathering materials for bathing or setting the table for a meal without any help from a caregiver are examples of tasks clients can perform. Taking small steps allows clients to experience success and minimizes the anxiety they may associate with being expected to abandon the sick role and become more independent.

Nurses identify character strengths with clients or discuss history, focusing on positive events involving success and independence, while avoiding excessive praise about the past activity (eg, statements such as "It was wonderful that you were able to do that, and it probably really helped you feel better, don't you think?"). This type of praise often increases anxiety for clients because they may perceive that health care providers expect

them quickly to regain independence. Instead, nurses provide positive reinforcement for the ability of clients to reminisce about the events (eg, "It's great that you can talk about that and describe what it was like for you."). Such responses help clients to talk about emotional events (instead of about physical feelings); they also help boost self-esteem. At the same time, they do not uproot clients from the "sick role" that is still so important.

Reducing Anxiety

Nurses encourage clients to engage in anxiety-reducing activities, including relaxation, meditation, and yoga. They frequently assess responses of clients to these therapies because some relaxation modalities (eg, progressive muscle relaxation) may cause clients to focus increasingly on bodily sensations and thus may be countertherapeutic. Quiet reading, arts and crafts, and low-impact aerobics may be alternative interventions (Figure 24.3).

Reestablishing Social Activities

Nurses plan for clients to participate in one social activity during the week between sessions. Such activities could be as simple as going to the grocery store or riding in the car with a friend. They should be activities that clients must perform outside the home for some time. The purpose is to provide a chance for clients to experience success at leaving the home and expanding their circle of experience. Nurses provide positive but gentle reinforcement for any activities.

Reestablishing Functional Family Processes

Care coordinators must assess family dynamics and functioning to determine what effects a client's illness has had on the family. They can hold a family meeting to discover and discuss the nature of problems. This must be done carefully to avoid making the family feel that the concerns of clients are invalid (see Chap. 15).

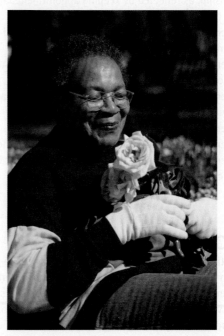

FIGURE 24.3 **This client with somatoform illness is benefiting from gardening and resting outdoors.**

Many times, relatives of clients with somatoform disorders have difficulty relating directly to one another. They may be uncomfortable verbalizing thoughts and feelings during the family meeting. Instead, they may focus on the client's symptoms or the problems that they and their loved one have experienced with medical care. Therapists also must work with family members to target needed supports for clients. Although dealing with relatives who have somatoform disorders can be exhausting, family members frequently have sufficient energy to participate. If family members are willing, therapists can schedule several sessions to provide support and to give suggestions about how to help clients.

Empathizing with clients about physical discomfort is important while simultaneously encouraging family members to assist clients to become more independent. One of the most effective interventions is to provide much empathy to clients within the family setting while providing suggestions for family interventions. For example, "As we can all see, Rose is having great difficulty with her back pain, but perhaps we can help her to do some small tasks even with the pain she is feeling."

> ### Think About It 24.1
> Review Case in Point 24.1. Imagine that both Rose and Andrew are 20 years younger and have three children, ages 16, 13, and 11 years. How might Rose's disorder affect the family?

▲ EVALUATION

Nurses determine whether treatment goals have been met by evaluating responses to interventions. Indicators of effective interventions include the following:

- The client's trust has been established within the therapeutic relationship, as reflected by keeping appointments and following the treatment plan.
- The client experiences fewer physical symptoms and visits to nonprimary health care providers.
- The client can discuss emotions and feelings rather than focusing on physical complaints.
- The client can make positive self-statements and manage ADLs with increasing independence.
- The client reports improvement in anxiety level.
- The client has engaged in social activities outside the home.
- The client and family can manage stressors without focusing on the client's physical status.

DISSOCIATIVE DISORDERS

Dissociation means altering self-awareness in an effort to escape an upsetting event or feeling. This normal method of self-preservation against emotionally overloaded situations happens when neither resistance nor escape is possible. It can include actively pretending to be somewhere or someone else, experiencing amnesia, or being able to "cut off" pain perception from body regions. The cognitive outcome is fragmented memory, which can lead to patchy or disorganized recall, seemingly illogical associations, and extreme affective reactions (eg, rage in response to relatively minor interpersonal "offenses").

Despite extensive published literature on dissociative disorders, dissociation remains poorly understood and controversial. Because of the lack of systematic study, little empirical information is available. Much of the research addresses dissociation as a symptom of anxiety disorders, personality disorders, and affective disorders rather than dissociation as the Axis I diagnosis. The field has advanced based on anecdotal experience, poorly designed studies, and polemical arguments. Published investigations have many methodologic flaws. The morass of literature on dissociative phenomena includes both advocates and critics.

Currently, most psychiatrists believe that dissociation is a legitimate phenomenon. They also believe that its most dramatic manifestation, **dissociative identity disorder** (DID), formerly known as multiple personality disorder, rarely occurs spontaneously but is easy to create. Student nurses reading this chapter are urged to keep an open mind and to understand that this area of psychopathology is poorly developed.

All humans have the capacity to dissociate. Acts of daydreaming or amnestic episodes constitute common examples (Hunter et al., 2004). In some cultures, voluntary experiences of trance or meditation are accepted practices and should not be considered psychiatric disorders (Cultural Spotlight 24.1).

> ## Cultural *Spotlight* 24.1
>
> ### Dissociative Cultural Phenomena
>
> Cultural considerations include the acknowledgment that trance states are seen in some cultures, including those from Indonesia, Malaysia, the Arctic, India, and Latin America. Indeed, dissociative phenomena occur around the world. They seem to be more prevalent in the less heavily industrialized, developing countries (Maldonado & Spiegel, 2004).
>
> Trance states function as part of a system of spiritual beliefs. In **dissociative trance**, a person's awareness of his or her immediate surroundings narrows. The person also may exhibit stereotyped behaviors, such as immobilization, collapse, or loud shrieking beyond his or her control. *Possession trance* in these cultures involves acquiring a new identity that is attributed to the influence of a spirit, power, deity, or other person. For diagnostic purposes, an individual must be experiencing dysfunction and stress, and the behaviors noted must not be a normal part of a broadly accepted collective cultural or religious practice (APA, 2000).
>
> Research shows that DID can be misdiagnosed in the Latino population because *ataque de nervios* is accepted as a diagnosis for this group, yet it has symptoms similar to DID. Amnesia is a predominant symptom of *ataque* and often is a culturally acceptable reaction to stress within the Latino community. The condition has a lifetime prevalence of 13.8% in Puerto Rico (Lewis-Fernandez et al., 2002). Although many Latinos consider it normal, it may be associated with other psychiatric disorders (Guarnaccia et al., 2005).

Conceptually, dissociation differs from repression in several different ways. *Repression* is hypothesized to result from intrapsychic conflicts (see Chap. 3). Dissociation is hypothesized to result from external trauma. Moreover, in dissociation, the information is kept out of awareness for a sharply delimited period, whereas in repression information is kept out of awareness for a long time (Maldonado & Spiegel, 2004). In other words, "repressed" memories in dissociation are specific to events.

When is dissociation a problem? Because mild states usually do not cause much difficulty in daily functioning, dissociation can be conceptualized on a continuum (Figure 24.4) or as a typology. In the continuum model, pathologic dissociation occurs when a person experiences more frequent or "deeper" states of dissociation. Everyday functioning deteriorates as a person moves from left to right along the continuum. In the typology model, pathologic dissociation represents a different kind of dissociative experience altogether. Each model seems to account for some of what is seen clinically (Putnam, 1997).

Dissociation leading to impaired functioning requires treatment. The degree of disruption of the self and the intensity and types of interventions vary.

Incidence and Prevalence

Fifty years ago, dissociative disorders were considered rare. During the 1980s and 1990s, the number of reported cases, especially of DID, increased precipitously and exponentially. Some experts assert that dissociative disorders may have been underdiagnosed in the past (Foote et al., 2006). A recent Finnish study found a 3.4% prevalence of dissociation in a nonclinical population (Maaranen et al., 2004). In Israel, where almost half of mental health professionals still doubt the existence of dissociative disorders, researchers using a Structured Clinical Interview found that 12% to 21% of 81 psychiatric clients met the *DSM-IV-TR* criteria for DIDs (Ginzberg et al., 2010). Other surveys demonstrate that transient experiences of depersonalization and derealization often occur in healthy people under conditions of fatigue or stress. The rate varies from lifetime estimates of 26% to 74% and from 31% to 66% during a traumatic event (Hunter et al., 2004).

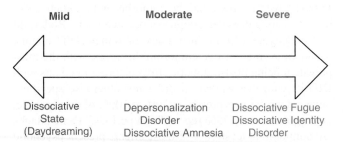

FIGURE 24.4 In the continuum model of dissociation, a range of behaviors from mild to severe may account for such experiences. The mild end includes everyday occurrences, such as briefly "zoning out" or daydreaming. The severe end includes fugue states and DID.

Etiology

The etiology of dissociative disorders is not known. Various substances or medical conditions can induce dissociative symptoms. For example, a seizure disorder or prolonged use of alcohol may cause amnesia. Clients experiencing such symptoms therefore must undergo a thorough medical evaluation before a definitive diagnosis of dissociative disorder is made.

These clients appear to be particularly susceptible to hypnotism and suggestion, with low sedation thresholds (APA, 2000; International Society for the Study of Dissociation [ISSD], 2005). The ability to dissociate is believed partly related to having the biologic capacity to do so when subjected to repeated stress (Fink, 1991). Physiologic studies suggest that excessive cortical arousal may precipitate dissociative reactions. Such arousal triggers reactive inhibition of signals in sensorimotor pathways through negative feedback relationships between the cerebral cortex and the brainstem reticular formation (Lowenstein & Putnam, 2005). Preliminary research on brain structures supports a hypothesis that the volumes of the hippocampus, parahippocampal gyrus, and amygdala are smaller in clients with DID than in control participants (Ehling et al., 2008). Further study is needed to determine whether structural changes are caused by or are the effects of cortical arousal.

Although the empirical literature does not support the popular contention that dissociative phenomena are more common in people who were abused as children, some clients with dissociative disorders have a background of family dysfunction. Those who connect history of abuse with dissociation believe the phenomenon stems from using "blocking" or amnesia to separate oneself from traumatic experiences. Over time, clients use dissociation as a form of coping with stressful events. Family dynamics found in abusive families may contribute to dissociative behaviors. Chapter 33 discusses dysfunctional family systems and the psychological consequences of child abuse.

Signs and Symptoms/Diagnostic Criteria

The *DSM-IV-TR* defines **dissociative disorders** as "a disruption in the usually integrated functions of consciousness, memory, identity, or perception"; the disturbance may be "sudden or gradual, transient or chronic" (APA, 2000, p. 519). This definition includes four disorders (*DSM-IV-TR* Box 24.2):

1. **Depersonalization disorder** is characterized by a recurring or persistent feeling that one is detached from one's own thinking. Affected clients feel that they are outside their mind or body, much like an observer.
2. **Dissociative amnesia** is characterized by loss of memory that is not organic and involves an inability to recall events or facts too extensive to be labeled as mere forgetfulness.
3. **Dissociative fugue** involves sudden travel away from home coupled with an inability to remember the past and confusion about identity or the adoption of a new identity.

DSM-IV-TR BOX 24.2

Dissociative Disorders

Dissociative Fugue

A. The predominant disturbance is sudden, unexpected travel away from home or one's customary place of work, with inability to recall one's past.

B. Confusion about personal identity or assumption of a new identity (partial or complete).

C. The disturbance does not occur exclusively during the course of Dissociative Identity Disorder and is not due to the direct physiologic effects of a substance (eg, a drug of abuse, a medication) or a general medical condition (eg, temporal lobe epilepsy).

D. The symptoms cause clinically significant distress or impairment in social, occupational, or other important areas of functioning.

Dissociative Amnesia

A. The predominant disturbance is one or more episodes of inability to recall important personal information, usually of a traumatic or stressful nature, that is too extensive to be explained by ordinary forgetfulness.

B. The disturbance does not occur exclusively during the course of Dissociative Identity Disorder, Dissociative Fugue, Post-Traumatic Stress Disorder, Acute Stress Disorder, or Somatization Disorder and is not due to the direct physiologic effects of a substance (eg, a drug of abuse, a medication) or a neurologic or other general medical condition (eg, Amnestic Disorder Due to Head Trauma).

C. The symptoms cause clinically significant distress or impairment in social, occupational, or other important areas of functioning.

Depersonalization Disorder

A. Persistent or recurrent experiences of feeling detached from, and as if one is an outside observer of one's mental processes or body (eg, feeling like one is in a dream).

B. During the depersonalization experience, reality testing remains intact.

C. The depersonalization causes clinically significant distress or impairment in social, occupational, or other important areas of functioning.

D. The depersonalization experience does not occur exclusively during the course of another mental disorder, such as Schizophrenia, Panic Disorder, Acute Stress Disorder, or another Dissociative Disorder, and is not due to the direct physiologic effects of a substance (eg, a drug of abuse, a medication) or a general medical condition (eg, temporal lobe epilepsy).

Dissociative Identity Disorder

A. The presence of two or more distinct identities or personality states (each with its own relatively enduring pattern of perceiving, relating to, and thinking about the environment and self).

B. At least two of these identities or personality states recurrently take control of the person's behavior.

C. Inability to recall important personal information that is too extensive to be explained by ordinary forgetfulness.

D. The disturbance is not due to the direct physiologic effects of a substance (eg, blackouts or chaotic behavior during Alcohol Intoxication) or a general medical condition (eg, complex partial seizures).

Note: In children, the symptoms are not attributable to imaginary playmates or other fantasy play.

Reprinted with permission from the *Diagnostic and Statistical Manual of Mental Disorders, Fourth Edition, Text Revision* (Copyright © 2000). American Psychiatric Association.

4. In DID, clients acquire two or more identities or personality states (**alters**) who take control over their behavior. Each alter has its own traits, behavior patterns, memories, and ways of engaging in interpersonal relationships. Clients usually have a primary personality, but alters can emerge (usually during times of great stress) with wildly different characteristics (Case Vignette 24.1). As with amnesia, DID involves an inability to recall important personal information that is too extensive to be labeled as forgetfulness. During periods of "altered" personality, clients may not be able to remember objective events or things that happened to them.

The *DSM-IV-TR* also includes a fifth category, *dissociative disorder not otherwise specified* (NOS). These disorders have a dissociative symptom as a primary feature but do not meet criteria for any of the four dissociative disorders. Examples include brainwashing, loss of consciousness

not attributable to a medical condition, and trance disorder. In this definition, trance disorder is not a normal part of a broadly accepted collective cultural or religious practice.

Comorbidities and Dual Diagnoses

Dissociative disorders may be comorbid with addictive behaviors, eating disorders, depression, and anxiety. Rodewald and colleagues (2011), in a study of female DID clients, found an average of five comorbid disorders, with the most prevalent being post-traumatic stress disorder in clients with DID or with dissociative disorder not otherwise specified. Severe depression is present in 70% to 100% of these people, and approximately 75% report "high periods." Panic attacks are common: at least 90% of these clients present psychotic symptoms (APA, 2000; ISSD, 2005). Dissociative disorders have been identified as the strongest predictor of multiple suicide attempts (Foote et al., 2008).

Case Vignette 24.1

Susan, a 20-year-old, part-time college student, is admitted to a psychiatric unit for evaluation of suicidal ideation. A psychological history reveals that Susan attempted suicide 2 years ago by cutting her wrists. When Susan was a child, an uncle physically and sexually abused her for approximately 7 years. Susan first sought psychiatric treatment at 17 years of age and was diagnosed with major depression with borderline personality disorder. Separate trials with several antidepressant medications failed to provide relief from her symptoms, which included self-destructive thoughts, feelings of hopelessness, and occasional mood swings.

During this hospitalization, Susan admits to hearing voices and having an imaginary companion who has "tried to protect her" since childhood. As her treatment progresses, she begins to exhibit different childlike behaviors and trancelike positions. Her subjective distress also increases, and she begins saying "I just want to die" and trying to cut and burn herself. During therapy, Susan exhibits two alternate personalities, "Betty" and "Barb." Barb, the older of the two "alters," tries to protect Betty, the abused child.

Reflection and Critical Thinking

- What issues may have contributed to a delayed or missed diagnosis in this client?
- What priorities are most important for Susan at this time? How can the nurse best intervene?

▲

Interdisciplinary Goals and Treatment

The treatment goal is for clients to learn how to control symptoms and distress. The best way to do so is a controversial subject that philosophically divides mental health care providers. One group of therapists believes that DID is a unique diagnosis, requiring involved exploration of alters and recovered memories and other distinct treatment modalities. The other group believes that well-meaning but misguided therapists induce the dramatic symptoms of DID—multiple alters and recovered memories—and that other diagnoses (eg, somatoform disorder, personality disorder) can explain the basic symptoms of these clients. This second group further believes that therapists must take care to avoid insinuating the presence of alters or a history of abuse in suggestible clients. Naturally, these diametrically opposed conceptual models yield very different treatment approaches (Lowenstein & Putnam, 2005).

Checkpoint Questions

3. Which disorder is characterized by sudden travel away from home coupled with an inability to remember the past and confusion about identity or the adoption of a new identity?

4. What is the overall treatment goal for the client with DID?

Individual Therapy

The onset of dissociative amnesia and dissociative fugue often is acute, and supporting clients in talking about recent events may prompt rapid recovery of memory. If talking alone is not effective, hypnosis may help prompt clients to reveal events and feelings and ultimately assist in restoring memory. However, many experts deny that hypnosis is an effective memory retrieval tool, and little empirical evidence substantiates its use as such. Indeed, most evidence suggests that hypnosis is not an effective method of recovering memory and that it increases suggestibility (Offshe & Watters, 1994). An interview using amobarbital sodium (Amytal Sodium, "truth serum") was once considered effective; however, this technique is no longer recommended because of poor outcomes (Maldonado & Spiegel, 2004; North & Yutzy, 1997).

Supporting clients with depersonalization disorder to talk about antecedent events surrounding feelings of anxiety and then planning behavioral techniques to cope with stressful situations are effective treatment strategies. Some experts advocate a modified cognitive–behavioral approach in the treatment of dissociative disorders (Fine, 1999). This therapy involves following a protocol of structured cognitive–behavioral interventions that promotes symptom relief for the client and also lays the foundation for subsequent intensive integration of the separate "ego states" into a unified whole. The primary goal is ensuring the stabilization and safety of the client while promoting relief of the dissociative symptoms.

Group Therapy

Although group therapy may be helpful for people with a dissociative process that is less severe than DID, the value of group therapy must be carefully assessed for clients with DID. Group work may be too intense and threatening for these clients, and the type of group should be evaluated carefully. In general, a highly structured group with a clear focus and time frame seems most useful.

As clients with dissociative disorder progress in their recovery, a 12-step group may be a helpful adjunct to individual therapy when their work includes recovery from addictions. However, because 12-step programs promote belief in a higher power, this concept must not overwhelm or threaten clients.

Psychopharmacology

Psychotropic medication is not a primary treatment for dissociative disorders (ISSD, 2005). However, antianxiety medications such as lorazepam may be helpful for short-term management of severe anxiety. Antidepressants also may be indicated, but clients should be evaluated individually for necessity and category of drug. The newer SSRIs can be effective for those with debilitating symptoms of comorbid depressive disorders, which occur frequently in this population (Maldonado & Spiegel, 2004).

Art Therapy

Art therapy may be a helpful adjunct when well timed and led by a trained professional who has knowledge of dissociative disorders. Art therapy encourages clients to tell their stories in a nonthreatening way; it is a safe alternative to acting out feelings destructively and can help clients and therapists gently to confront denial. For clients with DID, art can be a useful tool for promoting integration of alters. The different personalities can participate in a common activity and contribute toward a collective whole (Frye & Gannon, 1993). Other experts concur that art is invaluable as a form of therapy for clients with dissociative disorders, and it may also be useful as an aid in detecting the presence of a dissociative state or efforts to repress painful memories from a past trauma (Lev-Wiesel, 2005).

APPLYING THE NURSING PROCESS

Dissociative Disorders

▲ ASSESSMENT

Assessment of DID is imprecise. Examination of the client's behavior requires attention to multiple details. See Assessment Tool 24.2 for an inventory of questions.

Assessment with children and teens may be more difficult because symptoms may be subtler and dissociation may present in various forms. Children with dissociation may not recall information that their peers readily remember, such as the name of a teacher or important events. They may lie pathologically to cover up not knowing certain information. Trancelike states may result in attention problems at school. Difficulty concentrating is common, as are auditory hallucinations. Some experts assert that voices may be critical and abusive. Behavior problems may include aggression, anger, self-injurious behaviors, and sexual acting out.

▲ NURSING DIAGNOSIS

Possible nursing diagnoses for clients with dissociative disorders include the following (NANDA, 2007):

- **Disturbed Personal Identity** related to childhood trauma
- **Risk for Self-Mutilation** related to feelings of stress and use of maladaptive coping mechanisms
- **Risk for Suicide** related to feelings of pain and poor impulse control
- **Anxiety** related to fragmented identity and nonintegrated self
- **Ineffective Coping** related to perception of inability to control stressors and traumatic events
- **Ineffective Role Performance** related to amnestic episodes

▲ OUTCOME IDENTIFICATION AND PLANNING

Throughout the process of the client's recovery, the treatment team must maintain a sense of collaboration and congruence to provide a milieu of safety and consistency. As much as possible, the team should include the client in the planning to foster the development of empowerment and self-responsibility. Goals for clients, with integrated Nursing Outcomes Classification (NOC) labels, may include the following (Moorhead et al., 2008):

- **Distorted Thought Control:** The client will have fewer episodes of dissociation, depersonalization, use of alters, or fugue.
- **Identity:** The client will be able to recall recent and past events.
- **Coping:** The client will demonstrate adaptive coping strategies and gain emotional control.
- **Self-Mutilation Restraint:** The client will refrain from acts of self-harm.
- **Suicide Self-Restraint:** The client will control impulses and appropriately express feelings.

▲ ASSESSMENT TOOL 24.2 ▲

Inventory for Symptoms of Dissociation

- Does the client show inconsistent physical behaviors such as switching handedness, changing voices, or making frequent and marked changes in hairstyle on different occasions?
- Has the client ever been unable to remember how he or she wound up in a certain place? This behavior indicates a "blackout." In the absence of other symptoms of dissociative disorder, this finding could indicate alcohol abuse (see Chap. 30).
- Has the client written notes or created artwork of which he or she has no memory?
- Is there evidence of substance abuse or an eating disorder?
- What is the client's earliest childhood memory? For clients who report an abusive childhood, nurses should ascertain the type of abuse, its duration, and the number of people involved.

- Did the client have an imaginary childhood friend? If so, what was the nature of the relationship? Does the client still have conversations with this friend?
- Does the client have memory gaps? Are there periods that he or she cannot remember?
- Is the client sometimes accused of lying but does not think that he or she has lied?
- Does the client sometimes feel as if he or she is standing outside of himself or herself, as if watching another person?
- Does the client exhibit rapid changes in mood and thought process during one interview?
- Does the client express psychophysiologic complaints such as severe headache, chest pain, or a fluctuation in pain threshold?

▲ IMPLEMENTATION

Common labels from the Nursing Interventions Classification (NIC) for clients with dissociative disorders include, but are not limited to, **Behavior Management: Self-Harm, Body Image Enhancement, Delusion Management, Environmental Management: Violence Prevention, Hallucination Management, Reality Orientation,** and **Self-Esteem Enhancement** (Bulechek et al., 2008). All interventions involve establishing and maintaining a therapeutic alliance and helping clients correct distorted perceptions, learn new adaptive responses, practice new coping skills, and remain in the present (Kriedler et al., 2000).

The nurse's main role is to support and reinforce gains made in therapy. Specific techniques include the following:

- Educate clients about the recovery process. Clients may have idealistic fantasies of a "quick fix." They need to know that treatment may involve uncovering painful feelings and memories.
- Provide a safe, nonjudgmental environment to encourage clients to diminish defensive responses. A simple, structured environment is most helpful.

- Monitor the client's pace in uncovering memories. Manifestations that therapy is moving too fast may include attempts at self-mutilation, psychotic symptoms, and increased episodes of dissociation.
- Assist clients to learn "grounding" techniques, which bring clients into the present and remind them they are safe.
- Help clients identify times when strong emotions begin to be overwhelming. Keeping a journal of antecedents and developing a concrete plan for managing emotions are useful strategies.
- Assist clients to plan for discharge. One strategy is for clients to compile a list of people whom they can contact for support as needed. The list may include family members, friends, members of 12-step groups, and people staffing hotlines. Clients should post such lists where they can readily see them as a reminder of options and for a sense of control. Identifying safe places and comforting activities during stress helps clients continue to gain self-responsibility and self-control. See Therapeutic Communication 24.2.

Therapeutic Communication 24.2

The Client With a Dissociative Disorder

Jennifer, 24 years old, is experiencing an episode in which she does not know where she is or what is going on around her. The nurse is attempting to calm her down and orient her.

INEFFECTIVE DIALOGUE

JENNIFER: *(Crying and pacing)* Help me, help me!

NURSE: *(Looks frustrated)* Tell me what's wrong. How can I help?

JENNIFER: I'm afraid. I don't know what to do. Who are you?

NURSE: I'm the nurse. It's time for you to take your medications. *(Gives orders without providing an explanation)*

JENNIFER: Why do I need medication? I'm afraid you're trying to hurt me!

NURSE: You'll feel better if you cooperate. Please just take the medicine. *(Dismisses the client's feelings)*

JENNIFER: *(Begins to sob uncontrollably)*

EFFECTIVE DIALOGUE

JENNIFER: *(Crying and pacing)* Help me, help me!

NURSE: *(Remaining calm)* Tell me what's wrong. How can I help?

JENNIFER: I'm afraid. I don't know what to do. Who are you?

NURSE: I'm the nurse. My name is Elizabeth. I will be giving your medications today and helping you if you have a crisis or feel unsafe. *(Provides enough specific directions to orient to the "here and now")*

JENNIFER: What do I do now?

NURSE: A very important part of therapy is attending group. You should go to your groups according to your program schedule. *(Reinforces the schedule of the unit to convey structure and safety and to promote therapeutic involvement)*

JENNIFER: What if I don't remember what to do or where I am?

NURSE: I am here to help you know what to do next and to remind you where you are even if I have to tell you over and over again. Just ask me until your thoughts are clear enough for you to remember.

Reflection and Critical Thinking

- What assumptions did the first nurse make that led the interaction between her and Jennifer to go so poorly?
- Why is it important to orient the client with a dissociative disorder to the here and now?
- How can reinforcing a schedule and explaining the purpose of interventions help to ease dissociative symptoms?

Milieu Management

Clients with dissociative disorders may be hospitalized in psychiatric inpatient units when their symptoms interfere grossly with daily functioning, when they are out of touch with reality, or when they are a danger to self or others. All disciplines that work with clients with dissociative disorders are responsible for effective milieu management, but no other discipline is involved as much as nursing. Staff nurses set the tone of the unit and see that guidelines are upheld. For example, they expect clients to show involvement in the unit and exhibit appropriate behavior. Doing so conveys a sense of self-responsibility and ultimately empowerment as clients learn coping skills. They also convey that clients must verbalize, not act on, impulses related to violent and self-injurious behavior. This includes contracting with the client for safety (Stafford, 1993). As with all clients, physical restraints should be used only as a last resort because of the trauma they impose.

Other issues of concern include understanding that clients with DID may not easily accept new staff members or new peers (Stafford, 1993). People new to the milieu should give clients physical and psychological space to allow them to determine closeness. Also, staff should use touch judiciously with clients with DID and always ask first if a gesture of touch is acceptable. Because clients may have an exaggerated startle response, nurses must never touch them from behind. The best guideline is not to touch the client unless there is sound therapeutic rationale for doing so and the client's permission has been obtained.

Clients may practice new coping skills while hospitalized. These include calling a friend to discuss feelings of anxiety, focusing on topics that decrease anxiety; using reassuring self-talk; engaging in moderate exercise; and focusing on a favorite activity, such as painting, reading, singing, or watching a relaxing video (Benham, 1995).

Family Education

Dissociative disorders are difficult illnesses to explain and teach to family members. Clients frequently are misdiagnosed for years and may be treated for illnesses such as schizophrenia or bipolar disorder with psychotic features. Education is expedited when clients become aware of the gaps in time and memory.

Family education begins at diagnosis. Providing a simple explanation of the disorder, including its diagnostic criteria, is the best way to teach families about the illness. The most important feature that families need to learn is that the gaps in time and memory are critical safety issues for clients. For example, a client may get into the car and start driving without any idea of destination or reason for driving, ending up in an unknown place with strangers. Family members need to be aware of this possibility and prepared to activate an emergency search plan to locate and bring the client home quickly and safely.

▲ EVALUATION

Just as illness is a matter of degree, so too is recovery. In general, recovering clients slowly begin to trust people worth trusting. They have appropriate personal boundaries and begin to trust feelings. They also begin to try new activities with less fear and use new coping strategies to deal with anxiety.

SEXUAL DISORDERS

Disorders related to sexuality and gender identity are among the most intimate concerns any human can have. They can have significant consequences for self-concept, self-esteem, and overall quality of life.

Diverse sexual expressions involve many intrapersonal and extrapersonal factors: genetics, individual preferences, experiences, culture, and health. Because values and beliefs contribute to views regarding sexual expression, nurses must be aware of their own views and learn about the views of the clients with whom they work. In the event of a conflict of values, nurses should separate personal feelings and empathize with the sexual concerns and difficulties of clients. Empathy is essential for all therapeutic interactions. If nurses recognize that they cannot be accepting and supportive of a particular client, then they either should not work with that client or seek consultation from colleagues or supervisors on how to act professionally.

In general, sexual expression between two consenting adults that is not harmful (physically or psychologically) to either party, does not involve any force or coercion, and occurs in private is considered acceptable. Behaviors that violate these parameters (eg, pedophilia, incest, voyeurism) are not acceptable because they infringe on the will of others and are illegal.

Sexual Dysfunction

Sexual dysfunction refers to sexual expression "characterized by a disturbance in the processes that characterize the sexual response cycle or by pain associated with sexual intercourse" (APA, 2000, p. 535). In other words, it is a disruption of any of the phases of human sexual response (Box 24.2).

Few systematic epidemiologic data are available regarding the prevalence of sexual dysfunction. Results of existing research show wide variability. Differences stem from assessment methods, definitions used, and characteristics of the sample populations.

Etiology

Sexual dysfunction disorders can be *primary,* caused by various psychological and emotional conditions or a combination of psychological and medical conditions, or *secondary,* caused solely by a general medical condition or substance use. General medical conditions that may affect sexual function include injury, disease, menopause, or surgery. Substance abuse or use of some prescribed medications (including antihypertensives, antidepressants, and neuroleptics) also may contribute to sexual problems.

Changes in sexual functioning may interfere significantly with sexual expression and relationships. Clients may require referral for tests or therapy to determine the nature of the problem because there are so many potential causes.

Signs and Symptoms/Diagnostic Criteria

Sexual dysfunction is subdivided into (1) desire, (2) arousal, (3) orgasmic, or (4) pain disorders. In addition, they can be

BOX 24.2 Phases of Sexual Response

1. ***Excitement.*** *Men:* Sexual excitement is characterized by vasocongestion, which leads to rapid penile erection and scrotal tensing, thickening, and elevation. Shortening of the spermatic cords causes partial elevation of both testes, which increase in size. Men may partially lose and regain penile erection, which is normal. *Women:* The vasocongestion of sexual excitement leads to clitoral enlargement and vaginal lubrication. The vaginal orifice opens. Women may also experience nipple erection and breast enlargement.

2. ***Plateau.*** *Men:* The penile circumference thickens at the coronal ridge. Testes increase by approximately 50%. Fluid at the urethral meatus contributes to lubrication; it may contain active spermatozoa. Muscle contractions, breathing, heart rate, and blood pressure increase. *Women:* The clitoris retracts under its hood. The vagina expands while the uterus and cervix fully elevate. As in men, muscle contractions, breathing, heart rate, and blood pressure increase.

3. ***Orgasm.*** *Men:* Orgasm consists of expulsive contractions of the entire length of the urethra. Ejaculation is strongest with the first three or four contractions and then decreases. *Women:* Contractions occur very rapidly in the outer third of the vagina and labia minora.

4. ***Resolution.*** *Men:* Immediately after orgasm, vasocongestion rapidly disappears, with accompanying shrinkage in penis size. The scrotum and testes return to their normal position and size. Men also have a refractory period during which they cannot experience another erection. Length of the refractory period varies. *Women:* The clitoris returns to its normal size and position. The vagina relaxes. Women do not have a refractory period and may have multiple orgasms within a short time.

classified as lifelong or acquired, generalized or situational, or psychological or combined.

Desire Disorders

Hypoactive sexual desire disorder is characterized by persistently or recurrently deficient or absent sexual fantasies and desire for sexual activity. It may be global and encompass all sexual expression or situational and limited to one person or activity (eg, masturbation). These clients do not seek out sex, and they engage in it reluctantly if others initiate it. Hypoactive sexual desire frequently is associated with arousal or orgasm difficulties, as well as with depression. Some studies have found decreased testosterone levels in men with this problem. A lack of normative age- or gender-related data on frequency of sexual desire means that therapists must exercise clinical judgment in making this diagnosis. They should consider factors such as age in assigning it.

Sexual aversion disorder is characterized by persistent or recurrent extreme aversion to, and avoidance of, all (or most) genital sexual contact with a partner. The aversion may focus on a particular aspect (eg, genital secretions, penetration) or may be generalized to all sexual stimuli, including kissing and touching. When confronted with a sexual situation,

people with severe forms of this disorder experience panic attacks, anxiety, terror, faintness, nausea, palpitations, dizziness, and dyspnea. They may avoid sexual situations or potential sexual partners covertly (eg, going to sleep early, traveling, neglecting hygiene, abusing substances).

Arousal Disorders

In women, the arousal response includes pelvic vasocongestion, vaginal lubrication and expansion, and genital swelling. *Female sexual arousal disorder* is characterized by a persistent or recurrent inability to attain, or maintain until completion of the sexual activity, an adequate lubrication–swelling response.

In *male erectile dysfunction (ED),* clients have a persistent or recurrent inability to attain or to maintain an erection sufficient for satisfactory sexual performance. ED has different patterns. Some men report an inability to obtain any erection. Others complain of an adequate erection but losing tumescence during penetration. Others report erections sufficient for penetration that lose tumescence before or during thrusting (APA, 2000). ED is a common problem that increases with aging. One in 10 men is thought to have ED, but many are reluctant to discuss it (Case Vignette 24.2). It has no cure, but effective drug treatment is usually well tolerated.

Orgasmic Disorders

Female and *male orgasmic disorders* are marked by a persistent or recurrent delay in, or absence of, orgasm after normal

Case Vignette 24.2

George, 55 years old, is married with two teenage sons. After George arrives at the office for his annual examination, the nurse reviews his chart and sees that he was diagnosed with type 2 diabetes mellitus a few years ago but otherwise is healthy. Before the doctor performs the physical examination, the nurse asks George several questions related to his health. Toward the end of this interview, George looks down and quietly says, "I don't know how to say this. I'm not a man anymore." The nurse responds, "Tell me more about what you're experiencing."

George explains that he and his wife have not had sex for several months because he has trouble "getting turned on." He goes on to say that he felt badly when he could not satisfy his wife, and after a few times when he "couldn't do it," he stopped making sexual advances. Whenever his wife made sexual advances toward him, he "made some excuse." He asks the nurse, "Can anything be done to help me?"

Reflection and Critical Thinking

- What physical or medical factors might be contributing to George's sexual problems? What role might anxiety and emotions be playing?
- What measures should the nurse take next?

sexual excitement. **Premature ejaculation** is characterized by persistent or recurrent onset of orgasm and ejaculation with minimal sexual stimulation before, on, or shortly after penetration and before the client wishes it.

Men and women exhibit a wide variability in the type or intensity of stimulation that triggers orgasm. These diagnoses should consider the client's age and circumstances, as well as the adequacy of intensity and duration of sexual stimulation. Psychological or medical conditions may be the cause.

Pain Disorders

Dyspareunia (not from a general medical condition) is characterized by genital pain associated with sexual intercourse (men or women). Although most common during intercourse, it also may occur before or after. Intensity of symptoms can range from mild discomfort to sharp pain. **Vaginismus** (not resulting from a general medical condition) is characterized by recurrent or persistent involuntary spasms of the musculature of the outer third of the vagina that interferes with sexual intercourse. The physical obstruction caused by muscle contraction usually prevents coitus. These conditions tend to be chronic unless treated (APA, 2000).

Checkpoint Questions

5. Premature ejaculation is classified as what type of sexual dysfunction disorder?

6. What term describes genital pain associated with sexual intercourse in men or women?

Interdisciplinary Goals and Treatments

Sexual disorders affect many areas of life and frequently are intertwined with psychological disorders and physical conditions; they also may result from use of pharmacologic agents (Table 24.1). Professionals from many disciplines, including medicine, nursing, psychiatry, psychology, and social work, may contribute to treatment. The most effective strategy is a team approach with individual members working together to achieve optimal wellness for clients. Typical areas addressed include the following:

• Assessment of the couple affected by the sexual disorder
• Medication management as needed to improve sexual functioning or to provide symptom management or relief
• Education regarding "normal" sexual functioning
• Training in couple communication and sexual skills
• Couples counseling to address other issues that may exist in the couple's relationship

Treatment of specific sexual dysfunctions focuses mainly on targeting causative factors (which could be psychological, physical, or pharmacologic). For example, the goal in treating hypoactive desire disorder is to determine

and treat the cause, which could be childhood sexual abuse, hormonal imbalance, or depression (APA, 2000). Goals for aversion disorder may focus on managing anxiety symptoms; using medication, behavioral desensitization, and relaxation techniques; and uncovering and working through any underlying psychodynamic issues (eg, sexual abuse or related trauma) (APA, 2000).

Men with physiologic ED might be treated with medications, mechanical methods (eg, vacuum pump), or surgery (eg, penile prosthesis). Similarly, women with female orgasmic disorder might use a vibrator or vacuum pump (which causes engorgement of the clitoris) to facilitate orgasms. Therapy for both types of clients also might include encouragement to try activities other than intercourse for sexual fulfillment. In addition, men and women with arousal and orgasmic disorders may learn to find greater sexual pleasure by trying more foreplay, experimenting with different coital positions, and improving communication, especially about what sexual behaviors are pleasing and facilitate satisfaction. Encouragement to engage in sexual activities other than intercourse may be another way to obtain fulfillment.

When the cause of dysfunction is drug related, clients should consult with their health care provider about discontinuing the medications in question and request alternative treatment if possible. Providers may be able to prescribe a replacement drug without these side effects. If this is not possible, nurses explain the cause of the problem and encourage alterations in sexual activity as necessary. Such alterations could include longer foreplay before attempting coitus or taking another medication (if instructed by the physician) to block temporarily the action of the drug causing the sexual problem. For example, some antidepressants (especially SSRIs) cause decreased libido, ED, or anorgasmia in some clients. Cyproheptadine (Periactin), taken 1 hour before sexual intercourse, temporarily blocks the action of the SSRI, allowing the couple to enjoy sexual intercourse (Kaplan & Sadock, 2007).

Pharmacologic Therapy

Antianxiety medications sometimes are used with clients whose tension interferes with the ability to engage in sex. The SSRIs (eg, fluoxetine [Prozac]), tricyclic antidepressants, haloperidol (Haldol), lorazepam (Ativan), thioridazine (Mellaril), and monoamine oxidase inhibitors have been used to prolong sexual activity in men with premature ejaculation.

The U.S. Food and Drug Administration (FDA) has approved several medications for ED. Sildenafil (Viagra), vardenafil (Levitra), and tadalafil (Cialis) block the action of certain enzymes involved in the erectile response, achieving smooth muscle relaxation in the corpus cavernosum of the penis and allowing for the inflow of blood to the penis (National Institutes of Health, 2003). Vardenafil was found to effect erections in approximately 50% of clients who

TABLE 24.1 Psychological, Physical, and Pharmacologic Causes of Sexual Dysfunction*

Causes of Sexual Dysfunction	Types of Sexual Dysfunction
Psychological Causes	
Childhood or adult sexual abuse or trauma	Hypoactive sexual desire, sexual aversion, male and female sexual arousal disorder, male and female orgasmic disorder, vaginismus
Guilt	Female orgasmic disorder, male erectile disorder, female sexual arousal disorder, sexual aversion, vaginismus
Relationship stress, including anger or hostility toward partner and issues of control	Female orgasmic disorder, premature ejaculation, male orgasmic disorder, male erectile disorder, hypoactive sexual desire, sexual aversion, female sexual arousal disorder
Anxiety, fear, stress, including performance anxiety, fear of failure, fear of rejection, fear of pregnancy	Female orgasmic disorder, premature ejaculation, male orgasmic disorder, male erectile disorder, hypoactive sexual desire, vaginismus
Poor body image	Male erectile disorder, sexual aversion
Lack of knowledge, insufficient sexual technique	Female orgasmic disorder, male erectile disorder, dyspareunia
Cultural, religious, familial influences (past or present)	Female orgasmic disorder, male orgasmic disorder, male erectile disorder, sexual aversion
Negative attitude about sex	Male orgasmic disorder, male erectile disorder
Psychiatric illness, including anxiety (generalized) and depression	Female orgasmic disorder, male and female sexual arousal, hypoactive sexual desire
Major life changes	Hypoactive sexual desire
Physical Causes	
Infectious, inflammatory, and parasitic diseases	Female orgasmic disorder, hypoactive sexual desire, dyspareunia
Renal and urologic disorders	Male erectile disorder, dyspareunia, male and female sexual arousal disorder, hypoactive sexual desire
Local genital or pelvic pathology or trauma, congenital penile vascular or structural abnormalities	Female orgasmic disorder, male orgasmic disorder, male erectile disorder, dyspareunia, vaginismus
Endocrine disorders such as diabetes, Addison's disease, or hyperthyroidism	Female orgasmic disorder, male erectile dysfunction, hypoactive sexual desire, male and female sexual arousal disorder
Hormonal disorder	Hypoactive sexual desire, female orgasmic disorder, male erectile dysfunction, male and female sexual arousal disorder, dyspareunia
Neurologic disorders such as multiple sclerosis, Parkinson's disease, temporal lobe epilepsy, spinal cord disease, and amyotrophic lateral sclerosis	Male orgasmic disorder, premature ejaculation, female orgasmic disorder, male erectile disorder, male and female sexual arousal disorder
Surgical procedures such as perineal prostatectomy, abdominal–perineal colon resection, ileostomies and colostomies (sometimes), sympathectomy (frequently interferes with ejaculation), radical cystectomy, aortoiliac surgery, retroperitoneal lymphadenectomy	Female orgasmic disorder, male erectile disorder, hypoactive sexual desire
Radiation therapy	Male and female sexual arousal disorder
Aging	Female sexual arousal disorder, hypoactive sexual desire

(continues on page 478)

TABLE 24.1 Psychological, Physical, and Pharmacologic Causes of Sexual Dysfunction* (continued)

Causes of Sexual Dysfunction	Types of Sexual Dysfunction
Pharmacologic Causes	
Psychiatric Drugs	Male erectile disorder, hypoactive sexual desire, male and female sexual arousal disorder, male and female orgasmic disorder
Tricyclic antidepressants (eg, Tofranil, Vivactil, Elavil, Aventyl, Norpramin, Anafranil)	
Monoamine oxidase inhibitors (eg, Parnate, Actomal, Nardil, Eutonyl, Marplan)	
Lithium	
Amphetamines	
Neuroleptics	
Major tranquilizers (eg, Prolixin, Mellaril, Serentil, Trilafon, Stelazine, Reserpine, Haldol)	
Antidepressants (eg, Prozac, Asendin, Zoloft, Paxil)	
Antihypertensive Drugs	Male erectile disorder, male and female sexual arousal disorder
Catapres, Aldomet, Aldactone, Apresoline, Ismelin	
Commonly Abused Drugs	Female orgasmic disorder, male erectile disorder, male and female sexual arousal disorder, hypoactive sexual desire
Alcohol, nicotine, barbiturates, cannabis, cocaine, heroin, methadone, morphine	

* The nurse should be alert to the sexual consequences of every health issue with which the client may present. This is a list (not exhaustive) of psychological, physical, and pharmacologic causes of disrupted sexual performance. The list also presents the types of sexual dysfunction most often associated with the specific cause.

did not experience erections when taking sildenafil. Both sildenafil and vardenafil have similar half-lives and should be taken within 1 hour of having sex. Tadalafil has a longer half-life (17.5 hours) and may be taken from 30 minutes to 36 hours before having sex (Eli Lilly & Co., 2003).

Apomorphine (Uprima), another medication for the treatment of ED, is taken sublingually and produces erections in men more quickly (18 to 19 minutes after administration) than does sildenafil, vardenafil, or tadalafil. Because it is a dopamine receptor antagonist, apomorphine has also a different mechanism of action than sildenafil, vardenafil, and tadalafil. Apomorphine facilitates electrical impulses from the hypothalamus in the brain down through the spinal cord. It increases nitric oxide, which occurs naturally in the body, dilating blood vessels to get more blood flowing to the penis (Altwein & Keuler, 2001). Many other medications for the treatment of ED are in the development stages.

The "female Viagra" does not yet exist. Various herbal female sexual enhancers are available without a prescription to women. These products purport to enhance desire, excitement, and orgasm. Sildenafil (Berman et al., 2003), oral phentolamine (Rosen et al., 1999), and ephedrine (Meston, 2004) have been studied for their efficacy in treating female sexual arousal disorder (FSAD). The results of these studies suggest that all these drugs are effective for some women with FSAD. In fact, they are prescribed for women with FSAD; however, much more research is needed before the FDA approves them for such use.

> **Think About It 24.2**
> A 65-year-old man with a history of mild hypertension controlled by diet and diuretic therapy comes to the clinic for a routine physical examination. During the health history, the client states, "I've seen all these ads about Viagra and other medicines to help your sex life. Maybe I should try one." How should the nurse counsel this client?

Sex Therapy

Another treatment modality for sexual dysfunction is sex therapy. Sex therapy is a particular approach to sexual counseling practiced by master-level clinicians with specialized training in this mental health specialty. Most sex therapy currently combines cognitive and behavioral interventions with education about sexuality. Whereas the nurse generalist may be qualified to assess the client's sexual concerns and may be prepared to educate the client regarding normal sexual function, he or she generally is not prepared to provide sex therapy.

The American Association of Sex Educators, Counselors and Therapists (AASECT) is a not-for-profit, interdisciplinary professional organization whose members share an interest in promoting understanding of human sexuality and healthy sexual behavior. Their members include physicians, nurses, social workers, psychologists, allied health professionals, clergy members, lawyers, sociologists, marriage and family counselors and therapists, family planning specialists, and researchers, as well as students in relevant professional disciplines. The nurse interested in expanding his or her knowledge base in sex education can visit the AASECT web site at http://www.aasect.org.

Nursing Assessment

Collecting data about sexual values, practices, and concerns in a sensitive and professional way takes experience.

Students and inexperienced nurses should practice conducting interviews with colleagues, friends, or family until they are comfortable and confident about their skills. Throughout interviews, nurses maintain a composed, respectful, and matter-of-fact attitude. Focused and open-ended questions about less intimate material progress gradually to questions about more sensitive material (Assessment Tool 24.3).

▲ ASSESSMENT TOOL 24.3 ▲

Sexual Health History

I. Identifying data
  A. Age
  B. Sex
  C. Occupation
  D. Relationship status—single, married, number of times previously married, separated, divorced, cohabiting, serious involvement, casual dating (difficulty forming or keeping relationships should be assessed throughout the interview)
  E. Sexual orientation—heterosexual, homosexual, or bisexual (this may also be ascertained later in the interview)

II. Current functioning
  A. Unsatisfactory to highly satisfactory
  B. If unsatisfactory, why?
  C. Feeling about partner satisfaction
  D. Dysfunctions?—for example, lack of desire, erectile disorder, inhibited female arousal, anorgasmia, premature ejaculation, retarded ejaculation, pain associated with intercourse (dysfunction discussed later)
    1. Onset—lifelong or acquired
      a. If acquired, when?
      b. Did onset coincide with drug use (medications or illegal recreational drugs), life stresses (eg, loss of job, birth of child), interpersonal difficulties?
    2. Generalized—occurs in most situations or with most partners
    3. Situational
      a. Only with current partner
      b. In any committed relationship
      c. Only with masturbation
      d. In socially proscribed circumstance (eg, affair)
      e. In definable circumstance (eg, very late at night, in parental home, when partner initiated sex play)
  E. Frequency—partnered sex (coital and noncoital sex play)
  F. Desire/libido—how often are sexual feelings, thoughts, fantasies, dreams experienced (per day, week, etc.)?
  G. Description of typical sexual interaction
    1. Manner of initiation or invitation (eg, verbal or physical? Does same person always initiate?)
    2. Presence, type, and extent of foreplay (eg, kissing, caressing, manual or oral genital stimulation)

  3. Coitus? Positions used?
  4. Verbalization during sex? If so, what kind?
  5. Afterplay (whether sex act is completed or disrupted by dysfunction)? Typical activities (eg, holding, talking, return to daily activities, sleeping)?
  6. Feeling after sex: relaxed, tense, angry, loving
  H. Sexual compulsivity?—intrusion of sexual thoughts or participation in sexual activities to a degree that interferes with relationships or work, requires deception and may endanger the client

III. Past sexual history
  A. Childhood sexuality
    1. Parental attitudes about sex—degree of openness or reserve (assess unusual prudery or seductiveness)
    2. Parents' attitudes about nudity and modesty
    3. Learning about sex
      a. From parents? (Initiated by child's questions or parent volunteering information? Which parent? What was child's age?). Subjects covered (eg, pregnancy, birth, intercourse, menstruation, nocturnal emission, masturbation)?
      b. From books, magazines, or friends at school or through religious group?
      c. Significant misinformation
      d. Feeling about information
    4. Viewing or hearing primal scene—reaction?
    5. Viewing sex play or intercourse of person other than parent
    6. Viewing sex between pets or other animals
  B. Childhood sex activities
    1. Genital self-stimulation before adolescence; at what age? Reaction if apprehended?
    2. Awareness of self as boy or girl; bathroom sensual activities (regarding urine, feces, odor, enemas)?
    3. Sexual play or exploration with another child (playing doctor)—type of activity (eg, looking, manual touching, genital touching); reactions or consequences if apprehended (by whom?)

IV. Adolescence
  A. Age of onset of puberty—development of secondary sex characteristics, age of menarche for girl, wet dreams or first ejaculation for boy (preparation for and reaction to)

(continues on page 480)

ASSESSMENT TOOL 24.3   Sexual Health History (continued)

B. Sense of self as feminine or masculine—body image, acceptance by peers (opposite sex and same sex), sense of sexual desirability, onset of coital fantasies

C. Sex activities

1. Masturbation—age begun; ever punished or prohibited? Method used, accompanying fantasies, frequency (questions about masturbation and fantasies are among the most sensitive for clients to answer)

2. Homosexual activities—ongoing or rare and experimental episodes, approached by others? If homosexual, has there been any heterosexual experimentation?

3. Dating—casual or steady, description of first crush, infatuation, or first love

4. Experiences of kissing, necking, petting ("making out" or "fooling around"), age begun, frequency, number of partners, circumstances, type(s) of activity

5. Orgasm—when first experienced? (May not be experienced during adolescence.) With masturbation, during sleep, or with partner? With intercourse or other sex play? Frequency?

6. First coitus—age, circumstances, partner, reactions? (May not be experienced during adolescence.) Contraception and/or safe sex precautions used?

V. Adult sexual activities (may be experienced by some adolescents)

A. Premarital sex

1. Types of sex play experiences—frequency of sexual interactions, types and number of partners

2. Contraception or safe sex precautions used

3. First coitus (if not experienced in adolescence); age, circumstances, partner

4. Cohabitation—age begun, duration, description of partner, sexual fidelity, types of sexual activity, frequency, satisfaction, number of cohabiting relationships, reasons for breakup(s)

5. Engagement—age, activity during engagement period with fiancé(e), with others; length of engagement

B. Marriage (if multiple marriages have occurred, explore sexual activity, reasons for marriage, and reasons for divorce in each marriage)

1. Types and frequency of sexual interaction—describe typical sexual interaction (see above), satisfaction with sex life? View of partner's feelings

2. First sexual experience with spouse—when? What were the circumstances? Was it satisfying? Disappointing?

3. Honeymoon—setting, duration, pleasant or unpleasant, sexually active? Frequency? Problems? Compatibility?

4. Effect of pregnancies and children on marital sex

5. Extramarital sex—number of incidents, partner; emotional attachment to extramarital partners? Feelings about extramarital sex

6. Postmarital masturbation—frequency? Effect on marital sex?

7. Extramarital sex by partner—effect on interviewee?

8. Ménage à trois or multiple sex (swinging)

9. Areas of conflict in marriage (eg, parenting, finances, division of responsibilities, priorities)

VI. Sex after widowhood, separation, divorce—celibacy, orgasms in sleep, masturbation, noncoital sex play, intercourse (number of and relationship to partners), other

VII. Special issues

A. History of rape, incest, sexual or physical abuse

B. Spousal abuse (current)

C. Chronic illness (physical or psychiatric)

D. History or presence of sexually transmitted infections

E. Fertility problems

F. Abortions, miscarriages, or unwanted or illegitimate pregnancies

G. Gender identity conflict (eg, transsexualism, wearing clothes of opposite sex)

H. Paraphilias (eg, fetishes, voyeurism, sadomasochism)

Framing questions in a way that normalizes a wide range of sexual behaviors or problems helps clients feel more comfortable about sharing their unique experiences. For example, instead of asking "Do you sometimes have difficulty achieving an erection?" nurses could reframe the question as follows: "Men sometimes cannot have erections even when they really want to have intercourse. What is that like for you?" Nurses are also careful to use terminology that clients comprehend readily. Pictures, models, and diagrams may be helpful.

Sexual dysfunction is problematic not only for identified clients but also for their partners (Figure 24.5). Nurses may interview couples separately and together to obtain a complete picture of the difficulties. Nurses do not assume, however, that each partner will automatically be comfortable expressing feelings with the other present, or that it is acceptable for nurses to share one client's concerns, problems, or sexual history with the partner. Nurses always ask clients what they are comfortable with in this regard before proceeding (Therapeutic Communication 24.3).

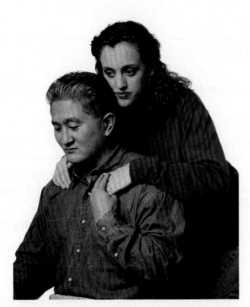

FIGURE 24.5 Problems in a sexual relationship can be devastating for couples. Interventions that focus on both partners can be particularly effective at resolving the physical issues and any emotional, psychological, or communication difficulties surrounding or stemming from them.

Information about the relationship itself includes how partners communicate with each other about sexual needs and preferences, how considerate each is of the other's wishes, as well as the sexual history of this partnership (eg, how soon did they become involved sexually, how satisfying has their sexual relationship been, have they experienced other sexual concerns such as infidelity or abusive sexual experiences, and what have been their best and worst times together sexually). Nurses also assess each partner's perception of problems as a whole, such as level of satisfaction in the relationship, strengths, support system, and willingness to work on problems.

Nursing assessments also include an understanding of cultural context and sexual orientation. Not all clients seeking help are heterosexual. Nurses also convey sensitivity about various lifestyle concerns (eg, homophobia, fear of hate crimes, disclosing or not disclosing a homosexual or bisexual orientation) when interviewing gay clients.

Nursing Interventions

Sharing intimate, potentially embarrassing information is difficult. The nurse's attitudes regarding sexuality powerfully influence the client's experience and response to treatment. Clients must not fear criticism or rejection from nurses. Thus, nurses refrain from negative verbal and nonverbal communications. Unconditional acceptance of clients facilitates a trusting and therapeutic relationship.

Providing information and helping clients gain insight are important. Nurses discuss sexuality and its expressions with clients, providing facts as necessary and encouraging

clients to ask questions and verbalize fears or concerns. In addition, nurses use this discussion as an opportunity to discuss the effects of health issues, medical or surgical treatments, or medications on libido, self-image, and sexual function.

Other areas in which nurses may provide teaching and counseling include relationship counseling and communication techniques for couples and referral to specialists in sexual counseling. Experts suggest that all too often, sexual partners are not encouraged to participate in the plan of care (Riley, 2002). Helping clients and partners achieve intimacy and satisfaction in their sexual relationship is an area where nurses play an important role. Nurses can encourage both people to actively collaborate in the plan of care. Regardless of the sexual dysfunction, improved communication skills and enhanced feelings of emotional intimacy will help both feel more satisfied. For example, a nurse may encourage the expression of feelings by both partners, model how to elicit feedback from each other, and instruct the couple on how to communicate clearly, honestly, and sensitively. Nurses may suggest activities that will encourage the development of new sexual patterns. They can clarify vague information or provide facts and dispel myths.

Advanced practice nurses (APNs) can explore deeper emotional issues or comorbid mental health problems with clients. For example, discussing underlying anxiety or history of childhood trauma may help clients gain insight into sexual problems. APNs also may discuss feelings that clients have directly related to the sexual problem, such as guilt, despair, anger, grief, loneliness, resentment, and depression. Any opportunity to verbalize feelings within a nonjudgmental, therapeutic context is helpful. APNs also can help clients overcome low self-esteem (Client-Centered Education 24.1).

> **Checkpoint Questions**
> **7.** What is the first step in caring for a client with a sexual problem?
> **8.** What feelings might a client with sexual dysfunction experience?

Paraphilias

Paraphilias are sexual expressions characterized by "recurrent, intense sexually arousing fantasies, sexual urges or behaviors generally involving (1) nonhuman objects, (2) suffering or humiliation of oneself or one's partner, or (3) children or other nonconsenting persons that occur over a period of at least 6 months" (APA, 2000, p. 566). To be considered paraphilias, the urges, fantasies, and behaviors also must cause clinically significant distress or impair social, occupational, or other important areas of functioning. For some clients, paraphilias are necessary for erotic arousal and sexual release (orgasm). For others, they are episodic (eg, during periods of stress). Although frequency

Therapeutic Communication 24.3

Respecting a Client's Wishes Regarding Sexual Issues

The nurse is working with Amy, a 30-year-old client, who mentions having sexual difficulties with her husband of 3 years.

INEFFECTIVE DIALOGUE	EFFECTIVE DIALOGUE
CLIENT: I don't know what he likes. Last week, he said our sex life is no good. I don't know what I'm doing wrong. *(Appears crestfallen)*	CLIENT: I don't know what he likes. Last week, he said our sex life is no good. I don't know what I'm doing wrong. *(Appears crestfallen)*
NURSE: Well, maybe nothing. Have you been arguing or under stress?	NURSE: Well, maybe nothing. Have you been arguing or under stress?
CLIENT: No more than usual.	CLIENT: No more than usual.
NURSE: What do you mean by usual?	NURSE: What do you mean by usual?
CLIENT: *(Shifts in her seat)* Well, I *am* always on his back about the time he spends with his friends. And he works so hard. It probably is my fault.	CLIENT: *(Shifts in her seat)* Well, I *am* always on his back about the time he spends with his friends. And he works so hard. It probably is my fault.
NURSE: It sounds like you two have problems both inside and outside the bedroom that you should address. Why don't we set up an appointment for both you and your husband to come in and discuss what's happening?	NURSE: Both members of a relationship can contribute to problems. They also can work together to solve them. *(Pauses)* Have you and your husband ever considered seeing a therapist together? You also could come here together to discuss issues.
CLIENT: *(Looks uncomfortable)* My husband would never feel comfortable talking about such things. I'd be embarrassed, too.	CLIENT: *(Pauses, seems to think it over)* I don't know how he'd feel talking about such things in front of other people. I'm afraid I'd be embarrassed in front of *him.*
NURSE: He might surprise you! How does Tuesday the 26th at 3:00 PM sound?	NURSE: These discussions take courage. Why don't you think about it? Maybe you can mention it to your husband and see how he reacts. Meanwhile, let's talk more about specific questions you have today.
CLIENT: Well . . . OK. *(The next day, the client calls and cancels the appointment.)*	CLIENT: *(Seems reassured and begins to discuss her relationship in more detail. Two weeks later, she calls to set up an appointment along with her husband.)*

Reflection and Critical Thinking

• Although the nurses in both examples proposed similar ideas, the outcomes were vastly different. Why do you think the second approach was more effective?
• What attitudes did the first nurse convey that may have contributed to the client's reluctance to pursue further discussion, with and without her husband?
• What are possible reasons it could be damaging to prematurely involve a client's sexual partner in treatment?

and intensity vary, these disorders tend to be lifelong and chronic (*DSM-IV-TR* Box 24.3).

Estimates regarding the general prevalence of paraphilias are unavailable. Although paraphilias rarely are diagnosed in general clinical facilities, the large commercial market in paraphiliac pornography and paraphernalia suggests that many people have these disorders. The most common presenting problems in specialty clinics are pedophilia, voyeurism, and exhibitionism. Approximately 50% of those with paraphilias seen clinically are married.

Paraphilias are diagnosed rarely in women, except for sexual masochism, in which the female-to-male ratio is estimated at 20:1 (APA, 2000).

Some clients are distressed by their problems; others experience distress only when someone interferes with their behaviors (eg, legal consequences). Some view their behaviors as an interesting part of their sexuality and seek to fulfill them with similarly interested partners (eg, sadomasochism). They may visit specialized prostitutes, read books or magazines about their paraphilias, search the Internet for

Client–Centered Education 24.1

Fostering Self-Esteem Related to Sexuality

In a society that places great value on sexuality and sexual performance, those experiencing sexual dysfunction may feel shame, despair, and guilt over their altered abilities to carry out their sexual roles. Male and female stereotypes persist and may add to feelings of decreased self-esteem. The partner of a client with sexual dysfunction may or may not be understanding and supportive and may increase the pressure to perform according to past abilities. Generalist nurses can help clients explore and overcome self-esteem issues. Some strategies for addressing these issues include the following:

- Listen for statements of self-worth and help the client explore his or her ideas about how sexual performance relates to self-judgments.

- Assist the client to differentiate a feeling (eg, loneliness) from a negative self-evaluation (eg, "I am unlovable").
- Help the client reexamine and reframe negative self-evaluations; teach the client to dispute negative self-evaluations.
- Encourage the client to view stereotypical measures of sexual performance as only one form of sexual expression.
- Encourage the client to include all his or her attributes, not just sexual performance, during self-evaluation.
- Encourage the client to focus on strengths and to increase activities in these areas.
- Help the client establish realistic goals and celebrate his or her successes.

---

information, or participate in paraphiliac subcultures. Some clients attend support groups that encourage responsible behavior.

Frequently, involvement in treatment is not voluntary but a consequence of criminal prosecution (court-ordered treatment). Some clients enter treatment at the insistence of their sexual partners. For example, when a husband tries to pressure his wife to assist him with cross-dressing and the wife is uncomfortable or not accepting, she may threaten to terminate the relationship unless he gets treatment. Treatment often is difficult and lifelong.

Clients, especially those who endanger the safety of others (pedophiles, violent sadists), may be prescribed drugs that reduce sexual desire and arousal. Cyproterone acetate (Androcur) and medroxyprogesterone acetate (Provera) reduce testosterone levels, which results in decreased deviant sexual behaviors. In addition, sertraline (Zoloft), fluoxetine (Prozac), and other SSRIs have been useful in reducing depressive symptoms and decreasing some paraphiliac behaviors (Bradford, 2001).

Other treatments for paraphilias include *satiation* (a technique in which sex offenders use their most erotic fantasies after orgasm in a boring, repetitive manner to extinguish their erotic quality); *signaled punishment* (a combination of aversion therapy and biofeedback of erections to deviant stimuli); and treatments aimed at the deficits of the person with paraphilia (eg, arousal to adult partners, assertive skills, ability to relate socially to adult partners, cognitions) (Kaplan & Sadock, 2007).

Checkpoint Questions

9. What is a paraphilia?

10. What two drugs may be used to decrease testosterone levels in an effort to decrease sexually deviant behavior?

Gender Identity Disorders

Gender identity disorders (GIDs) are characterized by a strong identification with the opposite gender and persistent discomfort with one's assigned sex. They lead to clinically significant distress or impaired social, occupational, or other functioning. People who identify with and live as if they are of the opposite sex are called **transsexuals**. Transsexuals are not to be confused with **transvestites**, who cross-dress for sexual arousal. Transvestites usually have no persistent desire for sex reassignment.

The number of U.S. transsexuals is unknown. European data suggest that roughly 1 in 30,000 adult men and 1 in 100,000 adult women seek sex reassignment surgery (SRS). In child clinic samples, approximately five boys for each girl are referred with this disorder. In adult clinic samples, men outnumber women by approximately 2 to 3:1 (APA, 2000).

Client advocates propose that the psychiatric diagnosis of GIDs unfairly stigmatizes transsexuals. They emphasize that cross-gender identity is a serious condition treatable with medical procedures. GIDs are also thought to be overly inclusive and to pathologize some ordinary behaviors.

Surgical techniques to create a vaginal barrel or penis are limited and expensive and may have unpleasant side effects. Murad and associates' (2010) meta-analysis of 28 studies shows that after sex reassignment, 80% of individuals with GID reported significant improvement in gender dysphoria and quality of life. Suicide rates decreased after reassignment but remained higher than those of the general population. The analysis found that 80% of SRS clients were satisfied with their new assigned sex and their physical appearance, and the majority had no doubts or regrets about their transformation. In male-to-female (MTF) hormone treatment in which breast enlargement is inadequate, surgical breast implants may be an option. Because of the expense

DSM-IV-TR BOX 24.3

Paraphilias

Exhibitionism

A. Over a period of at least 6 months, recurrent, intense sexually arousing fantasies, sexual urges, or behaviors involving the exposure of one's genitals to an unsuspecting stranger.

B. The person has acted on these sexual urges, or the sexual urges or fantasies cause marked distress or interpersonal difficulty.

Fetishism

A. Over a period of at least 6 months, recurrent, intense sexually arousing fantasies, sexual urges, or behaviors involving the use of nonliving objects (eg, female undergarments).

B. The fantasies, sexual urges, or behaviors cause clinically significant distress or impairment in social, occupational, or other important areas of functioning.

C. The fetish objects are not limited to articles of female clothing used in cross-dressing (as in Transvestic Fetishism) or devices designed for the purpose of tactile genital stimulation (eg, a vibrator).

Frotteurism

A. Over a period of at least 6 months, recurrent, intense sexually arousing fantasies, sexual urges, or behaviors involving touching and rubbing against a nonconsenting person.

B. The person has acted on these sexual urges, or the sexual urges or fantasies cause marked distress or interpersonal difficulty.

Pedophilia

A. Over a period of at least 6 months, recurrent, intense sexually arousing fantasies, sexual urges, or behaviors involving sexual activity with a prepubescent child or children (generally age 13 years or younger).

B. The person has acted on these sexual urges, or the sexual urges or fantasies cause marked distress or interpersonal difficulty.

C. The person is at least age 16 years and at least 5 years older than the child or children in Criterion A.

Note: Does not include an individual in late adolescence involved in an ongoing sexual relationship with a 12- or 13-year-old.

Sexual Masochism

A. Over a period of at least 6 months, recurrent, intense sexually arousing fantasies, sexual urges, or behaviors involving the act (real, not simulated) of being humiliated, beaten, bound, or otherwise made to suffer.

B. The fantasies, sexual urges, or behaviors cause clinically significant distress or impairment in social, occupational, or other important areas of functioning.

Sexual Sadism

A. Over a period of at least 6 months, recurrent, intense sexually arousing fantasies, sexual urges, or behaviors involving acts (real, not simulated) in which the psychological or physical suffering (including humiliation) of the victim is sexually exciting to the person.

B. The person has acted on these sexual urges with a nonconsenting person, or the sexual urges or fantasies cause marked distress or interpersonal difficulty.

Transvestic Fetishism

A. Over a period of at least 6 months, in a heterosexual male, recurrent, intense sexually arousing fantasies, sexual urges, or behaviors involving cross-dressing.

B. The fantasies, sexual urges, or behaviors cause clinically significant distress or impairment in social, occupational, or other important areas of functioning.

Voyeurism

A. Over a period of at least 6 months, in a heterosexual male, recurrent, intense sexually arousing fantasies, sexual urges, or behaviors involving the act of observing an unsuspecting person who is naked, in the process of disrobing, or engaging in sexual activity.

B. The person has acted on these sexual urges, or the sexual urges or fantasies cause marked distress or interpersonal difficulty.

Paraphilia Not Otherwise Specified

This category is included for Paraphilias that do not meet the criteria for any of the specific categories. Examples include, but are not limited to *telephone scatologia* (obscene phone calls), *necrophilia* (sexual activity with corpses), *partialism* (exclusive focus on part of body), *zoophilia* (animals), *coprophilia* (feces), *klismaphilia* (enemas), and *urophilia* (urine).

Reprinted with permission from the *Diagnostic and Statistical Manual of Mental Disorders, Fourth Edition, Text Revision* (Copyright © 2000). American Psychiatric Association.

and limitations of sophisticated surgeries, many clients seeking female-to-male (FTM) transformation undergo a double mastectomy with cosmetic chest resculpting and no attempt to create a penis (Ettner, 1999).

MTF hormone treatment results in less frequent erections, more rounded body contours, decreased testicular volume, and limited breast enlargement. FTM hormone treatment produces an increased sexual drive, amenorrhea, and hoarseness. Clients taking FTM hormone treatment who begin to lift weights may see a pronounced increase in muscle mass. FTM hormones also may increase the amount and coarseness of facial and body hair and cause frontal balding. Nurses discourage

clients from taking hormones without a physician's supervision and from purchasing black market hormones and quack "feminization pills."

Psychotherapy assists adults to find a workable, comfortable sexual identity. Transsexuals often have difficulty finding accepting partners; consequently, they may experience depression and anxiety related to their lack of an intimate connection. Support groups, as well as newsletters, magazines, and Internet chat rooms, can alleviate some distress and isolation by providing friends, correspondence, and a safe space to explore gender identity (Ettner, 1999). Those who undergo SRS usually first go through a period of 1 to 2 years of cross-living. During this time, psychotherapy to assist with the numerous adjustments necessary can be helpful.

Compulsive Sexual Behavior

A new clinical syndrome, *compulsive sexual behavior* (CSB; also called *sexual addiction* and *sexual impulsivity*) is appearing in the research and treatment literature more frequently. It is not in the *DSM-IV-TR* (APA, 2000). Characteristics of CSB include recurrent intense sexually arousing fantasies, sexual urges, or behaviors for at least 6 months that involve (1) compulsive cruising and multiple sex partners, (2) compulsive fixation on an unobtainable partner, (3) compulsive

masturbation, (4) multiple love relationships, or (5) compulsive sexuality in a relationship (Raymond et al., 2003). In addition, these fantasies, urges, or behaviors cause clinically significant social, occupational, or other distress or impairment. They are not the result of another medical condition or attributable to another psychiatric disorder.

Clients usually spend hours every day fantasizing or engaging in problematic sexual behavior. Examples include compulsively masturbating to pornography, viewing online pornography, or participating in online sexual chat rooms. Other examples include engaging in frequent anonymous sex in public places and picking up multiple partners each week in bars or bathhouses. Clients also report that they have tried to resist the urge to think about or act on the sexual behavior but find that eventually they give in. Frequently, clients engage in risky behaviors without regard for legal or occupational consequences (eg, an employee downloads pornography onto his computer at work). During the problematic behavior, clients experience temporary relief from their obsessive fantasies and compulsions, followed by guilt and remorse (Raymond et al., 2003).

SSRIs help reduce compulsive sexual behavior. Additional treatment strategies include individual and marital therapy, as well as self-help recovery groups based on the 12-step model (see Chap. 30).

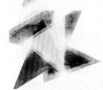

Reviewing and Applying Your Knowledge

Chapter Summary

- Somatoform disorders are characterized by complaints of severe physical symptoms or disabilities with no corresponding organic or physical pathology on testing or examination. They include somatization disorder, conversion disorder, hypochondriasis, pain disorder, and body dysmorphic disorder.

- Clients with somatoform disorders rely on physical symptoms to express emotional needs, such as gaining attention and forcing others to meet their dependencies.

- The highly elaborate self-diagnoses and symptoms of clients with somatoform illnesses are not responsive to reassurance, explanation, or standard treatment. Symptoms often enable clients unconsciously to assume the "sick role," which relieves them from social obligations and responsibilities.

- Somatoform disorders are difficult to treat and require an interdisciplinary, chronic care approach. Clinical treatments consist of individual, group, and family psychotherapies and a selection of limited somatic therapies, most often SSRI administration.

- Dissociative disorders include depersonalization disorder, dissociative amnesia, dissociative fugue, and dissociative identity disorder (DID, formerly called multiple personality disorder). The most severe is DID.

- Treatment modalities for dissociative disorders include individual modalities, group therapy, and art therapy.

- Nursing interventions for clients with DID include providing therapeutic communication, a consistent milieu for safety, and education of clients and family.

- Many factors influence the diverse scope of human sexual expression, including genetics, preferences, culture, life experiences, and health.

- Sexual dysfunction disorders can be primary (caused by various psychological and emotional conditions) or secondary (caused by a general medical condition or substance use).

- Treatment of specific sexual dysfunctions focuses mainly on targeting the causal factors (which could be psychological, physical, or pharmacologic) related to the particular disorder.

- Assessment of the client or client couple seeking help for sexual dysfunction includes review of the identified problem; examination of physical health, including medication and substance use; and exploration of the couple's relationship and communication skills.

- Generalist nurses provide education and counseling for clients seeking help with sexual dysfunction. APNs provide more in-depth interventions.

- Nurses encourage clients seeking help for sexual dysfunction to express their feelings about the problem. They should assess and address self-esteem issues.

- Paraphilias refer to sexual expressions characterized by recurrent, intense sexually arousing fantasies, urges, or behaviors generally involving (1) nonhuman objects or animals, (2) suffering or humiliation of self or partner, or (3) children or other nonconsenting persons. They persist for at least 6 months. Examples include exhibitionism, fetishism, frotteurism, pedophilia, sexual masochism, sexual sadism, transvestic fetishism, and voyeurism.

- Gender identity disorders manifest differently in children compared with adolescents and adults. Children may repeatedly state a desire to be, or insist that they are, the other sex. In adolescents and adults, the disturbance is manifested by symptoms such as a stated desire to be the other sex, frequently passing as the other sex, desire to live or be treated as the other sex, or the conviction that they have the typical feelings and reactions of the other sex.

Study Questions

1. When developing the plan of care for a client with a somatoform disorder, the nurse would expect to focus on which of the following first?

   a. Reducing the client's immediate symptoms.

   b. Enhancing the client's ability to see connections between emotion and body.

   c. Assessing the client for suicidal ideation.

   d. Establishing trust in the therapeutic relationship.

2. Bob, a man with somatoform disorder, has been in therapy for several weeks. When he arrives for therapy he states, "The pain in my arms and legs has been much worse this week." Which of the following responses will be most therapeutic?

   a. "Please tell me more about it."

   b. "You're focusing on your body again. Let's move on to another topic. How have you been feeling?"

   c. "Good morning, Bob. Are you ready to begin now?"

   d. "I notice you look better, though."

3. When caring for a client with a dissociative disorder, the nurse understands that a primary objective is to provide a therapeutic milieu. Which of the following milieus would the nurse judge to be most helpful to the client in the early stages of treatment? An environment that stresses

   a. Education and job training.

   b. Socialization and communication skills.

   c. Safety and structured activity.

   d. Intensive group therapy.

4. A client with DID has a history of pulling out her hair and scratching her face. Which of the following interventions would the nurse implement first?

   a. Use mitts to prevent further self-harm.

   b. Develop a "no self-harm" contract.

   c. Reorient the client to time and place with grounding techniques.

   d. Identify stress reduction strategies.

5. A 68-year-old male client complains that his erections are less rigid than before and that it takes him longer to achieve an erection. Which of the following responses would be most therapeutic?

   a. "What you describe sounds like normal age-related changes. Is this a concern for you?"

   b. "Erectile dysfunction is common, but many treatments are available, including drugs or surgery."

   c. "Is this causing a problem for your partner?"

   d. "That doesn't sound like a problem; it is very common in men your age."

Critical Thinking Questions

1. Describe major differences between somatization disorder and hypochondriasis. Discuss whether and how your treatment approach might differ between the two disorders and why (or why not).

2. Some states have laws mandating chemical castration of repeat sex offenders, particularly child molesters. Research this topic and provide arguments for and against chemical castration. Determine your own position on the subject. Consider points such as harmful side effects, whether chemical castration is cruel and unusual punishment, whether it is therapeutic treatment, and whether those undergoing chemical castration should receive a shorter sentence or parole.

References

Abramowitz, J. S., & Braddock, A. E. (2006). Hypochondriasis: Conceptualization, treatment, and relationship to obsessive-compulsive disorder. *Psychiatric Clinics of North America, 29,* 503–519.

Allet, J. L., & Allet, R. E. (2006). Somatoform disorders in neurological practice. *Current Opinion in Psychiatry, 19,* 413–420.

Altwein, J. E., & Keuler, F. U. (2001). Oral treatment of erectile dysfunction with apomorphine SL. *Urology International, 67*(4), 257–263.

American Psychiatric Association (APA). (2000). *Diagnostic and statistical manual of mental disorders* (4th ed., text rev.). Washington, DC: Author.

Aybek, S., Kanaan, R. A., & David, A. S. (2008). The neuropsychiatry of conversion disorder. *Current Opinion in Psychiatry, 21*(3), 275–280.

Barsky, A. J., Peekna, H. M., & Borus, J. F. (2001). Somatic symptom reporting in women and men. *Journal of General Internal Medicine, 16*(4), 266–275.

Becker, B. E. (1998). Clinical crossroads: The rehabilitative model for somatization disorder. *Journal of the American Medical Association, 279*(9), 656.

Benham, E. (1995). Coping strategies: A psychoeducational approach to post-traumatic symptomatology. *Journal of Psychosocial Nursing and Mental Health Services, 33*(6), 30–35.

Berman, J. R., Berman, L. A., Toler, S. M., Gill, J., & Haughie, S. (2003). Safety and efficacy of sildenafil citrate for the treatment of female sexual arousal disorder: A double-blind, placebo-controlled study. *Journal of Urology, 170*(6 Pt 1), 2333–2338.

Bowman, E. S. (2000, May). *Treating somatization related to child abuse.* Paper presented before the American Psychiatric Association, Chicago, IL.

Bradford, J. M. W. (2001). The neurobiology, neuropharmacology, and pharmacological treatment of the paraphilias and compulsive sexual behavior. *Canadian Journal of Psychiatry, 46,* 26–33.

Brown, R. J., Schrag, A., & Trimble, M. R. (2005). Dissociation, childhood interpersonal trauma, and family functioning in patients with somatization disorder. *American Journal of Psychiatry, 162*(5), 899–905.

Bulechek, G. M., Butcher, H. K., & McCloskey Dochterman, J. (2008). *Nursing interventions classification (NIC)* (5th ed.). St. Louis, MO: Mosby.

Creed, F. (2006). Can DSM-V facilitate productive research into the somatoform disorders? *Journal of Psychosomatic Research, 60,* 331–334.

Cunningham, S. J., Harrison, S. D., Feinman, C., & Hopper, C. (2000). Body dysmorphic disorder involving the facial region: A report of 6 cases. *Journal of Oral and Maxillofacial Surgery, 58*(10), 1180–1183.

Didie, E. R., Tortolani, C. C., Pope, C. G., Menard, W., Fay, C., & Phillips, K. A. (2006). Childhood abuse and neglect in body dysmorphic disorder. *Child Abuse and Neglect, 30,* 1105–1115.

Ehling, T., Nijenhuis, E. R., & Krikke, A. P. (2008). Volume of discrete brain structures in complex dissociative disorders: Preliminary findings. *Progress in Brain Research, 167,* 307–310.

Eli Lilly & Co. (2003). *Patient information: Cialis.* Indianapolis, IN: Author.

Epstein, R. M., Quill, T. E., & McWhinney, I. R. (1999). Somatization reconsidered: Incorporating the patient's experience of illness. *Archives of Internal Medicine, 159*(3), 215–222.

Ettner, R. (1999). *Gender loving care: A guide to counseling gender-variant clients.* New York, NY: W. W. Norton.

Fine, C. G. (1999). The tactical-integration model for the treatment of dissociative identity disorder and allied dissociative disorders. *American Journal of Psychotherapy, 53*(3), 361–376.

Fink, D. (1991). The comorbidity of multiple personality disorder and DSM-III-R Axis II disorders. *Psychiatric Clinics of North America, 14*(3), 547–566.

Foote, B., Smolin, Y., Kaplan, M., Legatt, M. E., & Lipschitz, D. (2006). Prevalence of dissociative disorders in psychiatric outpatients. *American Journal of Psychiatry, 163*(4), 623–629.

Foote, B. Smolin, Y., Neft, D. I., & Lipschitz, D. (2008). Dissociative disorders and suicidality in psychiatric outpatients. *Journal of Nervous & Mental Disease, 196*(1), 29–36.

Ford, C. V. (1995). Conversion disorder and somatoform disorder not otherwise specified. In G. O. Gabbard (Ed.), *Treatments of psychiatric disorders* (2nd ed., pp. 1736–1753). Washington, DC: American Psychiatric Press.

Frye, B., & Gannon, L. (1993). The use, misuse, and abuse of art with dissociative/multiple personality disorder patients. *Dissociation, 6*(2–3), 188–192.

Ginzberg, K., Somer, E., Tamarkin, G., & Kramer, L. (2010). Clandestine psychopathology: Unrecognized dissociative disorders in inpatient psychiatry. *Journal of Nervous & Mental Disease, 198*(5), 378–381.

Grant, J. E., Kim, S. W., & Crow, S. J. (2001). Prevalence and clinical features of body dysmorphic disorder in adolescent and adult psychiatric inpatients. *Journal of Clinical Psychiatry, 62*(7), 517–522.

Grant, J. E., Menard, W., Pagano, M., Fay, C., & Phillips, K. A. (2005). Substance use disorders in individuals with body dysmorphic disorder. *Journal of Clinical Psychiatry, 66*, 309–316.

Guarnaccia, P. J., Martinez, I., Ramirez, R., & Canino, G. (2005). Are ataques de nervios in Puerto Rican children associated with psychiatric disorder? *Journal of the American Academy of Child & Adolescent Psychiatry, 44*(11), 1184–1192.

Gunstad, J., & Phillips, K. A. (2003). Axis I comorbidity in body dysmorphic disorder. *Comprehensive Psychiatry, 44*(4), 270–276.

Han, C., Pae, C. U., Lee, B. H., Ko, Y. H., Masand, P. S., Patkar, A. A., & Jung, I. K. (2008). Fluoxetine versus sertraline in the treatment of patients with undifferentiated somatoform disorder: A randomized, open-label, 12-week, parallel-group trial. *Progress in Neuro-psychopharmacology & Biological Psychiatry, 32*(2), 437–444.

Holloway, K. L., & Zerbe, K. J. (2000). Simplified approach to somatization disorder: When less may prove to be more. *Postgraduate Medicine, 108*(6), 89–95.

Huber, M. (2000). Aspects of occupational disability in psychosomatic disorders. *Versicherungsmedizin, 52*(2), 66–75.

Hunter, E. C. M., Sierra, M., & David, A. S. (2004). The epidemiology of depersonalization and derealization. A systematic review. *Social Psychiatry and Psychiatric Epidemiology, 39*, 9–18.

International Society for the Study of Dissociation (ISSD). (2005). Guidelines for treating dissociative identity disorder in adults. *Journal of Trauma and Dissociation, 6*(4), 69–149.

Johns, M. (1999). Communicating effectively with a patient who has a somatization disorder. *American Family Physician, 59*(9), 2639–2640.

Kaplan, B. J., & Sadock, V. A. (2007). *Synopsis of psychiatry: Behavioral sciences/clinical psychiatry* (10th ed.). Philadelphia, PA: Lippincott Williams & Wilkins.

Katon, W., Sullivan, M., & Walker, E. (2001). Medical symptoms without identified pathology: Relationship to psychiatric disorders, childhood and adult trauma, and personality traits. *Annals of Internal Medicine, 134*(9, Pt. 2), 917–925.

Kriedler, M. C., Zupancic, M. K., Bell, C., & Longo, M. B. (2000). Trauma and dissociation: Treatment perspectives. *Perspectives in Psychiatric Care, 36*(3), 77–85.

Kroenke, K. (2006). Physical symptom disorder: A simpler diagnostic category for somatization-spectrum conditions. *Journal of Psychosomatic Research, 60*, 335–339.

Kroenke, K. (2007). Efficacy of treatment for somatoform disorders: A review of randomized control trials. *Psychosomatic Medicine, 69*(9), 881–888.

Leiknes, K. A., Finset, A., Moum, T., & Sandanger, I. (2007). Course and predictors of medically unexplained pain symptoms in the general population. *Journal of Psychosomatic Research, 62*, 119–128.

Lev-Wiesel, R. (2005). Dissociative identity disorder as reflected in drawings of sexually abused survivors. *The Arts in Psychotherapy, 32*, 372–381.

Lewis-Fernandez, R., Garrido-Castillo, P., Bennasar, M., Parrilla, E. M., Laria, A. J., Ma, G., et al. (2002). Dissociation, childhood trauma, and ataque de nervios among Puerto Rican psychiatric outpatients. *American Journal of Psychiatry, 159*, 1603–1605.

Lieb, R., Meinlschmidt, G., & Araya, R. (2007). Epidemiology of the association between somatoform disorders and anxiety and depressive disorders: An update. *Psychosomatic Medicine, 69*(9), 860–863.

Lowenstein, R. J., & Putnam, F. W. (2005). Dissociative disorders. In B. J. Sadock & V. A. Sadock (Eds.), *Kaplan & Sadock's comprehensive textbook of psychiatry* (Vol. 1, pp. 1829–1901). Philadelphia, PA: Lippincott Williams & Wilkins.

Maaranen, P., Tanskanen, A., Honkalampi, K., Haatainen, K., Hintikka, J., & Viinamaki, H. (2004). Factors associated with pathological dissociation in the general population. *Australian and New Zealand Journal of Psychiatry, 39*, 387–394.

Maldonado, J. R., & Spiegel, D. (2004). Dissociative disorders. In R. E. Hales & S. C. Yudofsky (Eds.), *Essentials of clinical psychiatry* (2nd ed., pp. 471–503). Washington, DC: American Psychiatric Press.

Margo, K. L., & Margo, G. M. (2000). Early diagnosis and empathy in managing somatization. *American Family Physician, 61*(5), 1282–1285.

Mayou, R., Kirmayer, L. J., Kroenke, K., & Sharpe, M. (2005). Somatoform disorders: Time for a new approach in DSM-V. *American Journal of Psychiatry, 162*(5), 847–855.

Meston, C. M. (2004). A randomized, placebo-controlled, crossover study of ephedrine for SSRI-induced female sexual dysfunction. *Journal of Sex and Marital Therapy, 30*, 57–68.

Moorhead, S., Johnson, M., Maas, M. L., & Swanson, E. (2008). *Nursing outcomes classification (NOC)* (4th ed.). St. Louis, MO: Mosby.

Murad, M., Elamin, M., Zumaeta, M., Mullan, R., Murad, A., Erwin, P., et al. (2010). Hormonal therapy and sex reassignment: A systematic review and meta-analysis of quality of life and psychosocial outcomes. *Clinical Endocrinology, 72*(2), 214–231.

NANDA International. (2007). *Nursing diagnoses: Definitions and classification (2007–2008).* Philadelphia, PA: Author.

National Institutes of Health. (2003). *Erectile dysfunction* (NIH Publication No. 04-3923). Bethesda, MD: Author.

North, C. S., & Yutzy, S. H. (1997). Dissociative and factitious disorders. In S. B. Guze (Ed.), *Psychiatric diagnosis* (pp. 285–289). Philadelphia, PA: Mosby.

Offshe, R., & Watters, E. (1994). *Making monsters: False memories, psychotherapy, and sexual hysteria.* New York, NY: Scribner's.

Phillips, K. A., Albertini, R. S., & Rasmussen, S. A. (2002). A randomized placebo-controlled trial of fluoxetine in body dysmorphic disorder. *Archives of General Psychiatry, 59*, 381–388.

Phillips, K. A., Coles, M. E., Menard, W., Yen, S., Fay, C., & Weisberg, R. B. (2005). Suicidal ideation and suicide attempts in body dysmorphic disorder. *Journal of the American Academy of Dermatology, 42,* 436–441.

Phillips, K. A., & Dufresne, R. G. (2002). Body dysmorphic disorder. A guide for primary care physicians. *Primary Care: Clinics in Office Practice, 29*(1), 99–111.

Phillips, K. A., Menard, W., & Fay, C. (2006). Gender similarities and differences in 200 individuals with body dysmorphic disorder. *Comprehensive Psychiatry, 47,* 77–87.

Putnam, F. W. (1997). *Dissociation in children and adolescents.* New York, NY: Guilford Press.

Raymond, N. C., Coleman, E., & Miner, M. H. (2003). Psychiatric comorbidity and compulsive/impulsive traits in compulsive sexual behavior. *Comprehensive Psychiatry, 44*(5), 370–380.

Riley, A. (2002). The role of the partner in erectile dysfunction and its treatment. *International Journal of Impotence Research, 14* (Suppl 1), S105–S109.

Rodewald, F., Wilhelm-Göling, C., Emrich, H., Reddemann, L., & Gast, U. (2011). Axis-I comorbidity in female patients with dissociative identity disorder and dissociative identity disorder not otherwise specified. *Journal of Nervous & Mental Disease, 199*(2), 122–131.

Roelofs, K., Keijsers, G. P., Hoogduin, K. A., Naring, G. W., & Moene, F. C. (2002). Childhood abuse in patients with conversion disorder. *American Journal of Psychiatry, 159*(11), 1908–1913.

Rosen, R. C., Phillips, N. A., Gendaro, N. C., & Ferguson, D. M. (1999). Oral phentolamine and female sexual arousal disorder: A pilot study. *Journal of Sex and Marital Therapy, 25,* 137–144.

Servan-Schreiber, D., Kolb, N. R., & Tabas, G. (2000). Somatizing patients: Part I. Practical diagnosis. *American Family Physician, 61*(4), 1073–1078.

Sharpe, M., & Carson, A. (2001). "Unexplained" somatic symptoms, functional syndromes, and somatization: Do we need a paradigm shift? *Annals of Internal Medicine, 134*(9, Part 2), 926–930.

Silverstein, B. (1999). Gender difference in the prevalence of clinical depression: The role played by depression associated with somatic symptoms. *American Journal of Psychiatry, 156*(3), 480–482.

Slaughter, J. R., & Sun, A. M. (1999). In pursuit of perfection: A primary care physician's guide to body dysmorphic disorder. *American Family Physician, 60*(6), 1738–1742.

Spence, S. A. (2000). Discrete neurophysiological correlates in prefrontal cortex during hysterical and feigned disorder of movement. *Lancet, 355*(9211), 1243–1244.

Stafford, L. L. (1993). Dissociation and multiple personality disorder: A challenge for psychosocial nurses. *Journal of Psychosocial Nursing and Mental Health Services, 31*(1), 15–20.

Stahl, S. (2003). Antidepressant and somatic symptoms: Therapeutic actions are expanding beyond affective spectrum disorders to functional somatic syndromes. *Journal of Clinical Psychiatry, 64*(7), 745–746.

Stone, J., Smith, R., Carson, A., Warlow, C., & Sharpe, M. (2006). La belle indifference in conversion symptoms and hysteria: Systematic review.*British Journal of Psychiatry, 188,* 204–209.

Sumathipala, A. (2007). What is the evidence for the efficacy of treatments for somatoform disorders? A critical review of previous intervention studies. *Psychosomatic Medicine, 69*(9), 889–900.

Sykes, R. (2006). Somatoform disorders in DSM-IV: Mental or physical disorders? *Journal of Psychosomatic Research, 60,* 341–344.

Taylor, S., Asmundson, G. J., & Coons, M. (2005). Current directions in the treatment of hypochondriasis. *Journal of Cognitive Therapy, 19*(3), 285–304.

Ward, N. S., Oakley, D. A., Frackowaik, R. S., & Halligan, P. W. (2003). Differential brain activations during intentionally simulated subjectively experienced paralysis. *Cognitive Neuropsychiatry, 8,* 295–312.

Web Resources

American Association of Sex Educators, Counselors, and Therapists: http://www.aasect.org

American Psychiatric Association: http://www.psych.org

American Psychological Association: http://www.apa.org

Gender Identity Disorder Reform Organization: http://www.GIDreform.org

International Society for the Study of Dissociation: http://www.issd.com

National Mental Health Association: http://www.nmha.org

Sex Addicts Anonymous: http://www.sa.org

Sex and Love Addicts Anonymous: http://www.sslaaf.org

Sexaholics Anonymous: http://www.sexaa.org

Sexual Compulsives Anonymous: http://www.sca-recovery.org

Sexuality Information and Education Council of the United States (SIECUS): http://www.siecus.org

Sidran Foundation: http://www.sidran.org

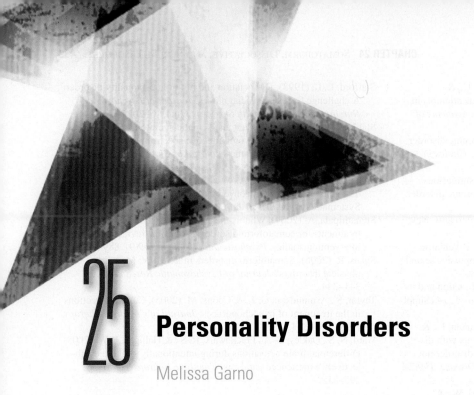

25

Personality Disorders

Melissa Garno

LEARNING OBJECTIVES

On completion of this chapter, you should be able to accomplish the following:

- Explain what is meant by *personality.*
- Define *personality disorder.*
- Discuss various theories about the etiology of personality disorders.
- Discuss factors that contribute to the variability of prognosis for clients with personality disorders.
- Identify clusters of personality disorders and the differentiating characteristics of their subtypes.
- Describe treatment options available for clients with personality disorders.
- Apply the nursing process to the care of clients with personality disorders.
- Discuss the importance of nursing self-care when working with clients who have personality disorders.

PERSONALITY

Personality comprises the sum of each person's unique bio-psychosocial characteristics. It consistently influences the person's inner experience and behavior across the lifespan. Personality is as essential to self-identity as physical appearance. It may even be considered the psychological equivalent of physical appearance because neither changes easily or quickly.

Since the earliest days of psychology and psychiatry, theorists have tried to explain the processes determining the formation of human personality (see Chap. 3). Psychoanalytic theories generally emphasize the importance of nurturance from immediate caregivers and loved ones in fostering positive personality traits. Biologic models stress the influence of genetic transmission combined with environmental exposures in the formation of personality. Social learning and cognitive–behavioral perspectives assert that people acquire personality characteristics through various cognitive processes interacting with the environment.

When personality development is stalled, disrupted, or somehow becomes negative, people are at risk for future problems. Clinical conditions currently referred to as *personality disorders* can occur.

OVERVIEW OF PERSONALITY DISORDERS

Personality disorder can be defined as a collection of personality traits that have become so fixed and rigid that they cause inner distress and behavioral dysfunction. It also can be explained as a lifelong behavioral pattern that negatively affects many areas of life, causes problems, and is not produced by another disorder or illness. The American Psychiatric Association (APA, 2000) defines personality disorder as "an enduring pattern of inner experience and behavior that deviates markedly from the expectations of the individual's culture."

Symptoms of personality disorders are serious. Clients with such disorders are at risk for psychiatric comorbidities, such as mood, anxiety, impulse control, and substance use disorders (Lenzenweger et al., 2007). See Cultural Spotlight 25.1.

Incidence and Prevalence

Establishing accurate statistics about the incidence and prevalence of personality disorders is challenging because many people with such illnesses do not seek professional help. In addition, diagnostic criteria for personality disorders have changed frequently, and the professional psychiatric community often questions or calls for reexamination of the different categories and types. Thus, actual rates remain less verifiable than with some other psychiatric disorders. Estimates are that at least 9.1% of Americans 18 years or older have a personality disorder (Lenzenweger et al., 2007).

Cultural *Spotlight* 25.1

Care in Diagnosis of Personality Disorders

Care providers must be cognizant of the client's cultural context before considering diagnoses of personality disorders. They need to think about whether certain behaviors or traits are reflections of customary expressions, habits, values, or political persuasions. For example, immigrants, members of minority groups, and others who have experienced actual discrimination may be more defensive, guarded, or suspicious of providers' motives than other clients. This does not mean that these clients have paranoid features; they are responding as anyone naturally would based on their history and experience. Women with cultural or religious backgrounds that expect or demand female submissiveness and deference to male decision making should not be thought to have dependent personality disorder. Such examples can be found for almost all of the different subtypes—the main point is not to immediately confuse what is "different" with what qualifies as a "disorder."

Etiology

Causes of personality disorders remain unknown and unverifiable. In fact, some experts support the position that what the *Diagnostic and Statistical Manual of Mental Disorders,* 4th edition, text revision (*DSM-IV-TR*; APA, 2000), refers to as "personality disorders" actually represents variants of normal personality structure (Samuel &Widiger, 2010; Widiger & Trull, 2007), or that there is inadequate separation between personality disorders and Axis I disorders (Lenzenweger et al., 2007; Krueger, 2005). Others claim that personal interaction with adverse environmental influences such as abuse, neglect, trauma, inadequate parenting, or a combination produces personality disorders (Lenzenweger, 2010; Tackett, 2006). Still others assert that nature, not nurture, is responsible. For example, evidence of a substantial genetic component to personality disorders is mounting. In twin studies, the heritability of personality disorders appears to be similar to the heritability of normal personality traits (Torgersen, 2009). Serotonin, norepinephrine, and acetylcholine are chemical messengers that contribute to the regulation of emotions (eg, sadness, anger, irritability) that commonly become problematic with some personality disorders (National Institute of Mental Health [NIMH], 2010). Other studies have identified different patterns of brain activity in people with borderline personality disorder (King-Casas et al., 2008). The truth may be that a combination of psychosocial and biologic factors is responsible for personality itself and personality disorders (Lenzenweger, 2010; NIMH, 2010).

Gender appears to be a major risk factor for some types of personality disorders. Females are at increased risk for avoidant, dependent, and paranoid personality disorders, whereas males are at higher risk for antisocial personality disorder. Additional risk factors include African American or Native American heritage, young adulthood, low socioeconomic status, and being divorced, separated, widowed, or never married (Grant et al., 2008; National Institute on Alcohol Abuse and Alcoholism [NIAAA], 2009).

Signs and Symptoms/Diagnostic Criteria

The *DSM-IV-TR* classifies personality disorders on Axis II of its system (see Chap. 1). The APA (2000) has done so to help ensure that health care providers do not overlook treatment of personality problems if more pronounced Axis I disorders overshadow them. Personality disorders manifest with symptoms in two or more of the following areas:

- Cognition—ways of perceiving and assigning meaning to self, others, and events
- Affectivity—the range, intensity, and appropriateness of emotionality
- Interpersonal behavior
- Impulse control (APA, 2000)

In addition, the behavior of clients with personality disorders endures, is inflexible, and pervades a wide range of personal and social contexts. Such behavior can be traced to adolescence or early adulthood. The enduring personality pattern cannot be better explained by another psychiatric disorder, substance abuse, intoxication, or a medical condition such as head trauma (APA, 2000).

Personality disorders fall into three clusters with descriptive similarities (APA, 2000):

- *Cluster A* represents disorders with odd or eccentric behavior as the core characteristic.

- *Cluster B* represents disorders with dramatic, emotional, or erratic manifestations.
- *Cluster C* represents disorders marked by anxious or fearful behaviors.

In total, there are currently 10 accepted personality disorders, divided across the three clusters.

Checkpoint Questions

1. How is personality defined?
2. According to the *DSM-IV-TR*, what four areas are involved in the symptomatology of personality disorders?
3. What cluster of personality disorders involves behavior that is odd or eccentric?

Cluster A

Clients with Cluster A personality disorders manifest signs and symptoms associated with the more adaptive end of the schizophrenic spectrum (see Chap. 29) (Pulay et al., 2009). Because the symptoms, management, and response to psychopharmacotherapy are similar to that of schizophrenia, disorders in this group are often referred to as the "schizophrenic spectrum cluster" (Ward, 2004). In addition to appearing odd or eccentric, those with these disorders often seem cold, withdrawn, suspicious, and irrational (*DSM-IV TR* Box 25.1). Cluster A personality disorders account for an estimated 5.7% of the population (Lenzenweger et al., 2007).

◢ DSM-IV-TR BOX 25.1 ◣

Cluster A Personality Disorders

Paranoid Personality Disorder

A. A pervasive distrust and suspiciousness of others such that their motives are interpreted as malevolent, beginning by early adulthood and present in a variety of contexts, as indicated by four (or more) of the following:
   1. Suspects, without sufficient basis, that others are exploiting, harming, or deceiving him or her
   2. Is preoccupied with unjustified doubts about the loyalty or trustworthiness of friends or associates
   3. Is reluctant to confide in others because of unwarranted fear that the information will be used maliciously against him or her
   4. Reads hidden demeaning or threatening meanings into benign remarks or events
   5. Persistently bears grudges, ie, is unforgiving of insults, injuries, or slights
   6. Perceives attacks on his or her character or reputation that are not apparent to others and is quick to react angrily or to counterattack
   7. Has recurrent suspicions, without justification, regarding fidelity of spouse or sexual partner
B. Does not occur exclusively during the course of Schizophrenia, a Mood Disorder With Psychotic Features, or

another Psychotic Disorder and is not due to the direct physiologic effects of a general medical condition.

Schizoid Personality Disorder

A. A pervasive pattern of detachment from social relationships and a restricted range of expression of emotions in interpersonal settings, beginning by early adulthood and present in a variety of contexts, as indicated by four (or more) of the following:
   1. Neither desires nor enjoys close relationships, including being part of a family
   2. Almost always chooses solitary activities
   3. Has little, if any, interest in having sexual experiences with another person
   4. Takes pleasure in few, if any, activities
   5. Lacks close friends or confidants other than first-degree relatives
   6. Appears indifferent to the praise or criticism of others
   7. Shows emotional coldness, detachment, or flattened affectivity
B. Does not occur exclusively during the course of Schizophrenia, a Mood Disorder With Psychotic Features,

another Psychotic Disorder, or a Pervasive Developmental Disorder and is not due to the direct physiologic effects of a general medical condition.

Schizotypal Personality Disorder

A. A pervasive pattern of social and interpersonal deficits marked by acute discomfort with, and reduced capacity for, close relationships as well as by cognitive or perceptual distortions and eccentricities of behavior, beginning by early adulthood and present in a variety of contexts, as indicated by five (or more) of the following:

1. Ideas of reference (excluding delusions of reference)
2. Odd beliefs or magical thinking that influences behavior and is inconsistent with subcultural norms (eg, superstitiousness, belief in clairvoyance, telepathy, or "sixth sense"; in children and adolescents, bizarre fantasies or preoccupations)

3. Unusual perceptual experiences, including bodily illusions
4. Odd thinking and speech (eg, vague, circumstantial, metaphorical, overelaborate, or stereotyped)
5. Suspiciousness or paranoid ideation
6. Inappropriate or constricted affect
7. Behavior or appearance that is odd, eccentric, or peculiar
8. Lack of close friends or confidants other than first-degree relatives
9. Excessive social anxiety that does not diminish with familiarity and tends to be associated with paranoid fears rather than negative judgments about self

B. Does not occur exclusively during the course of Schizophrenia, a Mood Disorder With Psychotic Features, another Psychotic Disorder, or a Pervasive Developmental Disorder.

PARANOID PERSONALITY DISORDER. People with *paranoid personality disorder* are suspicious and quick to take offense. They usually cannot acknowledge their negative feelings toward others and project these negative feelings on them. They may have few friends, look for hidden meaning in innocent remarks, be litigious and guarded, or bear grudges for imagined insults or slights.

Marital or sexual difficulties are common and often involve issues related to fidelity (Figure 25.1). People with paranoid personality disorder are quick to react with anger and counterattack in response to imagined attacks on their character or reputation. Despite their tendency to interpret the actions of others as deliberately threatening or demeaning, these people do not lose contact with reality (APA, 2000).

An estimated 2.3% of the general population meets the criteria for this disorder (Lenzenweger et al., 2007). A genetic contribution to paranoid traits and a possible genetic link between paranoid personality disorder and schizophrenia exist (Kendler et al., 2007).

SCHIZOID PERSONALITY DISORDER. Clients with *schizoid personality disorder* show indifference to social relationships, flattened affectivity, and a cold, unsociable, seclusive demeanor. They take pleasure in few, if any, activities. They usually never marry, have little interest in exploring their sexuality, and frequently live as adult children with parents or siblings. These lifelong loners often succeed at solitary jobs that others would find intolerable (APA, 2000). See Case in Point 25.1.

Less than 1% of the general population meets the criteria for schizoid personality disorder (Lenzenweger

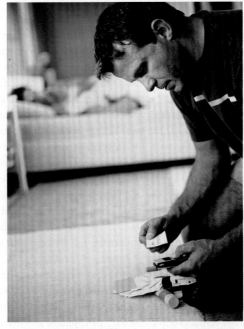

FIGURE 25.1 People with paranoid personality disorders frequently have conflicts and problems related to romantic relationships. Many such problems stem from lack of trust, jealousy, spying, suspicion, and stalking behaviors resulting from the underlying condition

et al., 2007), which is slightly more common in men than in women. Support for the heritability of this disorder exists (Kendler et al., 2007).

SCHIZOTYPAL PERSONALITY DISORDER. People with *schizotypal personality disorder* display an enduring

Case in Point 25.1

Margaret's Story

The parents of Margaret, 22 years old, bring her to therapy. They have become concerned that Margaret has no friends or social life and has become increasingly isolated. Margaret states she has no interest in friendships and prefers to be alone. She says she has never had a romantic attachment, doesn't really want one, and can't understand why this would concern anyone. Margaret is not working. She spends most of her time in her room, sewing needlepoint pillows.

The nurse notes that Margaret has a flat affect and seems cold and detached. When asked about what she hopes to get from therapy, Margaret responds, "I'm afraid of people. I might see some benefit to being less fearful of others. I would like a job, but I get so uncomfortable around others, I become nervous even thinking about it."

Key Assessment Findings

- **Consistent participation in solitary activities**
- **Absence of interest in romantic relationships**
- **No close friends or confidants**
- **Flat affect; cold, detached appearance**
- **Isolation; preference for being alone**
- **Lack of interest in forming friendships**

Nursing Diagnosis: Fear related to personality disorder as evidenced by statements "I'm afraid of people" and "I would like a job, but I get so uncomfortable around others, I become nervous even thinking about it."

NOC: Fear Self-Control: The client will verbalize a decrease in fear of others.

NIC: Coping Enhancement

- Establish a therapeutic relationship. Proceed slowly and emphasize the technical aspects of treatment in the beginning. Do not confront the client about her need for distance within the therapeutic relationship. Be consistent and stable. Provide calm reassurance and an atmosphere of acceptance. *The client's fear of others also includes a fear of the nurse. The outlined approach will help the client to sense the nurse's concern but will not press her beyond comfortable limits. The nurse can model safety and security in social relationships first within the therapeutic relationship.*

- Seek to understand the client's perceptions of her fears. Assist her to develop an objective appraisal of events. Explore her fears about others; use cognitive restructuring techniques to address irrational thought patterns. *Thought patterns predict behavior. Cognitive restructuring can replace faulty cognitions that lead to negative behaviors.*

- Encourage the client to examine unrealistic aspects of her fears. Explore her previous methods of dealing with problems; support the use of appropriate defense mechanisms and approaches. Encourage verbalization of feelings, perceptions, and fears. *Many clients with schizoid personality disorder have fears of unbearable dependency and fantasies about friendships. Examining these fears and fantasies is the first step toward helping the client to abandon them.*

- Provide appropriate social skills training. *Such training promotes a change in behavior that facilitates effective relationships.*

> 5/6/13: *The client began to discuss her fears and thought patterns.*
>
>   *D. Edwards, RN*

> 5/21/13: *The client explored past and current successful and unsuccessful interactions with others. She discussed her worries about other people interfering with her privacy and began to explore what she thinks would be the worst that could happen if she made a few friends.*
>
>   *D. Edwards, RN*

Nursing Diagnosis: Impaired Social Interaction related to personality disorder as evidenced by cold, detached appearance, absence of close friends or confidants, preference for being alone and solitary activities

NOC: Social Involvement: The client will demonstrate a beginning participation in social activities.

NIC: Behavior Modification, Social Skills

- Encourage the client to verbalize feelings associated with interpersonal problems. *Verbalization provides insight into underlying fears.*

- Assist the client to identify possible courses of action and their social/interpersonal consequences. *Such identification helps her begin to assume responsibility for thoughts, feelings, and behaviors and possible outcomes.*

- Identify a specific social skill that will be the focus of training; assist the client to role-play the skill. Provide feedback about performance. *Targeting training on one social skill prevents overwhelming the client. Role playing and providing feedback help to promote learning.*

> 6/11/13: *The client participated in role playing conversational techniques when meeting neighbors and visiting relatives. She successfully modeled respectful and kind greetings; she agreed to homework to help with practicing responses to questions.*
>
>   *v. Edwards, RN*

NIC: Socialization Enhancement

- Encourage the client to form one social relationship. Provide social skills training, as necessary. Encourage patience in developing

Case in Point 25.1 (continued)

Margaret's Story

relationships. Encourage family participation. *Initiating one relationship allows the client to focus on one thing at a time and avoid becoming overwhelmed. The development of a relationship takes time. Family involvement promotes better client outcomes.*

- Consider group therapy as a forum for beginning social interaction. Encourage honesty in presenting oneself to others; encourage respect for the rights of others. *The client may be able to experiment with social relationships within the safety of a group therapy setting. The therapist will need to protect the client from confrontation or criticism by other clients about her inability to participate or share. Honesty and respect for others facilitates trust.*

- Request and expect verbal communication. Help the client increase awareness of strengths and limitations in communicating with others. *Use of appropriate communication skills is necessary for successful relationships.*

- As therapy progresses, encourage the client to find an outside activity or job that allows some limited social interaction. *Even a moderate degree of social interaction can overwhelm the client. However, the client recognizes that her fears are preventing her from working. Her desire to work can become an important motivating force to continue therapy.*

> 7/12/13: The client reports use of coping strategies during encounters with family and neighbors. She mentions helping a neighbor with grocery shopping. She and her mother formed a "sewing bee" every other week with a family friend. This allows Margaret to practice interaction skills within a safe context and while doing an activity she enjoys. She has read literature about a group therapy session focusing on social skills and completed an online career inventory test.

EPILOGUE

It has been approximately 6 months since Margaret's first visit. Margaret continues to participate in therapy 1 to 2 times per week throughout this time. Initially, she was a bit reluctant to share information with the nurse, but her ability to express herself has gradually improved, especially during the past month. Margaret continues to struggle when interacting with others. "I don't feel as afraid as I used to be, but I still get really, really nervous around them." Margaret has agreed to continue therapy and begin group therapy in the hopes that she will become comfortable enough with others so that she can find a job.

---

and pervasive pattern of social and interpersonal deficits marked by extreme discomfort with and intolerance for close relationships. Their thought patterns are disturbed, with odd behavior, speech, and appearance. They may be suspicious, with ideas of reference without delusions of reference. In addition, they may be superstitious and believe themselves capable of unusual forms of communication, such as telepathy and clairvoyance. Schizotypal clients have a constricted or otherwise inappropriate affect. They generally lack friends or confidants other than first-degree relatives. They experience great social anxiety that does not diminish with familiarity and that seems associated with paranoid fearfulness rather than with low self-esteem (APA, 2000; Raine, 2006).

Estimates are that 3.3% of the general population has schizotypal personality disorder, with slightly higher incidences in males, and in lower income and unmarried populations (Lenzenweger et al., 2007; Pulay et al., 2009). It is genetically linked with schizophrenia. Evidence exists for dysregulation of dopaminergic pathways (Raine, 2006).

Cluster B

Clients with Cluster B disorders display dramatic, emotional, and attention-seeking behaviors (*DSM-IV-TR* Box 25.2). Their moods can be labile and shallow. They tend to become involved in intense interpersonal conflicts. Antisocial traits are more common in men, whereas borderline and histrionic

traits are more common in women (Wright, 2004). Cluster B personality disorders account for an estimated 1.5% of the population (Lenzenweger et al., 2007).

ANTISOCIAL PERSONALITY DISORDER. *Antisocial personality disorder* also encompasses *psychopathic personality* and *sociopathic personality*. Clients display aggression and irresponsibility that leads to frequent conflicts with society and subsequent involvement with the criminal justice system. Common associated behaviors include fighting, lying, stealing, domestic violence, substance abuse, and participating in confidence schemes (Figure 25.2). These people, although often superficially charming, lack genuine warmth (APA, 2000).

An estimated 1% of the general population meets the criteria for antisocial personality disorder (Lenzenweger et al., 2007). Males outnumber females by nearly 3 to 1. Although diagnosis of antisocial personality disorder is limited to clients older than 18 years, the person also must have a history of conduct disorder before 17 years (see Chap. 36) (APA, 2000; Gelhorn et al., 2007).

Antisocial personality disorder is difficult to diagnose and treat. One study found that these clients have less gray matter in the prefrontal cortex, the brain area that acts to control and regulate behavior (Raine, 2000). Findings support a genetic contribution to antisocial behaviors. Serotonergic

DSM-IV-TR BOX 25.2

Cluster B Personality Disorders

Antisocial Personality Disorder

A. There is a pervasive pattern of disregard for and violation of the rights of others occurring since age 15 years, as indicated by three (or more) of the following:
  1. Failure to conform to social norms with respect to lawful behaviors as indicated by repeatedly performing acts that are grounds for arrest
  2. Deceitfulness, as indicated by repeated lying, use of aliases, or conning others for personal profit or pleasure
  3. Impulsivity or failure to plan ahead
  4. Irritability and aggressiveness, as indicated by repeated physical fights or assaults
  5. Reckless disregard for safety of self or others
  6. Consistent irresponsibility, as indicated by repeated failure to sustain consistent work behavior or honor financial obligations
  7. Lack of remorse, as indicated by being indifferent to or rationalizing having hurt, mistreated, or stolen from another
B. The individual is at least age 18 years.
C. There is evidence of Conduct Disorder with onset before age 15 years.
D. The occurrence of antisocial behavior is not exclusively during the course of Schizophrenia or a Manic Episode.

Borderline Personality Disorder

A pervasive pattern of instability of interpersonal relationships, self-image, and affects, and marked impulsivity beginning by early adulthood and present in a variety of contexts, as indicated by five (or more) of the following:

  1. Frantic efforts to avoid real or imagined abandonment.
  2. A pattern of unstable and intense interpersonal relationships characterized by alternating between extremes of idealization and devaluation
  3. Identity disturbance: markedly and persistently unstable self-image or sense of self
  4. Impulsivity in at least two areas that are potentially self-damaging (eg, spending, sex, substance abuse, reckless driving, binge eating).
  5. Recurrent suicidal behavior, gestures, or threats, or self-mutilating behavior
  6. Affective instability due to a marked reactivity of mood (eg, intense episodic dysphoria, irritability, or anxiety usually lasting a few hours and only rarely more than a few days)
  7. Chronic feelings of emptiness
  8. Inappropriate, intense anger or difficulty controlling anger (eg, frequent displays of temper, constant anger, recurrent physical fights)

  9. Transient, stress-related paranoid ideation or severe dissociative symptoms

Histrionic Personality Disorder

A pervasive pattern of excessive emotionality and attention seeking, beginning by early adulthood and present in a variety of contexts, as indicated by five (or more) of the following:

  1. Is uncomfortable in situations in which he or she is not the center of attention
  2. Interaction with others is often characterized by inappropriate sexually seductive or provocative behavior
  3. Displays rapidly shifting and shallow expression of emotions
  4. Consistently uses physical appearance to draw attention to self
  5. Has a style of speech that is excessively impressionistic and lacking in detail
  6. Shows self-dramatization, theatricality, and exaggerated expression of emotion
  7. Is suggestible, ie, easily influenced by others or circumstances
  8. Considers relationships to be more intimate than they actually are

Narcissistic Personality Disorder

A pervasive pattern of grandiosity (in fantasy or behavior), need for admiration, and lack of empathy, beginning by early adulthood and present in a variety of contexts, as indicated by five (or more) of the following:

  1. Has a grandiose sense of self-importance (eg, exaggerates achievements and talents, expects to be recognized as superior without commensurate achievements)
  2. Is preoccupied with fantasies of unlimited success, power, brilliance, beauty, or ideal love
  3. Believes that he or she is "special" and unique and can only be understood by, or should associate with, other special or high-status people (or institutions)
  4. Requires excessive admiration
  5. Has a sense of entitlement, ie, unreasonable expectations of especially favorable treatment or automatic compliance with his or her expectations
  6. Is interpersonally exploitative, ie, takes advantage of others to achieve his or her own ends
  7. Lacks empathy: is unwilling to recognize or identify with the feelings and needs of others
  8. Is often envious of others or believes that others are envious of him or her
  9. Shows arrogant, haughty behaviors or attitudes

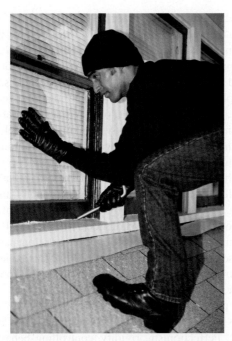

FIGURE 25.2 Criminal behaviors such as robbery are commonly associated findings with antisocial personality disorder.

dysregulation in the septohippocampal system may mediate low levels of behavioral inhibition. There also may be developmental or acquired abnormalities in the prefrontal brain systems and reduced autonomic activity. This may underlie the low arousal, poor fear conditioning, and decision-making deficits described in antisocial personality disorder. A genotype affecting monoamine oxidase A transcription is currently being studied as a predictor for antisocial personality disorder (Philibert et al., 2011). M**VIE** viewing **GUIDES**

BORDERLINE PERSONALITY DISORDER. By early adulthood, clients with *borderline personality disorder* (BPD) evidence instability in mood, impulse control, and interpersonal relationships. Their overall behavior is unpredictable and erratic. They tend to view people, circumstances, and overall life experience in terms of extremes—either all good or all bad. This tendency is referred to as **splitting** (APA, 2000).

Clients with BPD view themselves as victims and assume little responsibility for their own problems. Marked instability is particularly noticeable, with outbursts of unanticipated anger and rapid oscillations between depression and anxiety (Hunt, 2007; Tadić et al., 2009). Clients become intensely and inappropriately enraged if they believe others are ignoring them. They may impulsively try to harm or mutilate themselves, usually as cries for help or attempts to numb their emotional discomfort. Estimates are that 75% of people with borderline personality disorder attempt suicide, with almost 10% succeeding (Arvig, 2011). Marked and persistent identity disturbances also may emerge, with manifestations related to self-image, sexual orientation, long-term goals, and career choices (APA, 2000; Hunt, 2007). In addition, extreme

affective instability and emotional reactivity may manifest as intense dysphoria, irritability, anxiety, or all of these (Hart, 2007; Tadić et al., 2009). Such emotional episodes usually last just a few hours and rarely more than 1 day (APA, 2000).

An estimated 6% of the general population displays behaviors indicating BPD, with some researchers believing an overwhelming majority to be female (Hart, 2007; Hunt, 2007). However, recent studies show relatively equal prevalence among men and women (Grant et al., 2008). An overwhelming majority (up to 70%) of persons with BPD have been victims of sexual abuse or other violent crimes (NIMH, 2010). Research has implicated, but not well established, contributing biologic factors, such as abnormalities in the frontolimbic networks (Leichsenring et al., 2011). M**VIE** viewing **GUIDES**

HISTRIONIC PERSONALITY DISORDER. The 1.6% of the population thought to have *histrionic personality disorder* has a long-standing pattern of excessive emotionality and attention seeking (Lenzenweger et al., 2007). They strive constantly to be the center of attention by focusing exclusively on their own desires and interests during conversations with others. Other measures to gain attention include provocative dress and dramatic and highly emotional behaviors and displays (Figure 25.3). Despite their theatricality, their speech style is superficial and lacking in detail.

Because of feelings of insecurity, people with this disorder often engage in seductive behaviors to gain approval. Their extreme dependence on approval from others may cause their moods to appear shallow or excessively reactive to their surroundings. In addition, they can be naive, gullible, and easily influenced, while simultaneously given to temper tantrums as a result of low tolerance for frustration. Thus, people with this disorder often appear inconsistent and unpredictable. They usually blame failure or disappointment on others and tend to suppress or repress affect-laden material without acquiring any insight about their own inner experience and behavior (APA, 2000).

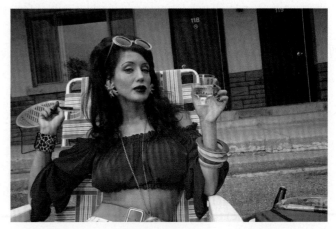

FIGURE 25.3 Some people with histrionic personality disorder dress provocatively and dramatically, often in an attempt to ensure that attention remains directed and focused on them.

This disorder is thought to occur more often in females, but there may be a bias toward diagnosing women with histrionic personality disorder.

NARCISSISTIC PERSONALITY DISORDER. Clients with *narcissistic personality disorder* have a lifelong pattern of self-centeredness, self-absorption, inability to empathize with others, grandiosity, and extreme desire for admiration. They feel that they are unusually special and often exaggerate their accomplishments to appear more important than they actually are. Despite such grandiose ideas, self-esteem is fragile. These clients are overly sensitive to what others think or say about them; however, they are particularly insensitive to the needs or feelings of others and lack empathy. In fact, they often feel entitled to special treatment from others; when it is denied, these clients can become demanding, angry, and offended (APA, 2000). Narcissists also can be haughty, arrogant, and capable of taking advantage of others to achieve their own ends. They are also often intensely envious of others but paradoxically they believe that others envy them (APA, 2000). Estimates are that over 6% of the adult population has this disorder, with a greater prevalence in men, younger adults, and single adults (Stinson et al., 2008).

Cluster C

Clients with Cluster C personality disorders are often anxious, tense, and overcontrolled. These disorders may coincide with Axis I anxiety disorders, often making differentiation among the disorders difficult (Lenzenweger et al., 2007). Cluster C personality disorders account for an estimated 6% of the population (Lenzenweger et al., 2007). See *DSM-IV-TR* Box 25.3.

AVOIDANT PERSONALITY DISORDER. People with *avoidant personality disorder* have a pattern beginning in early adulthood of social discomfort, timidity, and fear of negative evaluation. They are preoccupied with their perceived shortcomings and will risk forming relationships only if they believe acceptance is guaranteed. These clients often view themselves as unattractive and inferior; they frequently are socially inept. Consequently, they usually avoid occupations with social demands. They are reluctant to take risks or try new activities for fear of embarrassment, shame, or ridicule (APA, 2000).

Prevalence of the population estimated to have this disorder is 5.2% (Lenzenweger et al., 2007). Although clients with avoidant personality disorder also may be diagnosed with social phobia, there is one distinct difference; avoidant personality disorder pervades all social situations, whereas social phobia is confined to specific situations (eg, speaking or eating in public).

DEPENDENT PERSONALITY DISORDER. Clients with *dependent personality disorder* have a pervasive and excessive need to be taken care of, leading to submissive and clinging behavior and fears of separation (APA, 2000). In addition, they need so much approval from others that they have tremendous difficulty making independent decisions or starting projects. In effect, they do not trust their own judgment and often believe that others have better ideas.

People with dependent personality disorder fear abandonment, feel helpless when alone, and are miserable when relationships end. Consequently, they urgently seek another relationship to provide them with care and support. They may go to great lengths, even suffering abuse, to stay in a relationship. Because of their intense need to be taken care of, people with this disorder become extremely anxious if placed in a position of authority. As a result, they often have occupational difficulties (Ward, 2004) (Figure 25.4).

Estimates are that 0.5% of the population has dependent personality disorder (NIAAA, 2009). It is believed that women are diagnosed more often with it, partly from bias or social pressures to conform to gender roles.

OBSESSIVE-COMPULSIVE PERSONALITY DISORDER. Perfectionism, rigidity, controlling behavior, and extreme orderliness characterize people with *obsessive-compulsive personality disorder* (APA, 2000). These lifelong traits exist at the expense of efficiency, flexibility, and candor. Rigid perfectionism often results in indecisiveness, preoccupation with detail, and an insistence that others do things their way. Thus, they may have difficulty being effective at work and socially. People with obsessive-compulsive personality disorder also may have difficulty expressing affection and may appear depressed. M**O**VIE viewing **GUIDES**

Resisting authority and insisting that they and they alone are right are common behavioral patterns with these clients. Hoarding worthless objects, displaying stinginess, working excessively, showing stubbornness, and moralizing also occur to a high degree. Unlike Axis I obsessive-compulsive disorder (see Chap. 23), clients with obsessive-compulsive personality disorder do not have actual obsessions or compulsions. Instead, their inner struggle is to gain self-control through the control of others and the environment.

Males are diagnosed with this disorder twice as frequently as females, together comprising about 2.4% of the population (Lenzenweger et al., 2007).

Checkpoint Questions
4. What behavior would be typical in a client with a schizoid personality disorder?
5. How does a client with BPD view the world and others?
6. Which personality disorder is characterized by perfectionism, rigidity, controlling behavior, and extreme orderliness?

Comorbidities and Dual Diagnoses

People with personality disorders are at risk for other mental illnesses. Common psychiatric comorbidities include major depression (with or without psychotic features), anxiety disorders, and suicide crises. Clients with some Cluster B

DSM-IV-TR BOX 25.3

Cluster C Personality Disorders

Avoidant Personality Disorder

A pervasive pattern of social inhibition, feelings of inadequacy, and hypersensitivity to negative evaluation, beginning by early adulthood and present in a variety of contexts, as indicated by four (or more) of the following:

1. Avoids occupational activities that involve significant interpersonal contact, because of fears of criticism, disapproval, or rejection
2. Is unwilling to get involved with people unless certain of being liked
3. Shows restraint within intimate relationships because of the fear of being shamed or ridiculed
4. Is preoccupied with being criticized or rejected in social situations
5. Is inhibited in new interpersonal situations because of feelings of inadequacy
6. Views self as socially inept, personally unappealing, or inferior to others
7. Is unusually reluctant to take personal risks or to engage in any new activities because they may prove embarrassing

Dependent Personality Disorder

A pervasive and excessive need to be taken care of that leads to submissive and clinging behavior and fears of separation, beginning by early adulthood and present in a variety of contexts, as indicated by five (or more) of the following:

1. Has difficulty making everyday decisions without an excessive amount of advice and reassurance from others
2. Needs others to assume responsibility for most major areas of his or her life
3. Has difficulty expressing disagreement with others because of fear of loss of support or approval.
4. Has difficulty initiating projects or doing things on his or her own (because of a lack of self-confidence in judgment or abilities rather than a lack of motivation or energy)

5. Goes to excessive lengths to obtain nurturance and support from others, to the point of volunteering to do things that are unpleasant
6. Feels uncomfortable or helpless when alone because of exaggerated fears of being unable to care for himself or herself
7. Urgently seeks another relationship as a source of care and support when a close relationship ends
8. Is unrealistically preoccupied with fears of being left to take care of himself or herself

Obsessive-Compulsive Personality Disorder

A pervasive pattern of preoccupation with orderliness, perfectionism, and mental and interpersonal control, at the expense of flexibility, openness, and efficiency, beginning by early adulthood and present in a variety of contexts, as indicated by four (or more) of the following:

1. Is preoccupied with details, rules, lists, order, organization, or schedules to the extent that the major point of the activity is lost.
2. Shows perfectionism that interferes with task completion (eg, is unable to complete a project because his or her own overly strict standards are not met)
3. Is excessively devoted to work and productivity to the exclusion of leisure activities and friendships (not accounted for by obvious economic necessity)
4. Is overconscientious, scrupulous, and inflexible about matters of morality, ethics, or values (not accounted for by cultural or religious identification)
5. Is unable to discard worn-out or worthless objects even when they have no sentimental value
6. Is reluctant to delegate tasks or to work with others unless they submit to exactly his or her way of doing things
7. Adopts a miserly spending style toward both self and others; money is viewed as something to be hoarded for future catastrophes
8. Shows rigidity and stubbornness

Reprinted with permission from the *Diagnostic and Statistical Manual of Mental Disorders, Fourth Edition, Text Revision* (Copyright © 2000). American Psychiatric Association.

personality disorders are at increased risk for substance use disorders, affective disorders, anxiety disorders, and eating disorders (Grant et al., 2008; Saddock et al., 2009; Sansone et al., 2010; Tadić et al., 2009). Those with obsessive-compulsive and dependent personality disorders are believed to be at risk for depression. Those with narcissistic personality disorder can become suicidal if their grandiosity is threatened.

Implications and Prognosis

At one time, the prognosis for all personality disorders was considered grim because the consensus was that these conditions were untreatable. Current views emphasize that personality disorders are treatable because people continue to

grow and change throughout life. The treatment of personality disorders is thought to have a profound economic burden on society as a result of the high demands on psychiatric and health care services, as well as productivity losses due to the individual's disorder. Borderline and obsessive-compulsive personality disorders are associated with the greatest number of costs (Soeteman et al., 2008), and are often associated with physical injury and loss of productivity, respectively.

Prognosis varies widely, based on the degree of functional impairment and the client's motivation to change. People with little insight about how they contribute to troubled or unsatisfying relationships will likely make few efforts to alter their patterns of interacting. Those with greater

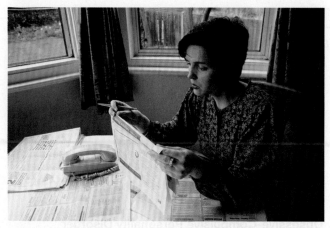

FIGURE 25.4 Clients with dependent personality disorder may have recurrent trouble getting or maintaining employment. They may be so afraid of taking charge or making decisions that they lose jobs as a result.

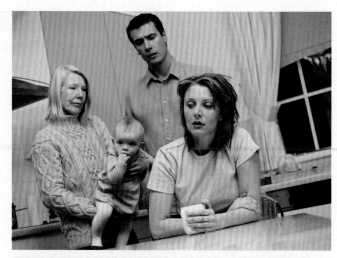

FIGURE 25.5 Many clients with personality disorders believe their problems exist outside themselves. They do not view themselves as the problem, which may result in resistance to psychiatric intervention. Often, they seek treatment after family members, employers, or legal systems have pressured them to do so.

distress may be more open to change resulting from therapy. As clinicians become more optimistic about and skillful in treating these disorders, it is hoped that more complete and reliable information will become available regarding their prognoses.

Interdisciplinary Goals and Treatment

Clients with personality disorders may resist psychiatric treatment. They may seek help when they become acutely uncomfortable with themselves, develop another psychiatric disorder, or are pressured to seek assistance by their families or the law (Figure 25.5).

Clients with BPD are at high risk for self-destructive behaviors, such as suicide attempts and self-mutilation. Emergency treatment is often initiated in response to these attempts at self-harm. They are estimated to account for 20% of psychiatric hospitalizations (NIMH, 2010). Although people with BPD are believed to be the most frequent recipients of psychiatric care in both inpatient and outpatient settings, the other disorders are also represented. For example, clients with paranoid and schizoid personality disorders may find that their families pressure them to seek treatment because of their odd behavior. Clients with schizotypal personality disorder may experience psychotic symptoms, requiring either inpatient or outpatient services. Many clients with antisocial, narcissistic, and borderline personality disorders also require treatment for substance abuse (Arvig, 2011).

Clients with personality disorders present themselves regularly to health care settings for other reasons. For example, they often arrive in trauma units or emergency departments following physical injury or other problems that have followed substance abuse or impulse-control difficulties. They may also present with other Axis I psychiatric disorders such as bipolar disorder, depression, anxiety disorders, and substance abuse (NIMH, 2010).

When a client with a personality disorder seeks treatment, identifying the specific type of disorder is considered less important than identifying and focusing on specific personality traits that influence treatment planning and health care (New York State Department of Health, 2006). Regardless of disorder, the principal objective of the interdisciplinary team should be to help clients maximize health-oriented behaviors.

Goals vary because personality disorders manifest in different ways. Long-term restructuring of personality requires years of psychotherapy, which is prohibitively costly and potentially unsuccessful. Thus, treatment is often short term. Also, as stated previously, many clients with personality disorders do not seek treatment unless a personal crisis compels them to do so, and they may terminate therapy quickly. Therefore, treatment frequently focuses on immediate problem solving, enhancement of coping, and improvement of social skills. Increased tolerance of anxiety without resorting to maladaptive coping mechanisms would be a positive outcome. Other goals include increased self-awareness and amelioration of the more destructive personality traits. Refer to Table 25.1 for goals of treatment for specific disorders.

Treating clients with personality disorders can be particularly stressful for all staff members because of clients' maladaptive and fixed ways of relating. A team approach that includes supportive and effective communication among everyone involved is thus recommended (Kerr et al., 2007; New York State Department of Health, 2006). Alcohol or drug abuse problems must be treated for therapy to progress. Brief hospitalization may be necessary during stressful periods or if suicide or other self-destructive behaviors are present.

Psychopharmacology

Pharmacologic agents such as atypical antipsychotics, antidepressants, or mood stabilizers are sometimes used as adjunctive treatment to control some symptoms in certain clients (Arvig, 2011). Antidepressants are used to treat affective dysregulation and impulsive behavior; lithium and

TABLE 25. 1 **Goals of Treatment for Specific Personality Disorders**

Personality Disorder	Goals
Cluster A	
Paranoid	Solve immediate crisis or problem.
Schizoid	Solve immediate crisis or problem.
Schizotypal	Complete social skills trainivng.
Cluster B	
Antisocial	Improve social relationships. Enhance insight into antisocial feelings and behaviors. If client is incarcerated, develop goals for life when released from custody.
Borderline	Prevent suicide. Function independently, maintain emotional balance, and engage in cognitive restructuring.
Histrionic	Prevent suicide. Gain insight into unrealistic expectations and fears.
Narcissistic	Develop a healthier sense of individuality. Recognize others as separate people. Improve coping mechanisms.
Cluster C	
Avoidant	Enhance social functioning. Solve immediate crisis or problem.
Dependent	Complete assertiveness training. Engage in cognitive restructuring.
Obsessive-compulsive	Experience specific symptom relief.

anticonvulsive mood stabilizers assist with behavior control; anxiolytics are used for both the acute and the chronic anxiety seen in certain personality disorders; and neuroleptics reduce acute, severe schizotypal symptoms, such as psychosis, anger, and hostility. In certain persons, such as those with borderline personality disorder, opioid antagonists are used to counteract the subjective numbing and physical analgesia felt during episodes of self-mutilation (APA, 2006).

Individual Psychotherapy

Most clients are likely to benefit from interpersonal interventions and individual psychotherapy. Studies have indicated that intensive therapies, such as inpatient and day treatment, are more effective than outpatient therapies (Bartak et al., 2010). Clients must be motivated to benefit from individual modalities, which may be insight oriented, supportive, or cognitive–behavioral (see Chap. 13). Because of the complexities associated with personality disorders (and usually comorbid issues), a combination approach may be indicated, depending on the client's motivation, progress, and

presenting symptoms. Through participation in individual therapy, affected clients gradually may develop insight into their problems and learn to acquire or generate emotional support and stability in more appropriate ways. In addition, cognitive–behavioral therapy with rational–emotive techniques, behavioral contracting, thought-stopping, positive coping statements, and covert rehearsal also may help clients make needed behavioral changes. Favorable outcomes have been seen in clients receiving cognitive therapy, with long-term reduction in personality disorder symptoms (Davidson et al., 2010).

Dialectical Behavioral Therapy

Another individual therapy approach, **dialectical behavioral therapy** (DBT), is used to treat clients with BPD (Linehan et al., 2006). The goal of DBT is to assist clients to overcome debilitating experiences with an "invalidating environment" by achieving stabilization, behavioral control, emotional calmness, effectiveness, joy, and wholeness. The therapist uses a dialectical approach of acceptance, validation, and problem solving to replace maladaptive behavior with skillful behavior through synthesis of inner contradictions and conflicts (Harned et al., 2010; Neacsiu et al., 2010). See Chapter 13 for more information (Evidence-Based Practice Spotlight 25.1).

Group Therapy

Group therapy focusing on cognitive behavioral and skills training can be beneficial for a variety of personality disorders (Blum et al., 2008). Specifically, groups can provide psychoeducational experiences that teach assertiveness skills, positive coping, relaxation techniques, and nonchemical coping (ie, no alcohol, street drug, or prescription drug abuse). Group therapy also can assist clients with borderline, avoidant, and dependent personality disorders to recognize how their personality disorders interfere with their relating in social contexts. Group therapy specifically assists clients with schizoid and avoidant personality disorders to reduce their patterns of social isolation. Peer groups can assist those with histrionic and antisocial personality disorders to modify and adopt more socially appropriate behaviors (Evidence-Based Practice Spotlight 25.2).

Family Education and Therapy

Clients with borderline, dependent, histrionic, and avoidant personality disorders may benefit from family treatment approaches. Relatives and significant others can be involved in treatment with the written consent of clients. Given the nature of some personality disorders (eg, paranoid personality disorder, obsessive-compulsive personality disorder), clients may not consent to family involvement. In such cases, the use of a family systems theoretical framework during the course of individual therapy may be beneficial to decrease overinvolvement and fusion. When clients and their families or significant others agree to engage in family therapy sessions, progress in reducing overinvolvement, acting out, and inappropriate dependence is possible (Case Vignette 25.1).

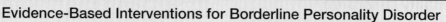

EVIDENCE-BASED PRACTICE SPOTLIGHT 25.1

Evidence-Based Interventions for Borderline Personality Disorder

Overview of Effective Treatment: Major recommendations for clients with BPD involve a combination of psychotherapy with adjunctive pharmacotherapy. Providers should give the client's potential for self-harm the highest priority when creating a management plan. Interventions should include maintaining a therapeutic alliance, providing education about BPD and its treatment, and monitoring progress. Plans should be flexible because of the frequency of comorbidities. The therapeutic relationship should be collaborative, integrating the client's preferences.

Pharmacotherapy may include SSRIs for affective dysregulation and impulse control problems (see Chaps. 16 and 27). Low-dose antipsychotics may help manage persistent anger and cognitive–perceptual symptoms, such as suspiciousness, referential thinking, paranoid ideation, illusions, derealization, depersonalization, and hallucinations (see Chaps. 16 and 29).

In addition to building a strong alliance with the client, other approaches include validating his or her suffering and experience, as well as helping the client take responsibility for actions. Additional components include managing feelings, promoting reflection rather than impulsive responses, diminishing the use of splitting, and setting limits on self-destructive behaviors.

What Has Not Been Shown Effective: Data are insufficient to support whether psychotherapy or pharmacotherapy is effective when used alone. Clinical experience indicates that clients benefit most from a combination of these two approaches. Team members should make efforts to always collaborate to prevent fragmentation of care.

Implications for Practice: Treatment should include open communication and collaboration among all health care team members. Transference and countertransference will likely pose problems. Risk management should address issues pertaining to suicide, boundary violations, and the likelihood of angry or impulsive behavior.

Reference

Oldham, J. M. (2005). *Guideline watch: Practice guideline for the treatment of patients with borderline personality disorder.* Arlington, VA: American Psychiatric Association. Retrieved from http://www.psych.org/psych_pract/treatg/pg/prac_guide.cfm.

EVIDENCE-BASED PRACTICE SPOTLIGHT 25.2

Evidence-Based Interventions for Antisocial Personality Disorder

Overview of Effective Treatment: Major recommendations begin with actively engaging people with antisocial personality disorder (APD) in treatment. Evidence shows that positive and reinforcing approaches to the treatment of APD are more likely to be successful than those that are negative or punitive. Provide consistent approaches to treatment across all levels of care in which the individual may be involved. Ensure that care is culturally appropriate for the individual. Discuss the implications of treatment with the person, the family, and relevant staff. Acknowledge the stigma and exclusion that have characterized care for people with APD. Emphasize that the diagnosis does not limit access to appropriate treatments for comorbid mental health disorders.

When working with women with APD, take into account the higher incidences of common comorbid mental health problems and other personality disorders and adapt interventions accordingly. Staff, in particular key workers, working with people with APD should establish regular one-to-one meetings to review progress, even when the primary mode of treatment is group based.

Pharmacologic interventions for comorbid mental disorders, in particular depression and anxiety, should follow current treatment recommendations for the comorbid disorder. For people with antisocial personality disorder who misuse alcohol or drugs, in particular opioids or stimulants, offer psychological interventions according to current treatment guidelines for substance use disorders.

Prevention of APD includes identifying children at risk and should focus on identifying vulnerable parents (parents with other mental health problems, or with significant drug or alcohol problems; mothers younger than 18 years, particularly those with a history of maltreatment in childhood; parents with a history of residential care; parents with significant previous or current contact with the criminal justice system). Early interventions consist of structured, supervised programs that target multiple risk factors of parenting, school behavior, and parental health and employment.

Family therapy should focus on engaging and supporting the family, engaging the support of the social and educational system, identifying maladaptive family interactions, and promoting new and more adaptive family interactions.

Reference

National Collaborating Centre for Mental Health. (2009). *Antisocial personality disorder. Treatment, management and prevention.* London, UK: National Institute for Health and Clinical Excellence. Retrieved from http://www.guideline.gov/content.aspx?id=14341&search=antisocial+personality+disorder#Section420.

Case Vignette 25.1

"I'm here because my wife has threatened divorce if I don't do something," says John, 38 years old. His wife, Gloria, accompanies him. She made the appointment 2 weeks ago; John obviously resents this. During the session, Gloria describes selfishness and miserliness from John. She reports that he insists on exact schedules for meals and sleep and refuses to allow her to shop for groceries or other articles unless she follows his precise instructions. She adds that he hoards worthless objects such as grocery bags, old clothes, used wrapping paper, and boxes. She also complains about a lack of affection. John says that Gloria is wasteful, scatterbrained, and disorganized. He says he closely monitors their finances because "we're hemorrhaging money." He complains that Gloria is too emotional and sentimental.

John stops therapy after two sessions, stating, "It ought to be obvious to any competent therapist that my wife, not me, needs help." Gloria continues individual therapy for about 6 months to explore whether she wants to stay married. She eventually files for divorce. Initially, John behaves as though nothing has changed. He stubbornly refuses to accept responsibility for any of the marital problems. He becomes more emotionally reactive when Gloria seeks half of their property and financial holdings.

In addition to the stress of the divorce, John is summoned to his manager's office to discuss problems with delegating work. Employees reporting to John have complained that he reserves all overtime for himself, thus increasing his salary at their expense. His boss states clearly that John must change his relationships with his workers and his overall work patterns.

The demands for personal and professional change are overwhelming for John, who becomes depressed. After a few

months, John entertains suicidal thoughts, feeling hopeless about taking control of his life. He seeks treatment. John receives the following diagnoses:

- Axis I: Major depression, single episode, severe 296.23
- Axis II: Obsessive-compulsive personality disorder, severe 301.4
- Axis III: Deferred
- Axis IV: Separation with impending divorce and job stress
- Axis V: GAF = 40 to 50 present; past 70

John's treatment regimen includes individual cognitive–behavioral psychotherapy combined with 100 mg of sertraline (Zoloft) daily for major depression. He is treated on an outpatient basis and readily contracts to refrain from self-harm. Through cognitive reframing, John learns to view the divorce and job difficulties as setbacks in what had been a fairly successful life. Because John experiences significant and timely relief from intense emotional pain, he decides to continue therapy even after he no longer requires antidepressants. He gains self-awareness and insight and wants to ensure as much as possible that he does not repeat previous behavior patterns. Although John does not like change, he decides that change from within appeals more to him than change imposed by external sources.

Reflection and Critical Thinking

- What features of John's case are common to all types of personality disorders?
- What challenges do health care providers face when working with clients who have symptoms that represent two or more disorders at one time?

Think About It 25.1

While preparing to meet a client, the nurse reviews the client's medical record, which reveals the following information: feels uncomfortable in social situations; shows evidence of social phobia; is extremely shy and fearful of others; verbalizes feelings of being unattractive and inferior to others; voices numerous shortcomings; has few relationships; is reluctant to try new things; states "Why should I, everyone will laugh at me." Her problems started in her early 20s. Evaluate the client's symptoms and determine the type of personality disorder that may be present. Suggest possible treatment outcomes and therapies that might be appropriate.

APPLYING THE NURSING PROCESS

Personality Disorders

▲ ASSESSMENT
Clients with personality disorders seldom seek psychiatric assistance unless they experience comorbid conditions.

Therefore, assessing for personality disorders in those with symptoms of depression and other mood disturbances, anxiety, psychosis, substance abuse, or suicide crisis is important. The co-occurrence of personality disorders can complicate the treatment and course of other diagnoses and subsequently reduce quality of life (Arvig, 2011).

No specific physical findings are associated with any personality disorders. Physical examination may reveal consequences and sequelae of various personality disorders. For example, clients (particularly with Cluster B disorders) may show signs of prior suicide attempts, such as self-inflicted scars. Substance abuse, a common comorbidity, may be reflected in physical signs and symptoms of alcoholism or various drug addictions (see Chap. 30).

▲ NURSING DIAGNOSIS
Because of the high rate of comorbidity, nursing diagnoses pertaining to other applicable psychiatric disorders, such as affective disorders, anxiety disorders, substance abuse, and even schizophrenia, need to be addressed to ensure optimal care. The following list contains some nursing diagnoses that reflect behavioral targets of intervention in clients with personality disorders (NANDA, 2008):

- Risk for Self- or Other-Directed Violence
- Risk for Self-Mutilation
- Ineffective Coping
- Disturbed Thought Process
- Anxiety
- Fear
- Impaired Social Interaction
- Social Isolation
- Chronic Low Self-esteem
- Ineffective Therapeutic Regimen Management
- Ineffective Family Coping

▲ OUTCOME IDENTIFICATION AND PLANNING

Personality disorders require a collaborative treatment approach. As stated previously, those with personality disorders may resist treatment or accept it for only short periods. Nurses need to consider this factor when developing a plan and setting goals with clients and family.

Major goals for the care of clients with personality disorders include the following (Moorhead et al., 2008):

- **Risk Control:** The client will experience physical safety.
- **Adherence Behavior:** The client will participate in therapy.
- **Symptom Control:** The client will exhibit improved coping and tolerance of anxiety.

▲ IMPLEMENTATION

Although standard care plans address the treatment of clients with personality disorders, nurses must individualize treatment to ensure the inclusion of comorbid issues. Ideally, the treatment plan synthesizes goals and approaches of all applicable psychiatric diagnoses. Effective approaches to the therapeutic relationship form the foundation of care for any person with a personality disorder. Table 25.2 outlines recommended approaches to interaction based on the client's personality type.

TABLE 25.2 Recommended Approaches to Personality Types

Cluster and Subtype	Recommended Approaches
Cluster A: Odd or Eccentric	
Guarded, suspicious, argumentative clients	Acknowledge their perception of the world without debate or agreement. Try to focus attention on treatment. Maintain a respectful, professional distance; clients may appreciate formal and "business-like" clinicians.
Aloof or uninvolved clients	Show that you understand their style and respect their privacy. Explain the rationale for personal questions, but do not push them to increase social involvement.
Idiosyncratic or eccentric clients	Provide a consistent approach that addresses complaints and beliefs; neither challenge them, nor reinforce their perspective.
Cluster B: Dramatic, Emotional, or Erratic	
Demanding clients	Set limits on interactions to minimize excessive and unrealistic demands. Refer clients, if needed, to programs that extend their social and health care support networks.
Dramatic, emotionally involved, and seductive clients	Demonstrate a supportive attitude. Maintain professional boundaries to prevent clients from provoking unhelpful responses.
Superior clients	Recognize and support their strengths and achievements, and show interest in their opinions. Demonstrate competence without challenging their need to feel superior.
Antisocial clients	Set realistic limits on visits; never tolerate aggressive behavior or anything that creates an unsafe environment. Consider a mental health consultation, which may help with development of an appropriate treatment plan.
Cluster C: Anxious, Fearful	
Orderly, controlled, and controlling clients	Clearly state the treatment approach and give the fullest details possible, with a discussion about treatment rationale and other options. Always avoid a struggle over who is in charge.
Anxiously avoidant clients	Show patience and availability; express empathy toward their fears.
Anxiously dependent and clinging clients	Consider providing more frequent but briefer appointments; scheduling interactions with them may help minimize excessive demands at inconvenient times. Forewarn clients of change, such as vacations and other absences.
Controlling, avoidant, and dependent clients	Directly address concerns about their behavior, suggesting that it may indicate underlying feelings about their illness and treatment. Encourage other staff to avoid feeling resentful toward clients who "act out" their frustration.

Adapted from New York State Department of Health. (2006). *Mental health care for people with HIV infection: HIV clinical guidelines for the primary care practitioner.* New York, NY: Author.

Nurses use many types of interventions to assist clients and their families. Common Nursing Intervention Classification (NIC) labels related to management of personality disorders include, but are not limited to, **Anxiety Reduction, Behavior Modification, Impulse Control Training, Limit Setting, Mutual Goal Setting,** and **Self-Responsibility Facilitation** (Bulechek et al., 2008). See Case in Point 25.2 for more information.

Promoting Participation in Treatment

Nurses help clients develop trust in themselves, others, and the environment. They use a straightforward, matter-of-fact manner while avoiding an overly warm approach. Nurses demonstrate punctuality, respect, and genuineness to clients. Nurses avoid interpreting the behavior of clients with personality disorders, who may experience interpretations as intrusive and controlling

Case in Point 25.2

Gail's Story

Coworkers escort Gail, 24 years old, to the emergency department (ED) after she "fell apart" and began crying loudly in her cubicle. The admissions nurse notes that Gail has superficial cuts on her arms. According to the colleague, Gail's behavior at work has been increasingly erratic during the past few weeks, with escalating reports of relationship troubles, long personal phone calls, sobbing at her desk, and poor performance. During the assessment interview, Gail is cooperative and calm. When asked about the cuts on her arm, Gail says that she did them on a particularly bad day when she had argued with her mother and fought with her boyfriend.

Review of Gail's history reveals several previous visits to EDs with minor injuries, cuttings, and emotional outbursts. A therapist diagnosed Gail with borderline personality disorder 4 years ago; since that time, Gail has been in and out of treatment. During the interview, Gail says that she has frequently left treatment because no one really understands her or has her best interests at heart. "But you seem different," she says to the nurse. "Maybe you will be the first person who can really help me."

Key Assessment Findings

- Diagnosis of BPD
- Self-mutilation
- Emotional outbursts and unprofessional behavior at work
- Four years of intermittent therapy
- Volatile personal relationships

Nursing Diagnosis: Self-Mutilation

NOC: Impulse Self-Control: The client will refrain from injuring herself.

NIC: Impulse Control Training
- Monitor client for changes in behavior or mood (Figure A). *Such observation optimizes safety and helps to prevent the client from participating in self-injurious behavior.*
- Discuss with the client the reasons for such monitoring. *Giving the client this information can help ensure her cooperation and also foster her understanding of why she is being observed frequently.*
- Engage the client in a "no self-harm" contract (Figure B). *Such a contract can encourage the client to assume self-control and reinforce limits. Feedback helps the client to differentiate inappropriate and appropriate responses as well as possible triggers and causes associated with behavior.*

NIC: Self-Mutilation Restraint
- Identify with the client situations that lead her to engage in cutting. *Knowledge of triggers helps the client determine appropriate methods to reduce their effects.*
- Design a behavior modification plan; assist the client to identify positive alternatives to cutting. *Planning fosters feelings of control over circumstances and impulses.*

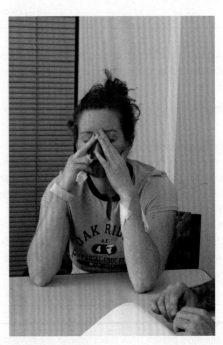

FIGURE A. Sudden bursts of anxiety or depression are common in clients with BPD. Ongoing assessment of their mood is important, particularly if they are dealing with self-mutilation or suicidal behaviors, to maintain safety.

Case in Point 25.2 (continued)

Gail's Story

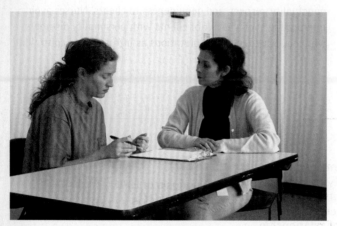

FIGURE B. The nurse solicits the client's agreement to engage in a no self-harm contract.

- Provide information about emergency hotlines to call if the urge to cut or harm oneself becomes overwhelming. *The team is obligated to put long-term measures in place to help ensure the client's safety.*

> 8/13/13: The client signed a no self-harm contract and refrained from self-mutilation and other harmful, self-inflicted behaviors during admission. She discussed behaviors and situations that lead to self-harm and agreed to implement the behavior modification strategies outlined.
>
> C. Hume, APRN

Nursing Diagnosis: Ineffective Coping related to insufficient resources, as evidenced by self-destructive behaviors inappropriate for context

NOC: Coping: The client will demonstrate use of adaptive coping skills.

NIC: Coping Enhancement
- Discuss the idea of keeping a journal with the client in which she writes about situations that cause emotional imbalance and subsequent feelings and behaviors. *A journal can provide insight about the client's responses.*
- Teach thought-stopping techniques (Figure C). Foster constructive outlets for emotions. *Cognitive restructuring leads to behavior changes. Constructive emotional outlets reduce the risk for acting out.*

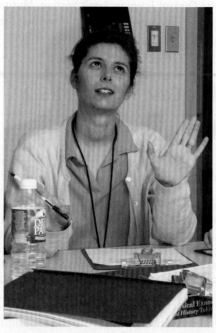

FIGURE C. The nurse teaches the client the technique of "thought-stopping" to help the client refrain from self-destructive behaviors.

- Assist the client to consider other coping strategies when stress, emotions, or feelings are intense, or when life circumstances are becoming overwhelming. Possibilities include exercise, relaxation techniques, discussion with trusted friends or health care providers, and cognitive restructuring. *Alternative coping technique must be available before the client can abandon former self-destructive strategies.*
- Arrange for longer-term follow-up care for the client that focuses specifically on care of clients with borderline personality disorder. Consider programs that implement a dialectical behavioral approach. *BPD can be difficult to manage and requires specialized techniques with proven success. Dialectical behavioral approaches have evidence-based support.*

> 8/15/13: The client agreed to try the journal. She mentioned wanting to resume yoga as a form of stress-relief and agreed to attend a follow-up session with a hospital-recommended dialectical behavioral therapist.
>
> C. Hume, APRN

EPILOGUE

Two months have passed since Gail's visit to the hospital. She has attended some sessions with the recommended therapist. Her behavior and situation have not improved dramatically, but she has had no further hospital admissions and so far has not engaged in any additional episodes of cutting.

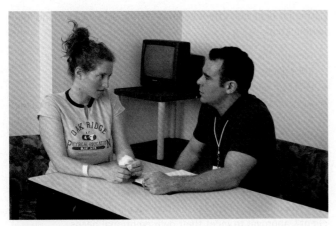

FIGURE 25.6 Clients with personality disorders may display manipulative and acting-out behaviors (eg, flirting, showing aggression, engaging in emotional displays) with nurses and other health care providers during treatment.

(Hazelton et al., 2006; Westwood & Baker, 2010). They use open-ended questions to assist clients to focus on their own behavior and its consequences. It is also important for nurses to be consistent and congruent with these clients; failure to do so may provoke increased manipulative and acting-out behaviors (Figure 25.6).

Nurses encourage clients to follow through with treatment for their disorder and comorbid issues. They also must encourage adherence to medication regimens for comorbid diagnoses. However, nurses should also monitor clients closely for prescription drug abuse (Arvig, 2011).

Enlisting the Family in the Treatment Plan

Relatives of clients with personality disorders have endured heartache, worry, concern, and possibly abuse. It is vitally important to include family members in the treatment plan, engage their help, acknowledge their experiences and efforts in coping with and caring for clients, provide support, and improve possible treatment outcomes for clients. See

Client-Centered Education 25.1 for specific teaching and intervention points.

Improving Coping Skills

Nurses encourage clients to assume responsibility for their thoughts, feelings, and behaviors without blaming, shaming, or punishing them. A good approach is to present the idea that behavioral change is within the realm of possibility, rather than to demand behavioral change. Nurses ask questions that assist clients to think through actual or intended behaviors. Doing so can help clients predict the consequences of their behaviors.

In addition to implementing techniques that will improve coping skills, nurses can suggest that clients learn how to manage stress better. Deep-breathing exercises, regular aerobic exercise, and progressive muscle relaxation are tools that clients can use to help dampen the negative effects of stress and possibly limit the need to use maladaptive coping strategies.

Reducing Inappropriate Behaviors

As stated previously, clients with personality disorders may display negative behaviors that can interfere with therapy, just as they interfere with interpersonal relationships. It may be necessary to tolerate a certain amount of acting-out behavior because clients may be testing if they can trust the therapeutic relationship. At times, however, nurses need to confront clients about their behaviors and set appropriate limits to move therapy forward.

Confronting the Client

Nurses intervene, using confrontation with clients who attempt to use manipulation or display other inappropriate behaviors. Doing so may assist clients to become more self-aware. Keys to using effective confrontation are as follows:

- Point out the manipulative or otherwise inappropriate behavior.
- Be specific when describing the behavior.

Client-Centered Education 25.1

Helping Families When Clients Have Personality Disorders

- Include the family in all treatment planning and goal-setting discussions. Members should feel like a part of the treatment team and that others value their expertise and experience.
- Address the client's social needs as well as clinical needs in the treatment plan.
- Explore expectations of the treatment plan with each family member and the client. Each family member may have different expectations.
- Assess and capitalize on the family's strengths in developing the treatment plan.

- Acknowledge and address the anxiety, depression, feelings of loss, and frustration family members may feel.
- Develop a crisis plan, including the professional response on which the family can depend.
- Make sure family members have relevant phone numbers for emergency services.
- Encourage clear communication among family members.
- Counsel the family in structured problem-solving techniques.
- Encourage family members to expand their system of social support.

- Remain calm and use a nonaccusatory, nonjudgmental, matter-of-fact manner.
- Stay focused on the actual behavior, rather than the client's explanation of it.

Nurses ensure that they use confrontation in a supportive setting. This technique is more effective when a nurse and client have made progress toward promoting trust (Therapeutic Communication 25.1).

Setting Limits

Nurses introduce limit setting when clients engage in manipulative, acting-out, dependent, or similarly inappropriate behaviors. This technique involves more than just telling clients to stop a particular behavior. Effective limit setting also involves the following steps:

- Identify the behavior the client needs to manage more effectively.
- Offer an appropriate behavioral substitute.
- Anticipate that the client will test the limit and even attempt to pit treatment team members against one another to force them to back down.
- Remain steadfast and consistent in limit setting.

Effective limit setting requires emotional maturity on the part of treatment team members. Limit setting almost always fails when nurses or other treatment team members need the client's approval to meet their own emotional needs.

Therapeutic Communication 25.1

Antisocial Personality Disorder

Stan Hopkins, 25 years old, is in police custody. He has been a mechanic since leaving the youth detention center, where he was incarcerated from 13 to 18 years of age for burglary, kidnapping, and assault with a deadly weapon. He was arrested 3 days ago for stealing valuables from customers. A psychiatric evaluation was requested after he was reportedly overheard saying that he would rather be dead than locked up again.

At the time of evaluation, the psychiatric liaison nurse from the mental health center's forensic services finds Stan slouched in his chair. Stan has the letters H-A-T-E and L-O-V-E tattooed on his hands. His beard is scraggly as he chews on a toothpick. He shows no signs of depression, mania, or psychosis.

INEFFECTIVE DIALOGUE

NURSE: The court asked me to evaluate you for suicide risk. Can you tell me how you feel? Do you feel like killing yourself? *(Tries immediately to assess suicide risk)*

CLIENT: Yeah, I do. I can't take being in jail again. I'd rather be dead.

NURSE: Mr. Hopkins, death can't possibly be better than 1 or 2 years in jail. *(Imposes her own opinion and challenges the client)*

CLIENT: To me it would. Especially since I didn't do anything wrong.

NURSE: But you stole jewelry from an elderly couple, didn't you?

CLIENT: No, I'm innocent. They were trying to steal from me!

NURSE: A couple in their 70s stole from you? Surely you see that doesn't make any sense. *(Continues to challenge the client; however, this will likely encourage more arrogant behavior)*

CLIENT: Listen, lady, it may not make sense to you, but you weren't there, were you? That old guy gave me the jewelry because they didn't have any money. He wasn't even going to do that, but I deserved to be paid, and I told him so. And if I have to go to jail because my lawyer says to cop a plea, then I'm going to hang myself!

NURSE: Hanging yourself won't do any good.

EFFECTIVE DIALOGUE

NURSE: Why do you think I was called to see you? *(Clarifies client's knowledge)*

CLIENT: That old couple didn't mind me taking the jewelry. They didn't have money to pay me for my work. They didn't mind. Now they've changed their story and here I am. With my record as a minor, they'll throw the book at me. My attorney says it's sealed, but I don't believe him. He just wants me to cop a plea, have no day in court, and get a minimal sentence of 2 to 3 years with a chance for parole in 18 months, I'd rather die.

NURSE: How would that help you? *(Tries to assist the client to predict the consequences)*

CLIENT: It wouldn't, but I wouldn't be in jail.

NURSE: So, you've had previous experiences with jail? *(Tries to learn what being in jail means to the client)*

CLIENT: I spent 5 years in juvenile detention. I swore I'd never go back.

NURSE: Why did you set yourself up for that possibility? *(Wants to assist client to identify antecedents and consequences of behavior)*

CLIENT: It really wasn't my fault! I didn't do anything! That old couple set me up.

NURSE: Why would they want to? *(Assists client to analyze his assertion logically)*

CLIENT: I don't know.

CLIENT: *(Showing frustration)* Are we finished yet? This is a waste of time. If they want to evaluate me, they should send a real psychiatrist.

NURSE: *(Tersely)* Mr. Hopkins, do you have a plan for how you would harm yourself?

CLIENT: Yeah. I plan on hanging myself right here if you don't leave.

NURSE: Thank you, Mr. Hopkins. I believe we're finished. *(Leaves quickly)*

NURSE: You are willing to die because of what you feel they did? *(Encourages client to evaluate his threat realistically)*

CLIENT: I wouldn't hurt myself. I just want you to know I don't want to go back to jail.

NURSE: I understand that you prefer not to go to jail. What do you think will happen if you keep threatening suicide? *(Assists client to identify consequences)*

CLIENT: I don't want to be put in with the psychos. Don't do that. I won't hurt myself.

NURSE: Can you give me that promise in writing? *(Assesses whether he will enter a behavioral contract to refrain from self-harm and also spells out the consequences if he continues to threaten or attempt suicide)*

CLIENT: Yeah, yeah.

Reflection and Critical Thinking

- Compare the questions the two nurses asked. Why were the second nurse's questions more effective?
- The first nurse failed to understand how communication techniques can feed into entrenched personality traits, in effect exacerbating them. Which traits did the client exhibit? How did they influence the outcome of the interview in the first example? How did the nurse in the second example avoid this pitfall?
- Discuss the issue of countertransference and how it may relate to the first nurse's encounter with the client.

Providing for Physical Safety

Most people with personality disorders and no other comorbidities rarely require psychiatric hospitalization. The exception is clients with BPD, who may require short-term hospitalization to provide crisis stabilization for attempted suicide (NIMH, 2010). Treatment approaches in such situations may include the following:

- Implementing a suicide watch as unobtrusively as possible to avoid providing increased attention and reinforcement for immature and often manipulative behavior (NIMH, 2010)
- Ensuring a safe environment while simultaneously discouraging clients from becoming dependent on and feeling entitled to hospitalization
- Behavioral contracting for personal safety to assist in providing for physical and psychological safety while simultaneously assisting clients requiring this measure to learn to accept responsibility for their behavior. The team can use this approach in both inpatient and outpatient treatment settings. It is often used to avert hospitalization when clients have restabilized quickly, as clients with BPD often do, and are cooperative and willing to accept or resume outpatient treatment.

▲ EVALUATION

Nurses evaluate care administered to clients with personality disorders based on whether clients reach higher levels of functioning. Reassessing client behaviors, examining responses to interventions, and revising goals, plans, and interventions accordingly may reflect only minimal client change or progress given the long-term nature of personality disorders. The following outcomes illustrate that doing all that is possible to administer effective treatment may still result in only modest changes in a client's overall level of functioning. Some client outcomes consistent with the preceding goals and treatment approaches include the following:

- The client demonstrates trust in the nurse and treatment team.
- The client attends group therapy and individual therapy regularly.
- The client models more adaptive coping skills and greater tolerance of stress.
- The client has no suicide crises.
- The client voices insight into thoughts, feelings, and behaviors.

Checkpoint Questions

7. What two techniques are associated with increased effectiveness of the therapeutic relationship?
8. What may result if the nurse fails to be consistent and congruent with clients who have personality disorders?

NURSE'S SELF-CARE

Clients with personality disorders can cause considerable difficulties for those who attempt to care for them (Daffern et al., 2010; Westwood & Baker, 2010). Consequently, others label them as complainers, drug seekers, grumps, or manipulators. In fact, they often trigger negative *countertransference* from their providers (displacement of negative feelings onto clients) (see Chaps. 3 and 13).

To ensure that nurses remain calm and objective, self-monitoring is essential (Westwood & Baker, 2010). Monitoring oneself in terms of expressing concern and setting boundaries has also been reported to increase the effectiveness of therapeutic relationships with clients with personality disorders. By practicing self-monitoring, nurses found that they were more effective in relationships with clients who have personality disorders and, as a result, were more helpful over time (Westwood & Baker, 2010).

Nurses may find it helpful to discuss their emotional reactions to clients who have personality disorders with knowledgeable and trusted colleagues (Bland & Rossen, 2005) (Figure 25.7). Doing so can help nurses to work through negative countertransference, resulting in their tolerating and accepting feelings of irritation and anger as natural reactions to clients with personality disorders. This realization can increase the nurse's own self-awareness and sense of emotional control. Identifying additional sources of support such as friends and family can also enhance and promote both personal and professional growth. Taking the necessary professional and personal time to

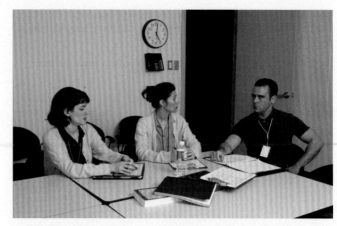

FIGURE 25.7 Ongoing discussions of emotional reactions to clients with personality disorders, as well as consistent reporting and conferring among members of the same treatment team, are essential to ensure consistency of care. They are also vital to ensuring the well-being of health care providers when working with challenging clients.

promote one's own emotional maturity and growth reaps benefits not only for nurses but also for all others with whom nurses have contact.

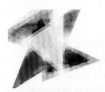

Reviewing and Applying Your Knowledge

Chapter Summary

- Personality disorder may be defined as a collection of personality characteristics that have become fixed and rigid to the point that the client experiences distress and behavioral dysfunction. Another definition refers to an enduring pattern of inner experience and behavior that deviates significantly from the expectations of the client's culture.

- Personality disorders can occur singularly or with other serious psychiatric disorders such as major depression, anxiety disorder, and substance abuse.

- The cause or causes of personality disorder are unknown. However, some speculate that personality disorders actually represent variants of normal personality, rather than disease processes. Others speculate that psychosocial factors such as abuse, neglect, or trauma cause personality disorders. Still others hypothesize that nature, not nurture, is responsible and point to growing evidence of a genetic component. Finally, there are those who think that a combination of biologic and psychosocial factors is responsible for the formation of personality and personality disorders.

- Determining an accurate prognosis for personality disorders is difficult. Based on reported clinical observations, some clients with personality disorders worsen with time, whereas others improve. Some clients drop out of treatment, preventing further follow-up; others refuse treatment, creating unknown variables in the study of these disorders.

- At one time personality disorders were considered untreatable. More recent evidence suggests otherwise. As optimism and knowledge about the treatment of these disorders grow, there is hope for more accurate and complete information about their prognosis.

- Ten types of personality disorders are organized into Clusters A, B, and C. Clients with Cluster A personality disorders typically are described as cold, withdrawn, suspicious, and irrational. Clients with Cluster B personality disorders display dramatic, emotional, and attention-seeking behaviors. Clients with Cluster C personality disorders often are anxious, tense, and overcontrolled.

- Clients with personality disorders may benefit from individual psychotherapy using supportive, insight-oriented, and cognitive–behavioral approaches. Group and family therapy also may benefit some clients with personality disorders.

- Nurses require skill in assessing, forming trust, setting limits, and using therapeutic confrontation to provide effective care for clients with personality disorders.

- Nurses must be aware that progress in treating personality disorders is usually slow and requires patience and maturity. For this reason, nurses must identify sources of personal and professional support to ensure their own health, survival, and growth.

Study Questions

1. Which of the following concepts would the nurse incorporate into the plan of care for a client being treated for a personality disorder?

   a. Psychoactive medications are prescribed to improve symptoms of the personality disorder.

   b. Self-monitoring by the nurse is necessary to ensure an effective therapeutic relationship.

   c. Group therapy, not individual therapy, is the preferred approach.

   d. Comorbid issues are not addressed because the personality disorder is the major cause of other psychiatric symptoms.

2. The nursing instructor teaches a group of students about the different clusters of personality disorders. For the instructor to determine that the teaching has been successful, which of the following disorder(s) would the students identify as belonging to Cluster C? Select all that apply.

   a. Avoidant personality disorder.

   b. Histrionic personality disorder.

   c. Borderline personality disorder.

   d. Antisocial personality disorder.

   e. Paranoid personality disorder.

   f. Obsessive-compulsive personality disorder.

3. A 20-year-old client displays behaviors such as fighting, lying, and stealing. The client has been arrested several times for attempted burglary and assault. Review of his medical record reveals that he was diagnosed with a conduct disorder at 15 years of age. The nurse suspects which personality disorder?

   a. Borderline personality disorder.

   b. Antisocial personality disorder.

   c. Narcissistic personality disorder.

   d. Histrionic personality disorder.

4. While interviewing a client diagnosed with schizoid personality disorder, the nurse notes that the client has a flat affect and is not communicative. The nurse accurately attributes this behavior to which of the following causes?

   a. The comorbid major depression associated with schizoid personality disorder.

   b. The failure to conform associated with schizoid personalities.

   c. The severely limited social interest associated with schizoid personality disorder.

   d. The paranoid delusions associated with schizoid personality disorder.

5. A client with narcissistic personality disorder is terminating treatment soon. The nurse considers the plan of care effective when the client exhibits which of the following outcomes?

   a. The client can see others as people.

   b. The client can make social contacts.

   c. The client no longer expresses suicidal thoughts.

   d. The client agrees to participate in assertiveness training.

Critical Thinking Questions

1. Do you know anyone whom you believe has a personality disorder? How has reading and studying this chapter altered or changed your opinion about this person?

2. Consider Case in Point 25.1. Do you think Margaret would have ever considered entering treatment if her parents had not made her go? Explain your position on the basis of what you have learned about personality disorders.

3. Consider Case Vignette 25.1. How are obsessive-compulsive personality disorder and obsessive-compulsive disorder similar? Which symptoms, if any, of each disorder did John present? Do you think John might need treatment again? Explain your position in terms of what you know about the mental illnesses of major depression and obsessive-compulsive personality disorder.

References

American Psychiatric Association (APA). (2000). *Diagnostic and statistical manual of mental disorders* (4th ed., text rev.). Washington, DC: Author.

American Psychiatric Association (APA). (2006). Practice guideline for the treatment of patients with borderline personality disorder. *Psychiatry Online*. Retrieved from http://www.psychiatryonline.com/content.aspx?aID=55433#55678. doi:10.1176/appi.books.9780890423363.54853

Arvig, T. (2011). Borderline personality disorder and disability. *American Association of Occupational Health Nurses Journal, 59*(4), 158–160. doi:10.3928/08910162-20110328-04

Bartak, A., Andrea, H., Spreeuwenberg, M. D., Thunnissen, M., Aiegler, U. M., Dekker, J., et al. (2010). Patients with cluster A personality disorders in psychotherapy: An effectiveness study. *Psychotherapy and Psychosomatics, 80*(2), 88–99.

Bland, A. R., & Rossen, E. K. (2005). Clinical supervision of nurses working with patients with borderline personality disorder. *Issues in Mental Health Nursing, 26*(5), 507–517.

Blum, N., St. John, D., Pfohl, B., Stuart, S., McCormick, B., Allen, J., et al.(2008). Systems training for emotional predictability and problem solving (STEPPS) for outpatients with borderline personality disorder: A randomized controlled trial and 1-year follow-up. *American Journal of Psychiatry, 165*, 468–478.

Bulechek, G. M., Butcher, H. K., & McCloskey Dochterman, J. (2008). *Nursing interventions classification (NIC)* (5th ed.). St. Louis, MO: Mosby.

Daffern, M., Duggan, C., Huband, N., & Thomas, S. (2010). Staff and patient's perceptions of each other's interpersonal style: Relationship with severity of personality disorder. *International Journal of Offender Therapy and Comparative Criminology, 54*, 611–624.

Davidson, K. M., Tyrer, P., Norrie, J., Palmer, S. J., & Tyrer, H. (2010). Cognitive therapy v. usual treatment for borderline personality disorders: Prospective 6-year follow-up. *British Journal of Psychiatry: The Journal of Mental Science, 197*, 456–462.

Gelhorn, H. L., Sakai, J. T., Price, R. K., & Crowley, T. J. (2007). DSM-IV conduct disorder criteria as predictors of antisocial personality disorder. *Comprehensive Psychiatry, 48*(6), 529–538.

Grant, B. F., Chou, S. P., Goldstein, R. B., Huang, B., Stinson, F. S., Saha, T. D., et al. (2008). Prevalence, correlates, disability, and comorbidity of DSM-IV borderline personality disorder: Results from the Wave 2 National Epidemiologic Survey on Alcohol and Related Conditions. *Journal of Clinical Psychiatry, 69*, 533–545.

Harned, M. S., Jackson, S. C., Comtois, K. A., & Linehan, M. M. (2010). Dialectic behavior therapy as a precursor to PTSD treatment for suicidal and/or self-injuring women with borderline personality disorder. *Journal of Traumatic Stress, 23*, 421–429.

Hart, B. G. (2007). Cutting: Unraveling the mystery behind the marks. *American Association of Occupational Health Nurses, 55*(4), 161–166.

Hazelton, M., Rossiter, R., & Milner, J. (2006). Managing the "unmanageable": Training staff in the use of dialectical behaviour therapy for borderline personality disorder. *Contemporary Nurse, 21*(1), 120–130.

Hunt, M. (2007). Borderline personality disorder across the lifespan. *Journal of Women and Aging, 19*(1–2), 173–191.

Kendler, K. S., Myers, J., Torgersen, S., Neale, M. C., & Reichborn-Kjennerud, T. (2007). The heritability of cluster A personality disorders assessed by both personal interview and questionnaire. *Psychology Medicine, 37*(5), 655–665.

Kerr, I. B., Dent-Brown, K., & Parry, G. D. (2007). Psychotherapy and mental health teams. *International Review of Psychiatry, 19*(1), 63–80.

King-Casas, B., Sharp, C., Lomax-Bream, L., Lohrenz, T., Fonagy, P., & Montague, P. R. (2008). The rupture and repair of cooperation in borderline personality disorder. *Science, 321*, 806–810.

Krueger, R. F. (2005). Continuity of axes I and II: Toward a unified model of personality, personality disorders, and clinical disorders. *Journal of Personality Disorders, 19*, 233–261.

Leichsenring, F., Leibing, E., Kruse, J., & New, A. S. (2011). Borderline personality disorder. *The Lancet, 377*(9759), 74–84. doi:10.1016/SO140-6736(10)61422-5

Lenzenweger, M. F. (2010). A source, a cascade, a schizoid: A heuristic proposal from the Longitudinal Study of Personality Disorders. *Development and Psychology, 22*, 867–881. doi:10.1017/SO954579410000519

Lenzenweger, M. F., Lane, M. C., Loranger, A. W., & Kessler, R. C. (2007). DSM-IV personality disorders in the National Comorbidity Survey Replication. *Biological Psychiatry, 62*, 553–564. Retrieved from http://www.ncbi.nlm.nih.gov/pmc/articles/PMC2044500

Linehan, M. M., Comtois, K. A., Murray, A. M., Brown, M. Z., Gallop, R. J., Heard, H. L., et al. (2006). Two-year randomized controlled trial and follow-up of dialectical behavior therapy vs. therapy by experts for suicidal behaviors and borderline personality disorder. *Archives of General Psychiatry, 63*, 757–766.

Moorhead, S., Johnson, M., Maas, M. L., & Swanson, E. (2008). *Nursing outcomes classification (NOC)* (4th ed.). St. Louis, MO: Mosby.

NANDA International. (2008). *NANDA International nursing diagnoses: Definitions and classification, 2009–2011*. Philadelphia, PA: Wiley-Blackwell.

National Institute of Mental Health (NIMH). (2010). *Borderline personality disorder* (NIH Publication No. 01-4928). Bethesda, MD: Author. Retrieved from http://www.nimh.nih.gov/health/publications/borderline-personality-disorder-fact-sheet/index.shtml

National Institute on Alcohol Abuse and Alcoholism (NIAAA). (2009). *Landmark survey reports the prevalence of personality disorders in the United States*. Bethesda, MD: Author. Retrieved from http://198.102.218.54/docs/doc08261.htm

Neacsiu, A. D., Rizvi, S. L., & Linehan, M. M. (2010). Dialectical behavior therapy skills use as a mediator and outcome of treatment for borderline personality disorder. *Behaviour Research and Therapy, 48*, 832–839.

New York State Department of Health. (2006). *Mental health care for people with HIV infection: HIV clinical guidelines for the primary care practitioner*. New York, NY: Author.

Philibert, R. A., Wernett, P., Plume, J., Packer, H., Brody, G. H., & Beach, S. R. (2011). Gene environment interactions with a novel variable monoamine oxidase A transcriptional enhancer are associated with antisocial personality disorder. *Biological Psychology*. Retrieved from http://www.ncbi.nlm.nih.gov/pubmed/21554924

Pulay, A. J., Stinson, F. S., Dawson, D. A., Goldstein ,R. B., Chou, S. P., Huang, B., et al. (2009). Prevalence, correlates, disability, and comorbidity of DSM-IV schizotypal personality disorder: Results from the Wave 2 National Epidemiologic Survey on Alcohol and Related Conditions. *Primary Care Companion Journal of Clinical Psychiatry, 11*(2), 53–67.

Raine, A. (2000). Brain differences in antisocial personality disorder. *Archives of General Psychiatry, 57,* 119–129.

Raine, A. (2006). Schizotypal personality: Neurodevelopmental and psychosocial trajectories. *Annual Review of Clinical Psychology, 2,* 291–326.

Saddock, B. J., Saddock, V. A., & Ruiz, P. (Eds.). (2009). *Kaplan and Saddock's comprehensive textbook of psychiatry* (9th ed.). Philadelphia, PA: Lippincott Williams and Wilkins.

Samuel, D. B., & Widiger, T. W. (2010). Comparing personality disorder models: Cross-method assessment of the FFM and DSM-IV-TR. *Journal of Personality Disorders, 24*, 721–745.

Sansone, R. A., Lam, C., & Wiederman, M. W. (2010). The abuse of prescription medications in borderline personality disorder: A gender comparison. *Primary Care Companion Journal of Clinical Psychiatry, 12*(6), ii: PCC.10l01001.

Soeteman, D. I., Hakkaart-van Roijen, L., Verheul, R., & Busschbach, J. J. (2008). The economic burden of personality disorders in mental health care. *Journal of Clinical Psychiatry, 69*, 259–265. Retrieved from http://www.ncbi.nlm.nih.gov/pubmed/18363454

Stinson, F. S., Dawson, D. A., Goldstein, R. B., Chou, S. P., Huang, B., Smith, S. M., et al. (2008). Prevalence, correlates, disability, and comorbidity of DSM-IV narcissistic personality disorder: Results from the Wave 2 National Epidemiologic Survey on Alcohol and Related Conditions. *Journal of Clinical Psychiatry, 69*, 1033–1045.

Tackett, J. L. (2006). Evaluating models of the personality-psychopathology relationship in children and adolescents. *Clinical Psychology Review, 26*(5), 584–599.

Tadić, A., Wagner, S., Hoch, J., Başkaya, O., von Cube, R., Skaletz, C., et al. (2009). Gender differences in axis I and axis II comorbidity in patients with borderline personality disorder. *Psychopathology, 42*, 257–263.

Torgersen, S. (2009). Personality and individual differences: The nature (and nurture) of personality disorders. *Scandinavian Journal of Psychiatry, 50*, 624–632. doi:10.1111/j.1467-9450.2009.00788.x

Ward, R. K. (2004). Assessment and management of personality disorders. *American Family Physician, 70*(8), 1505–1512.

Westwood, L., & Baker, J. (2010). Attitudes and perceptions of mental health nurses towards borderline personality disorder clients in acute mental health settings: A review of the literature. *Journal of Psychiatric and Mental Health Nursing, 17*, 657–662. doi:10.1111/j.1365-2850.2010.01579.x

Widiger, T. A., & Trull, T. J. (2007). Plate tectonics in the classification of personality disorder: Shifting to a dimensional model. *American Psychology, 62*(2), 71–83.

Wright, J. (2004). A survey of personality disorders. *American Family Physician, 70*(8), 1426.

Web Resources

Borderline personality disorder information and support: http://www.bpdcentral.com/index.php

Borderline Personality Disorder Research Foundation: http://www.borderlineresearch.org

Mental Health Sanctuary: http://www.mhsanctuary.com

National Education Alliance for Borderline Personality Disorder: http://www.borderlinepersonalitydisorder.com

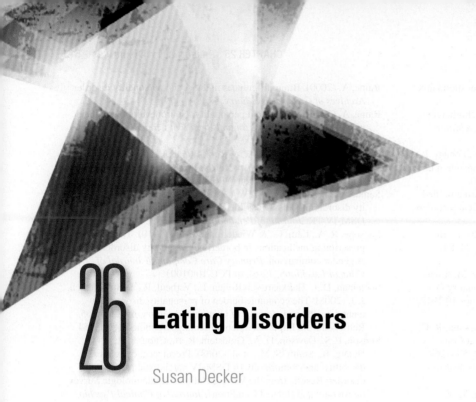

26 Eating Disorders

Susan Decker

KEY TERMS

amenorrhea
anorexia nervosa
binge eating
binge eating disorder
bulimia nervosa
eating disorders
emotional reasoning
purging
satiety

LEARNING OBJECTIVES

On completion of this chapter, you should be able to accomplish the following:

- Describe the incidence of and the populations at highest risk for eating disorders.
- Discuss possible etiologies for eating disorders.
- Differentiate anorexia nervosa, bulimia nervosa, and binge eating disorder.
- Describe the *DSM-IV-TR* diagnostic criteria for anorexia nervosa and bulimia nervosa.
- Outline interdisciplinary goals and common treatment modalities for clients with eating disorders.
- Apply the nursing process to the care of clients with eating disorders.

Healthy people need to regularly consume a rich variety of foods that are sufficient for energy needs, cellular growth and repair, and maintenance of sufficient weight. Depending on age, sex, physical condition, activity level, height, and other variables, most people normally should eat 1,500 to 2,500 calories each day, staggered over three meals and a few snacks. Eating, a normal response to hunger, should cease when the person attains **satiety** (comfortable fullness).

Sometimes, people develop problems related to normal food consumption and satiety. This chapter reviews disordered eating and the care and management of clients with food-related problems.

EATING DISORDERS: DEFINITION AND TYPES

Collectively, **eating disorders** are those in which eating:

* Is consistently below or above a person's caloric needs to maintain a healthy weight
* Is accompanied by anxiety and guilt
* Occurs without hunger or fails to produce satiety
* Results in physiologic imbalances or medical complications

The two most serious eating disorders are anorexia nervosa and bulimia nervosa. **Anorexia nervosa** is a life-threatening condition of disturbed body image, emaciation, and intense fear of becoming obese. **Bulimia nervosa** is a recurrent pattern of the uncontrollable consumption of large amounts of food (**binge eating**), followed by attempts to eliminate the body of the excess calories (**purging**) (Figure 26.1).

Incidence and Prevalence

Estimates of the combined prevalence of anorexia and bulimia nervosa are 1% to 4% of the general U.S. population (Kong, 2005). However, accurately determining the incidence of bulimia is particularly difficult because most clients with this disorder binge and purge in secret, and their weights may be relatively normal.

Historically, anorexia and bulimia have been diagnosed most frequently in white, affluent, well-educated adolescent and young-adult females. However, both disorders are becoming more widely distributed among social classes and cultures (Anderson & Yager, 2005). Although commonly thought of as disorders of youth, manifestations of eating disorders may persist well into middle or older adulthood (Agency for Healthcare Research and Quality [AHRQ], 2009; Mangweth-Matzek et al., 2006). Hospitalizations for eating disorders in boys and men seem to be growing (Woodside et al., 2001), although 89% of hospitalizations are still women (AHRQ, 2009). Recent studies have found an incidence ratio of two women to one man

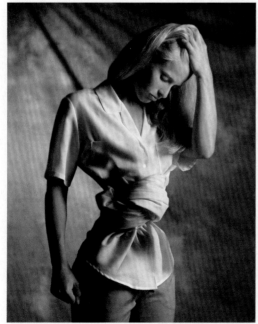

A

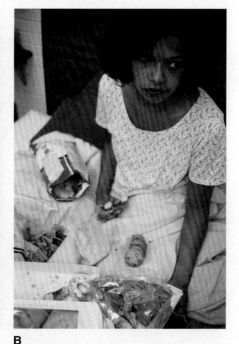

B

FIGURE 26.1 **(A)** Clients with anorexia nervosa are preoccupied with a fear of becoming obese. They increasingly restrict eating with the goal of becoming as thin as possible. No amount of weight loss satisfies the never-ending quest for thinness. The photo reflects the hollowness that many clients with this disorder report feeling, both internally and externally. **(B)** Clients with bulimia nervosa frequently consume large amounts of food during uncontrollable binges. To avoid weight gain, they then attempt to eliminate the excess calories through methods of purging.

for anorexia nervosa and a ratio of three women to one man for bulimia nervosa (Anderson & Yager, 2005). Popular emphasis on fitness, lean muscularity, and stringent weight requirements for certain sports (eg, wrestling, gymnastics) contribute to eating disorders in boys and men. Holm-Denoma and colleagues (2009) found that women who participated in sports had higher levels of eating disorder symptoms and that sports anxiety was a predictor of the drive for thinness. Additionally, eating disorders have a much higher incidence in the male homosexual population than in the male heterosexual population (Feldman & Meyer, 2007a; Russell & Keel, 2002). Boys and men with eating disorders may be less likely than girls and women to seek treatment.

Etiology

Why would people determinedly starve themselves when others view them as grotesquely thin? Why can't parents make their children with eating disorders eat? What would make some people ingest enormous amounts of food and then furtively vomit?

Causes of eating disorders vary and are influenced by impaired psychosocial functions, medical complications,

and psychiatric comorbidities (Wolfe et al., 2003). Multiple theories have been proposed to explain their development. The most accurate analysis is that eating disorders have a multifactorial etiology, developing from a complex interaction of individual, family, and sociocultural elements (Figure 26.2). A vulnerable personality, dieting that becomes uncontrolled, genetics, onset of puberty, major life changes or stressors, family functioning style, and sociocultural emphasis on slimness all may contribute to eating disorders.

Biologic Theories

The position of the Academy for Eating Disorders is that anorexia nervosa and bulimia nervosa are biologically based, serious mental illnesses (Klump et al., 2009) that are significantly heritable and are characterized by impairments in brain function and life activities. Because of the complexities of eating and supporting mechanisms, researchers have tried to address the effects of dieting on neurobiology and neuroendocrine systems as well as to identify biologic abnormalities in clients with eating disorders. Because eating behaviors can lead to neurobiologic changes and vice versa, teasing out cause from effect has been challenging. Whether

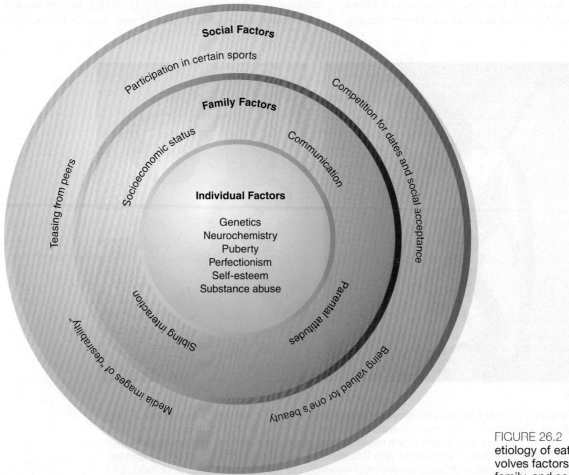

FIGURE 26.2 The multifactorial etiology of eating disorders involves factors at the individual, family, and social levels.

the biologic abnormalities seen in clients with eating dysfunction contribute to the disorders or are secondary to eating dysregulation remains unclear. What is evident is an association between several neurochemical disturbances and anorexia and bulimia.

Research findings strongly suggest that eating disorders may originate, at least in part, from hypothalamic, hormonal, neurotransmitter, or biochemical disturbances (Halmi, 2008; Kaye et al., 2009; Marken & Sommi, 2002; Monteleone et al., 2002; Wolfe et al., 2003). Both the noradrenergic and serotonergic systems help regulate eating, with norepinephrine activating and serotonin inhibiting hunger. Abnormalities in both the noradrenergic and serotonergic systems have been identified in anorexia as well as in bulimia. Meta-analysis of research provides significant evidence for the role of the serotonin system in the pathogenesis of eating disorders (Lee & Lin, 2010). Some research also suggests that dopamine, which regulates the rewarding property of food, may play a role (Frieling et al., 2010). Studies have found decreased levels of homovanillic acid, a major metabolite of dopamine, in the cerebrospinal fluid of clients with eating disorders. In addition, reduced levels of peptides (specifically, cholecystokinin) that help to regulate eating may contribute to the lack of satiety demonstrated by clients with bulimia during binges. Disturbances in leptin, a hormone secreted from adipose tissue, also have been implicated. However, current study findings are suggestive, more than conclusive. Additional research is needed before definitive statements about the complex biologic foundations of eating disorders can be made.

Evidence supporting a genetic element to eating disorders exists (Mazzeo & Bulik, 2009; Strober et al., 2000). Studies of twins and the sisters and daughters of people with eating disorders suggest a genetic link. Monozygotic twins have a concordance rate of 50% to 80% for eating disorders (Anderson & Yager, 2005). Studies suggest genetic susceptibilities on chromosomes 1, 2, and 13 (Halmi, 2008). Genetic vulnerability also may be related to hypothalamic dysfunction or family history of mood or anxiety disorders (Halmi, 2008). Wade and colleagues (2000) attribute 58% of cases of anorexia nervosa to genetics, with environmental factors also having a strong influence. However, the exact role of genetics in eating disorders remains speculative. Epigenetics, the means by which the environment affects altered gene expression, is of growing interest to researchers.

Studies from the National Institute of Mental Health suggest that anorexia, bulimia, and obsessive-compulsive disorder are associated with excessive levels of vasopressin, a brain hormone. Animal studies show that vasopressin, which is released in response to physical and emotional stress, prolongs behaviors learned under conditioned circumstances. In the same way that animals injected with vasopressin retain learned associations longer, vasopressin may enhance the conditioned obsessive-compulsive cycle of vigorous dieting, exercise, binging, and purging in people with eating disorders (Freund et al., 1993).

Psychosocial Theories

Supporters of behavioral theory argue that people with eating disorders initially may diet and lose weight, leading to an enhanced physical appearance, and gain approval for their weight loss. However, they may continue such dieting even after they have reached a normal or below-normal weight. As weight loss continues to a dangerous level, approval from others turns to concern. Regardless of the nature of interest from others, clients continue to receive attention centered on their weight. Thus, such attention may reinforce maladaptive eating behaviors. Disordered patterns eventually become autonomous, fueled by an ongoing drive for thinness and neurobiologic fear-conditioning of weight gain (Anderson & Yager, 2005).

Mood disorders, anxiety disorders, low self-esteem, perfectionism, perseverance, and avoidance appear to be predisposing factors for eating disorders (Anderson & Yager, 2005; Watson et al., 2011). Obsessive-compulsive disorder and eating disorders share many cognitive and behavioral similarities. Both psychiatric illnesses involve ritualistic behaviors, irrational thoughts and beliefs, and accompanying anxiety about the perceived catastrophe associated with not engaging in ritualistic activities. However, comorbid personality traits and symptoms may have wide variations (Steiger & Bruce, 2007). For example, bulimia occurs in people with marked psychopathology but also in those without other mental illnesses and with more circumscribed erosion of appetite/eating controls. Recent research (Watson et al., 2011) suggests that shape and weight overvaluation and conditional goal setting are important mediators of eating disorders. Rather than evaluating self-worth on many factors, persons with eating disorders evaluate primarily on shape and weight and perceive that an end state such as happiness can only be attained by reaching a certain goal, for example, a certain weight or clothing size.

Sociocultural Theories

Eating disorders are more prevalent in countries with an adequate food supply and where a thin-body ideal prevails. Western cultural contexts are thought to determine the differential risk in the development of eating disorders directly and indirectly (Bachner-Melman et al., 2009). Some social scientists argue that socialization of groups at high risk for eating disorders leads members to evaluate themselves against certain "idealized" standards of appearance, laying the groundwork for a negative body image. Clients who cannot naturally meet the ideal and begin to diet or exercise compulsively may progress toward an eating disorder. For example, before 1995, eating disorders were rare on the island of Fiji, where the cultural ideal of attractiveness was "plumpness" for women. However, within 5 years of the initiation of widespread access

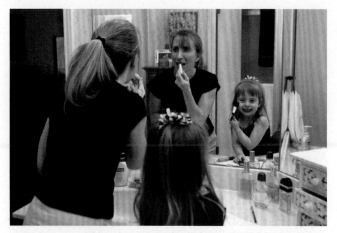

FIGURE 26.3 Children learn early about ways to enhance physical appearance and what society considers attractive. They also have a desire to act like influential adults. Families can supervise age-appropriate curiosity and imitative play while sending positive messages about their children's natural beauty and other virtues.

to television in Fiji, the incidence of eating disorders skyrocketed (Sorgen, 2002).

Most cultures highly value physical attractiveness, and people are subjected to images consistent with prevailing cultural norms from early ages. Notions of "femininity," "masculinity," "beauty," and "style" shape social conduct (Figure 26.3). Children learn from early ages that physical appearance can draw attention and praise or criticism from others.

Family-Based Theories

The families of clients with eating disorders have been portrayed negatively in the past. Some models projected images of such families as being overly concerned with external appearances and too involved with one another (being enmeshed; having poor personal boundaries; being overprotective, rigid, and unable to accept changes that accompany puberty; avoiding conflict; and displaying perfectionist tendencies). Despite the widespread acceptance of some of these notions that resulted from observational studies by Minuchin and colleagues (1975), reliable empirical literature to support these patterns of behavior is scant and has methodological shortcomings. Family advocates suggest that certain overprotective patterns, rather than helping to cause eating disorders, may be displays of normative behavior when children have a chronic and potentially life-threatening illness. Several studies suggest that some cases of eating disorders are associated with childhood physical or emotional abuse (Feldman & Meyer, 2007b; Mazzeo & Espelage, 2002) and childhood adversity (Johnson et al., 2002).

Although establishing causality may be impossible, studies provide some evidence to support disturbed patterns in families of clients with anorexia. The severity and extended course of anorexia nervosa places heavy demands on caregivers (Kyriacou et al., 2008). In such situations,

the appropriate hierarchy of "parent in charge of child" is reversed in terms of food and eating. These clients eat or not according to their desires, and parents exert very little influence over these behaviors. Feeling extremely helpless, parents often make extraordinary efforts to entice these children to eat. Caregivers may exhibit higher levels of expressed emotion in terms of criticism, hostility, and overprotection. It has been suggested that the level of expressed emotion may be related to illness duration; however, further research is needed to discern this relationship (Kyriacou et al., 2008).

> **Checkpoint Questions**
> 1. Why is accurately determining the incidence of bulimia so difficult?
> 2. Which neurotransmitter is associated with inhibition of feeding behavior?

Signs and Symptoms/Diagnostic Criteria

Before a primary eating disorder is diagnosed, other psychiatric illnesses, such as depression or schizophrenia, must be ruled out. With anorexia, a physiologic basis (eg, neoplasia) also must be eliminated.

Criteria for anorexia and bulimia from the *Diagnostic and Statistical Manual of Mental Disorders,* 4th edition, text revision (*DSM-IV-TR*) clearly delineate their clinical features (American Psychiatric Association [APA], 2000a; *DSM-IV-TR* Box 26.1). Eating disorders that do not meet full criteria for either of these problems are classified as *eating disorders not otherwise specified* (NOS).

Anorexia Nervosa

Although anorexia was described as early as the 17th century, health care professionals and the general public have become increasingly aware of it in recent decades. Typical signs and symptoms include a voluntary refusal to eat and typically a weight less than 85% of what is considered normal for height and age. Clients have a distorted body image and, to the bewilderment of others, view their bodies as fat. Some clients consider their whole bodies too fat, whereas others fixate on one or more particular parts (eg, stomach, legs) (Figure 26.4).

Although these clients consume little, they may be obsessed with food and spend time cooking for others, saving recipes, or talking about eating. They often obsessively pursue vigorous physical activity to burn "excess calories." Although at first the eating disorder may make clients feel "in control," eventually the disorder controls them.

In addition to psychological symptoms, clients experience the multiple physiologic consequences of starvation, some of which may be life threatening. Changes resulting from extreme weight loss may include **amenorrhea** (the absence or abnormal cessation of menstruation), lanugo hair, hypotension, bradycardia, hypothermia, constipation, polyuria, and electrolyte imbalances. Common laboratory

DSM-IV-TR BOX 26.1

Eating Disorders

Anorexia Nervosa

A. Refusal to maintain body weight at or above a minimally normal weight for age and height (eg, weight loss leading to maintenance of body weight less than 85% of that expected; or failure to make expected weight gain during period of growth, leading to body weight less than 85% of that expected).

B. Intense fear of gaining weight or becoming fat, even though underweight.

C. Disturbance in the way in which one's body weight or shape is experienced, undue influence of body weight or shape on self-evaluation, or denial of the seriousness of the current low body weight.

D. In postmenarchal females, amenorrhea, ie, the absence of at least three consecutive menstrual cycles. (A woman is considered to have amenorrhea if her periods occur only following hormone, eg, estrogen, administration.)

Restricting Type: During the current episode of Anorexia Nervosa, the person has not regularly engaged in binge-eating or purging behavior (ie, self-induced vomiting or the misuse of laxatives, diuretics, or enemas).

Binge-Eating/Purging Type: During the current episode of Anorexia Nervosa, the person has regularly engaged in binge-eating or purging behavior (ie, self-induced vomiting or the misuse of laxatives, diuretics, or enemas).

Bulimia Nervosa

A. Recurrent episodes of binge eating. An episode of binge eating is characterized by both of the following:

1. Eating in a discrete period of time (eg, within any 2-hour period) an amount of food that is definitely larger than most people would eat during a similar period of time and under similar circumstances

2. A sense of lack of control over eating during the episode (eg, a feeling that one cannot stop eating or control what or how much one is eating)

B. Recurrent inappropriate compensatory behavior in order to prevent weight gain, such as self-induced vomiting; misuse of laxatives, diuretics, enemas, or other medications; fasting; or excessive exercise.

C. The binge eating and inappropriate compensatory behaviors both occur, on average, at least twice a week for 3 months.

D. Self-evaluation is unduly influenced by body shape and weight.

E. The disturbance does not occur exclusively during episodes of Anorexia Nervosa.

Purging Type: During the current episode of Bulimia Nervosa, the person has regularly engaged in self-induced vomiting or the misuse of laxatives, diuretics, or enemas.

Nonpurging Type: During the current episode of Bulimia Nervosa, the person has used other inappropriate compensatory behaviors, such as fasting or excessive exercise, but has not regularly engaged in self-induced vomiting or the misuse of laxatives, diuretics, or enemas.

Reprinted with permission from the *Diagnostic and Statistical Manual of Mental Disorders, Fourth Edition, Text Revision* (Copyright © 2000). American Psychiatric Association.

---

abnormalities include increased serum cholesterol and carotene levels; decreased serum zinc and copper levels; increased blood urea nitrogen, cortisol, and growth hormone levels; anemia; leukopenia; and abnormal serum albumin. Low serum calcium levels may cause leg cramps. Repeated purging with laxatives can lead to permanent damage to the anal sphincter.

Families of clients with anorexia typically describe them as model children: compliant, obedient perfectionists who want to please adults with authority. They are usually high academic and athletic achievers. Symptoms frequently manifest after life changes, such as starting high school, moving to a new city or school, or going away to camp. Siblings of clients with anorexia are also at risk for eating disorders.

Bulimia Nervosa

Bulimia is characterized by episodic, uncontrolled, rapid ingestion of large quantities of food. It may occur alone or in conjunction with the food restriction of anorexia. Clients with bulimia nervosa compensate for excessive food intake by self-induced vomiting, obsessive exercise, use of laxatives and diuretics, or all of these behaviors. They may consume an incredible number of calories (an average of 3,415 per binge) in a short period, induce vomiting, and perhaps repeat this behavior several times a day (Figure 26.5).

Clients with bulimia may develop dental caries from the frequent contact of tooth enamel with food and acidic gastric fluids. Other physiologic complications include electrocardiogram (ECG) changes, parotid gland enlargement, esophagitis, gastric dilation, menstrual irregularity, and electrolyte imbalances.

The typical client with bulimia is a young, college-educated woman who achieves highly at work or school. Despite her achievements, she tends to be passive, dependent, and unassertive. Her family may be disorganized, noncohesive, in conflict, and characterized by confusing sex role expectations for women. Alcohol and substance abuse problems

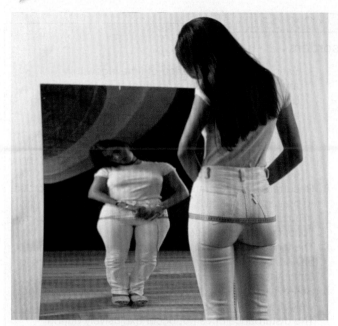

FIGURE 26.4 One of the hallmarks of anorexia nervosa is a distorted body image. Clients become fixated on their bodies and view themselves as fat even when objective evidence indicates otherwise. (Copyright © Oscar Burriel/Photo Researchers, Inc.)

are common, perhaps indicating increased impulsivity in this group (Wolfe et al., 2003). See Case Vignette 26.1.

Other Eating Disorders

Although this chapter focuses primarily on anorexia and bulimia, nurses should be aware of other eating disorders. **Binge eating disorder (BED),** an additional diagnostic category to the *DSM-IV-TR,* similarly affects males and females, many of whom are medically overweight or obese (Anderson & Yager, 2005). Characteristics of BED include recurrent eating binges; guilt, shame, and disquiet about binging; and marked psychological distress (Costin, 2002).

One of the most challenging current epidemics in Western countries involves overweight and obesity, conditions that result from the regular overconsumption of calories and sedentary lifestyles. Obesity has significant physical and psychological overtones and ramifications. Many researchers view obesity as the result of compulsive eating behavior. It certainly is associated with morbidity and is not a healthy state. Currently, obesity is not considered a psychiatric disorder in the *DSM-IV-TR;* however, because of the rapidly growing numbers of obese people of all ages (including pediatric clients), nurses need to be sensitive to their related emotional and psychological concerns and prepared to work with all clients to promote healthy lifestyles and knowledge of nutritious eating and effective eating behaviors.

Comorbidities and Dual Diagnoses

Numerous studies show an association between depression, anxiety, and eating disorders, but determining whether mood disorders lead to eating disorders or vice versa is difficult. Between 30% and 65% of clients with anorexia nervosa have a lifetime history of anxiety disorders, especially obsessive-compulsive disorder and social phobia, and between 50% and 68% have a lifetime prevalence of affective disorders,

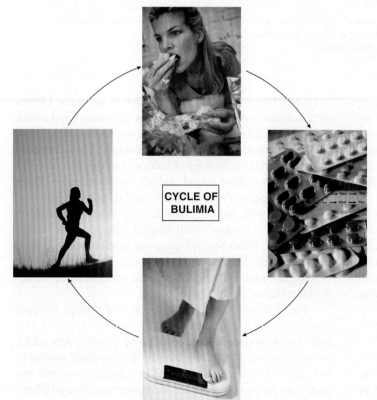

CYCLE OF BULIMIA

FIGURE 26.5 Clients with bulimia become trapped in recurring behaviors involving food and weight management. They ingest a vast number of calories at once and then take measures to purge themselves of their binge (eg, abuse of laxatives, diet pills, and diuretics). They monitor their weight several times a day; some exercise obsessively to burn off the calories.

Case Vignette 26.1

Kelsey, a high school sophomore, is 5'8" and weighs 115 lb (52.2 kg). A teacher refers her to the school nurse after hearing Kelsey vomit in the bathroom several times. The nurse initially notices that Kelsey's teeth are in poor condition. When the nurse asks about the vomiting, Kelsey looks embarrassed but confides that she is worried about gaining weight and forces herself to throw up after eating.

Upon questioning, Kelsey reports that she began trying to lose weight during the summer before her freshman year. Several of her friends were dieting, and Kelsey, although not overweight, gradually ate less and less. Between July and December, her weight dropped from 114 to 87 lb (51.7 to 39.5 kg). Her parents didn't worry at first but eventually became upset. Kelsey recalls that they tried to bribe her with food and fought about her refusal to eat. Right before that Christmas, Kelsey's mother took her to the family physician, who told Kelsey that she would be admitted to the hospital if she didn't eat. No other intervention occurred. The idea of being hospitalized and missing school frightened Kelsey, who always has been a straight-A student. She agreed to start eating and regained the lost weight over the next several months.

Kelsey can't remember exactly when she first thought of vomiting to control her weight. She learned that if she drank a lot of water after eating she could easily induce vomiting. With this discovery, she began eating larger amounts of food and then purging them. So that her family wouldn't be suspicious that food was disappearing quickly, she began buying, and then stealing, candy and cookies and hiding them in her room. Kelsey states that her parents have no idea what she is doing. The family has never discussed her weight since they took her to the doctor the previous year.

Kelsey reports that she sometimes wonders if she is crazy and that she is ashamed of her teeth. The nurse provides some basic information about anorexia nervosa and bulimia. Kelsey is relieved to hear that others have similar problems. The nurse explains that there is an association between frequent eating, vomiting, and dental caries but that Kelsey should not blame herself because she didn't develop eating problems on purpose.

With Kelsey's agreement, the nurse calls her parents in for a conference. She explains what is happening and that Kelsey needs assistance to cope effectively. Without blaming anyone, the nurse explains that it would help if the entire family met with a counselor experienced in eating disorders. The parents initially deny that Kelsey has a problem, emphasizing her excellent school performance and regular eating. They add that everyone in their family has poor teeth. However, after hearing in more detail about Kelsey's vomiting and stealing of food, they agree to attend a family session.

Reflection and Critical Thinking

- What biologic, social, family, and other factors may have contributed to Kelsey's development of an eating disorder?
- Was the intervention by the family physician appropriate? If not, how would you have modified this approach? How does your response relate to the importance of client teaching?
- What are the goals of family therapy? Based on the information provided, what factors may hinder the family's progress? What factors may assist their progress?

---

especially depression (Golden & Attia, 2011). For bulimia nervosa there is a high comorbidity for mood disorders (50% to 70%), anxiety disorders (13% to 65%), substance abuse (25%), and personality disorders (20% to 80%) (Golden & Attia, 2011). Anorexia nervosa and bulimia nervosa co-occur in 30% to 64% of clients (Marken & Sommi, 2002).

> ### Checkpoint Questions
> **3.** How do clients with anorexia nervosa view their bodies?
> **4.** How do families typically describe their relative with anorexia?
> **5.** What is the underlying cause of dental caries in clients with bulimia nervosa?

Implications and Prognosis

People with eating disorders rarely seek help, typically are not motivated to change, and often leave treatment (Nordbo et al., 2006). Many of them never seek or receive any intervention. Some recover spontaneously, whereas others have long-term problems. One study found that after 21 years, 50% of clients with anorexia nervosa had recovered fully, 25% had intermediate outcomes, 10% still met the criteria for anorexia nervosa, and 15% had died of anorexia-related complications (Zipfel et al., 2000). In a 5-year prospective follow-up study, 35% of clients continued to meet the full diagnostic criteria for anorexia nervosa (Fairburn et al., 2000).

Bulimia nervosa has higher rates of recovery than does anorexia nervosa. In a 10-year follow-up study of clients with bulimia, approximately 30% continued to engage in binge eating or purging behaviors. A 20-year longitudinal study found that adult roles in marriage and parenting were associated with significant decreases in disordered eating in women but not in men (Keel et al., 2007).

Interdisciplinary Goals and Treatment

The psychiatric field has long acknowledged the difficulties associated with treating clients who have eating disorders. Randomized, controlled studies to support interventions are scant. Care management is complex and frequently lengthy. Improvement often is gradual and characterized by "two steps forward, one step back." These clients may resist treatment because denial is typically strong.

Because of the complex nature of eating disorders, multimodality care is indicated (Kong, 2005). Individual and group psychotherapy, behavior therapy, cognitive–behavioral therapy (CBT), dialectical-pharmacologic behavior therapy (DBT), nutritional, and family therapy are used.

Psychopharmacology is also a component, although medications are usually not the primary intervention. See Evidence-Based Practice Spotlight 26.1 for current findings related to treatment modalities for specific eating disorders.

EVIDENCE-BASED PRACTICE SPOTLIGHT 26.1

Interventions for Eating Disorders

Disorders/ Behavior	Support for Treatment	Positive Effects— Consistent Evidence	Inconsistent Evidence—Unproven	Comments
Anorexia nervosa	Evidence-based treatments	*Psychosocial* Family therapy and renutrition are effective for younger clients, particularly with parental control of renutrition. CBT reduces relapse risk in adults after weight restoration. *Pharmacologic* Antidepressants (TCAs, SSRIs) elevate mood, but don't result in weight gain.	Family therapy not effective in adults with longer duration of illness. Individual psychotherapy Group therapy No evidence to support CBT during acute phase of illness before weight restoration No pharmacologic evidence for efficacy in weight gain Fluoxetine may play a role in relapse prevention in adults with anorexia nervosa Inconclusive evidence for efficacy of atypical antipsychotics	Many clients resist and display a limited response to treatment. Long-term monitoring and intervention may be necessary.
Bulimia nervosa	Evidence-based treatment	*Psychosocial* Individual or group CBT DBT (preliminary evidence) Combined CBT and fluoxetine Guided self-help *Pharmacologic* Fluoxetine 60 mg/day reduces core symptoms of binging and purging; medication-only trials suggest that although bulimic symptoms improve, they still persist.	*Not effective* Bupropion MAOIs *Some evidence* Trazodone, fluvoxamine, desipramine, topiramate; nutritional counseling alone	Combined CBT and fluoxetine led to greater improvements than fluoxetine only. Combined CBT and fluoxetine led to greater decreases in binging and purging than fluoxetine alone. Intervention includes treatment of co-occurring disorders, the establishment of regular nonbinge meals, and improvement of attitudes related to the disorder.
Binge eating disorder (BED) (overweight clients)	Evidence-based treatment	*Psychosocial* Individual or group CBT reduces binging and improves abstinence rates. DBT and guided self-help decrease binging. *Pharmacologic* SSRIs effective in short-term trials Low-dose imipramine in conjunction with standard dietary counseling and psychological support	CBT, DBT, and self-help not associated with weight loss *Some evidence* Promising results for weight reduction and reduced binge eating with such antiobesity medications as sibutramine, topiramate, and zonisamide	High placebo responses in BED are noteworthy. Possibly CBT, DBT, and guided self-help result in decreased binging but not weight loss. Perhaps clients distribute excess calories over nonbinge meals. Treatment strategies are similar to those for bulimia nervosa except that clients with BED present difficulties associated with being overweight.

Settings for Care

In many settings, nurses, physicians, psychotherapists, social workers, dietitians, and occupational therapists collaborate to form a treatment plan. Communication and consistency among team members are critical. The primary nurse often coordinates client care.

Treatment most commonly happens in community-based settings. In the current climate of health care reform, managed care and short-term treatments dominate. Settings for care increasingly include schools, community mental health centers, clinics, private offices, and day treatment centers.

Clients with anorexia nervosa are hospitalized more frequently than are those with bulimia. The primary reasons for hospitalization are low weight, depressed mood, low serum potassium level, lack of response to outpatient treatment, and family discouragement and demoralization. Other factors leading to inpatient admission include the client's desire for treatment and a diagnosis of maladaptive personality patterns such as an impulse disorder or borderline personality disorder (see Chap. 25).

Clinical and Dialectical-Pharmacologic Behavioral Therapies

Studies suggest that CBT may reduce relapse risk in adults with anorexia nervosa, but evidence of its effectiveness during the acute phase of illness is insufficient (AHRQ, 2006). Those with bulimia appear to have good response to CBT (Golden & Attia, 2011) in conjunction with interpersonal psychotherapy (Rigotti, 2000). One study showed that CBT was superior to interpersonal psychotherapy for improving symptoms of bulimia nervosa (Agras et al., 2000). A literature review indicates that pharmacotherapy and psychotherapy appear to play a role in the treatment of bulimia nervosa, but data support CBT as the intervention of choice (Golden & Attia, 2011; Mitchell et al., 2006).

Clinical trials indicate that CBT decreases the number of binge episodes in BED and leads to greater rates of abstinence for as long as 4 months after treatment (AHRQ, 2006). Results are mixed as to whether CBT improves self-rated depression.

DBT also has been found effective against bulimia nervosa. Medication trials with 60 mg/day of fluoxetine for 6 to 18 weeks reduced the core bulimic symptoms of binging and purging; this regimen is associated with prevention of relapse at 1 year (AHRQ, 2006).

Family Therapy

Family therapy may be part of inpatient or outpatient treatment. This modality assumes particular importance when clients are to return to a family home after discharge. Interventions focus on fostering open, healthy interaction patterns among members. Several randomized trials in which parents were empowered to help refeed the child with anorexia nervosa have shown short- and long-term success with weight restoration (Locke et al., 2005).

Family therapy is challenging because clients and families may deny the eating disorder. Even when they admit a problem, they may minimize its extent. These families also may have significant denial about other family problems or conflicts, which may be contributing to the eating disorder. To complicate matters, clients may not be thinking clearly and may be unable to reason effectively enough to participate meaningfully.

Behavior family systems therapy (BFST) is an approach that blends behavior modification, cognitive therapy, and family therapy. It relies on empirically tested behavioral and cognitive techniques (Robin et al., 1997, 1999). BFST for anorexia nervosa begins *after* the client is medically stable. It consists of four phases:

1. *Assessment:* The multidisciplinary team, consisting of dietitian, physician, psychologist, nurse, and other professionals, comes together to coordinate care with the client and family. Team members engage the family in treatment and check the client's weight weekly. They conduct history, behavioral, and social and functional analyses.
2. *Control rationale:* The therapist encourages parents to "take charge" of the client's eating and deals with their reactions. The therapist also coaches parents to develop an appropriate behavioral weight program.
3. *Weight gain:* The therapist begins to refine the weight-gain program and introduces non–food-related issues. He or she begins cognitive therapy interventions (eg, cognitive restructuring). Family psychotherapy and psychoeducation take place.
4. *Weight maintenance:* Control over food gradually returns to the client. Team members teach healthy ways of maintaining weight. Family interactions increasingly become the focus of treatment. The therapist fosters client individuation.

Children and adolescents with early-onset anorexia seem to respond well to family therapy, but this approach has not been found effective in adults with anorexia of long duration (AHRQ, 2006; Lock et al., 2006). See Evidence-Based Practice Spotlight 26.2.

Psychopharmacology

Difficulty with subject recruitment and high dropout rates have made it challenging to conduct randomized controlled trials of medication effectiveness (Golden & Attia, 2011). Medications are useful for some clients with eating disorders. Because one theory posits that a cause of eating disorders is disturbed serotonin regulation, researchers have studied the effectiveness of antidepressants. Study results have varied.

Pharmacologic therapy is not the primary intervention for anorexia in either youths or adults; however, antidepressants or antianxiety drugs may benefit clients with depressive, anxious, or obsessive-compulsive symptoms (APA, 2000b; Crow et al., 2009; Golden & Attia, 2011; Halmi, 2008).

EVIDENCE-BASED PRACTICE SPOTLIGHT 26.2

Interventions for Anorexia Nervosa

Overview of Effective Treatment: Family therapy has been shown effective for younger clients with a short duration of illness. One particular family therapy that encourages parents to oversee the young person's nutrition is associated with weight gain and psychological improvements. Tricyclic antidepressants (TCAs) have been associated with improved mood but not with weight gain. Cognitive–behavioral therapy (CBT) may reduce relapse risk for adults with anorexia nervosa after weight restoration. Fluoxetine may play a role in relapse prevention of anorexia nervosa in adults.

What Has Not Been Shown Effective: Studies provide no support for family therapy in adults with long duration of illness. In a summary of drug trials, no pharmacologic intervention for anorexia nervosa had a significant effect on weight gain. Evidence does not exist to determine whether

CBT works during the acute phase of the illness before normal weight has been restored.

There is inconclusive evidence for the efficacy of atypical antipsychotics.

Implications for Practice: Anorexia nervosa continues to be a difficult disorder to treat. People with it are resistant to intervention, frequently drop out of treatment, and often experience relapse. Medication trials have not demonstrated the effectiveness of medications to treat anorexia nervosa. Behavioral therapies appear to offer some benefit and may help prevent relapse. Because family therapy has been found effective with younger people who have anorexia nervosa, nurses should encourage parents to be closely involved in the treatment planning process, especially in taking control of renutrition.

References

Agency for Healthcare Research and Quality (AHRQ). (2006). *Management of eating disorders.* Rockville, MD: U.S. Department of Health and Human Services.

Golden, N., & Attia, E. (2011). Psychopharmacology of eating disorders in children and adolescents. *Pediatric Clinics of North America, 58,* 121–138.

Kaye, W., Nagata, T., Weltzin, T., Hsu, L. K., Sokol, M. S., McConaha, C., . . . Deep, D. (2001). Double-blind placebo-controlled administration of fluoxetine in restricting- and restricting-purging-type anorexia nervosa. *Biological Psychiatry, 49*(7), 644–652.

Pike, K., Walsh, B., Vitousek, K., Wilson, G. T., & Bauer, J. (2003). Cognitive behavior therapy in the posthospitalization treatment of anorexia nervosa. *American Journal of Psychiatry, 160*(11), 2046–2049.

Robin, A., Siegel, P., Moye, A., Gilroy, M., Dennis, A. B., & Sikand, A. (1999). A controlled comparison of family versus individual therapy for adolescents with anorexia nervosa. *Journal of the American Academy of Child and Adolescent Psychiatry, 38*(12), 1482–1489.

Walsh, B., Kaplan, A., Attia, E., Olmsted, M., Parides, M., Carter, J. C., . . . Rockert, W. (2006). Fluoxetine after weight restoration in anorexia nervosa: A randomized controlled trial. *Journal of American Medical Association, 295*(22), 2605–2612.

Although little evidence has shown that psychotropic medications contribute to weight gain in anorexia nervosa, data suggest that selective serotonin reuptake inhibitors (SSRIs), such as fluoxetine, help sustain recovery once weight is within 15% of normal (Rigotti, 2000). Summaries of drug trials indicate that no pharmacologic intervention for anorexia nervosa had a significant effect on weight gain, although antidepressants may be associated with improved mood (AHRQ, 2006). Some success has been shown in a controlled trial of olanzapine (Zyprexa) in treating low body weight and obsessive thinking in anorexia nervosa (Bissada et al., 2008).

Antidepressants do appear to have therapeutic benefits in many clients with bulimia (Golden & Attia, 2011), with a decrease in binge-purge behaviors reported as high as 75% (Work Group on Eating Disorders, 2000). Fluoxetine in particular has been found to be effective in the treatment of bulimia nervosa (Schatzberg et al., 2010) and is approved by the U.S. Food and Drug Administration for this purpose (Crow et al., 2009; Golden & Attia, 2011). Findings from the Fluoxetine Bulimia Nervosa Collaboration Study indicate that 60 mg/day of fluoxetine was superior to both placebo and lower doses (Marken & Sommi, 2002). The tricyclic antidepressants (TCAs) also have been

found to be effective in treating bulimia nervosa (Halmi, 2008; Rigotti, 2000), especially in combination with CBT. However, the SSRIs often are better tolerated and have greater cardiac safety than do the TCAs, especially in low-weight clients (Marken & Sommi, 2002). Clients who display obsessive-compulsive traits particularly may benefit from treatment with clomipramine (Anafranil) or fluoxetine (Prozac). Lithium, the TCAs, and anticonvulsants also have been reported useful in treating bulimia in adults. However, they are not recommended for treating children with bulimia.

In short-term medication-only trials, SSRIs appear to lead to reductions in symptoms of BED in overweight people (AHRQ, 2006). Low-dose imipramine in conjunction with dietary counseling and psychological support is also associated with decreases in binge eating and weight loss.

Checkpoint Questions

6. What are the four phases of behavior family systems therapy (BFST)?

7. Which drug is the only antidepressant approved by the FDA for treatment of bulimia?

APPLYING THE NURSING PROCESS

Eating Disorders

Eating disorders have complex accompanying physical and psychosocial problems, which makes their management greatly challenging. Sensitivity to the needs of clients with eating disorders helps nurses intervene constructively, even for those who resist treatment and persist in self-destructive behaviors. Forming an alliance with clients is crucial. A supportive but firm approach should engage clients in the therapeutic relationship. Case in Point 26.1 outlines nursing care for a client with anorexia nervosa.

▲ ASSESSMENT

Because clients with eating disorders may be secretive and unwilling to portray themselves as having problems, nurses must be skilled in eliciting feelings and thoughts. These clients may exhibit disturbances in many areas, so assessment can be complex. Knowledge of the etiology and diagnostic criteria of eating disorders and use of an organizational framework can provide needed guidance.

Health History

Assessment Tool 26.1 provides a comprehensive framework for organizing health history questions in key areas. Nurses ask questions designed to uncover various characteristics and problems. They must explore in depth any area of concern.

Case in Point 26.1

Jody's Story

Jody, a 20-year-old cross-country runner, is in her junior year of college. Her body fat is only 14%. Jody would like it to be even lower. The fastest runner on the team is very thin, and Jody runs extra miles every day to try to lose weight.

Jody's roommate is worried that Jody weighs herself several times a day, eats little, has stopped menstruating, and is often irritable and withdrawn. After hearing Jody vomiting in the bathroom several times, her roommate decides to confront Jody. She tells Jody what she has observed and explains that she wants to help. After responding with initial defensiveness, Jody admits, "I'm terrified that I will gain weight." She adds that she has low energy and leg pains. At her roommate's urging, Jody agrees to get an evaluation.

Jody meets with the family nurse practitioner. Although she is honest and forthcoming about her eating and exercise behaviors, Jody says that she doesn't really think she has a problem. The nurse practitioner replies, "I hear what you're saying and hope that this is not a problem. I am still worried about what I have seen and heard. I want to examine you and talk more about what is happening." Jody bursts into tears but agrees to the nurse practitioner's plan.

The nurse practitioner performs a physical examination, obtains some laboratory and diagnostic tests, and then continues her discussion with Jody. Jody reveals that her mother is controlling and that conflicts within the family never are handled in a straightforward way.

Key Assessment Findings

- **Cachectic appearance**
- **Height: 5′6″; Weight: 109 lb (49.4 kg)**
- **Heart rate: 50 bpm; blood pressure: 88/50 mm Hg**
- **Amenorrhea for the past several months**
- **Electrocardiogram: sinus bradycardia**
- **Laboratory tests: decreased hemoglobin and white blood cell count; low serum potassium, and calcium levels; decreased zinc and copper levels**
- **Reports of mother being controlling; family conflicts**

Nursing Diagnosis: Impaired Nutrition, Less Than Body Requirements related to fear of gaining weight as evidenced by reduced food intake, running extra miles to lose weight, dry skin and dull hair, vomiting, and abnormalities in laboratory test results

NOC: Nutritional Status: Food and Fluid Intake and **Nutritional Status: Nutrient Intake:** The client will gain 1 to 1.5 lb (0.45 to 0.68 kg)/week until she reaches 128 lb (58.1 kg) and will exhibit vital signs and electrolyte levels within acceptable parameters.

NIC: Eating Disorder Management
- Teach and reinforce concepts of healthy nutrition with the client and significant others. *They need to understand nutritional requirements to foster compliance and achieve positive outcomes.*
- Establish the amount of desired daily weight gain. Use behavior modification techniques to promote behaviors that contribute to weight gain and to limit weight loss behaviors as appropriate.

Develop a behavior modification contract for gradual weight gain that includes the following criteria:
- Ingesting 1,800 to 2,000 calories per day
- Limiting exercise to 30 minutes per day
- Establishing a system of rewards for compliance with contract (or restrictions for noncompliance). *A well-defined behavioral modification program that specifies desired weight gain will provide consistency, decrease power struggles, and enhance compliance.*
- Develop meal plans with the client. Meet with the school's dietitian to determine a plan that includes nutritious foods that the client likes. Establish expectations for appropriate eating behaviors, intake of food/fluid, and amount of physical activity. *Including the client in meal planning and expectations will enhance her sense of control.*

(continues on page 526)

Case in Point 26.1 (continued)

Jody's Story

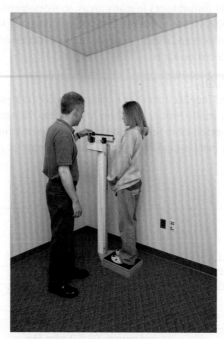

FIGURE A. **The nurse weighs the client daily.**

- Monitor the client's vital signs, food and fluid intake and output, and weight. Weigh the client daily at the same time and under the same conditions (Figure A). *Hypotension and bradycardia may result from starvation. Monitoring intake, output, and weight ensures the client's health.*
- Arrange for a family member or friend to supervise meals and remain with the client up to 1 hour after eating. Have this person observe the client during and after meals and snacks. *Direct observation will diminish the client's opportunities to avoid eating, to hoard or hide food, or to vomit.*
- Discuss with the client the need to avoid excessive exercise. Discuss the importance of exercise for physical and mental fitness, but that the client must stop relying on exercise for weight reduction (Figure B). *Clients with eating disorders may engage in excessive exercise to burn calories. By focusing on physical fitness, the client may begin to associate exercise with health promotion instead of weight loss.*
- Use a supportive, firm, nonjudgmental, and matter-of-fact approach in regulating eating behavior. *The client should not view a matter-of-fact approach as punishment. This approach also helps to alleviate guilt, leading the client to experience feelings of acceptance.*
- Encourage the client to use daily logs to record feelings, as well as circumstances surrounding urges to vomit or exercise to excess. *The client's participation promotes feelings of control. Record keeping provides the client with insight into her behaviors.*
- Provide support as the client begins to integrate new eating behaviors, changes in body image, and lifestyle alterations. *Support helps the client progress toward goal achievement and provides*

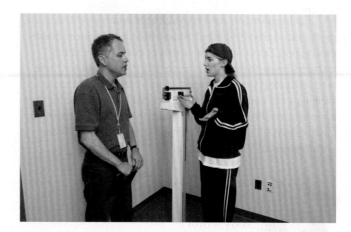

FIGURE B. **The nurse instructs the client that she needs to stop relying on exercise for weight reduction.**

reinforcement for positive behaviors, increasing the chances for successful outcomes.

Nutrition Management

- Ascertain client's preferences and collaborate with the dietitian related to calories and type of nutrients needed to meet the client's requirements (Figure C). *Incorporating the client's preferences along with necessary nutrients promotes compliance to achieve adequate nutrition.*
- Provide a liquid diet using supplements or through a nasogastric or nasoduodenal tube *as necessary* to maintain an adequate oral intake. *A liquid diet will provide adequate nutrition and fluid if the client is unwilling to eat and drink.*

NIC: Nutritional Monitoring

- Monitor trends in weight loss or gain and type and amount of usual exercise. *Monitoring for changes provides direct evidence of the client's compliance with the dietary plan.*

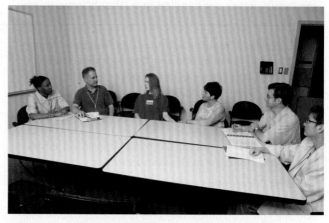

FIGURE C. **The interdisciplinary team works together to design a meal plan that is appropriate for the client's caloric and nutritional needs but that also includes the client's preferences to optimize the chances for success.**

Case in Point 26.1 (continued)

Jody's Story

- Assess the client for manifestations of poor nutrition in each body system. Note any changes in manifestations from the initial assessment, including the development of new manifestations. *Inadequate nutrition affects all body systems. Resolution of initial manifestations indicates improved nutritional status. The development of new manifestations may suggest a worsening of the client's status.*

NIC: Fluid/Electrolyte Management

- Monitor abnormal serum electrolyte levels. Evaluate the results of additional laboratory tests, including serum albumin, total protein, hemoglobin, and hematocrit. Assess for signs and symptoms of fluid and electrolyte imbalance. *The results of laboratory tests provide objective evidence of the client's nutritional status. Signs and symptoms of imbalances can provide additional evidence of abnormalities.*
- Keep an accurate record of intake and output. Give fluids as appropriate. *Intake and output monitoring is a valuable indicator of fluid balance. Fluid intake is necessary to correct possible dehydration.*
- Administer prescribed supplemental electrolytes as appropriate; monitor for side effects and for the client's response to therapy. *Electrolyte deficiencies are commonly associated with eating disorders and impaired nutrition. Supplements provide a means for replacing the electrolytes that are decreased, thereby reducing the client's risk for complications.*

> 4/12/13: The client has gained 1 lb/week during the last 3 weeks. Vital signs and electrolyte levels are within acceptable parameters. The client complies with daily nutrient, food, and fluid intake.
>
> K. Fenilworth, RN

Nursing Diagnosis: Disturbed Body Image related to fears of gaining weight as evidenced by low body fat percentage, behaviors involving limited eating and vomiting, and statements related to family conflicts and maternal control.

NOC: Body Image and Self-Esteem: The client will demonstrate a realistic appraisal of self.

NIC: Body Image Enhancement

- Use cognitive restructuring techniques; assist the client to review her own and others' bodies realistically. *The client can confront and substitute irrational beliefs with more realistic ones. External, objective feedback will help the client attain a healthier, more realistic body image.*
- Monitor the frequency of statements of self-criticism. Assist the client to identify aspects of her physical appearance about which she feels positive. Help her to separate physical appearance from personal worth (Figure D). *Self-criticism and negative self-perceptions promote an unrealistic body image. Evaluating changes in self-comments and self-descriptions, verbalizations*

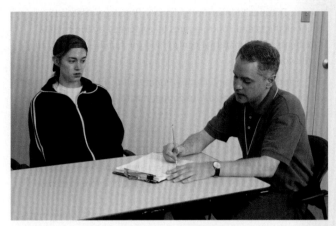

FIGURE D. During discussions of physical appearance and self-worth, the nurse documents the client's responses and works with her to separate her external elements from her internal personal worth.

of self-acceptance, and willingness to focus on positive attributes provides measures to evaluate progress toward goal achievement.

NIC: Self-Esteem Enhancement

- Assist the client to acknowledge the relationship between overly high self-expectations and feelings of inadequacy. Explore previous achievements and reasons for self-criticism or guilt. Encourage the client to identify strengths and resources. Reinforce her identified strengths. *Realistic self-expectations, positive reinforcement, and ongoing feedback will increase the client's sense of self-esteem.*
- Determine the client's locus of control and confidence in her own judgment. Encourage her to make decisions and choices independently. Convey confidence in the client's ability to handle situations. *Opportunities to practice independent functioning will help the client improve self-confidence and self-esteem.*
- Enhance the client's communication and socialization skills by promoting information, role-playing, and participation in group activities with peers. *Enhanced social skills will improve the client's peer relationships and contribute to improving her self-esteem.*

> 4/23/13: The client consistently describes herself in positive terms and demonstrates acceptance of self. She frequently verbalizes positive statements related to her internal picture of self and self-acceptance and body appearance. Statements are congruent among body reality, body ideal, and body presentation.
>
> K. Fenilworth, MSN

(continues on page 528)

Case in Point 26.1 (continued)

Jody's Story

Nursing Diagnosis: Interrupted Family Processes related to family conflicts and control issues as evidenced by the client's statements about maternal control and the family's inability to handle conflicts

NOC: Family Coping and Family Functioning: The client and family will demonstrate the ability to communicate directly and manage conflicts constructively.

NIC: Family Therapy
- Determine the client's usual roles within the family system and areas of dissatisfaction or conflict. *Families are highly individualized; knowledge of the specific roles of these family members provides a basis for intervention.*
- Progress discussion from least to most emotionally laden material. *Starting with the least emotionally laden material helps to establish rapport and trust.*
- Facilitate family discussion; help family members clarify what they need and expect from one another (Figure E). *Clarification of needs and expectations by members promotes sharing and awareness.*

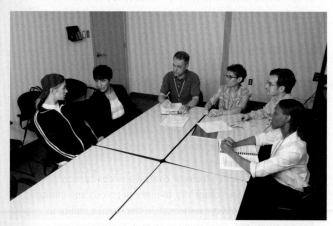

FIGURE E. The client's interdisciplinary team works with her and her mother to clarify expectations and facilitate improved communication.

- Assist family members to change by changing self as they relate to other family members; facilitate restructuring of family subsystems as appropriate. *Families are systems such that a change in one member ultimately affects all other members. Restructuring of family subsystems may be necessary to relieve conflict and improve communication.*

Family Integrity Promotion
- Determine typical family relationships, identify typical family coping mechanisms, and identify conflicting priorities among family members. *Identification of coping mechanisms provides opportunities to promote use of effective mechanisms while eliminating ineffective ones. Identification of conflicts aids in communicating and planning appropriate strategies to resolve them.*
- Explore ways for each member to increase autonomy. Role-model direct, constructive communication patterns for family members. *Children have more power to make decisions and accept responsibility for their own behavior. Role-modeling of open communication provides an example and gives family members permission to openly express their thoughts and feelings.*
- Encourage family members to openly identify and express conflicts. Encourage family members to speak for themselves by making "I," rather than "we," statements. *Communicating assertively fosters individuality and personal efficacy among family members. Family members need to learn to distinguish and be responsible for their own feelings, words, and actions.*

> 5/8/13: The client and family exhibit measures to communicate effectively and deal constructively with conflict. They consistently demonstrate role flexibility, ability to confront family problems, member involvement in decision making and problem solving, willingness to encourage age-appropriate autonomy and open communication, free expression of feelings and emotions, acceptance of change and new ideas, and ability to adapt to crisis.
>
> K. Fenilworth, RN

EPILOGUE

Jody agrees to undergo treatment as an outpatient at a local health care facility twice a week. Her roommate has agreed to provide support and also help in supervising Jody's mealtimes. After 4 weeks, Jody has gained approximately 1/2 lb (0.23 kg). The family nurse practitioner assesses Jody and finds that her vital signs remain low. Results of laboratory tests confirm leukopenia, anemia, hypocalcemia, and hypokalemia. An electrocardiogram also shows a prolonged QT interval. Jody's roommate reports that, although she hasn't directly observed it, she thinks that Jody is vomiting in secret at least once a day. Her roommate says, "Jody's mother has been calling every day and telling her to eat. Not long after the conversation, Jody is in the bathroom for a long time." Based on the findings, the family nurse practitioner decides that Jody should be admitted to the local acute care facility for evaluation and intensive treatment.

ASSESSMENT TOOL 26.1

Inventory for Clients With Eating Problems

Health Perception–Health Management

- How has your general health been?
- Do you have any health issues that need treatment?
- Have others been concerned about your health or your weight?
- Do you use laxatives or diuretics to control weight?

Nutrition–Metabolism

- Have you ever fasted to lose weight?
- Have you ever tried to vomit after eating?

Elimination

- Do you have to use laxatives to have a bowel movement?
- Do you have diarrhea often?

Activity–Exercise

- Do you feel weak or dizzy or have muscle cramping?
- Do you ever have palpitations?
- Do you follow a strict exercise regimen?
- Do you panic if you cannot exercise as much as you'd like?

Sleep–Rest

- Do you have difficulty sleeping?

Cognition–Perception

- Would you describe yourself as a perfectionist?
- Do you repeat things until you get them right?
- Have you ever been unable to get something out of your mind?
- Do you find yourself repeatedly thinking about the same things?
- How do you feel if you lose control, such as getting very angry or eating too much?
- What do you do when you feel you are losing control?
- Have you ever had times when you have eaten uncontrollably? What did you feel, and what did you do?

Self-Perception–Self-Concept

- What do you like best about your body?
- What do you like least about your body?
- If you could change how you look, how would you be different?
- What do you like best about yourself?
- What do you like least about yourself?
- How would you describe yourself to others?
- How would others (family, friends) describe you?
- What are your strengths?
- What are your weaknesses?

Roles–Relationships

- How is your relationship with your parents?
- How would you describe your family?
- Do you have many friends?
- Do you have a best friend?
- What do you like to do with your friends?
- What is school like?
- Do you study a lot?
- In what activities are you involved at school?
- Do you feel pressure to do well in school? If so, from whom?

Sexuality–Reproduction

- Have your periods become irregular or stopped completely? (for female clients)
- How do you feel about the body changes that occur at adolescence (eg, in females, breast development, menstruation, broadening of hips)?
- Is dating something that you enjoy?
- Have you had any sexual experiences?
- How do you feel about your sexual experiences (or lack of them)?

Coping–Stress Tolerance

- How do you make decisions about everyday things?
- How do you spend your free time? (For example, do you usually ask someone for advice or think things out for yourself?)
- Is your life right now pretty much the way you want it? If not, what would you change? What can you do to make these changes?
- What do you do to feel better when you are sad or upset?
- Have you ever felt like hurting yourself when you are down?
- Have you ever thought about committing suicide?
- Have you ever used alcohol or drugs to feel better?
- Have you ever stolen anything (eg, food or money)? If so, how do you feel about that?
- Do you get along with your parents? What happens when you argue with them? What do you argue about? What happens when you talk to them about a problem or concern?
- How do you get along with your siblings? Can you talk to them about your feelings and problems?
- Do your friends help you if you have a problem?

Values–Beliefs

- What is important to you?
- What do you care about?
- What is the meaning of life for you?

Nutrition

First and foremost, nurses start with an evaluation of nutritional status. They should review the client's history for previous high and low weights and for a chronology of recent weight fluctuations. Nurses also should question the rate of weight loss or gain and any associated circumstances, such as medical illness, psychiatric illness, situational crisis, or major life changes. Because clients may be reluctant to reveal details about dieting or binge-purge behaviors, nurses should ask clients to describe food and fluid intake for a typical day.

Elimination

Nurses ask clients about elimination disturbances, which commonly accompany eating disorders. Constipation may result from food restriction, self-induced vomiting, and slowed gastrointestinal motility. Excessive laxative use causes diarrhea and loss of protein, fluid, and potassium in stools. Long-term laxative use may lead to eventual reliance on laxatives for bowel elimination. Clients with severe weight loss may report polyuria.

Reproduction and Hormones

Nurses review areas of the history that may reveal problems with hormonal imbalances, which frequently result from excessive weight loss. For example, reproductive hormones regress to prepubertal levels in clients who have lost significant weight. Consequences include amenorrhea, breast atrophy, lanugo, and loss of axillary and pubic hair. Infertility accompanies amenorrhea, but this typically resolves once clients regain weight and menses resume.

Activity and Rest

Another concern is patterns of activity and rest. Assessment questions should cover types of exercise, involvement in organized sports (especially for students), difficulty sleeping, and fatigue or lack of energy. Often, patterns of exercise and rest are markedly disordered, with some clients engaging in compulsive activity at all times to burn calories. Some clients who exercise compulsively experience frequent insomnia. Early morning awakening is common.

Psychosocial

Clients with eating disorders typically lack awareness of the connection between their eating behaviors and underlying feelings, needs, and conflicts. They tend to exhibit intellectualization and all-or-nothing reasoning. They are more comfortable with abstractions than with recognizing and expressing feelings. These clients also tend to be perfectionists and to give up if something is not exactly right. They may overgeneralize and believe that

losing enough weight will solve all their problems. Emotional reasoning, a type of cognitive distortion, is characteristic (Table 26.1). **Emotional reasoning** means relying on emotions to determine reality. An example of emotional reasoning in clients with eating disorders is "I know I'm fat because I feel fat."

Clients with eating disorders experience considerable anxiety about obesity. Many have distorted body images, with even emaciated clients seeing themselves as fat although they are, in reality, alarmingly thin. They usually have a poor self-image despite achievements at school, sports, and work. Their expectations often are unrealistically rigid and high. They look to others for approval and perceive a lack of control over themselves and situations. They do not believe that their actions will lead to desired outcomes.

Clients with eating disorders frequently become isolated from family and friends. They often exhibit immature interactions and remain inappropriately dependent and childlike in their relationships with parents. They may stop dating and gradually abandon good friends. As the disorder persists, deficits in social skills increase. They often remain good students and spend much time alone studying. Isolation also may result from preoccupation with weight, food, and exercise.

Eating disorders are maladaptive attempts to meet life's demands, roles, and stresses. Clients may have difficulty in the following areas:

- Asking for help and nurturance
- Making decisions
- Meeting role expectations
- Expressing emotions
- Exerting control (perceived powerlessness)

Because clients with eating disorders may have compromised self-knowledge or self-awareness, their values and beliefs may be poorly defined. In addition, eating disorders emerge most often when clients are struggling to establish an identity and to formulate a philosophy about the meaning of existence. See Therapeutic Communication 26.1.

TABLE 26.1 Manifestations of Cognitive Distortions in Clients With Eating Disorders

Distortion	Explanations	Example
Catastrophizing/magnification	Giving an event or its consequences more merit than is realistic	"These jeans feel tight today. I know everyone can tell that I've gained 3 lb (1.4 kg)."
Dichotomous thinking	Reasoning by extremes; seeing everything as "black or white"	"If I'm not thin, I must be fat." "I've already eaten two slices of pizza and wrecked my diet. I might as well eat the whole thing."
Emotional reasoning	Relying on emotions to determine reality	"I know I'm fat because I feel fat."
Overgeneralization	Basing beliefs on one or a few, not necessarily related, considerations	"I don't have a boyfriend. It must be because I'm fat." "Liz is so thin and has the perfect life. I should lose weight so my life can be better."
Personalization	Overinterpreting an event as having personal significance	"Dad made a face when I grabbed a piece of candy from the jar. He must think I'm overweight."
Selective abstraction	Focusing on only some information while choosing to ignore other information	"I've lost 10 lb (4.5 kg), but I still can't fit into a size 8. I'm a failure."

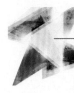

Therapeutic Communication 26.1

Moving with Resistance

Elise, a 16-year-old with bulimia nervosa, has come to the school mental health clinic at the insistence of her sister, who is concerned about Elise's purging. Elise presents with a sense of agitation, and during the interview she seems quite distracted. She asks for a glass of water. She stands, moves about, and generally appears unsettled and anxious. When asked if she wants to sit, she replies, "I prefer to stand."

INEFFECTIVE DIALOGUE

NURSE: Tell me why you are here.

ELISE: *(Walks toward door)* You know, I need a break. I'm going to sit out in the waiting room. If you want to talk to me there, that's fine.

NURSE: *(Looks at watch and shakes her head)* I don't think that's appropriate. Let's get started. We only have 40 minutes.

ELISE: *(Hand on doorknob)* Frankly, I don't think I need help, and this was a big mistake. I'm not nuts.

NURSE: *(Sighs and sits behind her desk)* Elise, you must want to be helped for something. You're here, aren't you?

ELISE: *(Getting defensive)* Well that wasn't my idea. My sister and boyfriend forced me. I am just fine.

NURSE: *(Notices Elise's behavior is defensive)* You're very defensive. There must be something behind all that defensiveness.

ELISE: Fine, then you have a good time trying to root around for what it is. *(Slams door on her way out)*

EFFECTIVE DIALOGUE

NURSE: What are some of the things that concern you?

ELISE: *(Walks toward door)* You know, I need a break. I'm going to sit out in the waiting room. If you want to talk to me there, that's fine.

NURSE: Before we step out, why don't we talk frankly for a minute. I guess that both you and I realize that this situation is stressful for you. It's hard to share important and personal information with a stranger. *(Remains patient with Elise, sensing that she is trying to express something other than her words)*

ELISE: I don't know, I guess you're going to get inside my head. Isn't that what psychotherapy does, shrink heads?

NURSE: I guess that depends on what you mean. What were you expecting today?

ELISE: *(Says with some exasperation but less tension)* I don't know. I guess I was expecting to lie down on some couch. I also thought that coming here meant that I was some kind of a nut.

NURSE: First of all, there are no couches. We'll talk for about 40 minutes and only about those things that *you* think are important. *(Trying to restore some sense of control to Elise)* You don't have to talk about anything that is too painful. That's your decision. We'll move at your pace. Is that OK with you?

ELISE: Yeah, I guess that will be fine.

NURSE: By the way, you said that you were afraid that you were "some kind of a nut." Are you worried that you'll be seen as unstable or "nuts" as you say? *(Redirecting Elise to what might be bothering her)*

ELISE: Yes, the thought had crossed my mind.

NURSE: What exactly are you worried about?

ELISE: My sister thinks I'm crazy. So does my boyfriend. They're convinced of it, and I'm beginning to wonder myself.

Reflection and Critical Thinking

- What types of communication did Elise exhibit in both scenarios? Assess the reason for Elise's fear of losing control. Why might she be anxious about this interview?
- What nonverbal cues did Elise and the nurse give in both scenarios?
- What methods of communication did the nurse use in the second scenario that ultimately were more effective than those used in the first?

Physical Examination

The behaviors associated with eating disorders involve manipulation or deprivation of foods and fluids, which can result in severely disturbed, even life-threatening metabolic processes. Nurses must be sure to obtain an accurate initial weight. A comprehensive physical examination may reveal numerous symptoms related to disturbances in nutrition and metabolism (Figure 26.6). Possible findings include dehydration, hypokalemia, cardiac dysrhythmia, hypotension, bradycardia, dry skin, brittle hair and nails, lanugo, frequent infections, dental caries, inflammation of the throat and esophagus, swollen parotid glands (from purging), amenorrhea, and hypothermia. A lowered pulse rate is a response to excessive exercise and starvation.

Laboratory Testing

Laboratory testing may be appropriate to assess for electrolyte abnormalities and cardiac dysfunction. Some clients with bulimia require an endoscopic examination to detect esophageal abnormalities incurred by frequent vomiting.

Laboratory studies are not diagnostic of eating disorders but help determine the extent of their harmful physiologic sequelae. They are especially important in cases of severe weight loss and in bulimia, in which serious volume, electrolyte, and cardiac rhythm disturbances are possible (Rigotti, 2000).

Abnormalities associated with anorexia nervosa include nutrition-related anemia, leukopenia, thrombocytopenia, bone marrow atrophy, and decreased chloride, calcium, magnesium, and phosphate levels (Hutter et al., 2009; Wolfe et al., 2003). Elevated blood urea nitrogen (BUN) levels may be related to dehydration or muscle wasting. Severe malnutrition may lead to elevated serum levels of hepatic enzymes and cholesterol. It is also associated with a sick euthyroid syndrome associated with reduced concentration of serum triiodothyronine (T_3). Decreased levels of follicle-stimulating hormone (FSH), luteinizing hormone (LH), estrogen, and progesterone are associated with secondary amenorrhea. Measurement of bone mineral density may be indicated for clients with a prolonged low weight state. In long-term starvation, dependence on gluconeogenesis is decreased, whereas use of ketone bodies as a cellular energy source is increased (Porth, 2009). In long-term starvation, depressed insulin levels and increased glucagon, cortisone, epinephrine, and growth hormones promote lipolysis in adipose tissue, thus liberating fatty acids to supply energy to cardiac and skeletal muscle cells and ketone bodies to sustain brain tissue. When the supply of adipose tissue is depleted, the breakdown of muscle and visceral protein is the last process to supply energy for life.

Laboratory studies in bulimia generally show fewer abnormalities (Rigotti, 2000; Wolfe et al., 2003). Repeated regurgitation may produce volume depletion, hypokalemia, and metabolic alkalosis with hypochloremia and increased concentration of serum bicarbonate. Laxative abuse may lead to hyponatremia, hypokalemia, and calcium and magnesium depletion. Diuretic abuse may cause hypochloremia, hyponatremia, and hypokalemia. Hypokalemia is particularly worrisome because it increases the risk for life-threatening cardiac dysrhythmias.

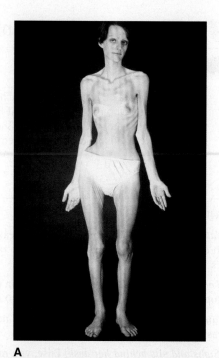

A

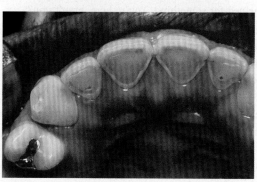

B

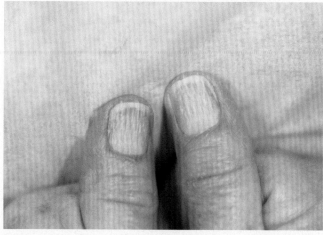

C

FIGURE 26.6 Physical examination of clients with eating disorders reveals characteristic findings. (**A**) This client with advanced anorexia nervosa has an obviously emaciated appearance. (**B**) The teeth of the client with bulimia nervosa who frequently self-induces vomiting may become eroded from frequent contact with digestive acids. (**C**) Clients also may have brittle, damaged hair and nails from poor nutrition, dehydration, and vitamin deficiencies.

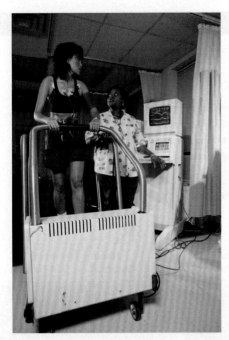

FIGURE 26.7 Clients with anorexia nervosa may undergo electrocardiogram studies. Nurses provide support during all forms of testing.

Electrocardiogram Studies

In anorexia nervosa, the cardiac muscle may atrophy, along with reduced left ventricular wall thickness and decreased cardiac output (Rigotti, 2000). Low-voltage ST segment depression, T-wave flattening, and prolonged QT intervals have been documented (Rigotti, 2000). Hypokalemia, which occurs in both anorexia nervosa and bulimia nervosa, contributes to prolonged ventricular repolarization and manifests as QT-interval prolongation or "U" waves (Wolfe et al., 2003) (Figure 26.7).

▲ NURSING DIAGNOSIS

Because of the multisystem nature of eating disorders, data analysis may suggest multiple nursing diagnoses. Clients who are medically unstable should have nursing diagnoses specific to their medical problems (eg, Deficient Fluid Volume, Decreased Cardiac Output).

Most nursing diagnoses for clients with eating disorders center on psychosocial problems. They may include the following (NANDA, 2007):

- **Imbalanced Nutrition: Less Than Body Requirements** related to refusal to ingest or retain ingested food, physical exertion in excess of caloric intake
- **Disturbed Thought Processes** related to all-or-none thinking, intellectualization, obsessions, overgeneralization, and malnutrition
- **Disturbed Body Image** related to unresolved psychosocial conflicts
- **Chronic Low Self-Esteem** related to unrealistic expectations from self or others, lack of positive feedback, striving to please others to gain acceptance

- **Powerlessness** related to belief that one's actions will not result in desired outcomes
- **Ineffective Coping** related to unmet developmental tasks (trust, autonomy), dysfunctional family system
- **Interrupted Family Processes** related to ineffective communication patterns, denial of problems and conflicts, unresolved issues of control, inability to manage conflict

▲ OUTCOME IDENTIFICATION AND PLANNING

Planning involves collaborating with the client and usually family to formulate an appropriate treatment approach and to set goals. Short-term goals focus on decreasing anxiety, stopping weight loss, restoring the person to an acceptable weight, and normalizing eating behaviors. Some identified desired outcomes, organized according to the Nursing Outcomes Classification (NOC), might include the following (Moorhead et al., 2008):

- **Nutritional Status: Food and Fluid Intake:** The client will have adequate dietary intake to meet body requirements and maintain weight that is appropriate to age and height.
- **Health Beliefs: Perceived Control:** The client will verbalize diminished fears and exhibit decreased anxiety regarding weight gain and loss of control.
- **Weight: Body Mass:** The client will not engage in binge eating or purging activities.
- **Impulse Self-Control:** The client will maintain an appropriate activity level.

Long-term goals focus on helping the client and, if possible, the family to resolve the psychological issues that precipitated the eating disorder and to develop more constructive coping mechanisms. Some identified desired outcomes, organized according to the Nursing Outcomes Classification (NOC), might include the following (Moorhead et al., 2008):

- **Body Image:** The client will verbalize adequate self-esteem.
- **Health Beliefs: Perceived Control:** The client will verbalize perceived control over actions.
- **Coping:** The client will recognize maladaptive coping behaviors and demonstrate adaptive coping behaviors.
- **Identity:** The client will recognize and verbalize emotions and needs.
- **Family Coping:** The family will demonstrate constructive communication patterns.
- **Family Support During Treatment:** The family will manage conflict constructively.

See Understanding Nursing Care 26.1.

▲ IMPLEMENTATION

The dynamics of eating disorders challenge nurses and other multidisciplinary care providers to establish relationships of open communication and trust with clients (Woolsey, 1998). Because many people with eating disorders never seek treatment, nurses commonly encounter the most severely ill clients in hospitals. Some clients are admitted to general psychiatric units or to units or facilities specializing in the treatment of eating disorders.

UNDERSTANDING NURSING CARE 26.1

EATING DISORDERS

Common Subjective Findings

Client denies existence of problem

Client reports preoccupation with weight

Feelings of sadness, worthlessness

Common Objective Findings

Underweight status

Poor skin turgor; lanugo

Bradycardia/hypotension/arrhythmias

Nursing Diagnosis: Disturbed Body Image

NOC	NIC
Body Image	Body Image Enhancement
	Emotional Support
	Support Group

Nursing Diagnosis: Imbalanced Nutrition: Less Than Body Requirements

NOC	NIC
Nutritional Status	Eating Disorders Management
Weight: Body Mass	Nutrition Management
	Weight Gain Assistance
Nutritional Status: Biochemical Measures	Electrolyte Management
	Electrolyte Monitoring
	Fluid/Electrolyte Management

Nursing Diagnosis: Chronic Low Self-Esteem

NOC	NIC
Depression Level	Hope Instillation
	Mood Management
Quality of Life	Self-Esteem Enhancement
	Values Clarification
Self-Esteem	Cognitive Restructuring
	Self-Esteem Enhancement
	Support System Enhancement

Indicators of Expected Outcomes

- Verbalizes satisfaction with appearance
- Reports a positive internal picture of self
- Moves toward congruence between self-perception and reality

Indicators of Expected Outcomes

- Improved food and fluid intake
- Improved weight-to-height ratio
- Stabilized vital signs
- Stabilized fluid and electrolyte levels

Indicators of Expected Outcomes

- Reports positive feelings of self-worth
- Describes self positively
- Verbalizes strengths and limitations

Families frequently are frustrated, angry, and scared after months of encouraging clients to eat. Temporarily removing clients from the home may relieve tensions and set the stage for behavior changes in clients and relatives (Box 26.1).

Nurses use many types of interventions to assist recovering clients and families. Common Nursing Interventions Classification (NIC) labels related to management of eating disorders include, but are not limited to, **Behavior Management, Eating Disorders Management, Nutrition Management, Nutrition Therapy, Self-Awareness Enhancement,** and **Weight Gain Assistance** (Bulechek et al., 2008).

Checkpoint Questions

8. What is the effect of excessive weight loss on the reproductive hormones of female clients with anorexia nervosa?
9. How does anorexia nervosa affect the heart?
10. What cognitive distortion is the client using when she says, "I've lost 8 pounds, but I still can't wear a size 3?"

BOX 26.1 Preventing Eating Disorders

When working with clients and populations who may be at risk for eating disorders, nurses should remember to discuss the "3 C's":

- **Communication**—How to recognize and express feelings
- **Conflict Resolution**—How to express needs when they are not being met
- **Coping**—What to do when the client cannot directly solve a problem

Restoring Nutritional Balance

Restoring nutritional balance is a priority for clients with severe eating disorders. Most experts believe that conducting meaningful psychotherapeutic interventions with these clients is impossible until they are nutritionally stable. Clearly malnourished clients should be under the care of an internist until they are in medically stable condition and no longer at risk for dangerous complications related to starvation.

Management necessitates a holistic approach. For example, because an increased workload resulting from an already compromised cardiac reserve can lead to congestive heart failure, refeeding very underweight clients means that nurses must carefully monitor cardiac function. Another important intervention is to carefully monitor electrolyte levels when refeeding clients with anorexia. They are at risk for development of a "refeeding syndrome" with accompanying hypokalemia.

Refeeding also involves establishing a contract that spells out expected behaviors, rewards, privileges, and consequences of noncompliance. Such contracts may be useful in preventing power struggles with clients. They typically address how much weight clients will gain and in what time frame. Typically, the priority is a healthy weight at which menses resumes and bone demineralization stops or is prevented.

The first goal is for clients *to stop losing weight.* Engaging them is important, as is giving clients the opportunity to eat independently. In inpatient settings, if supervision is needed, restricting access to bathrooms for 2 hours after meals may be necessary to prevent clients from engaging in self-induced vomiting.

When clients are in a medically stable condition, the treatment team may confer with the family to discuss the transition home. Clients should be integral parts of determining their treatment and care. If they believe that they have contributed to planning rewards and privileges, clients will perceive control over their environment and bodies and will be more likely to adhere to the regimen.

All health care team members must consistently carry out the terms of the contract. Even though clients may rebel against contract terms, it reassures them to know that consistent limits are being maintained and that they can trust the staff to help maintain control.

Hospitalized clients with anorexia frequently express frustration with the limitations placed on them regarding exercise. Examining the type of exercise may help in setting sound guidelines. Rigorous aerobic exercise is usually contraindicated when weight gain is a goal. However, allowing clients to engage in moderate resistance training (eg, weight lifting) would increase lean body mass as they gain weight and minimize increases in "fat weight," which is typically a great fear of clients (Figure 26.8). Developing a contract that allows clients to perform weight training would acknowledge the benefits of exercise in a healthy lifestyle, enable them to feel more in control, and help them develop a more positive body image while gaining weight (Michielli et al., 1994).

Nurses communicate caring to clients through a kind, firm, matter-of-fact approach. For example, when a client is upset that her activities are being restricted, the nurse responds, "When you gain 5 pounds, you will earn privileges to participate in more activities. This is your choice." Nurses avoid responding punitively, arguing about limits, bribing, cajoling, and being excessively vigilant and overprotective. Through their interactions, nurses convey to clients, "You are a worthwhile person, and I

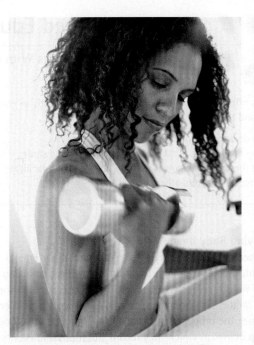

FIGURE 26.8 Some clients with eating disorders may have less anxiety as they gain weight during treatment if they are allowed to engage in moderate weight training.

care about you; I have expectations of you, and you are capable of meeting these expectations."

Think About It 26.1

At the start of a new school year, a group of teachers refers Paula, 16 years old, to the school nurse. Paula has had a noticeable weight loss during summer vacation, and faculty members are concerned that she may have anorexia. The nurse arranges a health conference with Paula and contacts Paula's parents. During the interview, Paula states, "I feel so fat and ugly." As part of the plan, the nurse uses a client contract approach with Paula. Describe how the nurse would use therapeutic communication in response to Paula's statement about being ugly and fat. Discuss the importance of a client contract in this situation.

Encouraging Realistic Thinking Processes

People with eating disorders tend to have perfectionistic personalities and to think in extremes (see Table 26.1). These traits help to explain the characteristic extreme fear of obesity. For example, a client who eats two cookies might conclude, "I couldn't control myself; I might as well give up and eat the whole bag of cookies." The client has defined rigid appropriate behaviors in terms of "walking on a tightrope," with the need for constant vigilance to keep from falling off. Clients must learn balance and moderation in thinking and behavior. Nurses reassure clients that life provides many opportunities and that they can move safely in many directions. They encourage clients to try new behaviors, explaining that although doing so may be frightening, clients gradually will become more confident about choices in all areas, including eating (Client-Centered Education 26.1).

Client-Centered Education 26.1

Teaching Points for Clients With Eating Disorders

Nurses offer the following suggestions to clients with an eating disorder and their family members:

- Provide unconditional love.
- Focus on the person rather than on the eating disorder.
- Give the client the power to make decisions and facilitate changes in matters other than eating.

- Demonstrate united support for one another and the plan for the client's treatment.
- Prepare for hospitalization if the client becomes medically unstable or for rehospitalization if he or she experiences a relapse.

Improving Body Image

Disturbed body image is related to disordered patterns of thought, such as overgeneralization (believing that losing sufficient weight will solve all her problems) and powerlessness. Social factors also influence body image. Nurses help clients recognize the influence of maladaptive thoughts by asking them to keep diaries in which they record situations and events that cause concern about physical appearance and weight. In discussing these situations, nurses and clients can begin to identify anxiety-provoking events and develop strategies for managing such situations without resorting to self-damaging behaviors. Such strategies include avoiding anxiety-provoking situations or people, or, if that is not possible, learning to desensitize oneself to certain situations. For example, clients might practice a form of progressive relaxation if they become agitated when they are at the mall, faced with images of extremely thin mannequins. Or they might try the cognitive technique of "disputation" if they have distorted thoughts about their bodies (see Chap. 3; Challenging Behaviors 26.1).

Fostering Self-Esteem

Low self-esteem in clients with eating disorders is associated with overly high self-expectations, a need for approval and acceptance from others, and possible deficiencies in social skills.

Nurses assist clients to recognize the association between overly high self-expectations and feelings of ineffectiveness. They help clients identify positive attributes and achieve self-approval. Along with undergoing individual therapy, clients may improve social skills by participating in group psychotherapy with others who have similar needs. Successful engagement with peers in recreational or occupational therapy activities also can enhance self-esteem.

Exploring Feelings of Powerlessness

Perception of control and autonomy increases as clients learn to express emotions and needs more directly, think less rigidly, and establish realistic self-expectations. Nurses encourage clients to assume responsibility for choices and decisions. For clients to take risks and grow, they must trust that nurses care about their well-being and will maintain appropriate limits. Nurses assure clients that they will gain the ability to exert appropriate behavioral controls and act autonomously.

Encouraging Effective Coping

Nurses encourage clients to discuss their feelings. Clients need to learn that strong emotions, especially "negative" ones, are acceptable and that they can be experienced and expressed without losing total control. Because clients may fear that

Challenging Behaviors 26.1

The Client With a Distorted Body Image

Situation: Your assigned client is Zoe Thin, 13 years old. She is diagnosed with anorexia nervosa. When you approach Zoe for lunch, she paces and says, "I can't stand this bulge in my tummy!"

Your Potential Feelings: Frustration, disbelief, lack of empathy.

What Is Going On? Zoe cannot perceive her body image accurately, even though she looks like a skeleton to you. She really is frightened about losing control and gaining weight. The thought of eating lunch makes her very anxious.

Strategy: Acknowledge Zoe's feelings of anxiety about eating lunch and show empathy for her fear. Provide a supportive, calm environment while she eats her lunch. Avoid discussing food and weight while Zoe eats. Acknowledge her efforts but avoid praise or flattery.

Nurse Action/Communication: You might say, "I know you think your tummy looks fat, but to me you look very thin. I can see that you're anxious about eating lunch, but that's a feeling I think you can deal with."

strong emotions will be overwhelming, nurses repeatedly distinguish between feelings and behaviors. They teach clients that the anxiety that follows strong feelings is normal and communicate that clients can learn ways to express those feelings without being hurtful toward self or others. Assertiveness training may be an adjunctive therapy that helps increase a client's ability to express feelings directly and constructively.

Restoring Family Processes

Some family therapists recommend focusing on four dysfunctional interaction patterns: enmeshment, overprotectiveness, conflict avoidance, and rigidity (Minuchin, 1974; Minuchin et al., 1975). Nurses can work with clients in these four areas in several ways.

Enmeshment and Overprotectiveness

When working with families, nurses help all members to make "I" instead of "we" statements. For example, one person should express "I feel sad" and "I am so angry!" as opposed to "We are all so upset!" Nurses encourage each member to speak for himself or herself, not for one another.

Parents in enmeshed families frequently try to protect their children by speaking for them (eg, "She feels happy most of the time."). Some relatives may not be accustomed to identifying and expressing their own feelings and need frequent prompting from nurses: "You look upset; what are you feeling right now?" Because enmeshed families typically have weak or inappropriate generational boundaries, nurses may ask siblings to sit together as a unit distinct from the parents. Such seating reinforces appropriate boundaries and helps to disrupt dysfunctional alliances that may exist between a parent and a child.

Conflict Avoidance and Rigidity

Families of clients with eating disorders tend to ignore or minimize conflicts. They may have unspoken rules that feeling sad or upset and having problems are unacceptable. Nurses help families to share and expose existing conflicts. If relatives try to avoid or deny conflict, nurses refocus them on the problem. They help families to express their conflict constructively—without shouting, threatening, accusing, or demanding—so that others can listen and respond.

Because clients with anorexia may be accustomed to diverting parental conflict, nurses ensure that parents talk to each other and instruct them not to involve clients directly.

For example, "Jane is not part of this conflict. This is between you and your wife. Keep talking to her, and don't involve Jane in it." Family members may have difficulty listening to one another's concerns and requests. Nurses model appropriate communication skills and help families repattern their communications.

Think About It 26.2

Linelle has anorexia nervosa. During a family meeting, the nurse asks Linelle a question and her mother answers for her. At a later family meeting, Linelle's parents begin to discuss their conflicts over past child-rearing decisions. Linelle gives her view of the events. The mother comments, "We are all so upset by this!" Discuss how the nurse would be most therapeutic at each of the meetings.

▲ EVALUATION

Evaluation of care involves determining if goals were met or if the client and family have made progress toward meeting them. Nurses evaluate the client's physical and psychosocial responses to interventions. Desired physical outcomes include weight gain, normal laboratory values and vital signs, and return of secondary sexual characteristics and menstruation. Desired psychosocial outcomes include a realistic perception of body image, direct expression of feelings, improved self-image, a sense of control over self and environment, and constructive family process.

As clients recover, they may feel guilty about and ashamed of their behavior while ill. Such feelings can persist long after clients attain normal weight. Nurses reassure clients that they could not have prevented their illness, and that their behavior during the disorder was an ineffective attempt to cope with stressors. Nurses also emphasize that clients now have increased coping skills and will not need to resort to previous destructive responses.

Nurses also evaluate the family's interaction patterns. Desired outcomes are that family members communicate directly with one another and deal openly with conflicts and that parents relinquish previous patterns of overcontrol and overprotectiveness to allow clients appropriate autonomy.

Even if a client and family appear to have met these goals, most clients require follow-up treatment to reinforce behavioral changes and to prevent a return of disordered eating. Follow-up should span at least 4 years because of the high rate of relapse.

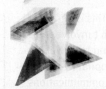

Reviewing and Applying Your Knowledge

Chapter Summary

- Anorexia nervosa and bulimia nervosa share many etiologic factors. Although multiple theories exist, most experts agree that eating disorders develop from a complex interaction of individual, family, sociocultural, and physiologic factors.

- Clients with eating disorders exhibit disturbances in many or all of the functional health patterns.

- Treatment of clients with eating disorders occurs in community-based and inpatient settings and is a complex and often lengthy process.

- Desired client outcomes include normalization of weight and eating patterns, improved self-esteem, and development of realistic thought processes, adaptive coping mechanisms, and constructive family processes.

- Most clients require follow-up treatment to reinforce behavioral changes and prevent a return of disordered eating.

Study Questions

1. A 21-year-old female client is 5'4" and weighs 145 lb (65.8 kg). She states that two or three times per week she consumes "too much" food and induces vomiting after she becomes sick. She reports that she has done this for several years. Which of the following would the nurse suspect?

   a. Anorexia nervosa.

   b. Binge eating disorder without compensatory behaviors.

   c. Bulimia nervosa.

   d. Eating disorder NOS.

2. A 17-year-old client admits to recent use of diuretics and laxatives to lose weight quickly. She is 5' tall, weighs 90 lb (40.8 kg), and has lost 15 lb (6.8 kg) in 3 weeks. The nurse is most concerned about which of the following possible physiologic consequences of the client's behavior?

   a. Dehydration.

   b. Hypokalemia.

   c. Hyponatremia.

   d. Anemia.

3. The multidisciplinary team is using behavior family systems therapy (BFST). Which of the following activities would be implemented in the weight maintenance phase?

   a. The family is engaged in treatment, and the client's weight is checked weekly.

   b. The therapist encourages the parents to take charge of the client's eating and coaches the family to develop an appropriate behavioral weight program.

   c. The therapist streamlines the weight-gain program and introduces non–food-related issues.

   d. The therapist fosters client individuation and encourages the client gradually to reassume control over food.

4. The nurse at a community mental health center has been coordinating the care of a client with anorexia nervosa. The 5'3", 16-year-old adolescent has maintained her weight at 110 lb (49.9 kg) for 6 months. This week, the client appears tired. Her weight has dropped to 104 lb (47.2 kg). Her laboratory test results reveal a potassium level of 2.3 mEq/L and a hemoglobin level of 12 mg/dL. The client states that she has been depressed, restricting foods, and using laxatives. Which of the following would the nurse do next?

   a. Ask the social worker involved in the client's care to arrange home visits.

   b. Call the physician to prescribe antidepressants and potassium supplements.

   c. Notify the physician of the findings and the need for inpatient care.

   d. Develop a contract that outlines consequences for dieting and using laxatives.

5. A client with an eating disorder has been involved in follow-up care for 4 years after her hospitalization for anorexia nervosa. Which of the following would be the most reliable indicator that the plan of care has been effective?

   a. The client has maintained her target weight for the past 3 years.

   b. The client reports that she has learned to accept her body.

   c. The client interacts with her peers.

   d. The client has moved into her own apartment.

Critical Thinking Questions

1. Can nursing interventions be therapeutic even if clients react emotionally to them?

2. An issue of concern when clients have eating disorders involves ways to help clients differentiate healthy eating and exercise patterns from the destructive manifestations that are occurring in these areas. What factors should nurses consider when discussing sports, activities, and exercise with clients?

3. What efforts can schools and their athletic programs make toward preventing eating disorders and identifying them in students? What obstacles may stand in the way of schools taking such measures?

References

Agency for Healthcare Research and Quality (AHRQ). (2006). *Management of eating disorders*. Rockville, MD: U.S. Department of Health and Human Services.

Agency for Healthcare Research and Quality (AHRQ) (2009). *Statistical brief #70: Health care cost and utilization project*. Rockville, MD: U.S. Department of Health and Human Services.

Agras, W. S., Walsh, B. T., Fairburn, C. G., Wilson, G. T., & Kraemer, H. C. (2000). A multicenter comparison of cognitive–behavioral therapy and interpersonal psychotherapy for bulimia nervosa. *Archives of General Psychiatry, 57*(5), 459–466.

American Psychiatric Association (APA). (2000a). *Diagnostic and statistical manual of mental disorders* (4th ed., text rev.). Washington, DC: Author.

American Psychiatric Association (APA). (2000b). Practice guidelines for the treatment of patients with eating disorders (revision). *American Journal of Psychiatry, 157*(1 Suppl.), 1–39.

Anderson, A., & Yager, J. (2005). Eating disorders. In B. J. Sadock & V. A. Sadock (Eds.), *Comprehensive textbook of psychiatry* (8th ed., Vol. 1, pp. 2002–2021). Philadelphia, PA: Lippincott Williams & Wilkins.

Bachner-Melman, R., Zohar, A., Elizur, Y., Kremer, I., Golan, M., & Ebstein, R. (2009). Protective self-presentation style: Association with disordered eating and anorexia nervosa mediated by sociocultural attitudes toward appearance. *Eating and Weight Disorders, 14* (1), 1–12.

Bissada, H., Tasca, G., Barber, A., & Bradwejn, J. (2008). Olanzapine in the treatment of low body weight and obsessive thinking in women with anorexia nervosa: A randomized, double-blind, placebo-controlled trial. *American Journal of Psychiatry, 165* (10), 1281–1288.

Bulechek, G. M., Butcher, H. K., & McCloskey Dochterman, J. (2008). *Nursing interventions classification (NIC)* (5th ed.). St. Louis, MO: Mosby.

Costin, C. (2002). An update on binge eating disorder. *Healthy Weight Journal, 16*(2), 20–23.

Crow, S., Mitchell, J., Roerig, J., & Steffen, K. (2009). What potential role is there for medication treatment in anorexia nervosa. *International Journal of Eating Disorders, 42*(1), 1–8.

Fairburn, C. G., Cooper, A., & Doll, H. (2000). The natural course of bulimia nervosa and binge eating disorder in young women. *Archives of General Psychiatry, 57*(7), 659–665.

Feldman, M. B., & Meyer, I. H. (2007a). Eating disorders in diverse lesbian, gay, and bisexual populations. *International Journal of Eating Disorders, 40*(3), 218–226.

Feldman, M. B., & Meyer, I. H. (2007b). Childhood abuse and eating disorders in gay and bisexual men. *International Journal of Eating Disorders, 40*(5), 418–423.

Freund, K., Graham, S., Lesky, L., & Moskowitz, M. (1993). Detection of bulimia in a primary care setting. *Journal of General Internal Medicine, 8,* 236.

Frieling, H., Römer, K., Schatz, S., Mittelbach, F., Wilhelm, J., De Zwaan, M., . . . Bleich, S. (2010). Epigenetic dysregulation of dopaminergic genes in eating disorders. *International Journal of Eating Disorders, 43* (7), 577–583.

Golden, N., & Attia, E. (2011). Psychopharmacology of eating disorders in children and adolescents. *Pediatric Clinics of North America, 58,* 121–138.

Halmi, K. (2008). Eating disorders. Anorexia nervosa, bulimia nervosa and obesity. In R. E. Hales, S. C. Yudofsky, & G. O. Gabbard (Eds.), *Textbook of psychiatry* (5th ed.). Washington, DC: American Psychiatric Publishing.

Holm-Denoma, J., Scaringi, V., Gordon, K., Van Orden, K., & Joiner, T. (2009). Eating disorder symptoms among undergraduate varsity athletes, club athletes, independent exercisers, and non-exercisers. *International Journal of Eating Disorders, 42* (1), 47–53.

Hutter, G., Ganepola, S., & Hofmann, W. (2009). The hematology of anorexia nervosa. *International Journal of Eating Disorders, 42* (4), 293–300.

Johnson, J., Cohen, P., Kasen, S., & Brook, J. (2002). Childhood adversities associated with risk for eating disorders or overweight problems during adolescence or early adulthood. *American Journal of Psychiatry, 159*(3), 394–400.

Kaye, W. H., Fudge, J. L., & Paulus, M. (2009). New insights into symptoms and neurocircuit function of anorexia nervosa. *National Review of Neuroscience, 10* (8), 573–584.

Keel, P., Baxter, M., Heatherton, T., & Joiner, T. (2007). A 20-year longitudinal study of body weight, dieting, and eating disorder symptoms. *Journal of Abnormal Psychology, 116*(2), 422–432.

Klump, K. L., Bulik, C. M., Kaye, W. H., Treasure, J., & Tyson, E. (2009). Academy for eating disorders position paper: Eating disorders are serious mental illnesses. *International Journal of Eating Disorders, 42* (2), 97–103.

Kong, S. (2005). Day treatment programme for patients with eating disorders: Randomized clinical trial. *Journal of Advanced Nursing, 51*(1), 5–14.

Kyriacou, O., Treasure, J., & Schmidt, U. (2008). Expressed emotion in eating disorders assessed via self report: An examination of factors associated with expressed emotion in carers of people with anorexia nervosa in comparison to control families. *International Journal of Eating Disorders, 41*(1), 37–46.

Lee, Y., & Lin, P. (2010). Association between serotonin transporter gene polymorphism and eating disorders: A meta-analytic study. *International Journal of Eating Disorders, 43* (6), 498–504.

Lock, J., leGrange, D., Forsberg, S., & Hewell, K. (2006). Is family therapy useful for treating children with anorexia nervosa? Results of a case series. *Journal of American Academy of Child Adolescent Psychiatry, 45*(11), 1323–1328.

Locke, J., Agras, W., & Bryson, S. (2005). A comparison of short- and long-term family therapy for adolescent anorexia nervosa. *Journal of American Academy of Child and Adolescent Psychiatry, 44* (7), 632–639.

Mangweth-Matzek, B., Rupp, C. I., Hausmann, A., Assmayr, K., Mariacher, E., Kemmler, G., . . . Biebl, W. (2006). Never too old for eating disorders or body dissatisfaction: A community study of elderly women. *International Journal of Eating Disorders, 39*(7), 583–586.

Marken, P., & Sommi, R. (2002). Eating disorders. In J. T. DiPiro, R. L. Talbert, G. C. Yee, G. R. Matzke, B. G. Wells, & L. M. Posey (Eds.), *Pharmacotherapy: A pathophysiologic approach* (5th ed., pp. 1155–1163). New York, NY: McGraw-Hill.

Mazzeo, S., & Bulik, C. (2009). Environmental and genetic risk factors for eating disorders: What the clinician needs to know. *Child and Adolescent Psychiatric Clinics of North America 18* (1), 67–82.

Mazzeo, S., & Espelage, D. (2002). Associations between childhood physical and emotional abuse and disordered eating behaviors. *Journal of Counseling Psychology, 49*(1), 86–100.

Michielli, D., Dunbar, C., & Kalinski, M. (1994). Is exercise indicated for the patient diagnosed as anorectic? *Journal of Psychosocial Nursing, 32*(8), 33–35.

Minuchin, S. (1974). *Families and family therapy.* Cambridge, MA: Howard University Press.

Minuchin, S., Baker, L., Rosman, B., Liebman, R., Milman, L., & Todd, T. (1975). A conceptual model of psychosomatic illness in children: Family organization and family therapy. *Archives of General Psychiatry, 32,* 1031–1038.

Mitchell, J., Agras, S., & Wonderlich, S. (2006). Treatment of bulimia nervosa: Where are we and where are we going? *International Journal of Eating Disorders, 40*(20), 95–101.

Monteleone, F., Brambilla, F., Bartolotti, F., & Maj, M. (2002). Serotonergic dysfunction across the eating disorders: Relationship to eating behavior, purging behavior, nutritional status and general psychopathology. *Psychological Medicine, 30*(5), 1099–1110.

Moorhead, S., Johnson, M., Maas, M. L., & Swanson, E. (2008). *Nursing outcomes classification (NOC)* (4th ed.). St. Louis, MO: Mosby.

NANDA International. (2007). *Nursing diagnoses: Definitions and classification (2007–2008).* Philadelphia, PA: Author.

Nordbo, R., Espeset, E., Gulliksen, K., Skarderud, F., & Holte, A. (2006). The meaning of self starvation: Qualitative study of patients' perception of anorexia nervosa. *International Journal of Eating Disorders, 39*(7), 556–564.

Porth, C. M. (2009). *Pathophysiology: Concepts of altered health states* (8th ed.). Philadelphia, PA: Lippincott Williams & Wilkins.

Rigotti, N. (2000). Approach to eating disorders. In A. Goorall & A. Mulley (Eds.), *Primary care medicine* (4th ed., pp. 1205–1211). Philadelphia, PA: Lippincott Williams & Wilkins.

Robin, A. I., Bedway, M., Siegel, P. T., Moye, A. W., & Gilroy, M. (1997). Therapy for adolescent anorexia nervosa: Addressing cognitions, feelings, and the family's role. In E. D. Hibbs & P. S. Jensen (Eds.), *Psychosocial treatments for child and adolescent disorders: Empirically based strategies for clinical practice* (pp. 239–259). Washington, DC: American Psychological Association Press.

Robin, A. I., Siegel, P. T., Moye, A. W., Gilroy, M., Dennis, A. B., & Sikand, A. (1999). A controlled comparison of family versus individual therapy for adolescents with anorexia nervosa. *Journal of the Academy of Child and Adolescent Psychiatry, 38*(12), 1482–1489.

Russell, C. J., & Keel, P. K. (2002). Homosexuality as a specific risk factor for eating disorders in men. *International Journal of Eating Disorders, 31*(3), 300–306.

Schatzberg, A., Cole, J., & De Battista, C. (2010). *Manual of clinical psychopharmacology* (7th ed.). Washington, DC: American Psychiatric Publishers.

Sorgen, C. (2002). *Overcoming eating disorders.* Retrieved from http://my.webmd.com/priority/article/1674.52649

Steiger, H., & Bruce, K. (2007). Phenotypes, endotypes, and genotypes in bulimia spectrum eating disorders. *Canadian Journal of Psychiatry, 52*(4), 220–227.

Strober, M., Freeman, R., Lampert, C., Diamond, J., & Kaye, W. (2000). Controlled family study of anorexia nervosa and bulimia nervosa: Evidence of shared liability and transmission of partial syndromes. *American Journal of Psychiatry, 157,* 393–401.

Wade, T., Bulik, C., Neale, M., & Kendler, K. (2000). Anorexia nervosa and major depression: Shared genetic and environmental risk factors. *American Journal of Psychiatry, 157*(3), 469–471.

Watson, H. J., Raykos, B. C, Street, H., Fursland, A., & Nathan, P. R. (2011). Mediators between perfectionism and eating disorder pathology: Shape and weight overvaluation and conditional goal setting. *International Journal of Eating Disorders, 44* (2), 142–149.

Wolfe, B., Betzger, E., & Jimerson, D. (2003). Eating disorders. In T. M. Buttaro, P. P. Bailey, J. Trybulski, & J. Sandberg-Cook (Eds.), *Primary care: A collaborative practice* (2nd ed., pp. 1237–1241). St. Louis, MO: Mosby.

Woodside, D. B., Garfinkel, P. E., Lin, E., Goering, P., Kaplan, A. S., Goldbloom, D. S., & Kennedy, S. H. (2001). Comparison of men with full or partial eating disorders, men without eating disorders, and women. *American Journal of Psychiatry, 158*(4), 570–574.

Woolsey, M. (1998). When food becomes a cry for help. *Journal of the American Dietetic Association, 98*(4), 395–398.

Work Group on Eating Disorders. (2000). *Practice guidelines for the treatment of patients with eating disorders* (2nd ed.). Arlington, VA: American Psychiatric Association.

Zipfel, S., Lowe, B., Reas, D. L., Deter, H., & Herzog, W. (2000). Long-term prognosis in anorexia nervosa: Lessons from a 21-year follow-up study. *Lancet, 355,* 721–722.

Web Resources

Eating Disorder Referral and Information Center: http://www.edreferral.com

Eating Disorders Resources: http://www.bulimia.com

National Association for Anorexia and Associated Disorders: http://www.anad.org

National Eating Disorders Association: http://www.edap.org

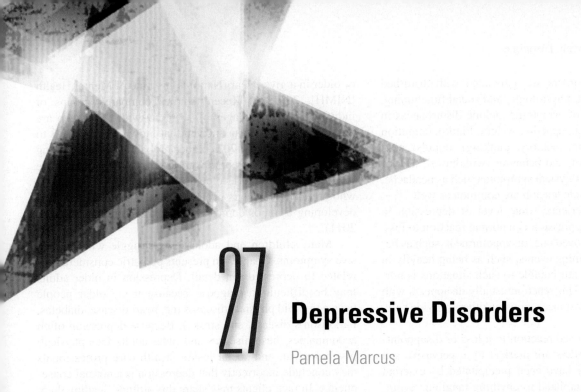

27

Depressive Disorders

Pamela Marcus

KEY TERMS

dysthymia
electroconvulsive therapy (ECT)
phototherapy
postpartum depression

LEARNING OBJECTIVES

On completion of this chapter, you should be able to accomplish the following:

- Discuss the incidence and prevalence of depressive disorders in the United States.
- Analyze different theories about the etiology of depressive disorders.
- List the symptoms of depressive disorders using criteria from the *Diagnostic and Statistical Manual of Mental Disorders,* 4th edition, text revision *(DSM-IV-TR).*
- Discuss interdisciplinary treatment modalities for clients with depressive disorders.
- Apply the nursing process to the care of clients with depressive disorders.

Depressive disorders are associated with disturbed psychological, physiologic, and social functioning. Wide-ranging groups of symptoms include disturbances in daily patterns (eg, sleep, appetite, weight, libido), cognition (attention/concentration, memory, thinking), impulse control (suicide, homicide), and behavior (withdrawal, lack of pleasure, fatigability). Physical symptoms such as headache, stomachache, and muscle tension are common as well.

Most people experience some level of depression in their lives. Transient depression is a normal reaction to loss, such as the death of a loved one; disappointment, such as being fired; or overwhelming events, such as being heavily in debt. Sadness directly attributable to such situations is normal and self-limiting. This reaction usually disappears with time, changes in circumstances, or when others provide help.

M VIE viewing GUIDES

Unlike the normal sad reaction to a loss or disappointment, depressive disorders are marked by a pervasive sad mood. The mood may have been precipitated by external events, or it may be unrelated to anything tangible. Symptoms can range from an overall dissatisfaction with life so persistent that some clients begin to recognize it as their usual state, to sudden and abrupt changes in functioning accompanied by apathy, hopelessness, and a decrease in the will to live. The risk for suicide that accompanies depressive disorders demands priority attention from health care providers. Chapter 34 discusses suicide in detail; suicide is discussed in this chapter as part of overall care for clients with depression.

It is important to note that alterations in mood are the main characteristics of bipolar disorders. Clients may swing from mania (elevated, expansive mood accompanied by frenetic activity) to depression. The salient features of bipolar disorder are discussed in Chapter 28, as is nursing management for clients with bipolar mania. The discussions in this chapter also apply to clients with bipolar illness experiencing depressive phases.

OVERVIEW OF DEPRESSIVE ILLNESS

Major depression is one of the most common illnesses of any type (medical or psychiatric), affecting people of all ages and backgrounds. It is currently the leading cause of U.S. disability in clients 15 to 44 years old, and it is projected to be the second leading cause of disability among all age groups by 2020. Public awareness of the scope of the problem and measures to prevent and treat it are crucial.

Incidence and Prevalence

Major depression affects approximately 14.8 million people 18 years or older (6.7% of the population) in any given year (Kessler et al., 2005). It can develop at any age, with average onset at 32 years. **Dysthymia** (chronic, mild depression) affects approximately 1.5% of the U.S. population 18 years

or older in a given year (National Institute of Mental Health [NIMH], 2011a,b). Recent studies compared groups of individuals from the ages of 18 to 59 with those who are over 60 years old. Data showed that individuals from 18 to 20 years of age had a 70% higher probability of developing a major depression, people who are 30 to 44 years old are 120% more likely to develop a major depression, and those who are 45 to 59 years of age have a 100% probability of developing a major depression over their lifetime (NIMH, 2011).

Many children and adolescents struggle with depressive symptoms. Chapter 36 presents pediatric considerations related to depression in detail. Depression in older adults may be difficult to diagnose because many older people have comorbid physical diseases (eg, heart disease, diabetes, Parkinson's disease, and stroke). Because depression often accompanies these diseases and older adults face physical, psychological, and social losses, health care professionals may conclude incorrectly that depression is a normal consequence. In fact, clients may share this attitude, leading them to fail to report troubling symptoms. See Chapter 37 for more information on depression in the elderly.

Depressive disorders are more prevalent in women than in men. Women have a 70% higher possibility of exhibiting a major depression than men (NIMH, 2011a,b). Genetics, sociocultural factors, hormones, and other elements may account for this disparity. Awareness in the general public and in the health care industry is also growing relative to depression that occurs during pregnancy and the postpartum period. This problem is discussed in this chapter.

Etiology

Depression, like all psychiatric illnesses, results from a combination or interaction of genes, environment, individual life history, development, and neurobiologic makeup. Definitive causes have not yet been discovered. Box 27.1 lists some identified risk factors for depression.

Genetic Factors

Decades of family studies have found an increased risk for depression in clients with first-degree relatives (parents, siblings, children) who have had depression (Kelsoe, 2005). Adoption studies show that the concordance rate for depression in monozygotic (identical) twins is 45% to 60%, whereas the concordance rate in dizygotic (nonidentical)

BOX 27.1 Risk Factors for Depression

- Gender: higher in women than in men
- Prior episode of depression
- Family history
- Stressful life event
- Current substance use
- Medical illness
- Few social supports

twins is 12% (Kelsoe, 2005). The difference in concordance rates supports the view that genetic factors contribute in some way to the development of depression in certain clients. Recent research has examined the relationship among genetic predisposition, major environmental stressors, and the development of depression (South & Krueger, 2011). Findings suggest that individuals with low levels of income had a higher level of psychiatric illnesses that involved internalizing syndromes, including depression. Other studies involving alteration in the serotonin transporter gene and early life stress events suggest that the presence of both may be predictive of the later development of depression (Colman & Ataullahjan, 2010; Nugent et al., 2011).

Physiologic Factors

Several areas of the brain seem to be especially affected in depressive disorders (Figure 27.1). The physiologic hypotheses most commonly discussed in relation to depressive disorders involve biologic amines and neuroendocrine stress responses.

BIOGENIC AMINES. Originally, the biogenic amine hypothesis held that depression resulted from a deficiency in *biogenic amines,* which are neurotransmitters synthesized by enzymes in the nerve terminal. This idea was first hypothesized when depression developed in clients being treated for hypertension with the biogenic amine-depleting agent reserpine. The monoamines that have been implicated in depression are norepinephrine (NE), dopamine (DA), and serotonin (5-HT). Disturbances in mood may result when absolute concentrations of NE, 5-HT, or both are deficient. Altered numbers, affinities, or both of 5-HT and NE receptors and uptake sites may affect metabolism. Recently, researchers have focused on possible involvement from second messenger systems, as well as "cross-talk" between the NE and 5-HT systems, in relationship to mood disorders (Bear et al., 2006; Pytliak et al., 2011; Thase, 2005). See also Chapter 2.

PSYCHONEUROENDOCRINE AND IMMUNE RELATIONSHIPS. The hypothalamic–pituitary–adrenal (HPA) axis is considered the "stress" axis. Its complex feedforward and feedback mechanisms interact with multiple body systems (see Chap. 39). The HPA axis and endocrine system are closely connected (Golden, 2007). The hypothalamus interacts with the central nervous system (CNS) on the pituitary gland through corticotropin-releasing hormone (CRH). CRH then stimulates the adrenal medulla, through the adrenocorticotropic hormone, to secrete catecholamines and cortisol. Both catecholamines and cortisol modulate the endocrine and immune systems (Bear et al., 2006).

Uncontrollable stressors lead to sustained hyperactivity of the HPA axis. The result is hypersecretion of adrenal glucocorticoids and CRH. In major depression, protracted elevation of glucocorticoid levels desensitizes the central glucocorticoid receptors and probably also those receptors located on macrophages, an important component of the immune response (Shelton, 2007). In fact, many aspects of cellular immunity are activated during depression, even though other immunologic markers are suppressed. Immune cells produce bioactive neuroendocrine hormones and have receptors for many of them (Uddin et al., 2011). The immune system may be thought of as a sensory organ for external stimuli such as bacteria, viruses, and tumors, whereas the CNS detects classic sensory stimuli.

The relationship between stress and its biologic effects has significant implications. People regularly exposed to traumatic, stressful, and unstable situations may be more likely to develop problems with mood as a result of overstimulation of the HPA pathways and endocrine system. This is an especially important consideration related to child development and the optimal environments in which children learn, live, and thrive (see Chap. 36).

Psychological Factors

Many therapists and counselors with clinical training in psychodynamic therapy continue to use this knowledge base extensively to guide treatment for depressive disorders. The preponderance of research on psychodynamic and psychoanalytic therapies for depression indicates that they are most effective when combined with psychotropic drugs (American Psychiatric Association [APA], 2010; NIMH, 2011a,b; Reynolds et al., 2006).

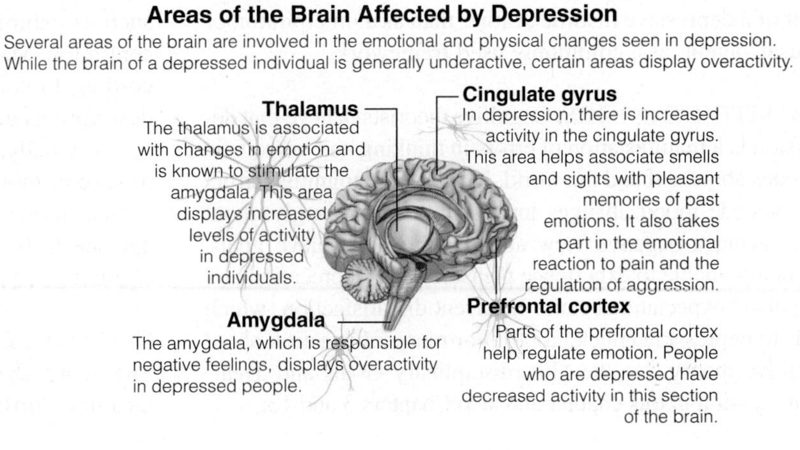

Areas of the Brain Affected by Depression

Several areas of the brain are involved in the emotional and physical changes seen in depression. While the brain of a depressed individual is generally underactive, certain areas display overactivity.

Thalamus
The thalamus is associated with changes in emotion and is known to stimulate the amygdala. This area displays increased levels of activity in depressed individuals.

Cingulate gyrus
In depression, there is increased activity in the cingulate gyrus. This area helps associate smells and sights with pleasant memories of past emotions. It also takes part in the emotional reaction to pain and the regulation of aggression.

Amygdala
The amygdala, which is responsible for negative feelings, displays overactivity in depressed people.

Prefrontal cortex
Parts of the prefrontal cortex help regulate emotion. People who are depressed have decreased activity in this section of the brain.

FIGURE 27.1 Brain regions involved in depressive disorders.

Briefly, psychodynamic theories postulate that clients with depression have unexpressed and unconscious anger about feeling helpless or dependent on others. They cannot express this anger toward the person or people on whom they feel dependent, so their anger turns inward. Psychodynamic theorists believe that such anger begins in childhood when basic developmental needs are not met. Children begin to see the world as hostile and unpredictable, blame themselves, and feel angry and inferior. Psychoanalytic theorists posit a link between unmet dependency needs in childhood and later mood disorders. Many therapists who treat clients with mood disorders use the psychoanalytic model during assessment (eg, related to feelings of helplessness, dependency needs, and anger) and then match findings with interventions that enhance functioning and self-perceptions.

LEARNED HELPLESSNESS. The original theoretical model of learned helplessness proposed that people susceptible to mood disorders have come to believe, based on experience, that they are ineffective and have no influence on factors that cause their suffering (Seligman et al., 1974). Behaviors that define learned helplessness include passivity, negative expectations, and feelings of helplessness, hopelessness, and powerlessness. These are also symptoms of major depression. Although learned helplessness as an etiologic (causal) factor in mood disorders has received less attention since the advent of molecular biology and the knowledge explosion in neurophysiology, many practitioners continue to use learned helplessness as a context from which to understand symptoms of depression and develop treatments.

More recent research conducted by scholars testing the "learned helplessness" hypothesis found that it failed to account for individuals' different reactions to situations that were thought to cause a learned helplessness reaction. Current research suggests that people's attributional styles contribute more to how they respond to adverse circumstances, and that their unique interpretations of life's events affect their potential for a "learned helplessness" response (Peterson et al., 1995). This later finding is consistent with cognitive theories of depression.

Nurses may find it helpful to view learned helplessness as relevant to the experiences of clients after the development of a depressive disorder, rather than as a precipitator, or "causal" agent, as a commonly used framework.

COGNITIVE FACTORS. Cognitive theorists believe that depression is a manifestation of errors in thinking and unrealistic attitudes about self and the world. In this view, cognitive errors that precede mood changes involve thinking wrongly about self, having a negative view about ability to achieve goals, and being unable to experience pleasure. Self-deprecation and unrealistic expectations cause recurrent dissatisfaction, which leads to depression (Beck, 2008). For more information about cognitive theory, see the "Interdisciplinary Goals and Treatment" section in this chapter and also Chapters 3 and 13.

> **Checkpoint Questions**
> 1. According to the monoamine hypothesis, which neurotransmitters are believed to be involved in depression?
> 2. What behaviors define learned helplessness?
> 3. According to cognitive theory, why do clients experience depression?

Signs and Symptoms/Diagnostic Criteria

Depressive illnesses can be categorized in various ways, depending on symptoms, severity, and persistence. If viewed on a continuum, mild reactive depression in response to grief or loss might be placed at the "normal" end, with suicidal depression or a depression with psychotic features at the opposite end.

The following paragraphs review criteria from the *Diagnostic and Statistical Manual of Mental Disorders,* 4th edition, text revision *(DSM-IV-TR)* for major depressive disorder and dysthymia (APA, 2000) *(DSM-IV-TR* Box 27.1).

Major Depressive Disorder

Clients with major depressive disorder demonstrate either a depressed mood or a loss of interest as well as an inability to derive pleasure from previously enjoyed activities. Other symptoms include recurrent thoughts of suicide, decreased or increased appetite, inability to concentrate, difficulty making decisions, feelings of worthlessness and self-blame, decreased energy, motor disturbances (agitation or severe slowness), disturbed sleep (insomnia or excessive sleeping), substance abuse, and social withdrawal. Clients may disregard grooming, cleanliness, and personal appearance due to a decreased energy and feelings of worthlessness. Stooped posture and dejected facial expression are nonverbal indicators of depression. Clients may appear disheveled, downcast, and tearful, and avoid eye contact. Conversely, they may be agitated (Figure 27.2); however, they usually do not exhibit bizarre or odd behaviors. Many clients resist attempts from others to engage them in the environment. They tend to exhibit withdrawn, isolated behavior

For diagnostic purposes, symptoms must be present most of the day nearly every day for at least 2 weeks, and they must cause significant distress or impair functioning, such as exhibiting an inability to work and decreased concentration. Major depressive disorder is classified further according to severity, longitudinal course of recurrence, and descriptions of the most recent episode.

Typically, major depressive episodes last several weeks to several months and are followed by periods of relatively normal mood and behavior. The average major depressive episode lasts approximately 4 months but may persist for 12 months or more without remitting.

Dysthymic Disorder

The word *dysthymia* comes from the Greek prefix *dys,* meaning "difficult" or "bad," and the Greek word *thymos,*

Depressive Disorders

Major Depressive Episode

A. Five (or more) of the following symptoms have been present during the same 2-week period and represent a change from previous functioning; at least one of the symptoms is either (1) depressed mood or (2) loss of interest or pleasure.

Note: Do not include symptoms that are clearly due to a general medical condition, or mood-incongruent delusions or hallucinations.

1. Depressed mood most of the day, nearly every day, as indicated by either subjective report (eg, feels sad or empty) or observation made by others (eg, appears tearful)

   Note: In children and adolescents, can be irritable mood.

2. Markedly diminished interest or pleasure in all, or almost all, activities most of the day, nearly every day (as indicated by either subjective account or observation made by others)

3. Significant weight loss when not dieting or weight gain (eg, a change of more than 5% of body weight in a month), or decrease or increase in appetite nearly every day.

   Note: In children, consider failure to make expected weight gains

4. Insomnia or Hypersomnia nearly every day

5. Psychomotor agitation or retardation nearly every day (observable by others, not merely subjective feelings of restlessness or being slowed down)

6. Fatigue or loss of energy nearly every day

7. Feelings of worthlessness or excessive or inappropriate guilt (which may be delusional) nearly every day (not merely self-reproach or guilt about being sick)

8. Diminished ability to think or concentrate, or indecisiveness, nearly every day (either by subjective account or as observed by others)

9. Recurrent thoughts of death (not just fear of dying), recurrent suicidal ideation without a specific plan, or a suicide attempt or a specific plan for committing suicide

B. The symptoms do not meet criteria for a Mixed Episode.

C. The symptoms cause clinically significant distress or impairment in social, occupational, or other important areas of functioning.

D. The symptoms are not due to the direct physiologic effects of a substance (eg, a drug of abuse, a medication) or a general medical condition (eg, hypothyroidism).

E. The symptoms are not better accounted for by bereavement, ie, after the loss of a loved one, the symptoms persist for longer than 2 months or are characterized by marked functional impairment, morbid preoccupation with worthlessness, suicidal ideation, psychotic symptoms, or psychomotor retardation.

Dysthymic Disorder

A. Depressed mood for most of the day, for more days than not, as indicated either by subjective account or observation by others, for at least 2 years.

   Note: In children and adolescents, mood can be irritable and duration must be at least 1 year.

B. Presence, while depressed, of two (or more) of the following:
   1. Poor appetite or overeating
   2. Insomnia or Hypersomnia
   3. Low energy or fatigue
   4. Low self-esteem
   5. Poor concentration or difficulty making decisions
   6. Feelings of hopelessness

C. During the 2-year period (1 year for children or adolescents) of the disturbance, the person has never been without the symptoms in Criteria A and B for more than 2 months at a time.

D. No Major Depressive Episode has been present during the first 2 years of the disturbance (1 year for children and adolescents); ie, the disturbance is not better accounted for by chronic Major Depressive Disorder, or Major Depressive Disorder, In Partial Remission.

   Note: There may have been a previous Major Depressive Episode provided there was a full remission (no significant signs or symptoms for 2 months) before development of the Dysthymic Disorder. In addition, after the initial 2 years (1 year in children or adolescents) of Dysthymic Disorder, there may be superimposed episodes of Major Depressive Disorder, in which case both diagnoses may be given when the criteria are met for a Major Depressive Episode.

E. There has never been a Manic Episode, a Mixed Episode, or a Hypomanic Episode, and criteria have never been met for Cyclothymic Disorder.

F. The disturbance does not occur exclusively during the course of a chronic Psychotic Disorder, such as Schizophrenia or Delusional Disorder.

G. The symptoms are not due to the direct physiologic effects of a substance (eg, a drug of abuse, a medication) or a general medical condition (eg, hypothyroidism).

H. The symptoms cause clinically significant distress or impairment in social, occupational, or other important areas of functioning.

Reprinted with permission from the *Diagnostic and Statistical Manual of Mental Disorders, Fourth Edition, Text Revision* (Copyright © 2000). American Psychiatric Association.

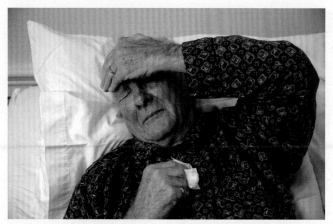

FIGURE 27.2 Mood-related symptoms of depression may vary in clients. This client is showing signs of agitated depression, with outward manifestations of grief and distress.

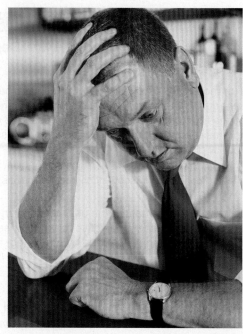

FIGURE 27.3 Clients with dysthymia may experience a pervasive dissatisfaction with life. They may have the illness for so long that they no longer recognize their unhappy mood as a deviation from normal.

meaning "mind." The *DSM-IV-TR* considers dysthymia a chronic depression in which symptoms, such as poor appetite or overeating, insomnia or excessive sleep, low energy, fatigue, low self-esteem, poor concentration, difficulty making decisions, and feelings of hopelessness are experienced by the individual. Diagnostic criteria include depressed or irritable mood most of the day, occurring more days than not for at least 2 years (1 year in children and adolescents). Within this time, the client has no more than 2 months without symptoms and has not experienced a manic or depressive episode (APA, 2000) (Figure 27.3).

Postpartum Depression

Following childbirth, approximately 85% of women experience hormonal fluctuations that result in transitory mood disturbances. These changes in mood may occur on a continuum from postpartum blues to postpartum psychosis (Massachusetts General Hospital Center for Women's Mental Health [MGH], 2012).

Postpartum depression (PPD) generally begins between the first 2 to 3 months up to the first year after delivery. For some women, mild symptoms may appear during pregnancy. Postpartum depression can occur in any woman who has recently delivered a child. The most common risk factors are a previous episode of PPD, depression during pregnancy, a history of depression or bipolar disorder, an increase in stressful events, inadequate support systems, and conflict in the marital dyad (MGH, 2012).

Postpartum psychosis is a severe psychiatric emergency. Women with this illness may harm their infants and/or themselves. Approximately 1 to 2 women in 1,000 develop a postpartum psychosis. Their symptoms occur within the first 48 to 72 hours up to the first 2 weeks after giving birth. The women experience symptoms that are similar to rapid cycling manic or mixed bipolar episodes, with the most common symptoms being dramatic mood swings, disorientation,

and disorganized or impulsive, erratic behaviors. They often experience destructive delusions concerning their infants and command hallucinations that instruct them to harm themselves or their babies. Nurses have a responsibility to assess for this condition and provide safety interventions in order to prevent infanticide or suicide (MGH, 2011).

In some women, the signs of postpartum depression are obvious, but many clients do not share their feelings out of embarrassment or fear of negative responses from others. Untreated PPD can pose dangers to women, their children, and entire families. Health care providers must regularly screen women for signs of PPD, which is treatable through mechanisms similar to those for all depressive disorders, once detected (Case Vignette 27.1).

Implications and Prognosis

Depression is highly treatable. Management tends to be more effective the earlier it is started, which also increases the likelihood of preventing recurrences (NIMH, 2012). Recent findings from the landmark STAR*D report also indicate that treatment is most successful for those in whom symptoms are eradicated, as opposed to merely controlled (Rush et al., 2006). See Evidence-Based Practice Spotlight 27.1.

As with many psychiatric illnesses, relapses are common and often tied to the adherence of clients to their treatment regimens. Outcomes depend on the severity of the disorder. Many clients with dysthymia never seek treatment. Clients with severe depression are at risk for suicide if their condition remains unaddressed (see Chap. 34).

Case Vignette 27.1

The Powers family consists of Leo, Greta, their two school-age children, and a new infant son. The couple has been married for 15 years. Leo is an accountant; Greta taught school before the children were born but has been a full-time homemaker for 10 years. The older children are doing well academically and are active in sports, music, and other extracurricular activities. The 5-month-old baby is thriving. Although Leo helps at night and on weekends, most housekeeping and child-related responsibilities are Greta's.

During the past 6 weeks, Greta has been in a "funk" that is worsening. Although the baby has started sleeping through the night, occasional insomnia for Greta has turned into difficulty sleeping almost every night. Unfortunately, she is sleeping for 3 to 4 hours during the day while the baby naps and is sometimes having difficulty waking to attend to him. Greta has been neglecting chores and meals, with the oldest child

taking on more duties and Leo cooking dinners. During the last 2 weeks, Greta has been neglecting personal hygiene and has stopped attending her children's games and school functions.

At Leo's urging, Greta visits her physician, who refers her to a mental health clinic because of the increasing evidence of postpartum depression. Leo goes with her to her first appointment. While the nurse is taking the history, Greta states tearfully, "What good am I? What kind of mother and wife am I?"

Reflection and Critical Thinking

- What immediately concerns you about the information provided?
- What measures can the family take immediately to help Greta? What long-term issues may be important to address?
- What other information would the nurse and health care team need to discuss and explore?

Interdisciplinary Goals and Treatment

Because of the significant challenges in caring for clients with depressive disorders, an interdisciplinary approach to provide comprehensive care is most effective. Many nurses work in acute care settings, step-down programs, day treatment programs, and community-based programs to provide the complex care necessary. These programs always have an interdisciplinary approach. In addition, many nurse practitioners work in outpatient clinics, seeing clients with mood disorders in psychotherapy and following them independently, while maintaining contacts with physician consultants and other professionals when necessary (Figure 27.4).

A combination of psychotherapy and medications is more effective than either approach alone in treating

depressive disorders (APA, 2010; NIMH, 2011a,b). Individual psychotherapeutic modalities are numerous. Family therapy also may help clients and their loved ones struggling with ongoing challenges related to chronic depression. In addition to psychopharmacologic strategies, somatic therapies such as electroconvulsive therapy may be alternatives for clients with refractory depression (see Chap. 18).

Cognitive–Behavioral Therapy

Cognitive–behavioral therapies are a common treatment for depressive disorders. They may be done individually or in group settings. The goal is to help clients identify and correct distorted, negative, and catastrophic thinking, thereby relieving symptoms. Behavioral modalities strive to modify

⚠ EVIDENCE-BASED PRACTICE SPOTLIGHT 27.1 ⚠

Findings From the Sequenced Treatment Alternatives to Relieve Depression (STAR*D)

Outcomes of the largest national study of treatment-resistant depression suggest that clients with persistent depression can improve after trying several strategies; however, the odds of overcoming depression diminish as they require additional treatment strategies. Those who become symptom-free have increased chances of staying healthy than do those who experience only symptom improvement. Clients who undergo many treatment steps

before becoming symptom-free are at increased risk for relapse within 1 year.

These findings emphasize the importance of health care providers conducting regular follow-up and paying attention to clients with chronic depression. Ongoing monitoring of symptoms and side effects of medications is crucial, because increased relapses correlate with poorer long-term outcomes.

From: Rush, A. J., Trivedi, M. H., Wisniewski, S. R., Nierenberg, A., Stewart, J. W., Warden, D., . . . Fava. M. (2006). Acute and longer-term outcomes in depressed outpatients who required one or several treatment steps: A STAR*D report. *American Journal of Psychiatry, 163*(11), 1905–1917.

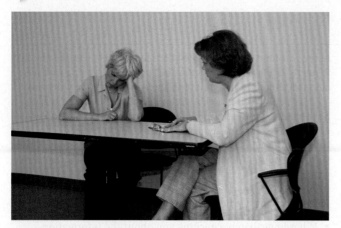

FIGURE 27.4 Nurse practitioners may assist clients with depression on an outpatient basis, monitoring medication regimens and providing counseling as appropriate.

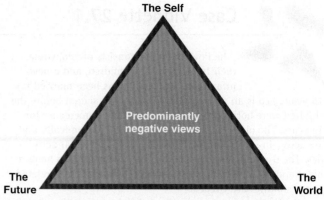

FIGURE 27.5 Beck's cognitive triad of depression. In this model, clients with depression see the future marked by continuing trouble, full of hardship, deprivation, and frustration. The client describes the world as negative, demanding, hostile, and full of obstacles. They view the self as deficient and inadequate and attribute unpleasant experiences to personal defects

maladaptation through homework assignments, structured schedules, and various other techniques

Aaron Beck (1972), who developed the first model of cognitive therapy, noticed that clients with depression tend to have a certain combination of similar negative attitudes, which he labeled the "cognitive triad" of depression (Figure 27.5). He also found that clients with depression tend to generalize by drawing global conclusions from a single, isolated event, and then ignoring incoming data that could provide contrary evidence. Therapeutic interventions focus on working actively with clients to change faulty thought patterns.

Psychopharmacology

Antidepressants are the drugs of choice for depressive disorders (including the depressive phase of bipolar disorder). With few exceptions, antidepressants have proven highly effective for all clients with depression. If one antidepressant is not effective, others are tried to determine which is optimal for a given client (University of Pittsburgh, 2008). The results of STAR*D studies provide the latest data regarding antidepressant therapy (http://www.edc.gsph.pitt.edu/stard).

In general, clients receive antidepressants for moderate or severe symptoms of depression, significant impairment in social or occupational functioning as a result of depression, or suicidal ideation. Strong indications for antidepressants include a history of a positive response to these medications; neurovegetative signs of depression, which include changes in appetite, changes in pattern of sleep, decrease in concentration, decrease in energy, and decrease in libido; unresponsiveness to psychotherapeutic interventions; recurrent depressive episodes; family history of depression; and client preference for drug therapy (APA, 2010; NIMH, 2011a,b).

In general, all antidepressants act at the level of the neuron. Their effects include changing the receptor itself, altering metabolism and breakdown of the neurochemical, or blocking reuptake of the neurochemical at the presynaptic receptor. These changes occur soon after the medication is administered; however, a reduction in depressive signs and symptoms usually takes between 2 and 6 weeks, depending on the drug. See Understanding Biologic Foundations 27.1.

Because each client is unique, the treatment team arrives at the medication of choice through trial and error. The ultimate effect of reducing depressive symptoms is almost identical for all classes of antidepressants. Thus, an antidepressant may be chosen based on its side effect profile and the client's unique needs and symptom constellation (APA, 2010). If a client has used an effective medication in the past, providers consider that drug for subsequent depressive episodes. Before assuming failure with any antidepressant, the client must remain on the drug long enough to ensure appropriate dose titration and achievement of a target dose range; this time frame is a minimum of 4 to 6 weeks (APA, 2010; Karch, 2007).

Often, antidepressant therapy is a long-term process, requiring patience from the client and clinician. This is often challenging when a client has a depressive disorder. Sometimes clients try several types and dosages of antidepressants before arriving at the optimal one. Encouragement and supportive nursing interventions are especially important during medication initiation with clients experiencing severe depression.

Some deterrents to maintaining antidepressant therapy include the length of time for clinical symptoms to subside and uncomfortable side effects that may be unacceptable to some clients. In addition, some medications (usually the TCAs) are potentially lethal, with a narrow therapeutic window. Providers must consider risk of overdose when prescribing these drugs to suicidal clients. Prescriptions for limited medication may be necessary for acutely at-risk clients. In most cases, TCAs are not considered for suicidal clients.

Antidepressants can precipitate mania in clients with bipolar disorder (see Chap. 28). They also can activate latent

Effects of Antidepressants on Neurotransmitters

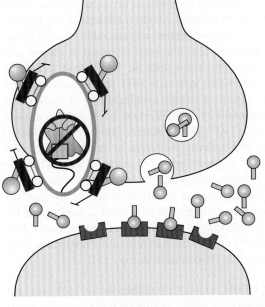

SSRIs. Selective serotonin reuptake inhibitors block the serotonin reuptake pump on the presynaptic neuron. Through blockade of this reuptake, more serotonin is available for longer periods at the synapses. Thus, neurotransmission of serotonin is enhanced, which helps mitigate depressive symptoms.

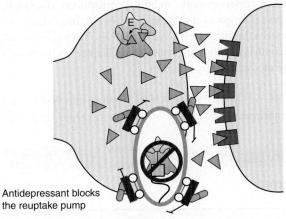

Antidepressant blocks
the reuptake pump

TCAs. Tricyclic antidepressants block the reuptake of norepinephrine and serotonin at the presynaptic neuron. They do their blocking at the noradrenergic level. By increasing the levels and availability of these neurotransmitters, problems with mood and energy decrease.

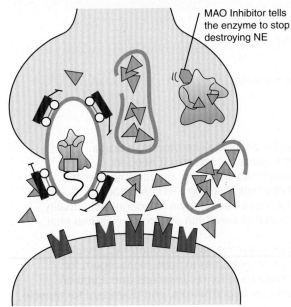

MAO Inhibitor tells
the enzyme to stop
destroying NE

MAOIs. Monoamine oxidase inhibitors work differently than SSRIs and TCAs. Their mechanism of action is to block the activity of monoamine oxidase, an enzyme that breaks down catecholamines, especially norepinephrine, in the neuron itself.

psychosis in some susceptible clients. Therefore, close symptom monitoring is critical. Abrupt discontinuation of antidepressants may cause severe rebound symptoms and a rapid return of the original depression. Thus, discontinuation proceeds with a very slow taper, guided by the elimination half-life of the parent compound and its metabolites and close symptom monitoring (APA, 2010; Karch, 2007).

Chapter 16 describes the mechanisms of action and full side effect profiles for each antidepressant group. The discussions that follow provide individual, class-specific side effects and special issues.

SELECTIVE SEROTONIN REUPTAKE INHIBITORS AND RELATED DRUGS. The SSRIs were the first-generation serotonergic agents; later generations include the serotonin antagonist and reuptake inhibitors (SARIs), which act as both 5-HT antagonists and reuptake blockers, and the serotonin norepinephrine reuptake inhibitors (SNRIs), which block reuptake of both 5-HT and NE. These medications are considered first-line drugs for depression, unless the client's history or medical condition warrants use of an alternative. For example, with certain gastrointestinal disorders (eg, chronic diarrhea, peptic ulcer disease), TCAs are a better first choice. Another example is a client with psychotic depression who begins electroconvulsive therapy as a first-line treatment.

The SSRIs have fewer side effects than do other antidepressants. Side effects most commonly affect the gastrointestinal system (nausea, vomiting, diarrhea) and CNS (headache, nervousness, anxiety, light-headedness) (APA, 2010; Karch, 2007). Loss of libido is also reported relatively frequently. The SSRIs have few to no anticholinergic or cardiotoxic side effects.

One possibly lethal reaction to the SSRIs is serotonin syndrome, which typically follows use of serotomimetic agents (SSRIs, TCAs, tryptophan, dextromethorphan, or meperidine) alone or with monoamine oxidase inhibitors (MAOIs). Serotonin syndrome also has been observed in clients who take a serotomimetic agent with St. John's wort, a popular herbal medication that increases 5-HT levels (see Chap. 16). The administration of certain combinations of these drugs results in hyperactivity of 5-HT in the CNS, leading to serotonin syndrome (APA, 2010; Karch, 2007). In particular, if a client is switching from fluoxetine to an MAOI, providers should allow a "washout" period of at least 5 weeks (half-life of fluoxetine) before beginning the MAOI. Conversely, if the client is switching from an MAOI to fluoxetine, the provider should allow a washout period of at least 2 weeks (half-life of MAOI). If switching to and from other SSRIs, the washout period should be at least the half-life of the alternative drug. See Understanding Psycopharmacology 27.1.

NOVEL (ATYPICAL) ANTIDEPRESSANTS. In general, the novel antidepressants, including trazodone (Desyrel), mirtazapine (Remeron), and bupropion (Wellbutrin, Zyban), are considered safer than the TCAs or MAOIs. They are considered second-line antidepressants. See Chapter 16 for details on these medications.

CYCLIC ANTIDEPRESSANTS. Before the SSRIs and novel antidepressants, TCAs were the first-line drugs for

UNDERSTANDING PSYCHOPHARMACOLOGY 27.1

Symptoms of and Treatment for Serotonin Syndrome

Symptoms

Confusion	Coma
Disorientation	Low-grade fever
Mania	Flushing
Restlessness or agitation	Rhabdomyolysis (rarely)
Myoclonus	Death (rarely)
Rigidity	
Hyperreflexia	**Treatment**
Diaphoresis	1. Immediately discontinue all serotonergic drugs.
Shivering	2. Give anticonvulsants for seizures if needed.
Tremors	3. Serotonin antagonist drugs (eg, cyproheptadine and propranolol) may help. Strong 5-HT2A antagonists, such as risperidone, have been shown to counteract lethality in a mouse model of serotonin syndrome (Nisijima et al., 2000).
Diarrhea	
Nausea	
Ataxia	4. Other drugs may also be used to counteract specific symptoms. Some examples include clonazepam for myoclonus, lorazepam for restlessness and agitation, chlorpromazine for hyperthermia, and diazepam for muscle rigidity.
Headache	
Autonomic instability	

depression. However, the other medications have fewer side effects and do not have the cardiotoxic effects or narrow therapeutic window of TCAs. In most cases, TCAs are used now only when SSRIs and novel antidepressants have been ineffective or when a client's prior success with TCAs is documented.

As a rule, TCAs are not used in clients at risk for suicide. Their narrow therapeutic window makes use dangerous. TCAs are also used cautiously in clients who are hypersensitive to any tricyclic drugs, or may be taking MAOIs, have had a recent heart attack, or are lactating. In addition, they are evaluated thoroughly and considered carefully in clients with preexisting cardiovascular disorders, closed-angle glaucoma, symptomatic benign prostatic hypertrophy, troublesome constipation, seizure disorders, impaired hepatic or renal function, or bipolar disorders, because TCAs may precipitate mania (APA, 2010; Karch, 2007).

MONOAMINE OXIDASE INHIBITORS. The MAOIs are used infrequently since the development of the SSRIs. They may be used to treat atypical depression or depression in clients who do not experience response to other drugs.

The MAOIs increase levels of tyramine. Therefore, if the client overdoses, takes other medications that interact with MAOIs, or eats foods that contain tyramine, NE will accumulate, leading to hypertensive crisis. This critical condition requires immediate medical intervention (Understanding Psycopharmacology 27.2). Other, less severe adverse effects include dizziness, vertigo, headache, constipation, nausea, dry mouth, and weight changes (APA, 2010; Karch, 2007).

Checkpoint Questions

4. Which drug class is inappropriate for use in a depressed, acutely suicidal client?

5. Which drug class typically is considered the first-line treatment for depressive disorders?

6. What condition may result if a client taking MAOIs ingests foods that contain tyramine?

Somatic and Integrative Interventions

Somatic therapies (see Chap. 18) may be used for depressive disorders. **Electroconvulsive therapy (ECT)** is most commonly employed when clients have depression that fails to respond to medications and other modalities. It involves the application of a small dose of electricity to the brain to induce a seizure and alleviate depressive symptoms. The exact mechanism of ECT remains unclear, but the seizure most likely modifies the neurochemical environment. This safe intervention has relatively few long-term side effects. Nevertheless, ECT may evoke strong fear and anxiety in clients and families, who may envision electrocution, death, or permanent intellectual changes. Resulting memory impairment can range from mild forgetfulness to severe confusion. This may persist for weeks or months after treatment but usually resolves.

Transcranial magnetic stimulation was approved by the U.S. Food and Drug Administration (FDA) in 2008 for use with individuals who have not responded favorably to antidepressants. This procedure involves the placement of a transcranial magnetic coil in contact with the client's head to stimulate superficial cortical neurons. Electrical stimulation of the superficial cortical neurons is accomplished by rapidly alternating MRI strength magnetic fields. Further research is necessary, because several studies have shown anywhere from no significant change to small or moderate improvement in the client's depression (APA, 2010).

Vagus nerve stimulation (VNS) has been approved by the FDA for use in clients who have not responded to antidepressant therapy and may benefit with long-term treatment. VNS is not indicated for use in the acute phase of treatment (APA, 2010). More information on the above procedures can be found in Chapter 18.

Phototherapy has proven effective for clients with symptoms of depression associated with a seasonal pattern. This condition, called *seasonal affective disorder,* may be related to lack of light and decreased melatonin production. See Chapter 18 for more information.

UNDERSTANDING PSYCHOPHARMACOLOGY 27.2

Hypertensive Crisis Alert

Symptoms of hypertensive crisis include:

- Occipital headache, which may radiate frontally
- Palpitations
- Neck stiffness or soreness
- Nausea
- Vomiting
- Sweating

- Dilated pupils
- Photophobia
- Tachycardia or bradycardia
- Chest pain
- Orthostatic hypotension, sometimes with falling
- Disturbed cardiac rate and rhythm

From Karch, A. M. (2007). *2007 Lippincott's nursing drug guide* (pp. 942–943). Philadelphia, PA: Lippincott Williams & Wilkins.

Many clients use complementary and alternative modalities to manage depressive symptoms (see Chap. 17). For example, St. John's wort is an herbal remedy many people take. Some clients choose options such as yoga, relaxation, acupuncture, and magnet therapies. The APA's (2010) practice guidelines endorse exercise as a means of augmenting psychotherapy and/or psychopharmacology.

APPLYING THE NURSING PROCESS

Depressive Disorders

Nurses frequently encounter clients whose primary diagnosis is depression. Because of its pervasiveness and frequent coexistence with other psychiatric and medical disorders, nurses may need to intervene for many additional clients with other primary diagnoses dealing with concomitant depression (see Chap. 39). This section focuses mainly on clients with depression that is so severe it requires ongoing monitoring and observation in a health care facility (Case in Point 27.1). Modifications to the assessments and interventions are appropriate as the client improves and is treated in an outpatient setting.

▲ ASSESSMENT

Nursing assessment involves systematic, thorough consideration of the client's safety, mental status, and psychological functioning. It also necessitates careful review of physiologic and psychomotor activity, as well as behavioral and social activity.

Several screening and follow-up tools are available for depression, which can and should be evaluated for across all settings and in all types of clients. Assessment Tool 27.1 reviews commonly used tools.

Safety

Safety is a priority for clients with depression. The focus of interventions may differ slightly, depending on the client's specific problems. Suicide is a primary concern for all clients with depression. Some clients may threaten to harm others and require a thorough violence assessment (see Chap. 32).

Suicide Risk

Suicide assessment is an examination that psychiatric–mental health nurses must learn, practice, and refine. Novice nurses should ask for assistance when learning how to do a suicide assessment and seek and obtain additional training and mentoring regarding the nuances and details.

Case in Point 27.1

Richard's Story

Richard is being admitted to a psychiatric hospital. His wife Louise accompanies him. Richard has a history of depression, with a suicide attempt 5 years ago. He had been in remission until losing his job 6 months ago. Since then, he has had increasing trouble with everyday tasks. "I can't seem to get started in the morning. I haven't been sleeping well at night," he reports. "I've lost about 25 pounds because I'm never hungry." Louise reports that her husband has been talking about what a failure he is and how much he has let everyone down. "I keep telling him that this is just a temporary setback, but no matter how much I reassure him, it doesn't matter." While she is talking, Richard begins to cry.

Richard has been taking his prescribed antidepressant but reports, "I don't think it's working anymore." Although he had been seeing a psychotherapist, he quit 2 years ago "when things were better" and hasn't gone back since.

The nurse asks Richard if he is having suicidal thoughts. He replies, "I don't want to kill myself, because I know how much it would hurt Louise and my son. But I can't imagine going on like this. There are days when I feel close to how I felt when I took those pills last time." Louise says, "We don't want things to get to that point again. That's why we're here for help."

Key Assessment Findings

- History of depression and suicide attempt
- Recent job loss
- Difficulty sleeping, lack of energy
- Weight loss
- Sad affect; crying during discussion
- Concerns over suicide

Case in Point 27.1 (continued)
Richard's Story

Nursing Diagnosis: Risk for Suicide related to previous history of suicide attempt and recent job loss as evidenced by statement "I can't imagine going on like this."

NOC: Suicide Self-Restrain: The client will refrain from attempting suicide.

NIC: Suicide Prevention
- Observe client closely on an ongoing basis. Remove all dangerous objects. *These measures help maintain safety.*
- Discuss with the client the reasons for such monitoring. *Giving the client this information can help ensure his cooperation and also foster his understanding of the close observation.*
- Spend regularly scheduled time with the client during the day. *Such interaction helps the client feel worthwhile and enables him to discuss issues of concern and any brewing problems.*

> 4/1/13: The client has been able to identify reasons to continue to live. He can identify his wife's support as a reason to work toward health. Safety is maintained. The client has not engaged in any suicidal behaviors during his admission.
> J. Hanson, APRN

Nursing Diagnosis: Hopelessness related to response to situational factors, as evidenced by lack of self-care, insomnia, weight loss, and statements about worthlessness.

NOC: Depression Self-Control and **Will to Live:** The client will verbalize reasons to continue participation in daily life and positive aspects.

NIC: Mood Management
- Discuss with the client both positive and negative aspects of his situation. *Clients with depression may not be able to recognize positive elements of their situation. Objective support from others can be useful to this process.*
- Assist the client to identify helpful support people. *Having resources to draw on may help the client recognize people he can turn to in difficult moments and provide validation of his worth and meaning to others.*
- Assist the client to consider other coping strategies when stress, emotions, or feelings are intense, or when life circumstances are becoming overwhelming. Possibilities include exercise, relaxation techniques, discussion with trusted friends or health care providers, and cognitive restructuring. *Alternative coping techniques must be available before the client can abandon self-destructive strategies.*
- Discuss with the physician and the nurse practitioner the possible need for medication dosage adjustments or a new pharmacologic approach. *The client's depressive symptoms may benefit from more intensive or stronger medications.*

> 4/1/13: The client verbalizes sleeping better at night. He has gained 4 lb since admission. The client identifies his wife and son as valuable sources of support. He is adhering to his new medication dosage.
> J. Hanson, APRN

EPILOGUE
Two months have passed since Richard was discharged from the hospital with stabilized symptoms of depression. He is adjusting well to his new medication dosage and has gained another 6 pounds. He and his wife have started to see a nurse psychotherapist clinical specialist to help them through this. Richard reports, "I still have bad days, but at least once in awhile I have a good day, now." He also reports better sleeping at night and that his therapist is helping to facilitate discussions with an employment counselor.

◢ ASSESSMENT TOOL 27.1 ◣
Scales and Screening Instruments for Depression

- *Hamilton Rating Scale for Depression (HAM-D-17):* This 17-item, observer-rated scale assesses depressive symptoms; it is one of the most widely used instruments for the clinical assessment of depressive states.
- *Hamilton Rating Scale for Depression (HAM-D-7):* This shorter version of the HAM-D-17 is a simpler and quicker method for assessing depression in clients.
- *Zung Self-Assessment Scale:* Clients self-rate 20 items to assess feelings, with a focus on clinical symptoms of depression within the past 2 weeks.

- *Beck Depression Inventory:* This 5-minute, 21-item scale assesses the intensity of depression in people 13 to 80 years of age.
- *Geriatric Depression Scale:* This 30-item, basic screening scale is used to evaluate depression in older adults.
- *Edinburgh Postnatal Depression Scale:* This is a 10 item self-administered test used to identify women who have symptoms of postnatal depression.

Factors that increase a client's risk for suicide include expression of current thoughts or plans about suicide, active mental illness (eg, severe depression, bipolar disorder, psychosis), substance abuse, history of suicidal attempts or behaviors, formulation of a plan, availability of means for completing suicide, disruption of important personal relationships, and failure at personal endeavors (NIMH, 2011a,b). It is a myth that forthright questioning about suicidal thoughts or plans increases the risk for suicide; direct, nonjudgmental questioning is most effective. In fact, clients often report feeling relieved that someone has asked them in detail about suicidal thoughts.

Chapter 34 reviews suicide, its assessment, and preventive interventions in detail. Nurses can briefly assess for suicide in clients with depression by asking the following questions:

- "When you feel depressed, what do you think about?"
- "Do you ever think about taking your own life?"
- "Do you have a plan for committing suicide?"
- "Do you have the means to carry out your plan?"
- "Have you ever rehearsed the plan?"
- "What interrupted your rehearsal?"
- "Would anything prevent you from killing yourself?"
- "What support people can you call for help when you are feeling like hurting yourself?"

Violence Risk

Although suicide may be more of a risk in depression than homicide, clients who are agitated, angry, or despairing may turn their feelings outward. Doing so increases the chances for harm to others. Nurses consider the following as warning signs for violence in clients with depression: ideas about or intent to harm others, history of violent behavior, severe agitation or hostility, and active psychosis, particularly with command hallucinations. See also Chapter 32.

Mental Status Examination

Mental status changes over time, sometimes rapidly. The frequency with which the Mental Status Examination is performed depends on the client's behavior, symptoms, medications, specific needs for ongoing monitoring (eg, the client who is on suicide precautions), and other environmental factors.

Clients with depression may be poorly groomed and disheveled, with a dejected facial expression. Because depression is mainly a manifestation of disturbed mood and affect, the client's emotional tone may be the most observable deviation from healthy behavior. In depression, affect may or may not be congruent with mood (ie, it may or may not match the observed mood). Affect is usually constricted but appropriate to content.

The thought content of clients with depression often involves issues of loss and abandonment, worthlessness, guilt, and hopelessness. Such clients may exhibit confusion, difficulty concentrating, and thought blocking. Clients may present with perceptual disturbances, such as hallucinations or delusions, particularly those of the persecutory type, especially if the depressive illness has psychotic features.

Depression can cause disturbed judgment, possibly related to anergia and withdrawal. Insight is often limited because clients cannot assess their situation objectively

Physiologic Stability

A primary nursing concern for clients with depression is physiologic integrity and function. Neurovegetative signs include either an increase or decrease in appetite, disturbed sleep patterns, decrease in energy, decrease in concentration, and a decrease in libido.

Nurses must fully assess for recent weight gain or loss, appetite changes, nutritional intake, and bowel habits. Early morning awakening is common, and sleep disturbances contribute to fatigue and exhaustion. Libido is usually lowered during depressive episodes.

▲ NURSING DIAGNOSIS

Common diagnoses for clients with mood disorders are as follows (NANDA, 2007):

- **Risk for Suicide** related to impaired judgment, hopelessness and distorted thinking
- **Risk for Violence** toward others related to history of aggression, perception of a threatening environment, inability to verbalize feelings, fear, agitation, and low tolerance level
- **Ineffective Health Maintenance** related to lack of concern for self, fatigue, and low self-esteem
- **Impaired Social Interaction** related to distorted thinking, feelings of low self-esteem, disorientation, or restlessness
- **Disturbed Thought Processes** related to biochemical imbalances, delusions, hallucinations, or psychological stress
- **Ineffective Therapeutic Regimen Management** related to lack of knowledge about medications and lack of incentive to maintain medication regimen upon discharge (Carpenito-Moyet, 2004).

▲ OUTCOME IDENTIFICATION AND PLANNING

The most important priority is maintaining the client's safety, as well as safety for others. Possible outcomes for clients, integrating labels from the Nursing Outcomes Classification (NOC), may include the following (Moorhead et al., 2008):

- **Suicide Self-Restraint:** The client will remain safe throughout the hospitalization and while receiving care in the outpatient setting, without harming self.
- **Aggression Self-Control:** The client will remain safe throughout the hospitalization and while receiving care in the outpatient setting, without harming others.
- **Self-Care Status:** The client will have adequate food and fluid intake, will maintain balanced rest, sleep, and activity, and will maintain personal care.
- **Social Interaction Skills:** The client will engage in appropriate social behavior.
- **Distorted Thought Self-Control:** The client will demonstrate logical, reality-based thought processes.
- **Will to Live:** The client will consistently maintain the medication regimen, including taking medications as ordered and

following up with his or her care provider for appropriate postdischarge visits and laboratory work.

▲ IMPLEMENTATION

Because many people with depression are hesitant to seek treatment, nurses commonly encounter the most severely ill clients in hospitals. Increasing numbers of primary care settings and general office units are implementing measures to screen and detect for depression in regular visits with clients (Figure 27.6). Nurses use many types of interventions to assist recovering clients and families. Common Nursing Interventions Classification (NIC) labels that are appropriate for individuals with depressive disorders are **Active Listening, Cognitive Restructuring, Coping Enhancement, Hope Instillation, Mood Management, Self-Esteem Enhancement, Spiritual Support, Suicide Prevention,**and **Teaching: Disease Process** (Bulechek et al., 2008).

Protecting the Client From Suicide

The first step is to assess the client's risk for suicide. If a client is at risk, nurses must immediately place him or her on suicide precautions with frequent or continuous one-to-one observation and reassessment. In addition, nurses place the client in a room central to the nursing station. The client is encouraged to participate in unit-based activities. At the same time, it is important to note that trying to force clients into activities for which they may not have the emotional or physical strength can add to their stress. In such cases, it is crucial that clients remain in line of sight of staff members in order to ensure their safety. The nurse removes all potentially dangerous objects (eg, glass, ties, belts, razors) from the environment. If the client needs these objects, nurses monitor use at all times. It is also important to note that the usual items that seem dangerous are not the only ones with which clients can commit suicide. They have been known to use glasses, combs, pens, and pencils inserted into their throat to kill themselves. Thus, the most important tool that staff members have in suicide prevention is vigilance

and client observation. Because the bathroom is the most common area for successful suicide completion in inpatient psychiatric settings, nurses must make sure to check the bathroom area when making client observational rounds.

Building a therapeutic relationship increases the likelihood that clients will convey suicidal thoughts to the nurse. Trust is established through brief, frequent contacts; empathy; and a nonjudgmental attitude of caring and respect. The nursing staff encourages clients to verbalize thoughts and feelings and discuss current stressors, particularly the precipitating factors that caused the suicidal thoughts or behavior at this time. It is important to ask clients to talk about suicidal thoughts or feelings when they surface. Then nurse and client explore the sadness, anger, hopelessness, or other feelings as well as events that may have precipitated those suicidal thoughts. Because suicidal clients are often ambivalent about dying, nurses encourage them to identify the types of thoughts or actions that will help them want to live or what interactions with others would keep them from committing suicide (see Chap. 34)

Although suicidal ideation often resolves when medications begin working, studies have shown that risk for suicide increases within the first 2 to 3 weeks after starting antidepressant medication, usually because the client's mood has not lifted as quickly as physical energy has returned. Therefore, this period is critical for monitoring the client's mood, suicidal feelings, response to medications, and energy. Nurses exercise extreme caution when assessing client's activities during the 2 to 3 weeks after initiation of medications if they are in a position to do so. Because most clients do not stay in hospitals for more than a few days, it is important that nurses convey the information of increased likelihood of suicidality during this time to clients and to responsible family members.

Managing the Potential for Violence

Nurses assess each client's level of risk for violence and, if necessary, place clients on violence precautions (see Chap. 32). Establishing geographic boundaries, such as room restriction or half-hall restriction, is part of ongoing monitoring. Also, clients likely will have "as-needed" medications ordered; nurses use them if aggressive or agitated behavior escalates. Other environmental approaches include reducing stimuli and opportunities for interaction with other clients in the milieu. Nurses remove all dangerous items from the client's room and monitor closely for use of any potentially harmful items.

Nurses help clients learn to recognize what triggers violent thoughts and behaviors. They teach clients not to act on these thoughts but to leave the situation and find a staff member to talk to about them. They help clients recognize and connect symptoms with any precipitating thoughts or circumstances so that the client can make the connection between them and determine other ways to respond. Nurses teach about medications and their potential positive effects on violent thoughts and behaviors.

Maintaining Physical Health and Personal Hygiene

Nurses monitor food and fluid intake and assess weight gain or loss, vital signs, and laboratory values. Clients with depression

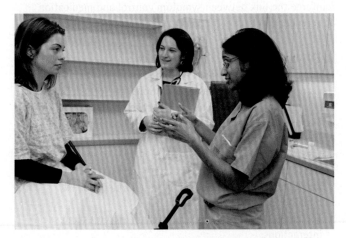

FIGURE 27.6 Screening for depression is becoming an increasing focus in primary care and office settings. The nurse is asking a postpartum woman how she is coping during a follow-up visit.

may have little or no interest in food; conversely, they may overeat. Nurses work with clients and nutritionists to devise menus that ensure appropriate caloric intake.

Balancing rest with activity can be a challenge. Clients may have little energy, sleep too much, or have disturbed sleep (Figure 27.7). Nurses should assess clients' subjective views of their sleep patterns and feelings of fatigue. It is helpful for both the nurse and the client to evaluate activity patterns. While in the inpatient setting, the nurse should encourage clients to spend time in common or recreational areas, instead of isolated areas, and provide opportunities for exercise. At bedtime, nurses encourage clients to drink warm milk, read, take a soothing bath, or engage in other activities that help induce sleep.

Clients with depression lack energy or interest. Nurses encourage independence in dressing, hygiene, and grooming but help with self-care (bathing, brushing teeth, choosing clothing) until attention, mood, and energy level are stabilized. The nurse should give positive reinforcement and encouragement when clients begin to show interest in their surroundings and appearance.

Enhancing Thought Processes
For clients with depression in an inpatient setting, nurses encourage sitting in the milieu, if appropriate and tolerated, to prevent isolation. If the client's anxiety is extreme, nurses should limit the client's interactions and contacts in the milieu but provide a comforting, low-stimulus environment in the client's room. The disturbed thought processes associated with depression can manifest as alterations in self-esteem. These clients often experience chronic, underlying low self-esteem and find it difficult to identify personal strengths. Nurses encourage clients to verbalize these feelings and discuss areas in which they display strengths and positive behaviors. They reinforce and validate constructive behaviors and thought patterns.

Agitation is extreme anxiety and disordered thinking. Clients with depression may display agitated or anxious behaviors. More often, the clinical picture for a client with severe depression is a reduction in activity, along with apathy and fatigue. Nevertheless, agitated depression can be challenging. Nurses

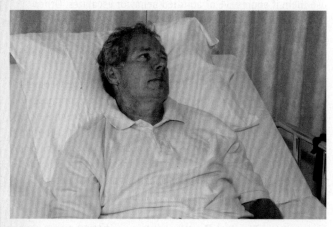

FIGURE 27.7 Clients with depression may struggle with sleep disturbances. They may sleep too much, or they may experience insomnia.

evaluate this symptom and explore associated feelings and underlying thoughts. Clients may present with hostility, apathy, and withdrawal. Exploring thoughts and feelings underlying withdrawn or hostile behavior is important because these may not be readily apparent. Nurses encourage clients to engage in milieu activities, such as exercising or playing cards, which may serve as outlets for excess energy.

Relaxation exercises, imagery, and progressive muscle relaxation may help clients with depression. These may be difficult for clients to concentrate on, or paradoxically, they may increase anxiety. Nurses evaluate the client's ability to tolerate such directed relaxation exercises and engage clients, if appropriate. Listening to music also may reduce anxiety.

Encouraging Treatment and Medication Adherence
Nurses provide information about the prescribed medication and needed aftercare, such as frequency of laboratory testing, discharge planning, and follow-up visits. They teach clients who are prescribed medications the importance of obtaining blood tests as directed by the prescribing provider. If possible, nurses help clients keep a notebook or cards on which to record information about medications, including mechanisms of action, dosages, side effects, and ongoing monitoring needs. They review information until clients are familiar with each medication and its actions.

To help link the importance of taking medication with relapse prevention, nurses list target symptoms and identify signs of relapse. They problem solve with clients about early management of symptoms so severity does not increase. Next, nurses explore what clients may perceive as barriers to obtaining medications, participating in follow-up with the psychiatric care provider, and undergoing necessary laboratory tests. Nurses work with clients to overcome these barriers.

Often clients become less vigilant and are apt to stop medication management and follow-up psychiatric care during periods of remission. Nurses work with clients and their families regarding the importance of adhering to the treatment regimen, especially during periods when symptoms are controlled. They reinforce the link between symptom control and medication adherence.

▲ EVALUATION
Improvement in symptoms is gradual but noticeable as medication and psychotherapeutic interventions take effect. Specific indicators that interventions are effective include the following:

* The client reports fewer or no suicidal thoughts.
* The client refrains from self-harm or acting aggressively toward others.
* The client ingests adequate calories and fluids, maintains a balance between rest and activity, and independently manages self-care.
* The client participates appropriately in activities and social interactions.
* The client expresses a positive sense of self-worth.
* The client adheres to the therapeutic regimen and discusses the importance of doing so after discharge.

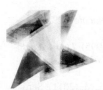

Reviewing and Applying Your Knowledge

Chapter Summary

- Depressive disorders are a significant problem in America. Suicide, which is closely associated, is an emergent national public health priority.

- The etiology of depressive disorders is complex and involves multiple interactions among genetic factors, physiologic factors, and psychological factors.

- Signs and symptoms and diagnostic criteria for the depressive disorders are highly specific.

- Depressive disorders are often unrecognized and, hence, go untreated; however, when clients receive appropriate treatment, outcomes are good. Multiple treatment modalities include individual, group, and family psychotherapies; pharmacotherapy; and somatic therapies.

- Psychiatric–mental health nurses must use the nursing process to assess, plan, implement, and evaluate care for people with depressive disorders.

Study Questions

1. A 35-year-old client with depression lost his job and most of his investments because of unethical business practices. He states his family would be better off without him because of the shame he has brought to them. Which response by the nurse would be most therapeutic?

   a. "Tell me more about the shame you feel."

   b. "Has your wife told you she wants a divorce?"

   c. "Are you thinking of killing yourself?"

   d. "You appear depressed."

2. A 30-year-old client with a history of depression returns to the mental health clinic for follow-up care. She takes 100 mg of sertraline daily. In addition, she states she tries to stay mentally and physically well by taking yoga classes, walking regularly, and taking vitamins and St. John's wort. She also relates that she is a lacto-ovo-vegetarian and gets most of her protein from cheese. Given this information, what should the nurse tell the client?

   a. "Avoid cheese. In conjunction with your medication, it can precipitate a severe hypertensive reaction."

   b. "You're doing a great job taking care of yourself. You've made several healthy lifestyle choices."

   c. "Stop taking St. John's wort. In conjunction with your medication, it can precipitate a serious reaction called serotonin syndrome."

   d. "You're doing a great job with your lifestyle choices. Do more intensive aerobic exercise, which has been shown to stabilize mood."

3. A 25-year-old client has been in inpatient treatment for severe depression for 3 weeks. He will be discharged soon, and the nurse is evaluating the effectiveness of the plan of care. Which outcome is the most appropriate indicator that the client's depression is resolving sufficiently for safe discharge?

   a. The client has resumed caring for his physical appearance.

   b. The client denies wanting to commit suicide.

   c. The client expresses a willingness to begin tapering his medication.

   d. The client sits in the public areas and speaks when addressed.

4. Which of the following variables would the nurse identify as exerting the greatest effects on relapse prevention for clients with depressive disorders?

   a. Strong social support.

   b. High socioeconomic status.

   c. Stress management skills.

   d. Medication adherence.

Critical Thinking Questions

1. During the past few months, a nurse has noticed that a friend seems unhappy and depressed. The friend has gained noticeable weight in a short time and seems to lack attention to her personal appearance, which is unusual. When the nurse has called to say "hi," the friend has reported that she was sleeping, even though the nurse is calling well before 8:00 P.M. What things might the nurse do to help ensure her friend's health? Could problems other than depression be causing symptoms?

2. A client comes to the mental health clinic complaining that his new medication is not working. When questioned, the client reports that he has been taking the drug for 9 days. What education needs are evident? How can the nurse intervene effectively?

References

American Psychiatric Association (APA). (2000). *Diagnostic and statistical manual of mental disorders* (4th ed., text rev.). Washington, DC: Author.

American Psychiatric Association (APA). (2010). *Practice guidelines for the treatment of patients with major depressive Disorder* (3rd ed.). Retrieved from http://www.psychiatryonline.com/pracGuide/pracGuideTopic_7.aspx

Bear, M. F., Connors, B., & Paradiso, M. (2006). *Neuroscience: Exploring the human brain* (3rd ed.). Philadelphia, PA: Lippincott Williams & Wilkins.

Beck, A. T. (1972). *Depression: Causes and treatment*. Philadelphia, PA: University of Pennsylvania Press.

Beck, A. T. (2008). The evolution of the cognitive model of depression and its neurobiological correlates. *American Journal of Psychiatry, 165*(8), 969–978.

Bulechek, G. M., Butcher, H. K., & McCloskey Dochterman, J. (2008). *Nursing interventions classification (NIC)* (5th ed.). St. Louis, MO: Mosby.

Carpenito-Moyet, L. J. (2004). *Nursing diagnosis: Application to clinical practice* (10th ed.). Philadelphia, PA: Lippincott Williams & Wilkins.

Colman, I., & Ataullahjan, A. (2010). Life course perspectives on the epidemiology of depression. *Canadian Journal of Psychiatry, 55*(10), 622–633.

Golden, S. H. (2007). A review of the evidence for a neuroendocrine link between stress, depression and diabetes mellitus. *Current Diabetes Review, 3*(4), 252–259.

Karch, A. M. (2007). *2007 Lippincott's nursing drug guide*. Philadelphia, PA: Lippincott Williams & Wilkins.

Kelsoe, J. E. (2005). Mood disorders: Genetics. In B. J. Sadock & V. A. Sadock (Eds.), *Comprehensive textbook of psychiatry* (8th ed., Vol. 1, pp. 1582–1594). Philadelphia, PA: Lippincott Williams & Wilkins.

Kessler, R. C., Chiu, W. T., Demler, O., & Walters, E. E. (2005). Prevalence, severity, and comorbidity of twelve-month *DSM-IV* disorders in the National Comorbidity Survey Replication (NCS-R). *Archives of General Psychiatry, 62*(6), 617–627.

Massachusetts General Hospital Center for Women's Mental Health. (2012). Postpartum psychiatric disorders. Retrieved from http://www.womensmentalhealth.org

Moorhead, S., Johnson, M., Maas, M. L., & Swanson, E. (2008). *Nursing outcomes classification (NOC)* (4th ed.). St. Louis, MO: Mosby.

NANDA International. (2007). *Nursing diagnoses: Definitions and classification (2007–2008)*. Philadelphia, PA: Author.

National Institute of Mental Health (NIMH). (2011a). *Any mood disorder among adults.* Retrieved from http://www.nimh.nih.gov/statistics/1ANYMOODDIS_ADULT.

National Institute of Mental Health (NIMH). (2011b). *Major depressive disorder among adults*. Retrieved from http://www.nimh.nih.gov/statistics/1MDD_ADULT.shtml. . .

National Institute of Mental Health (NIMH). (2012). *Depression*. Retrieved from http://www.nimh.nih.gov/health/publications/depression

Nisijima, K., Yoahino, R., Yui, K., & Katoh, S. (2001). Potent serotonin (5-HT)(2A) receptor antagonists completely prevent the development of hyperthermia in an animal model of the 5-HT syndrome. *Brain Research, 890*(1), 23–31.

Nugent, N. R., Tyrka, A. R., Carpenter, L. L., & Price, L. H. (2011) Gene-environment interactions: Early life stress and risks for depressive and anxiety disorders. *Psychopharmacology, 214* (1), 175–196.

Peterson, C., Maier, S. F., & Seligman, M. E. P. (1995). *Learned helplessness: A theory for the age of personal control*. New York, NY: Oxford University Press.

Pytliak, M., Vargrová, V., Mechirová, V., & Felsöci, M. (2011). Serotonin receptors—From molecular biology to clinical applications. *Physiological Research, 60*(1), 15–26.

Reynolds, C. F. III, Dew, M. A., Pollock, B. G., Mulsant, B. H., Frank, E., Miller, M. D., . . . Kupfer, D. J. (2006). Maintenance treatment of major depression in old age. *New England Journal of Medicine, 354*(11), 1130–1138.

Rush, A. J., Trivedi, M. H., Wisniewski, S. R., Nierenberg, A., Stewart, J. W., Warden, D., . . . Fava, M. (2006). Acute and longer-term outcomes in depressed outpatients who required one or several treatment steps: A STAR*D report. *American Journal of Psychiatry, 163*(11), 1905–1917.

Seligman, M. P., Friedman, R. J., & Katz, M. M. (Eds.). (1974). *Depression and learned helplessness in the psychology of depression: Contemporary theory and research*. New York, NY: John Wiley & Sons.

Shelton, R. C. (2007). The molecular neurobiology of depression. *Psychiatric Clinics of North America, 30*(1), 1–11.

South, S. C., & Krueger, R. F. (2011). Genetic and environmental influences on internalizing psychopathology vary as a function of economic status. *Psychological Medicine, 41*(1), 107–118.

Thase, M. E. (2005). Mood disorders: Neurobiology. In B. J. Sadock & V. A. Sadock (Eds.), *Comprehensive textbook of psychiatry* (8th ed., Vol. 1, pp. 1594–1603). Philadelphia, PA: Lippincott Williams & Wilkins.

Uddin, M., Koenen, K. C., Aiello, A. E., Wildman, D. E., de Los Santos, R., & Galea, S. (2011). Epigenetic and inflammatory marker profiles associated with depression in a community-based epidemiologic sample. *Psychological Medicine, 41*(5), 997–1008.

University of Pittsburgh. (2008). *Welcome to STAR-D*. Retrieved from http://www.edc.gsph.pitt.edu/stard

Web Resources

American Psychiatric Association: Healthy Minds. Healthy Lives: http://www.healthyminds.org

American Psychiatric Association: DSM-5: http://www.dsm5.org

Centers for Disease Control and Prevention. http://www.cdc.gov/ViolencePrevention/suicide

Edinburgh Postnatal Depression Scale: http://www.womensmental-health.org/quiz-are-you-suffering-from-postpartum-depression

Massachusetts General Hospital Center for Women's Mental Health: http://www.womensmentalhealth.org

Mayo Clinic: Postpartum Depression: http://www.mayoclinic.com/health/postpartum-depression

Mental Health Infosearch: http://www.mhsource.com

Mental Health Net: http://www.cmhc.com

National Depressive and Manic Depressive Association: http://ndmda.org

National Foundation for Depressive Illness: http://www.depression.org

National Institute of Mental Health (NIMH): http://nimh.nih.gov

National Mental Health Association: http://aoa.dhhs.gov/aoa/dir/181.html

Postpartum Education for Parents: http://www.sbpep.org

Postpartum Support International: http://www.postpartum.net

Society for Light Treatment and Biological Rhythms: http://www.sltbr.org

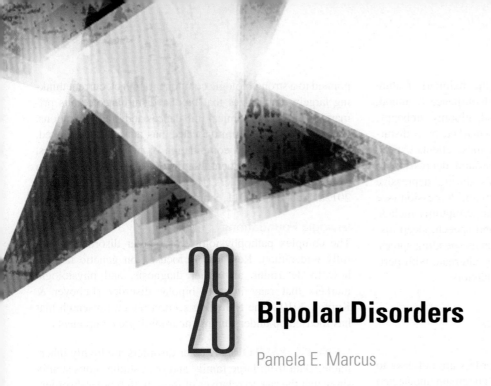

28

Bipolar Disorders

Pamela E. Marcus

KEY TERMS

cyclothymia
hypomania
manic episodes
rapid cycling
refractory mania

LEARNING OBJECTIVES

On completion of this chapter, you should be able to accomplish the following:

- Explain what is meant by *bipolar disorders.*
- Discuss the incidence and prevalence of bipolar disorders in the United States.
- Analyze various theories about the etiology of bipolar disorders.
- List symptoms of bipolar disorders using criteria from the *Diagnostic and Statistical Manual of Mental Disorders,* 4th edition, text revision (*DSM-IV-TR*).
- Outline interdisciplinary treatments for clients with bipolar disorders.
- Apply the nursing process to the care of clients with bipolar disorders.

As described in Chapter 27, the hallmark feature of depressive disorders is a disturbance in mood, in which the affected person feels sad, gloomy, unhappy, or "down." Bipolar disorders are also marked by a disturbance in mood. The difference is that these clients experience mood swings ranging from profound depression to extreme euphoria (mania). Symptoms during depressive episodes are consistent with those of major depression (see Chap. 27). During manic episodes the symptoms include grandiosity; rapid thoughts, actions, and speech; sleep disturbances; and impulsive behavior, such as spending sprees. Episodes of bipolar mood disturbances alternate with periods of normal mood and associated behaviors.

OVERVIEW OF BIPOLAR DISORDERS

Because the symptoms of bipolar disorders are not easy to pinpoint objectively, these disorders often remain undetected or misdiagnosed for up to 10 years after the onset of some depressive symptoms (National Institute of Mental Health [NIMH], 2010b; Schneck, 2011).

Incidence and Prevalence

Bipolar disorders affect approximately 2.6% of the U.S. population, with 82.9% of the cases reported to NIMH classified as severe bipolar disorder. The average age of clients experiencing their first manic episode is 25 years (NIMH, 2012b). Earlier age of onset is associated with worse outcomes, including rapid cycling in adulthood (Goldberg, 2011; Schneck, 2011). The lifetime prevalence of bipolar disorder, both types I and II, is 3.7% to 3.9% (Kessler et al., 2005). Rates of morbidity and mortality, particularly for bipolar depression, are associated with medical illnesses such as cardiovascular, cerebrovascular, and respiratory diseases, as well as with other psychiatric illnesses and substance use disorders (NIMH,. 2012a; Weiner et al., 2011). It is estimated that 25% to 50% of clients with bipolar disease attempt suicide at least once in their lifetime, with 15% completing suicide (American Foundation for Suicide Prevention, 2010; Wieseke et al., 2011).

Bipolar I disorder affects men and women equally; bipolar II disorder is more common in women (see later discussion) (Baldassano et al., 2005). Women are more likely to experience mixed mania and manic switches during treatment with antidepressants (Burt & Rasgon, 2004). Women also have higher rates of comorbid thyroid disease, bulimia, and post-traumatic stress disorder (American Psychiatric Association [APA], 2010; Baldassano et al., 2005). See Chapter 36 for a discussion of juvenile bipolar disorder.

Etiology

Before the early 1950s, psychologic theories regarding the etiology of most mental illnesses, including bipolar disorders, dominated. Extensive research and the success of specific and refined medications for treating disorders have clearly pointed to a strong biologic component. In fact, current thinking largely emphasizes that bipolar disturbance results primarily from neurochemical imbalances and brain alterations. Although a single definitive cause has not been pinpointed, scientists agree that a combination or interaction of genes, neurobiology, environment, life history, and development can result in bipolar disorders (Byerley & Badner, 2011; NIMH 2012a; Sklar et al., 2011; Smoller & Gardner-Schuster, 2007).

Biologic Foundations

The complex pathophysiology of bipolar disorders is not fully understood. Research is focused on genetic factors, how to determine an earlier diagnosis, and physiologic markers that may indicate bipolar disorder (Leboyer & Kupfer, 2010). The following section reviews research that has focused on understanding neurobiologic components.

GENETIC FACTORS. Bipolar disorders are highly inheritable. Data from large family and twin studies consistently show that the risk to relatives of those with bipolar disorders is greater than the risk to relatives of those without these disorders (Smoller & Gardner-Schuster, 2007). The estimate of inheritability is 80%, with over 25 genome-wide linkage studies (Byerley & Badner, 2011). Further research is ongoing. Current research projects are exploring the genome-wide association, a possible focus on chromosome 16 p, and other areas in the genome (Byerley & Badner, 2011; Sklar et al., 2011). An example of such research is exploring genes that are involved in both depression and bipolar disorder. The current hypothesis is that there may be an overlapping of genes in individuals with affective disorders that "turn on and off" depending on risk factors in the individual's environment (NIMH, 2010a) (see Chap. 2).

The complex mode of inheritance most likely involves multiple interacting genes. Dysregulation in the gene G protein receptor kinase 3 (GRK3), which is involved in dopamine metabolism, increases susceptibility to bipolar illness (Barrett et al., 2003). Baum et al. (2008) identified several genes in the etiology, implicating this disorder group as polygenic. The NIMH Science Update discusses the overlap genes in affective disorders. This update cites research from five different genome-wide association studies, showing genetic variations on chromosome 3 as well as a gene called *PBRM1*. The *PBRM1* gene is expressed more in the prefrontal cortex in individuals with bipolar disorder than it is in healthy individuals (NIMH, 2010a). Research is also focusing on genetic similarities between bipolar disorder and schizophrenia. This research is concentrating on the risk for disease and identifies a locus in ODZ4 and a calcium channel gene *CACNA1C* (Sklar et al., 2011). Ongoing genetic studies will continue to provide knowledge that may help identify people susceptible to mood disorders and possible medications that can target the genetic defects.

NEUROANATOMIC FACTORS. Various brain abnormalities seem to be associated with bipolar disorders (Understanding Biologic Foundations 28.1). Examples

UNDERSTANDING BIOLOGIC FOUNDATIONS 28.1

Brain Region Alterations in Bipolar Disorder

Prefrontal cortex

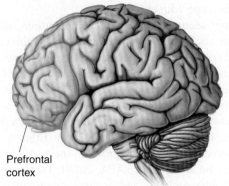

Prefrontal cortex

Fewer glial cells and abnormally sized neurons may be found in the brain. Activity in the prefrontal cortex may also be reduced.

Hypothalamus

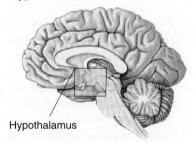

Hypothalamus

Increased numbers of neuropeptides may be found in the hypothalamus.

Cerebellum

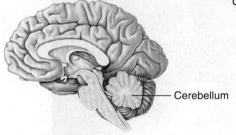

Cerebellum

The cerebellum, which helps control movements, may be smaller with less dense gray matter.

Amygdala and hippocampus

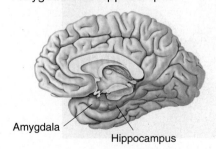

Amygdala

Hippocampus

The amygdala may show signs of enlargement, whereas the hippocampus may have less density and fewer neurons.

include volume reductions in the subregions of the prefrontal cortex, with amygdala and striatal enlargement and midline cerebellar atrophy (Strakowski et al., 2005). Other findings include enlarged lateral and third ventricles and white matter hyperdensities in 10% to 30% of affected clients (Savitz et al., 2005). Further evidence of structural pathology includes abnormal neuronal size and reduced glial cell density in the dorsolateral prefrontal cortices (Rajkowska et al., 2001). One study found a larger decline in hippocampal, fusiform, and cerebellar gray matter density over 4 years in clients with bipolar disorders compared with a control group (Moorhead et al., 2007).

NEUROTRANSMITTERS. Researchers once believed that absolute neurotransmitter levels (either too high or too low) in the synaptic cleft could explain mood disorders. Current belief is that these systems are far more complex (see Chap. 2). Investigators now focus on the neurotransmitter system functioning, such as increased sensitivity of the post-synaptic receptors. One hypothesis is that dysregulation in dopamine and serotonin systems combines with deficits in other systems (eg, GABA) to produce symptoms of mood disorders (Stockmeier, 2003).

Serotonin. A positron emission tomography study of clients with bipolar depression found increased serotonin in the thalamus, dorsal cingulate cortex, medial prefrontal cortex, and insula, and decreased serotonin at the level of the pontine raphe-nuclei (Cannon et al., 2006). It has become possible to determine the subpopulations of serotonin receptor sites. This has led to new understanding of the role of this neurotransmitter. Future research will concentrate on this area (Pytliak et al., 2011).

Dopamine. Various dopaminergic drugs have been found to trigger manic symptoms (eg, increased mood, energy, and talkativeness). Higher dopaminergic activity induced by reduced synaptic vesicle buffering capacity or higher dopaminergic receptor sensitivity may be associated with mania (Ackenheil, 2001).

GABA. Clients with bipolar disorder may have low plasma levels of GABA during depressive and manic phases. Expression of the GABA cell phenotype (GAD67) may be decreased in the hippocampus of clients with bipolar disorder, indicating decreased neurotransmission of GABA (Benes et al., 2007).

Intracellular Signaling. Studies have shown a relationship between signaling pathway abnormalities and altered neurotransmission. The G proteins are molecules that translate the signals emitted by cell membrane receptors and relay the signals to second-messenger systems (see Chap. 2). Studies have found increased G protein levels in clients with bipolar disorder, which suggests that this protein may be involved in its pathophysiology (Kapczinski et al., 2004).

Psychological Factors

Although current evidence and trends support biologic factors as the primary contributors to bipolar illness, psychosocial factors influence how people *respond* to their biologic makeup and whether problems emerge (see Chap. 3). Psychological and social issues also significantly influence how clients and families cope with chronic illness.

The following sections review the implications of psychological and social factors in treatment. Cognitive, interpersonal, and social rhythm theories can serve as frameworks from which health care providers can plan effective psychosocial interventions, which can foster adherence to treatment regimens (Miklowitz, 2006; NIMH, 2007). For example, clients with mania may neglect to take their medications when they feel well (Figure 28.1). Effective psychosocial interventions would provide methods for facilitating medication compliance (APA, 2010). Therapeutic relationships between clients and health care providers are essential to foster consistent individualized interventions during disease recurrences.

COGNITIVE FACTORS. From a cognitive viewpoint (see Chaps. 3 and 13), faulty beliefs about self and the world, specifically high-goal attainment beliefs, contribute to bipolar illness. An example of such a belief is that if people try hard enough, they can excel at anything. Another is that people can take risks without any consequences (Power, 2005). One dysfunctional attitude characteristic of bipolar disorder is goal-striving (Lam et al., 2004). Success in goal-striving

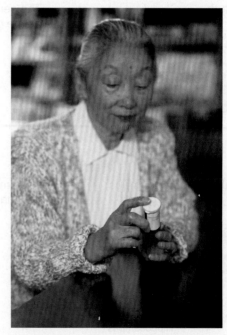

FIGURE 28.1 Ensuring adherence to medication regimens can be one of the most challenging aspects of care for clients with bipolar disorder. Frequently, clients fail to take their medicines during manic episodes because they are feeling so euphoric and energetic that they mistakenly believe they no longer need their drugs.

leads to euphoria. A positive feedback loop may lead to attempts to enhance the euphoria with increasingly driven behavior and disregard of feedback from others, disruption in normal routines, or both.

INTERPERSONAL AND SOCIAL RHYTHM MODEL. This approach is based on the social-psychodynamic models of Harry Stack Sullivan (1953) and Adolf Meyer (1957) along with the instability model of bipolar disorder (Goodwin & Jamison, 1990) and the Social Zeitgeber theory of mood disorders (Ehlers et al., 1993). It posits that psychosocial stressors trigger bipolar episodes by disrupting normal social rhythms. The subsequent result is disruption of circadian systems, leading to mania or depression (Hlastala & Frank, 2006) (see Chaps. 2 and 22). Disruption in the sleep–wake cycle has an effect on individuals without mood disorders. There is ongoing research that considers affective dysregulation during the day, which affects sleep at night. The circadian rhythm is disrupted as well as affect regulation (Leboyer & Kupfer, 2010). In addition, these stressors occur within an interpersonal context that is often interdependent with the illness (NIMH, 2010b).

Cognitive Functioning and Bipolar Disorder

Because bipolar disorder is a neuropsychologic disorder, it is important to understand the role cognitive functioning plays. Individuals with bipolar disorder may present with cognitive deficits in memory, concentration, and executive functioning (Leboyer & Kupfer, 2010; Shippee et al., 2011; Torres et al., 2011). These disruptions in brain functioning affect the ability to learn, work, and have long-term relationships (Shippee et al., 2011).

Checkpoint Questions

1. What brain areas are most associated with abnormalities linked to bipolar disorders?
2. What neurotransmitters are commonly shown to be involved with bipolar disorders?
3. Why are psychosocial interventions important in caring for clients with bipolar disorders?
4. According to cognitive theory, why do clients experience euphoria?

Signs and Symptoms/Diagnostic Criteria

Bipolar disorders can be classified according to severity and deviation from a euthymic (normal mood) state. This section reviews the *Diagnostic and Statistical Manual of Mental Disorders,* 4th edition, text revision (*DSM-IV-TR*) spectrum of bipolar disorders, which include bipolar I, bipolar II, and cyclothymic disorders (APA, 2000).

Bipolar I Disorder

Bipolar I disorder is characterized by one or more manic episodes, usually alternating with major depressive episodes (*DSM-IV-TR* Box 28.1). **Manic episodes** are periods of abnormally and persistently elevated, expansive, or irritable mood. During mania, clients exhibit extreme mood swings, with irritability or sudden outburst of misplaced rage. They have sleep disturbances, usually awakening earlier each day and feeling full of energy. Work output is decreased, with clients feeling distracted or restless. They may go on spending sprees or engage in sexually promiscuous behavior (Figure 28.2). Exaggerated self-esteem may lead to delusions of grandeur, elation, and other forms of excessive activity. Rapid "flights of ideas" lead to excessive and illogical rhyming, punning, and word associations, along with pressured speech.

Clients with mania may dress flamboyantly and exaggeratedly. They may choose bizarre clothing, jewelry, or makeup, usually in bright colors or "busy" patterns. Behavior is hyperactive and often intrusive. Initially, others may view these clients as sociable or fun to be around but eventually disengage because of hyperactivity and intrusiveness. Clients with mania tend to laugh and talk excessively, usually inappropriately. Because of feelings of euphoria, grandiosity, and power, they attempt to control the environment by invading personal space and ignoring environmental boundaries (eg, trying to go into the nurses' station). At the same time, they have little to no insight that their behaviors are inappropriate.

Manic episodes usually begin suddenly and last from a few days to a few months. While manic, clients tend not to realize that they are acting strangely and resist treatment. Abrupt mood shifts are common, with rapid changes from euphoria to anger or depression. Some clients have a hypomanic or relatively mild manic phase with severe depression (see *DSM-IV-TR* Box 28.1). Bipolar I disorders are coded based on the clinical picture during the most recent episode.

Symptoms found with bipolar depressive phases are consistent with those of major depression (see Chap. 27). For clients with bipolar illness, depressive symptoms tend to be far less responsive to conventional therapies than manic symptoms (Frye et al., 2004). The effects of bipolar depressive episodes in terms of duration and quality of life are substantially worse than are those of manic episodes (Calabrese et al., 2004).

Bipolar II Disorder

Bipolar II disorder is characterized by a major depressive episode (current or past) and at least one hypomanic episode. It differs from bipolar I disorder in that there is no history of a manic or mixed episode (*DSM-IV-TR* Box 28.2). **Hypomania** is a slightly less severe subcategory of mania. Differentiating points are that hypomania has no psychotic features and does not impair functioning to a level that necessitates hospitalization. Most hypomanic episodes in bipolar II disorder occur immediately before or after a major depressive episode.

Clients with bipolar II disorder have had an episode in which they experienced a persistently elevated, expansive, or

DSM-IV-TR BOX 28.1

Bipolar I Disorder

The client has one or more manic or mixed episodes and often one or more major depressive episodes [see *DSM-IV-TR* Box 27.1].

Manic Episode

A. A distinct period of abnormally and persistently elevated, expansive, or irritable mood, lasting at least 1 week (or any duration if hospitalization is necessary).

B. During the period of mood disturbance, three (or more) of the following symptoms have persisted (four if the mood is only irritable) and have been present to a significant degree:
   1. Inflated self-esteem or grandiosity
   2. Decreased need for sleep (eg, feels rested after only 3 hours of sleep)
   3. More talkative than usual or pressure to keep talking
   4. Flight of ideas or subjective experience that thoughts are racing
   5. Distractibility (ie, attention too easily drawn to unimportant or irrelevant external stimuli)
   6. Increase in goal-directed activity (either socially, at work or school, or sexually) or psychomotor agitation
   7. Excessive involvement in pleasurable activities that have a high potential for painful consequences (eg, engaging in unrestrained buying sprees, sexual indiscretions, or foolish business investments)

C. The symptoms do not meet criteria for a Mixed Episode.

D. The mood disturbance is sufficiently severe to cause marked impairment in occupational functioning or in usual social activities or relationships with others, or to necessitate hospitalization to prevent harm to self or others, or there are psychotic features.

E. The symptoms are not due to the direct physiologic effects of a substance (eg, a drug of abuse, a medication, or other treatment) or a general medical condition (eg, hyperthyroidism).

Note: Manic-like episodes that are clearly caused by somatic antidepressant treatment (eg, medication, electroconvulsive therapy, light therapy) should not count toward a diagnosis of Bipolar I Disorder.

Mixed Episode

A. The criteria are met both for a Manic Episode and for a Major Depressive Episode (except for duration) nearly every day during at least a 1-week period.

B. The mood disturbance is sufficiently severe to cause marked impairment in occupational functioning or in usual social activities or relationships with others, or to necessitate hospitalization to prevent harm to self or others, or there are psychotic features.

C. The symptoms are not due to the direct physiologic effects of a substance (eg, a drug of abuse, a medication, or other treatment) or a general medical condition (eg, hyperthyroidism).

Note: Mixed-like episodes that are clearly caused by somatic antidepressant treatment (eg, medication, electroconvulsive therapy, light therapy) should not count toward a diagnosis of Bipolar I Disorder.

Reprinted with permission from the *Diagnostic and Statistical Manual of Mental Disorders, 4th edition, text revision* (Copyright © 2000). American Psychiatric Association.

irritable mood clearly different from usual for at least 4 days. However, the hypomanic symptoms are not severe enough to cause marked social or occupational dysfunction or to require hospitalization.

Diagnosing bipolar II disorder sometimes is difficult, particularly if clients present for the first time with a depressive episode. Health care providers must carefully and accurately interview, gather health history data, and perform other assessments to determine whether clients have experienced a past hypomanic episode (Figure 28.3). Commonly, bipolar II is diagnosed after one nurse practitioner or physician has worked with a client for some time and become familiar with that client's presentation and symptom history.

Cyclothymic Disorder

Cyclothymia resembles bipolar I disorder, but symptoms are less severe. It almost is a "subclinical" bipolar I disorder. Clients experience repeated periods of nonpsychotic depression and hypomania for at least 2 years (1 year for children and adolescents). The opposing manifestations of depression and hypomania are seen in contrasting symptoms depending on the type of episode. For example, feelings of inadequacy, social withdrawal, hypersomnia, and diminished productivity during a depressive episode are replaced by inflated self-esteem, uninhibited social interaction, insomnia, and increased productivity during hypomania. Cyclothymia is diagnosed only if a client's symptoms have never met the criteria for a major depressive or manic episode (*DSM-IV-TR* Box 28.3).

Rapid Cycling

In **rapid cycling**, clients have four or more manic episodes for at least 2 weeks in a single year. The episodes are marked by either partial or full remission for at least 2 months or a switch to an episode of opposite type. Rapid cycling is associated with high risk of recurrence and resistance to conventional drug treatments. Clients with rapid cycling experience a greater severity of illness than do those without, and depressive symptoms are most prominent (Goldberg, 2011).

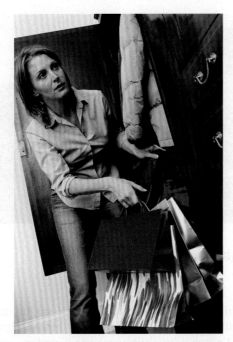

FIGURE 28.2 Clients with mania may go on shopping sprees, engage in risky sex, and behave in uncharacteristically unsafe and self-destructive ways. The consequences to their relationships, finances, and health can be catastrophic.

Implications and Prognosis

The implications of unrecognized, undiagnosed, and untreated bipolar illness are astounding. Costs are high, both to society and families. Estimated U.S. costs related to bipolar disorders were $24 billion in 1998 (Stimmel, 2004). The World Health Organization (WHO) lists bipolar disorder as the sixth leading cause of global disability (Woods, 2000).

Despite these facts, the prognosis for clients who receive care is good. In fact, bipolar disorders are very treatable. With psychotherapy, pharmacotherapy, and somatic therapies, most clients with these conditions can return to normal functioning.

Interdisciplinary Goals and Treatment

Caring for these clients can pose significant challenges. Most research studies report that a combination of psychotherapy and medications is more effective than either approach alone in treating bipolar disorder (Miklowitz et al., 2007). An interdisciplinary approach to long-term management is most common. Treatment settings generally best equipped for the complex and interdisciplinary care needed are acute care, step-down programs, day treatment programs, and community-based programs. In addition, many nurse practitioners who work in outpatient clinics encounter clients

---

DSM-IV-TR BOX 28.2

Bipolar II Disorder

A. Presence (or history) of one or more Major Depressive Episodes [see *DSM-IV-TR* Box 27.1].

B. Presence (or history) of at least one Hypomanic Episode.

C. There has never been a Manic Episode or a Mixed Episode [see *DSM-IV-TR* Box 28.1].

D. The mood symptoms in Criteria A and B are not better accounted for by Schizoaffective Disorder and are not superimposed on Schizophrenia, Schizophreniform Disorder, Delusional Disorder, or Psychotic Disorder Not Otherwise Specified.

E. The symptoms cause clinically significant distress or impairment in social, occupational, or other important areas of functioning.

Hypomanic Episode

A. A distinct period of persistently elevated, expansive, or irritable mood, lasting throughout at least 4 days, that is clearly different from the usual nondepressed mood.

B. During the period of mood disturbance, three (or more) of the following symptoms have persisted (four if the mood is only irritable) and have been present to a significant degree:
1. Inflated self-esteem or grandiosity
2. Decreased need for sleep (eg, feels rested after only 3 hours of sleep)
3. More talkative than usual or pressure to keep talking
4. Flight of ideas or subjective experience that thoughts are racing

5. Distractibility (ie, attention too easily drawn to unimportant or irrelevant external stimuli)
6. Increase in goal-directed activity (either socially, at work or school, or sexually) or psychomotor agitation
7. Excessive involvement in pleasurable activities that have a high potential for painful consequences (eg, the person engages in unrestrained buying sprees, sexual indiscretions, or foolish business investments)

C. The episode is associated with an unequivocal change in functioning that is uncharacteristic of the person when not symptomatic.

D. The disturbance in mood and the change in functioning are observable by others.

E. The episode is not severe enough to cause marked impairment in social or occupational functioning, or to necessitate hospitalization, and there are no psychotic features.

F. The symptoms are not due to the direct physiologic effects of a substance (eg, a drug of abuse, a medication, or other treatment) or a general medical condition (eg, hyperthyroidism).

Note: *Hypomanic-like episodes that are clearly caused by somatic antidepressant treatment (eg, medication, electroconvulsive therapy, light therapy) should not count toward a diagnosis of Bipolar II Disorder.*

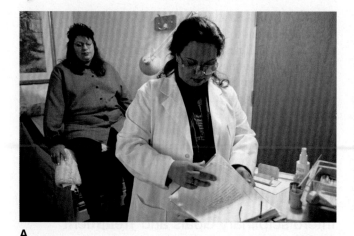

A

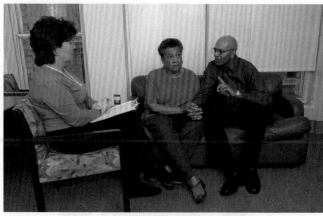

B

FIGURE 28.3 Thorough history taking and interviewing of (**A**) clients and (**B**) in some cases family is essential to the accurate diagnosis of bipolar illness.

with bipolar disorders and treat them independently, while maintaining contacts with physician consultants and other professionals as necessary.

Current research about treatments continues. The Systematic Treatment Enhancement Program for Bipolar Disorder (STEP-BD) is the largest ever interdisciplinary (including nursing) study of these disorders. It was designed to address key questions in areas of major clinical importance. The four primary objectives are as follows:

1. Implement common clinical practice procedures across a network of clinicians treating large numbers of bipolar clients in diverse treatment settings.
2. Determine the most effective strategies for treatment of bipolar depressive phases.
3. Determine which maintenance strategies most effectively prevent recurrences.
4. Provide a systematic means for translation of novel treatments and new findings into clinical practice.

Ancillary objectives of STEP-BD are to determine the benefit of specific interventions for bipolar clients with comorbid psychoactive substance use disorders, prognostic significance of common comorbidities, specific interventions for rapid cycling, specific treatment strategies for acute mania, best treatments for bipolar women who are or want to become pregnant, and the validity of proposed subtypes of bipolar illness.

Psychotherapy

Psychotherapy continues to be used extensively for bipolar disorder (APA, 2010; Miklowitz, 2006). Common modalities include psychoeducation, cognitive–behavioral therapy (CBT), family-focused treatment (FFT), and interpersonal and social rhythm therapy (IPSRT) (NIMH, 2007). This array of treatments can assist clients with medication adherence, ability to cope with environmental stress, and social–occupational functioning. See Evidence-Based Practice Spotlight 28.1.

DSM-IV-TR BOX 28.3

Cyclothymic Disorder

A. For at least 2 years, the presence of numerous periods with hypomanic symptoms and numerous periods with depressive symptoms that do not meet criteria for a Major Depressive Episode.

   Note: In children and adolescents, the duration must be at least 1 year.

B. During the above 2-year period (1 year in children and adolescents), the person has not been without the symptoms in Criterion A for more than 2 months at a time.

C. No Major Depressive Episode, Manic Episode, or Mixed Episode has been present during the first 2 years of the disturbance.

D. The symptoms in Criterion A are not better accounted for by Schizoaffective Disorder and are not superimposed on Schizophrenia, Schizophreniform Disorder, Delusional Disorder, or Psychotic Disorder Not Otherwise Specified.

E. The symptoms are not due to the direct physiologic effects of a substance (eg, a drug of abuse, a medication) or a general medical condition (eg, hyperthyroidism).

F. The symptoms cause clinically significant distress or impairment in social, occupational, or other important areas of functioning.

Reprinted with permission from the *Diagnostic and Statistical Manual of Mental Disorders, 4th edition, text revision* (Copyright © 2000). American Psychiatric Association.

⚠ EVIDENCE-BASED PRACTICE SPOTLIGHT 28.1 ⚠

Intensive Psychotherapy for Bipolar Depression

Overview of Effective Treatment: Results from STEP-BD indicate that clients taking medications for bipolar disorder are more likely to improve faster and stay well longer if they receive intensive psychotherapy. Results suggest that adding specific, targeted psychotherapy to medication may help increase clients' chances for lasting recovery. With 293 participants, researchers tested the effectiveness of three types of standardized, intensive, 9-month psychotherapy compared against a control group who received a three-session, psychoeducational program called collaborative care. The intensive therapies were as follows:

- Family-focused therapy, which required the participation of and input from relatives and focused on enhancing family coping, communication, and problem solving
- Cognitive–behavioral therapy, which focused on helping clients understand distortions in thought and activity and learn new ways of coping with the illness
- Interpersonal and social rhythm therapy, which focused on helping clients stabilize daily routines and sleep–wake cycles and solve key relationship problems

All participants were already taking medication for bipolar disorder; most were also involved in a STEP-BD medication study. Researchers compared time to recovery and stability over 1 year among clients in both groups.

After 1 year, 64% of those in the intensive psychotherapy groups had become well, compared with 52% of those in collaborative care therapy. Clients receiving intensive psychotherapy also became well on average 110 days faster than did those in collaborative care. In addition, clients who received intensive psychotherapy were one and a half times more likely to be clinically well during any month of the study year than were those who received collaborative care. Discontinuation rates among the groups were similar.

What Has Not Been Shown Effective: None of the three intensive psychotherapies was significantly more effective than the others, although rates of recovery were higher among those in family-focused therapy compared with the other groups.

References

Miklowitz, D. J., Otto, M. W., Frank, E., Reilly-Harrington, N. A., Wisniewski, S. R., Kogan, J. N., et al. (2007). Psychosocial treatments for bipolar depression: A 1-year randomized trial from the systematic treatment enhancement program. *Archives in General Psychiatry, 64,* 419–427.

National Institute of Mental Health. (2007). *Questions and answers about the STEP-BD depression psychosocial treatment trial.* Retrieved from http://www.nimh.nih.gov/trials/practical/step-bd/questions-and-answers.

Clinical trials have shown CBT, FFT, and psychoeducation to be most effective in relapse prevention, whereas CBT and IPSRT have the most efficacy in treating residual depression (Zaretsky et al., 2007). Studies also have shown that benefits of psychosocial interventions include increased clinical stability, fewer hospitalizations, improved medication adherence, and other functional and psychosocial gains, as measured by objective tests (Miklowitz, 2006; Zaretsky et al., 2007).

CBT, one of the most researched psychosocial interventions, is significantly effective for bipolar disorders (APA, 2010; Scott et al., 2006). Implementation may be with individuals or groups. The goal is to assist clients to identify and correct distorted, negative, and catastrophic thinking, thereby relieving symptoms (Beck, 1972; Beck et al., 1979). Mechanisms for modifying maladaptation include homework, structured schedules, and various other techniques (see Chap. 13). A focal area for bipolar disorders involves restructuring high-goal attainment beliefs. For example, some clients believe that they are invulnerable or cannot lose. Therapists work with them to monitor moods, recognize early signs of relapse, and develop action plans when depressed (Miklowitz, 2006).

One study (Lam et al., 2003) divided 103 clients with bipolar I disorder into two groups: one received 12 to 20 sessions of individual CBT, and the other did not. The group that received CBT had significantly lower relapse rates, fewer hospitalizations, improved medication adherence, and improved psychosocial functioning. Another study randomized 42 clients with bipolar disorder to CBT or a control group. The CBT group experienced fewer depressive relapses and more improvements in symptoms and functioning at the 6-month follow-up (Scott et al., 2001). A much larger multicenter study of 253 clients with bipolar disorder found that clients with fewer than 12 previous episodes did better with CBT, and that CBT was less effective for those with more episodes (Scott et al., 2006). STEP-BD demonstrated that out of 293 individuals who participated in a psychosocial treatment trial, those who participated in the intensive psychotherapies (FFT, CBT, and IPSRT) were more successive than collaborative care intervention (NIMH, 2007). See Chapter 13 for more information about CBT.

Checkpoint Questions

5. What is the difference between bipolar I and bipolar II disorders?
6. What characterizes rapid cycling?
7. What are common psychosocial treatment modalities for clients with bipolar disorder?

Psychopharmacologic Therapy

Mood stabilizers are the primary drugs used for bipolar disorders. They include lithium, anticonvulsants, and atypical antipsychotics (often combined with lithium or anticonvulsants) (see Chap. 16). Another important class is the class of medications used for **refractory mania** (ie, mania that fails to respond to conventional drug regimens).

MOOD STABILIZERS. Mood stabilizers are first-line drugs for treatment of bipolar disorders. They stabilize depressive and manic cycles. Some clients with bipolar disorders have significant depressive symptoms or depressive symptoms that do not respond to mood stabilizers alone. They may be prescribed antidepressants as well as mood stabilizers (see Chap. 27). The APA guideline (2010) recommends discontinuation of antidepressants as soon as possible in clients with bipolar disorders because these drugs may induce a switch to mania. Thus, close monitoring and follow-up are critical elements of care for clients with bipolar disorders who are taking antidepressants (Box 28.1).

Lithium. The therapeutic uses of lithium include the alleviation of acute mania and mania that follows depression (APA, 2010). Lithium is also used in the long-term management of bipolar illness (Goldberg, 2007). Lithium may also be used to reduce suicidal tendencies in clients with bipolar disorders (Cipriani et al., 2005). Its mechanism of action remains unknown. Research studies have shown that it may inhibit the proapoptotic glycogen synthase kinase 3 (GSK-3) (Jope, 2004) and capase (Li & El-Mallakh, 2000). Lithium may also inhibit inositol monophosphatase and inositol polyphosphatase, which, in conjunction with GSK-3, may alter growth

| BOX 28.1 | Antidepressants and Bipolar Disorders |

Health care providers should avoid use of antidepressants as monotherapy for clients with bipolar disorder (Goldberg, 2007). If clients can be treated with lithium alone, the risk for antidepressant-induced mania is avoided. However, if lithium is not sufficient, a combination of lithium and an antidepressant appears to reduce the risks for affective switch and for the induction of a long-term, rapid-cycling course.

In general, antidepressant treatments for unipolar depression are efficacious for bipolar depression as well. Antidepressants must be chosen carefully in clients who experience rapid shifts from mania to depression because some of them may trigger rapid mood switches to a manic state. Of the antidepressants, bupropion and the SSRIs carry less risk for inducing hypomania, mania, and rapid cycling than do the TCAs (APA, 2010). Tapering antidepressant medication after periods of sustained remission in clients with bipolar disorder is beneficial in limiting the risk for affective switch and acceleration of the cycle rate.

cone morphology with implications for synaptic formation (Eickholt et al., 2004). Lithium may affect other second-messenger systems, such as protein kinase C and calcium (McNamara & Lenox, 2004; Wasserman et al., 2004), and has been shown to normalize elevated intracellular sodium levels (Huang et al., 2007). See Understanding Psychopharmacology 28.1.

The importance of monitoring blood levels of lithium in clients taking it cannot be overstated. Lithium toxicity has a narrow therapeutic window. See Understanding Psychopharmacology 28.2 for related adverse effects. When clients start

UNDERSTANDING PSYCHOPHARMACOLOGY 28.1

Lithium

Use: Prevention and treatment of bipolar mania. Unlabeled uses include for bulimia, premenstrual syndrome, and prophylaxis of cluster headaches

Action: Unknown; alters sodium transport in neurons and muscle cells; increases uptake of norepinephrine and sensitivity of serotonin receptors; delays some second-messenger systems

What it does not do: May not improve depressive symptoms

What is needed to treat mania: (1) Medication compliance and (2) cognitive and environmental adjustments or modifications including structure, clarity, consistency, and reinforcements for appropriate behavior

Most common side effects: Lithium toxicity, headache, hyperkalemia, tachycardia-bradycardia syndrome, dermatologic problems (eg, pruritus, rashes), hypercalcemia, weight gain, and swollen or painful joints

Length of action: Mean, 24 hours (peak serum levels in 1–4 hours). Steady state reached in 5 to 7 days

Dosing: 150-, 300-, and 600-mg capsules. Lithobid, 300-mg slow-release tablets; Eskalith CR, 450-mg controlled-release tablets. Lithium citrate, 300 mg/5 mL liquid. Optimal response in acute mania is usually 600 mg tid or 900 mg bid. Obtain serum levels twice weekly in acute phase. Use lowest possible maintenance dose to alleviate symptoms and achieve serum level of 0.6 to 1.2 mEq/L. Obtain serum levels every 2 to 3 months. Monitor for side effects. Safety and efficacy in children younger than 12 years has not been established.

From: Karch, A. M. (2009). *2009 Lippincott's nursing drug guide*. Philadelphia, PA: Lippincott Williams & Wilkins.

UNDERSTANDING PSYCHOPHARMACOLOGY 28.2

Lithium Toxicity and Associated Serum Levels*

LITHIUM SERUM LEVEL	SYMPTOMS OF TOXICITY
1.5 mEq/L	CNS: lethargy, slurred speech, muscle weakness, fine hand tremors GI: nausea, vomiting, diarrhea, thirst GU: polyuria
1.5–2.0 mEq/L (mild to moderate toxicity)	CNS: coarse hand tremors, mental confusion, hyperirritability of muscles, drowsiness, incoordination GI: persistent GI upset, gastritis, salivary gland swelling, abdominal pain, excessive salivation, flatulence, indigestion CV: ECG changes (QT interval changes)
2.0–2.5 mEq/L (moderate to severe toxicity)	CNS: ataxia, giddiness, fasciculations, tinnitus, blurred vision, clonic movements, seizures, stupor, coma CV: serious ECG changes (arrhythmias), severe hypotension Respiratory: fatalities secondary to pulmonary complications GU: large output of dilute urine
>2.51 mEq/L (life-threatening toxicity)	Complex involvement of multiple organ systems and death

CNS, central nervous system; CV, cardiovascular; ECG, electrocardiogram; GI, gastrointestinal; GU, genitourinary.

*Toxic lithium levels are close to therapeutic levels (a small therapeutic window). Therapeutic levels in acute mania: 1 to 1.5 mEq/L. Therapeutic levels in maintenance: 0.6 to 1.2 mEq/L.

From: Karch, A. M. (2009). *2009 Lippincott's nursing drug guide.* Philadelphia, PA: Lippincott Williams & Wilkins.

therapy, practitioners must check their lithium levels twice weekly in samples drawn immediately before a dose and 8 to 12 hours after the prior dose (Karch, 2009). For maintenance therapy, lithium serum levels should be 0.6 to 1.2 mEq/L; serum levels should be monitored every 2 months once the client's condition is stabilized (APA, 2010; Karch, 2009).

Anticonvulsant Medications. Some anticonvulsants (divalproex and carbamazepine) are prescribed instead of lithium when clients do not experience a response to or have intolerable side effects from lithium.

Divalproex (Depakote) has been found particularly effective for clients with mixed mania, those who have experienced multiple episodes, and those with comorbid substance use disorders (Understanding Psychopharmacology 28.3) (APA, 2010; Goldberg, 2007). It was the only drug to demonstrate a significant reduction in alcohol-use symptoms in clients with dual-diagnosis bipolar disorder

UNDERSTANDING PSYCHOPHARMACOLOGY 28.3

Divalproex Sodium

Use: Treatment of bipolar disorders

Action: Unknown, but thought to increase level of GABA to brain neurons

What it does not do: May not improve depressive symptoms

What is needed to treat mania: (1) Medication compliance and (2) cognitive and environmental adjustments or modifications, including structure, clarity, consistency, and reinforcements for appropriate behavior

Most common side effects: Sedation, dizziness, drowsiness, unsteadiness, nausea and vomiting, tremors, and gastrointestinal problems; less commonly, increased body weight and metabolism and dose-related hepatic and hematologic effects; rarely, life-threatening pancreatitis and hepatic toxicity

Length of action: 6 to 16 hours (1–4 hours)

Dosing: Available in 125-mg delayed-release capsules, and 125-, 250-, and 500-mg enteric-coated tablets. Dosage depends on symptoms and clinical picture; initial dosage is low and increased gradually according to the client's specifics

From: Karch, A. M. (2009). *2009 Lippincott's nursing drug guide.* Philadelphia, PA: Lippincott Williams & Wilkins.

(Salloum et al., 2005). Carbamazepine (Tegretol) is used for acute mania and long-term maintenance therapy (APA, 2010). Researchers examined extended-release carbamazepine for its effect on mania and found it superior to placebo in improvement of manic symptoms in clients with bipolar I disorder (Weisler et al., 2004, 2005).

MEDICATIONS FOR REFRACTORY MANIA. Several medications from various classes are currently being studied as treatments for bipolar illness. Those mentioned here are used for mania refractory to lithium, divalproex, and carbamazepine (APA, 2010).

Lamotrigine (Lamictal), an anticonvulsant, has been found superior to placebo in preventing recurrences of depression in clients with long-term bipolar disorders. It has also been particularly effective for bipolar depression (APA, 2010). Potentially life-threatening side effects include Stevens–Johnson syndrome (Figure 28.4) and toxic epidermal necrolysis with multiorgan failure (Karch, 2009). Dizziness, ataxia, nausea, and minor rashes are other, less dangerous side effects. Clients taking lamotrigine require careful monitoring for dermatologic problems, particularly during introduction and titration. Topiramate (Topamax), another anticonvulsant, is being considered for refractory mania. Initial studies failed to find it effective in stabilizing acute mania; side effects included paresthesias, decreased appetite, dry mouth, and weight loss (Kushner et al., 2006).

Five atypical antipsychotics (olanzapine, risperidone, quetiapine, aripiprazole, and ziprasidone) have been approved by the U.S. Food and Drug Administration (FDA) for acute mania. Three of them are also indicated as adjunctive therapy to mood stabilizers for acute mania (APA, 2010;

Goldberg, 2007). A meta-analysis of randomized controlled trials of these five atypical antipsychotics found no significant differences in antimanic efficacy among them (Perlis et al., 2006). The same study found quetiapine and olanzapine to be superior to placebo for bipolar depression, whereas the other drugs demonstrated efficacy for maintenance treatment and for acute mania.

Although the novel antipsychotics have fewer motor side effects (eg, tardive dyskinesia, extrapyramidal syndrome) than traditional antipsychotics, significant clinical concerns for the second-generation drugs are metabolic effects and weight gain. Clozapine and olanzapine are associated with increased risks for diabetes mellitus and dyslipidemia (APA, 2010; Newcomer, 2005). Clozapine and olanzapine are also associated with the most weight gain among the atypical antipsychotics. Risperidone and quetiapine are associated with moderate weight gain, and ziprasidone and aripiprazole with minimal weight gain (Newcomer, 2005).

Symbyax, the first FDA-approved drug for bipolar depression, combines olanzapine (the active ingredient in Zyprexa) and fluoxetine (the active ingredient in Prozac). Symbyax is administered once daily in the evening, usually beginning with the 6 mg/25 mg capsule. Antidepressant efficacy was demonstrated with Symbyax in a dose range of olanzapine 6 to 12 mg and fluoxetine 25 to 50 mg.

Gabapentin (Neurontin), an antiepileptic agent, has demonstrated little efficacy in controlled studies. Its mechanism of action is thought to be related to its ability to inhibit polysynaptic responses and block pretetanic potentiation (Karch, 2009). Its few adverse effects include dizziness, insomnia, somnolence, ataxia, gastrointestinal upset, and fatigue.

Other novel treatments include calcium-channel blockers (including nimodipine) and omega-3 fatty acids (APA, 2010; Parker et al., 2006).

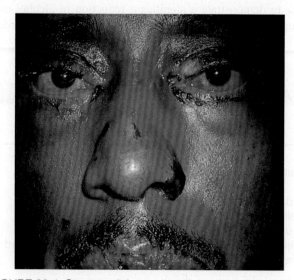

FIGURE 28.4 Stevens–Johnson syndrome is a potentially life-threatening side effect of lamotrigine, an anticonvulsant used with clients who have long-standing bipolar disorders. This client shows conjunctival and oral involvement.

Checkpoint Questions

8. Which drugs are considered first-line treatment for bipolar disorders?
9. Which drug has been found particularly effective in treating bipolar depression?
10. What are side effects of the anticonvulsant medications?
11. For maintenance therapy, what serum level of lithium is considered therapeutic?

Somatic Nonpharmacologic Interventions

Nonpharmacologic somatic interventions continue to be investigated as modalities for clients with bipolar disorders. Three examples include sleep deprivation, transcranial magnetic stimulation, and vagal nerve stimulation. Chapter 18 discusses these modalities in detail; see Box 28.2 for information about their application with clients who have bipolar illness.

BOX 28.2 Somatic Therapies for Bipolar Illnesses

Sleep Deprivation

Sleep deprivation (SD) has a strong and rapid effect on depressed mood in more than 60% of clients from all diagnostic subgroups of mood disorders, including bipolar illness (Wirz-Justice et al., 2005). Treatment can be total (clients stay awake all night) or partial (clients stay awake through the second half of the night). Improved mood is noticeable within hours; however, sleep following treatment can lead to relapse. Relapse prevention involves combining SD with other modalities, such as light therapy, selective serotonin reuptake inhibitors (SSRIs), lithium, or a short phase of sleep over 3 days following a single night of SD (Wirz-Justice et al., 2005).

Transcranial Magnetic Stimulation

Often used for seizures, transcranial magnetic stimulation (TMS) has been tested for its therapeutic effects in bipolar depression and mania. Studies have had mixed results (Dolberg et al., 2002; Nahas et al., 2003). Nahas et al. (1999) found an antimanic effect of right prefrontal TMS, whereas Kaptsan et al. (2003) found no significant differences between right prefrontal active TMS and right sham TMS. Results of a recent systematic review found no strong evidence of benefit for using TMS to treat depression, although the small sample sizes did not exclude the possibility of benefit (Martin et al., 2007). More research with larger sample sizes is needed.

Vagal Nerve Stimulation

Researchers have found that vagal nerve stimulation (VNS) alters the functional activity of the thalamus, hypothalamus, cingulate, and hippocampus (Chae et al., 2003) and increases the concentration of homovanillic acid, a dopamine metabolite, in the cerebrospinal fluid (Carpenter et al., 2004). Studies so far indicate that clients with unipolar and bipolar depression maintain improvements related to VNS for as long as 1 year after treatment (Rush et al., 2005).

APPLYING THE NURSING PROCESS

Bipolar Mania

Many nursing professionals work specifically with clients who have bipolar disorders. Studies often focus on the responses of these clients and their families to nursing interventions. Evidence-Based Practice Spotlight 28.2 examines the effectiveness of an educational intervention on compliance with medications, symptom level, and quality of life in outpatients with bipolar disorders who take lithium. The study reflects the high caliber of today's research and how it significantly contributes to nursing practice.

Bipolar disorders often coexist with other psychiatric and medical problems. Therefore, nurses should be prepared to encounter bipolar illness when working with clients who have other primary diagnoses.

PRACTICE & LEARN

Note: The following sections focus primarily on care of clients in the manic phase of bipolar disorder. Understanding Nursing Care 28.1 provides a visual depiction of common assessment findings, nursing diagnoses, outcomes and interventions, and indicators of success for clients experiencing mania. Chapter 27 outlines nursing care of clients with depression. The steps of the nursing process described there also apply to clients with bipolar disorder who are experiencing depressive episodes.

⚠ ASSESSMENT

Nursing assessment of manic behaviors involves systematic, thorough consideration of safety and mental status (including affect, thought processes, and intellectual functioning). It also necessitates careful review of physiologic, psychomotor, behavioral, and social activity (McColm et al., 2006; Miller, 2006).

Safety

Safety is a priority area to assess. Nurses perform both suicide and violence assessments for these clients (see Chaps. 32 and 34). Suicide is a primary concern for clients experiencing depressive phases. Agitated clients may threaten to harm others; clients with mania are at increased risk for accidents because of hyperactivity, loss of inhibition, and lack of judgment. In addition, they may be angry, hostile, and irritable, lashing out at others unexpectedly and getting into altercations.

Mental Status Examination

As discussed in Chapter 10, the Mental Status Examination (MSE) provides comprehensive and thorough information about a client's mental state. Mental status changes over time, sometimes rapidly. This can be especially pertinent in manic phases, which are marked by rapid fluctuations in all aspects of thought, mood, and behavior. See Assessment Tool 28.1 for a review of the MSE categories and common findings associated with mania.

Physiologic Stability

A primary concern for clients with bipolar disorders is physiologic integrity and function. Mania causes hyperactivity, resulting in an inability to sit still for the time needed to eat a meal. Clients with mania often neglect nutritional and fluid needs. Mania also leads to disturbed sleep, most often with lack of sleep for days or disturbed sleep–wake cycles. These clients may have patterns of brief napping and then extended activity. Many of them report feelings of hypersexuality and hyperarousal. They may become promiscuous, increasing risks for HIV, other sexually transmitted infections, and injuries.

Family Issues

Family may be worried about or angry with clients; they may also not understand the disease. Mania may lead families to feel

Client Education in Lithium Therapy

Overview of Effective Treatment: This study used a pretest/posttest experimental design to investigate whether psychoeducation about bipolar illness and medication to treat it can foster medication compliance. Researchers recruited clients with bipolar disorder who had been taking lithium for 10 years. Twenty-six subjects (14 experimental, 12 control) participated. The experimental group received three sessions of education about bipolar disorder and lithium. Topics included causative factors, clinical symptoms, goals of lithium therapy, and its side effects. Researchers collected data from both groups before and 3 months after intervention using a medication knowledge form, the Brief Symptom Inventory, and the WHO Quality of Life Scale. They also drew serum lithium levels. They analyzed data using the Wilcoxon signed rank and binomial tests.

After 3 months, the scores of the control group showed little difference from baseline. The study group had increased medication knowledge, decreased symptoms, and increased general health, physical function, and social domain of quality of life. Lithium levels in the study group increased after intervention, indicating increased regularity in lithium use. Lithium levels of the control group decreased. All these findings were statistically significant.

Implications for Practice: Psychoeducational programs may be beneficial nursing interventions for clients with bipolar disorder. Such programs may increase medication knowledge and compliance, as well as social adaptation and quality of life.

References

Dogan, S., & Sabanciogullari, S. (2003). The effects of patient education in lithium therapy on quality of life and compliance. *Archives of Psychiatric Nursing, 12*(6), 270–275.

UNDERSTANDING NURSING CARE 28.1

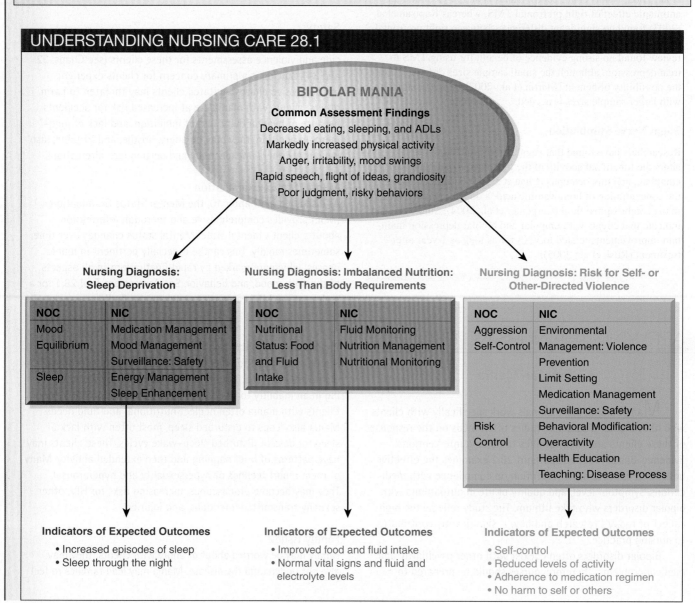

BIPOLAR MANIA

Common Assessment Findings
Decreased eating, sleeping, and ADLs
Markedly increased physical activity
Anger, irritability, mood swings
Rapid speech, flight of ideas, grandiosity
Poor judgment, risky behaviors

Nursing Diagnosis: Sleep Deprivation

NOC	NIC
Mood Equilibrium	Medication Management
	Mood Management
	Surveillance: Safety
Sleep	Energy Management
	Sleep Enhancement

Indicators of Expected Outcomes
• Increased episodes of sleep
• Sleep through the night

Nursing Diagnosis: Imbalanced Nutrition: Less Than Body Requirements

NOC	NIC
Nutritional Status: Food and Fluid Intake	Fluid Monitoring
	Nutrition Management
	Nutritional Monitoring

Indicators of Expected Outcomes
• Improved food and fluid intake
• Normal vital signs and fluid and electrolyte levels

Nursing Diagnosis: Risk for Self- or Other-Directed Violence

NOC	NIC
Aggression Self-Control	Environmental Management: Violence Prevention
	Limit Setting
	Medication Management
	Surveillance: Safety
Risk Control	Behavioral Modification: Overactivity
	Health Education
	Teaching: Disease Process

Indicators of Expected Outcomes
• Self-control
• Reduced levels of activity
• Adherence to medication regimen
• No harm to self or others

ASSESSMENT TOOL 28.1

Components and Findings of the MSE in Mania

Appearance and General Behavior

- Flamboyant, exaggerated behaviors
- Outlandish, extravagant, brightly colored, or sexually suggestive clothes
- Rushed or hurried behavior
- Reports of feeling better than ever
- Increased motor activity

Mood and Affect

- Affect may or may not be congruent with mood
- Very happy affect; laughter, giggling, or exaggerated displays of joy
- Inappropriate affect and mood for context

Thought Content and Process

- Superiority, competition, and self-aggrandizement
- Flight of ideas, ideas of reference, loose associations, tangential and bizarre conclusions

Perceptual Disturbances

- Hallucinations and delusions
- Anxiety
- Grandiose delusions involving power, wealth, fame, or knowledge

Judgment and Insight

- Outwardly impulsive, aggressive, and often dangerous behaviors
- Limited to no insight

"burned out," angry, and frustrated from trying to manage uncontrollable behaviors at home (Figure 28.5). Adherence to the medication regimen is the single most important factor in preventing relapse; however, many clients stop taking their drugs when they feel well. Assessing the family's knowledge about the disease and its treatment is essential, as is including them in care planning.

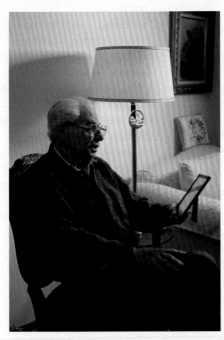

FIGURE 28.5 Family members may feel overwhelmed by the consequences and care involved when loved ones have bipolar illness. They may be unable to understand the behavior of relatives in the grips of illness or reconcile their behaviors with those under normal circumstances.

▲ NURSING DIAGNOSIS

Common nursing diagnoses for clients in the manic phase of bipolar disorder are as follows (NANDA, 2007):

- Risk for Self-Directed and Other-Directed Violence related to impulsivity and impaired judgment
- Ineffective Health Maintenance related to low attention threshold, hyperactivity, and lack of attention to self-care needs
- Impaired Social Interaction related to distorted thinking, disorientation, or restlessness
- Disturbed Thought Processes related to biochemical imbalances or psychologic stress
- Ineffective Therapeutic Regimen Management related to lack of knowledge about medications and lack of incentive to maintain medication regimen upon discharge

Nursing diagnoses for clients in the depressive phase are found in Chapter 27.

▲ OUTCOME IDENTIFICATION AND PLANNING

Some identified desired outcomes for clients with mania, organized according to the *Nursing Outcomes Classification* (*NOC*), include the following (Moorhead et al., 2008):

- Impulse Self-Control: The client will remain safe throughout hospitalization, without harming self or others.
- Aggression Self-Control: The client will demonstrate self-control in milieu activities and interactions with others, including maintaining appropriate boundaries and refraining from aggressive or risky behaviors.
- Self-Care Status: The client will have adequate food and fluid intake; will maintain balanced rest, sleep, and activity; and will maintain personal care.

- Social Interaction Skills: The client will engage in appropriate social behavior.
- Concentration: The client will demonstrate logical, reality-based thought processes.
- Compliance Behavior: The client will consistently maintain the pharmacologic regimen, including taking medications as ordered and following up with a care provider for appropriate postdischarge visits and laboratory work.

Outcomes for clients in the depressive phase can be found in Chapter 27.

▲ IMPLEMENTATION

Nurses use many types of interventions to assist recovering clients and families. Common *Nursing Interventions Classification* (*NIC*) labels related to management of mania include, but are not limited to, **Active Listening, Behavior Management/Overactivity, Behavior Management: Sexual, Cognitive Restructuring, Coping Enhancement, Guilt Work Facilitation, Limit Setting, Mood Management, Self-Esteem Enhancement, Simple Guided Imagery, Simple Relaxation Therapy,**

Socialization Enhancement, Spiritual Support, and **Teaching: Disease Process** (Bulechek et al., 2008).

Case in Point 28.1 describes a real-life episode of mania with nursing care, documentation, and outcomes. Interventions useful for clients in the depressive phase of bipolar disorder are found in Chapter 27.

Managing the Potential for Violence

Nurses assess risk for violence and, if necessary, place clients on violence precautions. Frequent assessments for risky or dangerous behaviors, such as running or throwing items, may be necessary (McColm et al., 2006). If clients are at risk for violence, establishing geographic boundaries, such as room or half-hall restriction, is part of ongoing monitoring. Also, clients likely will have "as-needed" medications ordered; nurses administer them if aggressive or agitated behavior escalates. Other environmental approaches include reducing stimuli and opportunities for interaction with other clients. Nurses remove all dangerous items from client rooms and monitor closely for use of any dangerous items.

Case in Point 28.1

Danielle's Story

Local police find Danielle, a 45-year-old woman, driving 80 miles per hour down the main street of the city. When stopped, Danielle is belligerent and shouts obscenities. She claims to be the "president's personal video assistant, and I have to finish this job before I meet him this morning!" Officers take Danielle to the local emergency department, where she is admitted involuntarily to the acute inpatient psychiatric unit.

Roger, Danielle's husband of 10 years, reports that Danielle has "been depressed off and on since she was 25 but has never been diagnosed with a psychiatric disorder." For the past 6 months, Roger has noticed that Danielle has been sleeping less. "She rarely takes time to eat. She is a wedding videographer and has been taking her camera out at night, filming scenes all over the city. She's become so short with the children lately." Roger says that Danielle is typically loving, caring, and nurturing. She normally enjoys her children and is very attentive to their activities and schoolwork.

The charge nurse observes Danielle in the milieu before the assessment. Danielle paces in the hallway, poking her head into rooms and asking clients what they are doing. She wears thickly applied makeup, scarves, and patterned clothes. She tries to engage others in an elaborate card game. When no one will play, Danielle curses and flings the cards across the room. The charge nurse approaches Danielle from the front and asks if they can talk. They go to a quiet room.

Throughout the interview, Danielle exhibits pressured speech and changes topics quickly. She dismisses her husband's concerns and states she's been doing "great, better than ever!" The charge nurse tries to discuss treatment goals, but Danielle's comments about what she expects are extravagant and unrealistic. "I'll win an Oscar for the video that I'm producing." Regardless of the topic, Danielle jokes briefly about it and returns to her plans for fame and fortune.

Key Assessment Findings

- Episodes of "depression"
- Elevation of mood for more than 1 week
- Decreased sleeping and eating; activities during nighttime
- Irritability, belligerence, extravagant and unrealistic expectations
- Statements of inflated self-esteem and grandiose ideas
- Risky behaviors (speeding while videotaping)
- Pressured speech; inability to focus on one topic at a time
- Flamboyant dress and exaggerated makeup
- Invasiveness with other clients

Case in Point 28.1 (continued)

Danielle's Story

Nursing Diagnosis: Risk for Other-Directed Violence related to impulsivity and impaired judgment as evidenced by risk-taking behaviors, irritability, anger, and belligerence

NOC: Impulse Self-Control: The client will demonstrate appropriate self-control behaviors to refrain from harming others.

NIC: Mood Management
- Evaluate mood initially and then at regular intervals; determine whether the client poses a safety risk to herself or others. Assess the client's level of risk for violence. Interact with her regularly. Assist her to consciously monitor mood, such as with a rating scale or journal. Help her identify thoughts and feelings underlying the dysfunctional mood. *Assessing mood and risk for violence helps staff members establish appropriate guidelines and interventions. Regular interactions convey caring and provide a chance for the client to discuss feelings. Awareness of mood changes helps the client identify possible related stressors.*
- Assist the client to express feelings appropriately; discuss anger management with her and determine appropriate behaviors when angry. Use limit-setting and behavior management strategies to help her refrain from intrusive and disruptive actions. Role model appropriate anger management; give the client feedback on her behavior. *Providing limits and outlets for anger gives the client a concrete framework for managing impulses. Role modeling and feedback reinforce constructive coping.*
- Use restrictive interventions. Limit the client's environment and remove dangerous objects. Use sedatives as needed. Physical restraint or seclusion is used only as a last resort. *Limiting interactions with others is the best approach to preventing violence if anger and outbursts escalate. Medication can be effective. Seclusion and restraint should be used only if all other methods fail.*
- Assist the client to identify precipitants of dysfunctional mood, differentiating what can and cannot be changed. Help her identify available resources, personal strengths, and abilities to modify such precipitants. Teach new coping and problem-solving skills as necessary. *Knowledge of precipitants helps the client develop strategies to prevent mood changes. Using personal strengths and abilities enhances her feelings of control.*
- Administer prescribed mood stabilizer (eg, lithium) as indicated; monitor for side effects (Figure A). Obtain serum lithium levels as appropriate. *Mood stabilizers are effective for bipolar disorders. Lithium has a narrow therapeutic window, thus the need to monitor serum lithium levels closely for possible toxicity.*

NIC: Behavior Management: Overactivity/Inattention
- Provide a structured and physically safe environment. Use a calm, matter-of-fact, reassuring approach. *A structured and safe environment and a calm, matter-of-fact approach help reduce the client's exposure to stressors and promote a therapeutic relationship.*

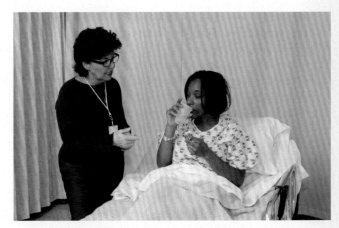

FIGURE A The nurse makes sure that the client takes her medicine as prescribed.

- Develop a behavioral management plan that all care providers implement consistently. Communicate rules, expectations, and consequences in simple language. Set limits on intrusive, interruptive behaviors. Praise desired behaviors; provide consistent consequences for both desired and undesired behaviors. *Consistency and clear communication about rules and expectations reduce power struggles and promote feelings of security for the client. Positive feedback for desired behaviors helps to reinforce them.*
- Redirect or remove the client from sources of overstimulation. Monitor and regulate level of activity and environment. *Overstimulation increases stress, possibly leading to undesired behaviors.*

> 4/6/13: The client refrains from harming others and uses appropriate strategies to control self and behavior. She often demonstrates the ability to identify harmful impulsive behaviors, identify consequences of impulsive actions to self and others, control impulses, use appropriate strategies for dealing with anger and frustration, and maintain self-control without supervision.

Nursing Diagnosis: Disturbed Thought Processes related to biochemical imbalance associated with psychiatric illness as evidenced by unrealistic, grandiose comments, pressured speech, and inability to focus on one topic

NOC: Distorted Thought Self-Control: The client will exhibit reality-based thinking and behavior that reflects appropriate thought content.

NIC: Reality Orientation
- Use a calm, forthright approach; provide clear directions for the client. Approach slowly and from the front; address her by name when initiating interaction. *Providing structure and expectations*

(continues on page 576)

Case in Point 28.1 (continued)

Danielle's Story

communicates that staff members are effectively managing the milieu, which should diminish power struggles and increase feelings of security for the client.

- Interrupt confabulation by changing the subject or responding to the feeling or theme, rather than the content. Engage the client in concrete, reality-oriented activities that focus on something outside the self. Involve her in a reality orientation group setting when appropriate. *Focusing on the present and encouraging participation in a reality orientation group promote logical thinking and reduce the possibility of distraction.*

NIC: Limit Setting

- Establish firm, reasonable expectations for behavior; communicate them clearly to the client. Identify, with her input as appropriate, undesirable behavior. Have all staff members enforce limits consistently. *Consistently implementing limits helps prevent the client from trying to split staff and will help her gain control of her behavior.*

- Avoid power struggles or trying to dissuade the client from grandiose, delusional ideas. Refrain from arguing or bargaining about established expectations and consequences. Accept manic behavior neutrally; do not respond with irritation or anger (Figure B). Avoid encouraging the client's jokiness; maintain a professional demeanor. Redirect her into productive or more appropriate activities. *Power struggles and arguments may contribute to increased mania. Not participating in the client's manic perceptions and thwarting her attempts to split staff help prevent escalation of mania. These clients are highly distractible; staff members can use this factor to their advantage by therapeutically redirecting energy when needed.*

- Modify behavioral expectations and consequences as needed. Decrease limit setting as the client's behavior approximates that which is desired. *Modification is necessary to accommodate for reasonable changes in the client's situation.*

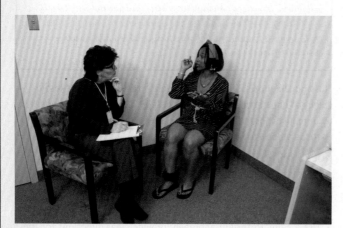

FIGURE B The nurse does not argue with or challenge the client, but she also does not encourage her delusional and grandiose beliefs. She communicates in a matter-of-fact therapeutic manner.

4/15/13: The client demonstrates an affect consistent with mood and begins to exhibit mood stabilization. She often demonstrates requests for validation of reality, appropriate interaction with others, logical flow of thought, and reality-based thinking.

Nursing Diagnosis: Risk for Imbalanced Nutrition, Less Than Body Requirements related to excessive physical activity, limited food and fluid intake, and inattention to physical needs

NOC: Nutritional Status: Food and Fluid Intake and Fluid Balance: The client will ingest a nutritionally adequate diet.

NIC: Nutrition Management

- Ascertain the client's food preferences. Monitor recorded nutritional intake for content and calories. *Offering foods the client likes increases the chances for success. Monitoring intake provides a basis for future interventions.*

- Frequently offer foods that the client can eat "on the run" (eg, crackers, fruits, cheese, sandwiches). Provide high-protein, high-calorie nutritious finger foods that she can readily consume. *The client may be too restless to sit for meals and too distracted to remember to eat. High-protein, high-calorie foods provide appropriate nutrients for energy needs.*

NIC: Nutritional Monitoring

- Weigh the client at specified intervals; monitor trends in weight loss or gain. *Weight is an objective measure of nutritional status.*

- Monitor vital signs, intake, and appropriate laboratory values, such as albumin, total protein, and hemoglobin and hematocrit levels. Assess for malnutrition. *The client with mania is at risk for physical complications secondary to fluid, electrolyte, and nutrient depletion.*

NIC: Fluid Monitoring

- Remind the client to drink frequently (Figure C). Obtain a sports bottle so that she can carry fluids with her. *She may be too physically active to remember to drink.*

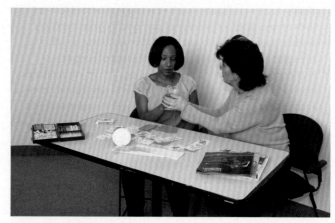

FIGURE C The nurse ensures that the client drinks adequate fluids.

Case in Point 28.1 (continued)

Danielle's Story

- Monitor intake and output, blood pressure, heart rate, and respiratory status. *These parameters provide objective evidence of fluid status.*
- Evaluate results of laboratory tests, especially serum electrolyte levels. *Results provide information about body fluid components and chemical indicators of nutritional status.*

> *4/15/13: The client ingests adequate nutrients to meet her needs. She demonstrates adequate oral food and fluid intake and no compromises in blood pressure, radial pulse rate, skin turgor, or mucous membranes.*

EPILOGUE

It has been a little over a week since Danielle was admitted to the psychiatric facility. She is receiving lithium; her serum lithium levels have remained within the therapeutic range. Danielle is also undergoing CBT. Her ability to maintain self-control is improving. In addition, her mood has stabilized and is congruent with her affect. She is beginning to demonstrate an understanding of her signs and symptoms and how they relate to her disorder. She states, "I can't believe I was acting so wildly. I'm just glad no one was hurt! I realize that I need to take care of myself. I can see how the medicine has helped me, and the therapy too." Danielle will be discharged 10 days after admission with follow-up at a community mental health center.

Developing a behavioral care plan with input from clients helps maintain self-control (Bisconer et al., 2006). Similar to a contract, a behavioral care plan details parameters for social interaction, such as which behaviors and comments are (or are not) appropriate. Nurses use the behavioral care plan to set limits on intrusive behaviors, such as entering another client's room without knocking, joining conversations when uninvited, and taking belongings without asking.

Nurses help clients learn to recognize what triggers violent thoughts and behaviors. They teach clients not to act on such thoughts but to leave the situation and find a staff member to talk to about them. Through role playing and feedback, nurses help clients learn to ask appropriately for what they need, instead of demanding that others assist them immediately or becoming angry when they don't.

Nurses educate clients about bipolar illness. They help clients recognize and connect symptoms with the disorder. They teach about medications and their potential positive effects on violent thoughts and behaviors.

Maintaining Physical Health and Personal Hygiene

Nurses monitor food and fluid intake and regularly assess weight, vital signs, and laboratory values. Small, light, high-protein meals that clients can eat while mobile help them consume sufficient calories. Clients with mania are at high risk for dehydration, which use of lithium exacerbates; thus, nurses monitor fluid intake carefully (Figure 28.6).

Balancing rest with activity can be a challenge (Miller, 2006). During manic phases, clients can go days without rest, which severely compromises physical health. Sleep is difficult because of hyperactivity. Nurses plan for clients to rest and calm down 1 hour before bedtime. They limit exposure to environmental stimuli, such as bright lights or loud music, before sleep and help clients identify activities that enhance relaxation. If needed, nurses gently but firmly enforce schedules. They

administer medications, as needed, for sleep and rest and teach appropriate use of such drugs and their side effects.

Clients with mania may neglect personal care and hygiene. In manic phases, they cannot focus long enough to complete simple tasks. Nurses encourage independence in dressing, hygiene, and grooming but help with self-care (bathing, brushing teeth, choosing clothing) until attention, mood, and energy level are stabilized. They establish (and post if necessary) a schedule for personal care. Nurses set limits for completion of morning care.

Enhancing Thought Processes

For all clients, nurses administer ordered as-needed medications to improve thought processes, which will stabilize most dramatically after therapeutic medication levels have been reached. At this time, clients can respond better to nonpharmacologic interventions. Until then, nurses assess the intensity of the thought disturbance and its effects on behavior. They closely observe while medications take effect because clients may hear command hallucinations regarding self-harm or harm toward others. Nurses do not argue with clients about the validity of hallucinations. Instead, they inform clients that they do not share the misperception (see Chap. 29). Another helpful strategy is to focus on a client's feelings about the hallucination, not the content itself ("You seem upset," not "Why would the voices tell you to hurt yourself?"). Nurses convey acceptance of and respect for clients while testing reality (Miller, 2006).

Clients with bipolar disorders have a limited attention span and disorganization from psychotic thinking. They may exhibit intrusive, loud, and agitated behaviors, which reflect a disturbed thought process and content. Nurses help clients focus on specific activities or statements. Limiting activities within the environment may be necessary until medications take effect. Nurses avoid direct confrontation; instead, they use gentle yet firm limit-setting techniques. They provide a quiet, safe environment

Intake and Output Chart

7:00 AM _11-18-09_ to 7:00 AM _11-19-09_

	Oral	I.V.		Blood	Other	Comments	Urine	Stool	Gastric tube	Drainage tubes		Vomitus	Other	Comments
						Intake				**Output**				
7-8	250					Force fluids to 1100cc/shift	300							
8-9														
9-10	120													
10-11	60													
11-12	100						250							
12-1	300													
1-2	240													
2-3	100						200							
8 hr Tot	1170						750							voiding 3 discomfort
3-4														
4-5														
5-6														
6-7														
7-8														
8-9														
9-10														
10-11														
8 hr Tot														
11-12														
12-1														
1-2														
2-3														
3-4														
4-5														
5-6														
6-7														
8 hr Tot														
24 hr Tot														
	Total intake						**Total output**							

FIGURE 28.6 An example of an intake and output sheet.

where clients can rest. For those who can tolerate limited activities, nurses provide physical outlets that are not tension producing, such as folding clothes or drawing.

Self-Esteem Issues

The disturbed thought processes associated with bipolar disorders can manifest as alterations in self-esteem. Clients with bipolar disorder often outwardly exhibit inflated self-esteem during manic phases. Nurses avoid validating grandiose statements (eg, "I'm the president's right-hand man!"). Instead, they encourage clients to discuss realistic self-perceptions and to identify positive elements. Nurses help clients connect grandiose statements to symptoms of bipolar disorder, thus increasing insight into the disease process.

Anxiety and Agitation

Agitation is extreme anxiety and disordered thinking. During this unstable state, clients can become violent. Clients with mania may present with highly anxious, agitated behaviors. Nurses assess these symptoms, maintain the medication regimen, and treat clients with as-needed medications. They evaluate the effects of the medications on the behaviors, while considering whether certain environmental triggers increase anxiety and reducing the client's exposure to them. Nurses limit client contact with others if agitation is extreme.

Relaxation exercises, imagery, and progressive muscle relaxation may help. These may be difficult for clients to concentrate on, or paradoxically, they may increase anxiety. Nurses evaluate each client's ability to tolerate such directed relaxation exercises and engage clients, if appropriate. Listening to music may also reduce anxiety.

Encouraging Treatment and Medication Adherence

Nurses assist clients with bipolar disorder to manage their medication regimens. They provide information about medications and needed aftercare, such as frequency of laboratory testing, discharge planning, and follow-up visits. For example, nurses instruct clients taking lithium that they will need to have their blood levels checked twice a week initially and every 2 months after achieving therapeutic levels. If possible, nurses help clients keep a notebook or cards on which to record information about drugs, including mechanisms of action, dosages, side effects, and ongoing monitoring needs. They help review information until clients are familiar with each medication and its actions.

To help link the importance of taking medication with preventing relapse, nurses list target symptoms and identify signs of imminent relapse. They problem solve with clients about early management of symptoms so severity does not increase. Nurses explore what clients perceive as barriers to taking the medications, obtaining medications, participating in follow-up with the psychiatric care provider, and undergoing necessary laboratory tests. Nurses work with clients to overcome these real or perceived barriers.

Treatment adherence is particularly problematic for clients with bipolar disorder. During mania, they often feel well or even better than well and thus do not perceive a need to take medicine. Nevertheless, many cases of relapse are related to failure to take medications during periods of relative stability or early relapse. Nurses address the issue of nonadherence matter of factly and discuss views and factors that may affect a client's ability or willingness to follow the therapeutic regimen. Often clients become less vigilant and apt to ignore medication management and follow-up psychiatric care during remissions. The client may feel stable and not see the need for taking the medications. Nurses work with clients and families regarding the importance of adhering to the treatment regimen by reinforcing the link between symptom control and medication adherence and sustaining a functional remission of symptoms (Client-Centered Education 28.1).

Think About It 28.1

Georgie Laine is a 32-year-old woman with a history of bipolar disorder. Approximately 2 months ago, she stopped taking lithium. After Georgie disappeared for 3 days, her family found her in a bar, claiming to be a millionaire, dressed provocatively, and buying everyone drinks. She is admitted to the psychiatric unit and has received two 300-mg doses of lithium carbonate. She is irritable and has been running up and down the hallway, asking men if they will lie down with her. She has also been entering other clients' rooms dressed in her underwear. Analyze this situation, predict the client's priority need, and describe measures to meet this need.

▲ EVALUATION

Improvement in symptoms is gradual but noticeable as interventions take effect. Specific indicators that interventions are effective include the following:

- The client refrains from acting aggressively toward others.
- The client ingests adequate calories and fluids, maintains a balance between rest and activity, and independently manages self-care.
- The client participates appropriately in milieu activities and social interactions.
- The client expresses a positive sense of self-worth without delusions of grandeur.
- The client demonstrates logical thought processes.
- The client reports reduced anxiety and agitation.
- The client adheres to the therapeutic regimen and discusses the importance of doing so after discharge.

Client–Centered Education 28.1

Helping a Loved One Who Has Bipolar Disorder

Family members of clients with bipolar disorders can experience a wide range of emotions about their loved ones, including frustration, anger, and helplessness. Nurses provide education and support to relatives so that they can better cope with their feelings and help clients. Points to incorporate include recommending that family members:

- Learn the warning signs of mania and depression. Suggest that they plan with their loved one, while he or she is well, what to do when they notice these symptoms. For example, the family may want to make arrangements for withholding credit cards and banking privileges.
- The client and the family should discuss and prepare an advance directive. This document should specify information such as current psychiatric health care providers; where the client should be hospitalized, if needed; which medications work and which ones have side effects that are bothersome to the client; and which family member(s) may discuss privileged information with the psychiatric mental health care providers.
- Support their family member in adhering to the treatment plan, taking medications as ordered, and seeing his or her mental health practitioner regularly.

- Offer to attend therapy sessions, if appropriate.
- Help the client refrain from using alcohol and drugs by encouraging him or her to seek help through local Alcoholics/Narcotics Anonymous Groups, local substance abuse treatment centers, or other supportive agencies that can provide assistance (see Chap. 30).
- Avoid interpreting their loved one's mood changes as rejection or an indication of their own inability to help. Remind them that this is the disease.
- Learn the warning signs of suicide. Tell them to take any threats or comments the person makes seriously and to seek help immediately from the person's mental health provider.
- Tell their loved one that his or her presence is deeply meaningful and important and that his or her suicide would be a tremendous loss.
- Share caregiving responsibilities with another family member or friend when the need is acute to prevent feelings of burnout.
- Understand that there is a difference between a good day and hypomania and between a bad day and depression. Let them know that their loved one can have good days and bad days that are not part of the illness.
- Take advantage of the help available from support groups.

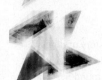

Reviewing and Applying Your Knowledge

Chapter Summary

• Bipolar disorders are a significant problem and emergent national public health priority in the United States.

• The etiology of bipolar disorders is complex and involves multiple interactions among genetic, physiologic, and psychologic factors.

• Signs and symptoms and diagnostic criteria for bipolar disorders are highly specific; broad classifications include bipolar I disorder, bipolar II disorder, and cyclothymia.

• Bipolar disorders are often unrecognized and go untreated; however, when clients receive appropriate treatment, outcomes are good. Multiple treatment modalities include individual, group, and family psychotherapies; pharmacotherapy; and somatic therapies.

• Psychiatric–mental health nurses must use the nursing process to assess, plan, implement, and evaluate care for people with bipolar disorder.

Study Questions

1. After a client diagnosed with bipolar I disorder has been taking lithium for 2 weeks, she complains of vomiting and diarrhea and is slurring her words. Which of the following would be the nurse's most appropriate action?

   a. Tell the client that these symptoms will disappear with time.

   b. Immediately call the physician to report the symptoms.

   c. Check the client's last serum lithium level.

   d. Immediately draw a blood glucose level from the client.

2. Which of the following activities would be most appropriate for a client with mania on an inpatient unit?

   a. Arts and crafts

   b. Playing a game of cards

   c. Walking with a staff member

   d. A cooking group

3. A client reports to the admissions nurse that he has not eaten or slept in the last week. He begins talking about finding a scientific formula that would turn candy into gold. The client tells the nurse that if nobody will go along with his plan, he will drive his car off a cliff. Based on this information, the nurse records the following information about mental status:

   a. Pressured speech, grandiosity, racing thoughts

   b. Grandiosity, insomnia, suicidal ideations

   c. Suicidal ideations, eating disorder, hyperactivity

   d. Flight of ideas, hypersomnia, grandiosity

4. A 25-year-old client has been in inpatient treatment for bipolar I disorder (manic episode) for 10 days. He will be discharged soon, and the nurse is evaluating the effectiveness of the plan of care. Which outcome is the most appropriate indicator that the client's mania is resolving sufficiently for safe discharge?

   a. The client has resumed caring for his physical appearance.

   b. The client denies wanting to harm self or others.

   c. The client exhibits appropriate levels of nutrition, fluid intake, exercise, and sleep.

   d. The client makes realistic statements about self and others.

5. Which of the following variables would the nurse identify as exerting the greatest effects on relapse prevention for clients with depressive or bipolar disorders?

   a. Strong social support

   b. High socioeconomic status

   c. Stress management skills

   d. Medication adherence

Critical Thinking Questions

1. Consider Case in Point 28.1. Is there any information other than that presented that you would want to learn from Danielle?

2. What thoughts do you have about the severity, longitudinal course, and chronicity of Danielle's symptoms?

3. What consequences and concerns might bipolar disorder pose for Danielle's children?

References

Ackenheil, M. (2001). Neurotransmitters and signal transduction processes in bipolar affective disorders: A synopsis. *Journal of Affective Disorders, 62,* 101–111.

American Foundation for Suicide Prevention. (2010). *Facts and figures: Special populations.* Retrieved from http://www.afs[.org/index.cfm?fuseaction=home.viewpage&page

American Psychiatric Association (APA). (2000). *Diagnostic and statistical manual of mental disorders* (4th ed., text rev.). Washington, DC: Author.

American Psychiatric Association (APA). (2010). *Practice guideline for the treatment of patients with bipolar disorder* (2nd ed.). Retrieved from http://www.psychiatryonline.org/guilelines.aspx. Retrieved 3/29/2012

Baldassano, C. F., Marangell, L. B., Gyulai, L., Nassir Ghaemi, S., Joffe, H., Kim, D. R., et al. (2005). Gender differences in bipolar disorder: Retrospective data form the first 500 STEP-BD participants. *Bipolar Disorders, 7,* 465–470.

Barrett, T. B., Hauger, R. L., Kennedy, A. D., Sadovnick, A. D., Remick, R. A., Keck, P. E., et al. (2003). Evidence that a single nucleotide polymorphism in the promoter of the G protein receptor kinase 3 gene is associated with bipolar disorder. *Molecular Psychiatry, 8,* 546–557.

Baum, A. E., Akula, N., Cabanero, M., Cardona, I., Corona, W., Klemens, B., et al. (2008). A genome-wide association study implicates diacylglycerol kinase eta (DGKH) and several other genes in the etiology of bipolar disorder [Electronic version]. *Molecular Psychiatry, 13*(2), 197–207.

Beck, A. T. (1972). *Depression: Causes and treatment.* Philadelphia, PA: University of Pennsylvania Press.

Beck, A. T., Rush, A. J., Shaw, B. F., & Emery, G. (1979). *Cognitive therapy of depression.* New York, NY: Guilford Press.

Benes, F. M., Lim, B., Matzilevich, D., Walsh, J. P., Subburaju, S., & Minns, M. (2007). Regulation of the GABA cell phenotype in hippocampus of schizophrenics and bipolars. *Proceedings of the National Academy of Sciences of the United States of America, 104,* 10164–10169.

Bisconer, S. W., Green, M., Mallon-Czajka, J., & Johnson, S. (2006). Managing aggression in a psychiatric hospital using a behaviour plan: A case study. *Journal of Psychiatric Mental Health Nursing, 13*(5), 515–520.

Bulechek, G. M., Butcher, H. K., & McCloskey Dochterman, J. (2008). *Nursing interventions classification (NIC)* (5th ed.). St. Louis, MO: Mosby.

Burt, V. K., & Rasgon, N. (2004). Special considerations in treating bipolar disorder in women. *Bipolar Disorders, 6,* 2–3.

Byerley, W., & Badner, J. A. (2011). Strategies to identify genes for complex disorders: A focus on bipolar disorder and chromosome 16P. *Psychiatric Genetics, 21*(4), 173–182.

Calabrese, J. R., Hirschfeld, R. M., Frye, M. A., & Reed, M. L. (2004). Impact of depressive symptoms compared with manic symptoms in bipolar disorder: Results of a U.S. community-based sample. *Journal of Clinical Psychiatry, 65,* 1499–1504.

Cannon, D. M., Ichise, M., Fromm, S. J., Nugent, A. C., Rollis, D., Gandhi, S. K., et al. (2006). Serotonin transporter binding in bipolar disorder assessed using [11C]DASB and positron emission tomography. *Biological Psychiatry, 60,* 207–217.

Carpenter, L. L., Moreno, F. A., Mitchel, A., Kling, M. A., Anderson, G. M., Regenold, W. T., et al. (2004). Effect of vagus nerve stimulation on cerebrospinal fluid monoamine metabolites, norepinephrine, and gamma-aminobutyric acid concentrations in depressed patients. *Biological Psychiatry, 56,* 418–426.

Chae, J., Nahas, Z., Lomarev, M., et al. (2003). A review of functional neuroimaging studies of vagus nerve stimulation (VNS). *Journal of Psychiatric Research, 37,* 443–455.

Cipriani, A., Pretty, H., Hawton, K., & Geddes, J. R. (2005). Lithium in the prevention of suicidal behavior and all-cause mortality in patients with mood disorders: A systematic review of randomized trials. *American Journal of Psychiatry, 162,* 1805–1819.

Dolberg, O. T., Dannon, P. N., Schreiber, S., & Grunhaus, L. (2002). Transcranial magnetic stimulation in patients with bipolar depression: A double blind, controlled study. *Bipolar Disorders, 4* (Suppl. 1), 94–95.

Ehlers, C. L., Frank, E., Kupfer, D. J., & Monk, T. H. (1993). Biological rhythms and depression: The role of Zeitgebers and Zeitstorers. *Depression, 1,* 293–295.

Eickholt, B. J., Williams, R. S. B., & Harwood, A. J. (2004). Mood stabilizers and the cell biology of neuronal growth cones. *Clinical Neuroscience Research, 4,* 189–199.

Frye, M. S., Gitlin, M. J., & Altshuler, L. L. (2004). Unmet needs in bipolar depression. *Depression and Anxiety, 19,* 199–208.

Goldberg, J. F. (2007). What psychotherapists should know about pharmacotherapies for bipolar disorder. *Journal of Clinical Psychology, 63,* 475–490.

Goldberg, J. F. (2010). Antidepressants in bipolar disorder 7 myths and realities. *Current Psychiatry, 9*(5), 41–48.

Goldberg, J. F. (2011). Ultra-rapid cycling bipolar disorder: A critical look. *Current Psychiatry, 10*(12), 42–52.

Goodwin, F. K., & Jamison, K. R. (1990). *Manic-depressive illness.* New York, NY: Oxford University Press.

Hlastala, S. A., & Frank, E. (2006). Adapting interpersonal and social rhythm therapy to the developmental needs of adolescents with bipolar disorder. *Development and Psychopathology, 18,* 1267–1288.

Huang, X., Lei, Z., & El-Mallakh, R. S. (2007). Lithium normalizes elevated intracellular sodium. *Bipolar Disorders, 9,* 298–300.

Jope, R. S. (2004). Inhibition of glycogen synthase kinase-3: A potential therapeutic target of lithium. *Clinical Neuroscience Research, 4,* 171–179.

Kapczinski, F., Frey, B. N., & Zannatto, V. (2004). Physiopathology of bipolar disorders: What has changed in the last 10 years? *Revista Brasileira de Psiquatria, 26*(Suppl 3), 17–21.

Kaptsan, A., Yaroslavsky, Y., Applebaum, J., Belmaker, R. H., & Grisaru, N. (2003). Right prefrontal TMS versus sham treatment of mania: A controlled study. *Bipolar Disorders, 5,* 36–39.

Karch, A. M. (2009). *2009 Lippincott's nursing drug guide.* Philadelphia, PA: Lippincott Williams & Wilkins.

Kessler, R. C., Bergland, P., Demler, O., Jin, R., & Walters, E. E. (2005). Lifetime prevalence and age-of-onset distributions of *DSM-IV* disorders in the national comorbidity survey replication. *Archives of General Psychiatry, 62,* 593–602.

Kushner, S. F., Khan, A., & Lane, R., & Olson, W. H. (2006). Topiramate monotherapy in the management of acute mania: Results of four double-blind placebo-controlled trials. *Bipolar Disorders, 8,* 15–27.

Lam, D. H., Watkins, E. R., Hayward, P., Bright, J., Wright, K., Kerr, N., et al. (2003). A randomized controlled study of cognitive therapy for relapse prevention for bipolar affective disorder: Outcome of the first year. *Archives in General Psychiatry, 60,* 145–152.

Lam, D., Wright, K., & Smith, N. (2004). Dysfunctional assumptions in bipolar disorder. *Journal of Affective Disorders, 79,* 193–199.

Leboyer, M., & Kupfer, D. J. (2010). Bipolar disorder: New perspectives in health care and prevention. *Journal of Clinical Psychiatry, 71*(12), 1689–1695.

Li, R., & El-Mallakh, R. S. (2000). A novel evidence of different mechanisms of lithium and valproate neuroprotective action on human SY5Y neuroblastoma cells: Caspase-3 dependency. *Neuroscience Letters, 294,* 147–150.

Martin, J. L. R., Barbanoj, M. J., Scholaepfer, T. E., Clos, S., Perez, V., Kulisevsky, V., & Gironell, A. (2007). Transcranial magnetic stimulation for treating depression. *Cochrane Database of Systematic Reviews, 2007*(2). CD003493.

McColm, R., Brown, J., & Anderson, J. (2006). Nursing interventions for the management of patients with mania. *Nursing Standard, 20*(17), 46–49.

McNamara, R. K., & Lenox, R. H. (2004). The myristoylated alanine-rich C kinase substrate: A lithium-regulated protein linking cellular signaling and cytoskeletal plasticity. *Clinical Neuroscience Research, 4*, 155–169.

Meyer, A. (1957). *Psychobiology: A science of man.* Springfield, IL: Charles C. Thomas.

Miklowitz, D. J. (2006). A review of evidence-based psychosocial interventions for bipolar disorder. *Journal of Clinical Psychiatry, 67*(Suppl 11), 28–33.

Miklowitz, D. J., Otto, M. W., Frank, E., Reilly-Harrington, N. A., Wisniewski, S. R., Kogan, J. N., et al. (2007). Psychosocial treatments for bipolar depression: A 1-year randomized trial from the systematic treatment enhancement program. *Archives in General Psychiatry, 64*, 419–427.

Miller, K. (2006). Bipolar disorder: Etiology, diagnosis, and management. *Journal of the American Academy of Nurse Practitioners, 18*(8), 368–373.

Moorhead, S., Johnson, M., Maas, M. L., & Swanson, E. (2008). *Nursing outcomes classification (NOC)* (4th ed.). St. Louis, MO: Mosby.

Moorhead, T. W., McKirdy, J., Sussman, J. E., Hall, J., Lawrie, S. M., Johnstone, E. C., et al. (2007). Progressive gray matter loss in patients with bipolar disorder. *Biological Psychiatry, 62*(8), 894–900.

Nahas, Z., Kozel, F. A., Li, X., Anderson, B., & George, M. S. (2003). Left prefrontal transcranial magnetic stimulation (TMS) treatment of depression in bipolar affective disorder: A pilot study of acute safety and efficacy. *Bipolar Disorders, 5*, 40–47.

Nahas, Z., Molloy, M. A., Hughes, P. L., Oliver, N. C., Arana, G. W., Risch, S. C., & George, M. S. (1999). Repetitive transcranial magnetic stimulation: Perspectives for application in the treatment of bipolar and unipolar disorders. *Bipolar Disorders, 1*(2), 73–80.

NANDA International. (2007). *Nursing diagnoses: Definitions and classification (2007–2008).* Philadelphia, PA: Author.

National Institute of Mental Health [NIMH]. (2007, April). *Questions and answers about the STEP-BD depression psychosocial treatment trial.* Retrieved from http://www.nimh.nih.gov/trial/practical/step-bd/questions-and-answers.

National Institute of Mental Health [NIMH]. (2010a, January 28). *Science update: Same genes suspected in both depression and bipolar illness: Increased risk may stem from variation in gene on/off switch.* Retrieved from http://www.nimh.nih.gov/science-news/2010/same-genes-suspected-in-both-depression-and-bipolar-illness.shtml

National Institute of Mental Health [NIMH]. (2010b, August 16). *Science update: Symptoms of bipolar disorder may go undiagnosed in some adults with major depression.* Retrieved from http://www.nimh.nih.gov/science-news/2010/symptoms-of-bipolar-disorder-may-go-undiagnosed-in-some-adults-with-major-depression.shtml

National Institute of Mental Health [NIMH]. (2012a). *Bipolar disorder.* Retrieved from http://www.nimh.nih.gov/health/topics/bipolar-disorder/index.shtml

National Institute of Mental Health [NIMH]. (2012b). *Statistics: Bipolar disorder among adults.* Retrieved from http://www.nimh.nih.gov/statistics/1BIPOLAR_ADULT.shtml

Newcomer, J. W. (2005). Second-generation (atypical) antipsychotics and metabolic effects: A comprehensive literature review. *CNS Drugs, 19*(Suppl. 1), 1–93.

Parker, G., Gibson, N. A., Brotchies, H., Heruc, G., Rees, A. M., & Hadzi-Pavlovic, D. (2006). Omega-3 fatty acids and mood disorders. *American Journal of Psychiatry, 163*, 969–978.

Perlis, R. H., Welge, J. A., Vornik, L. A., Hirschfeld, R. M. A., & Keck, P. E. (2006). Atypical antipsychotics in the treatment of mania: A meta-analysis of randomized, placebo-controlled trials. *Journal of Clinical Psychiatry, 67*, 509–516.

Power, M. J. (2005). Psychological approaches to bipolar disorders: A theoretical critique. *Clinical Psychology Review, 25*, 1101–1122.

Pytliak, M., Vargová, V, Mechirová, V, & Felsöci, M. (2011) Serotonin receptors—From molecular biology to clinical applications. *Physiological Research, 60*(1), 15–26.

Rajkowska, G., Halaris, A., & Selemon, L. D. (2001). Reductions in neuronal and glial density characterize the dorsolateral prefrontal cortex in bipolar disorder. *Biological Psychiatry, 49*, 741–752.

Rush, A. J., Sackeim, H. A., Marangell, L. B., et al. (2005). Effects of 12 months of vagus nerve stimulation in treatment-resistant depression: A naturalistic study. *Biological Psychiatry, 58*, 355–363.

Salloum, I. M., Cornelius, J. R., Daley, D. C., Kirisci, L., Himmelhoch, J. M., & Thase, M. E. (2005). Efficacy of valproate maintenance in patients with bipolar disorder and alcoholism: A double-blind, placebo-controlled study. *Archives of General Psychiatry, 62*, 37–45.

Savitz, J., Soms, M., & Ramesar, R. (2005). Neuropsychological dysfunction in bipolar affective disorder: A critical opinion. *Bipolar Disorders, 7*, 216–235.

Schneck, C. D. (2011). Bipolar phenomenology: Have we learned all we can learn? *American Journal of Psychiatry, 168*(1), 4–6.

Scott, J., Garland, A., & Moorhead, S. (2001). A pilot study of cognitive therapy in bipolar disorders. *Psychological Medicine, 31*, 459–467.

Scott, J., Paykel, E., Morriss, R., Bentall, R., Kinderman, P., Johnson, T., et al. (2006). Cognitive-behavioural therapy for severe and recurrent bipolar disorders: Randomised controlled trial. *British Journal of Psychiatry, 188*, 313–320.

Shippee, N. D., Shah, N. D., Williams, M. D., Moriarty, J. P., Frye, M. A., & Ziegenfuss, J. Y. (2011). Differences in demographic composition and in work, social, and functional limitations among the populations with unipolar depression and bipolar disorder: Results from a nationally representative sample. *Health and Quality of Life Outcomes, 9*(1), 90–99.

Sklar, P., Ripke, S., Scott, L. J., Andreassen, O. A., Cihon, S., et al. (2011). Large-scale genome-wide association analysis of bipolar disorder identifies a new susceptibility locus near ODZ4. *National Genetics, 43*(10), 977–983.

Smoller, J. W., & Gardner-Schuster, E. (2007). Genetics of bipolar disorder. *Current Psychiatry, 9*(6), 504–511.

Stimmel, G. L. (2004). The economic burden of bipolar disorder. *Psychiatric Services, 55*, 117–118.

Stockmeier, C. A. (2003). Involvement of serotonin in depression: Evidence from post-mortem and imaging studies of serotonin receptors and the serotonin transporter. *Journal of Psychiatric Research, 37*, 357–373.

Strakowski, S. M., Delbello, M. P., & Adler, C. (2005). The functional neuroanatomy of bipolar disorder: A review of neuroimaging findings. *Molecular Psychiatry, 10*, 105–116.

Sullivan, H. S. (1953). *The interpersonal theory of psychiatry.* New York, NY: Norton.

Torres, I. J., DeFreitas, C. M., DeFreitas, V. G., Bond, D. J., et al. (2011). Relationship between cognitive functioning and 6-month clinical and functional outcome in patients with first manic episode bipolar I disorder. *Psychological Medicine, 41*(5), 971–982.

Wasserman, M. J., Corson, T. W., Sibony, D., Cooke, R. G., Parikh, S. V., Pennefather, P. S., et al. (2004). Chronic lithium treatment attenuates intracellular calcium mobilization. *Neuropsychopharmacology, 29*, 759–769.

Weiner, M., Warren, L., & Fiedorowicz, J. G. (2011). Cardiovascular morbidity and mortality in bipolar disorder. *American Clinical Psychiatry, 23*(1), 40–47.

Weisler, R. H., Kalali, A. H., & Ketter, T. A. (2004). A multi-center, randomized, double-blind, placebo-controlled trial of extended-release carbamazepine capsules as monotherapy for bipolar disorder patients with manic or mixed episodes. *Journal of Clinical Psychiatry, 65,* 478–484.

Weisler, R. H., Keck, P. E., Swann, A. C., Cutler, A. J., Ketter, T. A., & Kalali, A. H. (2005). Extended-release carbamazepine capsules as monotherapy for bipolar disorder: A multicenter, randomized, double-blind, placebo-controlled trial. *Journal of Clinical Psychiatry, 66,* 323–330.

Wieseke, A., Bantz, D., & May, D. (2011). What you need to know about bipolar disorder besides disrupting lives, this illness can reduce life expectancy significantly. *American Nurse Today, 6*(7), 8–12.

Wirz-Justice, A., Benedetti, F., Berger, M., et al. (2005). Chronotherapeutics (light and wake therapy) in affective disorders. *Psychological Medicine, 35,* 939–944.

Woods, S. W. (2000). The economic burden of bipolar disease. *Journal of Clinical Psychiatry, 61*(Suppl 13), 38–41.

Zaretsky, A. E., Rizvi, S., & Parikh, S. V. (2007). How well do psychosocial interventions work in bipolar disorder? *Canadian Journal of Psychiatry, 52,* 14–21.

Web Resources

Child & Adolescent Bipolar Foundation: http://www.bpkids.org
Depression and Bipolar Support Alliance (DBSA): http://www.dbsalliance.org
Mental Health America (MHA): http://www.mentalhealthamerica.net
National Alliance for the Mentally Ill (NAMI): http://www.nami.org
National Institute of Mental Health (NIMH): http://http://nimh.nih.gov
Self assessment tool to determine level of symptoms and effectiveness of treatment: http://www.moodtracker.com
STEP-BD: http://www.stepbd.org, and http://www.stepbd.org/referencelist.html

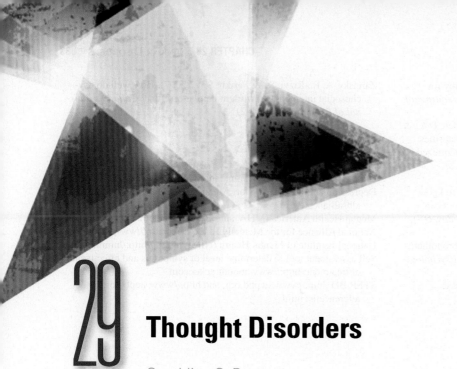

29

Thought Disorders

Geraldine S. Pearson

LEARNING OBJECTIVES

On completion of this chapter, you should be able to accomplish the following:

- Define schizophrenia.
- Compare other thought disorders with schizophrenia.
- Discuss proposed etiologies for schizophrenia.
- Identify signs and symptoms of schizophrenia.
- Explain the subtypes of schizophrenia.
- Compare the benefits and risks of antipsychotic medications.
- Describe the continuum of care for people with schizophrenia.
- Apply the nursing process to the care of clients with schizophrenia.

Thought disorders are serious and often persistent mental illnesses characterized by disturbances in reality orientation, thinking, and social involvement. Schizophrenia, the most prevalent thought disorder, is the main focus of this chapter, which also briefly addresses other closely related psychotic disturbances.

SCHIZOPHRENIA AND OTHER THOUGHT DISORDERS

Schizophrenia is a common and serious neurobiologic illness that affects 1% of people globally and approximately 2.5 million Americans (National Institute of Mental Health [NIMH], 2009). Experts currently view it as a metasyndrome, rather than a single disease, characterized by "multiple disease entities, multiple etiologic factors, multiple relevant pathophysiologic processes, multiple symptom dimensions, multiple protective and pathoplastic factors, all of which interact with the different current treatments to generate multiple different illness courses and individual outcomes" (Tandon et al., 2011, p. 5). Schizophrenia is a heterogeneous illness.

General hallmarks of thought disorders include disturbed thinking and preoccupation with frightening inner experiences (eg, delusions, hallucinations). Marked disturbances occur in affect (eg, flat, inappropriate), behavior (eg, unpredictable, bizarre), and social interactions (eg, isolation). These disturbances seem related to problems with brain circuitry.

The word *schizophrenia* historically referred to a "splitting off" of thoughts from emotions. However, the word has become confused with "split personality" or "multiple personality." Nurses must be careful not to confuse schizophrenia with dissociative disorders, in which clients actually display more than one personality (see Chap. 24). A more accurate interpretation of schizophrenia is a "disconnected mind." Such disconnection involves a lack of coherence in mental functioning, in which "thinking, feeling, perceiving, behaving, and experiencing operate without the normal linkages that make mental life comprehensible and effective" (Nasrallah & Smeltzer, 2003, p. 8). Currently schizophrenia is viewed as a complex illness with multiple etiologies and a variety of pharmacologic and psychosocial treatment choices. Much attention is being focused on prevention of this debilitating psychiatric illness (Tandon et al., 2011).

Schizophrenia is treatable. Unmanaged schizophrenia can devastate the lives of clients and severely disrupt families. Clients may become totally withdrawn from the environment with regressive behaviors, making it difficult to perform personal hygiene or activities of daily living, engage with others, or even notice physical illness or pain (Figure 29.1). Such severe, untreated symptoms can result in marked social, familial, and occupational dysfunction.

Stigma has long been cited as a major hurdle that keeps people with chronic psychiatric illness from fully

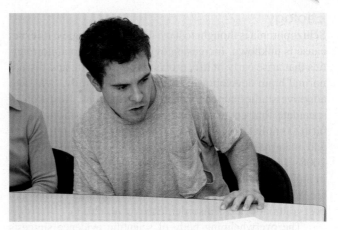

FIGURE 29.1 **Note the unkempt appearance, torn shirt, and disengagement of this client with active-phase schizophrenia.**

participating in life and seeking needed treatment services (Ross & Goldner, 2009). This is particularly true for people with schizophrenia and their relatives. Because schizophrenia has severe symptoms that are difficult to conceal, it is likely to result in stigmatization of clients and their loved ones. Those with schizophrenia suffer from the effects of the illness itself, inadequate clinical care and rehabilitation, and the stigma of shame and family burden. Many family members hide their relationships with people who have thought disorders or consider the illness to be a source of shame (Gonzalez-Torres et al., 2007). All family members may struggle with stigma when a relative suffers from schizophrenia.

Incidence and Prevalence

Symptoms of thought disorders usually emerge during late adolescence to the early 20s. However, schizophrenia has been diagnosed in children as young as 5 years and in people in their 40s. Schizophrenia occurs in all cultures, races, and social classes. In industrialized nations, a disproportionate number of affected people are in low socioeconomic groups. A possible explanation is that the illness interferes with productivity, limiting the occupational and earning potential and capacity for such clients and pushing them into low wage-earning thresholds. In addition, the stresses that those who live in poverty experience may trigger their vulnerability to schizophrenia (see Chap. 3).

Given its severity, prevalence, and enormous social, personal, and economic costs, it is remarkable how little attention schizophrenia receives. Estimates of its U.S. costs are $55.1 billion annually; this total includes direct (outpatient, medication, inpatient, and long-term care) costs of $22.7 billion and indirect costs of $32.4 billion (Wu et al., 2005). Schizophrenia is the most expensive of all chronic illnesses because it strikes people just at an age when they are ready to join the workforce and contribute to the economy. The chronicity of schizophrenia also contributes to lifelong intervention needs and risk of relapse that can necessitate expensive inpatient treatment interventions.

Etiology

Schizophrenia is thought to have multiple etiologies; its exact cause is unknown. Increasing evidence points to abnormalities that arise early in life, probably before birth, and disrupt normal brain development (Iritani, 2007). Family, twin, and adoptive studies support genetic contributions. Researchers speculate that environmental risks include gestational and birth complications, influenza epidemics, cannabis abuse, and maternal starvation during pregnancy (Tandon et al., 2008). Interestingly, there is a high rate of traumatic events in individuals diagnosed with schizophrenia. Similarly, there are high correlations between auditory hallucinations and post-traumatic stress disorder (Steel et al., 2011).

The overwhelming body of scientific evidence suggests that schizophrenia is a brain disease. Computed tomography scanning and magnetic resonance imaging have shown frequent enlargement of the lateral cerebral ventricles in people with schizophrenia (Nasrallah & Smeltzer, 2003). Sophisticated neurobiologic testing has shown specific brain alterations that make people with schizophrenia different. Examples include neurochemical imbalances, irregular patterns of certain neurons, and information-coordination difficulties. This chronic brain disorder structurally and functionally affects cortical and subcortical regions of the brain that influence cognitive, emotional, and motivational aspects of behavior (Kasai et al., 2002).

Despite the irrefutable evidence of a biologic basis for schizophrenia, researchers also suspect that psychosocial (ie, ecologic) factors influence vulnerability to thought disorders. They hypothesize that stress may activate (trigger expression of) a "schizophrenia gene" (although no such gene has been found) (see Chaps. 1 and 3). Because schizophrenia is most likely a group of disorders with heterogeneous causes, this chapter reviews biologic and psychosocial theories.

Biologic Theories

Current data about schizophrenia reveal a complex picture of brain dysfunction that includes genetic, neurologic, and metabolic disturbances and various neuropsychological deficits. These findings support the belief that schizophrenia is not one disorder but a group or collection of them. Ongoing research and improved assessment techniques are helping scientists test biologic theories more directly.

GENETIC INFLUENCES. Many studies strongly suggest a genetic contribution. Relatives of people with schizophrenia have a higher incidence of the disorder than that found in the general population. First-degree relatives (ie, parents, siblings, children) of clients with schizophrenia are at greater risk for the illness than are second-degree relatives (eg, grandparents, grandchildren, aunts, uncles, half-siblings). Schizophrenia is 13% more likely to develop in children with one parent who has schizophrenia than in those with unaffected parents; when both parents have schizophrenia, a child has a 46% risk for the illness (NIMH, 2006).

Studies of monozygotic (identical) twins have shown that if one develops schizophrenia, the likelihood that the other also will develop the illness is more than 50%. This result is significantly higher than for fraternal (nonidentical) twins. In addition, the incidence of schizophrenia in children adopted as infants by parents without schizophrenia, but whose biologic mothers had schizophrenia, equals the rate in children raised by their biologic mothers who had schizophrenia. Similarly, the incidence of schizophrenia in adopted children whose biologic mothers did not have schizophrenia equals the rate of schizophrenia in the general population (approximately 1%).

The exact mode of inheritance of schizophrenia has not been identified; opinion about its cause is divided. The monogenic hypothesis proposes that a single gene causes susceptibility. The more current polygenic hypothesis proposes that schizophrenia results from the interaction of many genes, and none of them individually is strong enough to produce schizophrenia. Genetic linkages have been established on numerous sites, with associated specific candidate genes. However, even with complete mapping of the human genome, it is unclear what combinations of genes result in schizophrenia. Ongoing research is attempting to identify susceptible genes that contribute to the pathophysiology (Tandon et al., 2008). Findings also suggest that an intermittent on/off switch triggers a gene involved as a chemical messenger to the brain. If the gene is turned on at increasingly high rates during development of the prefrontal cortex, the result is normal capacity for functions such as thinking and decision making. In people with schizophrenia, this event may not occur (Huang et al., 2007). Consequently, schizophrenia might be a developmental disease, influenced by maturation of the prefrontal cortex.

Schizophrenia may also develop from the interaction of genetic susceptibility with environmental stress or significant environmental risks. Although recent studies have failed to locate a single susceptibility gene, genetic influences increase the risk of schizophrenia but not of other psychotic disorders. Further research may clarify the genetic basis of schizophrenia. Most investigators agree that schizophrenia is best conceptualized as a "multiple-hit" illness, similar to cancer. In other words, a person may carry a genetic predisposition for it, but this vulnerability is not "released" unless other factors also intervene (see Chap. 2). Although most such factors are considered environmental (in that they are not encoded in DNA), most are also biologic and include factors such as birth injuries and nutrition (Kalat, 2006).

NEUROCHEMICAL AND NEUROANATOMIC CHANGES.

Research has focused on brain imaging and changes that accompany thought disorders. These changes involve the brain's structure, metabolism, blood flow, electrical activity, and chemistry.

Clients with schizophrenia have neurodevelopmental defects in brain circuitry and abnormal brain metabolism. Positron emission tomography (PET), which produces slice images of radioisotope density, has indicated relative metabolic underactivity of the frontal lobes (Figure 29.2). These

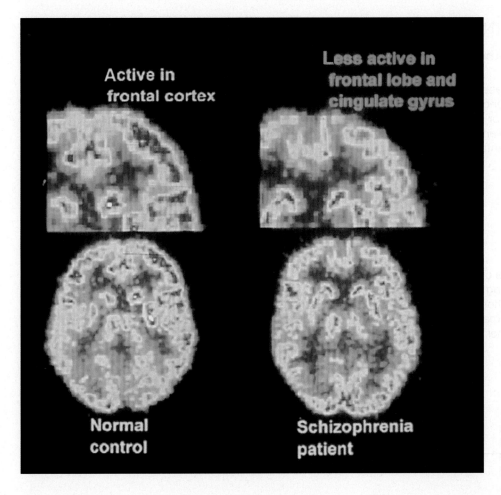

FIGURE 29.2 Positron emission tomography scan showing metabolic differences in a control subject (*left*) and a client with untreated schizophrenia (*right*).

PET scans have shown decreased basal ganglia activity, which antipsychotic (neuroleptic) medications can reverse. In schizophrenia, a structural or functional lesion disrupts the integrity of entire brain neural circuits (Buchanan & Carpenter, 2004).

The dopamine hypothesis of schizophrenia, the most enduring biochemical explanation, proposes that overactivity of dopamine results in the illness. In addition, an insufficiency of norepinephrine at certain central synapses of the brain, an imbalance between dopamine and norepinephrine, or both could be among the biologic causes. These biochemical differences in the nervous system of clients with schizophrenia cause them to process sensory information abnormally, resulting in disturbances of attention, inadequate social interaction, isolation, and hypersensitivity. While difficult to research, it is nonetheless believed that alterations in dopamine metabolism are associated with schizophrenia (Buchanan & Carpenter, 2004). Research also suggests that abnormal glutamatergic and cholinergic processes might contribute. Regardless of etiology, the pathophysiology of schizophrenia is complex (Tandon et al., 2011). See Understanding Biologic Foundations 29.1.

Several lines of evidence support speculation that schizophrenia results from early brain injury. For example, clients with schizophrenia are more likely than control subjects to have a history of birth injury and perinatal complications, which could result in subtle brain alterations and thereby set the stage for later illness. Others suggest that the maternal–fetal environment might also contribute, although exact mechanisms are unclear (Patterson, 2007). Neuroanatomic imaging and study may link schizophrenia to certain patterns of hemispheric brain dysfunction. These studies have suggested left hemisphere overactivation and consequent temporal abnormalities, as well as delays in sensory processing. Hallucinations have been correlated with accelerated glucose metabolism in the left temporal lobe. PET scans show relatively decreased metabolic activity in the frontal lobes and a low metabolic rate in the basal ganglia, both of which increase when antipsychotic medications are administered.

Other pathologic findings include dysfunctions of eye movements, impaired modulation of stimulus input that allows too much information to reach higher brain centers, laterality differences in which the left hemisphere may be less efficient than the right, impaired selective attention, and hypervigilance. Abnormalities of eye movement constitute a marker of particular significance because they are also found in nonaffected relatives of clients with schizophrenia. The same abnormalities also appear in related disorders, such as schizotypal personality disorder (Thaker et al., 1996) (see Chap. 25).

Neuroanatomic differences in clients with schizophrenia include several structural brain abnormalities. Cerebral

UNDERSTANDING BIOLOGIC FOUNDATIONS 29.1

The Dopamine Hypothesis of Schizophrenia

Normally, when dopamine is released in the brain, it follows normal neural pathways and connects appropriately to nerve cell receptor sites (see Chap. 2). Feedback and modulation are balanced, contributing to stable behavior and reality orientation.

In schizophrenia, excessive levels of dopamine bombard receptor sites, overstimulating brain areas that are involved with arousal and motivation. The disruption in normal neuronal communication may contribute to hallucinations, delusions, and other psychoses.

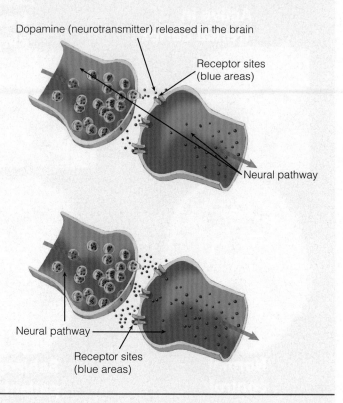

ventricular enlargement is the most consistently replicated finding, but sulcal enlargement and cerebellar atrophy are also reported. These abnormalities appear from the earliest stages of the illness and may be related to impairments in motivation, socialization, and complex problem solving. Ventricular enlargement is associated with poor premorbid functioning, negative symptoms, poor response to treatment, and cognitive impairment. Neuroanatomic studies also indicate a slightly decreased volume of the putamen, substantia nigra, and various portions of the limbic system, especially the temporal lobe and hippocampus. The limbic system, because of its role in the control of emotions, and the basal ganglia, because of their involvement in movement and movement disorders, have long been implicated in schizophrenia. Postmortem studies on clients with schizophrenia have found a decreased size of the limbic system. In some studies, the basal ganglia are reduced in volume. Other structural differences include cell loss, misalignment of cells, and altered membrane and intracellular structure (Buchanan & Carpenter, 2004).

Reduced numbers of neurons have been reported in several cortical areas. Frontal lobe abnormalities may account for some cognitive, attention-related, and affective symptoms. However, decreased frontal lobe size has been replicated less consistently than ventricular enlargement, with negative and positive studies appearing equally. More

research is needed before a definitive link can be made between frontal lobe size and schizophrenia.

Psychosocial Theories

According to the **vulnerability model** (sometimes called the **stress-vulnerability model**), under the stress of biologic and psychosocial factors, vulnerable people may be predisposed to "break down"—thus the archaic expression "nervous breakdown." No empirical evidence supports this model; professional consensus is that a complex interplay of environmental and biologic factors is responsible for the disease.

Risk factors (stressors) identified in the vulnerability model may include poverty, major life changes (eg, leaving home for college), substance abuse, and other environmental or interpersonal stressors. Moderators or buffers can include perceived social support, intact family, and a stable living environment (Browne, 2005).

Past views held that interpersonal influences, particularly disordered communication and interaction, contribute to schizophrenia. Although most researchers and clinicians acknowledge the influence of a supportive family and positive communication patterns in mental health, no prior or current evidence shows that family communication patterns cause schizophrenia. Theories of family communication and interaction as causes for this brain-based disorder have been discarded. A spokesperson for the National Alliance for the Mentally Ill (NAMI) says that major mental illness is a family problem only in the sense that the illness of one member affects the entire family (see Chap. 15). While family dynamics can influence the course of the illness, schizophrenia remains predominantly a brain-based disorder that makes people vulnerable to family stress and dysfunction. Family dynamics do not cause schizophrenia.

Checkpoint Questions

1. What is the ultimate result of the biochemical differences in the nervous systems of clients with schizophrenia?

2. What is the current professional consensus about the expression of schizophrenia?

Signs and Symptoms/Diagnostic Criteria

At one time, schizophrenia was conceptualized as being of two types: type I, in which positive symptoms prevailed, and type II, in which negative symptoms prevailed. However, recent studies have proposed more complex delineations of psychopathology. Indeed, the symptoms and signs are so diverse that they cover the entire range of human thought, emotion, and behavior. Students should approach this section knowing that it is not prudent to make simple distinctions or generalizations about schizophrenia. Much is to be learned; what may be "true" today may be found invalid tomorrow.

According to the *Diagnostic and Statistical Manual of Mental Disorders,* 4th edition, text revision (*DSM-IV-TR*), schizophrenia lasts at least 6 months and includes at least 1 month of two or more active-phase symptoms, such as bizarre delusions, hallucinations (eg, a running commentary of two voices conversing), disorganized speech, grossly disorganized or catatonic behavior, and negative behavior. These symptoms interfere markedly with social or occupational functioning (American Psychiatric Association [APA], 2000). The *DSM-IV-TR* (2000) delineates symptoms of schizophrenia as positive or negative.

Closely related psychotic disturbances include schizophreniform disorder, schizoaffective disorder, delusional disorder, brief psychotic disorder, and shared psychotic disorder. See *DSM-IV-TR* BOX 29.1. The diagnostic revisions proposed for *DSM-V* include elimination of schizophrenia subtypes. These have not been finalized (APA, 2011).

People with schizophrenia manifest alterations in cognitive functioning in all phases of the disorder. Cognition entails

---

DSM-IV-TR BOX 29.1

Thought Disorders

Schizophrenia

A. *Characteristic symptoms:* Two (or more) of the following, each present for a significant portion of time during a 1-month period (or less if successfully treated):
 1. Delusions
 2. Hallucinations
 3. Disorganized speech (eg, frequent derailment or incoherence)
 4. Grossly disorganized or catatonic behavior
 5. Negative symptoms, ie, affective flattening, alogia, or avolition

Note: Only one Criterion A symptom is required if delusions are bizarre or hallucinations consist of a voice keeping up a running commentary on the person's behavior or thoughts, or two or more voices conversing with each other.

B. *Social/occupational dysfunction:* For a significant portion of the time since the onset of the disturbance, one or more major areas of functioning such as work, interpersonal relations, or self-care are markedly below the level achieved prior to the onset (or when the onset is in childhood or adolescence, failure to achieve expected level of interpersonal, academic, or occupational achievement).

C. *Duration:* Continuous signs of the disturbance persist for at least 6 months. This 6-month period must include at least 1 month of symptoms (or less if successfully treated) that meet Criterion A (ie, active-phase symptoms) and may include periods of prodromal or residual symptoms. During these prodromal or residual periods, the signs of the disturbance may be manifested by only negative symptoms or two or more symptoms listed in Criterion A present in an attenuated form (eg, odd beliefs, unusual perceptual experiences).

D. *Schizoaffective and Mood Disorder exclusion:* Schizoaffective Disorder and Mood Disorder With Psychotic Features have been ruled out because either (1) no Major Depressive, Manic, or Mixed Episodes have occurred concurrently with the active-phase symptoms; or (2) if mood episodes have occurred during active-phase symptoms, their total duration has been brief relative to the duration of the active and residual periods.

E. *Substance/general medical condition exclusion:* The disturbance is not due to the direct physiologic effects of a substance (eg, a drug of abuse, a medication) or a general medical condition.

F. *Relationship to a Pervasive Developmental Disorder:* If there is a history of Autistic Disorder or another Pervasive Developmental Disorder, the additional diagnosis of Schizophrenia is made only if prominent delusions or hallucinations are also present for at least a month (or less if successfully treated).

(*continues on page 590*)

DSM-IV-TR BOX 29.1 Thought Disorders (continued)

Schizophreniform Disorder

A. Criteria A, D, and E of Schizophrenia are met.
B. An episode of the disorder (including prodromal, active, and residual phases) lasts at least 1 month but less than 6 months.

Schizoaffective Disorder

A. An uninterrupted period of illness during which, at some time, there is either a Major Depressive Episode [see *DSM-IV-TR* Box 27.1], a Manic Episode, or a Mixed Episode [see *DSM-IV-TR* Box 28.1] concurrent with symptoms that meet Criterion A for Schizophrenia.

Note: The Major Depressive Episode must include Criterion A1: depressed mood.

B. During the same period of illness, there have been delusions or hallucinations for at least 2 weeks in the absence of prominent mood symptoms.
C. Symptoms that meet criteria for a mood episode are present for a substantial portion of the total duration of the active and residual periods of the illness.
D. The disturbance is not due to the direct physiologic effects of a substance (eg, a drug of abuse, a medication) or a general medical condition.

Delusional Disorder

A. Nonbizarre delusions (ie, involving situations that occur in real life, such as being followed, poisoned, infected, loved at a distance, or deceived by spouse or lover, or having a disease) of at least 1 month's duration.
B. Criterion A for Schizophrenia has never been met.
C. Apart from the impact of the delusion(s) or its ramifications, functioning is not markedly impaired and behavior is not obviously odd or bizarre.

D. If mood episodes have occurred concurrently with delusions, their total duration has been brief relative to the duration of the delusional periods.
E. The disturbance is not due to the direct physiologic effects of a substance (eg, a drug of abuse, a medication) or a general medical condition.

Brief Psychotic Disorder

A. Presence of one (or more) of the following symptoms:
   1. Delusions
   2. Hallucinations
   3. Disorganized speech (eg, frequent derailment or incoherence)
   4. Grossly disorganized or catatonic behavior
B. Duration of an episode of the disturbance is at least 1 day but less than 1 month, with eventual full return to premorbid level of functioning.
C. The disturbance is not better accounted for by a Mood Disorder With Psychotic Features, Schizoaffective Disorder, or Schizophrenia and is not due to the direct physiologic effects of a substance (eg, a drug of abuse, a medication) or a general medical condition.

Shared Psychotic Disorder (Formerly Called Folie à Deux)

A. A delusion develops in an individual in the context of a close relationship with another person(s), who has an already-established delusion.
B. The delusion is similar in content to that of the person who already has the established delusion.
C. The disturbance is not better accounted for by another Psychotic Disorder (eg, Schizophrenia) or a Mood Disorder With Psychotic Features and is not due to the direct physiologic effects of a substance (eg, a drug of abuse, a medication) or a general medical condition.

Reprinted with permission from the *Diagnostic and Statistical Manual of Mental Disorders, 4th edition, text revision* (Copyright © 2000). American Psychiatric Association.

the entire gamut of skills necessary to process information correctly; it encompasses such important functions as memory, attention, and judgment. Through cognition, people learn about the world and their place in it. People with schizophrenia may have many cognitive difficulties at all stages of the illness, from prodromal to chronic (Sponheim et al., 2010).

Researchers have found three dimensions of psychopathology in schizophrenia: (1) disorganized, (2) psychotic, and (3) negative (Andreasen, 2000). For this discussion, the positive and negative symptoms are organized according to these three dimensions (Box 29.1).

The Disorganization Dimension

The *disorganization dimension* involves formal thought disorder, which affects the relationships and associations among the words people use to express thoughts (ie, the verbal form of thoughts). However, nurses must keep in mind that clients with mania or depression manifest thought disorder frequently and may have difficulties with cognition and cognitive processes (see Chaps. 27 and 28). None of the problems with cognition are believed to be disorder specific (Andreasen, 1999a). That said, many people with schizophrenia have disturbances in conceptual thinking that make their ideas difficult to follow. Manifestations include disorganized speech, disorganized or bizarre behavior, and incongruous affect.

DISORGANIZED SPEECH. Because thinking and speech are related intimately, disorganized thought is manifested by bizarre and convoluted speech. Historically, disorganized speech has been considered a primary characteristic of schizophrenia (Andreasen & Black, 2006). Researchers believe that clients cannot process complex thoughts or express coherent sentences because of malfunctioning in their information processing, which may be blocked, accelerated, or delayed because of alterations in brain structure and functioning (Andreasen, 1999b).

What you can see!

BOX 29.1 Positive and Negative Symptoms of Schizophrenia

Positive Symptoms

Positive formal thought disorder
- Derailment
- Tangentiality
- Incoherence
- Illogicality
- Circumstantiality
- Pressure of speech
- Distractible speech
- Clanging

Bizarre behavior
- Clothing, appearance
- Social, sexual behavior
- Aggressive, agitated behavior
- Repetitive, stereotyped behavior

Delusions
- Persecutory
- Jealous
- Guilt, sin based
- Grandiose
- Religious
- Somatic
- Delusions of reference
- Delusions of being controlled
- Delusions of mind reading
- Thought broadcasting
- Thought insertion
- Thought withdrawal

Hallucinations
- Auditory
- Voices commenting
- Voices conversing
- Somatic-tactile hallucinations
- Olfactory
- Visual

Negative Symptoms

Alogia
- Poverty of speech
- Poverty of content of speech
- Blocking
- Increased response latency

Affective flattening or blunting
- Unchanging facial expression
- Decreased spontaneous movements
- Paucity of expressive gestures
- Poor eye contact
- Affective nonresponsiveness
- Lack of vocal inflections

Avolition
- Impaired grooming and hygiene
- Lack of persistence at work or school
- Physical anergia

Anhedonia
- Few recreational interests or activities
- Little sexual interest or activity
- Impaired intimacy or closeness
- Few relationships with friends or peers

Attentional impairment
- Social inattentiveness
- Inattentiveness during testing

Harder to detect

The lack of a logical relationship between thoughts and ideas may be manifested by vague, diffuse, or unfocused speech (loose associations). Incoherent speech may involve the use of totally unrelated words (word salad). Some clients simply cannot get to the point (tangentiality). An example of loose associations follows:

> Let's see, there was one I would have liked if it wasn't for the instructor, well I go along with his, he was always wanted me to do the worse in the class, it seemed like, and I'd always get the bad, the grade, in my grading, and he tried to make other people like they were good enough to be in Hollywood or something, you know. I'd be the last one down the ladder. That, that's the way they wanted the grading to be in the first place according to whose, theirs, they, they have all different reasons that I, I think that they use that they want one, won't come out (Andreasen, 1985, p. 61).

Other examples of disorganized speech include *perseveration* (repeating oneself), distractibility, *clanging* (sound associations replace conceptual connections), *neologisms* (made-up words whose meaning is known only to the person), echolalia, and thought blocking. See Box 29.2.

People with schizophrenia may also use words in peculiar ways (Horwath & Cournos, 1999). For example, when a woman was asked why she was in the hospital, she replied, "Being unhealthy. In my head I feel like I'm a bleed." Clients may experience thought blocking, which is a sudden derailment or complete interruption in the flow of ideas. This disconcerting experience may leave clients feeling embarrassed or confused.

DISORGANIZED BEHAVIOR. Another aspect of disorganization is disorganized motor or social behaviors. People with schizophrenia may have profound psychomotor

Loose Associations

Nurse: What brought you to the hospital?
Client: I was home when a drum began beating. I flew too low.

Clanging

Nurse: Are you ready to take your stomach medicine?
Client: Peptobismuth, petrobismuth, peptibismark (for Pepto-Bismol); I'm gonna fly, cry, lie, buy, die.

Neologisms

Nurse: What are you holding?
Client: It's a fumebook. You know, a special temple to protect you.

Word Salad

Nurse: What would you like, Lucy?
Client: The thing that goes, the nails who made me barf.

retardation or excitement, and they may exhibit bizarre posture. Catatonic schizophrenia, in particular, is marked by episodes in which clients assume and maintain bizarre postures (Figure 29.3). In a catatonic stupor, clients may be unresponsive to questions or other stimuli, mute, and immobile, yet they may be fully conscious. Some clients may have a peculiar rigidity. They may allow others to move their limbs, but then they may hold them for hours in the position in which

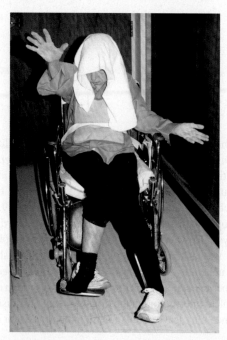

FIGURE 29.3 This woman with catatonic schizophrenia shows bizarre posturing and waxy flexibility. (Grunnitus Studio/Photo Researchers, Inc.)

they are placed. This is called *waxy flexibility.* In catatonic excitement, clients may show uncontrolled and aimless motor activity. They may engage in repetitive stereotypic movements with no apparent purpose, such as rocking back and forth for hours. Clients may also manifest normal mannerisms out of context, such as grimacing for no reason.

In addition, social behavior often deteriorates. Clients may withdraw from others and isolate themselves. They may become unkempt and wear the same clothing for weeks. Their surroundings may become cluttered and unfit for living. For example, they may refuse to bathe or clean up after themselves or their pets. Clients may also become "pack rats," hoarding papers and other nonessentials. In addition, they may exhibit socially inappropriate behaviors, such as defecating or masturbating in public.

INCONGRUOUS AFFECT. The final component of the disorganization dimension is incongruity or inappropriateness of affect (Andreasen & Black, 2006). In psychiatric terminology, *affect* refers to an observable behavior that expresses feeling or emotional tone in response to a certain stimulus. It refers to fluctuating changes in emotional "weather," whereas *mood* is a more sustained emotional "climate" (APA, 2000) (see Chap. 27). Clients with incongruent affect express themselves in a way that is not consistent with the situation or content of thought. They may smile or giggle for no apparent reason, or they may laugh uproariously while describing truly frightening or sad experiences.

The Psychotic Dimension

The psychotic dimension involves two classic symptoms that reflect confusion about the loss of boundaries between self and the external world: delusions and hallucinations. Delusions and hallucinations are real to clients with schizophrenia; people experiencing them are not simply "imagining things." These phenomena are physiologic events for clients, and important imaging studies have illustrated dramatic brain activity during hallucinations. See also Cultural Spotlight 29.1, which discusses the importance of context when considering psychotic manifestations in clients.

DELUSIONS. **Delusions** involve disturbances in thought content, rather than perception. They are firmly held false beliefs for which there is no support in reality, but that reasoning cannot correct. Delusions have varying themes and may be persecutory, grandiose, somatic, nihilistic, religious, or referential. Clients with paranoid schizophrenia usually have persecutory delusions. Examples include beliefs that neighbors, friends, or family are planning to harm them or are tormenting or ridiculing them; that others are spying on them; or that people or important organizations are controlling their bodies or minds. With grandiose delusions, clients falsely believe that they have great wealth, talent, influence, power, or beauty. Such clients may believe themselves to be famous or historically significant people, such as Napoleon or George Washington. Somatic delusions concern the body.

Delusions, Hallucinations, and Contextual Experience

When working with clients, health care providers must be cautious in differentiating psychotic symptoms from understandable and contextually oriented occurrences. For example, some religious people may discuss hearing the voice of God, seeing a spiritual vision, or having another experience that changed their view of the world or direction of their lives. Such a report or belief on the part of a client does not necessarily mean that he or she is experiencing a thought disorder. Spiritual or religious elements may be part of psychotic experiences, but assessment of the full spectrum of the client's symptoms and behaviors is necessary. Providers should not draw premature conclusions or dismiss strongly held religious beliefs because doing so can have damaging consequences on the therapeutic relationship (see Chap. 7).

Additionally, nurses and other providers must consider a client's life circumstances and contexts when listening to or exploring certain beliefs. For example, a client reports a lifelong fear that Hitler and the Nazis will return to try to rule the world. While such a belief might seem to indicate a delusion in some people, this concern would be totally understandable in a client who escaped from Poland in 1940 and lost many relatives in the Holocaust.

For example, clients might believe that they are incredibly ugly or that certain aspects of their appearance (eg, their noses) disgust others. Those with nihilistic delusions may believe that they are dead, dying, or no longer exist. With religious delusions, clients may believe that they have a special relationship with God or some other deity. In addition, they may think that they are the greatest sinners who ever lived or that they have a special mission from God. In referential delusions, clients believe that newspaper articles, television shows, or song lyrics are directed specifically at them.

Delusions are also accompanied by thought broadcasting, thought insertion, and thought withdrawal. In *thought broadcasting,* clients believe that others can perceive their thoughts (as though the thoughts are being aired out loud). Clients exhibiting *thought insertion* are convinced that their thoughts are not their own but rather the thoughts of others that have become implanted in their heads. In *thought withdrawal,* clients believe that their thoughts are somehow being removed from their heads.

The content and frequency of delusions vary according to culture. For example, in the United States clients may worry about the Federal Bureau of Investigation (FBI) or Central Intelligence Agency (CIA), whereas in other cultures they may worry more about demonic possession or possession by evil spirits (Andreasen & Black, 2006).

HALLUCINATIONS. Hallucinations are another manifestation of thought disorder (Challenging Behaviors 29.1). **Hallucinations** are sensory perceptions with a compelling sense of reality but no actual objective basis. During auditory hallucinations (the most common form), clients may hear the voice of God or close relatives, two or more voices with a running commentary about the client's behavior, or voices that command certain acts. Usually the voices are obscene, accusatory, or insulting. They may call clients names and make nasty remarks. Clients may hear voices with opposing views about the same subject, such as one voice giving commands to kill while another voice warns not to do so. Auditory hallucinations may also involve the sounds of bells, whistles, whispers, rustlings, and other noises; most often, however, they are of voices talking.

Challenging Behaviors 29.1

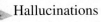

Hallucinations

Situation: Mr. Holland has a diagnosis of chronic schizophrenia. He has been hospitalized because of an exacerbation of symptoms, including hallucinations. When you approach him, he says: "The voices are telling me that you want to hurt me."

Your Potential Feelings: Anxiety, fear, nervousness about personal safety

What Is Going On? Mr. Holland is experiencing frightening, disturbing symptoms of psychosis. It is unlikely that he has personalized his fears to the nurse assigned to care for him that day. He is likely to experience all people as scary and threatening.

Strategy: Maintaining safety for yourself and the client is imperative. Maintain a nonthreatening stance, keep a physical distance away from Mr. Holland and, if possible, meet with him in an open space rather than a room with a closed door. Doing so allows him the freedom of retreating from the interaction and maintains your safety by allowing other staff on the unit to observe. Speak in a low, calm tone of voice. If Mr. Holland cannot tolerate a verbal interaction, let him know that you are available to talk when he wants to do so. Do not force him to talk or interact if he is actively hallucinating. Use peer support/supervision to ascertain the best technique in dealing with him.

Nurse Action/Communication: "I'm just checking in with you to see if there is anything you need right now. Please let me know if I can be helpful. Otherwise, I'll let you sit here quietly and will be at the nurse's station." Check his use of ordered PRN medication and offer it if appropriate.

Visual hallucinations (eg, monsters, frightening scenes) are less common than auditory hallucinations. They are likely to be threatening and are often accompanied by delusions and other sensory misperceptions. For example, clients with religious delusions may hear and see the Buddha or Christ beckoning them. Clients may also have tactile (touch), olfactory (smell), and gustatory (taste) hallucinations, but these are fairly uncommon. M**●**VIE viewing**GUIDES**

The Negative Dimension

The *DSM-IV-TR* (APA, 2000) lists three negative characteristic symptoms of schizophrenia: alogia, affective blunting, and avolition. Other common negative symptoms include anhedonia and attentional impairment. Negative symptoms account for substantial morbidity and impairment. They are most intractable and difficult to treat, and they reflect a deficiency of normal mental functioning.

Alogia is a poverty of thinking inferred by observing the client's language and speech (APA, 2000). People with alogia may have great difficulty producing fluent responses to questions and instead may manifest brief and concrete replies (Andreasen & Black, 2006). Spontaneous speech may also be reduced. Speech content may be empty and impoverished (poverty of speech). Sometimes the words themselves are adequate or even plentiful, but they convey little information because they are abstract, repetitive, or stereotypic (poverty of content).

Negative affect disturbances include **affective flattening or blunting**, which means a reduced intensity of emotional expression and response. The difference between flat and blunted affect is in degree. People with flat affect have no or minimal emotional expression (Figure 29.4). They may not react at all to circumstances that usually evoke strong emotions in others. People with blunted affect, on the other hand, have a significantly reduced intensity in emotional expression. They may react to circumstances but only slightly.

People with affective flattening or blunting fail to change their facial expressions in response to given circumstances. Movements lack spontaneity, gestures are slow and

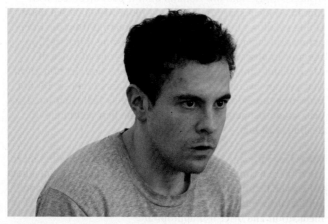

FIGURE 29.4 **Affective flattening.**

infrequent, voices lack inflection, and speech is considerably slow. Clients may appear wooden and robot-like; a loss of sense of self may accompany affective flattening. For example, a client may report that he or she has no feelings whatsoever and feels "dead" inside.

Complicating the picture of reduced intensity in emotional response is that up to 60% of people with schizophrenia report significant depressive symptoms (Andreasen, 1999a). However, depression is often difficult to recognize and diagnose because the symptoms of major depression and schizophrenia often overlap.

Avolition is the inability to start, persist in, and carry through any goal-directed activity to its logical conclusion (APA, 2000). In its most severe manifestation, avolition severely impairs social and occupational functioning. Clients seem to lose their will or drive. They cannot sustain work or engage in self-care. Some initiate projects and then disappear, abandoning endeavors for weeks or months. They may wander aimlessly or fail to show up to their jobs, if they have them. Others often accuse them of laziness, but avolition is not laziness; it is a loss of basic drive and capacity to formulate and pursue goals.

Anhedonia is loss of the capacity to experience pleasure subjectively. Clients may describe feeling empty and no longer able to enjoy activities (eg, hobbies, family, friends) that once gave them pleasure. This symptom is particularly tragic because clients are very aware that they have lost the capacity for pleasure. Researchers suggest that anhedonia should be further defined as anticipatory and consummatory (or in-the-moment) pleasure experiences. Individuals with schizophrenia may struggle more with anticipatory anhedonia (Gard et al., 2007). Clients also manifest an inability to concentrate. This attentional impairment may result from having to attend to multiple stimuli. For example, clients may be listening to inner voices and thus be unable to attend to external social interactions.

Other Symptoms

Lack of insight is a common symptom of schizophrenia. Clients may not believe that they are sick or that their behavior is at all odd or abnormal. Lack of insight is one of the most difficult aspects to treat. It may remain even if other symptoms, such as delusions and hallucinations, are brought under control.

Subtypes of Schizophrenia

Schizophrenia can be divided into five subtypes, largely based on the particular set of signs and symptoms that clients exhibit:

- *Paranoid*—Clients are preoccupied with delusions of persecution or grandeur (organized around a coherent theme), ideas of reference, or frequent auditory hallucinations. They may appear tense, suspicious, guarded, reserved, hostile, or aggressive.
- *Disorganized*—Clients demonstrate markedly regressed, disorganized, silly, inappropriate, and uninhibited

behavior; disorganized speech; flat or inappropriate affect; poor reality contact; poor grooming and social skills; a prominent thought disorder; and possibly grimacing, strange mannerisms, or other odd behaviors.

- *Catatonic*—Clients show motoric immobility or stupor, rigidity, excessive motor activity, extreme negativism, stupor, and peculiarities of movement, such as posturing, echolalia and echopraxia, mutism, and waxy flexibility.
- *Undifferentiated*—Behavior and speech clearly indicate schizophrenic psychosis but fail to meet the criteria of paranoid, disorganized, or catatonic types.
- *Residual*—Clients do not have active, positive symptoms, such as hallucinations and delusions, but continue to demonstrate negative symptoms, such as withdrawal from others or flat affect (APA, 2000).

Water Intoxication

Some clients with chronic schizophrenia drink excessive water, thereby inducing a state of **water intoxication**, characterized by polyuria and hyponatremia. When this condition becomes severe, it can result in seizures, coma, cerebral edema, and even death. The reasons for drinking excessive water are unknown, but possibilities include a response to delusional belief, changes in the secretion of antidiuretic hormone, or abnormalities in the hypothalamic region, which regulates thirst and fluid intake (Goldman, 2010).

Preventing water intoxication can be a challenge. Treatment includes restricting water intake, although clients can be very creative at finding it. Some have been known to drink from toilets in the absence of any other water source. Treatment of severe water intoxication involves the administration of furosemide (Lasix) and intravenous (IV) normal saline. IV hyperosmolar saline may be given cautiously in an emergency. Treatment is necessarily slow because too rapid replacement of saline may result in permanent brain damage.

Checkpoint Questions

3. What characteristic symptoms are associated with schizophrenia, according to the *DSM-IV-TR?*
4. What are the three dimensions of psychopathology in schizophrenia?
5. What is meant by the term *waxy flexibility?*
6. What term denotes disturbances in thought content involving firmly held false beliefs that reasoning cannot correct and for which there is no support in reality?
7. What are the five subtypes of schizophrenia?

Comorbidities and Dual Diagnoses

Estimates are that 50% to 75% of people with severe mental illness also have substance abuse problems, nicotine addiction, or both. When people with serious illness have a substance use disorder, they are referred to as having a **dual diagnosis**. Alcohol is the most abused substance, followed in frequency by cannabis and cocaine. More than 70% of

clients with schizophrenia smoke cigarettes (Hennekens et al., 2005). The combination of substance abuse and schizophrenia is associated with increased symptoms, more frequent relapses, less treatment compliance, homelessness, and violence (Compton et al., 2005). Cannabis abuse can make medication management of schizophrenia less effective (Zullino et al., 2008).

Whereas others often take substances for the pleasurable "high," those with severe mental illness usually take drugs to cope with their psychiatric symptoms (eg, hallucinations). This is called *self-medication.* Treatment programs often fail to address the dual needs of addicted people with schizophrenia; effective treatment addresses both disorders in an integrated manner. See Chapter 30 for a discussion of substance abuse and treatment.

In addition to substance abuse, clients with schizophrenia often are also diagnosed with anxiety disorders, specifically obsessive-compulsive disorder and panic disorder. See Chapter 23.

Differential Diagnosis

Numerous medical conditions can precipitate a thought disorder, psychosis, or delirium. Health care providers must assess thoroughly the medical status of every client, especially those with a rapid onset of psychotic symptoms. When psychosis is associated with a general medical condition, determining the etiology or causal relationship can be difficult. "If the association is purely coincidental, or if the general medical condition is partly or completely a consequence of the disturbed behavior, the psychiatric syndrome is a primary psychotic disorder. An inference that the nonpsychiatric condition may be causing a secondary psychotic syndrome is usually based on evidence of a pathophysiology that could plausibly alter brain function" (Nasrallah & Smeltzer, 2003, p. 73). See Box 29.3 for a list of conditions other than thought disorder that can alter thinking.

Cooper (2003) used research from a drug attitude scale to suggest that psychiatric nurses are often uncomfortable identifying drug-induced psychosis in clients with a dual diagnosis. He cited a lack of knowledge about the relationship between illicit drug use and psychosis. His research points to the need for psychiatric nurses to assess the potential physical conditions that could precipitate psychosis. This necessitates taking a thorough medical history on new clients and understanding the influence of past health issues on the present.

Implications and Prognosis

Clients with schizophrenia are at high risk for suicide. Approximately 10% to 15% of those with schizophrenia commit suicide; 50% attempt suicide at least once. Other risk factors for suicide in this population include depressive symptoms, young age at the disorder's onset, and absence of supportive family and friends (Mamo, 2007).

Clients with schizophrenia also have a higher mortality rate from accidents and medical illnesses. Identifying

---

BOX 29.3 Differential Diagnoses of Thought Disorders

- Lead toxicity and other environmental toxins
- Drug ingestion (recreational/illicit, over-the-counter, and prescription), including asthma medications, insulin, antihistamines, steroids, and antihypertensives
- Neurologic conditions (eg, meningitis, tumors, Parkinson's disease)
- Endocrine disorders (eg, thyroid dysfunction, Cushing and Addison diseases, pheochromocytoma)
- Seizure disorder
- Sensory deficits
- Sleep apnea
- Connective tissue disease (eg, systemic lupus erythematosus)
- Head trauma
- Metabolic/systemic imbalances (eg, fluid and electrolyte disturbances, hepatic encephalopathy, uremia, porphyria, Wilson's disease, hypoxia, hypotension, chronic pulmonary disease)
- Nutritional abnormalities (eg, vitamin B_{12} deficiency, pellagra, folate deficiency, Wernicke–Korsakoff syndrome, trace metal deficiencies, malnutrition)
- Neoplastic disorders
- Infections (eg, AIDS, neurosyphilis, viral hepatitis, mononucleosis, tuberculosis, systemic bacterial infections)
- Preoperative and postoperative states and intensive care unit psychosis

---

medical illness is extremely difficult when clients are psychotic or otherwise cannot communicate clearly their medical symptoms. High rates of smoking cigarettes can precipitate chronic respiratory disease. Weight gain with neuroleptic medications can cause metabolic syndrome, type 2 diabetes, and associated cardiac problems. The physical health risks associated with schizophrenia are as serious as the psychiatric symptoms of the disorder (El-Mallakh et al., 2010). Nurses are urged to take a leadership role in improving the physical health status of individuals with schizophrenia.

Long-term prognosis for people with schizophrenia remains guarded. Although antipsychotic drugs are used to manage acute positive psychiatric symptoms, induce remission, maintain stability, and prevent relapse, they are not without side effects. Adherence to medication and treatment regimens is a chronic problem for many with schizophrenia. Integration of medication management with psychosocial interventions and rehabilitative therapies offers the best chance of a positive long-term outcome (El-Mallakh et al., 2010). Although there have been cases in which a person has only one schizophrenic episode (during adolescence) and never has another, exacerbations and remissions typically mark the course of the illness. The pattern of symptoms in the first 5 years of the illness foreshadows the course of relapses and periods of functioning. Each psychotic episode leaves clients with a decreased level of functioning. Specifiers to describe the course of schizophrenia may be added after the first year of symptoms. These course specifiers include "episodic with

or without interepisode residual symptoms," "continuous," or "a single episode in full or partial remission" (APA, 2000).

The repeated admission of clients with schizophrenia to psychiatric hospitals is referred to as the *revolving door syndrome* (see Chap. 1). The two most predictive factors of repeated or "revolving door" admissions are substance abuse and failure to follow medication regimens.

Interdisciplinary Goals and Treatment

Both pharmacologic and psychosocial interventions are necessary to safeguard clients and promote their recovery. A combination of antipsychotic medications targeting the psychotic symptoms and psychosocial interventions aimed at social-cognitive deficits is generally thought to be the best model of care (Evidence-Based Practice Spotlight 29.1). In addition, mobilization of social supports and continuity of care, including discharge planning and ongoing care within the community, are essential interventions.

Overall goals of treatment for clients with schizophrenia include the following:

- Safety in all settings
- Stabilization on antipsychotic medication
- Client and family education about schizophrenia and its treatment
- Physical care of client
- Psychosocial support of client and family

The scope and breadth of needs are too great for any one professional to meet. An interdisciplinary team works together to provide the comprehensive care necessary to achieve desired outcomes. Professionals from psychiatry, nursing, psychology, and social work supply therapeutic services to clients with schizophrenia (see Chap. 12).

Case management and rehabilitation services are also essential to recovery (see Chap. 20). The most effective treatment model requires coordination of multidisciplinary care by a case manager. The case manager ensures that clients receive effective services, helps various care providers communicate with one another about interventions, functions as a liaison for and with family members, and works directly with clients to assess needs and arrange services. Clinical pathways, a tool that many case managers use, help the entire team monitor the client's progress over time (Table 29.1).

An optimal model of interdisciplinary treatment for those with schizophrenia includes assessment of current functioning, medication management, client and family education, skills training, family counseling, vocational training and rehabilitation, housing assistance, crisis intervention and brief inpatient services, continuity of care providers, and a network of ongoing social support. In 1992, the Agency for Healthcare Policy and Research and the National Institute of Mental Health funded the Schizophrenia Patient Outcomes Research Team (PORT) to develop and disseminate evidence-based recommendations for the treatment of schizophrenia. The team was developed in conjunction with

EVIDENCE-BASED PRACTICE SPOTLIGHT 29.1

Interventions for Schizophrenia

Overview of Effective Treatment: Antipsychotic medications have become the dominant mode of treatment for schizophrenia. Although use of these agents has both positive and negative aspects, research has shown that most clients receiving medication have fewer psychotic and negative symptoms. Limitations include significant side effects accompanied by the adverse effects of long-term use of neuroleptic medications.

Outcome studies have emphasized psychosocial treatment strategies, in conjunction with medication management, as preventing relapse and promoting overall functioning. Clients with strong social supports, including families, have a lower rate of relapse. Cognitive–behavioral therapy may also be helpful in preventing relapse. Specifically, cognitive interventions may be useful to assist with auditory hallucinations.

All relapse data are linked to the client's adherence to the prescribed medication regimen. When clients discontinue medication, there is a risk that the psychotic and negative symptoms associated with schizophrenia will reappear, regardless of psychosocial supports. Providing specialized care for people with early psychosis might decrease the number of inpatient readmissions.

What Has Not Been Shown Effective: No recent studies recommend the use of individual psychodynamic psychotherapy as an evidence-based treatment for clients with schizophrenia. In fact, sources suggest that this model of treatment is inappropriate for clients with schizophrenia. No studies can associate the effectiveness of family interventions in reducing families' levels of expressed emotion. Use of electroconvulsive therapy is not thought to be effective in managing the symptoms of schizophrenia.

Implications for Practice: Treatment of schizophrenia should be multidimensional and include medication management in conjunction with psychosocial interventions. Examples of interventions include psychoeducation about illness and side effects and support for activities of daily living. Nurses are in a key position to monitor the status of their clients with schizophrenia, noting that the key to relapse prevention involves maintaining contact with them and supporting them as they struggle with their illness. A strong need exists for nursing research involving specific intervention models that keep clients from experiencing relapses and maximize their functioning in the community.

References

Craig, T. K., Garety, P., Power, P., Rahaman, N., Colbert, S., Fornells-Ambrojo, M., & Dunn, G. (2004). The Lambeth Early Onset (LEO) Team: Randomized controlled trial of the effectiveness of specialized care for early psychosis. *British Medical Journal, 329,* 1067–1070.

England, M. (2006). Cognitive intervention for voice hearers. *Issues in Mental Health Nursing, 27,* 735–751.

Garety, P. A., Craig, T. K. J., & Dunn, G. (2006). Specialised care for early psychosis: Symptoms, social functioning and patient satisfaction—randomised controlled trial. *British Journal of Psychiatry, 188,* 37–45.

Hewitt, J., & Coffey, M. (2005). Therapeutic working relationships with people with schizophrenia: Literature review. *Journal of Advanced Nursing, 52,* 561–570.

Sadock, B. J., & Sadock, V. A. (2004). *Kaplan & Sadock's comprehensive textbook of psychiatry* (8th ed.). Philadelphia, PA: Lippincott Williams & Wilkins.

---

the University of Maryland School of Medicine and the Johns Hopkins University School of Public Health. The original and updated PORT recommendations, all evidence based, are statements about the care of people with schizophrenia The team's updated recommendations include addressing treatment of health conditions that disproportionately affect individuals with schizophrenia, including cigarette smoking, drug addiction, and antipsychotic-related weight gain (Kreyenbuhl et al., 2010). These can address other psychiatric and medical conditions, personal and social circumstances, and individual variations. The intervention categories are defined as follows:

- Antipsychotic medications
- Adjunctive pharmacotherapies for anxiety, depression, and aggression/hostility
- Electroconvulsive therapy
- Psychological interventions
- Family interventions

- Vocational rehabilitation
- Assertive community treatment/assertive case management (Lehman et al., 2004)

The PORT recommendations are based on substantial scientific evidence of efficacy; many of them focus on pharmacotherapies because considerably more research findings support the effectiveness of medications for clients with schizophrenia. Psychosocial modalities remain important, but less is known about which of these specific strategies are most helpful. Lack of empirical data signifies the need for more research about psychosocial interventions.

Checkpoint Questions

8. What is the typical course of schizophrenia?

9. What are the two most predictive factors of repeated admissions for clients with schizophrenia?

TABLE 29.1 **Clinical Pathway: Schizophrenic Disorder (295.1x, catatonic 295.2x, delusional 297.10, brief reactive psychosis 298.80)**

Patient Name: _____ Case Manager: _____ Physician: _____ Medical Record # _____

Admit date: _____ Expected LOS: _____ UR days certified: _____ Discharge date: _____

Actual LOS: _____

DAY/DATE:	0–8 HOURS	8–24 HOURS	DAY 2	DAY 3	DAY 4	DAY 5
ASSESSMENTS & EVALUATIONS	Nursing assessment Nutritional screening, wt Admit note, Precautions	H & P, Social Hx, RT/TA; Dr. Initial TX Plan/Admit Note Prec. Eval. AIMS Scale	Precaution Evaluation Document sleep patterns Observe/ document nonverbal behavior	Psych Eval done Social Hx done Precaution Evaluation	Assess readiness for discharge	Assess for goals achieved
PROCEDURES	Lab ordered-Admit profile UA, UDS, UCG, EKG, Other:	Lab done: UA, UDS, UCG, EKG Other:	Lab results checked Abnormals called to Dr.	Physician progress note r/t abnormal lab values		
CONSULTS	IT ordered Y/N FT ordered Y/N GT ordered Y/N	GT started Psych Testing Order Y/N	Schedule MTP meeting	IT started, FT started Psych Testing Done Home Contract		Psych Testing results
TREATMENT PLANNING	N1: _____ Axis III _____		RT/TA started School started	Master TX Plan Update/ Revise, RT/TA		
INTERVENTIONS	Assess S/H or Aggr. monitor anxiety stimulus	Monitor sleep pattern, orient × 4	Encourage group interaction	Give honest and consistent feedback	Encourage oral hygiene, adeq. fluid intake 2,000 mL	Assess client support net-work, output resources
MEDICATIONS	Meds ordered, Inf. Con.	Assess for EPS	Drug inter-action ✓'d, Dr. signs Inf. Con. ✓ for EPS	Meds evaluated/ readjusted Assess for EPS	Observe/ document response to Rx, ✓ for EPS	Discharge instructions for medication self-admin
LEVEL	Level ordered		Re-evaluate	Reevaluate	Reevaluate consider PHP	Reevaluate
TEACHING	Patient Rights Orient to Unit	Orient to Program	Goals setting, relaxation techniques	Meds reinforced; Altered perceptions as symptom	Coping skills for unusual perceptions	Teach family S/S of Rx non-compliance
NUTRITION/DIET	Type: _____	Chart daily intake	Chart daily intake	Chart daily intake	Chart daily intake	Chart daily intake
CARE CONTINUUM	Initial D/C Plans	Placement Search Outcome survey		Discharge Plan updated/rev		After care plan written Outcome survey

DAY/DATE:	0–8 HOURS	8–24 HOURS	DAY 2	DAY 3	DAY 4	DAY 5
CLIENT OUTCOMES	Controls violent impulses	ADLs w/assist, oriented × 3	Tolerates peer interaction	Improves insight	Uses adaptive coping skills	Goal-directed interactions

ADLs, activities of daily living; EKG, electrocardiogram; FT, family therapy; GT, group therapy; H & P, history and physical; Hx, history; IT, individual therapy; MTP, master treatment plan; r/t, related to; RT/TA, recreational therapy/therapeutic activities; S/H, suicide/homicide precautions; S/S, signs and symptoms; Signs Inf Con, signs informed consent; TX, treatment; UA, urinalysis; UDS, urine drug screen; UCG, urine test for pregnancy; ✓ for EPS, check for extrapyramidal symptoms.
Strategic Clinical Systems, Inc., 3715 Mission Ct., Granbury, TX 76049 (817) 326-4239. PsychPaths, Copyright © 1994. All rights reserved.
Authors: Darla Belt, RN, & Vickie Pflueger, RNC.

Psychopharmacologic Interventions

Because failure of clients to take prescribed medications is the primary cause of relapses of schizophrenia, adherence to a drug regimen is critical to successful treatment and relapse prevention. Antipsychotic (neuroleptic) medications are essential to treat symptoms during both acute and long-term phases of the illness. However, they do not cure schizophrenia. Early intervention with medication decreases some associated long-term comorbid, or coexisting, conditions. Medication also makes clients more amenable to other social, cognitive, and rehabilitative therapies.

Two categories of antipsychotic drugs are available to treat schizophrenia: traditional and atypical (Understanding Psychopharmacology Box 29.1). Traditional antipsychotics have been available since 1952 and most optimally manage mostly positive symptoms of schizophrenia. However, associated side effects (especially extrapyramidal side effects [EPSs]) are numerous and distressing; they often lead clients to become nonadherent. Neurobiology-based findings led researchers to develop the more recent atypical antipsychotics, which are effective against both positive and negative symptoms and less likely to induce EPSs. Older adults, who are particularly sensitive to EPSs, have better response to atypical antipsychotics (see Chap. 16).

Clients usually take antipsychotic drugs orally in liquid or tablet form, but intramuscular injections are also available for immediate action. In addition, some forms can be given in depot injections that release the medication over 2 to 4 weeks.

TRADITIONAL (CONVENTIONAL) ANTIPSYCHOTICS.

Traditional antipsychotics primarily treat hallucinations and delusions. This group includes chlorpromazine (Thorazine), fluphenazine (Prolixin), haloperidol (Haldol), trifluoperazine (Stelazine), thioridazine (Mellaril), thiothixene (Navane), and perphenazine (Trilafon). See Chapter 16 for a comprehensive discussion of their mechanisms of action and side effects.

The most common and distressing problem associated with traditional antipsychotics are acute **extrapyramidal side effects**, which may make clients feel worse than before they started taking medication, contributing to nonadherence. EPSs include *akathisia* (severe restlessness), *dystonia* (muscle spasms or contractions), chronic motor problems, and the pseudoparkinsonian symptoms of rigidity, masklike faces, and stiff gait (Karch, 2009).

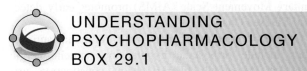

UNDERSTANDING PSYCHOPHARMACOLOGY BOX 29.1

Traditional and Atypical Antipsychotic Medications

MEDICATIONS	USUAL ADULT DAILY DOSAGE
Traditional (Conventional) Antipsychotic Medications	
High potency	
haloperidol (Haldol)	2–20 mg/day
fluphenazine (Prolixin)	2–20 mg/day
Medium potency	
thiothixene (Navane)	5–30 mg/day
trifluoperazine (Stelazine)	5–30 mg/day
perphenazine (Trilafon)	8–64 mg/day
molindone (Moban)	50–225 mg/day
loxapine (Loxitane)	25–100 mg/day
Low potency	
chlorpromazine (Thorazine)	200–800 mg/day
thioridazine (Mellaril)	150–600 mg/day
Long-acting depot antipsychotic medications	
depot haloperidol	50–200 mg as a monthly injection
depot fluphenazine	6.25–50 mg as injection every 2–3 weeks
Atypical (Novel) Antipsychotic Medications	
risperidone (Risperdal)	2–8 mg/day
clozapine (Clozaril)	150–600 mg/day
olanzapine (Zyprexa)	5–20 mg/day
quetiapine (Seroquel)	150–750 mg/day
ziprasidone (Geodon)	40–160 mg/day
aripiprazole (Abilify)	2–30 mg/day
paliperidone (Invega)	3–12 mg/day
asenapine maleate (Saphris)	5 mg/bid
iloperidone (Fanapt)	6–12 mg/bid
lurasidone (Latuda)	40–120 mg/day
olanzapine/fluoxetine (Symbyax)	6 mg/25 mg/day

EPSs are usually treated by reducing dosage, trying a different drug, or adding a medication that reduces or eliminates side effects (Understanding Psychopharmacology Box 29.2).

Tardive dyskinesia (TD) is a type of EPS characterized by abnormal, involuntary, irregular, choreoathetoid (writhing) movements, which may include lip smacking, neck twisting, facial grimacing, and chewing without food (Figure 29.5). TD can occur after several months to years of therapy with traditional antipsychotics; it develops in approximately one third of those who use these drugs. Treatment for TD usually involves decreasing or discontinuing the medication. Assessment by means of the Abnormal Involuntary Movement Scale (AIMS) promotes early detection of TD (see Chap. 16).

Other side effects associated with traditional antipsychotics include orthostatic hypotension; anticholinergic effects (eg, dry mouth, blurred vision, constipation, urinary retention); endocrine effects of amenorrhea, breast enlargement, galactorrhea, and male erectile dysfunction; photosensitivity; tachycardia; sedation; weight gain; and agranulocytosis (Buchanan & Carpenter, 2004). An associated life-threatening complication is neuroleptic malignant syndrome (NMS), marked by elevated temperature, severe EPSs (eg, rigidity, dystonia), autonomic dysfunction (eg, hypertension, tachycardia, diaphoresis), and an elevated creatine phosphokinase level. NMS requires immediate medical attention, transfer to an intensive care unit, and administration of bromocriptine and dantrolene (Buchanan & Carpenter, 2004).

UNDERSTANDING PSYCHOPHARMACOLOGY BOX 29.2

Medications Used for Side Effects of Antipsychotics

Anticholinergics—Used to treat parkinsonism and dystonia; may reduce akathisia
  benztropine (Cogentin) 1–6 mg
  trihexyphenidyl (Artane) 5–15 mg
Dopamine agonist—Used for its antiparkinsonian effect, without anticholinergic problems; may be less effective than anticholinergics
  amantadine (Symmetrel) 100–400 mg
Beta blocker (only central-acting not peripheral beta blockers)—Used to treat akathisia; contraindicated in clients with diabetes and asthma
  propranolol (Inderal) 30–100 mg
Benzodiazepines—Should not be used for clients with substance abuse; use with caution with clozapine because of the risk of respiratory depression and arrest
  clonazepam (Klonopin) 1.5–4 mg
  lorazepam (Ativan) 2–8 mg
Antihistamine—Used in IM form for rapid relief of acute dystonia; used to treat akathisia when sedation is needed
  diphenhydramine (Benadryl) 25–150 mg

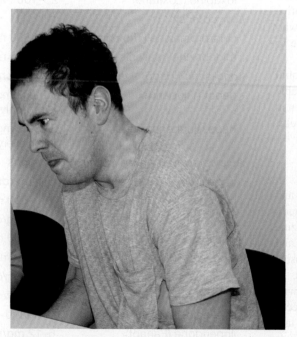
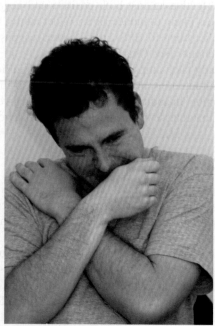

FIGURE 29.5 Clients with tardive dyskinesia may show involuntary movements such as sticking out their tongues or grimacing for no reason.

ATYPICAL (NOVEL) ANTIPSYCHOTICS. Atypical antipsychotics relieve both positive and negative symptoms of schizophrenia. They are also less likely to cause distressing EPSs. Atypical antipsychotics, discussed in depth in Chapter 16, include clozapine (Clozaril), risperidone (Risperdal), olanzapine (Zyprexa), quetiapine (Seroquel), ziprasidone (Geodon), aripiprazole (Abilify), paliperidone (Invega), asenapine maleate (Saphris), iloperidone (Fanapt), and lurasidone (Latuda). A combination medication of olanzapine and fluoxetine is marketed as Symbyax. See also Evidence-Based Practice Spotlight 29.2.

Since its U.S. release in 1989, clozapine (Clozaril) has been effective in treating refractory schizophrenia (ie, schizophrenia that does not respond to ordinary treatment). People with refractory schizophrenia make up approximately 30% of the total client population and are particularly prone to violence and suicide. Clozapine use has resulted in decreased negative symptoms, increased impulse control, reduced violence to self and others, and improved quality of life. Although not associated with EPSs or TD, clozapine has the potentially fatal side effect of agranulocytosis (1% to 2% incidence). Adverse reactions include lowered seizure threshold, hypotension, sedation, and elevated liver enzymes. Because agranulocytosis can be life-threatening, nurses provide extensive education to clients taking clozapine and their families, monitor weekly hematologic counts, and report and document any drop in white blood cell count. Another unpleasant side effect is weight gain. In general, clozapine is not used as a first-line agent because of the danger agranulocytosis poses.

Risperidone (Risperdal), an atypical antipsychotic approved for first-line treatment of thought disorders, effectively manages positive and negative symptoms with reduced EPSs and TD. The most commonly reported side effects are drowsiness, orthostatic hypotension, light-headedness, anxiety, dizziness, nausea, akathisia, constipation, and weight

---

△ EVIDENCE-BASED PRACTICE SPOTLIGHT 29.2 △

Clinical Antipsychotic Trials of Intervention Effectiveness (CATIE)

Purpose: To compare effectiveness of atypical antipsychotics with one another and with a traditional antipsychotic. The study involved long-term use, multiple comparisons, and real clients and was not sponsored by a pharmaceutical company.

Hypothesis: Researchers proposed that they would find significant differences in effectiveness among olanzapine, quetiapine, risperidone, ziprasidone, and perphenazine.

Design: The study included 1,493 clients 18 to 65 years diagnosed with schizophrenia. It excluded those with schizoaffective disorder, mental retardation, cognitive disorders, and serious and unstable medication conditions, as well as pregnant or breast-feeding women. It also excluded clients with a history of adverse reaction to one of the proposed treatments, treatment resistance, or only one schizophrenic episode. It allowed clients with comorbid medical illness and substance use and clients using other medications (except other antipsychotics).

This double-blind, controlled, randomized, three-phase study was done between January 2001 and December 2004 at 57 sites. Clients were randomized to olanzapine (7.5–30 mg/day), quetiapine (200–800 mg/day), risperidone (1.5–6 mg/day), ziprasidone (40–160 mg/day), or perphenazine (8–32 mg/day). Researchers added ziprasidone in January 2002 after receiving FDA approval for use.

Results
- No antipsychotic with a high degree of safety and tolerability causes a high degree of recovery in a substantial number of clients with schizophrenia.
- Appropriate dosing is critical to attaining optimum benefits from each agent.
- Studying long-term outcome is likely the best way of determining efficacy among agents.
- Client characteristics, such as length of illness, prior treatment, and treatment resistance could also be related to long-term outcome.

The study raised many questions:
- Should ziprasidone be used preferentially in clients with or even just at risk for metabolic problems?
- Should olanzapine be a preferred agent for clients who did not experience response to other agents?
- Should the conventional antipsychotics with lower risks of EPSs (such as perphenazine) be used more often?
- How would aripiprazole have compared to the agents in this study?

In summary, multiple treatment options should be available to people with schizophrenia. Also, conventional antipsychotics remain a viable option when planning treatment. Treatment should also be customized to each client.

References

Lieberman, J. A., Stroup, T. S., McEvoy, J. P., Swartz, M. S., Rosenheck, R. A., Perkins, D. O., . . . Hsiao, J. K. (2005). Effectiveness of antipsychotic drugs in patients with chronic schizophrenia. *New England Journal of Medicine, 353,* 1209–1223.

Stroup, T. S., Lieberman, J. A., McEvoy, J. P., Swartz, M. S., Davis, S. M., Capuano, G. A., . . . Hsiao, J. K. (2007). Effectiveness of olanzapine, quetiapine, and risperidone in patients with chronic schizophrenia after discontinuing perphenazine: A CATIE study. *American Journal of Psychiatry, 164,* 415–427.

gain. Olanzapine (Zyprexa), also approved for first-line use, has demonstrated an even lower incidence of EPSs than risperidone. Side effects are somnolence, nausea, light-headedness, dizziness, constipation, substantial weight gain, and headache (Karch, 2009). Quetiapine (Seroquel) is a relatively new atypical antipsychotic. Akathisia and EPSs have been reported rarely with its use, and older adults with psychoses seem to tolerate it well (McManus et al., 1999). Side effects include drowsiness, dizziness, postural hypotension, agitation, dry mouth, and weight gain (Karch, 2009).

In mid-2000, the U.S. Food and Drug Administration (FDA) approved the release of ziprasidone (Geodon), which is effective in treating negative, positive, and depressive symptoms of schizophrenia. Although side effects include somnolence, orthostatic hypotension, headache, nausea, constipation, dysphagia, and potential dysrhythmias, ziprasidone is considered weight neutral (ie, it does not make users gain weight). Most recently, aripiprazole (Abilify) for schizophrenia promises a much lower side-effect profile than other atypical antipsychotics. Paliperidone (Invega), an extended-release derivative of Risperdal, also has a side-effect profile lower than that of other atypical agents.

Although atypical antipsychotics are of great benefit to many people and usually do not have accompanying EPSs, a significant risk exists for the adverse effects of obesity, diabetes, and metabolic syndrome. Diabetes tends to develop within the first few months of treatment. Metabolic syndrome includes weight gain and hypertriglyceridemia, along with increased insulin, glucose, and low-density lipoprotein levels. Researchers are investigating a link between the use of atypical antipsychotics and abnormal glucose metabolism. They are also trying to determine whether some specific atypical antipsychotics pose greater or lesser risks for diabetic, metabolic, and cardiovascular alterations and complications than others. A key issue is that, regardless of the type of antipsychotic prescribed, nurses and other health care providers must be vigilant about careful baseline screening and follow-up monitoring to mitigate the risk of various complications that can develop (Bergman & Ader, 2005; Scheen & De Hert, 2007).

Psychosocial Interventions

Although pharmacotherapy is the staple of treatment for schizophrenia, it alone is not sufficient. Clients require additional strategies to address the many wide-ranging ramifications of the illness. Psychosocial care assists clients and families to cope with stress and problem solving; educates them about the illness, its treatment, and self-care; enhances medication compliance; and provides rehabilitative support to help clients master skills of independent living.

MILIEU MANAGEMENT. Milieu management refers to providing an environment rich with therapeutic possibility. Inpatients with thought disorders likely have impaired judgment and reality testing. Also, safety needs are paramount. Health care staff members assume responsibility for the well-being

and physical care of clients who cannot meet those basic needs. Symptom management and family education are ongoing in the milieu. Recreational and activity therapies can increase the client's social and occupational skills.

INDIVIDUAL AND GROUP THERAPY. Individual and group therapies that offer support, education, and behavioral and cognitive skills training (see the following section) are recommended to improve functioning and address specific problems, such as medication noncompliance or social isolation (see Chaps. 13 and 14). Conversely, individual and group therapies that focus on gaining insight into unconscious material are not recommended because these therapies may result in regression and transference, which can be harmful to these clients (Lehman et al., 2004). Rather, the goals of individual therapy are building a therapeutic relationship, helping clients stay oriented to reality, and assisting them to improve coping skills. This relationship can help clients experience guidance, support, and reinforcement for their health promotion efforts and successes.

Group therapy sessions focus on social skills, concentrating on appropriate interpersonal interaction. The therapist role-plays with clients, modeling and identifying suitable social actions and responses. Groups repeatedly act out various scenarios related to key social behaviors, during which clients receive feedback and support. Treatment also addresses practical matters, such as personal care, living skills, and money management.

COGNITIVE–BEHAVIORAL THERAPY. Cognitive–behavioral therapy (CBT) is an effective adjunct to antipsychotic medication and social skills training in managing symptoms of schizophrenia (England, 2007; Turkington et al., 2004). CBT aims to improve motivation, socialization, and reality testing through goal setting, increased coping and problem-solving skills, enhanced self-esteem, and improved control. Clients learn to replace distorted thoughts with rational and logical thoughts that have better outcomes. Clients also report learning rational self-talk. Evidence shows that CBT is most effective for positive symptoms and depression and less effective for negative symptoms (Turkington et al., 2004). It can be combined with family therapy and assertive community treatment programs (discussed later) targeting relapse prevention.

SOCIAL SKILLS TRAINING. Clear empirical evidence supports social skills training for people with schizophrenia. A review of studies evaluating interventions found that social skills training consistently resulted in improved social adjustment, independent living skills, cognitive measures, social competence, and skill acquisition (Landeen, 2001). It had no clear effects on employment status, relapse prevention, or psychopathology. Social skills training may improve the social competence of people with schizophrenia, resulting in improved adaptive functioning in the community (Velligan & Gonzalez, 2007).

VOCATIONAL REHABILITATION. Another aspect of psychosocial therapy involves employment training (Velligan & Gonzalez, 2007). Some clients with schizophrenia can be gainfully employed and should be offered vocational rehabilitation, particularly if they identify employment as a goal, have a history of successful employment and few psychiatric hospitalizations, and show good work skills. Vocational rehabilitation involves speedy placement in a real job, coupled with assistance and coaching from a therapist or job coach (Figure 29.6). The coach supports the client's transition back to work and encourages him or her to become involved in vocational educational services and counseling (Lehman et al., 1998).

Continuum of Care

People with schizophrenia require a seamless system of comprehensive care. Continuity must be preserved as clients move to and from various settings. Issues include medication and symptom monitoring, follow-up care, use of appropriate resources and services, and ongoing training and assistance with the skills needed for independent living.

DISCHARGE PLANNING. During an acute psychotic episode, care in the inpatient setting includes collaborative treatment planning with family members or friends who will be involved in the client's care in the community.

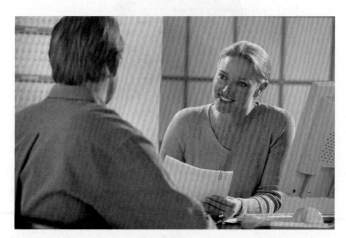

FIGURE 29.6 A job coach can be part of vocational rehabilitation for clients with schizophrenia. The coach can help the client to find appropriate educational and employment services, as well as help with job placement.

Introduction to community resources, arrangements for appointments with accessible community agencies, and information about phone help lines and how to contact care providers should be part of discharge teaching. Connecting clients and family members to NAMI support groups can provide an invaluable learning experience for them as well as an enormous source of emotional and social support. When clients are outpatients, needs are usually met through community mental health centers.

CARE IN THE COMMUNITY. The continuum of care in the community must provide for the client's extensive needs. Transportation, nutrition, social activities, substance abuse education, medication monitoring, psychoeducation, and access to decent, safe, and affordable housing are services that extend beyond traditional care boundaries but are essential in the client's rehabilitation. Employment is associated with better quality of life for clients with schizophrenia; employers should be prepared to give direct and constructive feedback to clients. These people are neither helpless nor frail and should not be regarded as such.

Unfortunately, deinstitutionalization from state hospitals has led to reinstitutionalization in jails, nursing homes, and shelters for many clients with long-term psychiatric problems; many other clients are living on the streets. The problems of those with schizophrenia, including substance abuse and medical illness, are complex. Clients require both physical and psychological assessment and management, medication monitoring, housing, rehabilitation, and community support. The Community Mental Health Center Act of 1963 brought about the construction of local community mental health centers where clients could receive services in their own communities. Community-based care for those with schizophrenia includes assertive community treatment (ACT), intensive case management (ICM), ongoing medication management, and housing, rehabilitation, social, and vocational supports (see Chap. 20). More effective than traditional approaches, ACT teams and ICM were developed to meet the client's multiple and complex health care needs (Salyers & Tsemberis, 2007).

Assertive Community Treatment. ACT is a program of individualized, consistent, comprehensive, and continuous services to clients with schizophrenia and other severe and persistent mental illnesses. A team, not an individual mental health worker, delivers services where people live, work, and play. Such services include helping clients with symptom management, medication monitoring, housing, vocational needs, parenting skills, nonpsychiatric medical care, and daily responsibilities and problems. ACT is designed for those clients "in greatest need" because of frequent relapse, repeated hospitalization, dual diagnosis, homelessness, incarceration, or resistance or avoidance of involvement in usual mental health services. ACT services reduce the most devastating outcomes of severe psychiatric illnesses, such as incarceration, repeated hospitalizations, and homelessness. This model of intensive community treatment is one of the best researched interventions available to people with schizophrenia. Research has shown that ACT substantially reduces psychiatric hospital use, increases housing stability, and can moderately improve symptoms and quality of life (Salyers & Tsemberis, 2007).

Intensive Case Management. ICM, another model of community care, involves assessment, referral, coordination, and integration of a cohesive program of services tailored to the client's needs. In addition, case managers serve as advocates for the client. A more useful model includes a case manager who is also a clinician with skills in helping to strengthen family coping.

Think About It 29.1

Kelsey Rilano, a 28-year-old client with a history of schizophrenia and substance abuse, is receiving treatment on an open inpatient unit. She had stopped taking medication at home and became increasingly psychotic, proclaiming that she was God and had special powers. Since resuming medication, her condition has improved; her team expects discharge within a few days. This is Kelsey's third hospitalization in 1 year. She once had an apartment and a job, but lately she has been homeless and unemployed. Propose how best to provide continuity of care for Kelsey after discharge.

APPLYING THE NURSING PROCESS

Schizophrenia and Thought Disorders

▲ ASSESSMENT

Nurses assess clients with thought disorders in various settings, from outpatient clinics, to homes, to inpatient units. They may assess clients with known histories of schizophrenia or those unknown to the mental health care system. Although formal assessment tools for schizophrenia exist, many nurses rely instead on interviews and direct observations.

Assessment begins with an interview and focuses on establishing signs and symptoms, degree of impaired thought processes, risk for self-injury or violence toward others, presence or absence of substance use or abuse, and available support systems. Nurses may wish to interview relatives or friends of clients as well to obtain all information regarding family history, previous episodes of psychotic symptoms, onset of symptoms, and thoughts of suicide or violent behavior.

Mood and Cognitive State

Nurses assess the client's mood, affect, and behavior, including the range of emotional expressiveness, motivation, and

interpersonal skills, while considering the client's cultural background. They are alert for signs and symptoms such as:

- Absence of expression of feelings
- Language content or conversation that is difficult to follow
- Pronounced paucity of speech and thoughts
- Preoccupation with odd ideas
- Ideas of reference (ie, believing that mundane objects have special meanings)
- Expressions of feelings of unreality
- Evidence of hallucinations such as comments that the way things appear, sound, or smell is different

In addition, nurses ask if clients have had difficulty concentrating or performing intellectual activities at a previous functional level. Ability to concentrate is necessary for effective participation in rehabilitation. Other signs and symptoms to assess include sleep disturbances, somatic complaints, and social withdrawal. Nurses also inquire about recent stressors, which can precipitate a psychotic episode in clients with thought disorders, and signs and symptoms of impending relapse. These warning signs include disrupted sleep cycle, significant mood changes (mostly depression), decreased appetite, and somatic complaints such as headache, malaise, and constipation (Figure 29.7). Relapse leads to client withdrawal, resistance, and preoccupation with psychoses.

Potential for Violence

Some clients with schizophrenia can become violent, directing injury either at themselves or others. Nurses assess potential for violence by inquiring about the following:

- History of violent or suicidal behavior
- Extreme social isolation

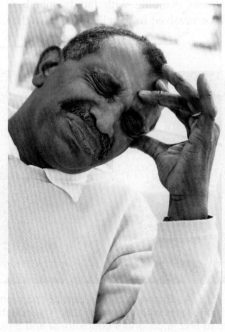

FIGURE 29.7 Headache may be a warning sign of a relapse of schizophrenia.

- Feelings of persecution or being "controlled" by others
- Auditory hallucinations that give orders to commit violent acts (command hallucinations)
- Concomitant substance abuse
- Medication noncompliance
- Feelings of anger, suspiciousness, or hostility

Nurses make other team members aware of a client's potential for violence; protecting clients and others from serious harm is a priority (Challenging Behaviors 29.2).

Assessing Social Support

Availability and responsiveness of a social support network and the client's role in the family and community are important factors in nursing assessment. The presence of caring, supportive family and friends influences recovery positively; its absence contributes to feelings of hopelessness. Assessing the availability of significant others helps nurses plan educational and other aspects of treatment.

Knowledge of Illness

Nurses assess the client's and family's knowledge of schizophrenia, its treatment, and the potential for relapse. Adherence to medication regimens and other therapeutic schedules is bolstered when clients and families understand the biologic basis of the illness, signs of recovery and relapse, and their roles in treatment. Clients and families benefit from awareness of not only the disease, but also treatments, goals of care, and types of available community services. Nurses assess whether clients and families are receiving all the services for which they are eligible.

PRACTICE & LEARN

▲ NURSING DIAGNOSIS

Nursing diagnoses that guide the nursing care of clients with schizophrenia include the following (NANDA, 2007):

- **Disturbed Thought Processes** related to biochemical imbalances, as evidenced by hypervigilance, distractibility, poor concentration, disordered thought sequencing, inappropriate responses, and thinking not based in reality
- **Disturbed Sensory Perception** (auditory or visual) related to biochemical imbalances, as evidenced by auditory or visual hallucinations
- **Risk for Other-Directed or Self-Directed Violence** related to delusional thoughts, hallucinatory commands, or panic, as evidenced by overt aggressive acts, threatening stances, pacing, or suicidal ideation or plan
- **Social Isolation** related to alterations in mental status and an inability to engage in satisfying personal relationships, as evidenced by sad, flat affect; absence of supportive significant others; withdrawal; uncommunicativeness; and inability to meet expectations of others
- **Noncompliance** with medication regimen related to health beliefs and lack of motivation, as evidenced by failure to adhere to medication schedule
- **Ineffective Coping** related to disturbed thought processes as evidenced by inability to meet basic needs
- **Interrupted Family Processes** related to shift in health status of a family member and situational crisis, as evidenced by changes in the family's goals, plans, and activities and changes in family patterns and rituals
- **Risk for Ineffective Family Management of Therapeutic Regimen** related to knowledge deficit and complexity of client's health care needs

▲ OUTCOME IDENTIFICATION AND PLANNING

Preparing the treatment plan is a collaborative effort between the entire mental health team and the client and family. No single treatment helps every client; rather, a plan must be tailored to each client's strengths, needs, and limitations. Although standardized nursing care plans exist for specific diagnoses, they must be individualized for each person. Case in Point 29.1 reflects such individualization for one client and his family.

Challenging Behaviors 29.2

Threatened Aggression

Situation: Your assigned client in your community health rotation is Mr. Eliche, who resides in a group home for adults with serious and chronic thought disturbances. You are visiting him for the third time, with your instructor and fellow students. You meet with him in the day room of the group home. The supervisor warns you that he has been upset recently and somewhat quiet. When you sit with him he struggles to maintain eye contact and turns away from you. When you ask him what is happening today, he says that he wants to kill his brother because he is "taking all my money." He speaks quietly but intently about obtaining a knife and "getting him."

Your Potential Feelings: Fear, anxiety, worry

What Is Going On? Mr. Eliche is experiencing a psychiatric emergency. His threats must be taken seriously.

Strategy: Directly inform Mr. Eliche that you need to speak with your instructor and the supervisor because what he is talking about is unsafe. Do not engage in a lengthy discussion with Mr. Eliche; instead, inform others about his statements. The clinical team can then decide if his behavior warrants further evaluation in a psychiatric emergency department or if he needs to be reevaluated for a medication change.

Nurse Action/Communication: Be as supportive as possible to Mr. Eliche but maintain safety of yourself and the other residents of the group home at all times. Rely on your supervisors to assist with planning interventions that will maintain this safety.

Case in Point 29.1

James's Story

The parents of James, 24 years old, bring him to the acute treatment center because of increasingly bizarre behavior, decreased sleep, and isolation. For the past 3 days, James has been pacing around the house, barely eating and sleeping, talking to himself, displaying odd mannerisms, and making strange statements. His parents add that James seemed to "have no facial expression" for 2 weeks prior to his unusual behavior. James states, "I just came here to help people."

Review of history reveals that James was treated with Prolixin and Cogentin when admitted to the hospital 2 months ago. The medications stabilized his psychoses, and James was discharged with instructions to receive follow-up care at a local community mental health center. His mother states that James stopped taking his medication several weeks ago because "he said the government was trying to control his mind. We can't force him to take his drugs because he gets very agitated."

When James was 2 years old, he suffered head trauma from an accident and resultant loss of consciousness. No family history of thought disorders is known. James has smoked marijuana and abused alcohol for at least 2 years. While the nurse is interviewing James, he admits that he hears voices that "tell me to do things," although he would not specify further. He says, "The voices scare me," as he looks over his shoulder, and he is easily distracted by noises in and outside the interview room. James makes clicking noises in quick succession before answering questions. His answers are often "hidden" in nonsensical language. He states he has "special powers," can break glass and blocks of ice with his fist, and can communicate with others through the radio.

James agrees to stay in the hospital for treatment after the nurse explains that this would be the best way to determine how to help him control the voices that scare him. James does not make eye contact but nods. He is admitted to a locked psychiatric unit.

Key Assessment Findings

- History of head injury with loss of consciousness
- Alcohol abuse for 2 years
- Previous hospitalizations; treatment with fluphenazine (Prolixin) and benztropine (Cogentin)
- Noncompliance with medication and community mental health center follow-up
- Auditory hallucinations
- Feelings of being controlled
- Disorganized speech
- Flat affect; lack of eye contact
- Distractibility
- Grandiose and persecutory delusions

Nursing Diagnosis: Risk for Self-Directed or Other-Directed Violence related to messages involved in auditory hallucinations as evidenced by client's statement of being afraid of the voices and inability to reveal content of voices

NOC: Suicide Self-Restraint and Impulse Self-Control: The client will refrain from harming himself or others.

NIC: Behavior Management: Self-Harm

- Assess the client's potential for violent behavior. Ask him directly if the voices tell him to hurt himself or anyone else. Communicate risks to other care providers. Maintain ongoing surveillance of the client and environment. *Preventing self- or other-directed violence is possible if health care providers heed warnings (eg, intimidating behaviors, threats). Continuing evaluation of the client and environment reduces the potential for injury.*

- Administer medication as ordered and needed (Figure A). Monitor for side effects and desired therapeutic effects. *Antipsychotic drugs are the most powerful tool in the treatment of schizophrenia. Even if a client receives depot injections, he may require more medication if psychotic symptoms escalate.*

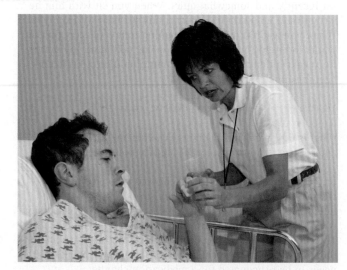

FIGURE A **The nurse is administering antipsychotic medication to help control symptoms, especially delusions and hallucinations.**

(continues on page 607)

Case in Point 29.1 (continued)

James's Story

- Assist the client to identify situations or feelings that may prompt self-harm. Give reassurance, comfort, and opportunity to discuss delusions. *Caring interventions help build a therapeutic relationship and may increase the likelihood that the client will reveal the content of his auditory hallucinations.*
- Communicate behavioral expectations and consequences. *Clear communication helps foster a therapeutic relationship and enhances the client's awareness and knowledge.*
- Instruct the client in appropriate coping strategies; teach and reinforce effective behaviors and appropriate expression of feelings. *Knowledge and reinforcement of coping strategies and behaviors help promote continued use by the client.*
- Place the client in a more protective environment if impulses/behaviors escalate. *Doing so can ensure the safety of the client and others.*

NIC: Suicide Prevention

- Be alert for signs of self-harm; keep the client in a protected environment with frequent observation until delusions and hallucinations subside. Determine the degree of suicidal risk and if the client has available means to follow through with a suicide plan. *Warning signs of self-directed violence may be covert; protecting, observing, and asking the client about them and any means to accomplish them may be the only preventive tools available.*
- Assign the client to a room near the nursing station. *Doing so facilitates observation.*
- Contract with the client as appropriate for "no self-harm." Implement necessary actions to reduce his immediate distress. Identify immediate safety needs when negotiating the contract; assist the client to discuss feelings about the contract (Figure B). Observe for signs of incongruence that may indicate lack of commitment. *Contracting reinforces behavioral expectations, promotes trust, and enhances overall safety. Identification of signs of incongruence aids in early detection and prevention of harm.*
- Interact with the client regularly; use a direct, nonjudgmental approach in discussing suicide; discuss plan for dealing with future suicidal ideation. *Frequent direct interaction helps convey caring and openness and provides an opportunity for the client to talk about feelings.*

NIC: Impulse Control Training

- Use a behavior modification plan; assist the client to identify problems or situations that require thoughtful action. Teach him to "stop and think" before acting impulsively. *Behavior modification helps reinforce positive problem-solving strategies to deal with the client's hallucinations and delusions.*
- Provide opportunities to practice problem solving; provide positive reinforcement for successful outcomes. *Positive reinforcement promotes the client's continued and appropriate use of strategies in the future.*

NIC: Environmental Management: Violence Prevention

- Determine with other team members a plan of action if violence appears imminent. Discuss the plan with the client; ask him to tell staff when or if he feels he may harm himself or others. *Having a plan will help staff more effectively manage violence. Engaging the client in the plan may help him gain control over his thought processes, increase the likelihood that he will comply with the plan, and help build a therapeutic relationship.*
- Place the client in the least restrictive environment that permits necessary observation. Remove other people from the vicinity of a violent or potentially violent client. *Use of the least restrictive environment protects the client's rights while maintaining unit safety.*

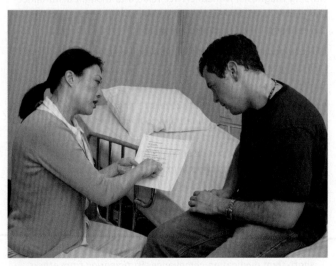

FIGURE B The nurse is reviewing the no-suicide contract with the client.

> 11/9/12: The client remains free from self-harm and refrains from harming others. He demonstrates impulse control and self-control, with no verbalizations of suicidal ideas or attempts to hurt self or others.
>
> M. Porter, APRN

Nursing Diagnosis: Disturbed Thought Processes related to possible neurochemical dysregulation as evidenced by non–reality-based thinking, auditory hallucinations, and delusions

NOC: Distorted Thought Self-Control: The client will demonstrate an increase in reality-based thinking with fewer hallucinations and delusions.

NIC: Delusion Management

- Focus on the client's underlying feelings, not the content, about the delusion. For example, "You seem troubled by these

(continues on page 608)

Case in Point 29.1 (continued)

James's Story

thoughts," not "Why would the government want to control your thoughts?" Avoid arguing about false beliefs; state doubt in a matter-of-fact manner. Avoid reinforcing delusions. Encourage the client to validate delusions with trusted others such as staff (reality testing) and to verbalize delusions to caregivers before acting on them. *Focusing on nondelusional content (eg, feelings) and discouraging an animated discussion of the delusional content (which would only end up reinforcing the delusion) will help the client see that his thoughts are not real. Asking the client to bring delusional content to the caregivers' attention provides opportunities for reinforcing reality-based thinking and may prevent bizarre or possibly violent behavior generated by delusions.*

- Provide recreational, diversionary activities that require attention or skill. *They help the client focus on something other than the delusions.*
- Monitor delusions for self-harmful or violent content; protect the client and others from potentially harmful delusional-based behaviors. *Monitoring is important for safety.*
- Continue giving medications as ordered and needed, observing for any side effects and desired therapeutic effects. *Antipsychotic drugs are the most powerful tool in the treatment of schizophrenia.*

NIC: Hallucination Management

- Keep the client in a safe, protected, restricted environment. Avoid excessive activity or stimulation. Provide appropriate surveillance/supervision. Maintain a consistent routine; assign consistent caregivers daily. Encourage the client to tell staff when he is hallucinating and to reveal the content of the hallucinations. Monitor hallucinations for harmful content. *Close observation of the client with active hallucinations in a secure environment is essential to maintain overall safety. Excessive sensory stimulation or changes in routine could overwhelm and agitate the client. Staff should be aware of any hallucinatory content, especially if it is potentially harmful.*
- Encourage the client to discuss rather than act on feelings and impulses. Focus on feelings about, rather than details of, the hallucination (eg, "You seem to be afraid," not "Why would the voices tell you to hurt yourself?"). *Focusing on the client's feelings, which are real, minimizes emphasis on the hallucination.*
- Do not argue with the client about whether the hallucinations are real; state, if asked, that you do not perceive the stimuli that the client perceives (Figure C). *Arguing with the client or expressing disbelief does not affect the client's belief in the reality of the hallucination and can disrupt trust and the therapeutic relationship. Expressing that you do not see, hear, or otherwise experience the hallucinatory stimuli indirectly encourages him to question the reality of the experience.*
- Use limit setting, area restriction, or other measures when the client cannot control behavior. *Measures to control behavior promote the safety and comfort of the client and others.*

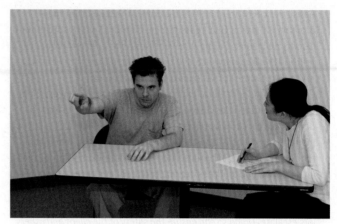

FIGURE C While discussing the client's hallucinations, the nurse provides reality orientation and avoids arguing or exploring the content in detail.

- Engage the client in reality-based activities. *Activities help to distract the client from the hallucinations and promote reality-based thought.*

> 12/15/12: *The client demonstrates reality-oriented thought with fewer hallucinations and delusions. He begins to consistently demonstrate recognition of hallucinations and delusions, fewer hallucinations and delusions, and more requests for reality validation.*
>
> M. Porter, APRN

Nursing Diagnosis: Nonadherence related to thought disturbance and delusions of being controlled as evidenced by statement of the "government trying to control his mind"

NOC: Adherence Behavior: The client will take prescribed medications.

NIC: Patient Contracting

- Encourage client to identify strengths and abilities; assist him to set realistic, attainable goals and to break them into small, manageable steps. Help him to notice even small successes. *Identification and participation enhance feelings of control. Breaking down goals prevents overwhelming the client and promotes feelings of accomplishment as he achieves each step.*
- Facilitate involvement of significant others in the contracting process if the client agrees; facilitate negotiation of contract terms if necessary (Figure D). Explain the rationale for medications. Discuss the possible use of depot injections to manage short-term medication compliance. *Participation from others provides additional support for the client. Flexibility in contract*

(continues on page 609)

Case in Point 29.1 (continued)

James's Story

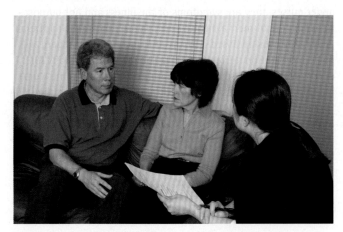

FIGURE D The team involves the client's parents in the medication adherence contracting process.

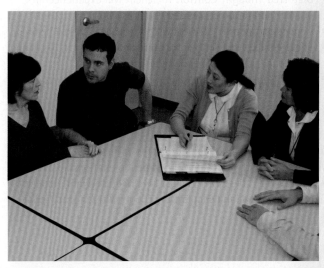

FIGURE E The nurse reviews key components of teaching for schizophrenia to the client and family

terms is necessary to meet changing needs. The client's refusal to take medication at home suggests that adherence most likely will remain an issue. Depot injections ensure the maintenance of therapeutic levels of neuroleptic medication for 2 weeks at a time.

- Encourage the client to identify appropriate meaningful reinforcers or rewards. *Appropriate rewards enhance the chances that the client will follow the contract.*

NIC: Self–Responsibility Facilitation

- Encourage verbalizations of feelings, perceptions, and fears about assuming responsibility. *An underlying knowledge of the client's status is important in individualizing strategies.*
- Initiate medication adherence therapy. Help the client achieve insight into the benefit of taking the drugs by helping him review the history of his illness, symptoms, and medication side effects; encourage him to consider the benefits versus the drawbacks of drug treatment. Encourage compliance and provide information about neuroleptic medication. *Medication adherence therapy, which involves medication education, support, and insight into the disorder, has been shown to increase long-term use of pharmacologic therapy.*

- Encourage independence, but assist the client with things he cannot perform. Set limits on manipulative behavior; refrain from arguing or bargaining about established limits. *Encouraging independence along with assistance and limit setting promotes responsibility for actions and enhances the client's feelings of control over the situation.*
- Teach the client and family about the disorder and the need to follow the treatment plan, including medication regimen and follow-up (Figure E). *Such instruction promotes improved understanding, which increases the chance for the plan to succeed.*

1/14/13: The client takes medications while hospitalized and exhibits a change in behavior reflecting effectiveness of the medication. He often demonstrates acceptance of diagnosis, adherence to appointments and follow-up, and appropriate beginning knowledge about the need for medications.

M. Porter, APRN

EPILOGUE

It has been 4 months since James was discharged home after a lengthy stay at the facility. He was referred to the local community mental health center for follow-up. He initially complied with his treatment plan; however, in the past 2 weeks, James has missed his appointments. His parents have called the center to report that James has stopped taking his medications. They are concerned because he is acting strangely and refuses to talk to them. His mother states, "He's really being bizarre. It's as if he's having a conversation with someone. When I ask him about it, he denies it. But I've heard him say several times that he'll take care of things." Personnel instruct the parents to bring James to an emergency facility for immediate evaluation.

Major goals for the care of clients with schizophrenia, organized according to the Nursing Outcomes Classification (Moorhead et al., 2008), are as follows:

- **Distorted Thought Control:** The client will experience improved thought processes and fewer psychotic symptoms.
- **Aggression Control:** The client will not engage in violent behavior.
- **Social Skills:** The client will acquire improved social skills and engage in satisfying social interaction.
- **Family Coping:** The client and family will gain knowledge about the disease process and treatment.

⚠ IMPLEMENTATION

Implementing a plan of care for clients with schizophrenia involves careful attention to the therapeutic relationship. Nurses who work with these clients must be straightforward, hopeful, and accepting and should view clients with unconditional

regard and dignity. They must work within the confines of each client's ability and willingness to participate. Furthermore, nurses demonstrate acceptance of clients and their actions without judgment. Although certain behaviors may disgust or anger nurses, they are symptoms of the illness and not purposefully directed at mental health staff. Failure to establish a therapeutic relationship based on trust and unconditional regard will make intervention difficult at best. Common interventions for clients with thought disorders organized according to the Nursing Interventions Classification (NIC) include, but are not limited to, **Active Listening, Anxiety Reduction, Complex Relationship Building, Delusion Management, Energy Management, Environmental Management: Violence Prevention, Family Integrity Promotion, Family Involvement, Hallucination Management, Self-Care Assistance, Socialization Enhancement,** and **Suicide Prevention** (Bulechek et al., 2008). See also Understanding Nursing Care 29.1.

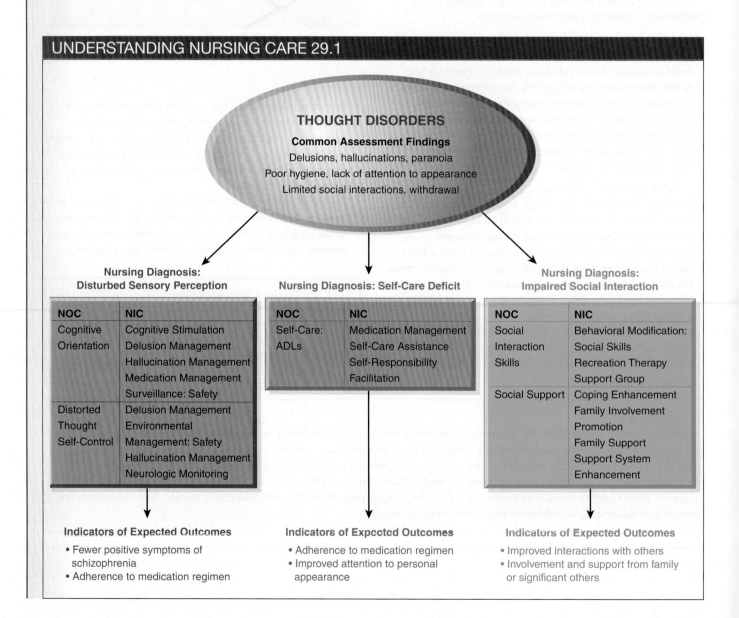

UNDERSTANDING NURSING CARE 29.1

THOUGHT DISORDERS

Common Assessment Findings
Delusions, hallucinations, paranoia
Poor hygiene, lack of attention to appearance
Limited social interactions, withdrawal

Nursing Diagnosis: Disturbed Sensory Perception

NOC	NIC
Cognitive Orientation	Cognitive Stimulation Delusion Management Hallucination Management Medication Management Surveillance: Safety
Distorted Thought Self-Control	Delusion Management Environmental Management: Safety Hallucination Management Neurologic Monitoring

Indicators of Expected Outcomes
- Fewer positive symptoms of schizophrenia
- Adherence to medication regimen

Nursing Diagnosis: Self-Care Deficit

NOC	NIC
Self-Care: ADLs	Medication Management Self-Care Assistance Self-Responsibility Facilitation

Indicators of Expected Outcomes
- Adherence to medication regimen
- Improved attention to personal appearance

Nursing Diagnosis: Impaired Social Interaction

NOC	NIC
Social Interaction Skills	Behavioral Modification: Social Skills Recreation Therapy Support Group
Social Support	Coping Enhancement Family Involvement Promotion Family Support Support System Enhancement

Indicators of Expected Outcomes
- Improved interactions with others
- Involvement and support from family or significant others

Addressing Disturbed Thought Processes and Sensory Perceptions

The focus of care in the early stages of treatment for clients with acute psychosis is improving reality testing. Although pharmacotherapy plays the major role in diminishing psychotic symptoms, nonpharmacologic interventions help as well.

Reinforcing Reality

Nurses reinforce and validate reality for clients with schizophrenia by involving them in present-oriented conversations and activities, describing real events, and clarifying facts (Challenging Behaviors 29.3). They apply this principle to delusions. For example, in response to the client's assertion that his body has turned to concrete, the nurse might reply, "I am looking at you, and your body looks like it is still made of flesh." However, it is important not to engage in arguments about delusions. Lengthy discussions may further strengthen the client's beliefs. No one can argue away perceptions of depersonalization, hallucinations, or delusions. These psychoses are real to clients. Rather, nurses state facts simply, concisely, and in a nonthreatening manner. They gently introduce doubt (eg, "No, Mr. L, I don't understand why the FBI would be interested in following you").

Reality-based activities, such as looking at pictures in a magazine or taking a walk, are therapeutic because they allow clients to interact in a satisfying interpersonal relationship and diminish the time spent in poor contact with reality. Often, clients cannot interact, but staying with them provides a vital link with the real world. Nurses do not permit clients to isolate themselves; doing so only increases withdrawal and poor reality orientation.

Understanding Language Content

Illogical, symbolic, and disorganized speech often holds a message that clients cannot express clearly. Nurses listen for themes and reflect back to clients the meaning deciphered. They do not dismiss verbal and nonverbal behaviors of clients as meaningless or nonsense. In effect, nurses try to decode the communication that clients offer and validate its meaning.

Much communication that clients present is confusing. Nurses must clarify and not assume they understand vague and ambiguous statements. They never pretend to understand or agree with a client's illogical or delusional thinking. Rather, they ask for clarification. At all times, nurses are role models for healthy, clear communication.

Intervening in Hallucinations

Clients who hallucinate are preoccupied and frightened by what they hear or see. Hallucinations are real to them, and nurses cannot argue away, dismiss, or ignore them. Nevertheless, nurses make it clear that they do not hear the voices or see the images.

Nurses do communicate concern that clients are bothered, upset, or frightened. For example, it is therapeutic to say, "No, I don't hear that voice saying bad things about you, but I imagine it is frightening for you to hear it. I would like to help you feel less frightened."

Nurses do not leave clients who are hallucinating alone; the nurse's presence is a reassuring and potentially calming force. Drawing clients into reality-based activities and conversation may distract them as well as reinforce reality (England, 2007). Some people with schizophrenia have found that elevated anxiety precedes hallucinations and therefore have developed skills to deal with anxiety. Other important interventions for managing hallucinations include using the following:

- Dismissal intervention (ie, telling the voices to go away)
- Various coping strategies (eg, jogging, telephoning, playing games, seeking out others, employing relaxation techniques)
- Competing stimuli (eg, listening to music or another's or one's own voice to overcome auditory hallucinations and visual stimuli to overcome visual hallucinations; the nurse might say, "Listen to my voice; don't listen to that other voice. You know me. I'm Barbara. I'm here with you now. Listen to me.")

Managing Violent Behavior

The first step in managing violent behavior is intervening before it occurs. Nurses are alert to inappropriate and possibly previolent behaviors such as irritability, intimidating behavior, refusal to cooperate with unit routines, motor restlessness, intense staring, loud speech, or overt threats. Nurses at this point do not overwhelm clients with too much talk or closeness. They avoid

Challenging Behaviors 29.3

The Client Who Is Hostile

Situation: Ms. Palmer has a diagnosis of chronic paranoid schizophrenia. You have worked with her for several weeks without difficulty, although her course of recovery during the hospitalization has been uneven. This particular morning she appears more disorganized than usual. When you greet her she says, "You remind me of my mother. I hated her. Get out of my sight."

Your Potential Feelings: Bewilderment, rejection, fear

What Is Going On? The client probably is frustrated with her symptoms not improving. Her sense of reality is impaired, and she may perceive people around her as threatening.

Strategy: The best intervention is "reality clarification." Assess whether Ms. Palmer is becoming more paranoid or psychotic or at risk for violence. If she seems more agitated than you have previously noted, notify your instructor and the head nurse on the unit. Otherwise, calmly point out to her that you are not really her mother and that you wonder if she is upset about something else. You might also ask if she is distressed about being in the hospital a long time. Say, "Tell me more about what is upsetting you." If Ms. Palmer is resistant to conversation, step away and return later to talk with her.

all but the most judicious touch because clients are likely to perceive physical contact as threatening and harmful.

It is usually appropriate to initiate urgent intervention when these behaviors are present. Clients may require chemical restraint, with oral medication being the most acceptable route. An intramuscular injection and seclusion are the next step if oral medication fails or clients refuse to take it. Physical restraint is the least acceptable intervention, fraught with danger of injury or even death (see Chap. 32). However, in some instances physical restraint may be unavoidable.

Enhancing Social Interaction

Although severe psychotic symptoms can subside with pharmacologic treatment, many clients still have severely restricted social lives. Impaired communication, lack of motivation, inattention to self-care, and difficulty establishing and maintaining relationships leave them isolated. The psychosocial approaches described earlier can help clients improve social functioning and enjoy a better quality of life. However, these interventions are usually not implemented until psychotic symptoms are controlled. Nurses can lay the groundwork for these interventions by establishing a therapeutic relationship and then implementing these measures as clients' thought processes improve.

Developing Trust

People with schizophrenia are likely to be anxious and fearful around others. Through therapeutic communication and trustworthy nonverbal behavior, nurses build trusting relationships with clients. This is accomplished through acceptance, a nonjudgmental attitude, and genuineness. Clients accurately perceive both a genuine desire to help and fear and repulsion; nonverbal behavior is usually more trustworthy than words.

Because of the illness, clients with schizophrenia have likely had unsatisfying or unsuccessful interpersonal relations and are unwilling or unable to take risks in encounters with others. Establishing rapport with clients becomes a gradual process built on consistent and pleasant interactions. With rewarding experiences, clients may be able to interact with more people. The ultimate message is that others can care for, not just take care of, the client.

Initiating Interaction

Nurses need to initiate interaction with clients, whose behavior often consists of withdrawal and isolation. The nurse's approach is nonthreatening and calm, giving clients plenty of space. For example, the nurse sits near the client but not so close as to threaten the client's personal space (Figure 29.8). This approach communicates that nurses are willing to respond to cues and progress at the client's pace.

Modeling Affect

Clients with schizophrenia often display flat, blunted, or inappropriate affect. Nurses model appropriate affect in their communication with clients and others through facial expressions and body language that match the tone or content of the message. For example, a nurse has a sad facial expression and

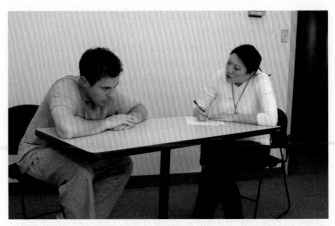

FIGURE 29.8 The nurse maintains a distance from the client that facilitates effective communication but does not threaten his personal space.

somber movements when discussing a sad event with the client. She does not reinforce inappropriate or bizarre behavior by smiling, laughing, nodding, or becoming angry with the client.

Promoting Medication Adherence

People with schizophrenia may fail to take medication as prescribed for several reasons. They may be disturbed by the medication's side effects, believe they do not need the drugs, think they do not have an illness, or believe that the medication is poison. Eighty percent of people with schizophrenia who stop taking their medication have a relapse within 1 year, compared with 30% who continue their regimen (Beebe, 2007). The most common causes of relapse and rehospitalization for "revolving-door" inpatients are medication nonadherence and medication nonresponse (ie, having little relief of symptoms from the medication).

Nurses are responsible for assessing and encouraging medication adherence (Therapeutic Communication 29.1). Accepting a diagnosis of schizophrenia is not a necessary condition for medication adherence. Research shows that client outcome is improved if psychoeducation is given to caregivers (McWilliams et al., 2011). Providing education to clients and family and promoting increased client autonomy and involvement will likely result in increased adherence to medication regimens. To do this, nurses must know the medication's action, use, dosage, route of administration, desired effects, side effects, toxic effects, contraindications, and nursing implications (see Understanding Psychopharmacology 29.1 and 29.2). Clients and families also must know this information, as well as how to intervene if an adverse reaction occurs.

For clients taking antipsychotics, nurses must be vigilant in monitoring their clients and ensuring periodic testing of glucose blood levels, lipids, and liver function. Other monitoring should include regular weights and heights with calculated basal metabolic index. It also includes assessing history of known risk factors for diabetes and heart disease, ensuring the presence of a fasting glucose test on clients' charts, regularly monitoring glucose levels, and referring clients with abnormal glucose or lipid levels to a medical specialist.

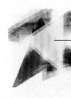

Therapeutic Communication 29.1

Disorganized Speech in Schizophrenia

Frank Oliver is a 41-year-old man with schizophrenia, disorganized type, continuous. Although he has had five prior psychiatric hospitalizations, Frank has been managing fairly successfully in the community through medication monitoring and ACT interventions. However, 2 weeks ago he experienced an acute psychotic episode and was hospitalized.

While administering 10 mg of Haldol, 1 mg of Cogentin, and 500 mg of Depakote to Frank, the nurse, Jenna Ivey, reviews his knowledge and beliefs about his medications.

INEFFECTIVE DIALOGUE

JENNA: Frank, you haven't done very well with taking your medications. Do you know what you're supposed to be taking?

FRANK: Depakote every day, Cogentin 300 mg every day, and a pink pill. Total containment.

JENNA: What do you mean by 'total containment?' And those amounts aren't right. At bedtime you take 10 mg of Haldol, 1 mg of Cogentin, and 500 mg of Depakote.

FRANK: Right. A precocious repercussion.

JENNA: Frank, that doesn't make sense.

FRANK: Make sense.

JENNA: OK, let's try again. Do you know why you take these medications?

FRANK: Doctors and policemen. You said to.

JENNA: I'm not a policeman, Frank. Why do you think that?

FRANK: Locked up. Upstairs. In, out.

JENNA: Do you mean because you're in a locked unit you feel like you're in jail? You're here for your own good, Frank.

FRANK: Not the light.

JENNA: I give up! We'll talk about this later, maybe tomorrow when you're feeling better.

FRANK: Okay.

EFFECTIVE DIALOGUE

JENNA: What are the names and amounts of these medicines that you take every day?

FRANK: Depakote every day, Cogentin 300 mg every day, and a pink pill. Total containment.

JENNA: You named two of them correctly, Frank, but you didn't have the amounts right. At bedtime you take 10 mg of Haldol, 1 mg of Cogentin, and 500 mg of Depakote. I want to ask you some questions about your medicines.

FRANK: Okay.

JENNA: How do these medicines help you?

FRANK: They help me accept that I'm not working right now. Makes me feel right when I see good people.

JENNA: What symptoms can they help with?

FRANK: Clean, work, happy, have no conflict or complaint. Sometimes my eye closes or pops out of my head. Automation.

JENNA: Is your eye bothering you?

FRANK: It's not fair for me to say right now.

JENNA: You don't want to answer that now?

FRANK: No.

JENNA: Frank, I need to know if you're having problems with your medicines so we can help you. And you need to know what to do if you have side effects. It would be good if we sat down together and talked more. Would you be willing to do that after I finish giving medicines to the others?

FRANK: Okay.

Reflection and Critical Thinking Questions

- In both dialogues, what therapeutic techniques did Jenna use to communicate with Frank? Identify any blocks or barriers to therapeutic communication.
- What statements did Jenna make in the first scenario that were less effective than the statements in the second scenario? Describe the effects of her statements.
- How does the conclusion of the conversation in the second scenario differ from the one in the first scenario?
- Describe Frank's communication style and themes. What do you think he was trying to say?
- What methods of communication did Jenna use in the second scenario that ultimately were more effective than those she used in the first?

Promoting Improved Coping

Stress management techniques such as breathing and relaxation exercises, imagery, nutritional improvement, and aerobic activity are useful measures to help clients with schizophrenia. Nurses teach clients to discover and practice the stress-relieving activities that work for them.

Learning their own signs of impending relapse is critical for clients and their families so they can contact a care provider for medication adjustments or implementation of other necessary interventions. Factors that promote recovery are adhering to medication, self-monitoring symptoms, understanding the illness and its treatment, having adequate housing, working at a vocation or job, receiving support from significant others, participating in community rehabilitation, and developing spirituality.

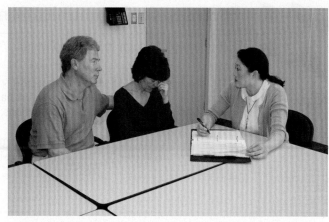

FIGURE 29.9 Many family members blame themselves for schizophrenia and other mental illnesses in their loved ones. Nurses must reinforce that relatives are not responsible for causing the disease. Referral to NAMI or support groups may also be helpful.

Checkpoint Questions

14. How should a nurse communicate with a client who is hallucinating?

15. What intervention is considered the least appropriate for a client with schizophrenia who is violent?

Strengthening Family Processes

Challenges and problems that families face when a relative has schizophrenia are immense. A client's inability to care for personal needs, difficulty managing money, social withdrawal, strange personal habits, suicide threats, and interference with schedules can be so extreme that families realistically fear for his or her safety, as well as that of other relatives. Family resources often deteriorate so much as to threaten well-being and stability. Chronic sorrow may develop in response to unending caregiver responsibilities.

The importance of social support is well documented in the research literature. Magliano and others (2003) conducted an extensive study of the effects of a social network on burden and pessimism in relatives of people with schizophrenia. They found a more supportive social network in relatives who reported lower levels of pessimism and burden about the family member with schizophrenia. Strengthening the social network is seen as a positive strategy for assisting such families.

Ritsner and colleagues (2011) found that psychosocial factors were strong predictors of subjective quality of life outcome when compared with disorder-specific changes. Their longitudinal research suggested that psychosocial supports were essential to health in clients with schizophrenia and schizoaffective disorder.

The literature has documented the effectiveness of psychoeducational programs for clients with schizophrenia and their families (McWilliams et al., 2011). Toprac and colleagues (2000) discuss the implementation of a Patient and Family Education Program (PFEP) to complement medication algorithms for the treatment of schizophrenia and other serious mental disorders. One of the best practices and treatment recommendations

specified by PORT involves giving family members education and support (Lehman et al., 2004). Teaching and encouraging the use of independent living skills promote independent functioning for clients. As their ability to accept more responsibility progresses, they receive greater responsibility. Clients and families learn to care for physical needs and to renew themselves through pleasurable activities, hobbies, and other interests.

Family members must understand that schizophrenia is a "no-fault" brain disease, with no reason for blame (Figure 29.9). Family-to-family education, now available in 40 states, has proved an effective means of education and support. Nurses promote measures that increase the family's social network and reduce stigma.

Clinical symptoms of schizophrenia and stigma are not the only barriers to recovery. Another barrier is hopelessness, including such attitudes from nurses and other health care providers. Care providers offer hope to clients and families through therapeutic relationships, successful experiences, family-to-family and client-to-client education, and symptom management skills.

Educating Clients and Families

Family members need education about schizophrenia and its treatment, access to help in crises, participation in decision making, information about resources, and respite care. The optimal approach to working with them is to recognize their contribution toward restoring health for clients (Beebe, 2007).

Nurses provide education (sometimes called *psychoeducation*) about the nature of schizophrenia, symptom management, necessity of medication adherence, signs of relapse, collaboration in treatment planning, and lifestyle accommodation. Education may also become treatment by seeking to develop insight and address therapeutic issues. For example, education can empower clients by increasing their sense of control and mastery over their lives and teaching coping and problem-solving skills (Kreyenbuhl et al., 2010). Families of consumers have come together to educate families of newly diagnosed people and one another in an effective nationwide program sponsored by NAMI (see Chaps. 1 and 15).

Teaching Symptom Management

People with schizophrenia must learn to monitor symptoms and recognize when they are worsening. Clients can learn how to deal with current behaviors and to detect early signs of relapse, which may be changes in mood, sleeping, or eating, or preoccupations. Significant others also can perform such monitoring.

Those with schizophrenia often lack insight into their illness. They may deny that anything is wrong, that medication has any helpful effect, or that certain triggers (eg, lack of sleep, stress) lead to relapses. However, clients who acknowledge and understand schizophrenia and its treatment can participate in their own care and recovery.

Clients with schizophrenia reported that insight means being able to recognize and control distortions in their perceptions and thoughts. They attributed such insight to taking medications. Other means of insight development were rational self-talk, labeling of unusual experiences as symptoms, and

information and feedback provided by family members (Baier & Murray, 1999).

▲ EVALUATION

Nurses base evaluation of the effectiveness of treatment on whether functioning has improved. Achieving this goal requires the availability of and access to appropriate community supports. Nurses reassess interventions continuously to determine whether clients have achieved therapeutic outcomes. During evaluation, they continuously evaluate for changes in client thinking, affect, and behavior. They redesign therapeutic plans as needed with clients and families. Outcomes that indicate improvement include the following:

- Decreased frequency of hallucinations and delusions
- Ability to recognize hallucinations or delusional thoughts
- More logical and reality-based thought processes
- Improved ability to concentrate
- Improved ability to interact with others
- Appropriate affect and mood

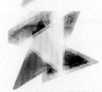

Reviewing and Applying Your Knowledge

Chapter Summary

- Schizophrenia, the most common and severe psychotic disorder, affects 1% of the population. It emerges most often during late adolescence and early adulthood.

- Other psychotic disorders include schizophreniform disorder, schizoaffective disorder, delusional disorder, brief psychotic disorder, shared psychotic disorder, and psychosis not otherwise specified.

- Schizophrenia is defined as a brain disorder, with clear deviations in the structure and function of affected clients. It is most likely a heterogeneous group of several distinct disorders of the brain with some common features, including thought disturbances and preoccupation with frightening inner experiences (eg, delusions and hallucinations), affect disturbances (eg, flat or inappropriate affect), and behavioral or social disturbances (eg, unpredictable, bizarre behavior or social isolation).

- The major theories of etiology are biologic, including genetic, neurochemical, and neuropathologic; viral; immunologic; and structural (ie, abnormalities of brain structure).

- People with schizophrenia manifest alterations in cognitive functioning (ie, memory, attention, and judgment). Researchers have found three dimensions of psychopathology in schizophrenia: disorganization, psychotic, and negative. Positive and negative symptoms of schizophrenia fall into these three dimensions.

- There are five subtypes of schizophrenia: paranoid, disorganized, catatonic, undifferentiated, and residual.

- Antipsychotic medications are the primary treatment for schizophrenia. Traditional antipsychotics primarily treat positive symptoms and are associated with numerous and distressing EPSs. Atypical antipsychotics treat both positive and negative symptoms and typically cause fewer side effects.

- Continuity of care is essential. It involves discharge planning and aggressive management in the community setting.

- Nursing interventions for clients with schizophrenia focus on safety, acceptance, medication education and adherence, intervention in hallucinations and delusions, social skills, monitoring of physical health status, self-care, and education.

Study Questions

1. Which of the following strategies would the nurse instruct the client to do as a measure to prevent relapse?

   a. Take additional medication on days when she is "feeling bad."

   b. Take stress management classes.

   c. Block hallucinations during daily activities.

   d. Report changes in sleeping, eating, and mood.

2. Which of the following would the nurse interpret as negative symptoms? Select all that apply.

   a. Poverty of speech

   b. Hallucinations

   c. Delusions

   d. Affective blunting

   e. Avolition

   f. Tangentiality

3. A client in a locked unit has been staring at a staff member, pacing and muttering under his breath. The nurse interprets this behavior to mean that the client

   a. wants to speak with the staff member, but his thinking is too disorganized to accomplish this.

   b. is having auditory hallucinations.

   c. feels threatened by the staff member and may become violent.

   d. is having visual hallucinations.

4. An 18-year-old client who has just begun taking Haldol comes to the nurse complaining of severe muscle spasms. The nurse assesses the client and notes that his heart rate is 104 beats per minute, his blood pressure is 160/90 mm Hg, and his temperature is 101°F. Based on these data, which of the following actions would the nurse do next?

   a. Check the chart for an "as-needed" order for an anticholinergic agent and administer it, recording the client's symptoms and the intervention.

   b. Immediately call the physician and report the findings because the client may be developing neuroleptic malignant syndrome.

c. Ask the client if he has been exposed to flu or cold viruses and administer acetaminophen for his elevated temperature.

d. Schedule an examination for later in the week with the physician, who will evaluate the client's cardiovascular status.

5. A client with schizophrenia has been in outpatient care through the mental health clinic. Which of the following observations best suggests that the plan of care has been effective?

a. The client has been compliant with taking her medications and attending therapy sessions.

b. The client reports that she no longer has hallucinations.

c. The client has resumed employment and attended community center social functions.

d. The client no longer believes that she has special powers.

Critical Thinking Questions

1. Consider Case in Point 29.1. If you just met James for the first time, what feelings would you most likely experience?

2. What factors would contribute to James's ability to achieve a more independent and satisfactory lifestyle?

3. Identify three interventions, in order of priority, for James. Provide rationales.

References

American Psychiatric Association (APA). (2000). *Diagnostic and statistical manual of mental disorders* (4th ed., text rev). Washington, DC: Author.

American Psychiatric Association (APA). (2011). *DSM-5 development*. Retrieved from http://www.dsm5.org/ProposedRevision/Pages/proposedrevision.aspx?rid=411#

Andreasen, N. C. (1985). *The broken brain: The biologic revolution in psychiatry*. New York, NY: Harper & Row.

Andreasen, N. C. (1999a). A unitary model of schizophrenia. *Archives of General Psychiatry, 56,* 781–787.

Andreasen, N. C. (1999b). Understanding the causes of schizophrenia. *New England Journal of Medicine, 340,* 645–647.

Andreasen, N. C. (2000). Schizophrenia: The fundamental question. *Brain Research Review, 31*(2–3), 106–112.

Andreasen, N. C., & Black, D. W. (2006). *Introductory textbook of psychiatry* (4th ed.). Washington, DC: American Psychiatric Publishing.

Baier, M., & Murray, R. L. (1999). A descriptive study of insight into illness reported by persons with schizophrenia. *Journal of Psychosocial Nursing, 37*(1), 14–21.

Beebe, L. H. (2007). Beyond the prescription pad: Psychosocial treatments for individuals with schizophrenia. *Journal of Psychosocial Nursing and Mental Health Services, 45*(3), 35–43.

Bergman, R. N., & Ader, M. (2005). Atypical antipsychotics and glucose homeostasis. *Journal of Clinical Psychiatry, 66*(4), 504–514.

Browne, G. (2005). Housing, social support and people with schizophrenia: A grounded theory study. *Issues in Mental Health Nursing, 26,* 311–326.

Buchanan, R. W., & Carpenter, W. T. (2004). Schizophrenia: Introduction and overview and other psychotic disorders. In B. J. Sadock & V. A. Sadock (Eds.), *Kaplan & Sadock's comprehensive textbook of psychiatry* (8th ed., pp. 1096–1109). Philadelphia, PA: Lippincott Williams & Wilkins.

Bulechek, G. M., Butcher, H. K., & McCloskey Dochterman, J. (2008). *Nursing interventions classification (NIC)* (5th ed.). St. Louis, MO: Mosby.

Compton, M. T., Weiss, P. S., West, J. C., & Kaslow, N. J. (2005). The associations between substance use disorders, schizophrenia-spectrum disorders, and Axis IV psychosocial problems. *Social Psychiatry and Psychiatric Epidemiology, 40*(12), 939–946.

Cooper, P. (2003). Psychosis: Do they know it's drug-induced? *Mental Health Nursing, 23*(2), 14–27.

El-Mallakh, P., Howard, P. B., & Evans, B. N. (2010). Medical illnesses in people with schizophrenia. *Nursing Clinics of North America, 45,* 591–611.

England, M. (2007). Efficacy of cognitive nursing intervention for voice hearing. *Perspectives in Psychiatric Care, 43*(2), 69–76.

Gard, D. E., Kring, A. M., Gard, M. G., Horan, W. P., & Green, M. F. (2007). Anhedonia in schizophrenia: Distinctions between anticipatory and consummatory pleasure. *Schizophrenia Research, 93,* 253–260.

Goldman, M. B. (2010). The assessment and treatment of water imbalance in patients with psychosis. *Clinical Schizophrenia and Related Psychoses, 4,* 115–123.

Gonzalez-Torres, M. A., Oraa, R., Aristegui, M., Fernandez-Rivas, A., & Guimon, J. (2007). Stigma and discrimination towards people with schizophrenia and their family members. A qualitative study with focus groups. *Social Psychiatry and Psychiatric Epidemiology, 42*(1), 14–23.

Hennekens, C., Hennekens, A., & Hollar, D. (2005). Schizophrenia and increased risks of cardiovascular disease. *American Heart Journal, 150*(6), 1115–1121.

Horwath, E., & Cournos, F. (1999). Schizophrenia and other psychotic disorders. In J. L. Cutler & R. Marcus (Eds.), *Psychiatry*. Philadelphia, PA: W. B. Saunders.

Huang, H.S., Matevossian, A., Shittle, C., Kim, S. Y., Schumacher, A., Baker, S. P., & Akbarian, S. (2007). Prefrontal dysfunction in schizophrenia involves mixed-lineage leukemia 1-regulated histone methylation at GABAergic gene promoters. *Journal of Neuroscience, 27*(42), 11254–11262.

Iritani, S. (2007). Neuropathology of schizophrenia: A mini review. *Japanese Society of Neuropathology, 27,* 604–608.

Kalat, J. W. (2006). *Biological psychology* (9th ed.). Belmont, CA: Wadsworth/Thomson Learning.

Karch, A. (2009). *2009 Lippincott's nursing drug guide*. Philadelphia, PA: Lippincott Williams & Wilkins.

Kasai, K., Iwanami, A., Yamasue, H., Kuroki, N., Nakagome, K., & Fukuda, M. (2002). Neuroanatomy and neurophysiology in schizophrenia. *Neuroscience Research, 43*(2), 93–110.

Kreyenbuhl, J., Buchanan, R. W., Dickerson, F. B., Dixon, L. B., & Schizophrenia Patient Outcomes Research Team (PORT). (2010). The Schizophrenia Patient Outcomes Research Team (PORT): Updated treatment recommendations 2009. *Schizophrenia Bulletin, 36,* 94–103.

Landeen, J. (2001). Review: Social skills training, supported employment programmes, and cognitive behaviour therapy improve some outcomes in schizophrenia. *Evidence Based Nursing, 4*(4), 115.

Lehman, A. F., Kreyenbuhl, J., Buchanan, R. W., Dickerson, F. B., Dixon, L. B., Goldberg, R., ... Steinwachs, D. M. (2004). The Schizophrenia Patient Outcomes Research Team (PORT): Updated treatment recommendations 2003. *Schizophrenia Bulletin, 30*(2), 193–217.

Lehman, A. F., Steinwachs, D. M., & the Co-Investigators of the PORT Project. (1998). *The Schizophrenia Patient Outcomes Research Team (PORT) treatment recommendations.* Rockville, MD: Agency for Healthcare Research and Quality.

Magliano, L., Fiorillo, A., Malangone, C., Marasco, C., Guarneri, M., & Maj, M. (2003). The effect of social network on burden and pessimism in relatives of patients with schizophrenia. *American Journal of Orthopsychiatry, 73,* 302–309.

Mamo, D. C. (2007). Managing suicidality in schizophrenia. *Canadian Journal of Psychiatry, 52*(6 Suppl 1), 59S–70S.

McManus, D. Q., Arvanitis, L. A., & Kowalcyk, B. B. (1999). Quetiapine, a novel antipsychotic: Experience in elderly patients with psychotic disorders. *Journal of Clinical Psychiatry, 60*(5), 292–298.

McWilliams, S., Hill, S., Mannion, N., Fetherston, A., Kinsella, A., & O'Callaghan, E. (2011). Schizophrenia: A five-year follow-up of patient outcome following psycho-education for caregivers. *European Psychiatry.* Retrieved from http://www.sciencedirect.com/science/article/pii/S0924933810001689. doi:10.1016/j.eurpsy.2010.08.012.

Moorhead, S., Johnson, M., Maas, M. L., & Swanson, E. (2008). *Nursing outcomes classification (NOC)* (4th ed.). St. Louis, MO: Mosby.

NANDA International. (2007). *Nursing diagnoses: Definitions and classification (2007–2008).* Philadelphia, PA: Author.

Nasrallah, H. A., & Smeltzer, D. J. (2003). *Contemporary diagnosis and management of the patient with schizophrenia.* Newtown, PA: Handbooks in Health Care.

National Institute of Mental Health (NIMH). (2006). *The numbers count: Mental disorders in America. A fact sheet describing the prevalence of mental disorders in America.* Retrieved from http://www.nimh.nih.gov/healthinformation/statisticsmenu.cfm

National Institute of Mental Health (NIMH). (2009). *Schizophrenia.* Retrieved from http://www.nimh.nih.gov/health/publications/schizophrenia/index.shtml

Patterson, P. H. (2007). Maternal effects on schizophrenia risk. *Science, 318,* 576–577.

Ritsner, M. S., Arbitman, M., Lisker, A., & Ponizovsky, A. M. (2011). Ten-year quality of life outcomes among patients with schizophrenia and schizoaffective disorder II. Predictive value of psychosocial factors. *Quality of Life Research.* Retrieved from http://www.springerlink.com/content/c1571881424u5206/fulltext.pdf .doi:10.1007/s11136-011-0015-4

Ross, C. A., & Goldner, E. M. (2009). Stigma, negative attitudes and discrimination towards mental illness within the nursing profession: A review of the literature. *Journal of Psychiatric and Mental Health Nursing, 16,* 558–567.

Salyers, M. P., & Tsemberis, S. (2007). ACT and recovery: Integrating evidence-based practice and recovery orientation on assertive community treatment teams. *Community Mental Health Journal, 43*(6), 619–641.

Scheen, A. J., & De Hert, M. A. (2007). Abnormal glucose metabolism in patients treated with antipsychotics. *Diabetes & Metabolism, 33*(3), 169–175.

Sponheim, S. R., Jung, R. E., Seidman, L. J., Mesholam-Gately, R. I., Manoach, D. S., O'Leary, D. S., ... Schulz, S. C. (2010). Cognitive deficits in recent-onset and chronic schizophrenia. *Journal of Psychiatric Research, 44,* 421–428.

Steel, C., Haddock, G., Tarrier, N., Picken, A., & Barrowclough, C. (2011). Auditory hallucinations and posttraumatic stress disorder within schizophrenia substance abuse. The *Journal of Nervous and Mental Disease, 199,* 709–711.

Tandon, R., Keshavan, M. S., & Nasrallah, H. A. (2008). Schizophrenia, "just the facts": What we know in 2008. 2. Epidemiology and etiology. *Schizophrenia Research, 102,* 1–18.

Tandon, R., Nasrallah, H. A., & Keshavan, M. S. (2011). "Just the facts": Meandering in schizophrenia's many forests. *Schizophrenia Research, 128,* 5–6.

Thaker, G. K., Cassady, S., & Adami, H. (1996). Eye movements in spectrum personality disorders: Comparison of community subjects and relatives of schizophrenic patients. *American Journal of Psychiatry, 153,* 362–368.

Toprac, M. G., Rush, A. J., Conner, T. M., Crismon, M. L., Dees, M., Hopkins, C., ... Shon, S. P. (2000). The Texas Medication Algorithm Project and Patient and Family Education Program: A consumer-guided initiative. *Journal of Clinical Psychiatry, 61*(7), 477–486.

Turkington, D., Dudley, R., Warman, D. M., & Beck, A. T. (2004). Cognitive–behavioral therapy for schizophrenia: A review. *Journal of Psychiatric Practice, 10,* 5–16.

Velligan, D. I., & Gonzalez, J. M. (2007). Rehabilitation and recovery in schizophrenia. *Psychiatric Clinics of North America, 30*(3), 535–548.

Wu, E. Q., Birnbaum, H. G., Shi, L., Ball, D. E., Kessler, R. C., Moulis, M., & Aggarwal, J. (2005). The economic burden of schizophrenia in the United States in 2002. *Journal of Clinical Psychiatry, 66*(9), 1122–1129.

Zullino, D. F., Waber, L., & Khazaal, Y. (2008). Cannabis and the course of schizophrenia. *American Journal of Psychiatry, 165,* 1357–1358.

Web Resources

National Alliance for the Mentally Ill: http://www.nami.org
Schizophrenia Society of Canada: http://www.schizophrenia.ca
Schizophrenics Anonymous: http://www.schizophrenia.com

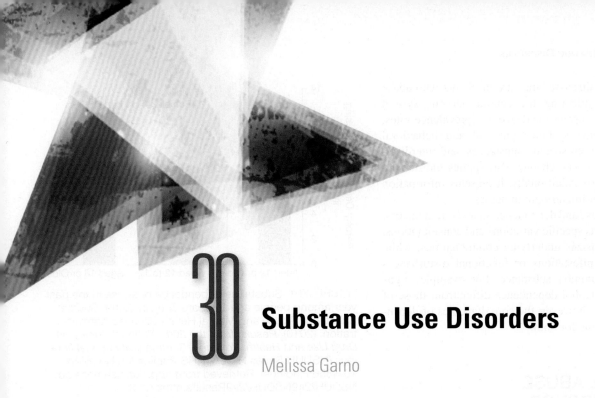

30

Substance Use Disorders

Melissa Garno

LEARNING OBJECTIVES

On completion of this chapter, you should be able to accomplish the following:

- Define substance abuse, substance dependence, tolerance, and withdrawal.
- Discuss the incidence of and current trends in substance use disorders.
- Describe etiologic factors involved in substance use disorders.
- Outline current diagnostic categories for various types of substance problems.
- Identify key information about alcohol and controlled substances relative to effects, signs of intoxication, and symptoms of withdrawal.
- Explain the importance of recognizing co-occurring disorders.
- Describe the effects of substance use disorders on physiology, behavior, family, and society.
- Identify the two main components of interdisciplinary treatment for clients with substance use disorders.
- Apply the nursing process to the care of the client who abuses or is dependent on substances.
- Discuss what is meant by an *impaired nurse* and how nurses should behave if they suspect substance problems in a colleague.

This chapter discusses the care of clients who abuse substances affecting the central nervous system (CNS). It examines current incidence and prevalence rates, etiology, classification systems, physical and behavioral changes associated with specific substances, and interdisciplinary interventions. The chapter also applies the nursing process to client care. Additionally, it presents information about the problem of impairment in nurses.

All drugs of abuse and dependence share certain factors; additionally, each has specific variations and considerations. This chapter emphasizes underlying commonalities, while also explaining manifestations or functional disturbances specific to each common substance. For example, signs and symptoms of alcohol dependence differ from those of cocaine dependence; however, the core dynamics of dependence remain the same for both.

SUBSTANCE ABUSE AND DEPENDENCE

Substance use disorders, as defined by the American Psychiatric Association (APA, 2000), is an umbrella term for substance abuse and substance dependence. **Substance abuse** means the repeated use of drugs (including alcohol) leading to functional problems. However, such problems involve neither compulsive use nor **withdrawal** (painful physical and psychological symptoms that follow discontinuance of a drug). **Substance dependence** is the correct term when a person uses alcohol or other drugs despite extreme negative consequences, such as significant impairments to daily living. Substance dependence also leads to **tolerance** (the body becoming less responsive to the drug with repeated exposure) and withdrawal when the client stops taking the substance in question.

The terms **addiction** and *dependence* are frequently used interchangeably. There is little consensus on what addiction actually means, but it usually refers to a behavior pattern characterized by overwhelming (compulsive) involvement with securing and using a drug and a high tendency of relapse after discontinuation. Addiction is often referred to as a "disease of perception" in that denial plays a major component. Addicted clients refuse to admit that they are powerless over their problem. They continue their habit despite its negative consequences, justifying such behavior and projecting its cause on external sources.

Incidence and Prevalence

Approximately 9% of the U.S. population 12 years and older has substance abuse or dependence (Substance Abuse and Mental Health Services Administration [SAMHSA], 2010b) (Figure 30.1). Highlights from the most recent National Household Survey on Drug Abuse are presented in Box 30.1; access to the full range of U.S. statistics on substance abuse and dependence can be retrieved from http://oas.samhsa.gov/NSDUH/2k9NSDUH/2k9Results.htm#Ch3. These data

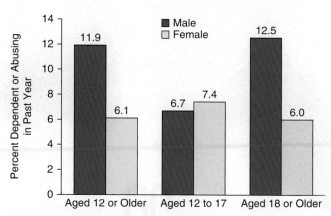

FIGURE 30.1 Substance dependence or abuse in the past year among people age 12 years or older, 2009. Source: Substance Abuse and Mental Health Services Administration. (2010). *Results from the 2009 National Survey on Drug Use and Health: Volume I. Summary of national findings* (NSDUH Series H-38A, HHS Publication No. SMA 10-4856 Findings). Retrieved from http://oas.samhsa.gov/NSDUH/2k9NSDUH/2k9Results.htm#7.1.2

serve as a valuable tool for states and community-based organizations to tailor programs to their specific demographic needs. They also indicate the extent of national substance problems.

Alcohol-Related Statistics

Drinking is most common among teens and young adults. In 2009, nearly 52% of Americans ages 12 and older reported using alcohol, with the highest use among those from 21 to

---

BOX 30.1 Key Facts from the 2009 *National Household Survey on Drug Abuse*

- Nearly 52% of Americans 12 years or older reported being current drinkers of alcohol.
- An estimated 21.8 million Americans 12 years or older (8.7% of the population) were current illicit drug users.
- The overall rate of current illicit drug use among those 12 years or older in 2009 (8.7%) was higher than the rate in 2008 (8.0%).
- In 2009, marijuana was the most commonly used illicit drug among persons 12 years and older at a rate of 21.8%; nonmedical use of prescription-type pain relievers, tranquilizers, stimulants, and sedatives ranked second at 16.7%.
- Current marijuana use increased from 6.7% in 2006 to 7.3% in 2009.
- From 2002 to 2009, there was an increase in the rate of current nonmedical use of prescription-type drugs among young adults ages 18 to 25 (from 5.5% to 6.3%).
- From 2002 to 2009, there were decreases in the use of cocaine (from 2.0% to 1.4%) and methamphetamine (from 0.6% to 0.2%) among young adults ages 18 to 25.

Substance Abuse and Mental Health Services Administration. (2010). *Results from the 2009 National Survey on Drug Use and Health: Volume I. Summary of National Findings* (NSDUH Series H-38A, USDHHS Publication No. SMA 10-4856 Findings). Retrieved from http://oas.samhsa.gov/NSDUH/2k9NSDUH/2k9Results.htm#Ch2.

25 years of age (70.2%). The prevalence of those reporting current alcohol use decreases with increasing age, from 66.4% of persons in their late 20s, to 50.3% of persons in their early 60s, and 39.1% of those ages 65 or older (SAMHSA, 2010b). Binge drinking also peaks among persons ages 21 to 25, with 46.5% of that age group consuming five or more drinks on one occasion (SAMHSA, 2010b). People who begin to drink early in life are at increased risk for long-term alcohol problems. Conventional wisdom has posited that college students particularly engage in heavy drinking. Although college students tend to drink in greater quantities than do nonstudents, they drink less frequently than do noncollege peers (SAMHSA, 2010b). Younger populations generally engage more frequently in binge drinking, whereas those who become dependent show more regular patters of heavy drinking (Anton, 2010). Studies have also shown that men are much more likely to drink in harmful ways than are women (SAMHSA, 2010b).

Drug-Related Statistics

The specific illicit drugs that had the highest levels of dependence or abuse in 2009 were marijuana, pain relievers, and cocaine. Since 2002, dependence or abuse has increased slightly for both marijuana and pain relievers. Cocaine abuse or dependence has declined (National Institute on Drug Abuse [NIDA], 2011c; SAMHSA, 2010b). The most frequently used illicit drug, and that preferred by the youngest population, is marijuana. The rate of hallucinogen abuse, including LSD, PCP, peyote, mescaline, psilocybin mushrooms, and ecstasy (MDMA), has remained steady since 2002, while the use of cocaine and crack has declined slightly. Nonmedical use of prescription drugs, primarily pain relievers, increased from 2002 to 2009. The majority of non-marijuana drug users include those who use psychotherapeutic drugs nonmedically. In 2009, an estimated 5.3 million persons used pain relievers, 2.0 million used tranquilizers, 1.3 million used stimulants, and 370,000 used sedatives (SAMHSA, 2010b).

The number of drug-related emergency department (ED) visits has increased significantly in recent years, from 2.5 million in 2004 to 4.6 million in 2009. The most recent statistics on drug-related ED visits include reports of drug abuse, adverse drug reactions, or other drug-related consequences. Forty-five percent of these visits involved drug abuse (nonmedical use of pharmaceuticals, illicit drugs, alcohol, and alcohol in combination with other drugs) (NIDA, 2011b). It is estimated that alcohol is a factor in about 60% of fatal burn injuries, drownings, and homicides; 50% of severe trauma injuries and sexual assaults; and 40% of fatal motor vehicle crashes, suicides, and fatal falls (National Institute on Alcohol Abuse and Alcoholism [NIAAA], 2010b).

Cultural and Ethnic Variations

Substance use disorders occur in all cultures and ethnicities. However, variations exist in patterns, preferences, and aspects of prevention, treatment, and rehabilitation. For example, 32% of Caucasians, 21% of Native Americans, 19% of African Americans, and 15% of Asian Americans report current drinking. The rate of drinking in Hispanics is 26%, but the average age of drinking in this group is older than in whites or Native Americans (NIAAA, 2006a; SAMHSA, 2010b). Cultural perceptions and expectations may influence differences in rates of use, peak age, and other factors.

Substance abuse seems to increase when people are exposed to drug use in their personal lives. Patterns of reporting by NIDA (2003b) reveal that perceptions of the harmfulness of drug use and the incidence of consequent use are more influenced by the increasing prevalence of drug use and personal observation of drug-related casualties and less influenced by concurrent mass media or drug prevention campaigns (NIDA, 2003b).

> **Checkpoint Questions**
>
> **1.** What does a client diagnosed with substance dependence experience that a client diagnosed with substance abuse does not?
>
> **2.** What are current trends in types of drugs used?

Etiology

Complex internal and external factors influence whether people engage in substances and to what degree they incur related problems. While some factors increase risks, others reduce them. For example, men are more likely to drink in harmful ways than women. Rates of use among African Americans and Hispanics peak later and persist longer into adulthood than in Caucasians. College students tend to drink less often but in greater quantities than noncollege peers (NIAAA, 2006b). Emerging multidimensional models strongly link substance use disorders to neurophysiology. Research and exploration reveals new information daily. Age, sex, ethnicity, and social setting affect use, as do availability of drugs, cost, and peer pressure. The U.S. culture also exerts an influence, with media depictions glamorizing alcohol and street drugs, and pharmaceutical companies promoting prescription and over-the-counter medications in widespread advertisements. Responses to specific drugs vary according to dosage, frequency, route of administration, and individual biologic, behavioral, social, and psychological factors.

Biologic Foundations

Strong familial links in substance use disorders have been identified (Thompson & Lande, 2007). Such patterns are likely to result from combinations of genetic predispositions, biologic influences, and learned behaviors (see Chaps. 2 and 3). Children of clients with alcoholism are 50% to 60% more likely to develop alcohol use disorders than are the general population (NIAAA, 2010a; Sadock & Sadock, 2008). Studies show similar links between heroin use and genetic ties within family systems (Trafton et al., 2007).

Between 40% and 60% of substance dependence is inherited (Anton, 2010). Studies supported by the National Institutes of Health have identified specific genes that increase the risk for alcohol dependency. To date, more than 20 genes have been identified as associated with alcoholism, although specific genes responsible for alcohol-related characteristics are still being studied (NIAAA, 2010a). Genes that code for brain chemicals and their receptors account for individual differences in response to substances (Anton, 2010). Genetic differences in neurotransmitter systems responsible for the brain's pleasure circuit can account for excessive substance use, as well as genetic differences in stress responses (Kilpatrick et al., 2007). A specific dopamine receptor has been identified that is responsible for motivation for reward seeking as well as the rewarding effects of cocaine (Bello et al., 2011). Increasingly, the elucidation of physiologic mechanisms involved with drug abuse and dependence is helping to explain the compulsion to use addictive substances despite negative consequences. Researchers have studied the effects of illicit drugs on reward pathways in the brain. Normally, the neurotransmitter dopamine sends pleasurable stimuli along a pathway involving the ventral tegmental area, nucleus accumbens, and prefrontal cortex (see Chap. 2). Drugs of abuse interfere with such neurotransmission. They may bind themselves to dopamine receptor sites, thus replacing dopamine's effects with their own. Or they may block the reuptake pumps that remove dopamine from the synapses, leading dopamine to accumulate there. Stimulation of receiving neurons initially results in mood-altering effects—depression or euphoria, depending on the drug used. With continued use and subsequent alterations in the normal neurotransmission related to dopamine, the brain may begin to produce less dopamine or the pleasure pathway may be destroyed. Cravings for stimulation of the pleasure pathway often lead to compulsive behaviors to obtain the chemicals of stimulation. Craving for the stimulus eventually becomes stronger than the reward. See Understanding Biologic Foundations 30.1.

Psychosocial and Behavioral Factors

Past theorists considered psychosocial and behavioral factors to be the primary cause of substance problems. Current experts view these factors as operating within the context of "vulnerability" in genetically susceptible people (see Chap. 3).

Individual personality factors associated with alcohol-related problems include antisocial behavior, poor self-regulation, poor self-control, anxiety, a tendency toward depression, and shyness (NIAAA, 2009). Affective disorders, such as depression and post-traumatic stress disorder, and psychological symptoms including sadness, hostility, anxiety, and social withdrawal are correlated with higher incidences of substance abuse (Tiet & Mausbach, 2007). Variations in problem-solving techniques and coping styles may also be associated with addictive disorders, with people who rely on cognitive and problem-solving skills being more prone to avoiding them (Weaver et al., 2000; Winter, 2001).

The stress response has also been investigated (see Chap. 24). Higher perceived stress is associated with greater severity of substance abuse, and chronic use has been hypothesized to change (perhaps permanently) the stress response and a person's coping styles (Anton, 2010). Alcohol's sedative properties affect individuals differently, depending on genetic makeup. Those who have a reduced sedative response to alcohol are at higher risk for alcohol use disorders (Hendler et al., 2011).

In summary, psychological and behavioral theories about substance abuse have revealed important information about individual coping styles and life stressors. However, psychological theories do not explain how people become addicted, how the addictive process is perpetuated, or the difficulty experienced by those attempting to stop.

Signs and Symptoms/Diagnostic Criteria

The *Diagnostic and Statistical Manual of Mental Disorders,* 4th edition, text revision (*DSM-IV-TR*) (APA, 2000) classifies substance use disorders into 12 categories, all of which share common subdiagnostic categories (dependence, abuse, intoxication, and withdrawal) with generic diagnostic criteria (*DSM-IV-TR* Box 30.1). Regardless of the type and subtype, clients with substance use disorders are impaired physically, socially, and psychologically at some time during their illness. They are also at risk for being socially ostracized because most cultures do not tolerate or accept the behaviors that result from chronic chemical impairment.

Alcohol-Related Disorders

Alcohol, also known chemically as **ethanol**, sometimes is abbreviated as ETOH. Technically, the substance is ethyl alcohol (C_2H_5OH). It is a legal drug; that is, its commercial distribution differs from the more tightly regulated sale of other drugs (ie, controlled substances).

The pharmacologic properties of ethyl alcohol produce mind- and mood-altering effects of CNS depression (similar to barbiturates). Alcohol is often mistaken for a stimulant; the reason for this misconception is that after drinking it, some people become more talkative, hyperactive, euphoric, self-confident, or aggressive. This behavior has been attributed to the disinhibiting effect produced by low doses of alcohol.

Alcoholic beverages include beer, wine, and distilled spirits. The alcohol content of a beverage is expressed as **proof** (concentration of ethyl alcohol). In the United States, proof is twice the ethanol concentration (eg, 100 proof is 50% ethyl alcohol, and 80 proof is 40% ethyl alcohol). A standard drink is defined as any drink containing 0.6 fluid ounce or 14 grams of "pure" alcohol. Examples of standard drinks include 12 ounces of beer (5% alcohol), 5 ounces of table wine (12% alcohol), or 1.5 ounces of liquor (40% alcohol). In contrast to other drugs that produce effects with small quantities, alcohol usually requires large quantities over an extended period to result in physical dependence. Excessive alcohol consumption can be described as either **binge drinking**, meaning five or more drinks on the same occasion

Dopamine Release. Dopamine (*red*) is a neurotransmitter involved in pleasurable sensations. As an electrical impulse arrives at the first neuron's terminal (*top*), vesicles move to the neural membrane and release dopamine into the synaptic cleft. Dopamine crosses the gap and binds to receptors on the second neuron (*bottom*). While dopamine is bound, various actions take place in the second neuron: enzymes are released or inhibited and ions exit or enter. New electrical impulses are generated, and neurotransmission continues.

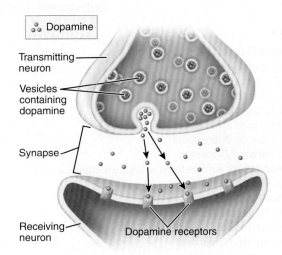

Dopamine Removal. Reuptake pumps (*yellow*) eventually remove dopamine from the synaptic cleft and pull it back into the original neuron. For normal neurotransmission, dopamine must not remain in the cleft.

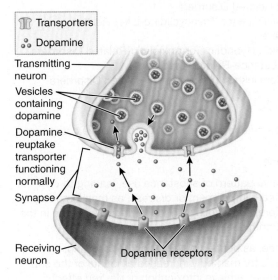

Addition of Cocaine. When cocaine (*blue*) enters the brain's reward pathway, it blocks the reuptake pumps that remove dopamine from the synapse. Dopamine accumulates in the synapse, causing feelings of intense pleasure. Unfortunately, prolonged cocaine use may lead the brain to begin to depend on its presence for normal function, "downregulating" its natural amount of dopamine. If the person stops using cocaine, insufficient dopamine is in the synapses, and the person experiences the opposite of pleasure—depression, fatigue, and low mood.

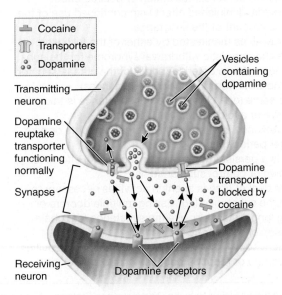

DSM-IV-TR BOX 30.1

Substance-Related Disorders

Categories

1. Substance-Related Disorders
   a. Substance Use Disorders
      i. Substance Dependence
      ii. Substance Abuse
   b. Substance-Induced Disorders
      i Substance Intoxication
      ii. Substance Withdrawal
2. Alcohol-Related Disorders
3. Amphetamine (or Amphetamine-Like)-Related Disorders
4. Caffeine-Related Disorders
5. Cannabis-Related Disorders
6. Cocaine-Related Disorders
7. Hallucinogen-Related Disorders
8. Inhalant-Related Disorders
9. Nicotine-Related Disorders
10. Opioid-Related Disorders
11. Phencyclidine (or Phencyclidine-Like)-Related Disorders
12. Sedative-, Hypnotic-, or Anxiolytic-Related Disorders
13. Polysubstance-Related Disorder
14. Other (or Unknown) Substance-Related Disorders

Criteria

Note: *These criteria apply to all 14 of the above categories.*

Dependence

A maladaptive pattern of substance use, leading to clinically significant impairment or distress, as manifested by three (or more) of the following, occurring at any time in the same 12-month period:

1. Tolerance, as defined by either of the following:
   a. A need for markedly increased amounts of the substance to achieve intoxication or desired effect
   b. Markedly diminished effect with continued use of the same amount of the substance
2. Withdrawal, as manifested by either of the following:
   a. The characteristic withdrawal syndrome for the substance (refer to criteria A and B of the criteria sets for Withdrawal from the specific substances)
   b. The same (or a closely related) substance is taken to relieve or avoid withdrawal symptoms
3. The substance is often taken in larger amounts or over a longer period than was intended
4. There is a persistent desire or unsuccessful efforts to cut down or control substance use
5. A great deal of time is spent in activities necessary to obtain the substance (eg, visiting multiple doctors or driving long distances), use the substance (eg, chain smoking), or recover from its effects
6. Important social, occupational, or recreational activities are given up or reduced because of substance use

7. The substance use is continued despite knowledge of having a persistent or recurrent physical or psychological problem that is likely to have been caused or exacerbated by the substance (eg, current cocaine use despite recognition of cocaine-induced depression, or continued drinking despite recognition that an ulcer was made worse by alcohol consumption)

Abuse

A maladaptive pattern of substance use leading to clinically significant impairment or distress as manifested by one (or more) of the following, occurring within a 12-month period:

1. Recurrent substance use resulting in a failure to fulfill major role obligations at work, school, or home (eg, repeated absences or poor work performance related to substance use; substance-related absences, suspensions, or expulsions from school; or neglect of children or household)
2. Recurrent substance use in situations in which it is physically hazardous (eg, driving an automobile or operating a machine when impaired by substance use)
3. Recurrent substance-related legal problems (eg, arrests for substance-related disorderly conduct)
4. Continued substance use despite having persistent or recurrent social or interpersonal problems caused or exacerbated by the effects of the substance (eg, arguments with spouse about consequences of intoxication, physical fights).

The symptoms have never met the criteria for dependence for this class of substance.

Intoxication

A. The development of a reversible substance-specific syndrome due to recent ingestion of (or exposure to) a substance. **Note:** Different substances may produce similar or identical syndromes.
B. Clinically significant maladaptive behavioral or psychological changes that are due to the effect of the substance on the central nervous system (eg, belligerence, mood lability, cognitive impairment, impaired judgment, impaired social or occupational functioning) and develop during or shortly after use of the substance.
C. The symptoms are not due to a general medical condition and are not better accounted for by another mental disorder.

Withdrawal

A. The development of a substance-specific syndrome due to the cessation of (or reduction in) substance use that has been heavy and prolonged.
B. The substance-specific syndrome causes clinically significant distress or impairment in social, occupational, or other important areas of functioning.
C. The symptoms are not due to a general medical condition and are not better accounted for by another mental disorder.

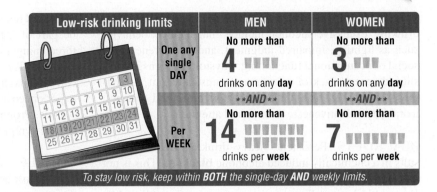

Low-risk drinking limits		MEN	WOMEN
One any single DAY		No more than **4** ▪▪▪▪ drinks on any **day**	No more than **3** ▪▪▪ drinks on any **day**
		AND	**AND**
Per WEEK		No more than **14** ▪▪▪▪▪▪▪ ▪▪▪▪▪▪▪ drinks per **week**	No more than **7** ▪▪▪▪▪▪▪ drinks per **week**

*To stay low risk, keep within **BOTH** the single-day **AND** weekly limits.*

FIGURE 30.2 Low-risk drinking limits. Source: National Institute on Alcohol Abuse and Alcoholism. (2010). *Rethinking drinking: Alcohol and your health: What are the risks?* Retrieved from http://rethinkingdrinking. niaaa.nih.gov/IsYourDrinkingPatternRisky/ WhatsLowRiskDrinking.asp

during 1 or more day in the past month, or **heavy drinking**, meaning five or more drinks on the same occasion on 5 or more days in the past month (SAMHSA, 2010b). Current national recommendations define low-risk drinking as no more than 4 drinks per day and 14 drinks per week for men, and no more than 3 drinks per day and 7 drinks per week for women (see Figure 30.2). Use in excess of these recommendations indicates heavy drinking and an increased risk for alcohol abuse (NIAAA, 2010b).

With increasing consumption, alcohol causes the following pattern (Figure 30.3):

1. Sedation
2. Impaired mental and motor functioning
3. Deepening stupor with a decreased stimulation response (including painful stimulus response)
4. Coma
5. Eventually, death from respiratory and circulatory collapse (Ries et al. 2009)

ALCOHOL CONCENTRATION IN THE BODY. Physical and behavioral manifestations of alcohol on the CNS relate directly to blood level and concentration in the brain. The **blood alcohol level (BAL)** is expressed as milligrams of alcohol per milliliter of blood. It is determined by a

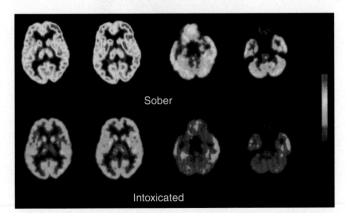

FIGURE 30.3 Alcohol drinking markedly reduces brain metabolism. Source: NIAAA, 2008. Retrieved from http://www .niaaa.nih.gov/Resources/GraphicsGallery/Neuroscience/ Pages/brain_activity.aspx

laboratory blood test, which may be used in medicolegal procedures to rule out intoxication in a comatose person. A breathalyzer also measures degree of intoxication. Use of handheld breathalyzers in home and other nonmedical settings has gained popularity.

Alcohol concentration in the blood depends on rates of absorption, transport to the CNS, redistribution to other parts of the body, metabolism, and elimination. Alcohol is absorbed through the mouth, stomach, and small intestine and delivered unchanged into the blood, where it circulates throughout the body, including the brain. In pregnant women, alcohol crosses the placenta into the fetal circulation. A person becomes intoxicated when circulating alcohol interferes with normal neurologic functioning (Ries et al., 2009).

Several factors can influence the rate of absorption of alcohol into the blood:

- Beverage substances, such as carbonation (CO_2) in champagne, can increase absorption.
- Drinking alcohol slowly over a long period may slow absorption and allow for metabolism by the liver. Because the body metabolizes alcohol at a steady rate, when a person drinks faster than the body can metabolize the alcohol, it accumulates in the blood.
- Food in the stomach (especially fatty food) slows absorption, whereas an empty stomach increases it.
- The drinker's emotional state may also affect absorption. For example, stress, fear, anger, and fatigue may increase or decrease absorption.

Body size affects the concentration of alcohol in the blood. The same amount of alcohol ingested by a 100-lb (45.3 kg) versus a 200-lb (90.7 kg) person results in greater blood alcohol concentration in the lighter person because the heavier person has more blood volume to dilute the alcohol. Body chemistry and cultural influences may also alter alcohol's behavioral effects.

Oxidation, which occurs mainly in the liver, eliminates 90% of the alcohol absorbed by the body. The remaining 10% is eliminated unchanged through fluids such as breath, sweat, and urine. The rate of drinking may vary, but alcohol is excreted at a fixed rate. The healthy liver metabolizes approximately 1 oz (29.5 mL) of alcohol per hour; the excess alcohol that the liver cannot metabolize continues to circulate in the blood.

INTOXICATION. Manifestations of intoxication after drinking excessive alcohol include maladaptive behavior such as fighting, impaired judgment, and interference with social or occupational functioning. Physiologic signs involve slurred speech, lack of coordination, unsteady gait, nystagmus, and flushed face. Other indicators are mood changes, irritability, talkativeness, or impaired attention.

BLACKOUTS. Persistent, heavy drinking frequently results in a chemically induced alcoholic **blackout**. This is not the same as passing out or fainting (losing consciousness). During blackouts, clients appear to function normally while drinking but later cannot remember what happened. The blackout may last a few or several hours. Clients may come out of the blackout and wonder "Where did I leave my car last night?" They may wake up in a strange place unable to remember leaving home and wonder "How did I get here?" or "Was I with someone?"

TOLERANCE. Prolonged heavy alcohol use results in physical and behavioral tolerance. Physical tolerance (tissue adaptation) means that changes occur in the cells of the CNS so that a person needs more of the substance to achieve the desired effect. Physically tolerant clients may experience symptoms of withdrawal after cessation or decreased consumption. Physical tolerance to alcohol never reaches the high-dose tolerance of opiates (see later discussion). Cross-tolerance to sedative-hypnotics and other CNS depressants is likely.

Behavioral tolerance to alcohol is manifested by the ability to mask the drug's effects. For example, clients with alcoholism acquire the ability not to slur words, to walk straight, and to function in ways that would not be possible in nondependent people who drink. The history of clients with alcoholism often reveals the ability to increase tolerance to alcohol and to maintain this increase for a long time, perhaps several years. Frequently, an irreversible drop in tolerance follows; clients become intoxicated with smaller amounts of alcohol.

WITHDRAWAL. *Alcohol withdrawal*, also referred to as *abstinence syndrome*, occurs after a reduction in or cessation of prolonged heavy drinking. The earliest signs include irritability and impatient behavior. A coarse tremor of the hands, tongue, and eyelids may follow, along with nausea and vomiting, general malaise or weakness, autonomic nervous system hyperactivity (eg, increased blood pressure and pulse), headache, paroxysmal sweats, anxiety, depressed or irritable mood, and orthostatic hypotension. Sleep disturbances, insomnia, nightmares, or hallucinations are other possibilities.

Alcohol withdrawal delirium, called **delirium tremens (DTs)**, is the most serious form of withdrawal syndrome. It occurs within 48 hours after cessation of, or reduction in, prolonged heavy drinking and can continue for as long as 1 week. Symptoms involve increased agitation, confusion, anxiety, delusions, coarse tremors, fever, diaphoresis,

increased heart rate, and precordial pain. Hallucinations may be part of DTs. The client may experience vivid, perhaps threatening auditory hallucinations, but consciousness is not clouded. The person's response to the hallucinations typically is anxiety or fear. Auditory hallucinations are usually experienced as voices but may be heard as hissing or buzzing sounds. Prompt and adequate sedation at the onset of withdrawal symptoms can prevent DTs.

COMPLICATIONS. Heavy consumption of alcohol adversely affects most body systems (Figure 30.4). Various medical conditions may signify alcohol problems. Clients may also develop cognitive disorders specifically associated with long-term alcoholism.

Nonspecific indicators of regular alcohol use include elevated mean corpuscular volume, gamma-glutamyltransferase (GGT), and carbohydrate-deficient transferrin levels. Although other conditions such as nonalcoholic liver disease, hyperthyroidism, and use of anticonvulsants can also elevate GGT levels, this combination of findings should raise suspicion of regular alcohol consumption of 6 to 8 oz/day (177.4 to 236.5 mL) (Compton, 2002). Care should be taken to note the coexistence of thyroid or seizure disorders to avoid confusion with these laboratory indicators of substance abuse.

Gastrointestinal problems such as esophagitis, gastritis, gastric ulcers, and acute or chronic pancreatitis result from

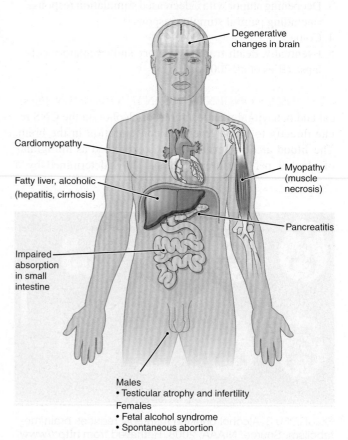

FIGURE 30.4 Chronic alcohol abuse has multisystemic complications.

the irritating effects of alcohol, the increased acid production that develops in response to alcohol's intake, and frequent vomiting after bouts of drinking. Cardiovascular problems such as mild to moderate hypertension, cardiomyopathy, or dysrhythmias result from the direct toxic effects of the substance and malnutrition. A high risk of cancer, especially of the mouth, pharynx, larynx, esophagus, pancreas, stomach, and colon, is associated with alcoholism. Hematopoietic complications include decreased white blood cell production, decreased granulocyte adherence, and thrombocytopenia, leading to compromised immune function.

Liver Damage. The liver is highly susceptible to alcohol's damaging effects because it is the primary organ that metabolizes alcohol. Alcohol is toxic to the liver, regardless of the person's nutritional status. Approximately 20% of heavy drinkers develop *alcoholic fatty liver* (steatosis), which can be reversed if they significantly reduce or stop alcohol consumption. In many cases, the only clinical symptom is an enlarged liver (hepatomegaly). *Alcoholic hepatitis,* a serious, sometimes reversible condition, involves inflammation and necrosis of the liver cells. Common clinical signs include swollen liver, nausea, vomiting, and abdominal pain. The presence of alcoholic hepatitis is a red flag that cirrhosis may soon follow. Up to 70% of alcoholic hepatitis clients eventually develop cirrhosis (NIAAA, 2005). In *cirrhosis,* the most serious and irreversible condition, the liver cells are destroyed and replaced by scar tissue. Clinical signs of cirrhosis include redness of the palms, contractures in the fingers, white nails, clubbing of the fingers and nails, liver enlargement or inflammation, and abnormal accumulation of fat in normal liver cells (Figure 30.5). Studies indicate that approximately 14% of clients with alcoholism develop cirrhosis if they drink

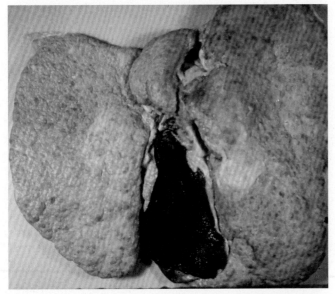

FIGURE 30.5 The surface of this liver with cirrhosis displays innumerable small nodules of hepatocytes separated by interconnecting bands of fibrous tissue. The dark structure is the gallbladder.

160 g/day of undiluted alcohol for 8 years. The survival rate for clients with late-stage cirrhosis is 60% for those who stop drinking and 35% for those who do not (Mann et al., 2004). Recent trends show an improvement in treatment outcomes for clients with cirrhosis with the increased use of interferon for chronic hepatitis and ursodeoxycholic acid for biliary cirrhosis. In addition, improved attention to general nutrition has been linked to improved outcome as well (Talawalker & Kamath, 2005).

Alcoholic Amnestic Disorder. Alcoholic amnestic disorder resulting from heavy, prolonged drinking is thought to be related to poor nutrition. Features include impaired ability to learn new information (short-term memory), recall remote information (long-term memory). neuropathy, unsteady gait, and myopathy.

Amnestic disorders related to thiamine deficiency include Wernicke's encephalopathy, a mild to severe decrease in mental functioning characterized by ophthalmoplegia (paralysis or weakness of one or more of the muscles that control eye movement), ataxia, nystagmus, and mental status changes. These symptoms improve with thiamine replacement. Approximately 80% to 90% of alcoholics with Wernicke's encephalopathy also develop Korsakoff's psychosis. Korsakoff's psychosis from thiamine deficiency is a chronic and debilitating syndrome characterized by persistent learning and memory problems. It also involves gait disturbances, short-term memory loss, disorientation, delirium, confabulation, and neuropathy. Korsakoff's psychosis is not reversible. **Wernicke–Korsakoff syndrome** is the coexistence of Wernicke's encephalopathy and Korsakoff's psychosis. See Chapter 31 for more information.

Alcoholic Dementia. Alcoholic dementia is associated with prolonged, chronic alcohol dependence. Signs include loss of intellectual ability severe enough to interfere with social or occupational functioning and impairments in memory, abstract thinking, and judgment. Degree of impairment may range from mild to severe and may include permanent brain damage (Figure 30.6).

Think About It 30.1

A 48-year-old man admitted to the ED has the following signs and symptoms: temperature, 101.5°F; pulse, 104 bpm; respirations, 28/minute; blood pressure, 178/94 mm Hg; profuse perspiration and tremulousness. Mental status examination reveals confusion, disorientation, visual hallucinations, and agitation. His neighbor, who accompanied him to the ED, states that the client stopped drinking 2 days ago after a long period of daily, heavy alcohol intake. Explain what substance-induced disorder you think this client is experiencing.

Controlled Substance Disorders

The Controlled Substances Act (Title II, Comprehensive Drug Abuse Prevention and Control Act of 1970; Public Law 91-513) regulates drugs other than alcohol. Congress

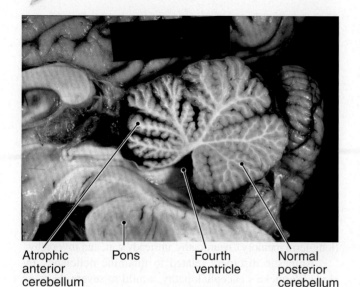

Atrophic anterior cerebellum   Pons   Fourth ventricle   Normal posterior cerebellum

FIGURE 30.6 This image shows the ravaging effects of chronic alcohol abuse on the brain. Compare the atrophied area of the anterior portion of the cerebellum with the normal posterior portion. Consequences of such damage include long-term memory and cognitive impairment.

implemented this law to decrease illegal use and abuse of drugs in the United States.

Controlled substances are categorized into classes, or categories, within which many symptoms, side effects, and withdrawal manifestations are similar (see *DSM-IV-TR* Box 30.1). There is often confusion about which drugs belong in which classification. An enormous amount of information is available about drugs of abuse. Table 30.1 presents eight major drug categories, examples of each, a description of intoxication effects, health consequences, and symptoms of withdrawal (Narconon International, 2010; NIDA, 2010a). The medical management of withdrawal syndromes for each category is based on the person's response to the drug, the dose and type of drug used, and the unique profile of associated withdrawal symptoms. Students should also consult the Web Resources section at the end of this chapter for more detailed information about specific drugs and their physiologic and behavioral effects.

STIMULANTS. Effects of stimulants include autonomic instability, irritability, anxiety, loss of coordination, and decreased muscle control. Symptoms of overdose for these types of drugs include agitation, hallucinations, and possible convulsions. Use of stimulants, even once, can have severe and life-threatening effects.

Amphetamines. Prescription forms of amphetamines are used for attention deficit/hyperactivity disorder in children, sleep disorders, and depression. Clients may abuse prescribed or illegal amphetamines to increase energy, alertness, or concentration; to elevate mood; or to suppress appetite (diet pills). Amphetamines primarily block the reuptake of norepinephrine and dopamine. Their stimulation of the peripheral nervous system leads to cardiovascular and temperature control problems. The effects of amphetamine use and overdose are similar to those of cocaine (see later discussion).

Methamphetamine. This highly addictive stimulant comes in many forms and can be ingested, smoked, snorted, or injected. The form of administration may alter the effects. This illegal substance is easy to produce and relatively cheap. Methamphetamine causes the release of high levels of dopamine, which can have toxic effects over time on nerve terminals. Long-term consequences of methamphetamine addiction include paranoia, hallucinations, depression, tooth decay, motor disturbances, cerebrovascular accident, and weight loss (Figure 30.7).

MDMA. Commonly known as "ecstasy," MDMA is also referred to as a "club drug" as a result of its use by attendees of bars, raves, and discos. MDMA has effects similar to methamphetamine. High doses can lead to malignant hyperthermia, with associated muscle breakdown, kidney and cardiovascular failure, and death.

Cocaine. Cocaine users generally smoke, inhale (snort), or inject the drug intravenously. Mixing the white powder with water or other drugs and substances can alter or enhance effects. After using cocaine, clients experience short-term increases in energy, alertness, confidence, and sociability. As the effects wear off, clients feel fatigued, annoyed, and depressed, with intense cravings for more of the drug.

A particularly addictive form is "crack," which is produced by boiling cocaine with water and baking soda until a precipitant remains. Clients then "crack" the hardened crystal into pieces and smoke them. Both the rush and the crash associated with crack use are more intense than those seen with regular cocaine.

Absorption of cocaine through the skin, mucous membranes, and blood–brain barrier is rapid. Use increases levels of dopamine in the synaptic clefts; prolonged cocaine use eventually leads to dopamine depletion. Subsequent increased blood levels of prolactin, norepinephrine, and serotonin lead to pervasive physical problems, such as tachycardia, hypertension, dilated pupils, elevated temperature, sleep disturbances, and anorexia.

Symptoms of cocaine intoxication depend on the route of administration and amount taken. Increased amounts result in agitation, restlessness, and tremors. Overdoses can cause convulsions and depression of the CNS and respiratory systems, which may be fatal. Symptoms of psychosis may also develop. Withdrawal symptoms are characterized by disturbed sleep, fatigue, lack of concentration, decreased sex drive, and depressed mood.

CANNABIS. Cannabis products include marijuana and hashish. They can be orally ingested or smoked. Use induces relaxation, pleasure, distortions of space and time, hunger,

TABLE 30.1 Commonly Abused Controlled Substances

Category (Examples/Street Names)	Effects of Intoxication	Health Consequences	Withdrawal Symptoms
Stimulants (*DSM-IV-TR* Categories: Amphetamine [or Amphetamine-Like]-Related Disorders and Cocaine-Related Disorders)			
Cocaine (blow, C, candy, coke, do a line, freeze, girl, happy dust, Mama coca, mojo, monster, nose, pimp, shot, smoking gun, snow, sugar, sweet stuff, white powder)	Increased heart rate, blood pressure, metabolism, mental alertness, energy, exhilaration	Rapid or irregular heartbeat, reduced appetite, weight loss, heart failure, insomnia, tremor, loss of coordination, irritability, anxiousness, restlessness, delirium, panic, paranoia, impulsive behavior, aggressiveness, psychosis	Duration varies among people and according to amount and frequency of use.
Crack cocaine (base, beat, blast, casper, chalk, devil drug, gravel, hardball, hell, kryptonite, love, moonrocks, rock, scrabble, stones, tornado)	Also with cocaine: increased temperature	Also with cocaine: chest pain, respiratory failure, nausea, abdominal pain, strokes, seizures, headaches, malnutrition, panic attacks	Nausea/vomiting, fatigue, muscle pain, long but disturbed sleep, sleeplessness, strong hangover, irritability, depression, violence, anxiety, panic attacks, lack of motivation, depersonalization, de-realization, paranoid delusions, intense cravings, exhaustion, mental confusion, intense hunger, agitation, shaking, depression, angry outbursts
Amphetamine (*Biphetamine*, *Dexedrine*: bennies, black beauties, crosses, hearts, LA turnaround, speed, truck drivers, uppers)	Also with MDMA: mild hallucinogenic effects, increased tactile sensitivity, empathic feelings	Also with MDMA: impaired memory and learning, hyperthermia, cardiac toxicity, renal failure, liver toxicity	
Methamphetamine (*Desoxyn*: beannies, blue devils, chalk, CR, crank, crystal, crystal meth, fast, granulated orange, ice, meth, Mexican crack, pink, rock, speckled birds, speed, tina, yellow powder)	Also with methamphetamine: aggression, violence, psychosis	Also with methamphetamine: memory loss, cardiac and neurologic damage, impaired memory and learning	
MDMA (*methylenedioxymethamphetamine*: Adam, bean, blue kisses, clarity, club drug, disco biscuits, E, ecstasy, hug drug, love drug, lover's speed, Mercedes, New Yorkers, peace, roll, white dove, X, XTC)			
Methylphenidate (*Ritalin*: crackers, one and ones, pharming, poor man's heroin, R-ball, ritz an ts, set, skippy, speedball, ts and ritz, ts and rs, vitamin R, West Coast)			

(continues on page 630)

629

TABLE 30.1 Commonly Abused Controlled Substances (continued)

Category (Examples)/Street Names	Effects of Intoxication	Health Consequences	Withdrawal Symptoms
Cannabinoids (DSM-IV-TR Category: Cannabis-Related Disorders)			
Marijuana (420, Aunt Mary, baby, bobby, boom, chira, chronic, ditch, ganja, grass, greens, hash, herb, Mary Jane, nigra, pot, reefer, rip, root, skunk, stack, torch, weed, zambi)	Euphoria, slowed thinking and reaction time, confusion, impaired balance and coordination	Cough, frequent respiratory infections, impaired memory and learning, increased heart rate, anxiety, panic attacks, tolerance, addiction	Withdrawal first appears in chronic users within 24 hr. Marijuana withdrawal is most pronounced for the first 10 days and can last up to 28 days.
Hashish (boom, chronic, gangster, hash, hash oil, hemp)			Irritability, anxiety, physical tension, decreased appetite and mood
Hallucinogens (DSM-IV-TR Category: Hallucinogen-Related Disorders)			
LSD (lysergic acid diethylamide: A, acid, black star, blotter, boomers, cubes, Elvis, golden dragon, L, micro-dot, paper acid, pink robots, super-man, twenty-five, yellow sunshine, ying yang)	Altered states of perception and feeling; nausea	Persisting perception disorder (flashbacks)	Psychotic-like episodes persist long after last use
Mescaline (beans, buttons, cactus, cactus buttons, cactus head, chief, love trip, mesc, mescal, mezc, moon, peyote, topi)	Also with LSD and mescaline: persistent mental disorders; increased body temperature, heart rate, blood pressure; loss of appetite, tremors, insomnia, numbness, weakness		
Psilocybin/psilocin (boomers, god's flesh, little smoke, magic mushroom, Mexican mushrooms, mushrooms, musk, sherm, shrooms, silly putty, simple simon)	Also with psilocybin: nervousness, paranoia		
Inhalants (DSM-IV-TR Category: Inhalant-Related Disorders)			
Solvents (paint thinners, gasoline, glues); gases (butane, propane, aerosol propellants, nitrous oxide), nitrites (isoamyl, isobutyl, cyclohexyl): laughing gas, poppers, snappers, whippets	Stimulation, loss of inhibition; headache; nausea/vomiting; slurred speech, loss of motor coordination; wheezing	Unconsciousness, cramps, weight loss, muscle weakness, depression, memory impairment, damage to cardiovascular and nervous systems, sudden death	Mild withdrawal syndrome
Opioids and Morphine Derivatives (DSM-IV-TR Category: Opioid-Related Disorders)			
Codeine (Empirin with Codeine, Fiorinal with Codeine, Robitussin A-C, Tylenol with Codeine: Captain Cody, schoolboy; [with glutethimide] doors & fours, loads, pancakes, syrup)	Pain relief, euphoria, drowsiness	Nausea, constipation, confusion, sedation, respiratory depression and arrest, tolerance, addiction, unconsciousness, coma, death	The worst symptoms pass within a few days, but it can take months to feel normal.

Substance	Effects	Additional/Withdrawal Effects
Fentanyl and fentanyl analogs (*Actiq, Duragesic, Sublimaze:* Apache, China girl, China town, dance fever, friend, goodfellas, great bear, he-man, jackpot, king ivory, murder 8, poison, tango and cash, TNT)	Also with heroin: staggering gait	Runny nose, sweating, muscle twitching, muscle pain, headaches, irregular heartbeat, nausea/vomiting, high blood pressure, fever, insomnia, dehydration, diarrhea, loss of appetite, yawning, weakness, stomach cramps, restlessness, lacrimation, rhinorrhea, perspiration, goose flesh, hot and cold flashes Also with heroin: dilated pupils, loss of appetite, tremors, panic, diarrhea
Heroin (*diacetyl-morphine:* Aunt Hazel, big H, black pearl, brown sugar, capital H, Charley, china white, dope, good horse, H, hard stuff, hero, heroina, little boy, mud, perfect high, smack, stuff, tar)		
Morphine (*Roxanol, Duramorph:* M, Miss Emma, monkey, white stuff)		
Opium (*Laudanum, paregoric:* ah-pen-yen, aunti, big O, black stuff, Chinese tobacco, chocolate, dopium, dover's deck, dream gun, hard stuff, hocus, joy plant, O, ope, pin yen, toxy, zero)		
Oxycodone HCL (*OxyContin:* Oxy, O.C., killer)		
Hydrocodone bitartrate, acetaminophen (*Vicodin:* vike, Watson-387)		

Dissociative Anesthetics (*DSM-IV-TR* Category: Phencyclidine [or Phencyclidine-Like]-Related Disorders)

Substance	Effects	Additional/Withdrawal Effects
Ketamine (*Ketalar SV:* bump, cat killer, cat valium, fort dodge, green, honey oil, jet, K, ket, kit kat, psychedelic heroin, purple, special K, special la coke, super C and vitamin K)	Increased heart rate and blood pressure, impaired motor function	Memory loss; numbness; nausea/vomiting; also, at high doses, delirium, depression, respiratory depression and arrest
PCP and analogs (*phencyclidine:* angel dust, belladonna, black whack, CJ, cliffhanger, crystal joint, Detroit pink, elephant tranquilizer, hog, magic, Peter Pan, sheets, soma, TAC, trank, white horizon, zoom)	Also with PCP: Possible decrease in blood pressure and heart rate, panic, aggression, violence	Mental instability

(continues on page 632)

TABLE 30.1 Commonly Abused Controlled Substances (continued)

Category (Examples/ Street Names)	Effects of Intoxication	Health Consequences	Withdrawal Symptoms
Depressants (*DSM-IV-TR* Category: Sedative-Hypnotic or Anxiolytic-Related Disorders)			
Barbiturates (*Amytal, Nembutal, Seconal, Phenobarbital*: barbs, reds, red birds, phennies, tooies, yellows, yellow jackets)	Reduced anxiety; feeling of well-being; lowered inhibitions; slowed pulse and breathing; lowered blood pressure; poor concentration;	Fatigue, depression, unusual excitement, fever, irritability, poor judgment, slurred speech, dizziness, confusion, impaired coordination, memory, judgment, respiratory depression and arrest, death;	Rapid heartbeat, shaky hands, insomnia or disturbed sleep, sweating, irritability, anxiety and agitation
Benzodiazepines (other than flunitrazepam) (*Ativan, Halcion, Librium, Valium, Xanax*: candy, downers, sleeping pills, tranks)	Also for barbiturates and benzodiazepines: sedation, drowsiness	Also for methaqualone: poor reflexes	
Flunitrazepam (*Rohypnol*: circles, forget-me pill, la rocha, lunch money drug, Mexican valium, pingus, R2, Reynolds, roche, roofies, rope, ruffles, wolfies)	Also for methaqualone: euphoria		
GHB(*gamma-hydroxybutyrate*: caps, cherry meth, ever clear, easy lay, fantasy, G, G-riffic, gamma hydrate, Georgia home boy, grievous bodily harm, liquid ecstasy, liquid X, soap, sodium oxybate)			
Methaqualone (*Quaalude, Sopor, Parest*: ludes, mandrex, quad, quay)			
Other Compounds			
Anabolic steroids(*Anadrol, Oxandrin, Durabolin, Depo-Testosterone, Equipoise*: abolic, anadrol, arnolds, bolasterone, dihydrolone, equipose, gym candy, juice, methyl testosterone, proviron, pumpers, stackers, therobolin, weight trainers, winstrol V)	No intoxication effects	Hypertension, blood clotting and cholesterol changes, liver cysts and cancer, kidney cancer, hostility and aggression, acne; in adolescents, premature stoppage of growth; in males, prostate cancer, reduced sperm production, shrunken testicles, breast enlargement; in females, menstrual irregularities, development of beard and other masculine characteristics	Mood swings, fatigue, restlessness, loss of appetite, insomnia, reduced sex drive, steroid cravings, depression, suicide attempts

If left untreated, some depressive symptoms associated with anabolic steroid withdrawal have been known to persist for 1 yr or more after the abuser stops using. |
| Dextromethorphan (DXM) (*found in some cough and cold medications*: robotripping, robo, triple C) | Dissociative effects, distorted visual perceptions to complete dissociative effects | For effects at higher doses see "Dissociative Anesthetics" | |

Sources: Narconon International. (2010). *Signs and symptoms of drug use.* Retrieved from http://www.narconon.org/drug-abuse/signs-symptoms-of-drug-abuse.html; and National Institute on Drug Abuse. (2010). *Commonly abused drugs.* Retrieved from http://www.nida.nih.gov/DrugPages/DrugsofAbuse.html.

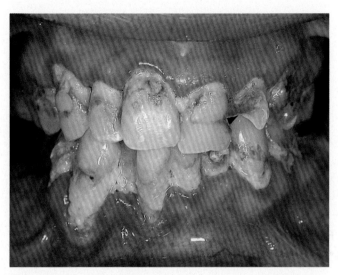

FIGURE 30.7 One of the ravaging physiologic effects of methamphetamine addiction is ruination of the teeth.

and food cravings. Effects last for a few hours after use. The long-term use of cannabis may lead to impairments of memory, attention, coordination, reaction time, and balance. Cannabis products do not have specific, well-defined withdrawal syndromes.

HALLUCINOGENS AND PHENCYCLIDINE. Hallucinogens and phencyclidine (PCP or "angel dust") share the effects of euphoria and alterations in perception, memory, and judgment. They also cause rapid emotional shifts, loss of coordination, irritation to the respiratory system, fatigue, insomnia, and autonomic instability. These dangerous drugs are often obtained under questionable circumstances with unknown dose ranges and mixtures. Clients who have experienced bad reactions to these drugs often show up intoxicated or in a dissociative state in EDs. Their altered judgment and perception may lead them to be physically aggressive or combative until the effects of the drug wear off.

OPIOIDS. These powerful drugs have been used for centuries to relieve pain and include opium, heroin, morphine, and codeine. When used clinically (eg, for cancer pain), opiates are safe and generally do not produce dependence, but improper and illegal use can quickly trigger addiction.

Heroin is the most commonly abused opiate and one of the most difficult and dangerous forms of addiction. It comes in white or brown powders often mixed with other substances to heighten or alter its effects. The most frequent form of administration is injection, a method that contributes to the ongoing spread of HIV and other diseases through shared needles and paraphernalia. The long-term effects of heroin include neurochemical and molecular brain alterations (Figure 30.8). Physical dependence and tolerance contribute to the compulsive nature of this addiction and its destructive effects on all parts of clients' lives. The need for more of the drug to achieve similar effects contributes

to preoccupation; financial, legal, employment, and relationship problems; physical incapacitation; and risk for overdose and death.

Reversal of opioid intoxication involves administration of naloxone (Narcan), an opioid antagonist. Abrupt cessation of opioid use leads to a dramatic withdrawal syndrome. Physical symptoms include severe cramping, tremors, panic, and chills. Medical supervision and management are often required through the withdrawal phase (see later discussion).

✓Similar to alcohol

SEDATIVES, HYPNOTICS, AND ANXIOLYTICS. Sedative-hypnotics are used medically to relieve anxiety and facilitate sleep. This class contains the most commonly prescribed drugs in the United States, including barbiturates, benzodiazepine, methaqualone, and other tranquilizers. With appropriate medical supervision, their use can be safe and appropriate. Clients may begin to abuse even prescription drugs, however, if they do not carefully follow their regimens or if they use these drugs with other substances or obtain multiple prescriptions from several physicians.

Sedatives, hypnotics, and anxiolytics cause sensory alterations, relaxation, impaired judgment, and behaviors similar to alcohol intoxication. Withdrawal symptoms may be acute and can include autonomic instability, coma, and death. Medical supervision of clients undergoing withdrawal from these drugs is required.

Two drugs within this category include Rohypnol and gamma-hydroxybutyrate (GHB). Colorless, tasteless, and odorless, their effects can be similar to the blackouts associated with alcoholism, with clients unable to remember what happened under the influence of these drugs. Rohypnol and GHB frequently are referred to as "date rape" drugs, used by unscrupulous criminals who slip them into drinks of unwitting (and unwilling) dates or acquaintances at bars or parties and then proceed to take advantage of the victim's incapacitation.

> **Checkpoint Questions**
> 3. List different forms of stimulants.
> 4. Identify the most commonly abused opiate and why it has such addictive and dangerous powers.
> 5. Explain why certain drugs are referred to as "date rape" drugs.

Comorbidities and Co-occurring Disorders

The terms *comorbidity* and **co-occurring disorder** describe clients with a coexisting substance use disorder and major psychiatric disorder. Common psychiatric illnesses linked with substance abuse include schizophrenia, schizophreniform disorder, antisocial personality disorder, anxiety disorders, and mood disorders (National Institute of Mental Health [NIMH], 2006). The substance use and psychiatric disorders are unrelated and meet *DSM-IV-TR* criteria. The presence of both disorders does not mean that one caused the

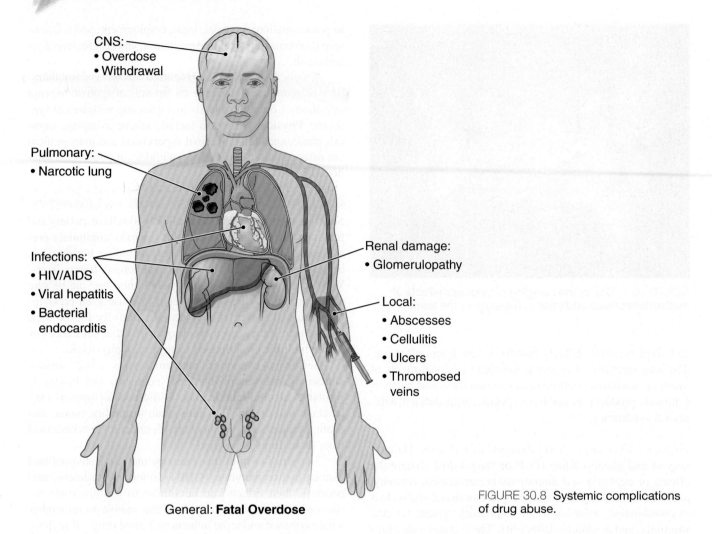

CNS:
• Overdose
• Withdrawal

Pulmonary:
• Narcotic lung

Infections:
• HIV/AIDS
• Viral hepatitis
• Bacterial endocarditis

Renal damage:
• Glomerulopathy

Local:
• Abscesses
• Cellulitis
• Ulcers
• Thrombosed veins

General: **Fatal Overdose**

FIGURE 30.8 Systemic complications of drug abuse.

other. Drug abuse may induce symptoms of another mental illness, or mental disorders can lead to drug abuse (NIDA, 2011a). The following are types of co-occurring scenarios:

• A client uses psychoactive substances to cope with symptoms or treatment of a major psychiatric disorder (eg, a client with schizophrenia uses alcohol for relief from the side effects of psychotropic medications). If this client did not meet the criteria for substance dependence, then treatment for the psychiatric illness would relieve both problems, and treatment and rehabilitation would focus primarily on the major psychiatric disorder.
• The client with psychoactive drug dependence presents with psychiatric symptoms as a result of intoxication, withdrawal, or other effects of the substance being used (eg, a client has a psychotic episode produced by cocaine). Treatment and rehabilitation would focus on substance dependence to alleviate the symptoms.
• The client with co-occurring disorders has two basically unrelated psychiatric disorders that may interact and exacerbate each other (eg, a client has bipolar disorder and alcohol dependence). Treatment and rehabilitation need to address both the psychiatric disorder and the substance dependence.

In 2005, approximately 5.2 million U.S. adults met the criteria for co-occurring disorders (Office of Applied Studies, 2008). In addition, 50% of those with a substance use disorder have had a co-occurring mental disorder in their lifetimes (NIMH, 2006). In clients with co-occurring disorders, both are considered primary, and the multidisciplinary care team must manage their complex relationship.

People with co-occurring disorders are often more difficult to treat and experience worse outcomes than other clients. The Drug Abuse Warning Network (DAWN) report revealed that when clients with co-occurring disorders visited the ED, equal numbers were treated and released as were admitted to inpatient units. Of those admitted, 40% were sent to psychiatric units, whereas 27% were referred to detoxification or other drug programs (DAWN of SAMHSA, 2005). Most people with co-occurring disorders receive no treatment at all. In this population, 34% receive treatment for the mental disorder only, whereas an alarmingly small percentage receives substance abuse treatment (4%) or dual treatment (8.5%) (Figure 30.9). Traditional modalities for co-occurring disorders (ie, substance dependence programs) have not been successful. NIDA (2011a) recommends evidence-based practices that combine psychopharmacologic, motivational, and behavioral

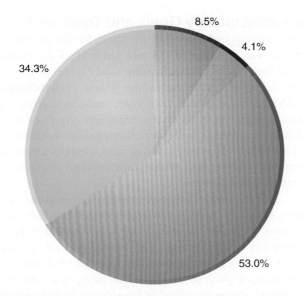

8.5%

4.1%

34.3%

53.0%

- ■ Treatment for Both Mental Health and Substance Use Problems
- ■ Substance Use Treatment Only
- ■ No Treatment
- ■ Treatment Only for Mental Health Problems

FIGURE 30.9 Past year treatment among adults 18 years or older with both serious psychological distress and a substance use disorder, 2005. From: Substance Abuse and Mental Health Services Administration (SAMHSA). (2006). *Results from the 2005 National Survey on Drug Use and Health: National findings* (NSDUH Series H-30, USDHHS Publication No. SMA06-4194). Rockville, MD: Author.

interventions at all levels of care, including multisystemic therapy (MST), brief strategic family therapy (BSFT), cognitive–behavioral therapy (CBT), modified therapeutic communities, integrated dual disorders treatment, dialectical behavior therapy (DBT), exposure therapy, integrated group therapy (IGT), and assertive community treatment (ACT) programs (NIDA, 2010b, 2011a). Ongoing research on the identification, treatment, and rehabilitation of clients with co-occurring disorders is needed to continue gathering evidence on best practices.

Implications and Prognosis

Use of alcohol and other drugs is associated with several other psychosocial problems. The incidence of alcohol-related fatalities or permanent disabilities is enormous. Social effects on families, especially children, are devastating. Destructive drinking patterns affect many U.S. teens. Prolonged substance use disorders and concomitant adverse behavior changes affect well-being and can evolve into a course of self-destruction. Ultimately, clients must learn to adapt to a life in which the substance is no longer the driving force—a challenging journey.

Perinatal Statistics and Risks

Drug and alcohol use and smoking are significant risk factors for poor perinatal outcomes. In 2005, approximately 17% of pregnant women reported smoking in the past month (SAMHSA, 2008). Young pregnant women were more likely than

older counterparts to smoke cigarettes and binge drink. Data indicate that women who reduce smoking and drinking during pregnancy revert to use of tobacco and alcohol after giving birth. Caetano et al. (2006) reported that rates of smoking and alcohol use in women during the year after giving birth were similar to those among all nonpregnant women.

The harmful effects of tobacco and alcohol on the human embryo and fetus are well documented (Centers for Disease Control and Prevention, 2010). Alcohol is a *teratogen,* meaning that it crosses the placenta when women drink during pregnancy and can cause adverse fetal effects. The most clearly alcohol-related birth defect is a specific pattern called **fetal alcohol syndrome** (FAS), the leading known preventable cause of mental retardation. Manifestations of FAS include the following:

- Prenatal and postnatal growth deficiency
- Facial malformations, including a small head circumference, flattened midface, sunken nasal bridge, and flattened and elongated groove between nose and upper lip (Figure 30.10)
- CNS dysfunction
- Varying degrees of major organ system malfunction

Behavioral and neurologic problems associated with fetal alcohol exposure may lead to poor academic performance and legal and employment difficulties in adolescence and adulthood.

Commonly used illegal drugs such as marijuana, cocaine, heroin, and methadone have similar teratogenic effects when taken during pregnancy and may cause dangerous withdrawal syndromes in newborns. Box 30.2 summarizes the potential adverse effects of maternal cocaine use during pregnancy.

Preventive and Public Health Strategies

Prognosis for recovery from substance use disorders varies with each client's circumstances. Even with effective treatments, 70% to 80% of individuals with substance abuse will relapse within the first year (Anton, 2010). Research continues into the factors that affect initial addiction, relapse, and

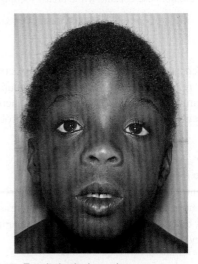

FIGURE 30.10 Fetal alcohol syndrome.

BOX 30.2 Consequences of Cocaine Use During Pregnancy

Increased Risks to Pregnancy

- Spontaneous abortion
- Abruptio placentae
- Stillbirth
- Uterine contractibility
- Prematurity

Maternal Risks

- Tachycardia, dysrhythmias, angina
- Seizures
- Cerebrovascular accidents
- Hypertension
- Anorexia resulting in weight loss
- Respiratory lung damage (if cocaine is smoked)
- HIV infection if intravenous route is used

Effects on Fetus

- Cerebral artery injury and infarction
- Acute hypertension
- Low birth weight
- Intrauterine growth retardation
- Decreased head circumference
- Decreased length
- Skull defects
- Increased cardiac anomalies
- HIV infection if intravenous route is used

Effects on the Newborn

- Increased risk for sudden infant death syndrome
- Abnormalities on the Brazelton Neonatal Behavioral Assessment Scale
- Poor suck-and-swallow pattern
- Fine motor tremors of hands, arms, legs
- Unusual response to stimuli
- Vomiting, poor feeding
- Weak pull-to-sit development
- Irritability, difficulty sleeping
- Intolerance to cuddling
- Difficult to comfort
- Seizures if mothers use cocaine while breast-feeding

recovery, such as personal resources, stressors, commitment, support for rehabilitation, and genetic makeup (NIAAA, 2011). Community-oriented programs and activities can help to prevent and contain alcohol and drug problems.

Checkpoint Questions

6. What is meant by the term *co-occurring disorder*?
7. What name is given to the condition that may result in an infant born to a mother who drinks alcohol during pregnancy?

Interdisciplinary Goals and Treatment

The two major objectives of treatment for clients with substance use disorders is (1) safe removal of the chemical from their bodies (**detoxification**) and (2) breaking through the denial that perpetuates the illness (**rehabilitation**). Although great strides have been made in diagnosis and treatment, more is necessary. Substance use disorders are difficult to manage, and most clients require several rounds of treatment before they attain success. Chances for recovery improve when certain medications are used in conjunction with behavior therapies.

Various interdisciplinary programs are available. Short-term programs (usually less than 6 months) include detoxification programs, short-term inpatient residential therapy, outpatient rehabilitation, and private-practice physician treatment. Long-term approaches may involve a medication maintenance program or residential therapeutic community treatment. Paraprofessional or lay services include programs such as Alcoholics Anonymous (AA), Cocaine Users Anonymous (CA), and Narcotics Anonymous (NA). See Box 30.3 for the principles that characterize effective drug abuse treatment.

Treatment should be based on the client's particular medical, social, and psychological needs. Some clients change their behaviors with only outpatient education. Others require intensive medical detoxification and long-term rehabilitation. Levels of care are related to client acuity and progress in intensity as follows:

- Early intervention, including assessment and education, possible opioid maintenance therapy
- Outpatient treatment, including psychosocial intervention and ambulatory detoxification
- Intensive outpatient/partial hospitalization/residential/inpatient treatment
- Medically managed intensive inpatient treatment

For each level, service recommendations involve the following six dimensions: acute intoxication/withdrawal potential; biomedical conditions and complications; emotional, behavioral, or cognitive conditions and complications; readiness to change; relapse, continued use, or continued problem potential; and recovery environment (American Society of Addiction Medicine, 2007).

Detoxification

Medically debilitated clients detoxify slowly. Withdrawal requires careful management. Providers consider the withdrawal time frame based on when clients will need the most support. Other factors influencing the length of detoxification include severity of dependence and overall health status.

Immediate goals of detoxification include providing a safe and humane withdrawal process, maintaining client dignity, and preparing clients for ongoing treatment after detoxification ends (See Evidence-Based Practice Spotlight 30.1). Principles of detoxification are as follows:

- Detoxification alone rarely is adequate for clients with substance dependence.

BOX 30.3   Principles of Addiction Treatment

1. **Addiction is a complex but treatable disease that affects brain function and behavior.** Drugs alter the brain's structure and how it functions, resulting in changes that persist long after drug use has ceased. This may help explain why abusers are at risk for relapse even after long periods of abstinence.

2. **No single treatment is appropriate for everyone.** Matching treatment settings, interventions, and services to an individual's particular problems and needs is critical to his or her ultimate success.

3. **Treatment needs to be readily available.** Because individuals with a drug addiction may be uncertain about entering treatment, taking advantage of available services the moment people are ready for treatment is critical. Potential patients can be lost if treatment is not immediately available or readily accessible.

4. **Effective treatment attends to multiple needs of the individual, not just his or her drug abuse.** To be effective, treatment must address the individual's drug abuse and any associated medical, psychological, social, vocational, and legal problems.

5. **Remaining in treatment for an adequate period is critical.** The appropriate duration for an individual depends on the type and degree of his or her problems and needs. Research indicates that most addicted individuals need at least 3 months in treatment to significantly reduce or stop their drug use and that the best outcomes occur with longer durations of treatment.

6. **Counseling—individual and/or group—and other behavioral therapies are the most commonly used forms of drug abuse treatment.** Behavioral therapies vary in their focus and may involve addressing a patient's motivations to change, building skills to resist drug use, replacing drug-using activities with constructive and rewarding activities, improving problem-solving skills, and facilitating better interpersonal relationships.

7. **Medications are an important element of treatment for many patients, especially when combined with counseling and other behavioral therapies.** For example, methadone and buprenorphine are effective in helping individuals addicted to heroin or other opioids stabilize their lives and reduce their illicit drug use. Also, for persons addicted to nicotine, a nicotine replacement product (nicotine patches or gum) or an oral medication (bupropion or varenicline) can be an effective component of treatment when part of a comprehensive behavioral treatment program.

8. **An individual's treatment and services plan must be assessed continually and modified as necessary to ensure it meets his or her changing needs.** A patient may require varying combinations of services and treatment components during the course of treatment and recovery. In addition to counseling or psychotherapy, a patient may require medication, medical services, family therapy, parenting instruction, vocational rehabilitation, and/or social and legal services. For many patients, a continuing care approach provides the best results, with treatment intensity varying according to a person's changing needs.

9. **Many individuals with drug addictions also have other mental disorders.** Because drug abuse and addiction—both of which are mental disorders—often co-occur with other mental illnesses, patients presenting with one condition should be assessed for the other(s). And when these problems co-occur, treatment should address both (or all), including the use of medications as appropriate.

10. **Medically assisted detoxification is only the first stage of addiction treatment and by itself does little to change long-term drug abuse.** Although medically assisted detoxification can safely manage the acute physical symptoms of withdrawal, detoxification alone is rarely sufficient to help addicted individuals achieve long-term abstinence. Thus, patients should be encouraged to continue drug treatment following detoxification.

11. **Treatment does not need to be voluntary to be effective.** Sanctions or enticements from the family, employment setting, and/or criminal justice system can significantly increase treatment entry, retention rates, and the ultimate success of drug treatment interventions.

12. **Drug use during treatment must be monitored continuously, as lapses during treatment do occur.** Knowing their drug use is being monitored can be a powerful incentive for patients and can help them withstand urges to use drugs. Monitoring also provides an early indication of a return to drug use, signaling a possible need to adjust an individual's treatment plan to better meet his or her needs.

13. **Treatment programs should assess patients for the presence of HIV/AIDS, hepatitis B and C, tuberculosis and other infectious diseases, as well as provide targeted risk-reduction counseling to help patients modify or change behaviors that place them at risk of contracting or spreading infectious diseases.** Targeted counseling specifically focused on reducing infectious disease risk can help patients further reduce or avoid substance-related and other high-risk behaviors. Treatment providers should encourage and support HIV screening and inform patients that highly active antiretroviral therapy (HAART) has proven effective in combating HIV, including among drug-abusing populations.

Adapted from National Institute on Drug Abuse. (2010). *Commonly abused drugs.* Retrieved from http://www.nida.nih.gov/DrugPages/DrugsofAbuse.html.

- Clinicians should use only those medication regimens or other detoxification procedures with established safety and efficacy. They must advise clients of any procedures they intend to try that have not been established as safe and effective.

- Providers should control clients' access to medication to the greatest extent possible during detoxification.
- Initiation of withdrawal should be individualized.
- Whenever possible, clinicians should substitute a long-acting medication for short-acting drugs of addiction.

EVIDENCE-BASED PRACTICE SPOTLIGHT 30.1

Evidence-Based Practice Guideline for Detoxification and Substance Abuse Treatment: An Overview of the Psychosocial and Biomedical Issues During Detoxification

Overview of Effective Treatment: Psychological dependence, co-occurring psychiatric and medical conditions, social supports, and environmental conditions critically influence the probability of successful and sustained abstinence from substances. Research indicates that addressing psychosocial issues during detoxification significantly increases the likelihood that the client will experience a safe detoxification and go on to participate in substance abuse treatment. Clients entering detoxification are undergoing profound personal and medical crisis. Withdrawal itself can cause or exacerbate current emotional, psychological, or mental problems. The detoxification staff needs to be equipped to identify and address potential problems. An initial evaluation will help staff foresee any variables that might complicate a safe and effective withdrawal. Health professionals should screen for medical and mental problems that may put the client at risk for a crisis such as infectious disease, suicide, or anger and aggression.

Proper nutrition during recovery improves to a significant extent the adverse effects of the substance abuse. Opioids are known to decrease calcium absorption and to increase cholesterol and body potassium levels. Magnesium deficiency is often seen in chronic alcohol dependence. Other nutrient deficiencies seen in alcohol abuse include protein, fat, zinc, calcium, iron, vitamins A and E, and the water-soluble vitamins pyridoxine, thiamine, folate, and vitamin B$_{12}$. Alcohol also contains calories (7 kcal/g)

that when consumed in excessive amounts may displace nutrient-dense foods. Cocaine is an appetite suppressant and may interfere with the absorption of calcium and vitamin D. Laboratory tests for protein, vitamins, and iron and the other electrolytes are recommended to determine the extent of liver function as well as supplementation. For clients who abuse alcohol, the administration of fluids to address dehydration should be the first step. Detoxification should include efforts to address nutritional deficits and to begin the client on a course of improved eating habits. Balanced meals consisting of low-fat foods, with an increased intake of protein, complex carbohydrates, and dietary fiber are recommended.

Strategies for engaging and retaining clients in detoxification include continually offering hope and the expectation of recovery. Education on the withdrawal process minimizes client anxiety. Using the client's support system promotes retention in detoxification. Motivation is enhanced by showing respect for client's decisions and focusing on client's strengths. During detoxification the client is usually not readily receptive to change. Therefore, it is not recommended that clinicians use direct confrontation in helping a person with a substance use disorder begin the process of detoxification and subsequent substance abuse treatment. In general, the basic concept is to try to move clients to the next stage of change. The clinician needs to identify any potential obstacles that might hinder the client's progress through the stages of change.

References

An overview of psychological and biomedical issues during detoxification. (2006, January 18). In Center for Substance Abuse Treatment (CSAT), *Detoxification and substance abuse treatment* (Treatment Improvement Protocol No. 45, pp. 19–41). Rockville, MD: Substance Abuse and Mental Health Services Administration (SAMHSA). Retrieved from http://www.guideline.gov/content.aspx?id=9117&search=detoxification#Section420.

- The intensity of withdrawal cannot always be predicted accurately.
- All means possible should be used to ameliorate signs and symptoms of withdrawal.
- Clients should begin participating as soon as possible in follow-up support such as peer group therapy, family therapy, individual counseling, 12-step programs, and drug recovery educational programs.

Understanding Psychopharmacology 30.1 lists medications currently used for detoxification. New medication treatments are developed continuously, so it is important to seek updated information. The SAMHSA website (see Web Resources section at the end of this chapter) is an excellent resource for regularly updated materials and guidelines.

ALCOHOL. Most clients can be detoxified from alcohol in 3 to 5 days. For clients with alcoholism, peak withdrawal symptoms develop the second day after the last ingestion of alcohol. Alcohol withdrawal is often assessed using the Clinical Institute Withdrawal Assessment—Alcohol, revised (CIWA-Ar). See Assessment Tool 30.1.

Medications commonly used to manage alcohol withdrawal include sedative-hypnotics, sympatholytics, anticonvulsants, and antipsychotics. The Center for Substance Abuse Treatment (CSAT, 2006) evidenced-based practice guidelines for medical treatment of alcohol withdrawal recommend benzodiazepines as first-line agents. All benzodiazepines are equally efficacious. Compared with non-benzodiazepine sedative-hypnotics, they have better overall documented efficacy, a greater safety margin, and lower abuse potential. The benzodiazepines reduce withdrawal severity, delirium, and seizures. The choice of benzodiazepine is guided by the following:

- Long-acting agents may be more effective in preventing seizures during withdrawal.
- Long-acting agents may contribute to a smoother withdrawal with fewer rebound symptoms.
- Short-acting agents may have a lower risk of oversedation.
- Certain benzodiazepines carry a higher risk for abuse.
- The cost of benzodiazepines varies significantly.

UNDERSTANDING PSYCHOPHARMACOLOGY 30.1

Medications Used for Detoxification

MEDICATION	INDICATION
For Alcohol	
Benzodiazepines	Decrease the likelihood and number of withdrawal seizures and episodes of DTs
Anticonvulsants: carbamazepine (Tegretol)	Prevent alcohol withdrawal seizures
Phenobarbital	Used for clients who are dependent on both sedative-hypnotics and alcohol
Beta-blockers: propranolol (Inderal)	Ameliorate autonomic nervous system hyperactivity
Antipsychotics: haloperidol (Haldol)	Decrease auditory, visual, or tactile hallucinations of DTs
Magnesium sulfate	Reduces seizure frequency
Vitamins	Treat nutrient deficiencies, particularly thiamine
For Opiates	
Clonidine (Catapres)	Treats some withdrawal symptoms; not effective for muscle aches, insomnia, or drug craving
Methadone	Relieves withdrawal from heroin, fentanyl, or any other opiate; prevents severe withdrawal symptoms
Buprenorphine	Produces mild opioid effects to reduce cravings
For Benzodiazepines	
Benzodiazepines: phenobarbital	Use decreasing doses of the drug of dependence; then substitute phenobarbital or another barbiturate for the addicting agent and the gradual withdrawal of the substitute medication; then substitute a long-acting benzodiazepine, such as chlordiazepoxide (Librium), tapered over 1 to 2 weeks
For Stimulants (Cocaine, Crack Cocaine, Amphetamines, and Methamphetamine)	
No specific treatment	Amantadine and modafinil currently being studied for reducing severity of withdrawal symptoms
For Marijuana	
Trazodone	Relieves persistent sleep difficulties
For Hallucinogens, PCP	
Benzodiazepines	Controls anxiety and promotes sedation secondary to residual symptoms (perceptual illusions and anxiety)
For Inhalants/Solvents	
Phenobarbital	Similar to indications for benzodiazepines

From: Center for Substance Abuse Treatment (CSAT). (2006). *Detoxification and substance abuse treatment* (Treatment Improvement Protocol Series 45; USDHHS Publication No. SMA06-4131). Rockville, MD: Substance Abuse and Mental Health Services Administration. Retrieved from http://www.ncbi.nlm.nih.gov/books/NBK14497.

Beta blockers, clonidine, and carbamazepine ameliorate withdrawal severity, but evidence to determine their effect on delirium and seizures is inadequate. Phenothiazines ameliorate withdrawal symptoms but are less effective than benzodiazepines in reducing delirium. These medications may be used as adjunctive therapy but are not recommended as monotherapy.

Considering that clients with alcoholism have developed physical tolerance to chemicals, dose determinations

ASSESSMENT TOOL 30.1

Clinical Institute Withdrawal Assessment of Alcohol Scale, Revised (CIWA-Ar)

Patient: _____ Date: _____ Time: _____ (24 hour clock, midnight = 00:00)

Pulse or heart rate, taken for 1 minute: _____ Blood Pressure: _____

NAUSEA AND VOMITING—Ask "Do you feel sick to your stomach? Have you vomited?" Observation.

0 no nausea and no vomiting
1 mild nausea with no vomiting
2
3
4 intermittent nausea with dry heaves
5
6
7 constant nausea, frequent dry heaves and vomiting

TREMOR—Arms extended and fingers spread apart. Observation.

0 no tremor
1 not visible, but can be felt fingertip to fingertip
2
3
4 moderate, with patient's arms extended
5
6
7 severe, even with arms not extended

PAROXYSMAL SWEATS—Observation.

0 no sweat visible
1 barely perceptible sweating, palms moist
2
3
4 beads of sweat obvious on forehead
5
6
7 drenching sweats

ANXIETY—Ask "Do you feel nervous?" Observation.

0 no anxiety, at ease
1 mild anxious
2
3
4 moderately anxious, or guarded, so anxiety is inferred
5
6
7 equivalent to acute panic states as seen in severe delirium or acute schizophrenic reactions

TACTILE DISTURBANCES—Ask "Have you any itching, pins-and-needles sensations, any burning, any numbness, or do you feel bugs crawling on or under your skin?" Observation.

0 none
1 very mild itching, pins and needles, burning or numbness
2 mild itching, pins and needles, burning or numbness
3 moderate itching, pins and needles, burning or numbness
4 moderately severe hallucinations
5 severe hallucinations
6 extremely severe hallucinations
7 continuous hallucinations

AUDITORY DISTURBANCES—Ask "Are you more aware of sounds around you? Are they harsh? Do they frighten you? Are you hearing anything that is disturbing to you? Are you hearing things you know are not there?" Observation.

0 not present
1 very mild harshness or ability to frighten
2 mild harshness or ability to frighten
3 moderate harshness or ability to frighten
4 moderately severe hallucinations
5 severe hallucinations
6 extremely severe hallucinations
7 continuous hallucinations

VISUAL DISTURBANCES—Ask "Does the light appear to be too bright? Is its color different? Does it hurt your eyes? Are you seeing anything that is disturbing to you? Are you seeing things you know are not there?" Observation.

0 not present
1 very mild sensitivity
2 mild sensitivity
3 moderate sensitivity
4 moderately severe hallucinations
5 severe hallucinations
6 extremely severe hallucinations
7 continuous hallucinations

HEADACHE, FULLNESS IN HEAD—Ask "Does your head feel different? Does it feel like there is a band around your head?" Do not rate for dizziness or light headedness. Otherwise, rate severity.

0 not present
1 very mild
2 mild
3 moderate
4 moderately severe
5 severe
6 very severe
7 extremely severe

ASSESSMENT TOOL 30.1 (continued)

AGITATION—Observation.

0 normal activity
1 somewhat more than normal activity
2
3
4 moderately fidgety and restless
5
6
7 paces back and forth during most of the interview, or constantly thrashes about

ORIENTATION AND CLOUDING OF SENSORIUM—Ask "What day is this? Where are you? Who am I?"

0 oriented and can do serial additions
1 cannot do serial additions or is uncertain about date
2 disoriented for date by no more than 2 calendar days
3 disoriented for date by more than 2 calendar days
4 disoriented for place/or person

Total **CIWA-Ar** Score _____
Rater's Initials _____
Maximum Possible Score 67

The **CIWA-Ar** is not copyrighted and may be reproduced freely. This assessment for monitoring withdrawal symptoms requires approximately 5 minutes to administer. The maximum score is 67 (see instrument). Patients scoring less than 10 do not usually need additional medication for withdrawal.
Sullivan, J. T., Sykora, K., Schneiderman, J., Naranjo, C. A., & Sellers, E. M. (1989). Assessment of alcohol withdrawal: The revised Clinical Institute Withdrawal Assessment for Alcohol scale (**CIWA-Ar**). *British Journal of Addiction, 84*, 1353–1357.

---

for alcohol withdrawal must be individualized so that clients can receive large amounts of medications rapidly if needed. Clients who are alcohol dependent require much larger than standard doses of sedatives to achieve desired effects. Providing only a fixed, standardized dose for all clients cannot adequately treat alcohol withdrawal (CSAT, 2006).

Individualizing therapy with withdrawal scales (eg, CIWA-Ar) leads to significantly less medication use and shorter treatment. For treatment based on symptom monitoring, suggested regimens include administering one of the following medications every hour when the CIWA-Ar score is 8 to 10 or more:

- Chlordiazepoxide, 50 to 100 mg
- Diazepam, 10 to 20 mg
- Lorazepam, 2 to 4 mg

For fixed-schedule regimens, one of the following medications may be given:

- Chlordiazepoxide, 50 mg every 6 hours for four doses, then 25 mg every 6 hours for eight doses
- Diazepam, 10 mg every 6 hours for four doses, then 5 mg every 6 hours for eight doses
- Lorazepam, 2 mg every 6 hours for four doses, then 1 mg every 6 hours for eight doses

When these regimens fail to control symptoms, additional medication can be provided (CSAT, 2006).

Long-term maintenance therapies for control of alcoholism include disulfiram (Antabuse), naltrexone (Depade, ReVia, and Vivitrol), acamprosate (Campral), and baclofen (Lioresal). Disulfiram interferes with alcohol degradation, resulting in severe flushing, nausea, and palpitations if clients drink, thereby discouraging them from doing so. Naltrexone blocks opioid receptors involved in the reward pathway stimulated by alcohol, thereby blocking the effects of alcohol. The result is a reduced craving for alcohol. Acamprosate acts on the GABA and glutamate neurotransmitter systems. Chronic alcohol dependence alters the levels and interaction of GABA and glutamate with their receptors, and treatment with acamprosate appears to normalize this system in the brain. The result of acamprosate therapy is reduced uncomfortable symptoms of abstinence, thereby aiding motivated clients to remain abstinent. Baclofen (Lioresal), another GABA receptor agonist, also decreases alcohol cravings and reverses withdrawal in clients with alcohol, cocaine, and opiate dependence (CSAT, 2006). Baclofen suppresses activity in the areas of the brain thought to react to triggers, thereby decreasing the obsession to use.

OPIOIDS AND OTHER DRUGS. Opioid maintenance or replacement drugs are useful for opiate-dependent clients who are not physically or psychologically ready for total abstinence. Maintenance therapy must be used in conjunction with other treatment methods to work toward the goal of eventually being chemically free. It is not a cure.

Methadone, naltrexone, and buprenorphine are medications used to assist with detoxification from and prevent relapse in opioid addiction. Methadone is a synthetic opiate used in the controlled replacement of illicit opiates, whereas naltrexone and buprenorphine are narcotic antagonists given to block the effect of opiates.

Methadone, a long-acting narcotic, is legally administered on a daily basis, substituting for the illegal use of shorter-acting opiates such as heroin. Heroin releases excess dopamine into the body, leading users to continuously seek more of the drug to occupy dopamine receptors in the brain. Methadone, which has pharmacologic properties similar to those of heroin, occupies and stabilizes the receptors for 24 to 36 hours, permitting discontinuation of heroin use. It effectively prevents withdrawal symptoms and cravings associated with heroin use. Methadone is administered in licensed clinics or by specially qualified physicians authorized to control its distribution and prevent diversion for illegal use.

The newest drug used to treat narcotic addiction is buprenorphine, a semisynthetic narcotic available in two forms: alone in the oral form of Subutex, and in combination as oral buprenorphine/naloxone (Suboxone). Buprenorphine (Subutex) produces mild opioid effects but not much euphoria. It satisfies cravings and enables opioid-addicted clients to abstain from illicit use without experiencing withdrawal. The combination drug Suboxone decreases client dependence on injectable opioids. Both forms have the potential for abuse. If oral Suboxone is crushed and injected, the naloxone (Narcan) component predominates and causes instant opiate withdrawal (CSAT, 2009).

Some drugs are used to help with withdrawal symptoms from addiction to other drugs of abuse. See Understanding Psychopharmacology 30.1 (CSAT, 2006).

Checkpoint Questions

8. What are the first-line agents used for treatment of alcohol withdrawal?
9. What are three examples of drugs used for replacement therapy?

Rehabilitation

Rehabilitation focuses primarily on the substance use disorder. Related problems such as unemployment, broken relationships, and legal problems cannot be resolved if addiction continues. Conversely, many problems that stem directly from substance abuse, such as physical illness, family quarrels, or financial difficulties, diminish with rehabilitation and continued abstinence. Emotional and social factors are treated concurrently with the substance use disorder.

After detoxification, rehabilitation interventions involve restoring physical and emotional stability, motivating clients to continue treatment, confronting their pathologic defenses and responses, improving their self-image, facilitating insight into problems, and planning for discharge and follow-up care. Table 30.2 lists common interdisciplinary rehabilitation interventions and important points about each.

An important aspect of any rehabilitation program is for clients to accept responsibility for their problem and to take needed actions toward their own recovery. Underlying the goal of discontinuing substance use and maintaining abstinence is behavioral change that will lead to greater

TABLE 30.2 Selected Interdisciplinary Interventions in Rehabilitation

Intervention	Description and Techniques
Breaking through defenses	Health care professionals must be ready for the defensiveness common in clients with substance use problems. They should help clients accept an objective reality; maintain a consistent, persistent approach that emphasizes there is no valid reason for clients to use substances; and keep clients focused on the substance problem without becoming sidetracked.
Understanding and accepting the disorder	Clients need to intellectually comprehend that they have a disease, not that they are weak or stupid. Health care providers can assist by providing educational materials, clarifying misinformation, explaining facts about drug effects and consequences, giving emotional support, and promoting abstinence.
Interacting with peers	Peer group identification and confrontation are powerful in recovery. Health care providers can assist clients to recognize and internalize that they are not alone in their suffering and that they can receive support and hope. Groups allow for confrontation by peers who attack pathologic defenses and help one another obtain insight into their behaviors.
Developing hope	Clients may feel hopeless, discouraged, and demoralized. They need help to realize that they can overcome their situation. Identifying with peers also in recovery is significant. Positive attitudes from health care providers also instill hope.
Resocializing	The lives of clients with addictions often revolve solely around themselves and their substance. Their social skills may be minimal or absent. Providers can assist clients to rebuild the capacity for relationships and to decrease self-centeredness.
Developing self-worth and opinions about self	Self-worth increases as clients begin to understand their illness. Providers can help clients take responsibility for changes in attitudes and actions and achieve satisfaction in successes and relationships. Clients may also need assistance to develop self-discipline, such as organizing and adhering to a daily routine. Health care providers can encourage positive efforts and motivation.

personal enrichment. Recovery is considered a lifelong process.

Researchers have extensively studied factors contributing to long-term sobriety after treatment (Hart & McGarragle, 2010; Pagano et al., 2009). Results have shown that the most helpful personal and lifestyle changes people in recovery can make are continued involvement in 12-step programs after treatment and development of a sober support network.

SELF-HELP GROUPS. The first, and perhaps most influential, substance abuse self-help group is Alcoholics Anonymous (AA). Two men who could not find help for their drinking—Dr. Bob, a surgeon, and Bill W., a New York stockbroker—founded AA in 1935. They discovered that by sharing their experiences and identifying with each other in their common problems with alcohol, they could overcome their compulsion to drink.

AA functions with a "12-step" model (Box 30.4). This model defines "hitting bottom" as an emotional and cognitive experience that impels people toward changing their behavior. According to 12-step theory, clients will not be compelled to alter their actions until the emotional and cognitive components of their attitude toward substance use have been transformed. "Hitting bottom" can bring about the distress necessary to challenge thought processes and substance-abusing behaviors. Research studies support that reflecting on the negative consequences of drinking is an important first step toward eventually making the final decision to become sober (Mohatt et al., 2008).

Many programs use a model similar to that of AA. They include Al-Anon (for families of substance abusers), Alateen (for teenagers who have a substance abuser in their life), NA (for narcotic abusers), CA (for cocaine abusers), and Adult Children of Alcoholics (ACOA).

BRIEF INTERVENTION. Traditional treatments for clients with substance use disorders require weeks to months. Nevertheless, brief intervention is an emerging strategy for addressing high-risk clients who do not display signs of chemical dependency but use substances in harmful or abusive ways. Brief interventions take minutes and require minimal follow-up.

Brief therapy focuses on immediate solutions to acute problems and is used most frequently for clients who abuse alcohol. The goal is to moderate alcohol consumption to sensible levels and to eliminate harmful behaviors (Heather, 2010). Sessions usually involve one to four therapy visits focused solely on increasing motivation to reduce substance use. Changing harmful patterns helps to minimize negative outcomes.

Client-Centered, Culturally Competent Care

Numerous factors prohibit people from seeking or receiving treatment for substance use disorders. Of the 17.6 million people in 2009 who needed but did not receive treatment, nearly 61% reported making no effort to get help. The six most often reported reasons for not obtaining treatment were (1) not ready to stop using, (2) no health coverage and could not afford cost, (3) possible negative effect on job, (4) concern that receiving treatment might cause neighbors/community to have negative opinion, (5) could handle the problem without treatment, and (6) not knowing where to go for treatment (SAMHSA, 2010b).

Improved understanding of the challenges and values of unique subcultures is necessary for services to be effective among diverse populations. One example is the homeless population (see Chap. 38). Glasser (2003) studied the effectiveness of current substance use therapies with the homeless, noting interventions that might enhance respect and dignity. The unique culture of the homeless is based on a synergistic relationship between resources and treatment, which is often threatened when basic needs for food and shelter remain unmet. Likewise, people who use limited resources for substances have little remaining for food and housing. Incorporating basic needs into treatment programs for homeless people acknowledges the barriers that they face.

Awareness of and respect for diverse cultural values are imperative in providing care congruent with a client's belief system. A working awareness of a client's cultural characteristics can serve to increase the effectiveness of interventions. The premise that culture can be curative (Castro & Alarcon, 2002) allows providers to offer culturally relevant and cohesive strategies when working with diverse populations. Providers must consider cultural variables such as

---

BOX 30.4 The 12 Steps of Alcoholics Anonymous

1. Admitted we were powerless over alcohol—that our lives had become unmanageable
2. Came to believe that a Power greater than ourselves could restore us to sanity
3. Made a decision to turn our will and our lives over to the care of God as we understood Him
4. Made a searching and fearless moral inventory of ourselves
5. Admitted to God, to ourselves, and to another human being the exact nature of our wrongs
6. Were entirely ready to have God remove all these defects of character
7. Humbly asked Him to remove our shortcomings
8. Made a list of all persons we had harmed, and became willing to make amends to them all
9. Made direct amends to such people wherever possible except when to do so would injure them or others
10. Continued to take a personal inventory, and when we were wrong, promptly admitted it
11. Sought through prayer and meditation to improve our conscious contact with God as we understood Him, praying only for knowledge of His will for us and the power to carry that out
12. Having had a spiritual awakening as the result of these steps, we tried to carry this message to alcoholics and to practice these principles in all our affairs

level of family orientation, tendency toward individualism or collectivism, degree of attention to social position, or posture toward need for harmony in relationships. For example, care for Asian Americans should incorporate the cultural need to "save face" and avoid the shame associated with improper behavior and failure to meet social obligations (Lee & Mock, 2005; Yu et al., 2009). By recognizing such cultural factors, providers can design treatments most likely to be effective.

APPLYING THE NURSING PROCESS

Substance Use Disorders

This discussion of the nursing process with clients who have a substance use disorder focuses on interventions that begin early in recovery and continue over time. Although rehabilitation is the setting of focus, nurses encounter

substance-related problems in all practice areas. A basic knowledge of the relationship between each step of the nursing process and recovery is vital to competent nursing practice. See Understanding Nursing Care 30.1 for a visual concept map that summarizes the care discussed in the following paragraphs. Case In Point 30.1 provides the story of Erica and her husband Paul, who is struggling with Erica's addiction to alcohol.

▲ ASSESSMENT

Assessment focuses on physical status and psychosocial circumstances. Assessment Tool 30.2 contains a typical inventory for gathering data relative to health history and physical examination for clients seeking treatment for substance use disorders.

Screening

Sometimes, a nurse strongly suspects drug or alcohol use in clients who have not admitted this problem. In such cases, a screening tool helps with identification. Many health care

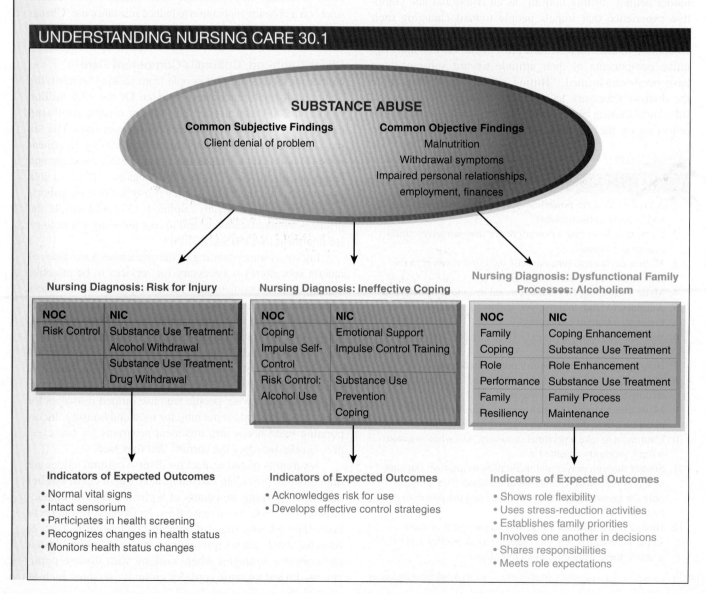

UNDERSTANDING NURSING CARE 30.1

SUBSTANCE ABUSE

Common Subjective Findings
Client denial of problem

Common Objective Findings
Malnutrition
Withdrawal symptoms
Impaired personal relationships,
employment, finances

Nursing Diagnosis: Risk for Injury

NOC	NIC
Risk Control	Substance Use Treatment: Alcohol Withdrawal
	Substance Use Treatment: Drug Withdrawal

Indicators of Expected Outcomes
- Normal vital signs
- Intact sensorium
- Participates in health screening
- Recognizes changes in health status
- Monitors health status changes

Nursing Diagnosis: Ineffective Coping

NOC	NIC
Coping	Emotional Support
Impulse Self-Control	Impulse Control Training
Risk Control: Alcohol Use	Substance Use Prevention
	Coping

Indicators of Expected Outcomes
- Acknowledges risk for use
- Develops effective control strategies

Nursing Diagnosis: Dysfunctional Family Processes: Alcoholism

NOC	NIC
Family Coping	Coping Enhancement
	Substance Use Treatment
Role Performance	Role Enhancement
	Substance Use Treatment
Family Resiliency	Family Process Maintenance

Indicators of Expected Outcomes
- Shows role flexibility
- Uses stress-reduction activities
- Establishes family priorities
- Involves one another in decisions
- Shares responsibilities
- Meets role expectations

Case in Point 30.1

Erica and Paul's Story

Erica, 38 years old, was arrested 2 days ago following an argument with another customer in a local bar. The judge ordered inpatient detoxification and treatment for alcoholism. This is Erica's fourth such admission in the past 7 years.

Six months ago, Erica's supervisor made her continued employment contingent on participation in a long-term, outpatient alcohol treatment program. She attended for 3 months until dropping out 1 week before the arrest. Paul reports, "I've thought about a legal separation until Erica can become sober, but I haven't been able to bring myself to move out. She's stopped doing anything to help with the house—she's drunk every day."

During the current admission interview, Erica expresses a need for treatment and discusses the negative effects of alcohol use. "I've been drinking a fifth of vodka and several beers every day. My last drink was 27 hours ago." The result of a blood alcohol level (BAL) drawn earlier is 0.05%. Review of history reveals a progressive decline in function, with increasing tolerance to and withdrawal symptoms from alcohol. Physical examination shows that Erica is underweight and deconditioned with gastric distress, mild cirrhosis, esophageal varices, and gum disease.

Key Assessment Findings

- **Daily and increasing alcohol ingestion**
- **Previous admissions for alcohol abuse treatment**
- **Aggressive and violent behavior, including arrest associated with drinking**
- **Employment problems related to alcohol**
- **BAL of 0.05 mg at 27 hours from last ingestion**
- **Underweight, deconditioned status**
- **Gastric distress with mild cirrhosis**
- **Esophageal varices**
- **Gum disease**
- **Family problems; abandonment of activities and responsibilities**

Nursing Diagnosis: Risk for Injury related to impending alcohol withdrawal as evidenced by blood alcohol level and timing of last ingestion

NOC: Risk Control: Alcohol Use: The client will exhibit minimal effects associated with alcohol withdrawal during the first week of detoxification.

NIC: Substance Use Treatment: Alcohol Withdrawal

- Minimize environmental stimuli during detoxification. Speak with a low, calm, reassuring voice. *A comfortable, quiet, non-threatening environment reduces anxiety-provoking stimuli.*
- Assess vital signs (Figure A). Look for indicators of impending withdrawal: tachycardia, hypertension, tremors, anxiety, sweating, hallucinations, and psychomotor agitation. *Monitoring vital signs and for the onset of withdrawal symptoms allows for timely intervention.*
- Institute seizure and fall precautions. *They promote the client's safety.*
- Administer sedatives as ordered. *They control the exaggerated sympathetic activity associated with withdrawal.*
- Monitor for covert alcohol consumption during detoxification. *Having to deal with uncomfortable feelings during sobriety may increase the client's anxiety and emotional discomfort, which may lead to relapse.*
- Continue frequent monitoring of vital signs, sensorium, and other variables. Provide verbal reassurance and reality orientation as appropriate. Report worsened condition immediately. Institute emergency procedures if the client shows signs of delirium. *Preventing alcohol withdrawal delirium is critical because of the associated mortality rate. Verbal reassurance and reality orientation help reduce anxiety associated with withdrawal and detoxification.*
- Listen to client's concerns about alcohol withdrawal. Encourage her to discuss feelings; assist with measures for effective coping. *Listening provides support and helps reduce anxiety and stress. Adaptive coping strategies must replace maladaptive ones for recovery.*

FIGURE A During withdrawal, the nurse assesses the client's vital signs to monitor for life-threatening changes.

7/18/13: *Effects associated with alcohol withdrawal have been minimized. Vital signs are within acceptable parameters, with no tremors, psychomotor agitation, or anxiety. BAL is within normal limits. Client is alert and oriented. She verbalizes that she recognizes improvement in overall health status.*

June Cusick, RN

(continues on page 646)

Case in Point 30.1 (continued)

Erica and Paul's Story

Nursing Diagnosis: Ineffective Health Maintenance related to continued alcohol abuse as evidenced by deteriorating health status, including cirrhosis, esophageal varices, underweight status, gum disease, and deconditioning

NOC: Personal Health Status and Substance Addiction Consequences: The client will demonstrate improved overall health status with adoption of health-seeking behaviors.

NIC: Nutrition Management

- Obtain an initial weight and periodically weigh the client. Encourage calorie intake appropriate for body type and lifestyle. *Weight is a valuable indicator of health status. These measures assist with tailoring a nutritional plan to the individual client.*
- Provide vitamin and mineral supplements. Encourage consumption of well-balanced meals with little refined sugar or caffeine. *Alcohol depletes essential nutrients, which must be replaced. Refraining from sugar and caffeine helps manage anxiety and mood swings.*
- Offer snacks as appropriate; provide easy-to-consume nutritious foods and drinks. *Snacks, liquids, and easily prepared foods facilitate intake and enhance the chances for success.*
- Monitor client's tolerance to intake; note any nausea or vomiting and characteristics of emesis. Consider small frequent meals. *Alcohol is highly irritating to the gastrointestinal tract. The client's history of esophageal varices increases her risk for hematemesis.*

NIC: Exercise Promotion

- Assist client to develop an appropriate and appealing exercise program; inform her about health benefits and physiologic effects of exercise. Provide positive feedback for efforts (Figure B). *Physical exercise increases stamina, helps balance mood, and aids in managing anxiety. Positive feedback promotes self-esteem and motivation for continued participation.*

NIC: Oral Health Restoration

- Instruct and assist client to perform oral hygiene after eating and as often as necessary. Encourage frequent rinsing of the mouth, using a soft toothbrush, and flossing between teeth twice daily; avoid the use of lemon-glycerin swabs. *Proper oral hygiene reduces the risk of further problems. Lemon-glycerin swabs are drying to the oral mucosa.*
- Assist client to select soft, bland, and nonacidic foods. *They prevent exacerbation of the already irritated oral mucosa.*
- Monitor client at least every shift for dryness of the oral mucosa. Monitor for signs and symptoms of glossitis and stomatitis. Arrange for dental care (Figure C). *Gum disease places a burden on the immune system.*

> 8/12/13: The client demonstrates improved physical fitness and energy level. She has gained 6 lb. Neurologic functioning is intact. She exhibits mild fatigue. The client is following her nutritional plan and has visited the fitness center twice each week, running on the treadmill and lifting weights for 30 minutes each time. The client is maintaining oral hygiene and has visited the dentist, with follow-up appointments scheduled.
>
> June Cusick, RN

Nursing Diagnosis: Dysfunctional Family Processes: Alcoholism related to long-standing history of alcohol abuse as evidenced by continued involvement in rehabilitation programs, continued and increasing alcohol consumption, and husband's statements about legal separation

NOC: Family Coping and Role Performance: The family will demonstrate balanced and adaptive family functional and mature interpersonal relationships.

NIC: Family Integrity Promotion

- Identify typical family relationships and coping mechanisms. Identify conflicting priorities among family members. *The family's relationships and coping mechanisms provide clues to develop an individualized plan of care.*

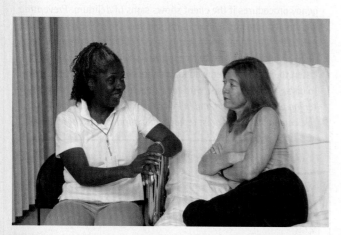

FIGURE B The nurse is discussing the benefits of healthy habits with the client, and encouraging the efforts she has made during her stay in rehabilitation.

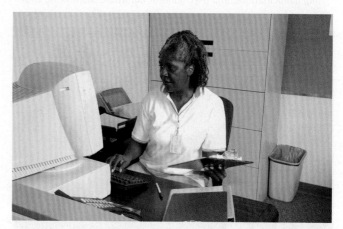

FIGURE C Based on the client's assessment findings, the nurse is making arrangements for a thorough dental evaluation.

Case in Point 30.1 (continued)

Erica and Paul's Story

- Teach family members effective communication skills and assertiveness. Help them to clarify what they want, expect, and need from one another. Explore topics to determine how each member can support and meet the needs of others. Help clients to recognize excessive dependency or unrealistic expectations. Refer family to support group for those dealing with similar problems. *Behavior that respects the rights and feelings of others leads to increased trust and intimacy. Self-awareness and insight into others improve relationships. Providing client and family support services and new tools for interaction will help them abandon older, less functional behaviors.*

NIC: Role Enhancement

- Help client and spouse explore appropriate expression of anger or other negative emotions. Collaborate with the family in problem solving. Teach problem-solving skills and conflict management techniques. Assist with conflict resolution. *Appropriate use of problem-solving techniques and conflict resolution help to build trust and respect for improving relationships.*

- Encourage client to assume functional parenting roles. Facilitate opportunity for client to role play new behaviors; facilitate discussion of expectations between client and spouse in reciprocal role. Explore potential problems (eg, power struggles) as client becomes more functional (Figure D). *The husband has been the responsible partner for many years. Although he may welcome the client's sobriety and involvement, it represents a change in his role, which may be difficult for him.*

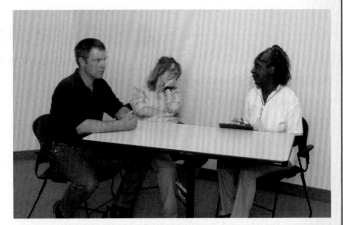

FIGURE D Ongoing discussions between the client and the spouse are vital during recovery from substance abuse. Long-standing dysfunctional patterns will take time to change and to improve. The nurse can facilitate ongoing discussions.

> 9/2/13: The family demonstrates a beginning ability to manage family function, roles, and relationships. They report use of stress-reduction activities. The spouse reports that the client is helping with some chores and tasks. The couple demonstrates respectful communication during interactions.
> Stewart Starkey, RN

EPILOGUE

Erica was discharged from the inpatient facility 5 months ago and has participated in an outpatient alcohol treatment program. Two weeks ago, she stopped by the local bar to say hello to some friends and began drinking. Later that same night, she fell down the steps and broke her wrist. Despite this setback, she continues to attend appointments. She has gained an additional 5 lb (2.2 kg) and is regularly visiting the gym. Her relationship with Paul remains challenging, particularly now that her wrist is broken and she cannot do as much at home. The spouses continue to attend counseling sessions for couples.

facilities include the easy-to-administer CAGE questionnaire in general assessments (Assessment Tool 30.3). A "yes" answer to any of the four CAGE questions indicates the need for further workup and referral.

Physical Examination

For clients with diagnosed substance abuse, the first days of treatment involve assessing for withdrawal signs and symptoms. Abrupt cessation of a drug toward which clients have developed tolerance and dependence likely will cause severe response. Withdrawal from alcohol and benzodiazepines can even be fatal as a result of seizures and cardiovascular symptoms. Withdrawal is characterized initially by irritability, strong urges to use the drug of choice, and elevated heart rate and blood pressure. For a guide to specific withdrawal problems based on drug category, refer to Table 30.1.

Assessment of baseline health status includes a physical examination, liver function studies, and possibly other diagnostic tests, depending on the preliminary findings. Use of alcohol and drugs impairs judgment, increasing the likelihood that clients have engaged in high-risk sexual behaviors. Drug abuse is one of the biggest contributors to the spread of HIV, through shared needles, cotton swabs, rinse water, and cookers used with injectable drugs, as well as engagement in high-risk sexual behaviors (SAMHSA, 2010a). Because substance abuse is a risk factor for sexually transmitted infections, clients may also undergo examination and testing for them.

Psychosocial Assessment

Psychosocial assessment focuses on the extent to which addiction has disrupted family, social, and work relationships. Another component is the identification of problem areas or relationships that may undermine treatment and recovery, as well as potential resources for support. For example, a client with alcoholism who works in a bar will face ongoing challenges to the avoidance of drinking. His or her treatment team will need aggressive solutions to help with this problem. A more common problem is the client whose spouse or partner also abuses substances or for some reason does not support the client's treatment. A thorough psychosocial assessment can

---

▲ ASSESSMENT TOOL 30.2 ▲

Substance Use Inventory

Health History Questions

Demographic Data

- Name:
- Age:
- Sex:
- Ethnic group:
- Marital status:
- Religious affiliation:
- Significant other:
- Reason for seeking care/motivation for treatment:

Current Substance Information

- What types of substances do you currently use?
  - Alcohol (specify beer, wine, whiskey)
  - Cocaine
  - Heroin
  - Marijuana
  - Sedative-hypnotics
  - Hallucinogens
- Which of the above drugs do you use in combination?
- What is the predominant substance of choice?
- Do you use any prescription drugs?
- What is the approximate amount of alcohol or drugs that you use?
  - How many six packs, quarts, fifths?
  - How many bags?
  - How many pills or hits daily?
- How do you take any drugs that you use?
- How frequently do you use substances? Daily, several times a week?
- Does use increase on weekends or other times?
- Do you engage in binge drinking?
- Have you ever tried to control or cut down drinking or substance use? How?
- When was your last drink or use of drugs?
- Have you developed tolerance? (explain)
  - When did it begin?
  - Has there been a change in tolerance?
- Are withdrawal symptoms present? (explain)
  - Is there a history of withdrawal?
  - Is there a history of seizures?
  - Is there a history of hallucinations? (explain)

Past Medical History

- Are there any present medical problems?
- Are there any chronic medical problems?
- Is there a history of any of the following: liver disease, hepatitis, diabetes, heart disease, anemia, drug overdose?

- Have there been any recent falls, injuries, accidents?
- Are you taking any prescribed medications?
- Do you have any known allergies?

Past Substance History

- Have you ever stopped drinking or using drugs?
- How long was the period of abstinence?
- Why did you abstain; what was the motivation?
- When did you start using substances?
- When did you first begin having difficulty in life circumstances because of substances?
- Have you ever been in treatment for substance abuse or dependency?
- What type of treatment did you have for substance abuse or dependency?
- How many times were you in treatment for the above?
- Is there a family history of alcohol abuse or dependency?
- Is there a family history of drug abuse or dependency?

Psychosocial History

- What is your spouse's, partner's, family's reaction to your use of substances?
- Do family members also abuse substances?
- Is substance use causing marital conflicts?
- Do you have children? How many, ages, and sex?
- Have children had school problems, health problems, or physical, emotional, sleeping problems?
- Is the family suffering from housing or nutritional problems because of substance use?
- What are your present living conditions?
- Do you live alone?
- What are your leisure activities or hobbies?
- Has your participation in these activities changed because of substance use?
- Have your friends changed or been lost because of substance use?
- Do social activities center on the substance use?
- What is your occupation and present place of employment?
- How long have you been with your present employer?
- Have you ever missed work from substance use?
- Have you abused substances while working?
- Is substance use jeopardizing work or business?
- How much time do you spend on substances?
- Do substances provide you with a source of income?
- Have you had any violations while intoxicated?
- Are any present legal offenses pending from substance abuse or dependency?
- Is present treatment court recommended?

ASSESSMENT TOOL 30.2 (continued)

Physical Examination

Area of Focus	Common Positive Findings/Indicators of Drug Problems
Vital Signs	
Blood pressure	Hypotension or hypertension
Pulse	Rapid, regular, irregular
Temperature	Elevated
Respirations	Rapid, shallow, depressed
Appearance	
Gait	Unsteady, normal, weaving, shuffling
Eyes	Conjunctival injection; bloodshot; dilated, pinpoint, pupils; lacrimation (tearing); vacant stare; poor eye contact; intense eye contact
Skin	Perspiration, cool, clammy, dry, bruises, needle tracks, scars, abrasions, gooseflesh, excoriations, reddened palms
Nose	Running (rhinorrhea), congested, red
Tremors	Fine or coarse, slight–moderate or severe
Grooming	Unkempt, unshaven, odor (alcohol, foul)
Mental Status/Behavior	
Speech	Slurred, incoherent, loud, monotone, hesitant, pressured, distracted
Attitude	Quiet, calm, demanding, agitated, irritable, impatient, vague, withdrawn, suspicious, anxious, tearful, happy, silly
Dominant mood—affect	Euphoric, depressed, angry, sad
Sensorium	Lack of orientation to time, person, place; changes in memory
Perception	Illusions, hallucinations, delusions, hallucinosis

identify such difficulties so the interdisciplinary team, with the client, can begin to plan possible solutions.

Clients are likely to underreport their habit and to minimize negative consequences. Questions about how drugs or alcohol have affected the client's life may reveal more pertinent data than direct questions about amount or frequency of use. Nurses also observe the family's nonverbal responses to the client's statements to determine incongruencies.

▲ NURSING DIAGNOSIS

Because of the wide-ranging physical and emotional needs of clients with substance use disorders, many nursing

▲ ASSESSMENT TOOL 30.3 ▲

The CAGE Questionnaire for Substance Abuse Screening

- Have you ever felt you should **C**ut down on your drinking?
- Have people **A**nnoyed you by criticizing your drinking?
- Have you ever felt bad or **G**uilty about your drinking?
- Have you ever had a drink (or **E**ye-opener) first thing in the morning to steady your nerves or to get rid of a hangover?

From Ewing, J. A. (1984). Detecting alcoholism: The CAGE questionnaire. *Journal of the American Medical Association, 252,* 1902–1907.

diagnoses may apply. Priority nursing diagnoses commonly applicable to this client population include the following (NANDA, 2008):

- **Risk for Injury** related to substance withdrawal
- **Ineffective Denial** related to dysfunctional defense mechanisms associated with substance abuse
- **Anxiety** related to sudden loss of maladaptive coping strategy (drug or alcohol use)
- **Ineffective Coping** related to dysfunctional behavior patterns secondary to substance abuse
- **Dysfunctional Family Processes: Alcoholism** related to substance abuse
- **Chronic Low Self-Esteem** related to doubts and anxiety about self-worth and abilities
- **Risk for Spiritual Distress** related to history of substance abuse
- **Deficient Diversional Activity** related to loss of primary activity (substance abuse)

▲ OUTCOME IDENTIFICATION AND PLANNING

Goals for recovery touch every aspect of the client's life. They vary according to the stage of recovery. Some identified desired outcomes, organized according to the *Nursing Outcomes Classification (NOC)*, might include the following (Moorhead et al., 2008):

- Risk Control: Withdrawal symptoms will be managed successfully.
- Knowledge: Substance Abuse Control: The client will acknowledge the substance problem and the need for treatment.
- Anxiety Self-Control: The client will identify and implement strategies for managing anxiety without using substances.
- Coping: The client will begin to develop adaptive coping strategies and will use them to manage stressors.
- Family Coping: The family will begin to rebuild damaged relationships.
- Self-Esteem: The client will identify positive aspects of self.
- Social Involvement: The client will develop alternative activities to replace time spent acquiring, using, or recovering from substance abuse.

▲ IMPLEMENTATION

Nurses use many types of interventions to assist clients in recovery and their families. Common *Nursing Interventions Classification* (*NIC*) labels related to management of substance use disorders include, but are not limited to, Anxiety Reduction, Emotional Support, Hope Instillation, Impulse Control Training, Nutrition Management, Spiritual Support, Substance Use Treatment: Alcohol Withdrawal, and Substance Use Treatment: Drug Withdrawal (Bulechek et al., 2008).

Managing Withdrawal

Detoxification is stressful and dangerous. Alcohol withdrawal delirium can be potentially fatal if not treated appropriately. Alcohol withdrawal occurs 24 to 48 hours after last ingestion, so clients require frequent observation for signs and symptoms of withdrawal on admission.

Nursing care during inpatient treatment of detoxification is critical. Nurses often play key roles in assisting clients through this potentially life-threatening experience (Figure 30.11). The first priority is protecting safety. The nurse frequently checks the client's vital signs and follows the facility's seizure and fall precautions. Monitoring symptoms over time provides data necessary for appropriate medication management.

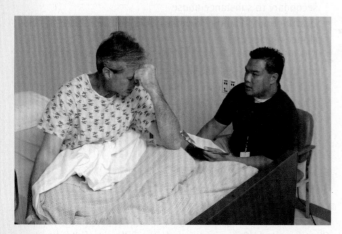

FIGURE 30.11 The highest nursing priority for the client undergoing detoxification and experiencing withdrawal is to help maintain safety.

Clients may experience frightening hallucinations or illusions during withdrawal. Medications may help ameliorate these symptoms. Nonpharmacologic nursing interventions for withdrawal-related sensory alterations include speaking in a low, calm, reassuring voice; providing reassurance about safety; and maintaining a comfortable, quiet, nonthreatening environment.

Breaking Through Denial

Denial, a defense mechanism (see Chap. 3), protects against painful or threatening realities. Moderate denial is normal and sometimes helpful. However, clients with substance problems cannot recover unless they first admit their problem. Doing so can be particularly challenging when clients are forced into treatment. Some clients who voluntarily enter treatment do so only to appease family, friends, employers, or the judicial system. Even clients who are fully committed to treatment may have problems overcoming denial.

Denial may involve obvious outright refusals to admit the existence or extent of a problem. It can also be subtle (Table 30.3). For example, a client might remark, "I drink a lot, but I've never been in trouble from it" or "I don't drink as much as my friends do." Denial may also manifest as minimizing or justifying the amount or frequency of use. Clients are unaware of being in denial; they are not purposefully lying. Denial arises from fear. When used to defend addictions, it is pathologic and results in perpetuating the problem.

Nurses begin to help clients relinquish denial first by establishing relationships built on trust. Treating clients respectfully, maintaining a nonjudgmental attitude, and examining personal attitudes toward substance use are critical components of care. To help clients confront denial, nurses respectfully but firmly present evidence of the severe dysfunction that has resulted from substance abuse. Examples might be job losses, financial problems, estrangement from family and friends, and legal difficulties. For example, a client may state that substance abuse was a way to deal with pressures at work. Instead of sympathizing with this rationalization, the nurse can point out that substance abuse probably compromised the client's job performance.

Another approach includes educating clients that substance abuse is a disease. Clients who feel weak or guilty about their problem may be more accepting of their situation if they recognize it as a disease, rather than a character flaw. Attendance at 12-step program meetings can provide more explanations of how substance abuse is a disease and also expose clients to stories and comments from others who have abandoned denial and begun recovery.

Nurses should also encourage clients to try to have an open mind about feedback that staff members and others provide. They can encourage clients to ask themselves the following questions when they challenge counselors or loved ones about their condition:

- Am I feeling defensive? What am I finding threatening?
- What will I lose if I accept their viewpoint?
- Why is this important to me?
- Have other people I trust said this to me?
- Is it possible that what they have said is true?

TABLE 30.3 **Forms of Denial**

Type	Explanation	Example
Simple denial	Refusing outright that one is chemically dependent	"I'm not addicted."
Minimizing	Admitting a problem but in such a way that it appears much less serious or significant than it actually is	"I wasn't that bad at the party." "Yes, I drink, but not that much." "I had a joint, but I was OK to drive." "I only drink beer, but I don't use drugs."
Rationalizing	Making excuses or giving reasons to justify addictive behavior; giving an inaccurate explanation of the cause of behavior	"I can't sleep, so I use pills." "I worked hard all week. I deserve to party." "I usually don't drive after I drink, but a friend needed a ride home. That's the last time I'm the nice guy!"
Intellectualizing	Avoiding emotional awareness or personal responsibility of a substance problem by analyzing the problem, or looking for causes of chemical dependency	"My family uses drugs; I have the genes to be addicted." "My childhood was so bad, it's a way of coping with my underlying feelings."
Blaming (projecting)	Maintaining that the responsibility for behavior lies somewhere else; placing the cause "out there," not within the person	"You'd drink too, if you were married to her!" "The cop was out to get me." "I lost my job; that's what made me use."
Diversion	Changing the subject to avoid a subject felt to be threatening	"You wouldn't expect me to walk in that condition, would you?" "Yeah, I got high last night. So what's for dinner?" "My drinking bothers you? Well you bother me!"
Bargaining	Cutting deals or setting conditions for when things will be right to deal with the problem	"I'll quit drinking if you quit smoking." "I'll quit smoking pot when there is less stress at work."
Passivity	Ignoring the situation, or being its victim	"I've tried to quit before, but it's stronger than me." "There's nothing I can do." "If only I had more willpower …"
Hostility	Becoming angry or unpleasantly irritable when the subject of addiction is mentioned; scaring or threatening people away from discussing it	"I'm lousy in bed when I'm drunk? Fine, no more sex." "Get off my back!" "You might not like that I deal drugs, but you like when I take you out to fancy dinners, don't you?"

Nurses should encourage clients to discuss their answers to these questions. Speaking openly with others helps expose maladaptive cognitive patterns and illogic that accompany addictive thinking. Nurses should also remember that breaking through entrenched thinking patterns takes time. See Therapeutic Communication 30.1.

Managing Anxiety

Substance use disorders compromise emotional maturation. Dealing with everyday events helps people to develop their coping skills. Clients using substances have stopped dealing with stressors in healthy ways and have stunted their emotional responses. As a result, their emotions and related behaviors may be immature. (Some clients display behavior associated with the age at which they began using the problematic substance regularly.) When clients begin recovery, they may experience anger, sadness, anxiety, frustration, and rejection. Not being able to

suppress these feelings with numbing substances, coupled with their compromised coping skills, may leave newly sober clients with anxiety and emotional discomfort. Overwhelming events or feelings may place such clients at risk for relapse.

Nurses should encourage clients to learn stress management techniques (see Chap. 24). Examples may include aerobic exercise, meditation, and deep breathing or relaxation. Being available for clients to talk to during rough patches and encouraging discussions with other staff members, supportive loved ones, or other recovering people are additional suggestions.

Teaching Effective Coping Strategies

All people use coping strategies during stressful situations. Immature and maladaptive examples include avoidance, repression, and blaming. Clients with substance use disorders typically have engaged in pathologic denial, projection, acting out, and complete avoidance. To experience recovery and

Therapeutic Communication 30.1

A Cocaine Abuser in Denial

Tom, 35 years old, was admitted 2 weeks ago to an inpatient substance abuse facility for detoxification and rehabilitation after cocaine use led to an automobile accident in which Tom killed a child. Tom has had no withdrawal symptoms; he reported that his most recent cocaine use was 2 days before admission. The nurse has been working with Tom since his admission and has observed his ongoing denial about the related circumstances (ie, Tom has expressed no feelings about the dead child). Tom also refuses to acknowledge the extent of his cocaine use and the many problems his dependency is creating.

INEFFECTIVE DIALOGUE

TOM: Like I've said before, the cocaine was just a pastime. It hasn't really caused any major problems for me.

NURSE: Oh, I see. You use it just for, sort of, recreation? Just to keep your mind off other things? How does it help do that? *(Nurse is reinforcing denial through nonconfrontation.)*

TOM: Well, when I'm high, I don't really have time to think, so there you have it!

NURSE: OK. I understand. But the cocaine must cause some trouble for you in your daily life, doesn't it?

TOM: Well, honestly, not really. I just take walks when I want some. My daughter doesn't really notice I'm gone because she's only 2. My wife doesn't even pay attention to me anymore, so that hasn't affected her either.

NURSE: It sounds like your life is about the same as it was before your cocaine use, then? *(The nurse ignores the content of Tom's message and rephrases or reframes the issue.)*

TOM: Yeah, I'd say so.

EFFECTIVE DIALOGUE

TOM: Like I've said before, the cocaine was just a pastime. It hasn't really caused any major problems for me.

NURSE: Tom, from what I understand, you were admitted because of a severe cocaine-related accident that killed a child. I would say that was a very serious consequence for not just you but others, too. *(Nurse uses confrontation with a recent example to help Tom face his cocaine use and its ramifications. The nurse avoids being judgmental but presents the view in a neutral, yet firm manner.)*

TOM: That's true. But the car was actually out of balance, and it was raining. I don't see how that was really my fault.

NURSE: The report states that you had white dust all over your shirt and that you were quickly moving straws and a bag around when the cops approached your car. *(The nurse does not accept Tom's excuse or blame of external factors for his actions. The nurse continues to focus on the cocaine problem.)*

TOM: You know, cops have their own way of seeing things. I had a bag of candy in the car for my daughter, and I also had some of those sipper drinks that have the straws glued onto the box. The cops will find anything to haul me in. I'm getting sick and tired of it.

NURSE: The drug test was done on that powder. It was pure cocaine. I know you saw those results the other day when we were together and your lawyer visited. Why are you continuing to avoid responsibility for your actions? *(The nurse confronts Tom again and also provides more facts.)*

TOM: Well, I . . . just don't know. I guess you have a point. *(Period of silence follows.)*

NURSE: This pattern has created a very difficult situation, and this isn't the first time. As much as you try to deny, it can't be an easy thing for you to go through—especially with a child's death. Can we explore what you mean when you say I have a point?

TOM: Well, maybe I contributed to the accident.

Reflection and Critical Thinking

- If you were Tom's nurse, how would you feel about his accident and the child's death? Would you have personal reactions and ideas about Tom based on these events?
- If you had been trying to work on Tom's denial, think of the feelings you might have had and explore them.
- How might you have intervened therapeutically or nontherapeutically, and how would you analyze your interventions?

personal growth, they must replace these strategies with more mature ones.

Nurses can help by teaching cognitive restructuring. Re-appraising situations diminishes the need for defensiveness. For example, a client may state that he always drinks too much during family get-togethers because he is uncomfortable around his father-in-law, who does not believe the client is good enough for his daughter. Using cognitive restructuring, the client learns to become aware of self-talk such as "He thinks I'm a failure" or "I'll never fit in." He can stop and replace these thoughts with positive statements, such as "I am a good and competent person" or "I get along well with most of my wife's family." Nurses can reinforce cognitive restructuring by suggesting that clients ask the following questions in stressful situations:

- What assertive, positive action can I take to make the situation less stressful to me?
- How can I look at this differently?
- What could I say to myself that would be more positive?
- Are others around me being negative? What can I do to avoid being affected by them?
- Are my expectations too high for this person or situation? What is more realistic?
- Am I blaming someone else for my problems?
- What can I do to take responsibility for my feelings and myself?

Improving Relationships

Substance use disorders affect entire families. Some relatives, usually spouses or children, assume the role of *enabler* or *codependent*. This term refers to a pattern of behavior, sometimes described as "controlling" or overly responsible, that relatives use in response to the stress and self-perpetuating crises associated with a client's substance problem. Enablers/codependents experience many self-defeating emotions and behaviors, such as feeling responsible for the problem, "walking on eggshells" around clients to avoid doing anything that might spur drinking or drug use, and assuming responsibilities that clients ignore or relinquish. Codependents function as rescuers, covering up and making excuses for clients. Because they protect clients from the full consequences of their behaviors, the net effect is to help perpetuate the addiction. Codependent relatives need attention from staff and counselors to learn to adjust to client sobriety to develop a less vigilant, more interdependent relationship. Nurses can recommend that family members begin their own recovery by attending support groups (eg, Al-Anon, Alateen). See Case Vignette 30.1.

Improving Self-Image

Each client enters recovery with a different personality and history. In most cases, clients' opinions of themselves are compromised because they no longer can hide from the devastation resulting from substance abuse and related problems. Guilt, shame, embarrassment, and despair are common early in recovery. Repairing damaged relationships, making amends

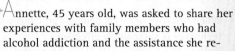

Case Vignette 30.1

Annette, 45 years old, was asked to share her experiences with family members who had alcohol addiction and the assistance she received from 12-step programs. This is her story:

Many years ago, to "save" my father from alcoholism, I was introduced to the 12 Steps of Alcoholics Anonymous through Al-Anon. In Al-Anon, I became conscious of my weaknesses and experienced the humility to accept that I was powerless over alcohol, that I could not save my father or make my husband well, whom I recognized was in the early stages of alcoholism.

The effects of alcoholism are pervasive; the entire family suffers. Because of my efforts to make things right, my continual failure to do so, my decreased view of myself following constant defeat, I became as sick as the alcoholic. My life was unmanageable. I decided to turn my will and life over to a Higher Power and in so doing embraced the 12 Steps.

Working the 12 Steps is not easy. It requires honesty and humility. It demands a commitment to grow, to stay on the journey no matter what. It necessitates trust that faithfulness will lead to wellness, and to the peace and joy that come when we accept the challenge to take responsibility, and to diligently work toward being the people we were created to be.

The wisdom of Al-Anon, along with the dynamic interaction that happens in the honest and caring environment of a support group, has helped give me the strength and courage to undergo a metamorphosis. Slowly I began to see that as we change, our situation changes. As we become integrated, we become more secure and loving and experience an inner harmony that affects all of our relationships. The family is the primary recipient of this blessed change.

There is more awareness than ever concerning alcoholism. What was once thought to be a disgrace is now known to be a disease of body, mind, and spirit. Tragically, my father died never knowing the serenity that can be found in Alcoholics Anonymous. Spiritually my husband was "reborn" and came to serenity through Alcoholics Anonymous. We have choices! Our choices make a difference.

Reflection and Critical Thinking

- What factors do you think contribute to the shame and stigma associated with substance use disorders?
- Commonly, people with parents who had alcohol problems develop similar problems themselves or become romantically involved with people struggling with addiction. What factors might contribute to this outcome?
- How can people who have struggled with addictions in their families help others? How can they stop the cycle in terms of future generations?

▲

to those who have been harmed, and maintaining sobriety are achievements that can help restore self-worth. Nurses can provide assistance by listening and communicating therapeutically, teaching communication and relationship skills, and encouraging ongoing participation in recovery programs.

Sources of poor self-images include negative self-talk and rumination (dwelling). Nurses can recommend the following strategies to help clients break these habits:

- When negative self-talk begins, consciously say, "Stop!" This technique is surprisingly effective.
- Replace the negative self-talk with positive, kind, optimistic statements.
- Set realistic goals for yourself and take pride in your achievements.
- Examine your values and beliefs and make your actions congruent with those values.
- Find personally rewarding activities.
- Volunteer your time to help others.
- Spend time with positive, healthy people; avoid people who can drag you down emotionally and spiritually.
- Participate in self-help groups.
- Don't compare yourself with others; you always will find someone who is better or worse off. Compare yourself with yourself instead.

An addiction occupies a major role in a substance abuser's life. It has been described as a "relationship." As destructive as such a relationship was, the client depended on it and may return to it for comfort. When the relationship is over, clients may feel relieved but also emotionally empty and spiritually bereft. Those caring for them must attend to these feelings of loss in the early stages of recovery and help establish new sources for emotional and spiritual connectedness.

AA addresses the spiritual aspect of recovery through its nondenominational reliance on a higher power, which each person defines differently and individually (see Chap. 7). Recovery programs that follow the 12-step model incorporate this concept. Nurses should recognize that clients recovering from substance use will experience spiritual distress. They can help by asking clients about their feelings, if they have relied on faith or spirituality in the past, and if they have someone with whom they can discuss spiritual issues. For clients who express a desire, nurses can also facilitate spiritual interventions that clients welcome (see Chap. 7). Listening attentively and using therapeutic communication techniques are invaluable tools when helping clients work through personal issues. Nurses also help clients explore culturally acceptable ways to feel connected.

Promoting Healthy Activities

Clients in recovery typically have devoted much time to their addiction. Substance use is integral to their existence and occupies most of their leisure time. In some cases, it also takes up work and family time. During treatment, clients may find themselves lonely, bored, idle, or conflicted about what to do with so much "free" time. They need to plan activities to minimize the temptation to revert to alcohol or drug use.

Nurses should encourage clients to develop health-promoting habits that can not only occupy time but also facilitate healing. Exercise programs, yoga, and meditation are examples. Clients can also resume pleasurable hobbies or pastimes that they once enjoyed before becoming addicted, or they may consciously develop new ones. Recommending attendance at 12-step meetings, particularly during times of the day formerly devoted to substance use, is integral to most recovery programs. Nurses should encourage clients to be aware of how boredom, loneliness, or past habits can be overwhelming triggers to resuming drinking or drug abuse and to plan accordingly.

▲ EVALUATION

Nurses evaluate the effectiveness of interventions using the following criteria:

- Has the client remained safe through substance withdrawal?
- Has the client refrained from using drugs, alcohol, or both?
- Has the client acknowledged his or her addiction and dependence?
- Does the client use healthy stress management techniques?
- Has the client identified alternative activities to drinking or taking drugs?
- Is the client participating in the treatment plan?

> **Checkpoint Questions**
> **10.** What is the priority when caring for the client experiencing withdrawal?
> **11.** What is the first step that the client with a substance dependence must make toward recovery?

IMPAIRED NURSES

With the pervasiveness of substance use disorders, it is not surprising that various health care workers themselves have problems. Nurses are no exception. An *impaired nurse* provides care while under the influence of substances affecting the CNS. Approximately 10% to 20% of nurses and nursing students have problems with substance abuse and addiction (Nauert, 2011).

Alcohol is the primary substance of abuse in nurses. Some nurses steal drugs from health care facilities; others legitimately obtain prescriptions for narcotic analgesics, minor tranquilizers, and hypnotics from physicians.

Possible indications of impairment include the following:

- Wearing long sleeves even in hot weather (to conceal needle marks)
- Weight loss

- Alcohol smell on the breath; frequent use of mints and mouthwash
- Deteriorating appearance and hygiene
- Unsteady gait
- Slurred speech
- Mood swings
- Forgetfulness or poor concentration
- Frequent absenteeism
- Illegible or incorrect charting
- Excessive medication errors

Many impaired nurses work for several years before any disciplinary action takes place. Peers may attribute unusual behaviors to stress or personal difficulties. Some coworkers choose to avoid conflict or fear lawsuits. Many nurses do not report impaired coworkers because of denial, lack of education, and professional stigma. Others keep silent for fear of the professional impact on the coworker's job (Esquibel, 2009). Ultimately, nurses need to report suspicions about colleagues to ensure client safety. Increasingly, state boards of nursing require nurses to report colleagues whom they suspect have substance use disorders. The first report should be to the impaired nurse's immediate supervisor, with as many documented facts as possible. All information must be kept confidential. Once the situation is investigated, the supervisor should share information with the suspected nurse in the presence of one witness. The intervention should be supportive and nonjudgmental. Research indicates additional need for educating nurses about addictive diseases, workplace policies on addiction and treatment, peer assistance programs, interventions, and referral options to help support nurses' recovery from addiction (Esquibel, 2009).

Many states now have *employee assistance programs* specifically for nurses that work with health agencies to confidentially treat impaired nurses and help them safely return to practice. After intensive treatment and ongoing attendance at support groups, a return to work can be negotiated. Probation can last for as long as 2 years. Recovering nurses are usually assigned to units without access to medications. They need to undergo random blood or urine drug screens.

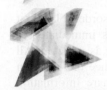

Reviewing and Applying Your Knowledge

Chapter Summary

- Substance use disorders include substance abuse and substance dependence. Substance abuse is taking alcohol or other drugs repeatedly so that functional problems result; however, it does not involve tolerance or withdrawal. Substance dependence is using alcohol or other drugs despite negative consequences, such as significant functional problems in daily living, with tolerance as substance use escalates and withdrawal when the drug of abuse is stopped.

- Substance abuse and dependence are among the most serious U.S. public health problems. Addictions to alcohol, marijuana, and prescription drugs continue to remain at steady levels. The use of methamphetamine, Rohypnol, GBH, inhalants, and anabolic steroids is growing.

- Substance use disorders are multidimensional and related strongly to neurophysiologic processes, with additional psychosocial and behavioral influences.

- The 12 categories of substance use disorders are alcohol, amphetamines, caffeine, cannabis, cocaine, hallucinogens, inhalants, nicotine, opioids, phencyclidines, sedative-hypnotics, and polysubstance abuse. All the categories may be subclassified as dependence, abuse, intoxication, and withdrawal.

- People with drug or alcohol dependence or abuse are impaired in multiple areas, including physically, socially, and psychologically, at some time during their disorder. Most cultures do not tolerate or accept associated behaviors. Signs and symptoms of abuse and dependence are specific to the drug used; however, functional impairment in several areas is a requisite for diagnosis.

- Many clients have co-occurring disorders—coexistence of a substance abuse disorder and a major psychiatric disorder.

- Interdisciplinary treatment of the client with a substance abuse disorder is critical to successful recovery. The two main components involve detoxification and rehabilitation. Various interdisciplinary programs include inpatient rehabilitation, outpatient programs, and private practice physician treatment. In addition, a wide network of 12-step treatment programs led by lay or peers and paraprofessionals exists throughout the world. These programs include AA, Al-Anon, ACOA, CA, and NA.

- Nurses play a critical role in the treatment and management of clients with substance abuse. Major issues include (1) managing withdrawal and maintaining safety,

(2) breaking through denial, (3) managing anxiety, (4) ¡teaching effective coping strategies, (5) improving family processes, (6) improving self-image, and (7) promoting healthy activities. Frequent reevaluation and assessment, with appropriate changes in care, are necessary to enhance treatment and ensure that clients successfully move toward healthier lifestyles that are free of substances of abuse.

- Chemical impairment in nurses is an all-too-common problem. Nurses are responsible for reporting suspected cases of impairment in colleagues to protect client safety.

Study Questions

1. When assessing a client, which of the following findings would alert the nurse to possible opiate abuse?

   a. Constricted pupils

   b. Liver disease

   c. Reddened eyes

   d. Reports of flashbacks

2. When interviewing a client with alcohol dependence, the nurse asks if she has ever experienced blackouts. The client asks the nurse to explain what blackouts are. Which of the following would the nurse use when describing blackouts to the client?

   a. Denying the unpleasant aspects and remembering only the pleasant experiences of drinking

   b. Being unable to perform work requiring concentration

   c. Having permanent amnesia for events that occurred while intoxicated

   d. Being unconscious from an overdose of alcohol

3. A client states that he snorts cocaine several times a day, spends all his money on obtaining the cocaine, and has been arrested once for threatening, abusive behavior. Which of the following would the nurse suspect?

   a. Substance withdrawal

   b. Withdrawal delirium

   c. Substance dependence

   d. Polysubstance abuse

4. The nurse would expect the physician to order which medication for a client undergoing withdrawal from narcotics?

   a. Barbiturates

   b. Anxiolytics

   c. Opiate-type drugs

   d. Anticonvulsants

5. When completing the initial interview of a client being admitted for detoxification, which of the following areas would be most crucial to assess?

   a. Reason for admission

   b. A complete physical history

   c. Type of drugs used

   d. Family history

Critical Thinking Questions

1. What information would you give to people who insist that addiction is simply a character flaw or a sign of weakness or stupidity? What measures can nurses take to better explain the cycle of substance dependency and to implement preventive and therapeutic community-oriented strategies against it?

2. What would be immediate priorities in planning care for a client admitted to an inpatient treatment facility for alcoholism? For opiate addiction?

3. Consider Erica and Paul from Case in Point 30.1. Discuss the possible longitudinal course of Erica's illness. How could a nurse work with this family to assist them to maintain optimal functioning, even during times of relapse?

References

American Psychiatric Association (APA). (2000). *Diagnostic and statistical manual of mental disorders* (4th ed., text rev.). Washington, DC: Author.

American Society of Addiction Medicine. (2007). *ASAM patient placement criteria for the treatment of substance-related disorders* (2nd ed.). Philadelphia, PA: Lippincott Williams & Wilkins.

Anton, R. (2010). Substance abuse is a disease of the human brain: Focus on alcohol. *Journal of Law, Medicine & Ethics, 38*, 735–744. doi:10.1111/j.1748-720X.2010.00527.x

Bello, E. P., Mateo Y., Gelman, D. M., Noain, D., Shin, J. H., Low, M. J., ... Rubinstein, M. (2011). Cocaine supersensitivity and enhanced motivation for reward in mice lacking dopamine D2 autoreceptors. *Nature Neuroscience*. Retrieved from http://www.niaaa.nih.gov/NewsEvents/NewsReleases/Pages/receptor_limits_rewarding_effects.aspx

Bulechek, G. M., Butcher, H. K., & McCloskey Dochterman, J. (2008). *Nursing interventions classification (NIC)* (5th ed.). St. Louis, MO: Mosby.

Caetano, R., Ramissety-Mikler, S., Floyd, L. R., & McGrath, C. (2006). The epidemiology of drinking among women of childbearing age. *Alcoholism: Clinical and Experimental Research, 30*(6), 1023–1030.

Castro, F. G., & Alarcon, E. H. (2002). Integrating cultural variables into drug abuse prevention and treatment with racial/ethnic minorities. *Journal of Drug Issues, 32*, 783–810.

Center for Substance Abuse Treatment (CSAT). (2006). *Detoxification and substance abuse treatment* (Treatment Improvement Protocol Series 45; USDHHS Publication No. SMA06-4131). Rockville, MD: Substance Abuse and Mental Health Services Administration. Retrieved from http://www.ncbi.nlm.nih.gov/books/NBK14497

Center for Substance Abuse Treatment (CSAT). (2009). *Buprenorphine: A guide for nurses* (USDHHS Pub. No. SMA09-4376). Rockville, MD: Substance Abuse and Mental Health Services Administration. Retrieved from http://buprenorphine.samhsa.gov/TAP_30_Certified.pdf

Centers for Disease Control and Prevention. (2010). *Alcohol use in pregnancy.* Retrieved from http://www.cdc.gov/ncbddd/fasd/alcohol-use.html

Compton, P. (2002). Caring for an alcohol-dependent patient. *Nursing, 32*, 58–63.

Drug Abuse Warning Network (DAWN of SAMHSA). (2005). *National estimates of drug-related emergency department visits.* Retrieved from http://www.oas.samhsa.gov/DAWN/2k5ed.cfm

Esquibel, K. S. (2009). *Registered nurses' perceptions of working with chemically impaired registered nurse colleagues.* Available from ProQuest Dissertations and Theses database. (UMI Number: 3360070)

Glasser, I. (2003). Bringing SA treatment to the homeless. *DATA: Brown University Digest of Addiction Theory and Application, 22*(8), 8.

Hart, K. E., & McGarragle, O. (2010). Perceived social support from counselors and client sobriety during aftercare: A pilot study of emotional and functional support. *Alcoholism Treatment Quarterly, 28*, 198–229. doi:10.1080/07347321003648216

Heather, N. (2010). Breaking new ground in the study and practice of alcohol brief interventions. *Drug & Alcohol Review, 2010, 29*, 584–588.

Hendler, R. A., Ramchandani, V. A., Gilman, J., & Hommer, D. W. (2011). Stimulant and sedative effects of alcohol. *Current Topics in Behavioral Neuroscience.* doi:10.1007/7854_2011_135

Kilpatrick, D. G, Koenen, K. C., Ruggiero, K. J., Acierno, R., Galea, S., Resnick, H. S., et al. (2007). The serotonin transporter genotype and social support and moderation of posttraumatic stress disorder in hurricane-exposed adults. *American Journal of Psychiatry, 164*, 1693–1699. doi:10.1176/appi.ajp.2007.06122007

Lee, E., & Mock, M. (2005). Asian families: An overview. In M. McGoldrick, J. Giodano, & J. Garcia-Preto (Eds.), *Ethnicity and family therapy* (3rd ed., pp. 269–289). New York, NY: Guilford Press.

Mann, R. E., Smart, R. G., & Govoni, R. (2004). *The epidemiology of alcoholic liver disease.* Retrieved May 4, 2007, from http://pubs.niaaa.nih.gov/publications/arh27-3/209-219.htm

Mohatt, G. V., Rasmus, S. M., Thomas, L., Allen, J., Hazel, K., & Marlatt, G. A. (2008). Risk, resilience, and natural recovery: A model of recovery from alcohol abuse for Alaska Natives. *Addiction, 103*, 205–215.

Moorhead, S., Johnson, M., Maas, M. L., & Swanson, E. (2008). *Nursing outcomes classification (NOC)* (4th ed.). St. Louis, MO: Mosby.

NANDA International. (2009). *NANDA International nursing diagnoses: Definitions and classification, 2009–2011.* Philadelphia, PA: Wiley-Blackwell.

Narconon International. (2010). *Signs and symptoms of drug use.* Retrieved from http://www.narconon.org/drug-abuse/signs-symptoms-of-drug-abuse.html

National Institute of Mental Health. (2006). *Mental health statistics.* Rockville, MD: Office of Consumer, Family and Public Information, Center for Mental Health Services.

National Institute on Alcohol Abuse and Alcoholism (NIAAA). (2005). *Alcoholic liver disease.* Retrieved from http://pubs.niaaa.nih.gov/publications/aa64/aa64.htm

National Institute on Alcohol Abuse and Alcoholism (NIAAA). (2006a). *National epidemiologic survey on alcohol and related conditions.* Retrieved from http://pubs.niaaa.nih.gov/publications/arh29-2/toc29-2.htm

National Institute on Alcohol Abuse and Alcoholism (NIAAA). (2006b). *Young adult drinking.* Retrieved from http://pubs.niaaa.nih.gov/publications/aa68/aa68.htm

National Institute on Alcohol Abuse and Alcoholism (NIAAA). (2008). *Alcohol and other drugs.* Retrieved from http://pubs.niaaa.nih.gov/publications/AA76/AA76.htm

National Institute on Alcohol Abuse and Alcoholism (NIAAA). (2009). *A developmental perspective on underage alcohol use.* Retrieved from http://pubs.niaaa.nih.gov/publications/AA78/AA78.htm

National Institute on Alcohol Abuse and Alcoholism (NIAAA). (2010a). *NIAAA: 40 years of research leadership.* Retrieved from http://pubs.niaaa.nih.gov/publications/AA79/AA79.htm

National Institute on Alcohol Abuse and Alcoholism (NIAAA). (2010b). *Rethinking drinking; Alcohol and your health: What are the risks?* Retrieved from http://rethinkingdrinking.niaaa.nih.gov/WhatsTheHarm/WhatAreTheRisks.asp

National Institute on Alcohol Abuse and Alcoholism (NIAAA). (2011). *Gene variants predict treatment success for alcoholism medication.* Retrieved from http://www.niaaa.nih.gov/NewsEvents/NewsReleases/Pages/Genevariantspredicttreatmentsuccessforalcoholismmedication.aspx

National Institute on Drug Abuse (NIDA). (2003a). *Drug abuse and AIDS.* Retrieved July 18, 2007, from http://www.drugabuse.gov/Infofax/DrugAbuse.html

National Institute on Drug Abuse (NIDA). (2003b). *Drug use among racial/ethnic minorities.* Retrieved from http://archives.drugabuse.gov/pdf/minorities03.pdf

National Institute on Drug Abuse (NIDA). (2010a). *Commonly abused drugs.* Retrieved from http://www.nida.nih.gov/DrugPages/DrugsofAbuse.html

National Institute on Drug Abuse (NIDA). (2010b). *Comorbidity: Addiction and other mental disorders.* Retrieved from http://www.drugabuse.gov/PDF/RRComorbidity.pdf

National Institute on Drug Abuse (NIDA). (2011a). *NIDA InfoFacts: Comorbidity: Addiction and other mental disorders.* Retrieved from http://www.nida.nih.gov/infofacts/comorbidity.html

National Institute on Drug Abuse (NIDA). (2011b). *NIDA InfoFacts: Drug related hospital emergency room visits.* Retrieved from http://www.nida.nih.gov/infofacts/hospitalvisits.html

National Institute on Drug Abuse (NIDA). (2011c). *NIDA InfoFacts: Nationwide trends.* Retrieved from http://www.nida.nih.gov/infofacts/nationtrends.html

Nauert, R. (2011, January 27). New approach addresses substance abuse among nurses. *Psych Central.* Retrieved from http://psychcentral.com/news/2011/01/27/new-approach-addresses-substance-abuse-among-nurses/22967.html

Office of Applied Studies. (2008). *Results from the 2005 National Survey on Drug Use and Health: National findings.* Retrieved from http://www.oas.samhsa.gov/NSDUH/2k5NSDUH/2k5results.htm#8.1.4

Pagano, M. E., Zetlner, B. B., Jaber, J., Post, S. G., Zywiak, W. H., & Stout, R. L. (2009). Helping others and long-term sobriety: Who should I help to stay sober? *Alcoholism Treatment Quarterly, 27,* 38–50.

Ries, R. K., Miller, S. C., Fiellin, D. A., & Saitz, R. (2009). *Principles of addiction medicine* (4th ed.). Philadelphia, PA: Lippincott Williams & Wilkins.

Sadock, B. J., & Sadock, V. A. (2008). *Kaplan & Sadock's synopsis of psychiatry: Behavioral sciences/clinical psychiatry* (10th ed.). Philadelphia, PA: Lippincott Williams & Wilkins.

Substance Abuse and Mental Health Services Administration (SAMHSA). (2008). *The NSDUH report: Pregnancy and substance use.* Retrieved from http://www.oas.samhsa.gov/2k3/pregnancy/pregnancy.cfm

Substance Abuse and Mental Health Services Administration (SAMSHA). (2010a). *The NSDUH report: HIV/AIDS and substance use.* Retrieved from http://oas.samhsa.gov/2k10/210/HIV-AIDS.htm

Substance Abuse and Mental Health Services Administration (SAMSHA). (2010b). *Results from the 2009 National Survey on Drug Use and Health: Volume I. Summary of national findings* (NSDUH Series H-38A, HHS Publication No. SMA 10-4856 Findings). Retrieved from http://oas.samhsa.gov/NSDUH/2k9NSDUH/2k9Results.htm#Ch2

Talawalker, J. A., & Kamath, P. S. (2005). Influence of recent advances in medical management on clinical outcomes of cirrhosis. *Mayo Clinic Proceedings, 80,* 1501–1508.

Thompson, W., & Lande, R. G. (2007). *Alcoholism.* Retrieved from http://www.emedicine.com/med/topic98.htm

Tiet, Q. Q., & Mausbach, B. (2007). Treatments for patients with dual diagnosis: A review. *Alcoholism: Clinical and Experimental Research, 31*(4), 513–536.

Trafton, J. A., Tracy, S. W., Oliva, E. M., & Humphreys, K. (2007). Different components of opioid-substitution treatment predict outcomes of patients with and without a parent with substance-use problems. *Journal of Studies on Alcohol and Drugs, 68*(2), 165–172.

Weaver, G. D., Turner, N. H., & O'Dell, K. J. (2000). Depressive symptoms, stress, and coping among women recovering from addiction. *Journal of Substance Abuse and Treatment, 18*(2), 161–167.

Winter, L. A. (2001). Personality and the use of coping resources in addicted populations. *Dissertation Abstracts International. Section B: The Sciences & Engineering, 61*(11B), 6155.

Yu, J., Clark, L. P., Chandra, L., Dias, A., & Lai, T. F. (2009). Reducing cultural barriers to substance abuse treatment among Asian Americans: A case study in New York City. *Journal of Substance Abuse Treatment 37,* 398–406. doi:10.1016/j.jsat.2009.05.006

Web Resources

American Academy of Addiction Psychiatry: http://www.aaap.org
American Society of Addiction Medicine: http://www.asam.org
Drug Enforcement Administration (DEA): http://www.usdoj.gov/dea/concern/concern.htm
National Council on Alcoholism and Drug Dependence: http://www.ncadd.org

National Institute on Alcohol Abuse and Alcoholism: http://www
.niaaa.nih.gov

National Institute on Drug Abuse: http://www.nida.nih.gov

Substance Abuse and Mental Health Services Administration: http://
www.samhsa.gov

The National Survey on Drug Use and Health (issued through SAM-
HSA), full report: http://www.drugabusestatistics.samhsa.gov/
nsduh.htm

Highlights of the DAWN report (issued through SAMHSA), full
report: https://dawninfo.samhsa.gov/default.asp

For an overview and tools to assess drinking patterns: http://www
.rethinkingdrinking.niaaa.nih.gov/Treatment improvement
protocols (through SAMHSA/CSAT): http://www.ncbi.nlm.nih
.gov/books/NBK14119/

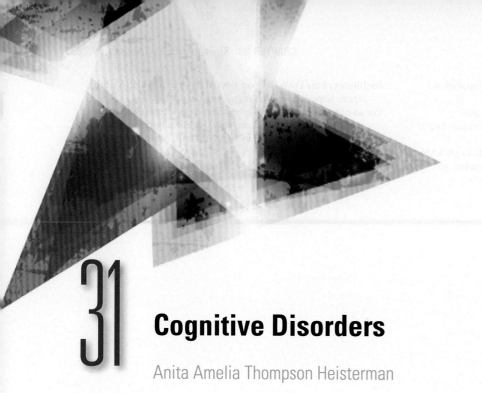

31

Cognitive Disorders

Anita Amelia Thompson Heisterman

LEARNING OBJECTIVES

On completion of this chapter, you should be able to accomplish the following:

- Define the term *cognitive mental disorder*.
- Discuss the incidence and significance of cognitive disorders.
- Identify clinical features or behaviors associated with cognitive disorders.
- Compare possible etiologies of various cognitive disorders, especially Alzheimer's disease.
- Explain the continuum of care and interdisciplinary treatment/management for clients and families dealing with cognitive disorders.
- Discuss common interventions for cognitive disorders.
- Apply the steps of the nursing process to care for clients with cognitive disorders.

Cognitive mental disorders are characterized by a disruption of or deficit in cognitive function, which encompasses orientation, attention, memory, vocabulary, calculation ability, and abstract thinking (see Chap. 10). Specific categories delineated by the American Psychiatric Association (APA, 2000) include the following:

1. Delirium, dementia, and amnestic and other cognitive disorders
2. Mental disorders resulting from a general medical condition (see Chap. 39)
3. Substance-related disorders (see Chap. 30)

This chapter focuses on delirium and dementia. Amnestic disorders are covered briefly, in line with their classification in the *Diagnostic and Statistical Manual of Mental Disorders,* 4th ed., text revision (*DSM-IV-TR*; APA, 2000).

ETIOLOGIC AND DIAGNOSTIC CHALLENGES OF COGNITIVE DISORDERS

Delirium usually results from an acute disruption in the homeostasis of the brain. Once the cause of disruption is eliminated or subsides, related cognitive deficits generally resolve in a few days to weeks. In contrast, *dementia* results from primary brain pathology that usually is irreversible, chronic, and progressive. Prognosis with dementia depends on whether a cause can be identified and reversed. For example, prompt oxygen treatment for dementia stemming from hypoxia can prevent further damage. A comparison of the characteristics of delirium versus dementia is shown in Table 31.1.

With most cognitive disorders, the brain is temporarily or permanently compromised. Usual consequences include disturbed perceptions, delusions, paranoia, and aggressive and disruptive behaviors. Clients may sense that their thinking is impaired and become frustrated, anxious, frightened, and distraught. High emotion may compound an already disordered state.

Most cognitive disturbances belong to one of the following categories:

- Primary brain disease
- Response of the brain to systemic (eg, metabolic, cardiovascular) disturbance
- Unique reaction of brain tissue to an exogenous substance
- Residual effects of or withdrawal from an exogenous substance (APA, 2000)

Many illnesses and medications can impair cognition. Any physical illness may present initially with neurologic symptoms, behavioral manifestations, or both. Thus, cognitive disorders may be difficult to diagnose and involve multiple visits to several practitioners, extensive laboratory and diagnostic tests, and many examinations over an extended period. Such intensive care usually is necessary to establish

TABLE 31.1 **Delirium Versus Dementia**

Characteristic	Delirium	Dementia
Onset	Rapid development	Gradual and insidious development
Duration	Brief duration of 1 month or less, depending on cause	Long, with progressive deterioration
Course	Diurnal alterations, more nocturnal exacerbations	Stable progression of symptomatology
Thinking and short-term memory	Disorganized and impaired	Short-term and long-term memory impairments, with eventual complete loss
Orientation	Markedly decreased, especially to environmental cues	Progressively decreases
Language	Rambling, pressured, irrelevant	Difficulty recalling the correct word; later may lose language
Perceptual disturbance	Environment unclear, progressing to illusions, hallucinations, and delusions	Often absent but can progress to paranoia, delusions, hallucinations, and illusions
Level of consciousness	Cloudiness that fluctuates; inattentiveness to hyperalert with distractibility	Not affected
Sleep	Day–night reversal, insomnia, vivid dreams and nightmares	May develop day–night reversal in later stages
Psychomotor actions	Sluggish to hyperactive; change of range unpredictable	Not affected initially, late in illness, restlessness with pacing
Emotional status	Anxious with changes in sleep; fearful if experiencing hallucinations; weeping; yelling	Depression/anxiety when insight into condition is present; late in pathology, anger with outbursts

what is causing or contributing to the cognitive decline so that health care providers can initiate appropriate treatment or management. Failure to treat a reversible condition may cause further damage, functional decline, or death.

Another complication is that multiple factors may underlie the clinical presentation of a cognitive disorder. For example, the same client may have Alzheimer's disease (dementia) and acute intoxication from overmedication (delirium). Or a client with the chronic problem of vascular dementia may experience delirium while hospitalized with pneumonia. Dementia itself is a risk factor for delirium. "*Cognitive decline* is not only a predisposing factor for delirium, but it has also been shown that delirium independently worsens cognitive function" in the following year (Leentjens & van der Mast, 2005). Thus, connecting the correct etiology and symptoms can challenge the most capable clinicians. As a practice standard, any change from the client's baseline functioning is a clue to investigate causes beyond the primary diagnosis.

DELIRIUM

Delirium is characterized by rapid onset of cognitive dysfunction and disrupted consciousness. It also is referred to as *intensive care unit psychosis, acute brain syndrome, acute confusion,* and *acute toxic psychosis.*

Incidence and Prevalence

Growing rates of delirium mirror the increasing older adult population and are expected to continue to rise. Delirium is the most common psychiatric syndrome in general hospitals, occurring in as many as 54% of elderly inpatients (Lin et al., 2010). It is associated with significantly increased morbidity and mortality both during and after hospitalization (Balas et al., 2007; McAvay et al., 2006; Rigney, 2006). Approximately 30% to 40% of clients older than 65 years experience delirium while hospitalized for a medical condition; another 10% to 15% have delirium on admission (Sadock & Sadock, 2007). Han et al. (2010) found that 76% of delirium clients presenting in the emergency department were not recognized as delirious, and dementia in 15 of 16 admitted clients remained unrecognized by hospital physicians. The prevalence of repeated episodes of acute confusion in nursing homes for those older than 75 years is 60%; more than 80% of clients with terminal illnesses experience delirium-related cognitive impairment (Sadock & Sadock, 2007).

Delirium related to surgery is common among all age groups. Estimates are that 30% of clients in surgical intensive care units, 40% to 50% of clients recovering from hip surgery, and more than 50% of postcardiotomy clients experience delirium (Sadock & Sadock, 2007).

Etiology

Any process, disorder, or agent that disrupts the integrity of the central nervous system (CNS) and diffusely impairs its cellular functioning can induce delirium (Box 31.1).

Researchers have postulated numerous risk factors: aging, postoperative status, metabolic disorders, drug withdrawal, and toxicity secondary to drugs or other exogenous substances.

Older adults are at significant risk for delirium, particularly those with preexisting cognitive impairment and postoperative clients. With aging, the neurologic system becomes more vulnerable to insults caused by underlying systemic conditions. Indeed, delirium often predicts or accompanies physical illness in older adults (Cole, 2004). This population also is at risk because of the number of medications (over-the-counter and prescription) many of them use (Figure 31.1). Medications, particularly those that exert effects on the CNS, are frequent causes of delirium (Gurwitz et al., 2003).

Any disturbance in any organ or system can disrupt overall metabolism and neurotransmission, leading to cognitive decline. Infections and fluid and electrolyte imbalances are common examples. Not surprisingly, medications are the primary exogenous offenders, especially in older adults. Often, an interplay of several factors leads to delirium (Foreman et al., 2003).

Checkpoint Questions
1. How does delirium differ from dementia?
2. What is a frequent cause of delirium in older adults?

Signs and Symptoms/Diagnostic Criteria

Clinical pictures of delirium vary. Nevertheless, the three salient features that comprise the main diagnostic criteria are (1) disordered cognition, (2) attention deficit, and (3) disturbed consciousness (*DSM-IV-TR* Box 31.1).

In delirium, *cognition* becomes disorganized. Clients appear confused and cannot reason, handle complex tasks, or problem solve. Associated speech may be pressured, rambling, bizarre, incoherent, or nearly absent. Impaired orientation and spatial ability may cause clients to confuse reality with imagery and dreams. Suspiciousness and persecutory delusions are common (Sadock & Sadock, 2007).

Clients may experience disturbed perceptions. Hallucinations usually are graphic and can induce anxiety verging on panic. Agitated clients can become combative to elude perceived threats. Mood alterations can lead to great lability, from irritability and dysphoria to euphoria (Sadock & Sadock, 2007).

Memory, particularly short term, becomes impaired. Another feature is an inability to focus or shift attention. Clients may have trouble attending to environmental stimuli. Attention problems usually are more pronounced at night. Clients may be disoriented to time, place, and person (Sadock & Sadock, 2007). In severe cases, they mistake the unfamiliar for the familiar. For example, they may identify and subsequently call health care providers by the names of siblings, spouses, or children.

BOX 31.1 Specific Causes of Delirium

Primary Brain Disease

- Head injury: concussion, contusion, hemorrhage, vascular obstruction
- Tumors

Systemic Diseases Secondarily Disrupting Brain Homeostasis

- Acid–base imbalance
- Cancer
- Cerebrovascular accident
- Dehydration
- Endocrine disorders: diabetes (hypoglycemia), hypothyroidism, or hyperthyroidism
- Epilepsy
- Fever from any cause
- Hypokalemia
- Hypoperfusion of the brain: myocardial infarction, dysrhythmia, congestive heart failure, vascular hypotension
- Hypoproteinemia
- Hypotension with cerebral ischemia
- Hypothermia or hyperthermia
- Hypoxia producing chronic obstructive pulmonary disease, anemia, gastrointestinal bleeding
- Infections: bacteremia, septicemia, urinary tract infection, upper respiratory infection
- Malnutrition
- Organ failure: hepatic, renal, pulmonary
- Postoperative state
- Sodium depletion
- Trauma: burns, hip fracture

- Uremia
- Vitamin deficiencies

Withdrawal of Exogenous Substances of Abuse

- Alcohol
- Barbiturates
- Sedative-hypnotics
- Tranquilizers

Brain Toxic Exogenous Substances

- Anticholinergic drugs
- Antidepressants: amitriptyline, doxepin
- Antidiarrheal agents: diphenoxylate
- Antidysrhythmic drugs: lidocaine, amiodarone, propranolol, digitalis
- Antihistamines
- Antihypertensives: methyldopa
- Antimicrobials
- Antiparkinsonian agents
- Antipsychotics: chlorpromazine, thioridazine
- Cimetidine
- Corticosteroids
- Digitalis glycosides
- Diuretics
- Narcotic analgesics: meperidine, pentazocine
- Neuroleptics
- Nonsteroidal anti-inflammatory agents: indomethacin
- Over-the-counter cold and cough medications
- Psychiatric medications: diazepam, flurazepam, tricyclic antidepressants, benzodiazepines
- Xanthines: caffeine, theophylline

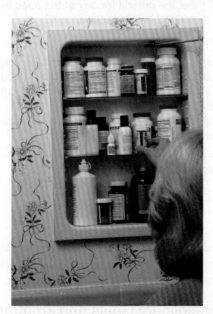

FIGURE 31.1 Older adults and other clients who use multiple medications are at risk for experiencing delirium. The confusion can develop as a side effect, an adverse reaction, an interaction among drugs or with foods or other substances, or as an idiosyncratic response.

Additional features of delirium include reduced consciousness, disrupted sleep–wake cycles, and abnormal psychomotor behaviors. Clients may fluctuate between alertness and somnolence. They may be drowsy during the day and nap sporadically at night, becoming extremely agitated on awakening (Sadock & Sadock, 2007). Psychomotor activity may range from hypoalert and hypoactive (typical of metabolic dysfunction) to hyperalert and hyperactive (common with drug withdrawal), to any combination. Hypoalert, hypoactive clients show minimal activity, appear stuporous, and are slow to respond. Others may mistakenly perceive them to have depression, missing the signs of delirium (Fick et al., 2007). Hyperalert, hyperactive clients are animated to the point of agitation and frequently have loud and pressured speech. They may remove intravenous (IV) lines and other tubes, "pick" at the air or sheets, or try (often successfully) to climb over side rails or the ends of beds. In addition, they often exhibit the classic, autonomic responses of dilated pupils, elevated pulse, and diaphoresis. See Case Vignette 31.1.

Implications and Prognosis

Delirium indicates an underlying medical problem and should be considered an urgent condition. Prognosis for

DSM-IV-TR BOX 31.1

Delirium

Delirium Due to a General Medical Condition

A. Disturbance of consciousness (ie, reduced clarity of awareness of the environment) with reduced ability to focus, sustain, or shift attention.

B. A change in cognition (such as memory deficit, disorientation, language disturbance) or the development of a perceptual disturbance that is not better accounted for by a preexisting, established, or evolving dementia.

C. The disturbance develops over a short period of time (usually hours to days) and tends to fluctuate during the course of the day.

D. There is evidence from the history, physical examination, or laboratory findings that the disturbance is caused by the direct physiological consequences of a general medical condition.

Substance-Withdrawal Delirium

A. Disturbance of consciousness (ie, reduced clarity of awareness of the environment) with reduced ability to focus, sustain, or shift attention.

B. A change in cognition (such as memory deficit, disorientation, language disturbance) or the development of a perceptual disturbance that is not better accounted for by a preexisting, established, or evolving dementia.

C. The disturbance develops over a short period of time (usually hours to days) and tends to fluctuate during the course of the day.

D. There is evidence from the history, physical examination, or laboratory findings that the symptoms in Criteria A and B developed during, or shortly after, a withdrawal syndrome.

Substance-Intoxication Delirium

A. Disturbance of consciousness (ie, reduced clarity of awareness of the environment) with reduced ability to focus, sustain, or shift attention.

B. A change in cognition (such as memory deficit, disorientation, language disturbance) or the development of a perceptual disturbance that is not better accounted for by a preexisting, established, or evolving dementia.

C. The disturbance develops over a short period of time (usually hours to days) and tends to fluctuate during the course of the day.

D. There is evidence from the history, physical examination, or laboratory findings of either (1) or (2):
1. the symptoms in Criteria A and B developed during substance intoxication
2. medication use is etiologically related to the disturbance

Delirium Due to Multiple Etiologies

A. Disturbance of consciousness (ie, reduced clarity of awareness of the environment) with reduced ability to focus, sustain, or shift attention.

B. A change in cognition (such as memory deficit, disorientation, language disturbance) or the development of a perceptual disturbance that is not better accounted for by a preexisting, established, or evolving dementia.

C. The disturbance develops over a short period of time (usually hours to days) and tends to fluctuate during the course of the day.

D. There is evidence from the history, physical examination, or laboratory findings that the delirium has more than one etiology (eg, more than one etiological general medical condition, a general medical condition plus substance intoxication or medication side effect).

Delirium Not Otherwise Specified

This category should be used to diagnose a delirium that does not meet the criteria for any of the specific types of delirium described in this section.

Examples include:

1. A clinical presentation of delirium that is suspected to be due to a general medical condition or substance use but for which there is insufficient evidence to establish a specific etiology.
2. Delirium due to causes not listed in this section (eg, sensory deprivation)

Reprinted with permission from the *Diagnostic and Statistical Manual of Mental Disorders, Fourth Edition, Text Revision* (Copyright (c) 2000). American Psychiatric Association.

recovery is good if the cause is recognized and managed promptly. With early identification and treatment, delirium usually lasts 3 to 5 days but may continue (rarely) for as long as 3 weeks. Bond and Neelon (2008) found that "in samples of hospitalized older medical surgical patients, delirium symptoms persisted at discharge and for up to 12 months." They further report that when delirium persists, it "results in longer hospitalization, institutional placement, rehospitalization, higher costs, impaired recovery, functional and cognitive decline, shorter life expectancy, and increased mortality." Failure to reverse the underlying cause may result in irreversible brain damage or death.

Interdisciplinary Goals and Treatment

Interdisciplinary goals are to identify clients at risk for delirium, recognize early signs, and quickly institute measures to correct underlying causes. In addition to early diagnosis and prompt treatment, therapeutic goals include managing acute

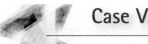

Case Vignette 31.1

Meredith, 75 years old and frail, is admitted to the hospital with a hip fracture resulting from a fall. She undergoes surgery on a general unit to repair the hip. Postoperatively, she initially appears alert and oriented, although she is in pain. She is receiving intravenous fluids and has an indwelling urinary catheter, both of which are to be discontinued in the morning.

The evening of the first postoperative day, Meredith tells the nurse that bugs are on the walls and that she wants to leave "this place." Upon further questioning, Meredith becomes mildly agitated and tells the nurse to "get out!" The nurse notifies the physician of the change in Meredith's mental status.

The physician orders computed tomography (CT) scanning to rule out a possible brain injury sustained in the initial fall. He also orders chest radiography and a urine culture. Results of the CT scan and chest radiography are normal; however, the urine culture reveals a urinary tract infection. The physician prescribes antibiotics to treat it and haloperidol, as needed, for the agitation.

Reflection and Critical Thinking

- What risk factors did Meredith have for experiencing delirium?
- How is Meredith's experience consistent with the etiology and clinical features of delirium? Could anything have been done to prevent this episode?

▲

confusion to maximize cognitive function, avoid injury, and prevent further decline.

Medical Interventions

Medical interventions focus on the underlying cause and thus vary. In cases of hypoperfusion or cerebral hypoxia, supplemental oxygen may significantly improve symptoms of delirium. Similarly, withdrawing medications or giving antibiotics for infections may lead to improvement.

Environmental Interventions

Team members must avoid use of physical and chemical restraints as much as possible. When these measures are absolutely necessary, they require utmost caution. The impetus for chemical or physical restraint clearly must be to protect clients from harm. Indeed, any type of restraint is a risk factor for, and may compound, delirium.

The team structures the environment to ensure safety as well as to maximize cognitive abilities and psychological comfort for clients. A fine balance exists between overstimulation and understimulation. Tailoring the environment to enhance the client's cognitive capability is essential. Providing a private room is beneficial, so that staff can minimize noxious and confusing environmental stimuli and maximize the services of supportive family or staff who can continually

remain with clients. However, the health care team cannot completely extinguish stimuli. Doing so may cause clients to withdraw and focus internally. Television often inundates clients with confusing sensory input, whereas soft music provides appropriate stimulation. Adequate lighting during the day and evening promotes realistic environmental perceptions. Clients should use any sensory aids (eg, glasses, hearing aids) that they normally require.

Client safety during episodes of delirium must not be compromised. Staff must be alerted if clients are at risk for wandering or leaving the premises. The propensity of clients with delirium to pull tubes, climb over side rails, or fall may require staff to institute one-on-one observation or encourage relatives to stay with clients at all times (Figure 31.2). Consistency from staff in terms of assignments and unhurried, daily routines is helpful, as are continuous visits by loved ones. Encouraging relatives to bring familiar objects from home (eg, personal effects, photographs) can increase the comfort level of clients with their current environment.

Cognitive and Psychosocial Interventions

Staff members can try to direct activity and cognitive focus by reorienting clients to the environment with calendars, clocks, and seasonal decorations. Ongoing interactions with clients are important. Therapeutic communication about the day's activities, repetition of explanations for the hospitalization, and reassurance that any hallucinations and delusions are part of the *transient* condition of delirium are helpful to clients.

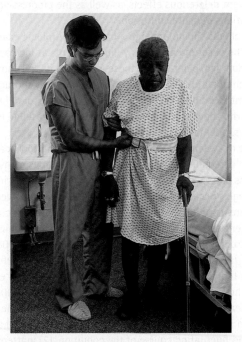

FIGURE 31.2 Clients with delirium may require one-on-one observation from a health care provider or relative to maintain their safety and prevent falls, aggressive behavior, or other negative consequences.

Clear and concise explanations for interventions also help to allay anxiety and promote orientation. Empathetic expressions of concern can ease clients' and relatives' fears. They also help to address the delirious symptoms of impaired memory and emotional problems. It is better to express empathy and choose interventions that allay anxiety than to be confrontational and, for instance, dispute possible delusions.

Team members must keep families informed and included in treatment plans. Relatives need to understand the biologic basis for the behavior that they witness in their loved ones. Helping them to understand the difference between delirium and dementia can be reassuring. Staff also should encourage relatives to join in efforts to reorient clients.

Checkpoint Questions

3. What are the components of cognition?
4. For approximately how long does delirium typically last?

APPLYING THE NURSING PROCESS

Delirium

▲ ASSESSMENT

Early assessment of acute confusion is essential nursing care for all hospitalized clients, particularly older adults. Nurses are in an ideal position to detect delirium. Prompt recognition and subsequent identification and treatment of underlying causes can prevent deleterious effects, as well as the progression and ramifications of acute confusion.

All clients should undergo a baseline neurologic examination at the onset of care for any illness. Clients at increased risk for delirium (eg, older adults, those with head injury) should have mental status examinations (MSEs) routinely throughout treatment (see Chap. 10). Nurses should evaluate for delirium in clients who show subtle or overt changes from baseline in mental status, orientation, or level of consciousness.

Use of systematic assessment and screening tools can enhance detection and management. Dementia has many dimensions and its symptoms wax and wane, particularly in the early stages. Because they are able to observe clients over time, nurses are in an ideal situation to provide more than a cursory assessment and make more in-depth evaluations on which to construct a meaningful plan of care (Devlin et al., 2008). The Delirium Observation Screening Scale (DOS) is a useful 25-item tool based on *DSM-IV-TR* criteria (Schuurmans et al., 2003). The Registered Nurses Association of Ontario (2003) has recommended the widely used Confusion Assessment Method (CAM) in its practice guidelines. The CAM focuses on (1) acute onset and fluctuating course of the condition, (2) inattention, (3) disorganized thinking, and (4) altered level of consciousness. Both the DOS and the CAM are specific to delirium. The Folstein Mini-Mental State Examination (MMSE) is excellent

for evaluating cognitive function; however, it does not differentiate delirium from dementia. It includes questions that test orientation, attention span, recall, and ability to execute simple instructions. The MMSE also can be used in conjunction with the DOS or CAM to test the client's improvement or deterioration (Assessment Tool 31.1). Once delirium is diagnosed and as treatment progresses, ongoing assessment of mental status is necessary to monitor the client's recovery.

In addition to experiencing cognitive changes, disoriented clients are likely to be anxious and emotionally distraught. Nurses assess for any changes in anxiety level. If anxiety escalates to overt agitation, clients can become dangerous to self and others. Carefully assessing anxiety and watching for signs of agitation (eg, increased motor activity, labile mood, combativeness) can alert staff to the need for interventions that increase psychological comfort and decrease the potential for danger.

Nurses also monitor the client's ability to perform daily self-care. Confused clients may be too distracted to eat or drink adequately; they may be inattentive to hygiene. Ongoing assessment of functional ability is necessary for their comfort and physical well-being.

▲ NURSING DIAGNOSIS

Nursing diagnoses common to clients with delirium include the following (NANDA, 2007):

- Acute Confusion related to delirium of known or unknown etiology
- Risk for Injury related to confusion and cognitive deficits
- Bathing/Hygiene, Toileting, Feeding, and Dressing/ Grooming Self–Care Deficit related to cognitive impairment
- Deficient Knowledge of family related to client diagnosis, progression, and prognosis

▲ OUTCOME IDENTIFICATION AND PLANNING

Planning is a collaborative effort of the entire treatment team in conjunction with family and clients (as able) Nurses must

---

▲ ASSESSMENT TOOL 31.1 ▲

Sample Mini-Mental Status Examination Questions

- What is the year?
- What is today's date?
- In what city (town) are we?
- Spell "globe" backward.
- Repeat the following statement: "A rolling stone gathers no moss."
- Write a sentence of your own choice. (Nurse evaluates whether sentence has a subject, predicate [verb], and object.)

Questions adapted from Folstein, M. E., Folstein, S. E., & McHugh, P. R. (1975). Mini-mental state: A practical method for grading the cognitive state of patients for the clinician. *Journal of Psychiatric Research, 12*(189), 189–198. Used with permission.

deliberately design the plan of care to meet each client's unique needs. General goals of care for clients with delirium, linked to the *Nursing Outcomes Classification* (*NOC*), are as follows (Moorhead et al., 2008):

- **Risk Control:** The client will remain physically safe.
- **Self-Care: Activities of Daily Living:** The client's basic needs will be met until self-care ability resumes.
- **Cognitive Orientation:** The client will return to baseline cognitive functioning.

Think About It 31.1

James Serby brings his 75-year-old wife, Helen, to the clinic. She has a history of Parkinson's disease and diabetes. Mr. Serby states that his wife hasn't seemed herself for the past few days. She is lethargic during the day and sometimes seems confused. He states her blood glucose levels have been elevated and that she frequently has been incontinent of urine. The nurse evaluates Mrs. Serby's mental status. The client is not sure of the day or year and has trouble with short-term memory. Is the client experiencing delirium or dementia? Provide support for your conclusion. Explain what Mrs. Serby's priority need is and why.

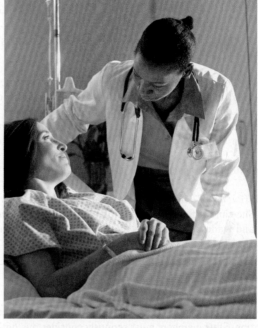

FIGURE 31.3 Addressing comfort, pain management, and other basic human needs is a core nursing intervention for clients with delirium.

▲ IMPLEMENTATION

Common *Nursing Interventions Classification* (*NIC*) labels related to management of delirium include, but are not limited to, **Anxiety Reduction, Delirium Management, Environmental Management: Safety, Fall Prevention, Reality Orientation**, and **Self-Care Assistance** (Bulechek et al., 2008).

Managing Symptoms of Delirium

Primary nursing interventions for delirium involve addressing the underlying cause and preventing further decline. Safety, hydration, nutrition, comfort, and pain management are core elements of care (Foreman et al., 2003). Simple physical and psychological comfort measures such as warmth, companionship, fluid provision, and reassurance are elemental (Figure 31.3).

Pain, too many stimuli, abrupt changes in routine, location, or room assignment, poor sleep, and insensitivity from others easily can worsen confusion and agitation. Nurses perform many activities to help promote a therapeutic milieu for those with acute confusion. In fact, environmental management is one of the most influential interventions for this condition. Confused clients are calmer when nurses eliminate stimuli that invite misinterpretation, such as abstract pictures or excessive noise. Conversely, cues such as clocks, recognizable photos, and calendars help restore orientation to time and place. One caveat is to avoid an understimulating environment, which also can be detrimental. The key is to remove difficult-to-interpret cues and replace them with simple, easy-to-recognize ones.

Confused clients also benefit from consistent routines implemented by familiar staff or family. Even though clients may be disoriented, they often recognize and are reassured by the presence of supportive relatives. Staff and family should reinforce the predictability of routines by telling clients what they are doing, what to expect, the time of day, and other relevant data as they proceed with activities. Consistency is stabilizing for these clients.

Directed activity may be helpful. Agitated clients may benefit from psychomotor tasks that distract them from anxiety. Bags with familiar items to "pack" and "unpack," Velcro to fasten and unfasten, and zippers to open and close provide sensory stimulation at a level adjusted to the client's compromised function. However, because inability to focus and attend to tasks is a hallmark of delirium, not all clients can or should participate in such activity.

Nurses approach clients calmly and empathetically, calling them by name and introducing themselves to facilitate attention and correct interpretation. They also are careful not to approach clients from behind, which allows minimal time to make adjustments. So that clients do not become frustrated, nurses avoid frequently quizzing them about orientation or posing questions that require decision making or abstract thinking. Instead, family and staff communicate in simple, direct sentences and focus on what is meaningful to clients.

Because clouded consciousness waxes and wanes, nurses never should assume that clients do not need or will not understand explanations. Recognizing their fears is helpful. Nurses may respond to fear with "It must be difficult to be so frightened, but I want you to know that I will not go far and I will do what needs to be done to keep you safe." Nurses must accept the sometimes bizarre behavior of clients with delirium and not demean or correct them for actions that they cannot control (Challenging Behaviors 31.1).

Challenging Behaviors 31.1

The Client Who Has Acute Confusion

Situation: Your assigned client has just arrived in the emergency department (ED). She is an 81-year-old woman who is emaciated, dirty, disheveled, and odiferous. She is yelling "Help me. Help me." At other times, she is difficult to arouse. She picks at her clothing and is attempting to get off the stretcher.

Your Potential Feelings: Anxiety, concern, repugnance

What Is Going On? The client is delirious from an unknown etiology. She cannot focus her attention, and her consciousness waxes and wanes. The top three culprits that cause delirium are medications, infections, and metabolic disturbances.

Strategy: The client needs immediate action to remain safe and to determine the etiology of her delirium. The multidisciplinary team assesses all biopsychosocial elements possible and institutes measures to reverse the acute confusion. The nurse assesses for pain.

Nurse Action/Communication: Assign someone to stay with the client. Do not use restraints. Move her away from some of the stimulation of the ED if possible. Explain procedures clearly and concisely and offer reassurance. You might say, "I imagine you are feeling quite afraid right now. You are in the emergency department of the hospital. We will keep you safe."

Occasionally, clients become so agitated that they need medication. Staff members must seriously consider this option when a client's behavior threatens the safety of self, family, or staff. Haloperidol (Haldol), a neuroleptic given either orally or by injection, is most commonly used for symptoms of delirium. It has minimal anticholinergic effects and does not cause the serious cardiovascular and respiratory side effects found with some other classes of antipsychotics. Extrapyramidal side effects are possible (Lacasse et al., 2006). Haloperidol is inexpensive and can be given orally in concentrated form at 1 to 2 mg every 2 to 4 hours. Older adults should receive 0.25 to 0.5 mg every 4 hours.

Atypical antipsychotics, including quetiapine (Seroquel), risperidone (Risperdal), olanzapine (Zyprexa), aripiprazole (Abilify), and ziprasidone (Geodon), occasionally are used to treat agitation related to cognitive disorders. Olanzapine (Zyprexa), risperidone (Risperdal), and ziprasidone (Geodon) are available as intramuscular injections. Although considered first-line treatments for agitation related to dementia, they have not yet been adequately and systematically studied to support short-term use over haloperidol for acute agitation in delirium (Alexopoulos et al., 2004). In fact, all antipsychotics, including Haldol, have warnings from the U.S. Food and Drug Administration (FDA) regarding potential cardiac events in older adults from prolongation of the Q-T interval. Expert consensus guidelines recommend tapering use of antipsychotics over 1 week once delirium has been stabilized (Alexopoulos et al., 2004).

For clients with hepatic dysfunction, lorazepam (Ativan) orally, intramuscularly, or intravenously may be used in doses from 0.5 to 2 mg. Lorazepam can affect respiratory and cardiac function; thus, nurses must monitor clients taking it. In some instances, lorazepam increases agitation and must be discontinued. Its use is most appropriate during alcohol withdrawal and for short-term treatment of anxiety (Alexopoulos et al., 2004).

Providing a Safe Environment

Because clients with clouded cognition are likely to misinterpret environmental clues, they are vulnerable to harm. Many also behave unsafely, such as pulling out tubes or wandering from units. Making the environment safe helps prevent harm that might result from confusion. Nurses place personal and familiar items (eg, call light, water pitcher, eyeglasses) close at hand so that clients are not injured while attempting to get them. Clients with delirium have sustained significant injuries by wandering into traffic, falling down stairs, or getting lost. Alerting staff and family to the possibility that clients may escape or wander and arranging for continuous observation if necessary helps prevent accidents.

Many clients with delirium, especially older adults, are injured climbing over raised bed rails. Beds should remain in the lowest position with rails down unless policy demands otherwise. Regular toileting may help prevent clients from attempting to get out of bed alone. Lighting needs to be bright enough so clients can see accurately. This is especially important at night and significant for older adults who need brighter light to see at all.

Nurses should not use restraints. Physical limitation may cause clients to become agitated and fearful, which increases stress and risk for injury. If restraints are the only option, nurses should identify the reason for use and find alternatives, such as providing the presence of loved ones, consistent caregivers, and attention to sleep, nutrition, toileting, and pain (O'Connell & Mion, 2003; Park et al., 2005). Because foreseeing all potential environmental dangers is impossible, nurses frequently check on these clients. At times, even this level of care is insufficient. Nurses may ask relatives to stay with loved ones, especially at night or during more agitated periods.

Assisting With Personal Care

The distractibility and cognitive disorganization of clients with delirium may seriously hamper their ability to maintain activities of daily living (ADLs). Potential consequences include poor nutrition and hydration, discomfort from wet clothing, skin breakdown, and immobility. Nurses must support the efforts of clients to carry out whatever ADLs they can, as well as assume

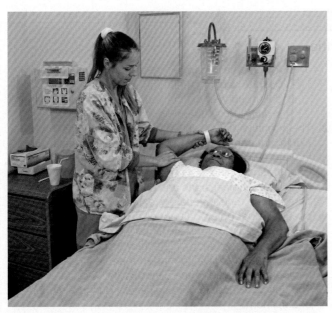

FIGURE 31.4 The nurse is performing passive range-of-motion exercises for a hospitalized client with episodic delirium to preserve overall health.

responsibility for those necessary activities that clients cannot manage. Establishing a routine to carry out activities also is helpful to confused clients. This routine should include regular toileting, offering fluids and food, and providing an opportunity for passive or active exercise (Figure 31.4).

Providing Client and Family Education

Clients who realize that their thinking is disordered may be frightened. Nurses must explain the nature of delirium. Clients and families need to realize that associated confusion and abnormal behavior have a biologic basis and are transient. Explaining the process, progress, and prognosis of delirium should alleviate some anxiety and apprehension. The team must continually update family as to the state of the underlying problem and the progress being made to resolve it. Relatives need to become partners with the team in planning care and implementing some interventions, such as reorientation.

▲ EVALUATION

As stated previously, signs and symptoms of delirium may fluctuate each day. A perspective on how well clients are recovering may evolve over several days. Because clients have varying baseline cognitive function, nurses evaluate each person's progress according to a previous level. Indicators of resolving confusion include the following:

*   Improved score on the chosen assessment scale (CAM, DOS, or MMSE)
*   Improved ability to communicate
*   Increased ability to focus attention
*   Increased ability to make decisions
*   Reduced delusional behavior
*   Improved ability to care for self
*   Decreased anxiety and agitation

> **Checkpoint Questions**
> **5.** What medication is used most commonly to treat the symptoms of delirium?
> **6.** Why should restraints be avoided as much as possible in clients with delirium?

DEMENTIA

Dementia is the term used for a syndrome characterized by several cognitive deficits that result from a general medical condition, use of a substance, or multiple biologic etiologies. Although there are several types, all forms of dementia affect memory and cognition.

Incidence and Prevalence

The U.S. National Institute of Neurological Disorders (National Institute of Neurological Disorders and Stroke [NINDS], 2007) reports that at least 6.8 million people have chronic cognitive impairment related to dementia; in some communities 50% of those 85 years or older have dementia. Given that those older than 85 years are the fastest-growing segment of older adults and that the large cohort born after World War II is now entering its seventh decade, incidence and prevalence of dementia are likely to increase.

Signs and Symptoms/Diagnostic Criteria

The clinical presentations of disorders within the subcategory of dementia do not differ significantly. All are characterized by ongoing multiple cognitive deficits, memory impairment severe enough to compromise social or occupational function, and decline from previous functioning (APA, 2000). The distinctiveness of the disorders arises from their differing origins (*DSM-IV-TR* Box 31.2).

Impaired Learning

Memory impairment significantly affects the relationships and work of clients with dementia. It encompasses the ability to learn and retain new material (short-term memory) as well as to recall previously learned information (long-term memory) (APA, 2000). Clients become repetitive and have difficulty remembering recent conversations, events, and appointments. They continually lose things. They may attempt to compensate for these lapses.

Compromised Ability for Complex Tasks

The chronic and degenerative nature of dementia causes significant deficiencies. Well-preserved social skills and attempts to conceal impairments often obscure clients' mental

DSM-IV-TR BOX 31.2

Dementia

Dementia of the Alzheimer's Type

A. The development of multiple cognitive deficits manifested by both
 1. Memory impairment (impaired ability to learn new information or to recall previously learned information)
 2. One (or more) of the following cognitive disturbances:
  a. aphasia (language disturbance)
  b. apraxia (impaired ability to carry out motor activities despite intact motor function)
  c. agnosia (failure to recognize or identify objects despite sensory function)
  d. disturbance in executive functioning (ie, planning, organizing, sequencing, abstracting)
B. The cognitive deficits in Criteria Al and A2 each cause significant impairment in social or occupational functioning and represent a significant decline from a previous level of functioning.
C. The course is characterized by gradual onset and continuing cognitive decline.
D. The cognitive deficits in Criteria Al and A2 are not due to any of following:
 1. Other central nervous system conditions that cause progressive deficits in memory and cognition (eg, cerebrovascular disease, Parkinson's disease, Huntington's disease, subdural hematoma, normal-pressure hydrocephalus, brain tumor)
 2. Systemic conditions that are known to cause dementia (eg, hypothyroidism, vitamin B_{12} or folic acid deficiency, niacin deficiency, hypercalcemia, neurosyphilis, HIV infection)
 3 Substance-induced conditions
E. The deficits do not occur exclusively during the course of a delirium
F. The disturbance is not better accounted for by another Axis I disorder (e.g., major depressive disorder, schizophrenia).

Vascular Dementia

A. The development of multiple cognitive deficits manifested by both
 1. Memory impairment (impaired ability to learn new information or to recall previously learned information)
 2. One or more of the following cognitive disturbances:
  a. aphasia (language disturbance)
  b. apraxia (impaired ability to carry out motor activities despite intact motor function)

  c. agnosia (failure to recognize or identify objects despite sensory function)
  d. disturbance in executive functioning (i.e., planning, organizing, sequencing, abstracting)
B. The cognitive deficits in Criteria A1 and A2 each cause significant impairment in social or occupational functioning and represent a significant decline from a previous level of functioning.
C. Focal neurological signs and symptoms (eg, exaggeration of deep tendon reflexes, extensor plantar response, pseudobulbar palsy, gait abnormalities, weakness of an extremity) or laboratory evidence indicative of cerebrovascular disease (eg, multiple infarctions involving cortex and underlying white matter) that are judged to be etiologically related to the disturbance.
D. The deficits do not occur exclusively during the course of a delirium.

Dementia Due to Other General Medical Conditions

A. The development of multiple cognitive deficits manifested by both
 1. Memory impairment (impaired ability to learn new information or to recall previously learned information)
 2. One (or more) of the following cognitive disturbances:
  a. aphasia (language disturbance)
  b. apraxia (impaired ability to carry out motor activities despite intact motor function)
  c. agnosia (failure to recognize or identify objects despite sensory function)
  d. disturbance in executive functioning (i.e., planning, organizing, sequencing, abstracting)
B. The cognitive deficits in Criteria Al and A2 each cause significant impairment in social or occupational functioning and represent a significant decline from a previous level of functioning.
C. There is evidence from the history, physical examination, or laboratory findings that the disturbance is the direct physiological consequence of a general medical condition other than Alzheimer's disease or cerebrovascular disease (eg, HIV infection, traumatic brain injury, Parkinson's disease, Huntington's disease, Pick's disease, Creutzfeldt–Jakob disease, normal-pressure hydrocephalus, hypothyroidism, brain tumor, or vitamin B_{12} deficiency).
D. The deficits do not occur exclusively during the course of a delirium.

Reprinted with permission from the *Diagnostic and Statistical Manual of Mental Disorders, Fourth Edition, Text Revision* (Copyright (c) 2000). American Psychiatric Association.

deterioration and mislead clinicians (Geldmacher, 2007). Family members often first recognize cognitive problems when loved ones have difficulties with routine activities: meal planning, managing checkbooks, driving, and using the telephone.

Impaired Reasoning

Dementia affects reasoning. Clients no longer seem able to respond to everyday problems at work or home. Ultimately, their thought processes degenerate so much that they show significant deficits in abstract thinking. They cannot cognitively adapt to new situations. This impairment severely limits their competence to adjust to the dynamics of life (APA, 2000). For example, if the bathroom at home floods, a client with dementia may be in a quandary about how to respond. Clients also may begin to exhibit uncharacteristic disregard for social conduct. For example, they may disrobe in public, exhibit inappropriate sexual behavior, suddenly use profanity, and strike out at others when frustrated. Families find such changes alarming and distressing.

Compromised Spatial Ability and Orientation

Because their ability to process sensory information diminishes, clients gradually begin to experience confusion, which affects attentiveness to the environment. As consciousness decreases, clients cannot concentrate, their attention span progressively declines, and they become distractible. They also may become disoriented. Eventually, they can no longer recognize or identify familiar objects (eg, parts of a telephone), a condition called **agnosia**. When sensory input falls below certain minimum requirements and when the brain is affected structurally so that it no longer perceives and interprets stimuli adequately, orientation decreases.

Disorientation and problems with spatial ability can make driving a point of contention. Relatives often recognize that affected clients are no longer safe drivers. Clients who continue driving may do so aimlessly for hours, unable to find their way home. Nevertheless, they usually have little insight into this declining ability.

Clients with dementia seem unable to organize items around the house. They get lost and cannot find their way around their neighborhood or home. They do not know where they are, how they came to be there, why they are there, or how they fit into the milieu. One man with early-stage dementia described his experience as having lost his "internal road map." Getting lost in a familiar place is often the incident relatives identify as the onset of dementia in loved ones.

Language Deficits

Frequently, clients with dementia have difficulty finding the words they want to use (**aphasia**) in conversation (Figure 31.5). This problem can result in a frustrating process of "charades," relying on others to guess the forgotten word (eg, referring to Thanksgiving as the time of the turkey or pumpkin). In addition, they may have difficulty following conversations.

Behavioral Problems

Behavior refers to individual responses to continual internal and external changes and to the brain's physiologic soundness. When something interferes with or interrupts brain integrity, maladaptive behavior often follows. This behavior is not to be confused with that of delirium, even though aberrant behavior is a hallmark of both conditions.

No key behavioral characteristic occurs in every client with dementia, but most changes become more pronounced

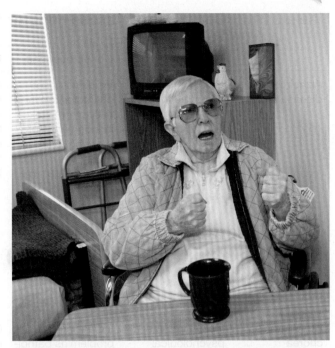

FIGURE 31.5 Aphasia, or difficulty finding words and language, is a hallmark finding with dementia. It can be one of the most frustrating and challenging symptoms for clients.

after sunset (a phenomenon known as **sundowning**). Clients may become more irritable and suspicious and misinterpret visual or auditory cues. Because of their diffuse cognitive impairment, they may experience illusions and hallucinations (see Chap. 29). Family members may report that loved ones have developed poor hygiene and become defensive or apathetic. Clients may find that they cannot perform motor tasks (eg, brushing the teeth, combing the hair) despite intact motor function, a condition known as **apraxia** (APA, 2000).

> ### Checkpoint Questions
> **7.** What term denotes the loss of the ability to recognize familiar objects?
> **8.** When do most behaviors become more pronounced in clients with dementia?

Types of Dementia

Table 31.2 compares the characteristics of the most common forms of dementia. Alzheimer's disease is discussed in the most detail below because of its frequency and growing emergence as a national health problem.

Alzheimer's Disease

Alzheimer's disease (AD) is the most prevalent form of dementia. Based on incidence and population studies, the Alzheimer's Association estimates that 5.4 million Americans had AD in 2011. Incidence and prevalence directly correlate with increased age. The illness occurs in 10% of people 65 years or older and rises to nearly 50% of those 85 years

TABLE 31.2 Comparative Assessment for Cognitive Disorders

	Cognition	Level of Consciousness	Memory	Appearance	Emotions
Alzheimer's disease	Global intellectual impairment	Insidious onset characterized initially by "mistakes in judgment," progressing to inability to comprehend, agraphia, aphasia, and finally to unresponsiveness	Clouding late in disease; short-term memory loss initially progressing to both short-term and long-term loss	Progressive loss of grooming habits as a result of forgotten social behaviors and decreasing coordination required to dress	Initially depression and anxiety about recognized regression, progressing to loss or severe dampening of emotions Subtle loss of interest in work Inability to recognize family members
Frontotemporal lobar degeneration (Pick's disease)	Intellect intact	Lack of insight into disease process	Not affected	Very poor hygiene	Dramatic personality changes Socially inappropriate behavior Flippant beyond reasonable propriety
Huntington's chorea	Insight into the psychological degenerative changes	Increasingly a problem as pathology progresses but without aphasia, agnosia, or apraxia	Choreiform movements	Disheveled	Mood swings from apathy to aggressive behavior Inappropriate behavior Despair about changes taking place Suicidal tendencies Decreased interest in job
Wernicke–Korsakoff syndrome	Cannot learn new information because of an inability to retain facts	Alert Cannot learn new or recall previously learned material	Suspended in time Recall limits to 2–3 min Extensive memory loss	Unsteady gait from peripheral neuropathies	Communication impaired related to memory gaps Confabulation
Vascular dementia	Not affected	Proceeds in a stepwise progression as ministrokes occur	Does not handle new situations well	Deterioration of hygienic standards	Depression or pseudodepression

or older. As the population continues to grow and age, the number of people with AD will likely reach 11 to 16 million by 2050 (Hebert et al., 2003). M**O**VIE viewing **GUIDES**

The incidence of AD is higher in women than in men, which may be because women outlive men. According to the National Institute on Aging (NIA, 2007), approximately 10% of cases are familial and result from mutations on chromosomes 1, 14, and 21. Familial AD (FAD) always has an onset before 65 years.

ETIOLOGIC FACTORS. Hallmark pathologic features of AD are neurofibrillary tangles and beta-amyloid plaques in the brain on postmortem examination (Understanding Biologic Foundations 31.1). In fact, AD is definitively

diagnosed according to these findings. The disease results in neuronal death and disrupted neurotransmission. Especially affected is acetylcholine (ACh), a critically important neurotransmitter for memory and cognition. Clinical studies with *acetylcholinesterase inhibitors* (drugs that inhibit the enzyme that destroys ACh) have shown efficacy in slowing AD (Birks et al., 2000; Birks & Harvey, 2006). Thus, neuronal destruction and resulting disruption of ACh transmission are involved in the elusive etiology of AD.

Extensive research continues to unravel the mysterious etiology of AD. Because of confusion regarding the type of dementia in participants, existing research was inadequate. New diagnostic criteria for AD, issued in 2011 by the NIA, and new Alzheimer's Association criteria for research

UNDERSTANDING BIOLOGIC FOUNDATIONS 31.1

Neurologic Alterations in Alzheimer's Disease

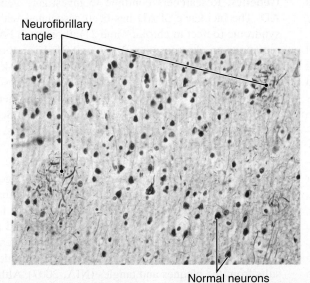

Neurofibrillary tangle

Normal neurons

Neurofibrillary tangles. The microscopic study image shows normal neurons versus the characteristic tangles of AD.

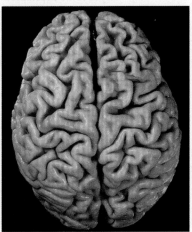

NORMAL

AD

Cortical atrophy. Compare the normal brain on the left with the brain ravaged by AD on the right.

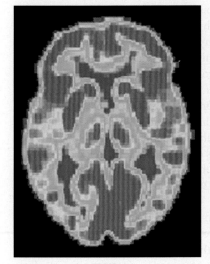

NORMAL

AD

Brain scans. Dark bluish purple areas signify areas of lost brain activity. Compare the multicolored normal brain scan on the left with the vast bluish regions found in the client with AD on the right.

participant selection will assist in refining research studies. Multiple and diverse studies are investigating the role of genetics, inflammation, oxidative stress, vascular changes, metabolism, beta-amyloid and tau proteins, lifestyles and diet, education levels, hormones, and growth factors. The etiology of AD may be a combination of genetic vulnerability and exposure to environmental and psychosocial stressors. Research supported by the NIA has focused not only on etiology, but also on risk and protective factors and efforts to slow disease progression. The known risk factors include age, family history, presence of the apolipoprotein E4 (*apoE4*) gene, and mild cognitive impairment.

Ultimately, researchers may find that interacting etiologies are responsible for AD. Certainly, the course of the illness varies widely. A person may have biologic markers for AD but show no symptoms and function well (Snowdon, 2003). AD is considered to be clinically heterogeneous; that is, symptomatology varies during its average 8- to 10-year course. Various groups have attempted to stage the progressive functional decline of AD (Box 31.2). Doing so helps clients, family members, and health care providers to

plan for the extensive management necessary for those with the illness.

Genetics. Researchers continue to investigate genetics in AD. The incidence of AD has been associated with Down syndrome (defect in chromosome 21); those with FAD have mutations on chromosomes 1, 14, and 21. Even those with nonfamilial or sporadic AD seem at increased risk if they carry the apolipoprotein E (*apoE*) gene on chromosome 19. This gene has three forms, and having an *apoE4* gene from both parents seems to increase risk (NIA, 2007). Searching for clues to the formation of beta-amyloid plaques, investigators also are looking at other chromosomes.

Oxidative Stress. Oxidative stress is cellular damage caused by *oxygen-free radicals*. Some researchers believe that aging results from oxidative stress. They are attempting to determine if free radicals contribute to the tangles and plaques that lead to neuron death in AD. Results have been inconclusive; it is unclear whether oxidative stress precedes or results from the plaques and tangles (NIA, 2007). Although it is yet to be replicated, one study demonstrated some benefit of vitamin E, an antioxidant, in slowing the progression of AD (Tabet et al., 2000). Two animal studies found that antioxidants combined with behavioral enrichment enhanced cognition in dogs (Milgram et al., 2004, 2005). The practice guidelines of the Quality Standards Subcommittee of the American Academy of Neurology support the use of up to 1,000 IUs of vitamin E twice a day (Doody et al., 2001). Many clinicians empirically prescribe 400 to 800 units of vitamin E with cholinesterase inhibitors to people diagnosed with dementia.

Immunology. Some studies showing abnormally high antibody titers in clients with AD raised the possibility of an immunologic etiology. Researchers thought that immunization could prevent beta-amyloid plaques, leading to a vaccine for AD. However, clinical trials were discontinued because of subsequent inflammation in the brains of some participants. Research continues with the discovery that passive immunization removed beta-amyloid from the brains of immunized mice (NIA, 2007). Similar investigations into the tau proteins that make up neurofibrillary tangles have revealed that a modified piece of tau given as a vaccine to mice helped eliminate tau from the brain (NIA, 2007). Investigators have found that specific forms of tau and beta-amyloid must be present to create conditions leading to AD. Beta-amyloid seems to trigger various changes that lead to tau alterations, causing an atmosphere that creates tangles that contribute to neuron death (NINDS, 2007).

Hormones. Researchers have explored hormones, specifically estrogen, and nerve growth factors. Although initial animal studies suggested that hormone replacement therapy in postmenopausal women protected against cognitive decline, later evidence found that women taking combined estrogen

---

BOX 31.2 Stages of Alzheimer's Disease

Mild

The client:
- Frequently repeats himself or herself
- Regularly misplaces articles
- Cannot recall familiar words to use in conversation
- Withdraws from formerly enjoyed activities
- Is aware of and frustrated with own "forgetfulness"
- Changes are not readily apparent to others and often are denied or excused by family.

Moderate

The client:
- Has decreased ability to carry out ADLs and IADLs
- Encounters difficulty finding way around neighborhood and home
- Is disoriented to time and place
- Shows disruptive behaviors (wandering, pacing)
- Has hallucinations and delusions
- Cannot perform complex motor activities
- Shows problems with visual perception (and thus is susceptible to accidents)
- Needs supervision frequently
- Displays temperament fluctuations, from composed and tranquil to screaming and argumentative
- Deterioration is apparent to friends and family.

Severe

The client:
- Has lost capacity for self-care and use of language
- Has only minimal long-term memory
- Must have 24-hour, 7-day-a-week care

and progestin were at significantly increased risk for dementia (Schumaker et al., 2003). Investigation into *nerve growth factors* (proteins that regulate neuronal maturation, survival, and repair) led to the development of memantine (Galantamine), a drug that is beneficial for cognition and function in moderate to severe AD (McShane et al., 2006).

Inflammation. Vascular disease and AD share risk factors, so investigators continue to study the relationship between neuron death from stroke and from AD (NIA, 2007; NINDS, 2007). Studies by the NIA (2007) found that the inflammatory response following stroke led to rapid formation of beta-amyloid. With a possible relationship between inflammation and AD, some researchers believe that anti-inflammatory medications (eg, ibuprofen, aspirin) may help prevent AD. Although studies have not clearly supported this notion (Tabet & Feldman, 2003), and guidelines do not support nonsteroidal anti-inflammatory drugs (NSAIDs) as treatment (Doody et al., 2001), some clinicians empirically prescribe them for clients with AD and no evidence of vascular dementia. Researchers are studying other medications used for cardiovascular treatment as preventive drugs against AD (NINDS, 2007). Reports from the longitudinal Honolulu Asia Aging Study indicate increased formation of plaques and tangles in the brains of those with high cholesterol levels. Reducing cholesterol levels with statins has been shown to prevent pathogenesis associated with AD (Scott & Laake, 2001).

Diet. There is increasing emphasis on the role of diet in prevention of—not treatment of—AD. Studies advocate for the Mediterranean diet, which is rich in polyunsaturated fats, fish, nuts, cruciferous vegetables, fruits, and dark green leafy vegetables. Longitudinal studies reported fewer cases of AD in healthy elderly people following dietary patterns similar to those of the Mediterranean diet, whereas participants who regularly consumed foods high in saturated fat suffered an increased incidence of AD (Scarmeas et al., 2006, 2009; Solfrizzi et al., 2010). In 2011, Bayer-Carter et al. found low levels of beta-amyloid 42 (a primary biomarker of AD) in the cerebrospinal fluid of healthy cognitively intact participants who adhered to a 4-week low-saturated-fat, low-glycemic-index diet.

PREVENTIVE FACTORS. Research has not been limited to biologic etiologies. Incidence of AD is higher among people living in industrialized areas and from lower socio-economic groups (NIA, 2007). Many factors could account for these findings, including environmental toxins, diet, lifestyle, and stress. Several large epidemiologic studies and research initiatives (Abbott et al., 2004; Larson et al., 2006; Podewils et al., 2005; Weuve et al., 2004) have shown a lower incidence of cognitive decline in people who regularly exercise. Researchers also are investigating the roles of leisure, education, and cognitive stimulation. Frequent participation in cognitively stimulating activities may be associated with decreased incidence of AD (Snowdon, 2003)

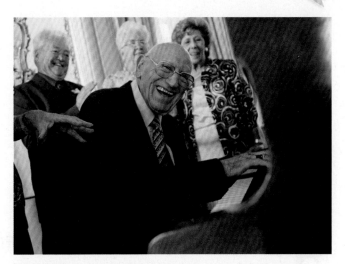

FIGURE 31.6 Ongoing participation in cognitively stimulating activities may be protective against the development of AD.

(Figure 31.6). Similarly, a high level of education may be a protective factor. Although education may stimulate neuronal connections, the finding also could result from the degree of exposure to risk factors associated with socioeconomic status. The herb ginkgo biloba has many promising properties, including increasing blood supply, reducing blood viscosity, modifying neurotransmitters, and reducing the density of oxygen-free radicals (see Chap. 17). Its efficacy in improving memory is inconclusive and requires further research (Birks & Grimley-Evans, 2007).

Vascular Dementia

The second most common form of dementia is vascular dementia. Although its overall incidence is considerably less than that of AD, some researchers allege that it is the most common dementia in men and in those older than 85 years. Risk factors for vascular dementia parallel those for stroke: hypertension, smoking, hyperlipidemia, atrial fibrillation, and diabetes. Computed tomography scanning and magnetic resonance imaging (MRI) often verify the brain disease in this particular dementia. On examination clients may have carotid bruits, funduscopic abnormalities, or enlarged heart chambers (Sadock & Sadock, 2007).

In vascular dementia, cognitive deficits arise from multiple infarcts in the cortex and white matter of the brain following hemorrhage or stroke. Clients experience a faster onset with vascular dementia than with AD, and a stepwise or fluctuating progression, rather than a steady and gradual deterioration. They show focal neurologic signs. Specific symptoms depend on the affected brain sectors and the extent of damage. Frequently, accompanying neurologic evidence of cerebrovascular disease includes paresis (limb paralysis) or headaches. Clients with vascular dementia also experience impaired memory, aphasia, apraxia, agnosia, and difficulties with executive functioning. Mixed dementias (both vascular and AD) are common (NINDS, 2007).

Lewy Body Disease

Lewy body disease is sometimes mistaken for AD because of clinical similarity but is associated with earlier and more prominent visual hallucinations, parkinsonian features, and disturbed behaviors. The exact incidence is unknown because only four population studies have been conducted, but the estimated prevalence of Lewy body disease is 22% of all dementias (Rahknone et al., 2003). On autopsy, Lewy inclusion bodies in the cerebral cortex confirm diagnosis. A distinguishing characteristic is significant adverse reactions to antipsychotic drugs (NINDS, 2007).

Parkinson's Disease

Parkinson's disease progresses slowly and has no known cure. This neurodegenerative illness affects 1 million Americans. Although its predominant feature is immobility, cognitive decline runs concurrently in more than 30% of clients (NINDS, 2007). Decreasing numbers of brain cells in the substantia nigra result in depletion of dopamine (Understanding Biologic Foundations 31.2). Clients exhibit involuntary muscle movements at rest, overall slowness, and rigidity. Most often, they have postural instability and disturbed gait. Intellectual deficits vary, but their progression is insidious.

UNDERSTANDING BIOLOGIC FOUNDATIONS 31.2

The Pathophysiology of Parkinson's Disease

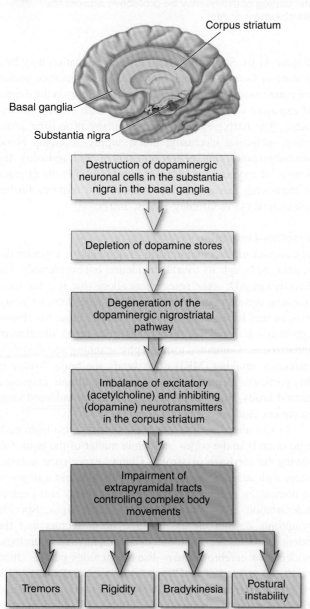

Diminished numbers of dopaminergic neurons in the substantia nigra of the brain result in the manifestations of Parkinson's disease. One such manifestation is dementia, which develops in more than 75% of clients with the illness.

Unlike other types, Parkinson's dementia does not impair language capabilities. It does impair memory retrieval and executive function. Although Parkinson's dementia is unique and different from AD, some who have Parkinson's disease also have AD.

Huntington's Disease

Huntington's disease, a hereditary disorder associated with dementia, results from a faulty gene for a protein called huntingtin. Because it is autosomal dominant, children of an affected parent have a 50% chance of inheriting the trait-carrying gene. Men and women are affected equally. The disease inevitably develops in those with the trait in their 30s or 40s. Time from onset to death is approximately 15 years (NINDS, 2007). Prenatal and presymptomatic testing for Huntington's is possible but not always available. Moreover, the test has a high-anxiety quotient for at-risk people because currently there is no cure.

Clients with Huntington's disease experience *chorea,* or involuntary, jerky, arrhythmic movements that intensify with stress. At one time, the illness was commonly referred to as Huntington's chorea. Clumsiness, muscle weakness, and gait disturbance are also present (NINDS, 2007). Chorea usually peaks 10 years after onset and then stabilizes or decreases. This particular dementia causes no aphasia, agnosia, or apraxia but does result in memory deficits, slowed thinking, problems with attention, and deficient judgment. Cognitive symptoms often begin as mild emotional manifestations (eg, irritability) and progress to anxiety and depression (NINDS, 2007). As the frontal lobe deteriorates, clients become labile, impulsive, easily frustrated, irritable, hostile, and aggressive. The illness becomes increasingly relentless, and clients often exhibit mood or intermittent explosive disorders.

Human Immunodeficiency Virus Dementia

Human immunodeficiency virus (HIV) dementia is seen more frequently in a younger population than are the other dementias because HIV is more prevalent in younger people. Although dementia occurs in as many as 75% of those with HIV, other causes such as infections, tumors, and adverse drug reactions need consideration (Sadock & Sadock, 2007). MRI of the brain often reveals some type of pathologic change, and clients usually manifest other symptoms accompanying HIV. Clinicians should be alert for mild cognitive decline or neurologic symptoms such as headaches, vision changes, and neuropathies that might signal CNS involvement in clients with AIDS (Sadock & Sadock, 2007).

Those with HIV dementia show memory loss, poor judgment, and decreased executive function. At times, motor movements are delayed. Progression of HIV dementia differs from other forms with a predictably steady mental deterioration. Some clients with HIV dementia have daily episodes of memory loss and confusion alternating with mental clarity. Problems also can stabilize for months to years before downward progression ensues. Antiretroviral drugs used to treat HIV/AIDS can delay onset and reduce symptoms (NINDS, 2007).

Frontotemporal Lobar Degeneration

Frontotemporal lobar degeneration (FTLD), formally known as Pick's disease, accounts for approximately 5% of progressive dementias. Onset is at 40 to 60 years of age; studies show that FTLD occurs slightly more often in men, usually those with an affected first-degree relative (Sadock & Sadock, 2007). FTLD is highly heritable and researchers have identified five possible genes involved (Rohrer et al., 2009). PET scans and MRI can indicate which portion of the brain is involved, but to discriminate FTLD from other forms of dementia, more research is needed to pursue biomarkers for conclusive diagnosis. Because the frontal lobes are affected, changes in behavior, personality, and judgment, rather than memory, are the presenting symptoms, followed by progressive speech decline and motor disorders (Braaten et al., 2006). Whereas careful behavioral assessment and also data collection from clients and caregivers remain the cornerstones of diagnosis, conclusive diagnosis of FTLD happens only on autopsy (Dickson et al., 2011; Josephs, 2008). General microscopic findings include atrophy of the frontotemporal regions of the brain, in contrast to the more parietal–temporal distribution of AD (Sadock & Sadock, 2007). Investigators do not clearly understand why this atrophy occurs, but they believe it to explain aberrant behaviors seen with FTLD. In beginning stages, people with Pick's disease have *less* disorientation and memory loss than do those with AD and *more* personality changes, including loss of social constraints (resulting in frequent social and behavioral problems).

Creutzfeldt–Jakob Disease

With a global incidence of approximately one new case per 1 million people per year, this rare, rapidly progressive, and ultimately fatal disease results from a protein-like agent called a *prion* (NINDS, 2007). Symptoms ensue after age 60. Although 5% to 10% of U.S. cases are thought to be genetic, the disease is thought to spread through contact with contaminated human brain tissue or from improperly sterilized neurosurgical tools. Ingestion of certain neurologic parts of cows infected with a prion similar to the one causing Creutzfeldt–Jakob disease has been the source of contamination in British and U.S. outbreaks. This type is a variant of the classic Creutzfeldt–Jakob disease and is more common in adults younger than 60 years. Both forms are termed "spongiform" because of the spongy appearance of the cerebral and cerebellar cortex (NINDS, 2007). In older adults, the disease may be misdiagnosed as AD, but symptoms are initially more suggestive of a psychiatric illness other than dementia (NINDS, 2007).

Clients with Creutzfeldt–Jakob disease pass through three distinct stages. Initially, mental abnormalities progress to a rapidly deteriorating dementia. Then, jerking, seizure-like activity appears, with ataxia, dysarthria, and other cerebellar signs. Extrapyramidal signs, sensory disruption, and seizures are other manifestations during the middle phase. Coma marks the final phase, with clients dying of infections and respiratory problems (NINDS, 2007).

Implications and Prognosis

Prognosis for people with dementia is poor. Currently, no cures are available; however, certain interventions appear to delay or slow progression of some forms and symptoms.

Interdisciplinary Goals and Management

Clients and families truly need participation from an entire health care team for a comprehensive management regimen. Overall goals for clients with dementia include physical care, a safe environment, behavior management, and psychosocial support and education of clients and caregivers. See Evidence-Based Practice Spotlight 31.1.

Clients with dementia benefit from as early a diagnosis as possible to promote interventions that slow illness progression. Early diagnosis also gives relatives time to adjust and rearrange their lives as they increasingly assume the caregiver role. The health care team interacts most intensively with clients during early stages, when clients are still aware of and thus most frustrated and depressed about cognitive losses. As the disease becomes more incapacitating,

health care providers expand their involvement with relatives, often forming close-knit partnerships. These alliances promote the physical health and safety of clients and support the whole family.

As they lose cognitive abilities, clients develop more extensive and demanding needs. Families need teaching from physicians and nurses on how to care for loved ones who can no longer independently handle ADLs. Relatives (most often spouses or daughters) usually assume the role of primary caregiver. In doing so, they take on an exhausting and constant job for people who show decreasing appreciation and, with time, no longer even recognize them. This is not only *physically* but also *emotionally* stressing. Health care providers must be resources to families for innovative care tactics, referrals to community offerings for respite and home health care, information about support groups, and group or personal counseling. Such support helps family members to care for loved ones and delays or permanently avoids the institutionalization of clients.

Medical and Supportive Interventions

Family caregivers need to know how to meet the physical needs of loved ones as self-care capabilities diminish. Some families need minimal information and guidance; others require more tangible assistance (eg, home health aides).

⚠ EVIDENCE-BASED PRACTICE SPOTLIGHT 31.1 ⚠

Nonpharmacologic Treatment of Dementia-Related Agitation

Overview of Effective Treatment: Interventions based on understanding the meaning of behavior and a comprehensive biopsychosocial assessment allow nurses to modify the environment and adapt nursing care to client needs. Major practice recommendations support assessing patterns of agitated behaviors, avoiding triggers for these behaviors, implementing general communication techniques, and using specific interventions, including sensory enhancement/relaxation, social contact, behavior therapy, structured activities, and environmental modifications. These have been found to decrease agitation and reduce the need for physical and chemical restraints. The strongest evidence based on randomized controlled studies supports the use of individualized music that stimulates remote memory and sensation.

What Has Not Been Shown Effective: Restraints have not been shown effective in preventing injury or reducing dementia-related agitation. In fact, increased agitation and injury have been associated with restraint use. The current standard of care is restraint free, requiring both institutional policies and individualized care of clients with cognitive impairments. Although antipsychotic medications are effective for short-term management of agitation, they are not without risk.

Implications for Practice: Physical and chemical restraints are associated with increased risk to people with cognitive impairment. Comprehensive assessment and individualized care along with environmental modifications are evidence-based nursing interventions that can significantly improve the care and reduce agitated behaviors in people with dementia.

References

Agency for Healthcare Research and Quality (AHRQ). (2007). Efficacy and comparative effectiveness of off-label use of atypical antipsychotics. A summary for clinicians and policymakers (AHRQ Publication No. 07-EHC003–2). Available at http://www.effectivehealthcare.ahrq.gov

Gerdner, L. (2007). *Individualized music for elders with dementia.* Iowa City, IA: University of Iowa Gerontological Nursing Interventions Research Center, Research Dissemination Core.

McGonigal-Kenney, M. L., & Schutte, D. L. (2004). *Non-pharmacologic management of agitated behaviors in persons with Alzheimer disease and other chronic dementing conditions.* Iowa City, IA: University of Iowa Gerontological Nursing Interventions Research Center, Research Dissemination Core.

Park, M., Hsiao-Chen Tang, J., & Ledford, L. (2005). *Changing the practice of physical restraint use in acute care.* Iowa City, IA: University of Iowa Gerontological Nursing Interventions Research Center, Research Dissemination Core.

Thiru-Chelvam, B. (2004). *Bathing persons with dementia.* Iowa City, IA: University of Iowa Gerontological Nursing Interventions Research Center, Research Dissemination Core.

Changing the environment often can assuage or exacerbate behavioral problems as dementia progresses. Sometimes, however, behavioral problems are best managed pharmacologically. Behaviors that warrant medication include extreme agitation, depression, and disinhibition. Clients with dementia taking any medications require careful monitoring because the drugs actually can cause or compound behavioral problems. Sometimes, merely lowering a dosage, discontinuing the medication, or substituting another drug resolves issues.

Psychopharmacologic Interventions

One finding in AD is diminished cholinergic neurotransmission, resulting in too little ACh in the cholinergic system. Although the cause of this problem remains unknown, it happens early in the disease. Compelling evidence shows that drugs that inhibit ACh destruction or increase cholinergic activity can slow deterioration of memory and function in mild to moderate AD. Systematic reviews of two such drugs, rivastigmine and donepezil, support their efficacy for treatment of AD and dementia related to Parkinson's disease (Birks et al., 2000; Maidment, 2008; Maidment et al., 2006; Wattmo et al., 2011).

Cholinesterase inhibitors increase availability of ACh by interfering with the enzyme that breaks it down. These centrally acting drugs help elevate the level of ACh by decreasing the binding sites of acetylcholinesterase, which lengthens the potential for cholinergic activity. These drugs are effective as long as some cells still produce ACh (Sunderland et al., 2004). Thus, they are most efficacious for mild to moderate AD. Even then, their effects on cognition are modest, with only small improvements and possible slowing of deterioration. However, clinical evidence suggests that cholinesterase inhibitors provide significant benefits by improving function for clients and decreasing burden for caregivers (Geldmacher, 2007).

Tacrine (Cognex) was the first centrally acting, noncompetitive acetylcholinesterase inhibitor to be created. The liver rapidly absorbs and metabolizes tacrine, making it vulnerable to toxicity and requiring ongoing monitoring of liver function, especially the level of alanine aminotransferase (ALT), every week for the first 18 weeks of use of tacrine. Because of the potential for liver toxicity, tacrine is no longer used. Rivastigmine (Exelon), galantamine (Reminyl), and donepezil (Aricept) are more widely used cholinesterase inhibitors. Rivastigmine now has an FDA warning because of cardiac complications noted in two large clinical trials. The most common drug is donepezil. In some people, donepezil delays the progression of dementia for 6 to 12 months. It has a longer duration than tacrine, does not require monitoring of liver function, and is administered only once a day at bedtime. Clients usually start with 5 mg/day, increasing to 10 mg/day after 4 to 6 weeks. Higher doses may not help all clients, and donepezil has an increased risk of cholinergic side effects (nausea, diarrhea,

insomnia). Donepezil can cause irregular heartbeats in clients with heart conditions (Sunderland et al., 2004). See Chapter 16 as well.

> **Think About It 31.2**
> A client with AD was initially prescribed tacrine. However, his physician has discontinued use of tacrine because of possible liver problems and has ordered donepezil. Develop a teaching plan for the client's family about donepezil, including the differences between it and tacrine.

Memantine has a detectable effect on cognitive function and functional decline measured at 6 months in people with moderate to severe AD (McShane et al., 2006). Twenty milligrams a day seems to prevent neurodegenerative changes (Sunderland et al., 2004). Other drugs thought to have some neuroprotective promise (discussed earlier) for people with early signs or family history of AD are anti-inflammatory medications such as ibuprofen; statins (for lipid control); antioxidants, particularly vitamin E; and ginkgo biloba. However no evidence of the effectiveness of any of these medications is available.

Psychosocial Interventions

Because of dementia's grim prognosis, clients and family need support from the interdisciplinary team to endure the shock of its initial diagnosis. They also need guidance for the future. In early stages, clients may need emotional support to deal with their fear, grief, depression, and cognitive losses. Caregivers need progressive help from professionals to deal with their own exhaustion, depression, and frustration. Family needs to participate in care planning and receive education about available assistance with the physical care they render.

Psychoeducational approaches have been shown to enhance caregivers' coping (Hepburn et al., 2003, 2007). Although perceived caregiver burden may not change significantly, psychosocial interventions are associated with significant reduction in caregiver psychological distress, as well as improved caregiver knowledge and client mood (Brodaty et al., 2003; Farran et al., 2004). These data are vital because enhanced caregiver coping and self-care may help delay or prevent institutionalization of clients with dementia, as well as caregiver morbidity. See Evidence-Based Practice Spotlight 31.2.

> **Checkpoint Questions**
> **9.** What is the hallmark pathologic feature of AD?
> **10.** What is the second most common form of dementia?
> **11.** What hereditary disease is associated with dementia?
> **12.** Which class of drugs has been proven to be moderately successful in slowing the cognitive decline of dementia?

EVIDENCE-BASED PRACTICE SPOTLIGHT 31.2

Interventions for Cognitive Disorders

Disorders/ Behavior	Support for Treatment	Positive Effects— Consistent Evidence	Inconsistent Evidence—Unproven	Comments
Delirium	Evidence-based treatments	*Psychosocial:* Expert consensus guidelines support individual and environmental comfort measures to manage agitation	Not enough controlled studies to show psychosocial interventions as consistently effective	Treatment consists of removing the underlying cause of delirium
		Pharmacologic: Haloperidol, Ativan		Haloperidol and Ativan are effective in treating psychotic symptoms and agitation for short-term use only.
Dementia	Evidence-based treatments	*Psychosocial Individual:* Sensory enhancement/ relaxation, social contact, behavior therapy, structured activities, environmental modifications, music therapy	Validation therapy	Individual psychosocial interventions based on expert consensus guidelines, level C Randomized trials, level B
		Caregiver: Support and psychoeducation		Meta-analysis, level A
		Pharmacologic Cholinesterase inhibitors: donepezil (Aricept), rivastigmine (Exelon) NMDA receptor antagonist: Memantine (Namenda)	Statins Antioxidants Anti-inflammatories Vitamins such as B_{12}, B_6, and folate	Best for early stage; tacrine (Cognex) rarely used because of hepatic effects. Galantamine (Reminyl) less used because of cardiac effects. Best for midstage; reduces memory loss and may improve function, but does not change the course of the illness. If memory unchanged after 6 months, treatment is successful.
		Antipsychotics: typical: haloperidol; atypical: olanzapine, risperidone, quetiapine		There is midlevel but no strong evidence to support off-label use of atypical antipsychotics for dementia-related agitation/ psychosis. All atypical agents increase risk of death in elderly; olanzapine and risperidone increase risk of stroke for elderly.
	Promising treatments		Ginkgo biloba	
Specific considerations based on type of dementia				Treatment varies slightly with the type of dementia. For vascular dementia, agents that treat the underlying cause (statins, antihypertensives) may prevent further deterioration. Antipsychotics should not be used for Lewy body dementia.

APPLYING THE NURSING PROCESS

Dementia

▲ ASSESSMENT

The first step in determining nursing approaches to management is assessment. Clients require screening for any underlying, treatable physical problems that accentuate or are comorbid with dementia. Any condition in Box 31.3 can confound diagnosis. All potentially reversible and treatable causes must be ruled out before a diagnosis is made. Doing so necessitates extensive history taking, thorough physical assessment (including neurologic and mental status examinations), and diagnostic testing (Assessment Tool 31.2). If screening procedures reveal treatable illnesses, action should be initiated to resolve them. Treating underlying illnesses expedites recovery from any delirium, improves overall health and delays further decline, and eliminates symptoms that can obscure dementia and thus prevent timely diagnosis. Once clients have been evaluated and treated for underlying medical conditions, nurses can proceed with assessment of cognitive functioning.

Behavior

Nurses assess various components of behavior and function (Assessment Tool 31.3). A functional assessment with a screening tool that measures not only physical ADLs but also instrumental ADLs (IADLs) can be useful for determining the level of impairment and degree of assistance needed. An example is the Functional Assessment Questionnaire (FAQ).

Assessment of the client's ability to perform ADLs is one of the most important parameters in the detection of dementia. Clients may have minimal to no insight about when decline in cognition and function or behavioral changes began. Family must be involved in supplying information because they may be

---

BOX 31.3 Differential Diagnosis for Dementia

- Drug withdrawal (benzodiazepines, alcohol, opioids, cocaine)
- Endocrine disturbance (thyroid disorder, Cushing's syndrome, Addison's disease)
- Heavy metal toxicity (lead, mercury, arsenic)
- Infections (HIV/AIDS, neurosyphilis, viral hepatitis, systemic)
- Bowel impactions
- Metabolic disruption (fluid and electrolyte imbalances, hepatic encephalopathy, uremia, porphyria, hypoxia, hypotension, chronic obstructive pulmonary disease)
- Neoplastic
- Neurologic disease (Parkinson's disease)
- Nutritional (deficiencies in vitamin B_{12}, folate, or thiamine; malnutrition)
- Pain
- Seizures
- Sensory deficits or overload
- Trauma

---

more reliable sources. Nurses question clients and family in a nonjudgmental, nonthreatening way and recognize that denial is common. Clients may try to cover up gaps in memory, and family may rationalize disruptive behavior as "quirks."

Mental Status

Several tools to assess mental status are available (Assessment Tool 31.4). An example is the Short, Portable Mental Status Questionnaire (SPMSQ) developed by Pfeiffer. The MMSE remains the gold standard for assessment of memory. Its excellent reliability and validity make it widely used in various clinical settings, including primary care. Scores below 23 indicate a need for further evaluation in high school graduates; scores below 26 should prompt further investigation in those with higher education levels. Although the MMSE does not assess abstract thinking, nurses can assess it by asking clients to interpret a proverb such as "a rolling stone gathers no moss." Failure to adequately explain such a saying may indicate problems with abstract reasoning, concentration, or executive functioning. However, nurses need to consider first whether clients would be familiar with a particular proverb based on age and culture.

Another useful and simple clinical tool is the Clock Draw Test, first developed by Shuman in 1986. Nurses ask clients to draw a clock, put numbers on it, and put the hands at a specified time (Figure 31.7). This simple test of executive functioning, visuospatial skills, and general organization can measure cognition over time (Levenson et al., 2005).

Perceptual Problems

Nurses may discover perceptual problems by observing behavior and exploring odd or unusual comments of clients. Family members may provide invaluable associated data. They can contribute information about unusual behavior and relate any episodes of hallucinations (eg, a client verbalized fears and concerns about seeing bugs that no one else saw).

Orientation

Nurses must ask such questions about orientation to person, place, time, and date skillfully so as not to insult clients' intelligence. They phrase questions conversationally or inform clients that some basic questions are part of the examination. Nurses also should ask family members if clients become more restless, agitated, or confused in the evening (sundowning).

Memory

Incidents evoking remote memory usually are easy to elicit from clients, but more recent events may prove problematic. Nurses can assess recent memory by evaluating responses of clients to questions involving events of the previous hour, day, or week. Use of the MMSE, described previously, can provide ongoing objective data about short-term memory.

Family

Family members, as indicated previously, are vital resources for historical data. They often can provide much information

ASSESSMENT TOOL 31.2

Screening Tests for Dementia

Test	Clinical Importance
1. White blood cell count with differential	1. Infection
2. Complete blood count with differential; hemoglobin (Hb)	2. Anemia and hematocrit (Hct)
3. Erythrocyte sedimentation rate (ESR)	3. Infection or vasculitis
4. Urine examination and toxicology test	4. Urine examination and toxicology test
a. Sugar and acetone	a. Diabetes
b. Leukocytes	b. Infection
c. Barbiturates and other toxic substances	c. Toxicity
d. Albumin	d. Renal failure
e. Porphyria screen	e. Renal failure
f. Heavy metals (lead, mercury, manganese, aluminum, arsenic); can be done as serum test as well	f. Heavy metal intoxication
5. Serum tests	5. Serum tests
a. Blood urea nitrogen	a. Renal failure
b. Creatinine	b. Diabetes, hypoglycemia
c. Glucose	c. Thyroid disease
d. Triiodothyronine (T_3), thyroxine (T_4)	d. Evaluation for imbalance, including Na^1, K^1, Ca^{21}, Cl^2, PO_4; parathyroid-induced changes in calcium, phosphate
e. Electrolytes	
f. Mg^1, Br^1	e. Bromides still are present in some common drugs and overuse may inadvertently lead to toxicity
g. Copper	f. Wilson's disease
h. Serum folate level, ferritin, iron	g. Nutritional problems, thiamin deficiency, iron deficiency
i. Vitamin B_{12}	
j. Aspartate aminotransferase (AST)	h. Dementia, delirium, malnutrition
k. Bilirubin	i. Increased in hepatic disease
l. Venereal Disease Research Laboratory (VDRL) or rapid plasma reagin (RPR)	j. Increased in hepatic disease
m. Drug levels—specific search for evidence of drugs	k. Syphilis
n. Human immunodeficiency virus (HIV)	l. Barbiturate, ethanol (ETOH), other drug overdose
o. Lactate dehydrogenase (LDH)	m. Present in AIDS dementia
p. Parat hyroid hormone	n. Elevated in myocardial infarction, hepatic disease, and CNS damage
6. Routine radiographs	o. Associated with a variety of cognitive disorders
a. Chest	6. Routine radiographs
b. Skull	a. Infection, heart failure
7. Electroencephalogram (EEG)	b. Evidence of increased intracranial pressure, fractures
8. Computed tomography (CT) scan	7. Ictal phenomena
9. Magnetic resonance imaging (MRI)	8. Brain tumor, subdural hematoma, infection, hemorrhage
10. Spinal tap—cerebrospinal fluid (CSF)	9. More sensitive for detection of vascular changes than CT
11. Ultrasound—carotid or Doppler	10. Infection, hemorrhage
12. Single-photon emission computed tomography (SPECT)	11. Detect vascular dementia
	12. Highlights brain activity, helps in differential diagnosis of dementias

Compiled from Sadock, B. J., & Sadock, V. A. (2007). *Kaplan & Sadock's synopsis of psychiatry* (10th ed.). Philadelphia, PA: Lippincott Williams & Wilkins; and from Gauthier, S. (2007). *Clinical diagnosis and management of Alzheimer's Disease* (3rd ed.). Boca Raton, FL: Abingdon Oxon Taylor Francis.

ASSESSMENT TOOL 31.3

Questionnaire for Dementia

Subjective Data

Behavioral Changes (Often Asked of the Family)

Is there a change in behavior? If so,
a. How does the present behavior differ from former behavior?
b. When was this change in behavior first recognized?

Emotional Changes

- Are any of the following present: depression, anxiety, paranoia, agitation, grandiosity, confabulation?
- Does the client have insight into the fact that "things are not right?"
- Is the client complaining of many physical ailments for which there are no bases?
- Are certain previous personality traits becoming predominant or exaggerated?

Social Changes

- Is the client exhibiting embarrassingly loud and jocular behavior?
- Is there sexual acting-out beyond the bounds of propriety?
- Has the client shown signs of short temper, irritability, or aggressiveness?
- Is there an increasing inability to make social judgments?

Intellectual Behavior

- Has the ability to remember recent events decreased?
- Has the ability to problem solve decreased? (This might be especially apparent in the work or job area.)
- Do new environments or even old environments result in the client's disorientation?
- Is it difficult for the client to carry out complex motor skills? Do his or her efforts result in many errors?
- Are any of the following language problems present?:
  - Has the client's language changed?
  - Does the client's language ramble and wander from the point of the conversation?
  - Is the point of the conversation never clearly stated?
  - Is there difficulty comprehending complex material?
  - Does the client have trouble remembering names of people and objects?
  - Does the client have difficulty writing?

Functional Capacity

- Are there any changes in the client's ability to perform ADLs?
- Is there difficulty transferring or ambulating?
- Is there difficulty bathing, dressing, or grooming?
- Is there difficulty eating or toileting?
- Are there any changes in the client's ability to perform instrumental ADLs?

- Is the client able to make a grocery list, shop for food, and handle money?
- Is the client able to use the telephone?
- Can the client prepare a meal and complete housekeeping tasks?

Objective Data

Level of Consciousness

Is the client confused, sleepy, withdrawn, adynamic, apathetic?

Appearance

Is there decreased personal hygiene?

Attention

- Does the client have decreased ability to repeat digits after the interviewer?
- Do other stimuli in the environment easily distract the client from the interviewer?
- Does the client focus on only one of the stimuli in the environment, and is he or she unable to turn attention from the one stimulus?

Language

- Outflow of words decreases.
- Patterns of repetitive, tangential, or concrete speech appear.
- Writing skills decrease more rapidly than the spoken word.

Memory

Test the client's ability to remember four unrelated words and recent events. (Confabulation and anger often will be used by the client to move the interviewer away from questions related to memory.)

Constructional Ability

The client is instructed to copy a series of line drawings; the client often is unable to do this, or the ability to do so declines dramatically over time.

Cortical Function

- The client's ability to perform arithmetic is faulty and reveals many errors.
- Proverb interpretation—usually, the client gives only a concrete interpretation of the proverb.
- Similarities—the client often denies similarities between two objects and instead gives a concrete answer. For example, when asked, "What is the similarity between a tiger and a cat?" the client may reply, "One is small and one is large. There is no similarity."

ASSESSMENT TOOL 31.4

Testing for Cognitive Deficits

Focus of Test	Name of Test	What Is Measured	Analysis Potential
Intelligence, verbal performance	Wechsler Adult Intelligence Scale—Revised (WAIS-R)	Crystallized and fluid intelligence	Notes if client can pay attention and use memory
Memory	Wechsler Memory Scale–Revised California Verbal Learning Test		Alzheimer's Sensitive in early dementia If single finding, may indicate amnestic disorder
Language skills	Boston Diagnostic Aphasia Examination	Aphasia subtest—word-finding ability (common in dementia)	Alzheimer's Single finding may indicate focal deficit
Conceptualization	WAIS-R Similarities Subtest	Abstract versus concrete thinking	
Visuospatial skills	Benton Visual Retention Test Block Design subtest of the WAIS-R		Alzheimer's
Attention	Digit Span Subtest of the WAIS-R		Single finding may indicate delirium disorder, focal frontal lesion

Zarit, S. H., & Zarit, J. M. (2007). *Mental disorders in older adults: Fundamentals of assessment and treatment.* New York, NY: Guilford Press.

concerning a client's ability to carry out ADLs and IADLs. Interactions between family and client during the interview also can reveal the condition of the client's social skills and family dynamics.

Nurses must assess family members, especially caregivers, for signs of stress or burnout. Although this issue might not be pertinent during early stages of dementia, it becomes paramount as clients progressively degenerate and demands for physical care mount. It also becomes a factor as the role of "caregiver" increasingly becomes dominant, while the roles of spouse, companion, confidante, and lover fade. Loss of these roles can result in loneliness and depression. Early detection of caregiver and family stress may help prevent elder abuse and neglect, preserve family relationships, and prevent caregiver morbidity.

Education

Nurses must determine the needs of clients and family for information and instruction about the illness, its management, and support. Caregivers can provide better assistance when they know what to expect as the disease progresses and how to address common problems. Burnout, guilt, and frustration may be ameliorated when family members understand the commonality of and how to handle their feelings. Use of psychoeducational approaches has been demonstrated effective in enhancing family coping and reducing caregiver depression and anger (Coon et al., 2003; Hepburn et al., 2003).

▲ NURSING DIAGNOSES

There are as many nursing diagnoses for clients with dementia as there are possible symptoms. Although nursing diagnoses must reflect the uniqueness of each client, a plan of care might include the following (NANDA, 2007):

- Chronic Confusion related to cerebral degeneration
- Self-Care Deficit related to cognitive and motor impairments
- Risk for Injury related to cognitive and psychomotor impairments reducing ability to adapt to changing environment
- Caregiver Role Strain related to the ongoing and mounting needs of the client as evidenced by expressions of sadness, guilt, despair, and stress
- Interrupted Family Processes related to degenerative cerebral changes in a family member

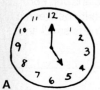   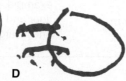

A   B   C   D

FIGURE 31.7 A useful and simple test of mental status is the Clock Draw Test. The example in A would be rated as excellent, whereas B would be good, C would be fair, and D would be poor.

▲ OUTCOME IDENTIFICATION AND PLANNING

Planning care for clients with dementia is most effective when family, clients, and team members collaborate to determine the most realistic goals. Those involved also should include measures that encourage family cohesiveness and stability. The family needs to decide what responsibilities different members can assume and what respite interventions they can initiate to prevent exhaustion. Major goals for the care of clients with dementia, organized according to the *Nursing Outcomes Classification (NOC)*, are as follows (Moorhead et al., 2008):

- **Health Maintenance:** The client's physical needs will be met.
- **Cognitive Orientation:** The client's environment will be safe and protected.
- **Distorted Thought Control:** The client will have infrequent episodes of agitation.
- **Caregiver Well-Being:** The caregivers will take measures to ensure adequate respite and find ongoing avenues for support.
- **Family Coping:** The client's caregivers and family will have psychosocial support and resources for respite care.

▲ IMPLEMENTATION

Interventions for clients with dementia and their families are numerous and range the entire holistic spectrum. Some common *Nursing Interventions Classification (NIC)* labels include, but are not limited to, **Caregiver Support, Coping Enhancement, Dementia Management, Environmental Management, Reality Orientation, Respite Care,** and **Support Group** (Bulechek et al., 2008).

Case in Point 31.1 describes nursing care for a client and family facing Alzheimer's disease.

Managing the Client's Health

Nursing actions facilitate optimal functioning and prevent further decline by promoting physical health, environmental stability, and emotional well-being. They also play an important role in caregiver teaching concerning appropriate care of the client in home settings. Because exogenous substances can initiate or exacerbate aberrant behavior, nurses must be sensitive to the response of clients to prescribed medications. In addition to knowing the side effects and toxic reactions of specific drugs

Case in Point 31.1

Betty's Story

Betty, 76 years old, lives with her daughter and son-in-law. She moved in with them 11 years ago, following the death of her husband. Betty has many friends and has stayed active. Her daughter Audrey and son-in-law Linc have accompanied Betty to a doctor's appointment.

Audrey reports to the nurse that she is concerned about her mother's behavior. "I'm not surprised that she forgot my birthday last week because she's having difficulty recalling when she'll celebrate hers! Lately she's forgotten other things, like bingo games. She's also been avoiding her weekly bridge game with friends, telling me she's too tired or doesn't feel like it." Audrey reports that Betty, normally an early riser and fastidious, has been staying in bed late and spending days in her pajamas. "I asked her about this, thinking she wasn't feeling well. She told me angrily, 'Why can't I enjoy my old age? Why should I be busy every minute?'" Audrey relates that a few months ago, Betty got lost coming back from a grocery trip. After meandering over several back roads, it became clear that she was lost, and she called Linc for help. Upon questioning by the nurse, Betty states that she just wanted to go for a drive.

Betty undergoes physical, neurologic, mental status, and functional evaluations, a battery of laboratory tests, and a computed tomography scan. She uses some words inappropriately and scores 22 on the Mini-MSE. No other significant findings appear. The physician gives a diagnosis of dementia of Alzheimer's type: late onset, uncomplicated. Because the disease is in an early stage, she prescribes donepezil (Aricept).

The nurse is discussing with the family the prognosis and needs for future care. Betty is very upset. Initially, she denies her problem but then cries and admits that she has been concerned about her mental functioning. Discussion centers on the need for support and that eventually Audrey and Linc may need help for Betty to remain at home. All agree that Betty should remain as active as possible and continue bridge and cognitively stimulating activities.

Key Assessment Findings

- Impaired memory; forgetfulness
- Disturbed executive function (inability to find way home from grocery store)
- Cognitive deficits
- Decreased involvement in social activities (bridge games)
- Below normal score on Mini-MSE
- New diagnosis—dementia of Alzheimer's type: late onset
- Therapy with donepezil (Aricept)

(continues on page 686)

Case in Point 31.1 (continued)

Betty's Story

Nursing Diagnosis: Anticipatory Grieving related to recent diagnosis of dementia as evidenced by changes in current status, initial denial of problems, and reaction to diagnosis

NOC: Grief Resolution: The client will verbalize feelings about diagnosis and potential decline in functional ability.

NOC: Psychosocial Adjustment: Life Change: The family will set realistic goals, maintain productivity, and use effective coping strategies.

NIC: Grief Work Facilitation

- Assist the client to identify and express fears and feelings. Help her deal with her initial reaction. Listen carefully and empathetically. Communicate acceptance. Include significant others (Figure A). *Encouraging the client to express feelings and listening empathetically help her release sadness and fear. They also help her to feel that others care.*
- Instruct the family about the phases of grieving; support the client's progression through them. *Loss of cognitive function is one of the most frightening changes a person can face. The family needs time to process their feelings.*
- Help the client identify existing coping strategies and consider new ones. Examples include living in the present, meditating, praying, and practicing deep breathing or relaxation. *Establishing a plan for stress management can help the client during times of fear and anxiety. Stress reduction techniques also may increase feelings of well-being.*

NIC: Anticipatory Guidance

- Assist the family to identify available resources. *Doing so reveals additional support. Options allow the family to find solutions for problems, which enhances feelings of control.*
- Rehearse techniques needed to cope with upcoming crises as appropriate. *Practicing techniques facilitates their use when needed.*

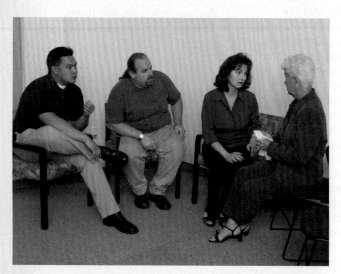

FIGURE A. The nurse encourages the client and family to share feelings about the diagnosis of AD and gives acceptance and support.

> 9/13/13: The client begins to verbalize feelings associated with her condition. The family discusses the reality of the situation and unresolved conflicts. They plan to share the news and ask for support from a few relatives and close friends. They also plan to seek solace from a spiritual advisor and to continue recreational and other enjoyable activities for as long as possible.
>
> B. Morita, RN

Nursing Diagnosis: Risk for Injury related to cognitive impairment as evidenced by progressive changes in memory and executive function

NOC: Personal Safety Behavior: The client will remain free from injury.

NOC: Safe Home Environment: The family will adjust the home as necessary to ensure it is in optimal condition to maintain safe and independent living for the client.

NIC: Environmental Management: Safety

- Identify danger areas and safety hazards in the home. Instruct the family to make garages and basements unavailable to the client because dangerous items often are stored there. Teach them to lock medications, poisons, cleaning agents, and other toxic fluids in secure containers or rooms. Ensure that doors leading outside are locked or have alarms installed. Instruct the family to secure windows and any doors on the upper floors of the home. *Decreasing cognitive skills increases the client's risk for injury. Keeping certain areas off-limits and the rest of the house safe and secure optimizes the client's freedom at home while protecting her.*
- Modify the environment to minimize hazards and risks. Plug electrical outlets and remove electrical items that pose hazards. Move the thermostat on the hot water heater to its lowest setting. Remove all electrical appliances from counters and control knobs from the stove and oven. *Making the home safer should give the family some peace of mind about the client's safety. Monitoring the home is the best intervention for maintaining safety. Interventions will help prevent accidental burns or fires.*
- Recommend appropriate protective and adaptive devices (Figure B). *Protective devices limit mobility or access to harm; adaptive devices increase environmental safety.*
- Provide emergency phone numbers; have the family keep them readily available. *Quick access is crucial during a crisis.*

Nursing Diagnosis: Chronic Confusion related to Alzheimer's disease as evidenced by memory impairment, forgetfulness, and client's statements about changes in mental functioning

NOC: Cognition: The client will exhibit adequate mental functioning with assistance.

Case in Point 31.1 (continued)

Betty's Story

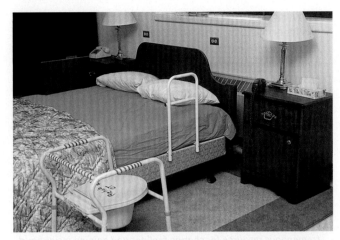

FIGURE B. The family installs guard rails along the client's bed to protect against falling or wandering at night. They place a commode in her bedroom as well so that she does not have to leave her room during sleep (and risk injury) if she develops the urge to eliminate.

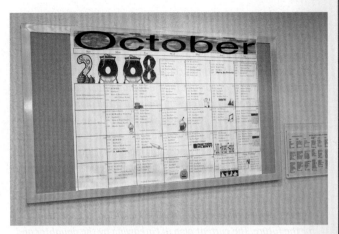

FIGURE C. The nurse works with the family to establish a calendar that lists all of the month's events so that they can be more organized while integrating the client's situation into their lifestyle. The month and year are displayed in large letters and numbers to reinforce time orientation for the client.

NIC: Dementia Management

- Control environmental stimulation. Help establish a calming atmosphere. Encourage the family to remove household clutter and to provide adequate lighting without glare. Create predictability and simplify choices. Assist the family to establish a daily routine for grooming, meals, and activities; teach them to ask relatives and friends to visit, but to do so one or two at a time. *Controlled stimulation will help the client feel secure at home. Simple choices and tasks that she can complete successfully prevent frustration and loss of self-esteem. Nonglare lighting is less disruptive and helps decrease perceptual difficulties. Limiting visitors allows the client to continue socializing but in a controlled way.*
- Introduce self when initiating contacts with the client; address her distinctly by name. Speak slowly in a clear, low, warm, and respectful tone of voice. *These measures prevent startling the client. Using her name helps reorient her as needed.*
- Use distraction, not confrontation, to manage behavioral problems. *Confrontation increases the client's frustration and stress.*
- Provide space for the client to pace or wander safely; provide finger foods if the client cannot sit and eat. *Providing space minimizes the risk of injury; finger foods can help promote adequate nutrition.*
- Encourage one-to-one and group activities geared to the client's cognitive abilities and interests. When giving directions, do so one at a time. *Limiting choices and activities minimizes overstimulation, which can increase anxiety. Individual simple directions prevent the client from becoming overwhelmed.*
- Use symbols to locate areas or important items. *Symbols may be easier for the client to comprehend than the written word.*

NIC: Cognitive Stimulation

- Orient the client to person, place, and time. Provide environmental memory cues. Cut out pictures from magazines and place them on cabinets and drawers to illustrate contents. Provide a large-print calendar in a conspicuous spot and record all appointments there (Figure C). Encourage the client to review the calendar daily. Reinforce and repeat information. *Environmental cues will help jog the client's memory and keep her as independent as possible for as long as possible. Repetition promotes awareness.*

> 10/7/13: The family participates in a thorough home evaluation and demonstrates substantially adequate lighting and handrails, use of personal alarm system, accessible assistive devices, and furniture arrangement to reduce risks. No injuries or problems have occurred since the initial visit. They also have posted emergency numbers and a hotline in key locations. The client is maintaining adequate cognitive function with assistance. She demonstrates only mild compromise in attentiveness, concentration, and cognitive orientation. She can identify self, place, and time and respond to cues.
>
> B. Morita, RN

Nursing Diagnosis: Decisional Conflict related to uncertainty about future health and resources

NOC: Decision Making: The family will verbalize appropriate plans for the future.

(continues on page 688)

Case in Point 31.1 (continued)

Betty's Story

NOC: Participation in Healthcare Decisions: The family will identify available support for achieving outcomes.

NIC: Decision–Making Support

- Establish communication; facilitate articulation for goals of care. *Communication is important for the therapeutic relationship; knowledge of goals facilitates an individualized plan of care.*
- Provide information as requested. Describe options available for care, including full-time nursing at home, adult day care centers, nursing homes, and other long-term facilities (Figure D). Help the family explore the advantages or disadvantages of each option. Supply all information as requested but avoid portraying a hopeless prognosis. Respect the client's right to receive or not receive information. *Family members need information so they can plan for the future. The current plan of caregiving by the daughter and son-in-law alone will not be feasible if the client needs more than their resources allow. The client still may be in denial; the health care team needs to respect her right to not receive information.*
- Help the client clarify values and make important decisions while cognitive function is high. Encourage her to provide advance directives. *Facilitating decisions now helps ensure that others can carry out the client's wishes if she cannot make necessary legal decisions.*

Nursing Diagnosis: Interrupted Family Processes related to changes in client's health status as evidenced by progressive cognitive changes and changes in usual roles

NOC: Family Coping: The family will demonstrate positive coping measures to deal with changes.

NIC: Family Process Maintenance

- Identify effects of role changes on family processes. Promote family cohesion. Help family members, including the client, identify their feelings about role and health status changes. Help them resolve any guilt feelings. Identify effective coping mechanisms;

encourage their use as family adjusts to changes. Discuss strategies for normalizing family life. *Open communication about the effects of AD will help family members. The client may feel guilt about not being able to help more or becoming a "burden" on the family; caregivers may have resentment about increased responsibilities.*

- Minimize disruptions by facilitating family routines and rituals. *Encouraging normal activities reduces feelings of guilt or anxiety related to the client's current condition.*
- Discuss existing social support mechanisms; assist the family to use them. Help them resolve any conflicts; suggest attending an Alzheimer's support group. Identify home care needs and how these might be incorporated into the family lifestyle (Figures E and F). *Helping the family resolve feelings and identify appropriate coping behaviors will decrease stress. Support groups are a tremendous resource for sharing feelings and gaining insight and help. Incorporating home care needs minimizes disruptions.*

Nursing Diagnosis: Risk for Caregiver Role Strain related to increasing requirements for care as evidenced by progressive nature of disorder

NOC: Caregiver Stressors: The caregiver will identify need for assistance in caring for her mother.

NOC: Caregiver Emotional Health and Caregiver Physical Health: The daughter will obtain essential respite and support to maintain her own functioning while caring for her mother.

- Determine the caregiver's level of knowledge and acceptance of role. Provide practical support. Explore her reaction and help her identify stressors, tasks, or behaviors that are most frustrating or anxiety producing. Help her develop a plan for managing them. Provide support for her decisions. Give information about the disease and local support groups. *Helping the caregiver become aware of her feelings, strengths, the progressive nature of AD, and available supports will empower her to manage the increasing demands of caregiving while protecting her emotional state. Thinking through and planning ahead will help her manage responsibilities.*
- Teach techniques to improve the security of the client. *Techniques for client security reduce the risk of injury to the client and caregiver.*
- Explore with the caregiver how she is coping; teach stress management techniques and health care maintenance strategies to sustain her physical and mental health. *Determining coping and providing instruction about stress management and health care maintenance strategies enhance her ability to provide the necessary care.*
- Give encouragement to the caregiver during setbacks for the client. *Setbacks can promote guilt, frustration, and anxiety. Encouragement helps preserve the caregiver's self-esteem.*

NIC: Emotional Support

- Provide emotional support. Make supportive or empathetic statements. *Emotional support helps to reduce feelings of anxiety in stressful situations.*

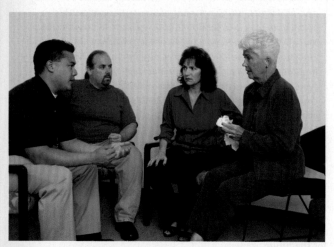

FIGURE D. The nurse discusses various options for short-term and long-term care with the family.

Case in Point 31.1 (continued)

Betty's Story

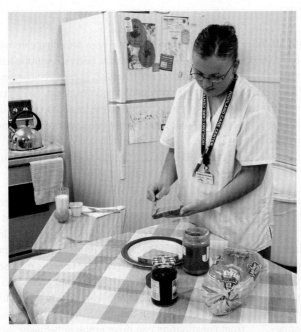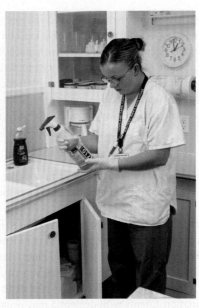

FIGURES E AND F. The family arranges for ongoing visits from a home health aide, who provides assistance with meals and housecleaning. Such help is often necessary to account for the extra demands that the client's illness places on the entire family.

- Encourage the caregiver to get adequate rest and to maintain her own physical, emotional, and spiritual health. Help her recognize that caregiving is stressful. Encourage her to express feelings of anxiety, anger, or sadness. Encourage her not to feel ashamed or guilty if she experiences impatience, frustration, sadness, or anger. *Deep breathing, meditation, and visualization, as well as physical exercise and adequate rest, can help the caregiver manage feelings of anxiety and stress. Finding sources for personal comfort and happiness will help her maintain an identity separate from her caregiving role. She then can come to understand that these emotions are natural when caring for someone who may be unhappy, ungrateful, or difficult.*

NIC: Respite Care
- Monitor the caregiver's endurance. Establish a plan for respite care. Encourage her to set realistic limits on what and how much she can do. Counsel her to avoid becoming isolated and to accept help from others. *The caregiver cannot perform total full-time care alone.*
- Coordinate volunteers for in-home services. Arrange for substitute caregivers. Identify community resources for respite care or other family members or friends who can regularly relieve the caregiver for a few hours at a time (Figure G). *Respite is essential to prevent burnout, which is common among full-time caregivers, especially those who are socially isolated or have no relief from their duties.*

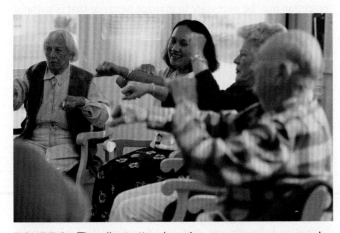

FIGURE G. The client attends a day program once a week so that her daughter has an outlet for respite care.

12/16/13: *The family has established plans that assist them to manage their new reality. They involve a cousin and a nephew to provide respite care 2 days a week. They arrange for a nursing home health aide to visit once a week to assist with various tasks and for Betty to attend an adult day care facility once a week. They continue to enjoy normal family routines and attend support meetings. The daughter reports mild compromise in life satisfaction and sense of control. She verbalizes no feelings of resentment and says that she can currently balance her caregiving responsibilities.*

B. Morita, RN

(continues on page 690)

Case in Point 31.1 (continued)

Betty's Story

Epilogue

Nine months have passed since Betty was first diagnosed with AD. Since then, Audrey and Linc have been providing care with support from family, friends, the local Alzheimer's association, and health services. However, in the past month, Betty's condition has deteriorated. She has become increasingly confused, with mood fluctuations, and cannot dress or wash herself. She also has become incontinent of urine, mostly at night. Audrey reports, "She tried to make tea yesterday and left the stove on. Sometimes, she doesn't recognize me." Two days ago, Betty got out of bed during the night, fell, and fractured her hip. She was admitted to the local hospital for treatment. Linc says, "My wife is so exhausted. Her mother needs so much care. I don't think Audrey can handle this anymore. We're meeting with a social worker to make a decision about moving Mom to a nursing home."

that clients receive, nurses also must be alert to possible drug interactions, and ensure correct administration by a responsible caregiver.

Nurses assess for any symptoms of physical illness. Prompt recognition and appropriate intervention may stop an episodic illness from becoming comorbid, or a comorbid illness from accelerating mental dysfunction. Nurses and caregivers pay particular attention to nutrition and hydration, as well as to bowel and bladder elimination. Clients with dementia may resist or neglect eating, and poor hydration usually accompanies poor diet. Nurses and caregivers need to offer foods and fluids throughout the day. Giving food in small portions or offering finger foods may increase the likelihood of eating.

Constipation or impaction from insufficient bulk or water can have serious consequences if not treated promptly. Clients may be unable to articulate feelings of fullness; caregivers should keep a record of bowel movements to monitor regularity. Insufficient fluids can lead to urinary stasis and urinary tract infections. Monitoring fluid intake so that clients receive at least 2,000 mL/day (unless contraindicated by renal or cardiac disease) helps prevent infection and maintain health.

Enhancing Sensory Capabilities

For clients with trouble interpreting the environment, sensory aids, such as eyeglasses and hearing aids, can be instrumental in helping them feel more in control. Nurses can provide reading material in large type, if necessary, and speak to clients directly and carefully to further maximize ability to process sensory input. Caregivers also need to be aware that sensory disturbances are not limited to sight and hearing but also may involve perception of pain and temperature. Thus, caregivers must take precautions with hot liquids and bath water to avoid burning clients. Diminished or altered pain perception further emphasizes the need for surveillance by staff of the client's physical condition.

Meeting the Client's Physical Needs

The ability of clients to care for themselves decreases as the severity of dementia increases. The health care team and family need to reevaluate continually the client's capacity for self-care.

Caregivers can help by enhancing the environment to facilitate the limited ability of clients to perform ADLs and IADLs and by fulfilling unmet needs themselves. Sometimes, clients display aberrant behavior because of unmet needs. An underlying medical problem may be undetected, or clients may be in pain. As ability to communicate decreases, caregivers and health care staff need to observe clients carefully to try to discern the meaning behind their actions. Something as basic as discomfort from constipation can drive problem behavior, which may subside after a basic need has been met.

Encouraging Appropriate Behaviors

Clients with dementia often cannot change their behavior. Therefore, the most successful nursing intervention may be to change what clients experience. Consideration of the client's experiences and remote memories can aid in restructuring the environment to make it less formidable and frightening for the client. It is normal to seek the comfort of home when confused or frightened. As the client's condition deteriorates, home will be associated with 40- to 60-year-old memories, and the newest decorating and technology will likely confuse and frighten the client, possibly eliciting a fight-or-flight response. Some progressive technologies, such as wireless phones and televisions without dials, are not possible to avoid. Pharmacologic intervention may be necessary to manage behavior that is harmful to clients, their family, or the health care team.

Modifying the Environment

Clients with dementia face multiple dangers resulting from impaired cognitive abilities. Safety concerns include falls, poisoning, wandering and getting lost, and injury to self or others from dangerous objects. Starting fires and getting burned also are fairly common. All of these situations are worsened by the client's inability to respond quickly to emergencies. Environmental modification can be the key to managing behavior and keeping clients safe. Pathologic changes in the brain decrease the ability of clients to interpret the environment accurately. Many clients overreact, especially when multiple cues bombard them. Decreasing noise, choices, pain, and overstimulating interactions can help clients maintain stable, appropriate behaviors. Simply

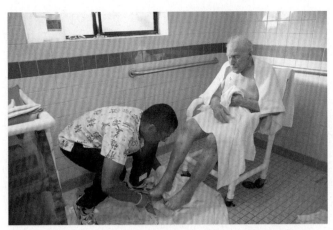

FIGURE 31.8 Bathing and hygiene can be activities during which clients with dementia become particularly agitated, fearful, or confused. Care providers should take measures to preserve safety and comfort, such as ensuring the client's warmth and performing a sitting shower bath to minimize symptoms.

controlling environmental light may decrease hallucinations or illusions. Instituting routines and simplifying choices help easily confused clients.

Times when personal care is being given, such as bathing, seem especially to agitate clients with dementia. There often is a way to modify the environment to provide positive experiences for clients. Sometimes, changing the site of the bath or giving a bed bath instead of a shower or tub bath in the bathroom of the home or the institution is helpful (Figure 31.8). Adapting bath time to the client's usual schedule, rather than the institutional routines, may be helpful (Thiru-Chelvam, 2004).

The goals of care for people with dementia are to enhance function and prevent further decline. Preservation of function requires nurses to encourage clients to perform their own ADLs, rather than to do these tasks for them. Cueing and prompting are two strategies designed to preserve functioning. For example, a nurse might put toothpaste on a toothbrush and hand it to the client as a cue to brush the teeth. The nurse may lay out clothing in the order in which the client should put it on.

Prompting involves verbal step-by-step directions, but only as much direction as clients need. Such interventions provide assessment data as well.

Enhancing environmental cues may be beneficial for clients. Clocks and calendars strategically placed may help keep clients oriented. Reality orientation, sensitively applied, can be beneficial, but care must be taken to avoid frustrating clients and causing more problems. Although validation therapy has not been found consistently useful for those with cognitive impairment (Neal & Briggs, 2003), validating and attending to the feeling behind the content of communication is a vital component of psychiatric nursing care.

Management of disruptive behaviors exhibited by clients, such as wandering, attempting to leave, entering others' rooms, and hoarding items, can challenge nurses as well as family caregivers. At times, efforts to intervene in such behaviors seem only to result in further agitation and even aggression (Challenging Behaviors 31.2). Formal research into nonpharmacologic interventions has been hindered by the need for a common language and a systematic approach (Cohen-Mansfield, 2003). Although such investigations are now being conducted to determine which interventions are consistently most helpful, empirical evidence suggests a multimodal, individualized approach to be most effective (Werner, 2003). All behavior has meaning and should be viewed as an attempt by clients to communicate a need. Therefore, attempting to discern and respond to the need expressed by clients may help calm them. For example, if a client is wandering, the nurse should walk with her (Figure 31.9). If a client is taking clothing from another person's room, the nurse should attempt to distract him by giving him laundry to sort and fold. The more nurses know about their clients' former routines, occupations, and lifestyles, the more individualized care can be. Developing creative and flexible interventions and providing safe alternatives to potentially harmful behaviors is a key to less disruptive behavior. To help guide care, evidence-based practice guidelines for nonpharmacologic management of agitated behaviors are available at http://www.dissemination-core@ iuiowa.edu (McGonigal-Kenney & Schutte, 2004).

Challenging Behaviors 31.2

The Client Who Is Disruptive

Situation: Your assigned client is an 81-year-old woman with Alzheimer's disease. She has been wandering in and out of other client rooms, taking their clothing and belongings. When you attempt to redirect her, she yells "Get out of my way. I am trying to do my work" and takes a swing at you.

Your Potential Feelings: Fear, frustration, surprise

What Is Going On? The client cannot perceive reality and may believe she is home and that the clothing belongs to her or a

family member. She may think you are an intruder or are attempting to harm her.

Strategy: Step back, literally and figuratively, and determine what the client is attempting to communicate through her behavior. Formulate a response based on your assessment.

Nurse Action/Communication: You might say, "I have some laundry I need to put away. Can you come help me sort and fold it?" Walk with her to her room and provide her with some towels to fold.

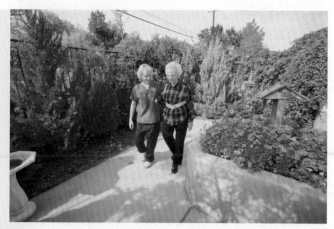

FIGURE 31.9 Some nursing homes and long-term care facilities have outdoor areas where nurses, visitors, and health care personnel can walk with clients who have dementia and are pacing or wandering.

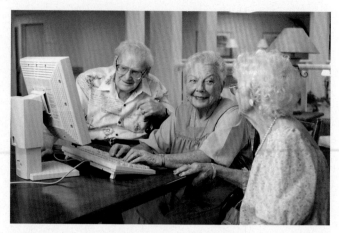

FIGURE 31.10 Adult day care centers can provide respite outlets for family members who have to work or need a reprieve from the ongoing work involved in preserving the health and safety of clients with dementia. They also may provide a socialization outlet, particularly for clients with mild to moderate problems.

Those caring for clients with cognitive disorders can monitor their interactions with them. Usually, caregivers with a calm demeanor have more success handling or interacting with clients manifesting problems. An attentive, gentle approach is especially helpful when personal care is required. In fact, Werezak and Morgan's (2003) investigations led them to suggest that the psychosocial environment is the most important element of care for people with dementia.

At times, there may seem to be no way to resolve the emotional frustration, agitation, or outbursts of clients who are angry with their environment and those in it. Caregivers might find it beneficial to redirect or distract clients. They can do so by asking to see personal items, such as photographs, and then talking about illustrated family members and life events (Therapeutic Communication 31.1).

Performing Pharmacologic Interventions

Cholinesterase inhibitors are moderately successful at slowing the cognitive decline of dementia (Birks, 2008; Birks et al., 2000; Birks & Harvey, 2006). Health care teams must determine which medication is best for each client and educate family members about dosages, schedules, and possible side effects (Declercq, 2009). Team members also must take responsibility for assessing the client's response and any possible side effects.

Preserving the Family Unit

Family members must be prepared for the personal toll that their new role as caregivers may take. Nurses can provide information concerning creative ways to care for loved ones, including providing counseling and information about respite care. Day care for clients is one possibility that allows relatives to rest from their extensive caregiving activities and allows them to continue with their own daily routines and responsibilities (Figure 31.10). Through day care, a spouse or child may be able to retain a job and income and have the energy to care for the client during evening and weekend hours. Some communities have overnight respite care to give the caregiver welcomed "downtime."

Family support groups and individual family counseling may help some families experiencing stress or having difficulty coping. As previously noted, one of the most effective interventions is to educate family members about the necessary skills of caregiving. Nurses empower families when they work with relatives to increase their problem-solving skills. Showing family members that they have options and linking them to community-based services are tremendous contributions.

Although many families wish to keep their loved ones at home as long as possible, all must recognize that long-term care is an option. Only the family can make this decision, but professional care providers should tactfully raise this issue occasionally.

▲ EVALUATION

Outcomes for clients may focus less on improving cognition and more on maintaining current functioning for as long as possible and on successful adaptations by clients and family to the ongoing decline. When evaluation of the plan of care reveals that interventions are no longer effective or feasible, the health care team and family (and clients, if possible) need to devise different interventions. Indicators of an effective care plan include the following:

- The client's physical needs are met.
- The client is well nourished and well hydrated.
- The client does not sustain injuries.
- Episodes of wandering or agitation are infrequent and managed successfully.
- The caregiver reports satisfaction with his or her quality of life and has social supports and respite care options in place.

Therapeutic Communication 31.1

A Client with Dementia

Annie Tepsin, a 64-year-old woman with dementia, comes to the day care center three times a week. Today, Annie's husband tells Roy Smith, the nurse, that Annie was awake most of the previous night. After her husband leaves, Annie begins to follow Roy in and out of the day room, activity room, kitchen, and sunroom. Around 10:30 AM, she asks Roy, "Are we going to eat soon?"

INEFFECTIVE DIALOGUE	EFFECTIVE DIALOGUE
ROY: It's too early to eat, Annie. You eat at 11:30, just after ceramics.	ROY: It's too early to eat, Annie. Lunch is at 11:30, just after ceramics.
ANNIE: *(Walks with Roy out of the day room)* When will I eat? Do I eat soon?	ANNIE: *(Walks with Roy out of the day room)* When will I eat? Do I eat soon?
ROY: *(Looks at watch and shakes his head)* You don't eat until later. I have to go into the sunroom to work on the plants.	ROY: *(Stops, looks directly at Annie, and smiles)* Annie, you eat at lunch time, 1 hour from now. Let's go into the sunroom. You can help me water the plants. *(Remains patient with Annie, sensing that she is trying to express something other than her words)*
ANNIE: *(Follows Roy to the sunroom)* When will I eat?	
ROY: *(Sighs and continues to water the plants)* Annie, are you hungry?	ANNIE: *(Helps Roy bring plants to the sink in the sunroom)* When did you say I will eat?
ANNIE: NO! I'm not hungry! Why do you ask that?	ROY: *(Stops watering the plants, looks at Annie, and smiles)* Annie, are you hungry? *(Uses positive and "cueing" nonverbal behavior)*
ROY: *(Notices Annie's behavior is beginning to escalate and feels puzzled as to why she is getting upset)* Annie, go back to the other room and look at your memory book. *(Points to Annie's pocketbook)* It's in your purse. I'll walk you there. *(Walks Annie to the day room, sits her at a table and tells another nurse to keep an eye on Annie)*	ANNIE: NO! I'm not hungry! Why do you ask that? *(Gets louder)*
	ROY: *(Realizes Annie's behavior is beginning to escalate)* Annie, I remember seeing a picture of you in your garden. Would you show me that picture again? I think it's in your memory book in your purse. *(Points to Annie's pocketbook)* Would you show me the picture of you in your garden?
ANNIE: *(Sits at the table, looking confused and sad)*	ANNIE: *(Looks at her purse and then rummages through it and pulls out a little photo book)* You want to see my pictures?
	ROY: Yes, Let's go sit on the sofa and look at them. *(Goes over and sits down, patting the cushion for Annie to sit. Annie comes over and begins thumbing through the book, telling Roy about the pictures.)*

Reflection and Critical Thinking

- What types of communication did Annie exhibit in both scenarios? Assess the reason for Annie's repetitive speech. Why might she be more hungry, tired, or insecure this morning?
- What nonverbal cues did Roy give in the first scenario? How did these differ from his actions in the second scenario? What were the results of the differences?
- What methods of communication did Roy use in the second scenario that ultimately were more effective than those he used in the first?

AMNESTIC DISORDERS

Amnestic disorders include conditions with *short-term memory loss* as the hallmark. Memory deterioration is so great that it prevents clients from functioning at previous levels of social and occupational performance and seriously deters them from learning new information. They typically cannot recollect events as recent as 2 minutes earlier; they may have difficulty recalling events or knowledge that they formerly knew. Acuity of remote memory recall varies, and clients become adept at confabulation to hide deficits.

Brain damage leaves clients disoriented to time and place to some degree but not to personhood (APA, 2000). They have a superficiality of emotions that precludes deep ties with others. They frequently adopt a blandness of affect. Progression of symptomatology depends on the underlying etiology and its severity.

Classifications of amnestic disorders are listed in *DSM-IV-TR* Box 31.3. Like dementia, the symptomatologies share commonalities; etiologies are the differentiating factors.

Wernicke's syndrome and Korsakoff's syndrome co-occur so frequently that they present a classic picture and thus often are combined and referred to as Wernicke–Korsakoff syndrome. By itself, Wernicke's produces ataxia, confusion, and paralysis of some ocular motor muscles. Both syndromes result from compulsive ingestion of alcohol that supersedes nutritional intake (see Chap. 30). Indeed, this syndrome usually is found in 40- to 70-year-old clients with alcoholism and a history of steady and progressive alcohol intake. In time, they develop a vitamin B_1 (thiamin) deficiency that directly interferes with glucose production (the brain's main nutrient), resulting in symptomatology (Sadock & Sadock, 2007). Clients have great difficulty with recent memory, specifically learning *new* information. Because they cannot recall recent events, they fill in memory gaps with fabricated or imagined data (**confabulation**). This is truly a case of anterograde amnesia. Clients have no awareness of their memory defect, nor do they care.

The prognosis for people experiencing amnestic disorders varies greatly. As with other cognitive disorders, etiology determines duration and severity. With Wernicke–Korsakoff syndrome, administration of thiamin can help alleviate some ataxia. Generally, however, memory impairment remains.

Checkpoint Questions

13. What is the hallmark of amnestic disorders?

14. What is confabulation?

NURSE'S SELF-CARE

Nurses working with clients who have dementia may experience challenging feelings that arise from knowing there is, as yet, no cure for the ongoing cerebral degeneration. Those who work with clients who have dementia deliver highly stressful care. In nursing homes especially, staff members face arduous work environments with intense labor and client demands. Debilitating illnesses, the psychological overlay of dying and death, and emotional responses of family members struggling with their own fears and guilt challenge the physical stamina and mental acumen of the most dedicated and experienced nurses.

To preserve "self," nurses overcome with responsibilities may begin to burn out. Some nurses may begin to approach client care with a "policy-only" mentality and sequester themselves emotionally from situations or interactions. They may personally develop problems with substances and health and may engage in frequent absenteeism, tardiness, and turnover.

Nurses who find themselves burning out must recognize the signs of this stress reaction and take steps to intervene before becoming locked into a pattern. Those who notice signs of burnout should seek help from health care professionals and their supervisors.

DSM-IV-TR BOX 31.3

Amnestic Disorders

Amnestic Disorder Due to a General Medical Condition

A. The development of memory impairment as manifested by impairment in the ability to learn new information or the inability to recall previously learned information.

B. The memory disturbance causes significant impairment in social or occupational functioning and represents a significant decline from a previous level of functioning.

C. The memory disturbance does not occur exclusively during the course of a delirium or a dementia.

D. There is evidence from the history, physical examination, or laboratory findings that the disturbance is the direct physiological consequence of a general medical condition (including physical trauma).

Substance-Induced Persisting Amnestic Disorder

A. The development of memory impairment as manifested by impairment in the ability to learn new information or the inability to recall previously learned information.

B. The memory disturbance causes significant impairment in social or occupational functioning and represents a significant decline from a previous level of functioning.

C. The memory disturbance does not occur exclusively during the course of a delirium or a dementia and persists beyond the usual duration of substance intoxication or withdrawal.

D. There is evidence from the history, physical examination, or laboratory findings that the memory disturbance is etiologically related to the persisting effects of substance use (eg, a drug of abuse, a medication).

Reprinted with permission from the *Diagnostic and Statistical Manual of Mental Disorders, Fourth Edition, Text Revision* (Copyright (c) 2000). American Psychiatric Association.

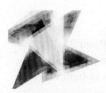

Reviewing and Applying Your Knowledge

Chapter Summary

- Cognitive disorders appear throughout the general population. They are especially prominent among older adults.

- Possible etiologies of cognitive disorders include primary brain disease, systemic disturbances, influences of exogenous substances, and withdrawal and residual effects of exogenous substances.

- Aberrant behaviors associated with cognitive disorders may include deficits in the sensorium, attention span, orientation, perception, and memory.

- Symptoms of cognitive disorders may be approached in terms of acute onset and chronic progression.

- Gathering and analyzing assessment data for a client with a cognitive disorder require participation of family members or friends who have been in close contact with the client.

- Continuum of care involves the collaborative efforts of the entire interdisciplinary health care team.

- Goal-setting for the client with an organic disorder focuses on eliminating the organic etiology, preventing acceleration of symptoms, and preserving dignity. Preserving optimal levels of functioning and preventing further decline are key goals.

- Specific nursing interventions strive to maintain the client's optimal physical health, structure the environment, promote socialization and independent functioning, and preserve the family unit.

Study Questions

1. Delirium develops in a 78-year-old man recovering from emergency hip surgery. He seems to be hallucinating and is mildly confused. Which of the following would the nurse do first?

   a. Loosely apply a vest restraint.

   b. Obtain an order for haloperidol.

   c. Arrange for an unlicensed assistant to sit with the client.

   d. Move the client to a room close to the nurse's station.

2. An 82-year-old woman with no history of neurologic dysfunction is admitted to the hospital with a possible bowel obstruction. She has been vomiting for several days. In addition to managing her medical care, nurses are monitoring the client for signs of delirium. Which of the following assessment findings would suggest that delirium may be developing in the client?

   a. The client removes her IV line and tries to climb over the side rails to get out of bed.

   b. The client has trouble finding the right word when speaking.

   c. The client requests pain medication frequently.

   d. The client is not sleeping well at night.

3. A 70-year-old woman with dementia, Alzheimer's type, lives at home with her husband, who is her full-time caregiver. The nurse is teaching the husband about interventions to prevent injury. Which of the following suggestions would be most appropriate?

   a. Put childproof caps on bottles containing cleaning fluids.

   b. Put cleaning fluids on a high shelf.

   c. Lock cleaning fluids in a cabinet in the kitchen.

   d. Store cleaning fluids in plain bottles in the garage.

4. The nurse questions the wife of a client with dementia to assess if she is at risk for depression or anxiety related to her caregiving activities. Which of the following statements or questions would be most useful in eliciting information?

   a. "You must feel overwhelmed by your caregiving responsibilities. Tell me about it."

   b. "Why don't you tell me about what your usual day is like?"

   c. "Do you feel stressed by your caregiving responsibilities?"

   d. "Do you wish you had more help with your husband?"

(continues on page 696)

5. A client with early-stage Alzheimer's disease is started on donepezil. The nurse is evaluating the caregiver's understanding of the medication and determines that the caregiver has understood the instructions when she makes which of the following statements?

   a. "My husband will only need to take this medication once a day."

   b. "This medicine will not affect his stomach and can be taken between meals."

   c. "This medication will prevent my husband's memory problems from worsening."

   d. "This medication may cause urinary retention. I'll monitor his intake and output."

Critical Thinking Questions

1. Reread Case Vignette 31.1 and Case In Point 31.1. Compare how the memory of each client is affected. What are the differences and similarities in behavior?

2. Compare and contrast the prognoses for both clients.

3. What nursing interventions would be appropriate for each client?

4. Would you work with the families differently? How and why?

References

Abbott, R. D., White, R., Ross, G. W., Masaki, K. H., Curb, J. D., & Petrovich, H. (2004). Walking and dementia in physically capable elderly men. *Journal of the American Medical Association, 292*(12), 1447–1453.

Alexopoulos, G. S., Streim, J., Carpenter, D., & Docherty, J. P.; Expert Consensus Panel for Using Antipsychotic Drugs in Older Patients. (2004). Using antipsychotic agents in older patients. *Journal of Clinical Psychiatry, 65*(Suppl. 2), 5–99; discussion 100–102; quiz 103–104.

American Psychiatric Association. (2000). *Diagnostic and statistical manual of mental disorders* (4th ed., text rev.). Washington, DC: Author.

Balas, M. C., Deutschman, C. S., Sullivan-Marx, E. M., Strumpf, N. E., Alston, R. P., & Richmond, T. S. (2007). Delirium in older patients in surgical intensive care units. *Journal of Nursing Scholarship, 39*(2), 147–154.

Bayer-Carter, J., Green, P., Montine, T., Vanfossen, B., Baker, L., Watson, G., et al. (2011). Diet intervention and cerebrospinal fluid biomarkers in amnestic mild cognitive impairment. *Archives of Neurology, 68*(6), 743–752.

Birks, J. (2008). Cholinesterase inhibitors for Alzheimer's disease. *Cochrane Database of Systematic Reviews, 2008*(1). Retrieved from EBSCO*host*.

Birks, J. S., & Grimley-Evans, J. (2007, April 18). Ginkgo biloba for cognitive impairment and dementia. *Cochrane Database of Systematic Reviews, 2007*(2). CD003120.

Birks, J. S., Grimley-Evans, J., Iakovidou, V., & Tsolaki, M. (2000). Rivastigmine for Alzheimer's disease. *Cochrane Database of Systematic Reviews, 2000*(4). CD001191.

Birks, J. S., & Harvey, R. (2006, January 25). Donepezil for dementia due to Alzheimer's disease. (Cochrane Review). *Cochrane Database of Systematic Reviews, 2006*(1). CD001190.

Bond, S., & Neelon, V. (2008). Delirium resolution in hospitalized older patients with cancer. *Cancer Nursing, 31*(6), 444–451.

Braaten, A. J., Parsons, T. D., McCue, R., Sellers, A., & Burns, W. J. (2006). Neurocognitive differential diagnosis of dementing diseases: Alzheimer's dementia, vascular dementia, frontotemporal dementia, and major depressive disorder. *International Journal of Neuroscience, 116*(11), 1271–1293. doi:10.1080/00207450600920928

Brodaty, H., Green, A., & Koschera, A. (2003). Meta-analysis of psychosocial interventions for caregivers of people with dementia. *Journal of the American Geriatrics Society, 51*(5), 657–664.

Bulechek, G. M., Butcher, H. K., & McCloskey Dochterman, J. (2008). *Nursing interventions classification (NIC)* (5th ed.). St. Louis, MO: Mosby.

Cohen-Mansfield, J. (2003). Non-pharmacologic interventions for psychotic symptoms in dementia. *Journal of Geriatric Psychiatry and Neurology, 16*(4), 219–224.

Cole, M. G. (2004). Delirium in elderly patients. *American Journal of Geriatric Psychiatry, 12,* 7–21.

Coon, D. W., Thompson, L., Steffan, A., Sorocco, K., & Gallagher-Thompson, D. (2003). Anger and depression management: Psychoeducation skill training interventions for women caregivers of a relative with dementia. *Gerontologist, 43*(5), 678–689.

Declercq, T. (2009). Withdrawal versus continuation of chronic antipsychotic drugs for behavioural and neuropsychiatric symptoms in elderly patients with dementia. *Cochrane Database of Systematic Reviews, 2009*(2). Retrieved from EBSCO*host*.

Devlin, J., Fong, J., Howard, E., Skrobik, Y., McCoy, N., Yasuda, C., & Marshall, J. (2008). Assessment of delirium in the intensive care unit: Nursing practices and perceptions. *American Journal of Critical Care, 17*(6), 555–566.

Dickson, D., Kouri, N., Murray, M., Josephs, K. (2011). Neuropathology of frontotemporal lobar degeneration-tau (FTLD-Tau). *Journal of Molecular Neuroscience, 44*(3), 141–153.

Doody, R. S., Stevens, J. C., Beck, C., Dubinsky, R. M., Kaye, J. A., Gwyther, L., et al. (2001). Practice parameter: Management of dementia (an evidence-based review). Report of the Quality Standards Subcommittee of the American Academy of Neurology. *Neurology, 56*(9), 1154–1166.

Farran, C., Gilley, D., McCann, J., Bienias, J., Lindeman, D., & Evans, D. (2004). Psychosocial interventions to reduce depressive symptoms of dementia caregivers: A randomized clinical trial comparing two approaches. *Journal of Mental Health & Aging, 10*(4), 337–350.

Fick, D. M., Hodo, K. M., Lawrence, F., & Inouye, S. K. (2007). Recognizing delirium superimposed on dementia: Assessing nurses' knowledge using case vignettes. *Journal of Gerontological Nursing, 33*(2), 40–47; 48–49.

Folstein, M. E., Folstein, S. E., & McHugh, P. R. (1975). Mini-mental state: A practical method for grading the cognitive state of patients for the clinician. *Journal of Psychiatric Research, 12*(189), 189–198.

Foreman, M. D., Mion, L. C., Trygstad, L., & Fletcher, K. (2003). Delirium: Strategies for assessing and treating. In: M. D. Mezey, T. Fulmer, & I. Abraham (Eds.), *Geriatric nursing protocols for best practice* (2nd ed., pp. 116–140). New York, NY: Springer.

Gauthier, S. (2007). *Clinical diagnosis and management of Alzheimer's Disease* (3rd ed.). Boca Raton, FL: Abingdon Oxon Taylor Francis.

Geldmacher, D. (2007). Treatment guidelines for Alzheimer's disease: Redefining perceptions in primary care. *Primary Care Companion to Journal of Clinical Psychiatry, 9,* 2.

Gurwitz, J. H., Field, T. S., Harrold, L. R., Rothschild, J., Debellis, K., Seger, A. C., et al. (2003). Incidence and preventability of adverse drug events among older persons in the ambulatory setting. *Journal of the American Medical Association, 289*(9), 1107–1116.

Han, J. H., Wilson, A., & Ely, E. W. (2010). Delirium in the older emergency department patient: A quiet epidemic. *Emergency Medical Clinics of North America, 28*(3), 611–631.

Hebert, L. E., Scherr, P. A., Bienias, J. L., Bennett, D. A., & Evans, D. A. (2003). Alzheimer disease in the U.S. population: Prevalence estimates using the 2000 census. *Archives of Neurology, 60*(8), 1119–1122.

Hepburn, K. W., Lewis, M., & Sherman, C. W. (2003). The savvy caregiver program: Developing and testing a transportable dementia family caregiver training program. *Gerontologist, 43*(6), 908–915.

Hepburn, K., Lewis, M., Tornatore, J., Sherman, C., & Bremer, K. (2007). The savvy caregiver program: The demonstrated effectiveness of a transportable dementia caregiver psychoeducation program. *Journal of Gerontological Nursing, 33*(3), 30–36.

Josephs, K. (2008). Frontotemporal dementia and related disorders: Deciphering the enigma. *Annals of Neurology, 64*(1), 4–14.

Lacasse, H., Perreault, M. M., & Williamson, D. R. (2006). Systematic review of antipsychotics for the treatment of hospital-associated delirium in medically or surgically ill patients. *Annals of Pharmacotherapy, 40*(11), 1966–1973.

Larson, E. B., Wang, L., Bowen, J. D., McCormick, W. C., Teri, L., Crane, P., & Kukull, W. (2006). Exercise is associated with reduced risk for incident dementia among persons 65 years of age and older. *Annals of Internal Medicine, 144*(2), 73–81.

Leentjens, A., & van der Mast, R. (2005). Delirium in elderly people: An update. *Current Opinion in Psychiatry, 18*(3), 325–330.

Levenson, J. L., Collins, J., & Puram, D. (2005). Images in psychosomatic medicine: The Clock-Drawing Test. *Psychosomatics, 46,* 77–78.

Lin, R., Heacock, L., & Fogel, J. (2010). Drug-induced, dementia-associated and non-dementia, non-drug delirium hospitalizations in the United States, 1998–2005: An analysis of the national inpatient sample. *Drugs & Aging, 27*(1), 51–61.

Maidment, I. (2008). Cholinesterase inhibitors for Parkinson's disease dementia. *Cochrane Database of Systematic Reviews, 2008*(1). Retrieved from EBSCO*host*.

Maidment, I., Fox, C., & Boustani, M. (2006, January 25). Cholinesterase inhibitors for Parkinson's disease dementia. *Cochrane Database of Systematic Reviews, 2006*(1). CD004747.

McAvay, G., Van Ness, P. H., Bogardus, S. T., Zhang, Y., Leslie, D. L., Leo-Summers, L. S., et al. (2006). Older adults discharged from the hospital with delirium: 1-year outcomes. *Journal of the American Geriatrics Society, 54*(8), 1245–1250.

McGonigal-Kenney, M. L., & Schutte, D. L. (2004). *Nonpharmacologic management of agitated behaviors in persons with Alzheimer disease and other chronic dementing conditions.* Iowa City, IA: University of Iowa Gerontological Nursing Interventions Research Center, Research Dissemination Core.

McShane, R., Arreosa Sastre, A., & Minakaran, N. (2006, April 19). Memantine for dementia. *Cochrane Database of Systematic Reviews, 2006*(2). CD003154.

Milgram, N. W., Head, E., Zicker, S. C., Ikeda-Douglas, C., Murphey, H., Muggenburg, B. A., et al. (2004). Long-term treatment with antioxidants and a program of behavioral enrichment reduces age-dependent impairment in discrimination and reversal learning in beagle dogs. *Experimental Gerontology, 39*(5), 753–765.

Milgram, N. W., Head, E., Zicker, S. C., Ikeda-Douglas, C., Murphey, H., Muggenburg, B. A., et al. (2005). Learning ability in aged beagle dogs is preserved by behavioral enrichment and dietary fortification: A two year longitudinal study. *Neurology of Aging, 26*(1), 77–90.

Moorhead, S., Johnson, M., Maas, M. L., & Swanson, E. (2008). *Nursing outcomes classification (NOC)* (4th ed.). St. Louis, MO: Mosby.

NANDA International. (2007). *Nursing diagnoses: Definitions and classification (2007–2008).* Philadelphia, PA: Author.

National Institute of Neurological Disorders and Stroke (NINDS). (2007). *The dementias: Hope through research.* Retrieved from http://www.ninds.nih.gov

National Institute on Aging (NIA). (2007). *Alzheimer's Disease Education and Referral Center. Progress report on AD 2005–2006.* Retrieved from http://www.nia.nih.gov/ Alzheimers

Neal, M., & Briggs, M. (2003). Validation therapy for dementia. *Cochrane Database of Systematic Reviews, 2003*(3). CD001394.

O'Connell, A. M., & Mion, L. C. (2003). Use of physical restraints in the acute care setting. In: M. D. Mezey, T. Fulmer, & I. Abraham (Eds.), *Geriatric nursing protocols for best practice* (2nd ed., pp. 116–140). New York, NY: Springer.

Park, M., Hsiao-Chen Tang, J., & Ledford, L. (2005). *Changing the practice of physical restraint use in acute care.* Iowa City: University of Iowa Gerontological Nursing Interventions Research Center, Research Translation and Dissemination Core.

Podewils, L. J., Guallar, E., Kuller, K. H., Fried, L. P., Lopez, O. L., Carlson, M., et al. (2005). Physical activity, APOE, genotype and dementia like findings from the Cardiovascular Health Cognition Study. *American Journal of Epidemiology, 161*(7), 639–651.

Rahknone, T., Eloniemi-Sulkava, U., Rissanen, S., Vafanen, A., Viramo, P., & Sulkava, R. (2003). Dementia with Lewy bodies according to the consensus criteria in a general population aged 75 years or older. *Journal of Neurology, Neurosurgery and Psychiatry, 74*(5), 720.

Registered Nurses Association of Ontario. (2003). *Screening for delirium, dementia and depression in older adults.* Toronto, Ontario, Canada: Author.

Rigney, T. S. (2006). Delirium in the hospitalized elder and recommendations for practice. *Geriatric Nursing, 27*(3), 151–157.

Rohrer, J., Guerreiro, R., Vandrovcova, J., Uphill, J., Reiman, D., Beck, J., ... Rossor, M. (2009). The heritability and genetics of frontotemporal lobar degeneration. *Neurology, 73*(18), 1451–1456. doi:10.1212/WNL.0b013e3181bf997a

Sadock, B. J., & Sadock, V. A. (2007). Delirium, dementia, and amnesic and other cognitive disorders and mental disorders due to a general medical condition. In: B. J. Sadock & V. A. Sadock (Eds.), *Kaplan and Sadock's synopsis of psychiatry: Behavioral sciences/ clinical psychiatry* (10th ed., pp. 319–349). Philadelphia, PA: Lippincott Williams & Wilkins.

Scarmeas, N., Luchsinger, J., Schupf, N., Brickman, A., Cosentino, S., Tang, M., & Stern, Y. (2009). Physical activity, diet, and risk of Alzheimer disease. *Journal of the American Medical Association, 302*(6), 627–637.

Scarmeas, N., Stern, Y., Mayeux, R., & Luchsinger, J. (2006). Mediterranean diet, Alzheimer disease, and vascular mediation. *Archives of Neurology, 63*(12), 1709–1717.

Schumaker, S. A., Legault, C., Rapp, S. R., Thal, L., Wallace, R. B., Ockene, J. K., et al. (2003). Estrogen plus progestin and the incidence of dementia and mild cognitive impairment in postmenopausal women: The Women's Health Initiative Memory Study: A randomized controlled trial. *Journal of the American Medical Association, 289*(20), 256–262.

Schuurmans, M. J., Shortridge-Baggett, L. M., & Duursma, S. A. (2003). The Delirium Observation Screening Scale: A screening instrument for delirium. *Research and Theory for Nursing Practice, 17*(1), 31–50.

Scott, H. D., & Laake, K. (2001). Statins for the prevention of Alzheimer's disease. *Cochrane Database of Systematic Reviews, 2001*(4). CD003160.

Snowdon, D. A. (2003). Healthy aging and dementia: Findings from the Nun Study. *Annals of Internal Medicine, 139*(5 Pt 2), 450–454.

Solfrizzi, V., Frisardi, V., Seripa, D., Capurso, C., Vendemiale, G., Pilotto, A., & Panza, F. (2010). Dietary patterns and protection against Alzheimer disease and cognitive decline. *Archives of Neurology, 67*(10), 1285–1286. doi:10.1001/archneurol.2010.244

Sunderland, T., Mirza, N., & Linker, G. (2004). Cognitive enhancers. In: A. F. Schatzberg & C. B. Nemeroff (Eds.), *Textbook of psychopharmacology* (3rd ed., pp. 639–650). Washington, DC: American Psychiatric Publishing.

Tabet, N., Birks, J., & Grimley-Evans, J. (2000). Vitamin E for Alzheimer's disease. *Cochrane Database of Systematic Reviews, 2000*(4). CD002854.

Tabet, N., & Feldman, H. (2003). Ibuprofen for Alzheimer's disease. *Cochrane Database of Systematic Reviews, 2003*(2). CD004031.

Thiru-Chelvam, B. (2004). *Bathing persons with dementia.* Iowa City, IA: University of Iowa Gerontological Nursing Interventions Research Center, Research Dissemination Core.

Wattmo, C., Wallin, Å. K., Londos, E., & Minthon, L. (2011). Long-term outcome and prediction models of activities of daily living in Alzheimer disease with cholinesterase inhibitor treatment. *Alzheimer Disease & Associated Disorders, 25*(1), 63–72.

Werezak, L. J., & Morgan, D. G. (2003). Creating a therapeutic psychosocial environment in dementia care: A preliminary framework. *Journal of Gerontological Nursing, 29*(12), 18–25.

Werner, P. (2003). Nursing care adaptations, behavioral interventions, environmental changes and sensory enhancement: Conceptual, process and outcome issues. In: D. P. Hay, D. T. Klein, L. K. Hay, G. T. Grossberg, & J. S. Kennedy (Eds.), *Agitation in patients with dementia: A practical guide to diagnosis and management* (pp. 91–102). Washington, DC: American Psychiatric Publishing.

Weuve, J., Kung, J. H., Manson, J., Bretcher, M. M., Ware, J. H., & Goldstein, F. (2004). Physical activity, including walking and cognitive function in older women. *Journal of the American Medical Association, 292*(12), 1454–1461.

Zarit, S. H., & Zarit, J. M. (2007). *Mental disorders in older adults: Fundamentals of assessment and treatment.* New York, NY: Guilford Press.

Web Resources

Alzheimer's Association: http://www.alz.org

Alzheimer's Disease Education and Referral (ADEAR) Center: http://alzheimer's.org

Children of Aging Parents (CAPs): *http://www.aoa.dhhs.gov/coa/dir/77.html*

Eldercare Locator: *http://www.aoa.dhhs.gov/elderpage/locator.html*

SEVEN

Psychiatric Emergencies

32

Anger and Aggression

Kevin Ann Huckshorn

KEY TERMS

aggression
anger
dangerousness
hostility-related variables
impulsivity
intent
restraint
seclusion

LEARNING OBJECTIVES

On completion of this chapter, you should be able to accomplish the following:

- Define broad factors that can increase risk for anger, aggression, and violence.
- Discuss the role that health care environments can play when conflict, aggression, and violence occur, including staff beliefs, attitudes, and behaviors.
- Discuss legal issues relevant to aggression and violence in people with psychiatric disorders.
- Describe various interventions to manage anger and aggression.
- Apply the nursing process to the care of clients who demonstrate aggressive and violent behavior in health care settings.

This chapter explores angry, aggressive, and violent behaviors in adults. It especially emphasizes those with psychiatric diagnoses who are receiving inpatient care, although most of the content applies to all clients across all settings. The chapter explains terms relevant to a conceptual understanding of the causality of aggression. It presents related psychobiologic, social, and environmental contributors. It reviews therapeutic options and the steps of the nursing process for managing anger and aggression. For information on the problems of community violence, abuse, and working with victims of these phenomena, see Chapter 33.

DEFINITIONS

Aggressive behavior usually involves anger and physical or verbal threats or actions. **Anger** is an emotional response to perceived frustration, shame, or humiliation. It can be positive when people direct it toward actual injustices or if it motivates them to organize and institute constructive and beneficial change. Anger loses any positive effect when it turns inward, flails ineffectively with little or no cause, bullies those with less strength or power, harms or hurts the self or others physically or emotionally, or rages out of control. The ways in which humans deal with anger tend to persist over time. Those with anger problems early in life are likely to continue to have challenges dealing with this difficult emotion unless they receive some help.

Health care providers generally view anger negatively in people with mental illness, whether their anger is justified or not. This point is one of the main themes of this chapter. When people depend on others for care, those giving that care often meet expressions of anger with disbelief, irritation, frustration, and a desire to provide consequences so that "clients" will "learn" (National Executive Training Institute [NETI], 2007). However, no research findings show that long-term learning results from punishing practices. Examples of such practices include taking away privileges, using seclusion or restraint, or forcing people to do things.

Aggression means intentional behavior with the potential to cause destruction or harm; it may manifest as verbal threats or attacks, negative use of objects, or physical assaults on known people, strangers, or self (Anderson & Bushman, 2002). Aggression toward self includes suicidal gestures and self-harm, although the latter can have other causes, such as maladaptive coping (see Chaps. 25 and 34) (NETI, 2007). Aggression against others ranges from verbal threats to homicide. *Violence* denotes physical aggression by one or more people against others (Citrome, 2007).

Hostility-related variables are regular and predictable emotions, attitudes, and behaviors in humans confronted with frustrating circumstances, unfair application of rules, unjust practices, discrimination, shaming, or humiliation. Irritability, resentment, and impulsivity have been linked with conflict, aggression, and the potential for medical conditions such as essential hypertension, cardiovascular disease, and atherosclerotic heart disease (Fredrickson et al., 2000; Matthews et al., 2004; Siegman et al., 2000).

POTENTIAL CONTRIBUTORS TO ANGRY, AGGRESSIVE, OR VIOLENT BEHAVIORS

Primarily, anger and aggression are emotional responses. Clearly, some people are more predisposed to aggressive and violent reactions and behaviors than others. Concurrent with one of the overarching themes of this book, a combination of genetic/biologic factors and life experiences can result in problems with anger and violence. The following sections review several possible contributors.

Psychiatric Illness

Aggressive behaviors, including physical violence, occur across all clinical diagnostic categories. They are rare in people with psychiatric diagnoses as compared with the general population (American Psychiatric Association [APA], 2000). Nevertheless, some psychiatric symptoms have a potential for related aggression. For example, clients with thought disorders may experience command hallucinations and delusions that others are imminently going to harm them (see Chap. 29). Such symptoms may lead to violence, especially if clients feel under immediate threat (Citrome, 2007; NETI, 2007). Box 32.1 lists some examples of psychiatric diagnoses and associated patterns of aggression or violence.

The deinstitutionalization movement of the late 20th century resulted in public state hospitals discharging thousands of people, many of whom had nowhere to go and whose illnesses were in varying states of control. Outcomes since have been mixed. One negative consequence is the growth in homelessness (see Chap. 38). More than 700,000 U.S. adults are homeless on any given night (Cunningham & Henry, 2007). In addition to chronic health problems, approximately 50% of homeless people have mental illness. The simple calculation is that 186,078 adults with serious and persistent mental illness (SPMI) are homeless each night. Becoming homeless often creates a chaotic living environment in which people have one of two choices: to become victims of violence or to actively defend themselves to survive. Homeless people are often involved in traumatic experiences such as attempted robberies, sexual assaults, and muggings. Poor nutrition, increased substance abuse, and increased severity of disease also may contribute to aggressive responses in homeless people with SPMI.

Medical Conditions

One factor that might increase risk for aggression and violence is a medical condition that causes or leads to psychiatric symptoms. Clients who experience increasing anxiety, irritability, agitation, and thought problems and also have a predilection for intent to injure self, others, or property present a complicated diagnostic dilemma. First, they require a

---

BOX 32.1 Psychiatric Diagnoses and Patterns of Aggression or Violence

- **Antisocial personality disorder (adults):** Callous, cynical, contemptuous of the feelings and rights of others, irresponsible, exploitative, lacks empathy, often violent
- **Attention-deficit/hyperactivity disorder:** Predominantly hyperactive-impulsive type with low frustration tolerance, temper outbursts, intrusive, oppositional behavior
- **Bipolar disorders (especially bipolar I manic episodes):** Irritability, agitation, and violent behavior during manic or psychotic episodes; highly comorbid with alcohol abuse, which worsens the prognosis
- **Conduct disorder (children):** Aggressive conduct that threatens or causes physical harm to other people or animals
- **Delusional disorder, persecutory type:** Persecutory delusions (eg, of being conspired against, cheated, spied on, maliciously maligned, poisoned or drugged); often resentful and angry and may become violent toward those whom they believe are threatening or harmful to them
- **Dementia:** Generalized irritability and low frustration tolerance, confusion, destructive attempts at self-protection
- **Dissociative identity disorder:** Aggressive behavior toward self (self-mutilation, suicide attempts) and toward others
- **Impulse-control disorders** (eg, intermittent explosive disorder): Discrete episodes of failure to resist aggressive impulses resulting in serious injury to self, assaults on others, or destruction of property
- **Oppositional defiant disorder** (children): Negativistic, hostile, defiant, spiteful, blaming behavior directed at adults or peers, primarily by verbal aggression
- **Paranoid personality disorder:** Pervasive distrust and suspiciousness that others will exploit, harm, or deceive oneself even with no evidence of such; overly vigilant; holds grudges, unwilling to forgive perceived insults or slights; may attack others suddenly
- **Post-traumatic stress disorder:** Irritability, hypervigilance, and outbursts of anger
- **Schizophrenia, paranoid type:** Persecutory ideation, which may predispose the person to suicidal behavior, or anger and violence toward others
- **Substance-related disorders:** Aggressive episodes that result from the direct physiologic effects of the drugs of abuse or the medication

Source: American Psychiatric Association. (2000). *Diagnostic and statistical manual of mental disorders* (4th ed., text rev.). Washington, DC: Author.

---

differential evaluation for any contributing medical condition. Health care providers must review their health history, conduct a physical examination, and proceed with pertinent laboratory tests to ascertain whether psychotic, manic, depressive, or anxiety symptoms are related primarily to a general medical condition (APA, 2000). Nurses must investigate all appropriate medical causes of psychiatric symptoms. The totality of medical disorders that can induce psychiatric symptoms is broad and beyond the scope of this chapter. See Box 32.2 for a summary.

Traumatic Life Events

Impulsivity, viewed as a symptom of an underlying brain disorder or a pervasive personality trait, includes actions performed with little or no regard for consequences (Fish, 2002; Greenberg & Hollander, 2003). Impulsive characteristics include unpredictable behavior, hypervigilance that results in threats toward others for mild offenses, irresponsibility, low tolerance for frustration, poor problem solving, disturbed relationships, restlessness, and general disregard for social rules and customs. Traumatic experiences, such as a history of physical, sexual, or emotional abuse, neglect, or chaotic family life, can significantly alter the developing brain. Such alterations may damage areas that help control angry and aggressive responses. They also may contribute to a neurochemical environment that predisposes people to substance abuse, which further compromises the ability to cognitively reason or process stress (Saxe & Johansson, 2003).

Traumatic events involve direct threats of death, severe bodily harm, or psychological injury (Rosenberg et al., 2001). They are personal experiences of interpersonal violence (Jennings, 2004a; Moses et al., 2003; National Association of State Mental Health Program Directors Research Institute, Inc. [NASMHPD], 2006). Estimates are that 36% to 81% of the general population has experienced some kind of significant traumatic event, with even higher rates for those who seek public mental health and substance abuse treatment (Cusack et al., 2004; Frueh et al., 2000). Differences in traumatic experiences appear linked to gender, with men more commonly exposed to combat, physical attacks, being threatened with a weapon, and kidnapping, and women more likely exposed to sexual violence, neglect, and physical abuse in childhood (Rosenberg et al., 2001). Many people who experience trauma develop post-traumatic stress disorder (PTSD) (see Chap. 23). The chronic, debilitating symptoms of PTSD have serious adverse effects on social, familial, and occupational functioning. The disorder is associated with significant social maladjustment, poor quality of life, medical comorbidity, physiologic arousal, general symptom severity, and psychiatric comorbidity (Cusack et al., 2003).

Adults and children in the criminal and juvenile justice systems commonly report histories of physical and sexual abuse. Both childhood abuse and neglect increase the likelihood of being arrested as a juvenile by 53%, as a young adult by 38%, and for violent crime by 38% (Jennings, 2004b). In 1998, 92% of incarcerated girls reported sexual, physical, or severe emotional abuse in childhood (Jennings, 2004b). Boys who experience or witness violence are 1,000 times more likely to commit violence (van der Kolk, 1998). Thus, severe social problems seem to be positively correlated with histories of trauma and abuse.

The theme of *traumatic life experience* and its correlation with violence and aggression appear more than coincidental to many scholars and researchers (Cusack et al., 2003; Jennings, 2004b). Empirical findings are only now becoming widely published. Van der Kolk, a pioneer in the field, was

BOX 32.2 Selected Medical Conditions Associated With Aggression and Violence

Chronic Pain

Bone and joint diseases (eg, severe arthritis, rheumatism)

Neurobiologic Disorders

Brain tumors
Traumatic brain injury
Neurotransmitter imbalances
Seizure disorder
Parkinson's disease
Multiple sclerosis
Huntington's disease
Dementia

Infectious Diseases

Neurosyphillis
Meningitis
Herpes simplex encephalitis
HIV encephalopathy

Endocrine Disorders

Hyperthyroidism
Hypothyroidism
Hyperparathyroidism
Hypoparathyroidism
Adrenal disorders

Diabetes mellitus
Pancreatic tumors
Progressive hypoglycemia

Metabolic Disorders

Hyponatremia
Hypernatremia
Chronic renal failure
Hepatic encephalopathy
Porphyria
Systemic lupus erythematosus

Vitamin Deficiencies

Wernicke's encephalopathy
Pernicious anemia
Folate deficiency

Exogenous Toxins

Alcoholic hallucinosis
Hallucinogens
Illicit stimulants
Amphetamine-induced psychosis
Inhaled solvents
Heavy metals
Medications

the first to explore the overall human response to trauma. He postulates that the "earliest and possibly most damaging psychological trauma is the *loss of a secure base*" and that great damage results both psychologically and developmentally (1987, p. 32). He emphasizes the damage that can occur when abusive or neglectful parenting interferes with childhood attachment. Children with disrupted attachments often have lifelong psychobiologic consequences characterized by extreme overreactions to many events, poor tolerance of anxiety, depression, passivity, poor socialization, numbed effect, hypervigilance, trouble modulating anger or aggressive feelings, and self-destructive behavior. In later life these children, depending on the severity of the trauma and the developmental stage in which it occurred, may be prone to psychiatric illness and find it difficult to form or maintain stable relationships or employment. Such problems set the stage for the perpetuation of impulsive, hostile, and violent outcomes.

Biologic Factors and Temperament

Temperament is the sum total of a person's constitutional or biologic personality dispositions. It is partly genetic, evident early in life, and somewhat stable across situations and over time (see Chap. 36). Temperament is thought to remain consistent throughout the lifespan. Although most associated studies focus on infants and children, some researchers have

found that adults at risk for adjustment problems had difficult temperaments as preschoolers. The temperament most relevant to potential aggression is negative emotionality.

Negative emotionality is manifested by irregularity in biologic functions; behavioral inhibition, including shyness, fearfulness, and withdrawal from new or novel situations; slow adaptability; and an intense and negative mood (Figure 32.1). For example, on the first day of preschool, the

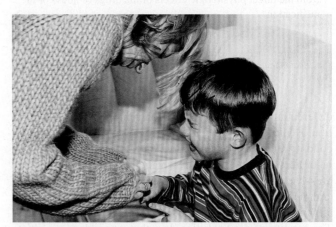

FIGURE 32.1 Negative emotionality early in life may be a predictor of violent or aggressive reactions in adolescence and adulthood

child with negative emotionality stands silently alone, while his or her peers freely explore the environment and interact with one another. Studies have found that a predisposition to negative emotionality increases the likelihood of impulsive, antisocial, and aggressive behavior (Scarpa & Raine, 1997; Vitaro et al., 2006). Although negative emotionality may be difficult to change, health care providers and nurses can encourage people with this trait to become more positive thinkers and to gain confidence and positive emotional experiences.

Social–Environmental Factors

Researchers often apply Bandura's (1973) social learning theory to explain aggressive behavior that people learn from exposure to aggressive models or as the result of random positive reinforcement of direct experience. As discussed earlier, exposure to aggression may occur in families characterized by abuse, violence, and trauma (Maxwell & Maxwell, 2003). Subcultures such as gangs or exposure to violent television shows, movies, and video games also may contribute.

Findings about aggressive video games indicate that children, especially boys, who prefer them are more aggressive and show less prosocial behavior than those with a low preference for them (Huesmann, 2007; Huesmann et al., 2003). Some researchers and theorists believe that television, video, and movie violence portrays coercive behavior that results in the attainment of some material reward, social recognition, or successful retaliation against enemies. In essence, the media glorifies violence and teaches people how to aggress.

Brink (2001) believes that the acceptance of violence, greed, and lust as natural, everyday experiences is negatively influencing society. Children identify with heroes portrayed in movies or on television as "violent men and women, who shoot, knife, and karate-kill" (p. 6). The theory of *cognitive priming* suggests that violent video games may have been a contributing factor in school shootings by adolescent boys who played such games (Anderson & Dill, 2000; Bensley & Van Eenwyk, 2001). Violent video games activate an aggressive cognition, making it more likely for people to act on previous aggressive thoughts toward others (Barlett et al., 2007; Konijn, 2007). In addition gangs may promote violent crime as a means of achieving recognition and status. Aggressive sports and war also may lead to imitation of aggressive behavior (Challenging Behaviors 32.1).

Checkpoint Questions

1. What are some medical illnesses or problems that may contribute to aggressive behavior?
2. What theory suggests that violent video games may contribute to violence in those who play them?

HEALTH CARE ENVIRONMENTS AND ANGRY AND AGGRESSIVE CLIENT BEHAVIOR

Aggression and violence in health care environments continue to escalate, not only in inpatient mental health facilities, but also in emergency care, long-term care, and home care. Nurses who experience injuries in the workplace may lose time from work and incur financial as well as psychological costs, including post-traumatic stress responses (Love & Morrison, 2003). Such evidence has led to increased interest in methods of preventing violence in health care settings and a better understanding of nurse–client interaction styles in all care settings.

Challenging Behaviors 32.1

The Client Who Is Hostile and Profane

Situation: Your assigned client is 15 years old and has attention-deficit/hyperactivity disorder and oppositional defiant disorder. This is his first partial hospitalization admission. You have been asked to do his intake assessment. As soon as you begin to ask him questions, he says to you: "F— off. I don't need any m—f—help!"

Your Potential Feelings: Anger, repugnance

What Is Going On? To understand what's happening, focus on what the client might be feeling that leads him to express himself with hostility and profanity. He may be very frightened and confused at having been admitted to a psychiatric program. He may be trying to establish control through intimidation and devaluation. Rude language, as offensive as you might find it, is often part of adolescent culture.

Strategy: This situation calls for responding primarily to the possible feelings behind the hostile and rude language.

Nurse Action/Communication: Maintain a calm and supportive attitude. The client does not know you personally, so avoid taking his projected hostility and profanity personally. You might say: "It's pretty scary to be in this situation. Tell me about what's going on with you." The client might respond with more rude and profane language, but your willingness to ignore it and remain concerned can result in the client feeling understood and able to express further feelings and information.

Considerations for Inpatient Settings

Nurses who show sincere and consistent respect and empathy for a client's immediate situation and personal suffering are more likely to succeed in defusing frustration and anger than are nurses who interact in an authoritarian or uncaring manner (Carlsson et al., 2004). Interpersonal precursors linked with escalating client violence include confusion or anger about the behavior of other clients (eg, disputes over cigarettes or food) and aversive stimulation from staff or the environment. Examples of staff behavior that can contribute to frustration and anger in clients include the following:

- Rules that prevent clients from leaving activities
- Power disputes over medications
- Blocked access to phones, televisions, or rooms
- Denials of requests in general
- Threats of or actual physical restraint
- Ignoring clients or making fun of them
- Ordering clients to do or not to do something

Most clients well understand the power differential in inpatient settings. This difference can cause much anguish and frustration (Figure 32.2); at times, it can lead to violence. In addition, either overstimulation from turmoil or understimulation from a lack of engaging activities may promote conflict (Nijman et al., 1999). Overall, avoidance of power struggles, use of empathy, and mediation of conflicts are the best practices against aggressive or violent confrontations with clients (NETI, 2007).

Outpatient Factors

Most clients receiving outpatient care are well enough that they are not experiencing problems that would lead to displays of anger and aggression. One important factor is for such clients to continue with their treatment to avoid relapses and symptoms that may cause behavior to escalate.

During outpatient visits, nurses need to help clients understand the importance of adherence with their treatment regimens and the potential results of nonadherence. The ability to provide choices in treatment and to listen to the

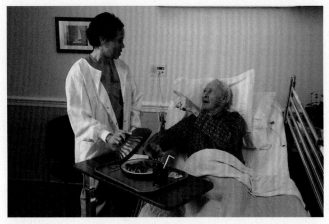

FIGURE 32.2 **Power differentials during hospitalization, as well as illness itself, can lead to angry outbursts in clients.**

concerns of clients is paramount. Psychotropic medications have significant side effects that make adherence difficult. Concerns from clients about weight gain, fatigue, drooling, dry mouth, decreased libido or sexual performance, and psychomotor changes need thorough discussion and documentation, with appropriate referrals to prescribing practitioners. Proper involvement of family and significant others is crucial in ensuring treatment adherence, minimizing symptom breakthrough, and deterring recidivism.

LEGAL ISSUES RELATED TO DANGEROUSNESS AND INTENT

Violent acts are the primary focus for legal assessment of dangerousness in all clinical settings, including forensic settings. **Dangerousness** is defined as behaviors that carry a high risk of harm or injury to self or others. It usually includes a *temporal* aspect; in other words, there is some sense of a time frame in which this dangerous behavior will occur. The sooner or more pending the time frame, the more dangerous the person may seem.

In general, involuntary commitment occurs only when a police officer, physician, or a court deems a client diagnosed as mentally ill as imminently dangerous to self or others (see Chaps. 6 and 19). Forty-three states are implementing the requirement for the least-restrictive treatment alternative by permitting commitment to outpatient treatment settings rather than to inpatient care when possible (NASMHPD, 2006). In general, criteria for involuntary outpatient commitment reflect that clients do not require continuous hospitalization, could be treated more appropriately in an outpatient program (or a combined inpatient and outpatient program), will adhere to a prescribed treatment plan, and are not likely to become dangerous or experience further deterioration if they follow the prescribed treatment plan. Outpatient commitment often is a matter of controversy; some consider it coercive because it compels clients to participate under threat of court sanctions and interferes with basic civil rights (Bazelon Center for Mental Health Law, 2003).

Regarding the rights of clients in hospitals and clinics, voluntary clients may refuse any treatment, although staff at the facility may then ask clients to leave. In most states, involuntary clients have a right to refuse antipsychotic drugs unless they are found incompetent. In any case, qualified personnel can administer medications legally in an emergency (ie, client is dangerous to self or others).

Intent is an important criterion when evaluating and differentiating accidental from deliberate harm or injury to others or property. Evaluation of *intent* requires thoughtful and sophisticated analysis because labeling clients as intentionally aggressive segregates them from others and may unfairly lead others to view and treat them as antisocial. People who seek mental health services have complicated and individual histories. It is often easy for staff to label them in one way and then impossible to reverse that clinical determination (see Chap. 8).

As a result of the *Tarasoff* decision (*Tarasoff v. Board of Regents of the University of California,* 1976), it is mandatory in most states for health care personnel to report any clear threat from clients about intent to harm specific people. Psychiatrists, psychotherapists, and other mental health care providers must warn authorities (if specified by state law) and potential victims of possible dangerous actions of their clients, even if clients protest. Most mental health agencies include this caveat in admission paperwork. The *Tarasoff* decision is not a specific law, but rather a legal principle based on interpretation of laws and precedents. It continues to be controversial. Each state may differ in its interpretation of the law regarding the duty to warn. Most mental health professional codes of ethics also address the duty to warn (see Chap. 6).

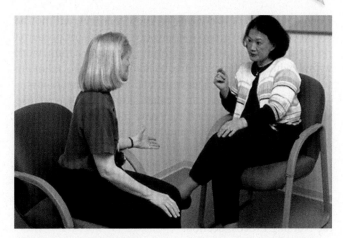

FIGURE 32.3 Sometimes just giving some focused attention to upset clients can calm simmering emotions and solve problems that would otherwise lead to anger.

> **Checkpoint Questions**
> 3. What types of behaviors by health care personnel are most likely to contribute to aggressive or violent responses from clients?
> 4. What are the roles of dangerousness and intent in terms of legal issues related to inpatient care?

INTERDISCIPLINARY MANAGEMENT OF AGGRESSION AND VIOLENCE

Overall goals for aggressive or violent clients are for them not to threaten or harm anyone and to gain insight into and skill at managing aggressive impulses. Achieving such goals requires specific treatment strategies. Providers should use the more restrictive strategies carefully and only when danger is imminent (NETI, 2007). In general, they should not use involuntary medications at the same time as seclusion or restraint. They should try only one of these interventions first, giving it some time to work, before trying something else.

Verbal Interventions

People want others to listen to and understand their concerns and complaints. Receiving care in a mental health facility is difficult at best and does not generally involve consistently individualized attention. In fact, many consumers note that they have felt ignored, disrespected, or coerced into certain activities during admission (NETI, 2007).

Verbal interventions are especially important when interacting with clients whose behavior is escalating as a result of conflict, regardless of the reason. Everyone has his or her own story. Often just giving some focused attention to upset clients and sincerely listening to them to try to meet their immediate needs can de-escalate a situation (Figure 32.3). Such verbal communication is most effective when used early. Waiting until clients are losing control is too late in most circumstances.

Skilled mental health nurses are familiar with the people they are helping and immediately respond to any behavioral change or escalation, no matter how minor. "Knowing" clients as quickly and as well as possible can help prevent violence or manage conflicts (NETI, 2007). One way to improve familiarity with hospitalized clients is to do a minirounds following shift report. Having face-to-face verbal communication early in the shift facilitates the exchange of crucial information about mental status and, at least, ensures that nurses are aware of the names and faces of people in their care.

Five important steps in communicating with clients to prevent the escalation of aggressive behavior include (1) making personal contact, (2) discovering the source of distress, (3) relieving the distress, (4) keeping everyone safe, and (5) assisting with alternative behaviors and problem solving. These strategies are discussed in more detail in the Nursing Process section.

Limit Setting

Limit setting occurs when someone in authority (often, nurses) *respectfully reminds* clients of the boundaries of acceptable behavior (as opposed to *disrespectfully demanding cooperation*) and sets limits as warranted (Lowe et al., 2003). A helpful strategy is to first find out what is upsetting the client, often by asking the client to come with the nurse to discuss this (and therefore removing him or her from the general population). Next, it is important to assess how important the client's need, request, or demand is and to meet it if possible. If the "demand" cannot be met, nurses should focus on underlying issues. Generally, nurses can simplify the feelings generating demands into separate issues. For example, clients may be afraid or bored. They might feel ignored or that they are not getting any better. Some clients may be concerned about other aspects of their lives. Nurses can intervene effectively by listening and following up on whatever is troubling clients. Sometimes just asking, "What is going on? What are you worried about?" is sufficient.

Clients may find it reassuring to know that they will not be allowed to be destructive to themselves, others, or property. Being reminded of established limits gives them a framework within which to function freely and adequately, maintain self-esteem, learn new behaviors, and gain self-awareness.

Verbal intervention can escalate situations when a nurse and client are strangers or if they have had previous unpleasant interactions. Involving another person who knows and has a relationship with the client can be key (Figure 32.4). Nurses also need to understand that in mental health settings, it is best to "get to know" everyone in their care as soon as possible. Additional guidelines for communicating with clients whose behavior requires limit setting can be found in the Nursing Process section.

Cognitive–Behavioral Interventions

Cognitive–behavioral techniques can be useful in assisting clients to confront dysfunctional and irrational thinking, test the reality of their thinking and behavior, and learn to use more positive and assertive responses in interactions (see Chaps. 3 and 13). Examples for angry and aggressive clients include guided discovery and anger management.

Guided Discovery

The "guided discovery" technique has been successful with clients who have depression or anger control problems (Rickelman & Houfek, 1995). In this approach, clinicians use specific learning experiences to teach clients how to recognize the connection between their thoughts, feelings, and behaviors; identify and replace automatic negative thinking with positive thinking; and substitute dysfunctional expectations and appraisals with reality-based interpretations. These strategies also are known as cognitive reframing or cognitive restructuring.

Anger Management

Anger management training often is done in groups. Clients learn how their thoughts and feelings are separate events. For instance, feelings do not necessarily translate into

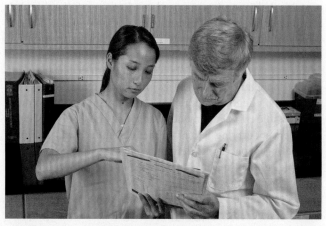

FIGURE 32.4 This nurse is consulting with another health care provider about a mutual client new to the nurse.

actions. Perceptions of events do not necessarily influence emotions or behaviors. Clients can learn to manage angry responses to events by changing their thoughts about them (Dunbar, 2004). Often, people believe that feelings dictate their behavior. The important learning here is that feelings are just feelings and can be managed. In essence, feelings and behavior are two different states.

Cognition or thoughtful review of situations should dictate behaviors in all circumstances. Clients need to learn how to identify and monitor their own anger cues, behavioral and physiologic signals related to anger arousal, signs of impending loss of control, and how to rechannel aggressive responses early.

Assaultive clients tend to experience anger and behavioral responses as automatic, reflexive, deeply ingrained reactions. They have used them often, and the link between feelings and behaviors has become a pattern in previous confrontative episodes. Many people actually use the statements "you made me angry" or "you made me upset." In truth, no one has the power to make anyone else "feel" anything. An essential component of anger management is learning that one's own personalities and life experiences lead to reactions that can be controlled.

Less anger is aroused when clients can define situations as "problems calling for solutions," rather than as "threats calling for attacks." The further a person has progressed into a provocation, the less likely he or she is to initiate anger control. Defining a situation as a problem needing a solution is not an easy skill. Clients who experience some success in using cognitive problem-solving methods rather than emotional reactionary responses may begin to take pride in new ways of coping with anger. In many situations, learning how to take a time-out when certain feelings or emotions surface is an effective skill that clients can practice in everyday living (Case Vignette 32.1).

Behavior Therapy: Token Economy

A key expectation in mental health treatment settings is that clients will act or behave in socially appropriate ways. The rationale for the use of a token economy involves identifying positive interpersonal and self-care behaviors that providers can reinforce by dispensing a predetermined number of tokens to clients, contingent on improvements in their behavior (McMonagle & Sultana, 2004). Desired behavior results in the client receiving tokens, whereas undesired behavior can result in losing tokens or in no action.

Currently, use of token economies is under national review. Studies have not found these historic, behavioral programs very effective. They may create "compliance" in inpatient environments, but sustaining results following discharge into the community is difficult. Most troubling, these programs may lead to conflict and aggressive behavior. In many situations, implementation of token-based interventions by different staff across shifts is idiosyncratic at best. In general, token economies are not noted for teaching people "illness self-management." They also do not address

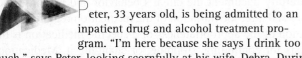

Case Vignette 32.1

Peter, 33 years old, is being admitted to an inpatient drug and alcohol treatment program. "I'm here because she says I drink too much," says Peter, looking scornfully at his wife, Debra. During the interview, he is sarcastic and noncommunicative, ridiculing Debra's comments and belittling her.

Debra relates that Peter drinks half a bottle of vodka and several beers daily and takes amphetamines occasionally. "He's been injured in several fights at bars and has slapped or pushed me on several occasions. He's grown extremely controlling, not letting me have the car keys or money." Peter blames his wife for his current circumstances. However, the employee assistance program manager at Peter's company referred him to treatment when he failed a random urine-screening test for drugs. Peter's continued employment is contingent on his recovery from alcohol and drug abuse. He has not had a drink for 72 hours and shows no signs of alcohol withdrawal syndrome.

Peter is admitted to an open unit and oriented to the facility and the milieu activities. He complains about the "rinky-dink" recreation area and laughs openly at other clients. Another male client yells at him from across the room, "What's your [expletive] problem?" Before Peter can answer, the nurse asks him if he would like to play basketball. He agrees, and the psychiatric technician takes Peter outside to play. The other clients resume their game of pool.

After 30 minutes, Peter returns and appears calmer. The nurse asks to speak with Peter. She questions him about his relationship with his wife and his history of fighting. He says, "Debra just does such silly stuff that gets me so frustrated. Other people, too. Fighting in bars is just a way for me to let off steam. But I guess it's kind of stupid, though." He acknowledges that it isn't right to hit his wife. "I just can't control my anger. I think she might leave me if this continues. I watched my dad do the same things, and my mom took us and left."

Peter also admits that he has gotten into trouble at work several times for "mouthing off." "That's probably why I haven't been promoted to supervisor yet." The nurse says, "I hear you saying that your anger is causing you trouble in many areas of your life and that you would like to be able to control your anger better." "Yes," says Peter, "that's correct."

Reflection and Critical Thinking

- What is your initial response to Peter? How can nurses manage their own emotions when working with emotional clients?
- What potential problems are nurses at risk for encountering with Peter?
- What alternative treatments might be most effective? Should family interventions be part of the plan at this point?

---

individual daily concerns and tend to treat entire client populations as one homogenous group.

Group and Family Therapy

Group therapy may be helpful for clients who use angry or antisocial behaviors because it gives them an opportunity to receive feedback from others about their interactive style. Problem solving among peers and peer pressure for socially acceptable behavior may have a stronger influence for such clients than one-to-one therapy. In addition, family therapy may be indicated when clients' aggressive and violent behaviors are specific to or exacerbated by interactions with their families or significant others. During sessions, the health care provider, client, and family can discuss strategies for anger deceleration and problem solving.

Group and family therapies only work with people who can interact effectively with others and who have sufficient cognitive and verbal skills to express themselves. Most people with mental illness have these skills, but capabilities vary. In some cases these skills surface only after psychiatric symptoms are somewhat stabilized.

Prevention of Vapor Lock and Meltdown

Greene's (2001) theory about children who lose behavioral control and experience an "inflexible–explosive episode" seems applicable to adults also. Such people may lack two essential skills: flexibility and frustration tolerance. According

to Greene (2001), inflexible–explosive episodes have three phases.

In the first phase, *vapor lock* leads people to feel frustrated or overwhelmed, rendering them unable to think clearly and rationally until someone helps them. During vapor lock, people may be capable of some rational thought, so interventions to facilitate rationale thought are essential.

The second phase is called the *crossroads*. At this time, appropriate interventions from parents, caregivers, or health care providers may facilitate "communication, collaborative problem-solving, and resolution" (Greene, 2001, p. 22). Greene suggests the following interventions during crossroads:

1. Acknowledge the person's frustration about the incident.
2. Stay calm.
3. Use empathy and take the person's perspective. Empathy helps keep the person from overreacting when frustrated.
4. Invite the person to solve the problem with you (eg, "Let's think of how we can work this out.").
5. If the person is stuck, assist him or her to generate alternative solutions.

If frustration escalates, clients may enter a third phase called *meltdown*, or "disintegrative rage." Behaviors may become more verbally and physically aggressive and destructive (Greene, 2001). Clients may be highly anxious, with little or no cognitive capacity for learning (see Chap. 23). Verbal de-escalation may be ineffective; clients may require more structured limit setting. Early interventions to prevent meltdown are essential.

Pharmacologic Intervention

If aggression escalates and clients do not respond to other methods, health care providers may administer prescribed medications. Although the U.S. Food and Drug Administration has not approved one specific medication for treating aggression, several classes of psychotropic drugs have been used to manage acute aggressive episodes and chronic aggressive behavior (Bender, 2003; Brieden et al., 2002;

Glick et al., 2001; Hollander et al., 2003; Reist et al., 2003; Schur et al., 2003). Health care personnel must observe and carefully document the client's behavior and responses before and after the initiation of the medication regimen. Evaluation of the appropriateness of a specific medication is the basis for continuing, stopping, or changing it. Medications may not be advisable if assaultive clients are potentially under the influence of an unknown substance.

Understanding Psychopharmacology 32.1 reviews examples of medications used to treat aggressive behavior. Chapter 16 also discusses many of these medications in detail; the reader is referred to that chapter for more information.

UNDERSTANDING PSYCHOPHARMACOLOGY 32.1

Typical Medications Used to Treat Aggressive Behavior

TYPE	DOSAGE RANGE	INDICATIONS	CAUTIONS
Antipsychotics			
haloperidol (Haldol)	0.5–5 mg PO two to three times daily, adjust as necessary; maximum dose 100 mg/day; for acute psychosis, 2–5 mg IM, which may be repeated every hour or every 4–6 h if symptoms are controlled	Active psychosis, thought disorder, dangerous and destructive behaviors, agitation, hostility, paranoia	Tolerance to sedative effects: akathisia mistaken for increased agitation
chlorpromazine (Thorazine)	Psychosis: 10–25 mg two to four times daily; increase dose by 20–50 mg daily, every 3–4 days PRN	See haloperidol	Orthostatic hypotension
clozapine (Clozaril)	Maximum: 1,500 mg/day; 300–900 mg daily	Clients with schizophrenia who cannot tolerate or do not have adequate response to standard antipsychotic agents	Dose-related seizures, leukopenia, agranulocytosis Discontinue if white blood cell count falls below 2,000/mm^3 or granulocyte count falls below 1,000/mm^3
risperidone (Risperdal)	3–6 mg/day (older adults should start slowly)	Delusions, hallucinations, depression, apathy	Insomnia, agitation, increased anxiety, headache, extrapyramidal reactions (eg, tremors, dystonia, oculogyria)
Sedatives and Hypnotics			
Benzodiazepines			
lorazepam (Ativan)	1–10 mg/day; for anxiety, 2–3 mg two or three times daily; for insomnia, 2–4 mg at bedtime, total daily dosage should not exceed 10 mg	Acute agitation, aggression, insomnia	Paradoxical rage; tolerance to sedative effect
clonazepam (Klonopin)	Initially 0.5 mg three times daily; may be increased by 0.5–1.0 mg every 3 days	Aggression and anxiety	Hyperactivity

UNDERSTANDING PSYCHOPHARMACOLOGY 32.1

Typical Medications Used to Treat Aggressive Behavior (continued)

TYPE	DOSAGE RANGE	INDICATIONS	CAUTIONS
Others			
chloral hydrate	Sedative: 250 mg three times daily Hypnotic: 500–1,000 mg 15–30 min before bedtime, total daily dosage should not exceed 2,000 mg	Used primarily as a bedtime sedative in sufficient dosage to induce sleep; may be used PRN to achieve sedation in agitated clients Central antimuscarinic effects (antiparkinsonian action)	Tolerance to sedative effect
diphenhydramine (Benadryl)	25–50 mg every 4–6 h; daily dosage should not exceed 300 mg	Central antimuscarinic effects (antiparkinsonian action)	Hemolytic anemia, reduced white blood cell count, blood platelet destruction
buspirone (BuSpar)	Maximum dose: 20–60 mg/day in divided doses; should not exceed 60 mg	Chronic aggression (eg, head injury, dementia); aggression related to anxiety	Paradoxical aggressiveness
Tricyclics			
amitriptyline (Elavil)	Initially 25 mg two to four times daily; may be increased cautiously PRN and as tolerated by 10–25 mg daily every week in equally divided doses; not to exceed 150 mg/day	Recent severe head injury when agitation has not responded to behavioral techniques	Orthostatic hypotension, cardiac dysrhythmias, seizures
trazodone (Desyrel)	50 mg three times a day, may be increased by 50 mg daily at intervals of 3 or 4 days PRN; not to exceed 400 mg daily	Depression (with or without anxiety)	Confusion, muscle tremors, excitement, priapism in men
Selective Serotonin Reuptake Inhibitors			
fluoxetine (Prozac)	Initially 20 mg daily; if no improvement after 3 wk of treatment, dose may be increased by 20 mg/day PRN; not to exceed 80 mg/day	Irritability, aggression, brain injury	Drug-induced seizures (0.2%), serum sickness–like syndrome (2%–3%)
sertraline (Zoloft)	50 mg daily; may increase every week to a maximum of 200 mg/day	Clients with personality disorders and impulsive aggression; aggression after closed-head injury	Headaches, nausea, diarrhea, insomnia, and male sexual dysfunction
Mood Stabilizer			
lithium	300–1,200 mg/day Therapeutic plasma levels: 0.6–1.0 mEq/L	Impulsive aggression; aggression and irritability related to mania; useful with prison populations or clients with mental retardation	Monitor plasma levels, potential fatal toxicity, leukocytosis, hypothyroidism, diabetes insipidus–like syndrome
Anticonvulsants			
carbamazepine (Tegretol)	100–200 mg/12 h; may be increased every week by 200 mg daily PRN; not to exceed 1,200 mg daily	Irritability and aggression related to complex seizure disorders and other organic brain disorders	Bone marrow suppression, hematologic abnormalities, hepatotoxicity

(continues on page 710)

UNDERSTANDING PSYCHOPHARMACOLOGY 32.1

Typical Medications Used to Treat Aggressive Behavior (continued)

TYPE	DOSAGE RANGE	INDICATIONS	CAUTIONS
valproic acid (Depakene)	Initially, 15 mg/kg every 24 h; dose increased cautiously by 5–10 mg/kg per 24 h every 7 days PRN; usual dose from 1,000–1,600 mg in divided doses; not to exceed 60 mg/kg daily	Episodic explosiveness related to brain injury	Bizarre behavior, hallucinations, drug-induced hepatitis with jaundice, pancreatitis
propranolol (Inderal)	20 mg three times daily or 60 mg every 3–4 days to maximum dose of 640 mg/day	Chronic or recurrent aggression related to organic brain disorders or injuries; irritability and aggression not directly related to psychotic ideation; hypertension	Onset of action 4–6 wk, aggravation of arterial insufficiency, bronchospasm, hyperglycemia, hypoglycemia, insomnia, nightmares
pindolol (Visken)	10–60 mg two times daily	See propranolol	See propranolol
mitroprolol (Lopressor)	100–450 mg one to two times daily	See propranolol	See propranolol

---

Checkpoint Questions

5. What is the overall goal of treatment for aggressive and violent clients?
6. What is another name for guided discovery?
7. What three phases are associated with inflexible–explosive episodes?

Restraint and Seclusion

Several important terms are relevant to the discussion of *restraint* and *seclusion*. The Centers for Medicare and Medicaid Services (CMS) of the U.S. Department of Health and Human Services (2006), formerly known as the Health Care Financing Administration, uses the following definitions:

- A **restraint** is any manual method or physical or mechanical device, material, or equipment attached to a person's body that restricts freedom of movement or normal access to one's body. Restraint methods include manual and mechanical methods and the use of drugs.
- A *drug used as restraint* is a medication used to control behavior or to restrict freedom of movement and is not a typical or standard treatment for the person's medical or psychiatric condition.
- **Seclusion** is the involuntary confinement of a person in a hazard-free room or area that is locked and where the person can be directly observed. Seclusion also includes putting a person in an unlocked room where the client thinks he or she must stay or face consequences from staff.

Related Controversies

Use of restraint, seclusion (R/S), or both in behavioral health treatment facilities remains controversial. Proponents view R/S as a necessary intervention to ensure safety in volatile situations in which client behaviors pose a risk of physical harm to self or others. Opponents note that R/S procedures often are used inappropriately as punishment or for staff convenience, resulting in physical or emotional trauma and, sometimes, death (NETI, 2007). Over a decade ago, the National Alliance on Mental Illness (NAMI) (2000) published the report *Cries of Anguish,* highlighting client abuse, neglect, and deaths linked to R/S incidents in 24 states and the District of Columbia from October 1998 to March 2000.

In the past, staff frequently secluded or physically restrained agitated, angry, and hostile clients in psychiatric institutions until they became demonstrably calmer. Although previously seen as an acceptable way to manage crises and keep clients and staff safe, R/S as a therapeutic intervention is currently under intense scrutiny. National mandates are in place to reduce the use of these dangerous procedures (NETI, 2007), and best practice models for implementation of any programs to reduce restraint and seclusion incidents suggest that reduction measures should be accompanied by movement toward a prevention model. Because client aggression can often result from a coercive environment (Goren et al., 1993), such a model includes involvement of every staff member in the creation of a problem-solving environment that is not punitive.

Consensus is growing that use of R/S in treatment settings should be reduced and ultimately eliminated (NAMI,

2003). "Restraint minimization" is a focus of ongoing discussion worldwide (Evans et al., 2002; NETI, 2007). One reason is that no evidence shows that R/S has any therapeutic benefit or leads to positive behavior change. In fact, use of R/S may foster distrust between clients and staff and impede recovery (Mohr et al., 2003). Also, when in seclusion, clients describe feeling neglected, fearful, isolated, out of control, vulnerable, bad, and punished (Martinez et al., 1999). These feelings are not conducive to developing trust or a therapeutic relationship. Children especially recall these events as confusing and report them as traumatic to watch or experience (Mohr et al., 1998). Likewise, a "milieu" in which R/S is a threat or punishment cannot be called therapeutic. Many professionals dispute applying the term "intervention" to either restraint or seclusion. They consider use to be a "safety measure of last resort" and a therapeutic failure.

R/S creates significant psychological risks for psychiatric clients, retraumatizing those who may have a history of trauma, dehumanizing them, and causing loss of dignity (NETI, 2007). In addition, nurses and other staff may be at risk for assault by some clients during a restraint procedure, resulting in physical injury, psychological suffering, lost work time, and financial costs (NETI, 2007).

Moreover, the literature is clear that use of restraints is a potentially dangerous procedure that affects the cardiorespiratory and other systems and has the potential for adverse physical consequences, including death. Possible causes of restraint-related death include asphyxia, cardiac complications, blunt trauma to the chest, strangulation or choking, and aspiration (Huckshorn, 2006; Mohr et al., 2003). Nunno's (2006) review of the deaths of 45 children in residential care found that 64% were the result of asphyxiation.

Another important concern is the physical evaluation of clients. Those undergoing R/S often are left alone and unattended for lengthy intervals. Health care providers often neglect to pay attention to physical status, including evaluating for the presence of medical problems. Consequently, many regulatory boards and professional organizations, including The Joint Commission, have released position statements supporting more stringent standards for use of R/S (D'Orio et al., 2007; International Society of Psychiatric Nurses, 1999; NASMHPD, 1999a, 1999b).

> **Think About It 32.1**
> As part of a class assignment, you are to debate the issues surrounding the use of R/S. You will not know which side you will be assigned until just before the debate. Compose arguments for and against the use of these procedures.

Standards in Behavioral Health Care

Because of the risks of R/S, a primary guideline is that use should be limited to emergencies in which the risk of a client physically harming self, staff, or others is imminent. Furthermore, R/S should be applied only when other less-restrictive methods to ensure client safety have failed. Nonphysical interventions are the first choice. When de-escalation fails and R/S is implemented, R/S should be discontinued as soon as possible. Coercion, discipline, convenience, and retaliation by staff are unacceptable reasons for placing clients in R/S. These events need to be reviewed with such factors in mind. The Joint Commission (2009) standards note that leaders of psychiatric treatment facilities should create a milieu "that minimizes circumstances that give rise to restraint and seclusion use and that maximizes safety when restraint or seclusion is used." It also emphasizes the need to raise awareness among staff about how clients perceive the R/S experience.

In December 2006, the main regulatory agency of the federal government, the CMS, issued its Final Rule governing clients' rights. The Final Rule included a new single standard for restraint and seclusion, combining these practices for acute, medical, and behavior management purposes, and adopted the restraint and seclusion definitions and death reporting requirements established by the Children's Health Act (Le Bel, 2008). The new standard also identified new staff training requirements for safe application, practice competencies, and understanding how to recognize physical distress and monitor physical well-being. Students should be aware that the same standards for R/S apply whether the psychiatric client is in a mental health facility or a medical facility. See Box 32.3 for more guidelines for use of R/S.

Outpatient Management

Early discharge of violent or potentially violent people is a growing and urgent concern for health professionals, families, and the general populace. The shift to outpatient care management mandates development of realignment strategies to fit inpatient education and treatment into an implemented plan of care that reinforces and maintains a "seamless" continuity of treatment when the client is discharged. This approach includes the following:

- A comprehensive client database that the hospital and community care systems can use to articulate services based on client needs: Treatment protocols can be designed so that inpatient interventions, such as cognitive therapy or anger management groups, can be continued in community outpatient settings. Discharge planning for clients who have been violent may involve intensive case management and strong links with community centers that provide mental health services, treatment for substance abuse, social and welfare services, and probation and other criminal justice services.
- Organization of pertinent observational data and interaction incidents into useful client assessment data: For example, for the potentially violent client, such data might include any behavioral patterns typical of the client escalating into violence and any particular interventions that were successful in helping the client regain self-control.

BOX 32.3 Summary of Standards for Restraint and Seclusion (R/S)

Who Can Issue Orders for R/S?

A physician with specialized training and experience in the diagnosis and treatment of mental diseases, or a licensed independent practitioner (LIP) with specialized training and experience in the use of emergency safety interventions and permitted by the state and facility, may issue orders for R/S. State definitions of LIP vary. Psychologists and advanced practice nurses may be able to order R/S, depending on licensure and scope of practice. According to the CMS (2006), if a client's treating physician has not ordered R/S, staff members must consult him or her as soon as possible. Orders for R/S are not to be written as "standing" or on an "as-needed" basis (Joint Commission, 2004).

What Is the Maximum Duration of R/S That Can Be Ordered?

Verbal and written orders for R/S are limited to 4 hours for clients ages 18 years and older, 2 hours for children 9 to 17 years, and 1 hour for children younger than 9 years of age (Joint Commission, 2004). If additional time is necessary, staff must obtain a new order from the physician, LIP, or another person qualified and authorized by the organization. The client requires regular reevaluation.

When Must a Client Placed in R/S Be Evaluated and by Whom?

The Joint Commission (2004) requires a physician or LIP to conduct face-to-face evaluation of the client *within 1 hour* of initiation of R/S and to assess the need for ongoing R/S. He or she works with client and staff to identify ways to help the client gain behavioral control, evaluates and revises the plan of care, and provides a new written order, if necessary (Joint Commission, 2004). If the client is no longer in R/S when the original verbal order expires, the physician or LIP evaluates the client in person within 24 hours of initiation of R/S (Joint Commission, 2004).

The 1-hour rule has sparked much debate within the mental health community. Most advocacy organizations support it and contend that in emergencies involving R/S, physicians are ultimately responsible and accountable for responding to clients. Opponents, mostly providers or treatment facilities, contend that some rural hospitals do not have a qualified physician or LIP on hand to evaluate a client face-to-face within 1 hour of R/S.

What Factors Are Considered in Assessing and Monitoring Safety While a Client Is in R/S?

Qualified staff members assess the client at the initiation of R/S and every 15 minutes thereafter, focusing on the following (Joint Commission, 2004, p. PC-52):

- Signs of injury associated with the application of R/S
- Nutrition and hydration
- Circulation and range of motion in the extremities
- Vital signs

- Hygiene and elimination needs
- Physical and psychological status and comfort (this includes recognizing when to contact a medically trained LIP or emergency medical services to evaluate or treat physical status)
- Client's readiness for discontinuation of R/S. Early in the process, staff members explain to the client the rationale for R/S and the behavior criteria that he or she must meet for discontinuation; they assist the client to meet the behavior criteria.

Staff members must observe the client continuously as long as he or she is in R/S. They must have direct eye contact with the client, although this can occur through a window or doorway if their presence in the room is likely to increase the client's agitation (Joint Commission, 2004). Based on the client's condition and wishes, staff members may use video and audio monitoring equipment after the first hour (Joint Commission, 2004). According to The Joint Commission (2004), staff members authorized to initiate and monitor R/S should demonstrate competence in recognizing how factors such as age, developmental status, sex, ethnicity, and history of physical or sexual trauma may influence reactions to physical contact. For example, the client may prefer a staff member of the same sex (unless his or her history indicates previous abuse by someone of the same sex). All staff with direct client contact must receive continuing education and training in proper and safe application of R/S procedures, as well as nonphysical interventions (Joint Commission, 2004).

What Type of Debriefing Is Done?

Within 24 hours after the R/S episode, staff who participated, the client, and the client's family (if appropriate) hold a debriefing to discuss the circumstances and factors resulting in the use of R/S and ways to prevent future episodes (Joint Commission, 2004). Other topics include what might have been handled differently and whether staff members addressed the client's physical well-being, psychological comfort, and right to privacy. Staff also may counsel the client for any trauma resulting from the R/S. If indicated, the team modifies the client's treatment plan.

What Type of Reporting Is Required?

Staff members record the R/S incident in the clinical/case record and include information about age, sex, health status, and history of trauma before R/S (Joint Commission, 2004). They document fully the circumstances that led to R/S, including nonphysical interventions, rationales for the restraint used, particular behavior criteria identified for discontinuing R/S, and length of each R/S episode. They report assessment and monitoring data, as well as debriefing with client and staff. They also report any injuries and related treatments, as well as any deaths. The hospital must report to CMS any client's death that results while he or she was in R/S or instances in which it is reasonable to assume that a client's death is a result of R/S (CMS, 2001; Joint Commission, 2004).

• Collecting outcome data: In the ever-changing health care system, nurses must document client outcomes related to nursing interventions, including which of the client's symptoms improved and to what extent. Close monitoring of medication effects and of client compliance with the treatment plan is essential.

A Note on Other Settings

Of recent interest to future psychiatric and school nurses is the situation in the U.S. public school system. In 2009 the U.S. Government Accountability Office (GAO) was asked to investigate R/S practices in public schools. The investigation found "hundreds of cases of alleged abuse and death related to the use of these methods on school children during the past two decades" and cited specific examples of death and injury to children (GAO, 2009). Following the release of the GAO report in May 2009, the U.S. Department of Education directed each state to review its current policies and guidelines regarding the use of R/S in schools to ensure that every student is safe and protected and, if appropriate, to develop or revise its policies and guidelines. Permanent legislation is still pending in this area as of this writing and students are encouraged to keep abreast of changes and regulations.

Checkpoint Questions

8. Orders for restraint and seclusion are limited to what time frame?

9. After initiation of R/S, face-to-face evaluation of the client must be done within what time frame and by whom?

10. When is debriefing done? Who is involved?

APPLYING THE NURSING PROCESS

Angry, Aggressive, or Violent Behavior

⚠ ASSESSMENT

Watching for behavioral cues and listening carefully for tone in communication enable nurses to prevent angry and hostile feelings from escalating. Clients may reveal behavioral clues through comments, actions, or mood. Alternatively, a client's history may indicate a potential for violence (Box 32.4).

Nurses may see signs of escalating aggressiveness in the following features:

• *Thinking and perception:* Is the client making aggressive statements? What is his or her view of the world and others? Does the client suffer from potentially harmful delusions or hallucinations? (For example, a wife is convinced that her husband is trying to kill her and the "voices" she hears in her head tell her to kill him.)

• *Motor activity and body language:* Does the client exhibit increased psychomotor agitation (fidgeting, pacing) along with a tense posture, clenched fists, or a tightened jaw?

BOX 32.4   Risk Factor Profiles for Violent Behavior

Demographic

• Young age
• Male sex
• Lack of employment
• Limited education

History

• Violence to self or others
• Antisocial behavior
• Arrests for criminal acts
• Violence within family of origin (eg, physical abuse, sexual abuse)
• Aggressive childhood behavior, including cruelty to animals

Psychiatric Diagnosis

• Antisocial personality disorder
• Substance abuse
• Psychoses (especially paranoid schizophrenia and violence-prone delusions or hallucinations)
• Schizoaffective disorder
• Impulsive aggression

Medical

• Traumatic brain injuries
• Other central nervous system dysfunctions

Social–Environmental

• Association with antisocial peers
• Low residential stability
• Living with and financially dependent on family members(s)
• Living in a violent milieu
• Access to lethal weapons

Cognitive

• Negative perceptions and appraisals of impending events as aversive and anger inducing

Behavioral

• Poor impulse control
• Escalating anger or agitation
• Coercive, exploitative interaction style
• Antisocial and criminal acts
• Statement of intent to harm self or others

• *Mood or affect:* Has the client's affect or verbalization increased, or has the way in which he or she expresses wants and needs changed noticeably? (For example, the client speaks loudly with an angry tone of voice that he wants the staff to let him out of the hospital.)

• *Physical state:* Does the client have seizures, delirium, or brain lesions that may influence sudden violent behavior with no warning?

• *Context:* Does the client have a history of violence? A history of outbursts against self or others may include past involvement in being secluded or restrained, repeated criminal behavior or suicide attempts, and use of alcohol, other addictive drugs, or hallucinogenic drugs that diminish control over behavior (Littrell, 1998; NETI, 2007).

All these questions should be asked on admission to the service. See also Assessment Tool 32.1.

▲ NURSING DIAGNOSIS

The nursing diagnoses primarily relevant to potentially aggressive and violent clients are **Risk for Self-Directed Violence** and **Risk for Other-Directed Violence** and **Ineffective Coping** related to psychopathology, poor impulse control, or history of violence (NANDA, 2007).

▲ OUTCOME IDENTIFICATION AND PLANNING

Most potentially violent clients require direct, one-to-one assistance from staff to meet goals. Clients will not know how to manage expectations without education, prompting, and support. Examples of such goals, incorporating labels from the *Nursing Outcomes Classification* (*NOC*), include the following (Moorhead et al., 2008):

- **Impulse Control:** The client will contract with staff to avoid acting on violent impulses and ask staff for help when these situations occur.

- **Aggression Control:** The client will report feelings of impending loss of personal control and ask for help from staff.
- **Abusive Behavior Self-Restraint:** The client will discuss feelings of anxiety, anger, frustration, and aggression and describe effective ways that work to prevent these feelings from escalating in a *personal safety plan.*
- **Coping:** The client will state awareness of typical appraisals of precipitating events, ways to reframe thoughts and behavioral responses more constructively, and awareness of personal competencies in problem solving and coping.

▲ IMPLEMENTATION

Nurses and other mental health care professionals must weigh carefully the principles of safety and provide the least restrictive environment possible. At the same time, they need to effectively prevent aggression and violence and safely deal with these behaviors when they happen. Staff members must maintain caring and concern and use a nonauthoritarian approach directed at mediating conflicts and finding win–win answers. Even floridly psychotic clients whose tension increases before violence may respond positively to nonjudgmental interpersonal contact. Nurses planning care for clients with angry, aggressive, or violent behavior must address immediate needs, such as identifying specific triggers, developing a safety plan with clients, otherwise preventing behavior from escalating, and ensuring the safety of other clients and staff.

▲ ASSESSMENT TOOL 32.1 ▲
Assessment of Violence and Homicidal Ideation

Violence Assessment

Assess ideas about violence or intent to harm others:

- "Is there anyone who you have been thinking about hurting?"
- "Have you had ideas that you would want to hurt someone?"
- "Do you feel anger toward anyone in particular?"

Assess history of violent behavior:

- "Have you ever felt violent like this before?"
- "Have you ever lost control and been violent toward another person?"
- "Can you describe that situation?"
- "How many times in the past have you been violent toward someone?"
- "What types of things do you do when you are feeling violent?"
- "Did you hurt anyone while you were in the hospital before?"
- "What happened?"

Assess seriousness and severity of past violent behavior:

- "How serious were you in your intent to kill or hurt _____?"
- "What did you do to carry out your plan?"

- "Did your actions result in injury or death to the other person?"
- "Did anything happen as a result of your behavior?"

Assess severe agitation or hostility:

- "How are you feeling right now?"
- "Do you feel angry about anything in particular?"
- "What things are causing you to feel irritated or angry now?

Assess mental status for active psychosis (see Mental Status Examination in text in Chapter 10)

Assessment of Homicidal Ideation

Assess whom the client wishes to harm:

- "Do you feel as though you would want to harm or kill another person?"
- "Who is it that you would wish to harm or kill?"

Assess whether the client has an active plan and methods or means:

- "Do you have a plan developed to kill or hurt _____?"
- "Are these weapons (or other methods) available to you in your home?"

Nurses use many types of interventions to assist clients and families. Common *Nursing Interventions Classification* (*NIC*) labels include, but are not limited to, **Anger Control Assistance, Behavior Management, Environmental Management: Violence Prevention, Impulse Control Training,** and **Support Groups** (Bulechek et al., 2008).

Maintaining the Safety of Clients and Staff

Nurses must be concerned for the safety of clients, others in the immediate environment, and themselves. Some general guidelines for safety awareness include the following:

- Get to know everyone in your care on your shift. Make rounds immediately following shift report, introduce yourself, and ask if there is anything you can do to help.
- Do not make promises to talk to someone and not follow through.
- If you get into a "situation":
  - Take a position just outside the client's personal space (slightly out of arm's reach).
  - If possible, stand on the client's nondominant side (usually the side on which he or she wears a wristwatch).
  - Keep an open posture with your hands in sight.
  - Keep the client in visual range.
  - Make sure the door of a room is readily accessible. Avoid letting the client get between you and the door.
  - Be friendly, concerned, and avoid being demanding unless the danger is imminent. If the latter, it is perfectly acceptable to say "Please stop that now" authoritatively.
  - Retreat from the situation and summon help if the client's aggression escalates to imminent violence.
  - Avoid being alone with an escalating client.
- Call a colleague (who knows the client better than you) to help you in any troubling situation.
- Create a safety plan on admission with the client to find out what helps him or her calm down and what upsets him or her.
- Find out the point of conflict. Try to either empathize or remove the source of conflict.

Defusing Anger and Aggression Through Verbal Interventions

Simply speaking in a therapeutic manner can help defuse anger and foster insight for clients. Conversely, engaging in power struggles by subtly or overtly trying to establish authority can escalate aggression (NETI, 2007). When using verbal interventions, nurses follow these steps:

1. *Make contact:* Appear calm and in control. Speak in a normal, nonprovocative, and nonjudgmental tone. Be alert to verbal and nonverbal behavior that indicates the feelings of clients. Ask what clients are feeling. State your observations of what you see clients doing behaviorally and how you think they might be feeling. Check your understanding.
2. *Discover the source of distress:* Attempt to discover their concerns and respond with empathy, interest, and willingness to help. Encourage clients to describe and clarify their experience to increase awareness of and triggers for problematic feelings. Use open-ended questions, which elicit meaningful descriptions. Yes-or-no questions are useful for specific information, such as "Are you feeling angry?" However, a series of yes-or-no questions may seem like an interrogation. Avoid using "why" questions, which may seem accusatory and lead clients to feel defensive. Listen and paraphrase the responses of clients. Ask if your understanding is correct.
3. *Relieve the distress:* Often, nurses are aware of only the deficit side of various disturbing behaviors and the affect of an angry person. They may not be cognizant of the client's competency to prevent anger escalation by maintaining control and rebuilding constructive functioning. If possible, talk with clients about their ideas for a plan of action that would help deal with the situation. Doing so affirms the client's competence and provides information for further problem solving (Greene, 2001). Discussing the following is useful:
   - What does the client want?
   - What has the client tried in the past?
   - How well did it work?
   - What can the nurse (you) do to help the client right now.

Recognizing what has been tried and how well it worked can help clients avoid repeating mistakes, make adaptive choices, and avoid limit-setting situations.

See Box 32.5 for additional, situation-specific interventions to prevent escalation of client aggression.

Setting Limits to Prevent Violent Behavior

Setting firm but fair limits sometimes helps clients to establish appropriate boundaries and can increase feelings of security. Before setting a limit, nurses need to describe the problematic behavior; communicate what would be more helpful, and offer some specific alternatives. Examples include walking with nurses, having some one-to-one time, making a phone call, and listening to music. Clients must have the chance to "save face" and can often de-escalate when they are sincerely and respectfully presented with alternatives to their intended behavior.

Nurses state their wishes (the limit) in a matter-of-fact manner, not as advice, bribery, or punishment. The "limit" tells clients specifically what they are to do or not to do in the situation. Also, nurses help clients understand the reason for the limit.

In escalating situations, nurses may need to express consequences for clients who test the limit or continue inappropriate behavior. However, outlining consequences often **sounds like a threat and can escalate situations further.** This is a very important point, because limit setting requires skill, both as to when and how such an intervention should be implemented. Dangerous situations can arise when limit setting is done in a way that makes clients feel threatened or that they are being treated unfairly. Nurses should reserve this measure for real emergencies. The demeanor of nurses is extremely important throughout this kind of negotiation and must combine competence and compassion.

BOX 32.5 Situation-Specific Interventions to Prevent Escalation of Client Aggression

- When the client asks questions in a demanding way, such as "Why isn't my doctor here?" or "Why can't you give me my medication now?", avoid becoming defensive or authoritarian. Address the client's concern in a factual, respectful, and supportive manner. Studies by nurse researchers indicate that anger in hospitalized clients tends to escalate when they are confronted with an authoritative, superior attitude on the part of nurses and other health care staff (Love & Morrison, 2003).
- When the client makes refusals, such as "I'm not going to take that medicine," or "I'm not going to group," remain calm and avoid a power struggle with the client. Useful responses include a supportive acknowledgment of the client's concern and asking the client to explain the reasons behind the refusal (Carlsson et al., 2004). After hearing the client's story, explain the consequences of the refusal and help the client toward solutions or alternatives.
- When the client directs verbal anger at you, allow the client to "vent," then express understanding. For example, "I can see that you are disappointed" (or whatever feeling the client is expressing). Work with the client toward constructive solutions.
- When the client uses intimidation like "I'm going to sue everyone who works on this unit," avoid trying to justify the situation or defend your actions. Show empathy for the client's feelings. For example, "I know you're frustrated at having to wait for your treatment." Receiving the nurse's understanding may help calm the client.
- When the client's behavior continues to escalate toward violence, assess the need for limit setting.

Nurses must use limit setting uniformly because unjust or idiosyncratic use of directives or rules tends to incite anger in most people in any setting. When clients test a limit, they usually experience some anxiety. Having staff respond predictably to ensure safety and protection fosters security and confidence.

Teaching Anger Management and Coping Skills

Anger is the common emotion that leads to aggression and violence. It results from many variables, including personality, experiences, temperament, low frustration tolerance, poor coping skills, and negative thought patterns. Many people, not just those with psychiatric disorders, have difficulty dealing with anger or other troubling feelings. Different events trigger different people to anger. Shame and humiliation are particularly difficult feelings, and nurses should make every effort to avoid events that could trigger these emotions in clients (NETI, 2007). Clients also can learn to control anger by recognizing what triggers their anger, how behaviors contribute to volatile situations, and how self-talk can either help or hinder adaptive coping.

Nurses may want to suggest that clients keep a journal to obtain insight into patterns of behavior. Clients can write about their angry feelings and consciously try to identify precursors to feeling out of control or enraged (Figure 32.5). Often, clients can identify situations that trigger anger and are thereby empowered to implement other strategies that will modulate angry responses before acting on them. One such strategy is *cognitive restructuring* or changing the automatic self-talk that feeds into negative feelings, including anger. Nurses assist clients to begin to recognize the self-talk that encourages anger. For example, a client may say to himself, "This person is trying to make me look bad. I want to hurt this guy." A nurse can teach the client to recognize this thought and replace it with a more acceptable one such as "This isn't my problem, it's his. Relax."

Another effective method for controlling aggression is to teach assertiveness skills. Although typically an intervention for clients with traits of dependency and passivity, assertiveness training also can benefit aggressive clients by teaching them appropriate tools for meeting their needs without infringing on the rights of others. Assertive statements follow a pattern:

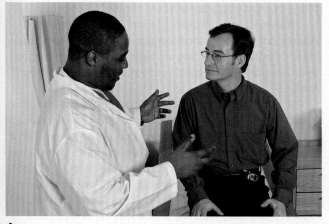

A

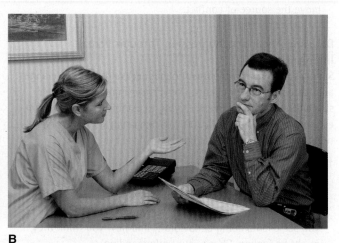

B

FIGURE 32.5 Clients learning cognitive techniques to control anger may learn to recognize triggers and feel more empowered to implement strategies to modulate responses before acting on them. **(A)** This client is learning to step away from volatile situations and gain control over his feelings. **(B)** Later, he sits down with a nurse to review his journal entries about his feelings and methods that worked to channel them successfully

1. "When. . . ." (Concretely describe the other person's behavior.)
2. "The effects are. . . ." (Objectively describe the effect of the other person's actions.)
3. "I feel. . . ." (Honestly describe feelings.)
4. "I prefer. . . ." (Respectfully suggest desired outcome or behavior.)

A correlate to assertiveness training is teaching better communication and problem-solving skills. Empathic communication can help chronically angry clients improve their relationships. Clients can learn about making "I" statements ("I feel hurt by your remarks") instead of "you" statements ("You hurt my feelings") to avoid making judgments by relating feelings rather than opinions and to develop better listening skills. Clients should learn to ask for feedback to enhance their ability to communicate. Nurses can include family or loved ones of clients in this process.

Finally, nurses can instruct clients in *personal feeling management,* also known as *sensory modulation techniques* (NETI, 2007). All humans have "sensory diets" that lead them, often unconsciously, to seek out certain experiences that make people feel better. Some people work out or run, some listen to music or play the piano, and others find a bath or quiet time to help calm and relax them. The point is that everyone is different and that nurses need to discover the client's personal experiences in seeking natural opportunities. In many situations, clients do not know what their "sensory diets" are and need help to identify these activities. Consultation with an occupational therapist is generally required to successfully create a sensory plan (Champagne & Stromberg, 2004).

Another set of anger de-escalation strategies is set forth in "The Four S Model" (Delaney et al., 2000), an intervention framework for use by nursing and other staff in daily interactions with clients. The purposes of the model's intervention strategies are to stabilize acute symptoms, restore functionality, establish a support network, and plan for symptom management (Chabora et al., 2003). The four S's are safety, support, structure, and symptom management:

- *Safety* involves securing the physical and emotional well-being of clients without the use of R/S. It includes such interventions as reducing environmental stimuli and enlisting staff to help calm clients in a "show of support" when needed.
- *Support* includes being available to clients, listening and talking with them helpfully, acknowledging and praising their strengths, offering various comfort measures (eg, blankets, warm showers, fresh air), and using verbal de-escalation when needed.
- *Structure* techniques (similar to limit setting) restore clients' positive behavior and may include restating behavioral expectations, negotiating a safety contract, and assisting clients in constructive problem solving.
- *Symptom management* addresses specific symptoms and negative consequences. It includes various stress management

and relaxation strategies, diversionary activities (ie, soft music, journaling, playing cards, reading, watching television), and social skills and medication education (Chabora et al., 2003).

> ### Checkpoint Questions
> 11. What five areas are crucial to assessing clients for signs of escalating aggression?
> 12. What three steps should nurses implement when managing potentially aggressive clients?

▲ EVALUATION

When evaluating care for clients with angry, aggressive, or violent behavior, nurses consider the following to evaluate indicators of success:

- Did implementation of the plan of care (or personal safety plan) prevent an escalation of aggressive behavior, although emotions may have been intense?
- Was everyone's safety maintained (including the "observers of the incident")?
- Did health care personnel follow the institution's written policies and procedures for dealing with aggressive behavior?
- Did the client (and nursing staff) learn any new problem-solving techniques or resources for handling aggressive behaviors in the future?
- Was the client's dignity respected? Did staff avoid the development of a win–lose situation or avoid shaming or humiliating the client?

Expected outcomes for clients include the ability to report feelings of loss of control and to ask for help from appropriate staff. Clients need to learn to discuss the antecedents to their feelings of anxiety, anger, shame, being treated unfairly, and frustration. They must describe effective ways to prevent the escalation of these feelings. They verbalize awareness of cognitive appraisals of precipitating events, ways to reframe thoughts and behavioral responses more constructively, and awareness of personal competencies in problem solving and coping. Clients use assertive communication skills and can maintain self-control of aggressive and violent inclinations as evidenced by a calm demeanor and no aggressive and violent behavior. They are optimistic about using more constructive cognitive skills and changing methods of coping with anger in future frustrating situations.

Again, these outcomes do not just occur. When they happen, it is through active treatment, such as daily one-to-one and group interventions and constant oversight by treatment team members. Before discharge, clients and family members (or significant others) verbalize knowledge of available community support services, such as ongoing anger management groups, and their intent to use phone numbers of a crisis hotline or other resources if needed.

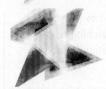

Reviewing and Applying Your Knowledge

Chapter Summary

- Determinants of aggressive and violent behavior include psychological, environmental, medical, biologic, and sociocultural factors.

- Events linked with client violence on inpatient units include a coercive interaction style from staff, idiosyncratic enforcement of rules, long wait times, overcrowding, no active treatment, boredom, delayed discharge placement, indifference from staff, and shaming or humiliation.

- Health care providers can use literally hundreds of interventions to defuse conflict. The identification of which will be most effective depends mainly on "knowing the client," being empathetic, and having the skills and creativity to come up with de-escalation solutions.

- Three major types of psychiatric interventions include verbal negotiation, pharmacotherapeutics, and physical restraint and seclusion. Health care providers need to avoid the latter two interventions when possible. They should make all efforts to help clients learn to "self-sooth" and to teach illness management in ways that clients can transfer to community living.

- Other therapeutic strategies with reported success in helping clients toward greater self-awareness and positive management of anger include cognitive therapy, behavior therapy, anger management groups, and group/family therapies.

- Assessment data for clients with anger or violent symptoms focus on past history of aggressive or violent behavior, substance abuse, homelessness, history of traumatic life events, how clients handle anger or anxiety, cognitive patterns, problem solving, and communication.

- When planning therapeutic interventions, the nurse and client choose desired outcomes based on the client's issues, needs, and current skills in maintaining self-control of aggressive and violent inclinations.

- Evaluation requires a close examination of client and nursing efforts toward meeting behavioral outcomes and what additional therapeutic interventions might be more effective.

Study Questions

1. Which of the following events on a psychiatric unit is most likely to precipitate aggressive or violent behavior in a violence-prone client (Mr. A.)?

   a. A psychiatric technician asks Mr. A. if he would like some juice during snack time.

   b. A nurse asks Mr. A., who is frowning and pacing, if he is feeling upset about something.

   c. A nurse reminds Mr. A. that it is time to take his medication, which he has been doing willingly.

   d. Another client on the unit picks up Mr. A's pack of cigarettes and says that they are his.

2. When preparing a group presentation about the emergency use of seclusion and restraint, which of the following would the nurse be least likely to incorporate into the discussion?

   a. It is not necessary to immediately try to involve the client in conversation to find out why he or she is upset.

   b. Specific written policies and procedures clearly directing the use of restraint or seclusion should be available in mental health institutions.

   c. Justification for emergency use of seclusion and restraint is legally based on professional clinical judgment and professional standards of care, including documented signs describing the emergence of imminently dangerous behavior that could result in serious harm to self or others.

   d. A professional nurse should act as a leader to direct the actions of staff in implementing emergency seclusion and restraint procedures for a client whose behavior is violent and out of control.

3. Which of the following medications would the nurse expect to administer most commonly to a client with aggressive behavior associated with acute psychoses?

   a. Diazepam

   b. Haloperidol

   c. Lithium

   d. Fluoxetine

4. Which intervention is most appropriate for the nurse to implement with an aggressive client exhibiting an early level of anger escalation?

a. Administer ordered sedative medication.

b. Place the client in seclusion.

c. Use a physical restraint.

d. Talk with client to discover the source of distress and relieve the distress.

5. Which of the following statements would reflect that anger management training for a violence-prone client has been ineffective?

a. The client has gained awareness of thoughts, feelings, and behaviors related to anger arousal.

b. The client thinks that "others make him feel angry" and as a result blames them for his resultant behaviors.

c. The client reappraises arousal situations as a personal problem that has a solution, rather than as a threat calling for an attack.

d. The client gains awareness of others' points of view and the consequences of his or her own emotional and behavioral responses.

Critical Thinking Questions

1. Is limit setting appropriate for all clients who are potentially violent?

2. With staff shortages and decreased lengths of hospital stay, what increased client safety concerns occur in hospitals?

3. What kinds of community support resources need to be in place to accommodate commitment to outpatient treatment settings and preventive commitment?

References

American Psychiatric Association (APA). (2000). *Diagnostic and statistical manual of mental disorders* (4th ed., text rev.). Washington, DC: Author.

Anderson, C. A., & Bushman, B. J. (2002). Human aggression. *Annual Review of Psychology, 53,* 27–51.

Anderson, C. A., & Dill, K. E. (2000). Video games and aggressive thoughts, feelings, and behavior in the laboratory and in life. *Journal of Personal and Social Psychology, 78,* 772–790.

Bandura, A. (1973). *Aggression: A social learning analysis.* Morristown, NJ: Prentice Hall.

Barlett, C. P., Harris, R. J., & Baldassaro, R. (2007). Longer you play, the more hostile you feel: Examination of first person shooter video games and aggression during video game play. *Aggressive Behavior, 33*(6), 486–497.

Bazelon Center for Mental Health Law. (2003). *Criminalization of people with mental illness: The role of mental health courts in system reform.* Washington, DC: Author.

Bender, K. J. (2003). Consensus on treatments for aggression in youth. *Psychiatric Times, 20*(7).

Bensley, L., & Van Eenwyk, J. (2001). Video games and real-life aggression: Review of the literature. *Journal of Adolescent Health, 29*(4), 244–257.

Brieden, T., Ujeyl, M., & Naber, D. (2002). Psychopharmacological treatment of aggression in schizophrenic patients. *Pharmacopsychiatry, 35,* 83–89.

Brink, P. (2001). Violence on TV and aggression in children (Editorial). *Western Journal of Nursing Research, 23*(1), 5–7.

Bulechek, G. M., Butcher, H. K., & McCloskey Dochterman, J. (2008). *Nursing interventions classification (NIC)* (5th ed.). St. Louis, MO: Mosby.

Carlsson, G., Dahlberg, K., Lutzen, K., & Nystrom, K. (2004). Violent encounters in psychiatric care: A phenomenological study of embodied care knowledge. *Issues in Mental Health Nursing, 25*(2), 191–217.

Centers for Medicare & Medicaid Services (CMS). (2006). *Hospital conditions of participation: Patients' rights* (No. 42 CFR Part 482). Baltimore, MD: U.S. Department of Health and Human Services.

Chabora, N., Judge-Gorny, M., & Grogan, K. (2003). The Four S Model in action for de-escalation: An innovative state hospital–university collaborative endeavor. *Journal of Psychosocial Nursing and Mental Health Services, 41*(1), 23–28.

Champagne, T., & Stromberg, N. (2004). Sensory approaches in inpatient settings: Innovative alternatives to seclusion and restraint. *Journal of Psychosocial Nursing, 42,* 35–44.

Citrome, L. L. (2007). *Aggression.* Retrieved from http://www.emedicine.com/Med/ topic3005.htm

Cunningham, M., & Henry, M. (2007). *Homelessness counts.* National Alliance to End Homelessness. Retrieved from http://www.endhomelessness.org/content/article/detail/1440

Cusack, K. J., Frueh, B. C., & Brady, K. T. (2004). Trauma history screening in a community mental health center. *Psychiatric Services, 55*(2), 157–162.

Cusack, K. J., Frueh, B. C., Hiers, T. G., Keane, T. M., & Mueser, K. T. (2003). *The impact of trauma and posttraumatic stress disorder upon American society* (Report to the President's Commission on Mental Health. Unpublished subcommittee report.). Washington, DC.

Delaney, K. R., Pitula, C. R., & Perraud, S. (2000). Psychiatric hospitalization and process description: What will nursing add? *Journal of Psychosocial Nursing and Mental Health Services, 38*(3), 7–13.

D'Orio, B., Wimby, G., & Haggard, P. J. (2007). Reducing risk associated with seclusion and restraint. *Psychiatric Times.* Retrieved from http://www.psychiatrictime.com/print.jhtml;jsessionid=ZULDQ1ZD5UIZAQSNDLPSK

Dunbar, B. (2004). Anger management: A holistic approach. *Journal of the American Psychiatric Nurses Association, 10*(1), 16–23.

Evans, D., Wood, J., & Lambert, L. (2002). Physical restraint: Part 2. Minimisation in acute and residential care facilities. *Best Practice: Evidence Based Practice Information Sheets for Health Professionals, 6*(4), 1–6.

Fish, K. (2002). Assessment of impulsivity among psychiatric inpatients. *Journal of Psychosocial Nursing and Mental Health Services, 40*(6), 30–35.

Fredrickson, B., Maynard, K., Helms, M., Haney, T., Siegler, I., & Barefoot, J. (2000). Hostility predicts magnitude and duration of blood pressure responses to anger. *Journal of Behavioral Medicine, 23*(3), 229–243.

Frueh, B. C., Dalton, M. E., Johnson, M. R., Hiers, T. G., Gold, P. B., Magruder K. M., & Santos, A. B. (2000). Trauma within the psychiatric setting: Conceptual framework, research directions, and policy implications. *Administration and Policy in Mental Health, 28*(2), 147–154.

Glick, I. D., Murray, S. R., Vasudevan, P., Marder, S. R., & Hu, R. J. (2001). Treatment with atypical antipsychotics: New indications and new populations. *Journal of Psychiatric Research, 35*(3), 187–191.

Goren, S., Singh, N., & Best, A. (1993). The aggression-coercion cycle: Use of seclusion and restraint in a child psychiatric hospital. *Journal of Child and Adolescent Psychiatric Nursing, 9*, 27–36.

Greenberg, J., & Hollander, E. (2003). Brain function in impulsive disorders. *Psychiatric Times, 20*(3), 81–85.

Greene, R. W. (2001). *The explosive child.* New York, NY: HarperCollins.

Hollander, E., Tracy, K. A., Swann, A. C., Coccaro, E. F., McElroy, S. L., Wozniak, P., et al. (2003). Divalproex in the treatment of impulsive aggression: Efficacy in cluster B personality disorders. *Neuropsychopharmacology, 28,* 1186–1197.

Huckshorn, K. A. (2006). Re-designing state mental health policy to prevent the use of seclusion and restraint. *Administration and Policy in Mental Health, 33*(4), 482–491.

Huesmann, L. R. (2007). The impact of electronic media violence: Scientific theory and research. *Journal of Adolescent Health, 41*(6, Suppl 1), S6–S13.

Huesmann, L. R., Moise-Titus, J., Podolski, C. L., & Eron, L. D. (2003). Longitudinal relations between children's exposure to TV violence and their aggressive and violent behavior in young adulthood: 1977–1992. *Developmental Psychology, 39,* 201–221.

International Society of Psychiatric Nurses. (1999). *The use of restraint and seclusion: Position statement.* Middleton, WI: Author.

Jennings, A. (2004a). *Criteria for building a trauma-informed mental health service system* (Unpublished draft papers). Rockville, ME: Author.

Jennings, A. (2004b). *The damaging consequences of violence and trauma: Facts, discussion points, and recommendations for the behavioral health system.* National Technical Assistance Center. Alexandria, VA: National Association of State Mental Health Program Directors.

The Joint Commission. (2004). Provision of care, treatment and services. In *2010 Comprehensive accreditation manual for behavioral health care.* Oak Brook Terrace, IL: Author.

Konijn, E. A., Bijvank, M. N., & Bushman, B. J. (2007). I wish I were a warrior: The role of wishful identification in the effects of violent video games on aggression in adolescent boys. *Developmental Psychology, 43*(4), 1038–1044.

Le Bel, J. (2008). Regulatory change: A pathway to eliminating seclusion and restraint or "regulatory scotoma"? *Psychiatric Services, 59*(2), 194–196.

Littrell, K. (1998). Current understanding of violence and aggression: Assessment and treatment. *Journal of Psychosocial Nursing, 36*(12), 18–24.

Love, C. C., & Morrison, E. (2003). American Academy of Nursing Expert Panel on Violence Policy recommendations on workplace violence (adopted 2002). *Issues in Mental Health Nursing, 24*(6–7), 599–604.

Lowe, T., Wellman, N., & Taylor, R. (2003). Limit-setting and decision-making in the management of aggression. *Journal of Advanced Nursing, 41*(2), 154–161.

Martinez, R. J., Grimm, M., & Adamson, M. (1999). From the other side of the door: Patient views of seclusion. *Journal of Psychosocial Nursing, 37*(3), 13–22.

Matthews, K., Gump, B. B., Harris, K. F., Haney, T. L., & Barefoot, J. C. (2004). Hostile behaviors predict cardiovascular mortality among men enrolled in the Multiple Risk Factor Intervention Trial. *Circulation, 109,* 66–70.

Maxwell, C. D., & Maxwell, S. R. (2003). Experiencing and witnessing familial aggression and their relationship to physically aggressive behaviors among Filipino adolescents. *Journal of Interpersonal Violence, 18*(12), 1432–1451.

McMonagle, T., & Sultana, A. (2004). Token economy for schizophrenia (Cochrane Review). *The Cochrane Library, Issue 1.* Chichester, UK: John Wiley & Sons.

Mohr, W. K., Mahon, M. M., & Noone, M. J. (1998). A restraint on restraints: The need to reconsider the use of restrictive interventions. *Archives of Psychiatric Nursing, 12*(2), 95–106.

Mohr, W. K., Petti, T. A., & Mohr, B. D. (2003). Adverse effects associated with physical restraint. *Canadian Journal of Psychiatry, 48*(5), 330–337.

Moorhead, S., Johnson, M., Maas, M. L., & Swanson, E. (2008). *Nursing outcomes classification (NOC)* (4th ed.). St. Louis, MO: Mosby.

Moses, D. J., Reed, B. G., Mazelis, R., & D'Ambrosio, B. (2003). *Creating trauma services for women with co-occurring disorders: Experiences from the SAMHSA Women With Alcohol, Drug Abuse and Mental Health Disorders Who Have Histories of Violence Study.* Delmar, NY: Policy Research Associates.

NANDA International. (2007). *Nursing diagnoses: Definitions and classification (2007–2008).* Philadelphia, PA: Author.

National Alliance on Mental Illness (NAMI). (2000). *Cries of anguish: A summary of reports of restraints and seclusion abuse received since the October 1998 investigation by the* Hartford Courant. Retrieved from www.nami.org/update/hartford.html

National Alliance on Mental Illness (NAMI). (2003). *Seclusion and restraints: Task force report.* Arlington, VA: Author.

National Association of State Mental Health Program Directors (NASMHPD). (1999a). *Position statement on services and supports to trauma survivors.* Alexandria, VA: Author.

National Association of State Mental Health Program Directors (NASMHPD). (1999b). *Position statement on seclusion and restraint.* Retrieved from http://www.nasmhpd.org/general__files/position__statement/posses1.htm

National Association of State Mental Health Program Directors Research Institute, Inc. (NASMHPD). (2006). Data element: Does the mental health code allow the use of outpatient civil commitment? In *State Mental Health Agency Profiling System 2005.* Alexandria, VA: Author.

National Executive Training Institute (NETI). (2007). *Training curriculum for reduction of seclusion and restraint. Draft curriculum manual.* Alexandria, VA: National Association of State Mental Health Program Directors (NASMHPD), National Technical Assistance Center for State Mental Health Planning (NTAC).

Nijman, H. L., Campo, J. M., Ravelli, D. P., & Merckelbach, H. L. (1999). A tentative model of aggression on inpatient psychiatric wards. *Psychiatric Services, 50,* 832–834.

Nunno, M., Holden, M., & Tollar, A. (2006). Learning from tragedy: A survey of child and adolescent restraint fatalities. *Child Abuse & Neglect, 30*(12).

Reist, C., Nakamura, K., Sagart, E., Sokolski, K. N., & Fujimoto, K. A. (2003). *Journal of Clinical Psychiatry, 64*(1), 81–85.

Rickelman, B. L., & Houfek, J. (1995). Toward an interactional model of suicidal behaviors: Cognitive rigidity, attributional style, stress, hopelessness, and depression. *Archives of Psychiatric Nursing, 9*(3), 158–168.

Rosenberg, S. D., Mueser, K. T., Friedman, M. J., Gorman, P. G., Drake, R. E., Vidaver, R. M., et al. (2001). Developing effective treatments for posttraumatic disorders among people with severe mental illness. *Psychiatric Services, 52,* 1453–1461.

Saxe, G., & Johansson, R. (2003). *A trauma informed approach to extreme behaviors in intensive child mental health programs.* Boston, MA: Boston University School of Medicine.

Scarpa, A., & Raine, A. (1997). Psychophysiology of anger and violent behavior. *Psychiatric Clinics of North America, 20*(2), 375–394.

Schur, S., Sikich, L., Findling, R. L., Malone, R., Crismon, M. L., Derivan, A., et al. (2003). Treatment recommendations for the use of antipsychotics for aggressive youth (TRAAY). Part I: A review. *Journal of the American Academy of Child and Adolescent Psychiatry, 42*(2), 132–144.

Siegman, A., Townsend, S., Civelek, A., & Blumenthal, R. (2000). Antagonistic behavior, dominance, hostility, and coronary heart disease. *Psychosomatic Medicine, 62*(2), 248–257.

Tarasoff v. Board of Regents of the University of California, 17 Cal 3rd 425, 551 P. 2d 334, 131 Cal Rptr. 14 (1976).

U.S. Government Accountability Office (GAO). (2009). *Seclusion and restraints: Selected cases of death and abuse at public and private schools and treatment centers* (No. GAO-09–719T). Washington, DC: Author.

Van der Kolk, B. A. (1987). *Psychological trauma.* Boston, MA: American Psychiatric Press

Van der Kolk, B. A. (1998). Psychology and psychobiology of childhood trauma. *Praxis der Kinderpsychologie und Kinderpsychiatrie, 47*(1), 19–35.

Vitaro, F., Barker, E. D., Boivin, M., Brendgen, M., & Tremblay, R. E. (2006). Do early difficult temperament and harsh parenting differentially predict reactive and proactive aggression? *Journal of Abnormal Child Psychology, 34*(5), 685–695.

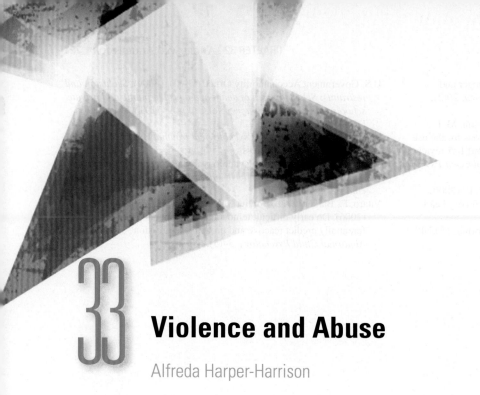

33

Violence and Abuse

Alfreda Harper-Harrison

LEARNING OBJECTIVES

On completion of this chapter, you should be able to accomplish the following:

- Understand the scope and sources of community violence.
- Describe an organizational model for the multiple conditions that support community violence.
- Explain key factors that increase risk for the development of violent responses in young people.
- Identify the dynamics of intimate partner violence and the nurse's role in recognizing, screening, and assisting its victims.
- Discuss the effects of maltreatment on child development.
- Identify the scope of elder abuse and key prevention strategies.
- Define rape and sexual assault.
- Describe the phases of the rape trauma syndrome and treatment approaches.
- Apply the nursing process to the care of the trauma survivor.
- Understand the importance of self-clarification before intervening with clients who have experienced abuse and assault.

Concerns about violence and personal safety are part of every person's reality. Significant advances have been made in understanding violence and developing effective prevention methods. However, addressing community violence effectively demands involvement from many players, including health care professionals, families, educators, community leaders, law enforcement officials, legislators, faith-based organizations, and the media. To join this effort and assist victims appropriately, nurses must understand the public health approach to violence, know the dynamics underlying aggressive behaviors (see Chap. 32), and use skill in formulating responses.

Violence is defined as threatened or actual physical force by one person or group against another. It may be criminal or noncriminal, but violence causes or is likely to result in psychological or physical injury or death (Citrome, 2007). Unfortunately, violence erupts in many forms.

This chapter focuses on the topics of youth violence, family violence, and rape and sexual assault. It explores a model of violence that is central to adapting a public health approach to prevention and treatment and to caring for victims of violence or abuse. For a discussion of how to approach clients who display violent or aggressive behavior, see Chapter 32.

THE ECOLOGICAL MODEL OF VIOLENCE

The causes of violence are multifactorial. Internal factors certainly are relevant to understanding why people commit violent acts. However, violence is better understood as a complex occurrence, and curbing its origins and spread involves understanding it as a social phenomenon with roots in individuals, families, communities, and society at large.

As with other complex phenomena (see Chap. 3), an **ecological model** of the phenomena of violence has great explanatory power. This model identifies and orders the multiple levels of influence that place people at risk of becoming victims or victimizers (Tolan et al., 2003). It orders relevant factors at the level of the individual/peer, family, and community. The broader culture of the child and family also contributes to risk. The levels of influence have been categorized as follows:

1. Societal influences and macrosystem
2. Microsystem
3. Individual factors

The ecological approach not only orders within each level specific factors that contribute to risk, but also illustrates how the factors interact to increase the risk of people engaging in violence. See also Chapter 3.

Societal Influences and Macrosystem

In the broadest view, societal beliefs and cultural norms can foster violence within families and communities. A culture forms not only by active endorsement of particular values

but also by passive acceptance of certain phenomena. U.S. culture sends powerful messages about the acceptance of violence and often appears to condone violent and aggressive behavior in its tacit and sometimes active portrayal of violence in the media and its reluctance to curb firearm proliferation. The reader of any media source will encounter stories of shootings or other violent acts on a daily basis.

Homicide had been among the top 15 causes of death since 1965, rising as high as 13th in 2001, but had fallen to 16th in 2010 (Centers for Disease Control and Prevention [CDC], 2006b). Nonetheless, U.S. homicide rates surpass those of all other Western nations (U.S. Department of Justice [DOJ], 2007b). Young adults have the highest rates of both homicide victimization and offending (DOJ, 2007b). Despite such disturbing statistics, violent images and content permeate U.S. popular culture, which increasingly is targeted toward younger populations. An examination of approximately 2,500 children's television programs revealed that nearly 70% contained some form of physical violence (Wilson et al., 2002). Evidence of the relationship between youths viewing violence, identifying with aggressive characters and behaving aggressively, and suffering negative effects from violent video games is growing (Gentile & Stone, 2005; Huesmann, 2007; Huesmann et al., 2003).

Although self-defense is a common justification for gun ownership, suicide, homicide, and accidental deaths in the home outnumber deaths associated with self-defense by a margin of 40 to 1 (American College of Physicians, 1998). In 2004, 66% of all homicides were committed with firearms (DOJ, 2007a).

The macrosystem includes the formal and informal social structures and societal influences that make up the world of children and their families: neighborhoods, schools, workplaces, churches, and social service agencies. Living in a poor inner city increases the likelihood of exposure to events such as stabbings, assaults, and shootings. Children exposed to violence are more likely to develop symptoms of overall distress, nervousness, and depression (Jaycox et al., 2002). Exposure also increases the likelihood of a child being a victim of violence, which may be a risk factor in the development of violent behavior (Brook et al., 2003; Leeb et al., 2007). Researchers continue to examine the link between community violence exposure and delinquent activity. Some suggest that a violent community draws highly aggressive youth together through experiences that support their involvement in violence (Figure 33.1) (Halliday-Boykins & Graham, 2001).

Microsystem

The microsystem represents the family environment, including such factors as family dynamics, parenting style, and socioeconomic status. Ideally, families should foster a protective atmosphere that serves as the first center of learning for infants and toddlers to build secure attachments that stay with them for the rest of their lives. Conversely, being raised in a low-income family with scant social support actually

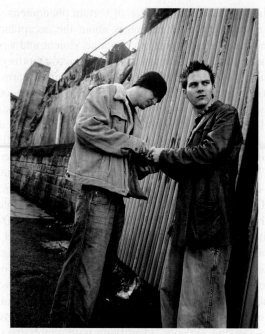

FIGURE 33.1 Living in a rough community may draw teens looking for acceptance, distraction, and identification together, leading to potentially delinquent and violent behaviors.

can become a risk factor because of time constraints that may prevent close supervision of children (Costello et al., 2003). However, poverty alone is not a direct cause of child behavior problems. The picture is much more complex.

Much research on violence and the family involves child maltreatment. A picture emerges of the maltreated child's family life as one of stress, chaos, and negligence (Gauthier, 2003; Leeb et al., 2007). A family in emotional and economic turmoil and living in a violent neighborhood faces a social context that increases the risk for all members to become victims or perpetrators of violence.

Individual Factors

Finally, both biologic and neurodevelopmental factors within people increase their potential for violence. This level often is termed *ontogenic,* indicating a view of development as an ongoing interaction between a person's emerging capabilities and the environmental response. For instance, attachment behaviors, which are critical to subsequent mastery motivations and social learning, result from the infant's innate behaviors to elicit parental responses and how parents meet that attachment-seeking behavior. Insecure or faulty attachments between infants and their primary caregivers often are viewed as a launching pad for subsequent problems with social learning and regulating behavior, a precursor to delinquency (Schore, 2001). This example illustrates one way in which sequences of development can enhance or impede how children eventually negotiate their environment, especially any skill grounded in social learning, such as problem solving.

PUBLIC HEALTH APPROACH TO VIOLENCE PREVENTION

The ecological approach to community violence recognizes that multiple factors interact to increase a person's potential for violence. Just as violence has many causes, it follows that the solutions rest with a public health approach. A **public health approach** holds that the multiple causes of violence require multiple solutions addressing each level of the problem. Interventions must include community-based efforts to identify sources, data collection on risk and protective factors within a population, and community-based interventions that reduce risk and enhance protective factors. In addition, evaluating and monitoring the interventions and providing public education about those that are effective are essential (Dodge, 2001; Hahn et al., 2007).

The Center for Mental Health Services (CMHS) (2001) details a national plan for preventing school violence that is a good example of the public health approach. This plan begins by detailing the epidemiology of school violence and providing a thorough literature review on causes and patterns of adolescent violence. Its analysis reveals that specific situations (eg, poverty, discrimination, alcohol), as well as events arising from interpersonal disputes or criminal actions (eg, muggings, robberies), can cause adolescent violence. After a review of risk and protective factors, the plan describes how programs must develop interventions that simultaneously involve the family, child, school, peer groups, and community. Finally, the plan evaluates current interventions and their effectiveness, compiling a list of exemplary and model programs.

In addition, the Task Force on Community Preventive Services has reviewed findings of universal, school-based programs intended to prevent violent behavior at all grade levels (pre-kindergarten through high school). Strong evidence shows that such programs decrease rates of violence consistently at all grade levels (Hahn et al., 2007).

> **Checkpoint Questions**
> 1. According to the ecological model of violence, what three levels of influence place a person at risk for becoming a victim or victimizer?
> 2. What is meant by a public health approach to violence prevention?

YOUTH VIOLENCE

Violence among U.S. youth has reached almost epidemic proportions. The statistics speak for themselves:

- Homicide is the second leading cause of death for 15- to 19-year-olds and the leading cause for African Americans in this age group (Anderson et al., 2001).
- In 2003, 5,570 people aged 10 to 24 years were murdered, an average of 15 each day. Of these victims, 82% were killed with firearms (CDC, 2007b).

- In an average month, public secondary schools experience 525,000 attacks, robberies, and shakedowns and 125,000 threats against teachers, more than 5,000 of whom are harmed (CDC, 2002). These violent acts exact a toll on victims, families, and communities and on national resources.
- In 2004, more than 750,000 people aged 10 to 24 years were treated in emergency departments for injuries sustained from violence (CDC, 2007b).

Less obvious ramifications include the 6% of teens who report not going to school on one or more days in the 30 days preceding the nationwide survey because they felt unsafe at school or on their way to and from school (CDC, 2007b). Being afraid to attend school creates absences and anxieties that place a cost on school performance and, ultimately, development (Figure 33.2).

Risk and Protective Factors for Youth Violence

What accounts for the ever-increasing incidence of youth violence? In line with the ecological model, four categories of risk factors have been identified: individual, family, peer/school, and environment. Experts agree that one factor in isolation rarely causes a teen to pick up a gun and shoot someone. Rather, the risk factors are additive: the more that a person is exposed to violence from various categories, the greater is the likelihood of violence erupting (Commission for the Prevention of Youth Violence, 2000). Fortunately, certain aspects can serve as protective factors against the risk factors to which people are exposed.

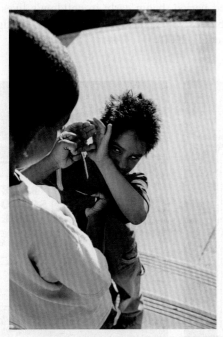

FIGURE 33.2 Violence and bullying can cause many children to fear going to school. This problem may lead to increased absences, poor performance, and social problems. Physical illness in children is another concern because of a hyperactive stress and immune response.

Individual Risk Factors

Individual factors that contribute to youth violence are numerous. Particular neurobiologic patterns create risk. For example, researchers are finding increasingly that low serotonin levels are related to aggression in young men (Holmes et al., 2001). The idea of a biologic predisposition to antisocial behavior also has received considerable attention. Although sorting the contributions of biologic versus environmental influences is difficult, evidence suggests that for youths with early-onset behavior problems, particular temperamental, physiologic, and attentional factors may underlie their problems with self-regulation (Sourander et al., 2007). For instance, aggressive infants often show low reactivity; they later become toddlers who display little fear at new situations and a muted response to social rewards such as praise (Frick et al., 2003). These predispositions set the stage for early aggression, which is a strong risk factor for later aggressive behavior (Broidy et al., 2003). Finally, early experiences of neglect and abuse may cause changes in brain chemistry and the neurotransmitters crucial to behavioral regulation, creating a risk for future aggressive responses.

Another set of individual risk factors could be grouped as behavioral influences. Included are aggressive youths' predispositions to particular cognitive biases, such as the belief that violence is a legitimate method of handling conflict, or to misread situations so that they attribute hostile intent to benign situations (Muris et al., 2002). For example, when shoved or pushed by a peer accidentally, aggressive youths are quick to assume that the peer had malicious intent. Often, their aggressive response is based on misreading the situation. Other risk factors include emotional or psychosocial problems, academic problems, and alcohol or drug abuse. When these factors are taken together, a profile emerges of multiple, early precursors to youth violence.

Family Risk Factors

The family exerts a tremendous influence on development. Attachment problems, family stress, and inappropriate parenting styles contribute to persistent behavior problems. Particularly harmful to a child's development are neglectful or disengaged parents, a situation that contributes to attachment problems and a continuing lack of emotional support (Campbell et al., 2000; Tremblay et al., 2004). Other influences may include poor monitoring of children, exposure to violence, and poor family functioning. Although one may think that dealing with a problem child calls for stringent parenting, research demonstrates that harsh parenting, which usually is accompanied by parents' anger and control-oriented interactions, predicts the persistence of behavioral difficulties in kindergarten children (Cole et al., 2003).

Peer Risk Factors

Peer associations and peer status become risk factors for youth violence in several ways. In grade school, aggressive children frequently use aggression for control and social gain. In the process, they create a class of victims who may experience long-term maladjustment. In the teen years, peers become a major force. Association with teens who condone antisocial or aggressive behavior becomes a strong predictor for violent behavior (Dahlberg & Potter, 2001). In this case, academic failure of group members may follow, which compounds risk. Associations with peers can take the form of gang involvement, which is associated with both gun involvement and disproportionate criminal and violent offenses (Commission for the Prevention of Youth Violence, 2000). In a sophisticated study testing the multiple factors of the ecological risk model, gang involvement emerges as one of the strongest risk factors for youth aggression, with gangs depicted as "setting the stage for deviance training" (Tolan et al., 2003).

Neighborhood Risk Factors

As mentioned, a youth's macrosystem (neighborhood and community) can become a risk factor for violence. Living in a violent neighborhood increases the risk that the child will be involved in aggressive interchanges, affording the opportunity for him or her to think through aggressive sequences and increasing the sense that aggression is a legitimate response to conflict. Over time, this way of thinking becomes characteristic and supports aggressive behavior (Guerra et al., 2003).

Protective factors offset risk. Nevertheless, poverty creates known contributors to violent behavior. As the CMHS (2001) points out, living in poverty segregates people from mainstream society and, in doing so, isolates youth from seeing possible opportunities to escape. In poor neighborhoods, unemployment is high and people are moving about looking for jobs, further disconnecting them from support systems and increasing their sense of isolation. These factors, family instability, and lack of support all increase the risk for violence (CMHS, 2001).

Protective Factors

Scientists have studied children who have overcome adversity to understand resiliency and the factors connected to the ability to thrive even in adverse life conditions. These *protective* factors include some innate characteristics, such as solid intelligence, as well as acquired features, such as self-regulatory abilities, self-esteem, and strong parental monitoring (Buckner et al., 2003; Self-Brown et al., 2006). A child with a secure parental attachment enters school with many advantages and is likely to embark on a career of school success (Valentino et al., 2011). Children who enter school with emotional security and a sense of well-being are ready not only for learning academics but also critical social skills (eg, respecting the rights of others, giving and receiving support). Children with these social aptitudes function better in school. Finally, a community can be a protective factor when it provides good schools, recreational outlets, and laws and surveillance that limit youths' access to guns, alcohol, and drugs (Figure 33.3).

Public Health Approach to Youth Violence

Since the early 1990s, youth violence prevention has received tremendous attention from government agencies, scientists, community activists, and health professionals. Scores of programs have demonstrated short-term positive outcomes; a few have shown long-term efficacy (Hahn et al., 2007). As interventions proliferate, governmental and community activists and scientists agree that programs must be evidence based; they must address multiple risk factors over a sustained period, begin early in children's lives, and involve all parties with a stake in the outcomes (Dodge, 2001; Thornton et al., 2000).

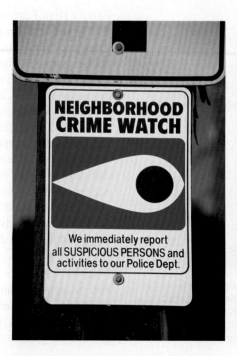

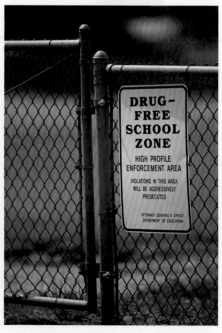

FIGURE 33.3 Communities can take measures to fight against violence and poverty through town watches, drug-free initiatives, and other efforts that increase supervision and intervention for children.

Nurses' Role in Youth Violence Prevention Efforts

Nurses participate in violence prevention at several levels. Some nurses have developed model prevention programs aimed at at-risk youth and community-based parenting programs to teach how to deal effectively with hard-to-manage children (Gross & Grady, 2002). Nurses have been key participants in school-based programs that address the mental health needs of youth. They have participated in many successful home-visiting programs that provide support and education to mothers at risk (Olds et al., 2002). Nurses also have been involved in comparative reviews of violence prevention programs, examining their efficacy and addressing future needs (Cooper et al., 2000). Nurses are in a prime position to identify children at risk by virtue of their work in primary care and health clinics. In these settings, they also can educate families about firearm safety, substance abuse, and violence prevention. Through these and future efforts, nurses are meaningful participants in violence prevention.

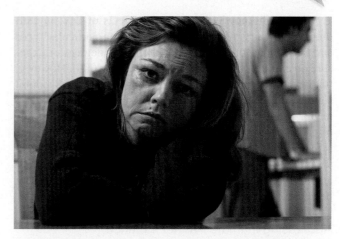

FIGURE 33.4 Intimate partner violence has physical, psychological, and social ramifications. Many victims do not know where to turn or how to receive help. Health care providers must provide front-line assistance through regular screening, teaching, and treatment efforts.

> **Checkpoint Questions**
> **3.** How does poverty contribute to youth violence?
> **4.** Public health prevention programs are based on what concept?

FAMILY VIOLENCE

Intimate Partner Violence

The World Health Organization has declared violence a major public health problem, with intimate partner violence (IPV) being one of the most common forms of violence against women (Krug et al., 2002). In the United States, IPV (also called *domestic violence*) has reached epidemic proportions and is the predominant cause of injury to women, more common than rapes, mugging, and automobile accidents combined. Nearly 5.3 million incidents of IPV occur each year among U.S. women 18 years or older; 3.2 million occur among men. Approximately 1.5 million women are raped or assaulted annually by an intimate partner (CDC, 2006a). Although IPV occurs against men, women are significantly more likely to be victims. IPV results in nearly 2 million injuries and 1,300 deaths nationwide every year (CDC, 2006a). It taxes society in both human and financial terms.

Defining the Scope of Intimate Partner Violence

The term *domestic violence* calls to mind physical aggression between a husband and wife. In Western society, intimate relationships exist between people of the same and opposite sex, married and unmarried. In addition, there are many ways to inflict harm on another person, with physical aggression being just one method.

Clinicians and researchers have assembled a set of uniform definitions for **intimate partner violence**. Intimate partners are current or former spouses or nonmarital partners (dating or same-sex partners). Violent acts include physical and sexual violence, as well as threats and psychological–emotional abuse. Physical violence includes acts used with enough force potentially to cause death, disability, or injury, as well as scratching, pushing, shoving, burning, or using restraint on another's body (Figure 33.4). These uniform definitions are important for researchers but also for nurses charged with detecting IPV. Screening for IPV will be effective only if health care professionals evaluate clients for both psychological and physical injury and have an accurate perspective on the broad range of actions and relationships considered IPV.

Cost to Children

IPV threatens and often destroys family life. Children often witness IPV, with worldwide estimates at 50% to 64% of cases (Krug et al., 2002). Although systematic national investigation of children's exposure to IPV has been exceedingly scant, one five-state study found that, on average, children lived in the households of 75% of adult female assault victims (Fantuzzo et al., 1997).

Children in homes with IPV are at risk for a range of emotional, physical, and behavioral symptoms. They demonstrate higher levels of depression and lower levels of self-esteem; these effects are pronounced in boys especially (Reynolds et al., 2001). In addition, these children are at risk for physical violence themselves. The link between marital conflict and child maltreatment has received much attention since the early 1990s. Children of battered women are at an increased risk for abuse. In sum, studies comparing children exposed to IPV with children from nonviolent homes indicate that this exposure:

- Adversely affects a range of child functioning
- Produces different adverse effects at different ages
- Increases the risk of child abuse
- Is associated with other risk factors, such as poverty and parental substance abuse

Although knowledge about the effects of IPV on children is growing, information is lacking on particular types and frequencies or the influence of various degrees of exposure on children's functioning (Mohr et al., 2000). However, findings have shown that children of abused mothers exhibit significantly more internalizing, externalizing, and total behavior problems than do children of the same age and sex of nonabused mothers (McFarlane et al., 2003). Routine screening for abuse of all women at the time of well-child visits could promote early detection and treatment for IPV against women and has the potential to interrupt and prevent behavioral problems for their children.

Addressing Intimate Partner Violence

Although scientific and public interest in IVP has intensified during the past decade, a coordinated response to the problem has been slow to develop. The Surgeon General has identified family violence as a priority public health issue and has called for an organized approach to screen for, treat, and prevent further violence (U.S. Public Health Service, 2003). However, the inability of health care, judicial, and religious systems to handle IPV effectively is well documented. The health care community in particular has been slow to participate. Of particular concern has been health professionals' long record of poor screening and identification of IPV.

PROBLEMS WITH DETECTION AND SCREENING.
The literature confirms that a significant factor in the underdetection of IPV rests with professional behavior (Cantu et al., 2003). Health care practitioners often fail to identify and intervene with abused women. They are vigilant in assessing health history, surgeries, dietary and bowel patterns, sexual activities, and current physiologic functioning, but not IPV. The underlying dynamics of poor screening practices are complex and include both biases and knowledge deficits.

Health care professionals may hold assumptions about IPV—biases that create barriers to screening. For instance, they may believe that IPV is a personal matter and that they have no role in this private controversy. They may believe that IPV is restricted to particular socioeconomic groups and remain naive about its prevalence (Falsetti, 2007; Gunter, 2007).

Knowledge deficits also result in a failure to identify and intervene with abused women. One survey found that most advanced practice nurses (APNs) working in women's health received little education or training on how to identify and manage cases of suspected abuse. Those APNs who received instruction in their basic or advanced nursing program were most likely to feel prepared to screen for IPV (Hinderliter et al., 2003).

IMPORTANCE OF SCREENING. Screening for IPV must be systematic and direct (Assessment Tool 33.1). Including questions that identify IPV in triage and entry point protocols significantly increases the identification of abused women (Kelly, 2007). Screening also is critically important because the way in which the immediate aftermath of violence is handled is an important determinant of the survivor's psychological response.

Diagnosis and treatment of IPV are ethical duties. Several states have developed protocols for health care professionals to minimize physical and psychological trauma and facilitate protection and support services in cases of IPV. Standards for identification, treatment, and evaluation of IPV are in place. Recently, a review of literature exposed a lack of research supporting the relationship between universal screening and decreased disability or premature death (Berg, 2004). However, support for universal screening remains high because it is relatively easy, and if IPV is left undetected, the consequences are high (Ferris, 2004). The American College of Emergency Physicians' (2007) policy statement on IPV emphasizes the need to evaluate clients presenting to the emergency department (ED) for IPV; develops multidisciplinary approaches for identification, treatment, and referral; and recognizes the necessary special services and resources. The Joint Commission (2012) mandates that hospitals have objective criteria and uniform standards for identifying and assessing possible victims of abuse and neglect.

Nurses' Role

In the health care system, nurses see women in various settings and often are the first point of contact in primary care offices and EDs. Considering their key role, it is critical that nurses screen for IPV. In the new health care arena, a vital link for assessing and intervening is the primary health care provider. Both physicians and nurses, through the normal course of providing care to women, are likely to encounter victims of physical, sexual, and psychological violence (Cantu et al., 2003). Suspicion should be raised to assess for victimization and safety and to supply needed information about available community services.

As they assume their appropriate role in the effort to screen and treat victims of IPV, nurses face barriers common to all health professionals. Time is a persistent problem. In numerous surveys, professionals report that time constraints pose the major barrier to IPV screening. However, such screening can be simple. Two basic questions are "Has a past or current partner ever caused you to be afraid?" and "Has a past or current partner ever physically hurt you?" (Hinderliter et al., 2003). Screening tools of various lengths are available (see Assessment Tool 33.1), but short tools demonstrate significant success in detecting abuse (Punukollu, 2002). In posing these questions, nurses are sensitive to the client's reluctance to reveal abuse. They have readily available information and avenues for referral.

In summary, significant barriers to screening for IPV remain, and myths and education may affect practices. Health care professionals must recognize these barriers if they are to improve their screening practices. As nurses increase their presence in the primary care arena, they will become pivotal in identification and referral of IPV clients. Their efforts must focus on the achievement of universal screening, both from a legislative and a practice perspective.

▲ASSESSMENT TOOL 33.1▲

Intimate Partner Violence Documentation Form

Explain to Client: The majority of what you tell me is confidential and cannot be shared with anyone without your written permission. However, I am required by law to report information pertaining to child or adult abuse and gunshot wounds or life-threatening injuries.

STEP 1—Establish total privacy to ask screening questions. Safety is the first priority. Client must be alone, or if the client has a child with her, the child must not be of verbal age. ONLY complete this form if YOU CAN assure the client's safety, privacy, and confidentiality.

STEP 2—Ask the client screening questions.

"Because abuse is so common, we are now asking all of our female clients:

Are you in a relationship in which you are being hurt or threatened, emotionally or physically?

___ Yes ___ No

Do you feel unsafe at home?"

___ Yes ___ No

If both screening questions are NO in Step 2, and you are not concerned that the client may be a victim, sign and date the form in the signature block directly below. Provide information and resources as appropriate.

Signature _____ Title _____ Date _____

If both screening answers are NO and you are concerned that the client may be a victim, go to Step 5. If the client answers YES to either question, proceed to Step 3 below. Sign and date the signature block on the back of the form after completing Step 6.

STEP 3—Assess the abuse and safety of the client and any children.

Say to client: "From the answers you have just given me, I am worried for you."

       "Has the relationship gotten worse or is it getting scarier?"   ___ Yes ___ No

       "Does your partner ever watch you closely, follow you, or stalk you?"   ___ Yes ___ No

Ask the following question in clinic settings only. Do not ask in home settings:

"If your partner is here with you today, are you afraid to leave with him/her?"   ___ Yes ___ No

"Is there anything else you want to tell me?" _____

_____

_____

_____

Name: _____

ID No: _____

Date of Birth: _____

DH 3202, 2/03
Stock Number: 5744-000-3202-2

(continues on page 730)

ASSESSMENT TOOL 33.1   Intimate Partner Violence Documentation Form (continued)

"Are there children in the home?"   ___ Yes ___ No

If the answer to the question above is "yes," say to client: "I'm concerned for your safety and the safety of your children. You and your children deserve to be at home without feeling afraid."

"Have there been threats of abuse or direct abuse of the children?"   ___ Yes ___ No

STEP 4—Assess client's physical injuries and health conditions, past and present.

Observations/Comments/Interventions:

_____

_____

_____

_____

_____

_____

_____

_____

_____

_____

STEP 5—If both screening answers are NO, and you ARE CONCERNED that the client may be a victim:

a. Say to the client: "All of us know of someone at some time in our lives who is abused. So, I am providing you with information in the event you or a friend may need it in the future."

b. Document under comments in Step 6.

STEP 6—Information, referrals, or reports made.

Yes   No
___   ___   1. Client given domestic violence information including safety planning
___   ___   2. Reviewed domestic violence information including safety planning
___   ___   3. State Abuse Hotline (1-800-96-ABUSE) and State Domestic Violence Hotline number (1-800-500-1119) given to the client
___   ___   4. Client called hotline during visit
___   ___   5. Client seen by advocate during visit
___   ___   6. Report made. If yes, to whom: _____

Comments

_____

_____

_____

_____

_____

_____

Signature _____ Title _____ Date _____

Source: Florida Department of Health.

Child Maltreatment

Child maltreatment is a major public health crisis. In 2004, approximately 872,000 children were victims of maltreatment (Child Welfare Information Gateway, 2006). *Maltreatment* is a general term for a wide range of acts of commission and omission that result in injuries or death. For this discussion, **maltreatment** is behavior toward another person that is (1) outside the norms of conduct and (2) involves a significant risk of physical or emotional harm. Four categories are recognized, the various forms of which often do not occur in isolation but overlap:

* Physical abuse: scaldings, beatings with objects, severe physical punishment, and Munchausen syndrome by proxy (see Chap. 24)
* Sexual abuse: incest, sexual assault by a relative or stranger, fondling of genitals, exposure to indecent acts, sexual rituals, or involvement in pornography
* Neglect: deficiencies in caregiver obligation that harm the child's psychological health, physical health, or both
* Emotional maltreatment: acts such as verbal abuse and belittlement, acts designed to terrorize a child, and lack of nurturance or emotional availability

Effects on Child Functioning

SOCIAL FUNCTIONING. Maltreated children tend to be attached less securely to their mothers or primary caregivers than nonmaltreated children. Interactions with caregivers are less frequent and characterized by more negative effects for maltreated children (Springer et al., 2003). In addition, maltreated children have increased difficulties with peers. They generate fewer quality solutions to interpersonal problems and have difficulty understanding complex social roles. Their social involvement and sophistication in play also are decreased. They display decreased socially competent behaviors in interactions, initiate fewer positive interactions with peers, are both withdrawn and aggressive with other children, and show inappropriate responses to peer distress. Because of these difficulties, maltreated children are not popular; they have fewer friends, and their peer group is more likely to reject them (Brown, 2003).

BEHAVIORAL FUNCTIONING. Parents report that maltreated children display significant oppositional and aggressive behavior. Teachers agree that such preschoolers display significant behavior disorders and conduct problems (Brown, 2003; Springer et al., 2003). Observations of maltreated and nonmaltreated preschoolers show that maltreated children display fewer peer interactions, engage in fewer prosocial behaviors, and are more aggressive.

According to parent report, school-age maltreated children display significantly more problem behaviors overall, are more aggressive and less compliant, and show more internalization of problems and disturbed behavior than do other children (Brown, 2003). Their teachers confirm these reports. Investigations of school discipline records show significantly increased referrals to the principal, suspensions, and overall behavior problems in maltreated children (Springer et al., 2003; Tenney-Soeiro & Wilson, 2004). Other findings indicate that maltreated children display more developmental delays as infants; have increased sensitivity to aggressive stimuli; have a greater frequency of running away, being expelled, and using drugs; and are diagnosed more frequently with oppositional or conduct disorders (Leeb et al., 2007) (Case Vignette 33.1).

EMOTIONAL AND INTELLECTUAL FUNCTIONING. In general, older maltreated children display more emotional maladjustment and psychiatric symptoms than do children who have not been maltreated (Springer et al., 2003). They also tend to be more depressed or hopeless than their peers who have not been maltreated (Springer et al., 2003; Toth & Cicchetti, 2010).

In addition, symptoms of post-traumatic stress disorder (PTSD) are more common in maltreated children (see Chap. 23) (De Bellis & Thomas, 2003; Scott et al., 2003) (Box 33.1). Finally, maltreated children show difficulty with

Case Vignette 33.1

Dan, 10 years old, has a history of extreme maltreatment. He has just been transferred to a new psychiatric unit. While reviewing the transfer records, the nurse notes that Dan had been doing well before his admission to the previous hospital. Last month, however, he again began to have violent outbursts.

On this unit, Dan is calm for the first 2 weeks. Nurses note that he is a bit distant, displaying poor social skills and tending to instigate other children. He also tends to isolate himself in his room. The plan is to include Dan in the unit activities, to begin to build trusting relationships, and to continue to assess him.

One day another child touches Dan as they go toward the group room. Dan becomes angry and starts yelling that he has been touched inappropriately. Dan goes into the group room and remains loud and irate, which the nurse identifies as his pattern when he is stressed and anxious. The group leader tries to engage Dan in the activity, but Dan continues to be disruptive and eventually is taken out of group. The nurse decides to give Dan a time-out, but Dan continues to yell about the injustice of being singled out. He does not understand what he did wrong.

BOX 33.1 Child Maltreatment and Post-Traumatic Stress Disorder

The deleterious effects of sexual abuse in childhood include fear and anxiety, anger and hostility, shame and guilt, inappropriate sexual behavior, and depression. Other stress-related symptoms include somatic complaints (eg, stomachaches, headaches), sleep disturbances, nightmares, withdrawal from peers and adults, difficulty concentrating, increased arousal or hyperalertness, and intrusive thoughts and flashbacks of the experience.

Some children may develop post-traumatic stress disorder (PTSD; see Chap. 23). Children manifest PTSD in their play as well as in the symptoms of PTSD described earlier. For example, children frequently reenact the traumatic experience in their play. In addition, children's play may reflect themes or aspects of the trauma such as fear, helplessness, or intrusion. Whereas traumatic nightmares in adults frequently include repetitions of the event, in children nightmares may not include recognizable trauma-related content. The following is a vignette of a child with PTSD after childhood sexual abuse.

Tommy, age 6 years, was referred for therapy when his first-grade teacher complained that he was "unmanageable" in the classroom. She described him as "moody," explaining that some days were worse than others. She noted he had difficulty staying on task, frequently left his seat, and disturbed other children by taking their supplies, verbally teasing them, or aggressively hitting and punching them. Tommy was not well liked by his peers, who tended to avoid him and exclude him from their games.

At home, his parents stated he had frequent nightmares, had difficulty following directions, and seemed to be aggressive with his younger sister and neighborhood children.

During an interview with his parents, the therapist learned that Tommy's biologic father had sodomized him when Tommy was 3 years old. Tommy's mother thought he had forgotten the experience. Tommy's stepfather related that he and Tommy had a good relationship and Tommy called him "Dad." In therapy, Tommy frequently drew big dinosaur-like monsters that were after him and with whom he battled. As Tommy progressed in therapy, he remembered his father "hurting him in his behind," and he expressed fear that his father would come for him one day.

Gradually, as Tommy began to feel safe again, his behavior in school improved. His drawings began to reflect smaller monsters and larger more powerful figures of himself. He began to play more appropriately with peers and his nightmares decreased significantly. Until he dealt with the powerful feelings of helplessness and fear that his sexual abuse generated, Tommy continued to reenact the aggression he experienced and the fear he felt.

Tommy displays some of the symptoms of PTSD, which are presented in Chapter 23. In considering a diagnosis of PTSD, clinicians evaluate if the symptoms in each group have been present for 1 month and if they have caused significant social or occupational impairment.

---

empathy and emotional recognition and have a more aggressive response bias (Brown, 2003).

The current empirical knowledge base about the effects of maltreatment on intellectual functioning suggests that scores on cognitive measures tend to be significantly lower for maltreated children than for their peers who have not been maltreated. This difference appears more pronounced in measures of verbal intelligence and language (Scott et al., 2003). Children who are maltreated are often hypervigilant, on edge, and have impaired ability to control their impulses. Moreover, they tend to make attributions about their environments that suggest that their worldview is one of constant danger from which they must protect themselves. Such children are often quite challenging to treat, because much of their behavior has its origins in their maltreatment during crucial years of their development. Often they are unable to put their fears into words because of their attenuated verbal intelligence, because they have no memory of their maltreatment, or both.

HEALTH AND PHYSICAL FUNCTIONING. Several studies suggest that maltreated children are at risk for impaired physical growth and development. In addition, there is evidence of increased heart rate in response to everyday scenes; more documented scars, skin wounds, and neurologic soft signs; and greater drug use. Maltreated children often have a history of feeding and sleeping problems, physical handicaps, and serious health problems at birth; early

developmental delays; developmental disabilities or mental retardation; and more illnesses, "accidents," and hospitalizations early in life (Tenney-Soeiro & Wilson, 2004).

With respect to physical health as adults, various somatic symptoms consistently are increased in adults with a history of physical or sexual abuse (Springer et al., 2003). They include nightmares, back pain, frequent or severe headaches, pelvic pain, eating binges or self-induced vomiting, fatigue, breast pain, abdominal pain, sleeping difficulties, irritable bowel syndrome, and fibromyalgia (see Chap. 24).

Nurses' Role

Health care professionals are legally required to report child maltreatment. They must report any suspected cases of child abuse to their local child protection agency. During routine assessments and physical examinations, nurses question any scars, bruises, and marks on children. A child may be reluctant to discuss an injury. Health care providers ask specific questions, such as when and how it happened (Figure 33.5). If nurses have any question about the origin of an injury, they consult members of the multidisciplinary team, and they thoroughly question the parent or guardian. Such conversations are difficult. They begin with general questions about the parents' understanding of the problem, noting any discrepancies between their explanation and the physical findings. As the interview proceeds, nurses pose more specific questions about discipline practices.

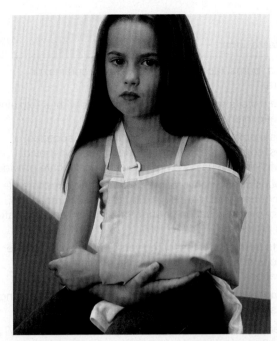

FIGURE 33.5 In cases of suspected child maltreatment, health care providers patiently but thoroughly investigate with the child about the source of injuries and try to gauge if the explanation is plausible.

It is beyond the scope of this chapter to review how to conduct an interview or examination when a nurse suspects abuse. Nurses are alert to any signs or symptoms of abuse but also operate within the scope of their knowledge, consulting with more experienced team members and examiners as necessary.

The treatment of maltreated children is a complex issue involving collaboration among many disciplines, social service agencies, and the criminal justice system. Effective treatment programs recognize the multidimensional nature of the origin of family violence. Treatment and interventions aim at variables operating at all levels of the problem: individual psychopathology, family dysfunction, stress, and lack of social support.

Checkpoint Questions

8. What are the four categories of child maltreatment?
9. Symptoms of what psychiatric disorder are commonly associated with child maltreatment?

Elder Abuse

Elder abuse is the mistreatment of older adults. It occurs in homes and institutional settings, including hospitals and long-term care facilities. This problem is found in all socioeconomic groups. In the United States, approximately 500,000 older adults experience abuse and neglect in their domestic setting each year; many incidents are unreported (CDC, 2007a). Women outnumber men as victims. Prevalence and incidence are not known, partly because of inconsistent definitions of elder abuse. Elder abuse may include one or a combination of the following: physical abuse, physical neglect, sexual abuse, psychological abuse or neglect, financial abuse, and violation of personal rights (Table 33.1).

Causes

Theories on the causes of elder abuse vary. Increasing societal violence and caregiver stress are possible factors. Elder abuse may result from complex interactions among victims, caregivers, life stresses, and social systems (Miller, 2009).

Sociocultural factors include demographics, ageism, poverty, and disability. The number of U.S. older adults is increasing, especially among the oldest old (see Chap. 37). With increased life expectancy and modern medical technology, older adults may have extended periods of disability and dependency. Current trends in family size have resulted in fewer or more distant relatives available to provide care for frail, older adults. Hospitals discharge clients after shorter stays and with greater physical care needs, which places greater stress on family caregivers. Because families (ie, spouses and children) provide most care to older adults, they are most likely to be the perpetrators of elder abuse. Those without support networks or knowledge of community resources are at highest risk for elder abuse.

Caring for older adults with disabilities can be demanding and stressful, especially when clients have cognitive impairments (see Chap. 31). Chances for elder abuse increase when caregivers have personal problems or inadequate support. Caregivers at risk for becoming abusive have a history of psychological illness, substance abuse, being abused, violent behavior, or role conflict and feeling overwhelmed in the caregiver role.

Nurses' Role

Nurses must be aware of elder abuse so that they can make appropriate assessments to identify potentially dangerous situations and actual cases of mistreatment. Nurses suspect mistreatment when older adults have delayed seeking treatment for injuries, fail to explain or give improbable reasons for injuries, or have frequent admissions for dehydration. Nurses who make home or residential visits to clients assess the environment for cleanliness and safety.

In all settings, nurses assess communication between caregivers and older adults. Agitation, fear, and reticence from elder clients are possible indicators of mistreatment. Suspicious caregiver behaviors include humiliating comments, frequent interruptions, use of an unfeeling voice, and a lack of caring (Miller, 2009) (Assessment Tool 33.2).

Once nurses have detected elder abuse, they are responsible for reporting the mistreatment. Each state has its own guidelines to follow. Usually, after nurses have reported the abuse, a state protective services worker meets with the victim (Miller, 2009). The adult protective worker has knowledge about resources for managing the abuse and begins to develop plans for the older adult's care and safety.

Interventions for elder abuse can be primary, secondary, or tertiary and involve a multidisciplinary approach (Miller, 009). Primary interventions help prevent

TABLE 33.1 Types of Elder Abuse

Type	Definition	Manifestations
Physical abuse	Intentional infliction of bodily harm	Bruises, burns, lacerations, dislocations, sprains, or fractures
		Frequent visits to emergency departments with unexplained traumatic injuries
		Unreasonable descriptions of how injuries happened
		Depressed, anxious, withdrawn, or confused behavior
		Passivity or anxious behavior to please health care providers
Physical neglect	Intended or unintended failure by a caregiver to meet the older adult's basic needs	Malnourishment, dehydration, poor hygiene, pressure ulcers, contractures, perineal excoriation, fecal impaction, signs of overmedication or undermedication, and untreated health problems
		Reports from clients that caregivers leave them in unsafe situations or that they cannot obtain medical care or medications
		Substandard housing in disrepair with poor housekeeping
		Depression, poor self-esteem, and apathy
Sexual abuse	Sexual activity without consent or the ability to provide consent	Reddened or traumatized genitals, genital pain, sexually transmitted infections, bruises, scratches, or abrasions
		Depression, anxiety, and withdrawal
Psychological abuse	Infliction of mental anguish by yelling, verbally assaulting, or threatening, humiliating, and intimidating the person	Restlessness, insomnia, hand tremors, or worsening in chronic health conditions
		Depression, anxiety, paranoia, and confusion
		Fear of strangers in their home environment
Psychological neglect	Failure of the caregiver to meet the older adult's emotional needs	Isolating the elder from contact with other people or not providing a stimulating environment, socially and cognitively
		Similar behaviors to victims of psychological abuse
Financial abuse or material exploitation	Use of, or taking the possessions of, an older adult for personal or monetary gain without consent or through unwarranted power	Theft, mismanagement of funds, improper financial advice, or use of the older adult's money for personal benefit
Violation of personal rights	Taking unlawful advantage of the older adult's rights	Loss of privacy
		Not being given opportunities to be involved in decision making

mistreatment through education. Health care providers and the public should be informed about the scope of the problem. Caregivers require education about how to provide care and manage related stressors. Secondary intervention aims at minimizing harm through early identification of mistreatment, which involves protocols or tools for screening. Tertiary intervention includes rehabilitation of both victim and abuser. Examples include counseling and psychotherapy.

Checkpoint Questions

10. Who are the most likely perpetrators of elder abuse?
11. When assessing the interaction between an older adult client and caregiver, what are three possible assessment findings in the older adult that might suggest mistreatment?

RAPE AND SEXUAL ASSAULT

Rape is forced or coerced sexual penetration (oral, anal, or vaginal) of a nonconsenting person. **Sexual assault** is forced or coerced sexual acts on a nonconsenting person. **Statutory rape** is rape of a minor (age varies among states). With statutory rape, consent is not an issue; minors are considered incapable of giving consent because of their vulnerability and dependence on adults or older peers.

Rape and sexual assault are acts of violence. These forced sexual behaviors shatter the victim's sense of self, safety, and predictability. Criminal statutes on rape vary, but all states define rape as a crime. In 2005, there were 69,370 completed rapes, 58,060 attempted rapes, and 61,530 sexual assaults (DOJ, 2005). This statistic does not include statutory rape.

The preceding statistics reflect reported and attempted rapes; however, most cases are unreported (DOJ, 2005).

ASSESSMENT TOOL 33.2

Elder Assessment Instrument (EAI)

	Very Good	Good	Poor	Very Poor	Unable to Assess
I. General Assessment					
1. Clothing					
2. Hygiene					
3. Nutrition					
4. Skin integrity					
5. Additional comments:					

	No Evidence	Possible Evidence	Probable Evidence	Definite Evidence	Unable to Assess
II. Possible Abuse Indicators					
6. Bruising					
7. Lacerations					
8. Fractures					
9. Various states of healing of any bruises or fractures					
10. Evidence of sexual abuse					
11. Statement by elder re: abuse					
12. Additional comments:					
III. Possible Neglect Indicators					
13. Contractures					
14. Decubiti					
15. Dehydration					
16. Diarrhea					
17. Depression					
18. Impaction					
19. Malnutrition					
20. Urine burns					
21. Poor hygiene					
22. Failure to respond to warning of obvious disease					
23. Inappropriate medications (under/over)					
24. Repetitive hospital admissions due to probable failure of health care surveillance					
25. Statement by elder re: neglect					
26. Additional comments:					
IV. Possible Exploitation Indicators					
27. Misuse of money					
28. Evidence of financial exploitation					
29. Reports of demands for goods in exchange for services					
30. Inability to account for money/property					
31. Statement by elder re: exploitation					
32. Additional comments:					

(continues on page 736)

ASSESSMENT TOOL 33.2   Elder Assessment Instrument (EAI) (continued)

V. Possible Abandonment Indicators						
33. Evidence that a caretaker has withdrawn care precipitously without alternate arrangements						
34. Evidence that elder is left alone in an unsafe environment for extended periods of time without adequate support						
35. Statement by elder re: abandonment						
36. Additional comments:						
VI. Summary						
37. Evidence of abuse						
38. Evidence of neglect						
39. Evidence of exploitation						
40. Evidence of abandonment						
41. Additional comments:						

VII. Comments and Follow-Up

_____

_____

_____

Adapted from Fulmer, T., & Cahill, V. M. (1984). Assessing elder abuse: A study. *Journal of Gerontological Nursing, 10*(12), 16–20; and Fulmer, T., Street, S., & Carr, K. (1984). Abuse of the elderly: Screening and detection. *Journal of Emergency Nursing, 10*(3), 131–140.

Common reasons for not reporting these crimes include the belief that rape is a private and personal matter and fear of reprisal from the perpetrator.

Types of Rape

Rape by a Stranger

A popular conception is that the rapist is a stranger who surprises the victim. However, rape by a stranger accounts for only about 15% of total rapes. In 85% of cases, the survivor knows the rapist (eg, acquaintance, close friend, lover, family member, neighbor).

Date Rape and Acquaintance Rape

Most rapes involve people who know each other. Survivors of date rapes include women of all ages: the 50-year-old woman who accepts an offer from a coworker for assistance with installing a ceiling fan, the 20-year-old coed who becomes drunk at a party and passes out, and the 70-year-old woman who accepts a ride from a kindly looking church member.

Date or acquaintance rapes are no less traumatic or repugnant than other types; the serious physical and emotional consequences should not be minimized because the victim knows the perpetrator. Research shows that survivors of date rape experience more self-blaming behaviors because they believe they should have suspected the rapist or feel foolish for having trusted the rapist. A sense of betrayal frequently is an issue.

Ascertaining the incidence of these rapes is difficult because victims often do not report them. According to the National Crime Victimization Survey (DOJ, 2005), approximately 48% of victims are raped by a friend or acquaintance, 30% by a stranger, 16% by an intimate, and 2% by another relative. Date rape does not happen just on the first date; it may occur during any stage of a relationship. In a study of the victimization of college women (National Institute of Justice, Bureau of Justice Statistics, 2002), 20% reported either a rape incident (10%) or an attempted rape incident (10%). In other words, women have a 20% risk of being raped or sexually assaulted while attending college. In 96% of these cases, a classmate (35.5%), friend (34.2%), boyfriend or ex-boyfriend (23.7%), or acquaintance (2.6%) perpetrated the rape.

Marital Rape

Currently, marital rape is a crime in all states; however, 33 states have exemptions for prosecuting husbands for rape. These exemptions usually are related to the use of force. If the wife cannot show evidence of force by her husband (eg, bodily injuries), she cannot claim that he raped her. To intervene effectively in cases of marital rape, nurses should familiarize themselves with the laws in their state.

Rape Trauma Syndrome

Burgess and Holmstrom (1974) described the rape trauma syndrome, a two-phase process experienced by all rape survivors. The first phase, which may last days or weeks, is the *acute phase of disorganization.* As clients begin to respond to the rape, fear, anxiety, disbelief, anger, and shock are common. Physical responses include sleep disturbance, nightmares, body aches and pains related to the rape, fatigue, and loss of appetite. These vary according to the nature of the rape and the victim's perception of the incident. Ritual behaviors associated with ensuring safety (eg, checking window and door locks repeatedly), hyperalertness to potential danger (eg, scanning the environment continually for the rapist), and an increased startle response may be present.

Some survivors openly express their feelings; others exhibit a controlled response (Figure 33.6). Both responses are normal, and nurses should not assume that the rape did not affect (traumatize) survivors who have a more stoic response. One interpretation of this behavior is that clients feel out of control and therefore control the one thing they can—their own reaction.

Acute-phase emotional responses may include increased irritability, difficulty concentrating, and obsessive thoughts about the rape or some aspect of it. Tearfulness, anger, humiliation, shame, and guilt also are common. Shame and guilt frequently are related to self-blame from reviewing and assessing behavior associated with the rape. Family, friends, and professional helpers may reinforce these feelings inadvertently by questioning the survivor's actions or implying the survivor is to blame.

All of these symptoms may lead clients to feel like they are "going crazy." The world no longer makes sense. Clients no longer feel safe but vulnerable and out of control of the environment, feelings, and behaviors (Case Vignette 33.2).

The second phase of the rape trauma syndrome is the *long-term process of reorganization.* In this phase, clients work toward integration and resolution of the experience. Healthy integration and resolution involve regaining empowerment and reconnecting with others. Most survivors benefit substantially from professional help during this phase. In therapy, they can learn ways to feel safe again and to manage disturbing symptoms. Furthermore, they can remember and work through associated feelings. Gradually, survivors begin to reassert control and gain a new sense of relative safety—a new worldview.

Additional Ramifications of Rape

Survivors of rape may exhibit psychiatric disorders. PTSD is a possible diagnosis. To manage symptoms (eg, anxiety, fear), clients may find alcohol or drugs helpful. The use of these substances may lead to abuse or actual dependence.

In addition, rape survivors may experience depression, anxiety disorders (eg, phobias, agoraphobia, panic disorder), and sexual dysfunction disorders.

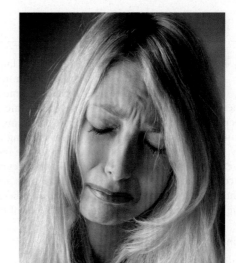

A

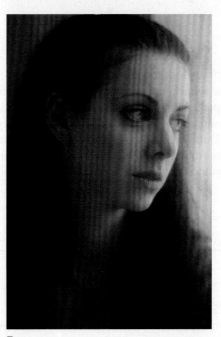

B

FIGURE 33.6 Responses to rape and sexual assault vary widely. Some react very emotionally (**A**); others are stoic (**B**). Nurses respond to both types of reactions with empathy and support.

Treatment for Survivors of Rape or Sexual Assault

Acute care after rape or sexual assault usually occurs in the ED. Long-term treatment occurs in outpatient settings such as rape crisis centers, victim services agencies, and the offices of mental health professionals. Treatment approaches vary and frequently are used in combination.

Case Vignette 33.2

A nurse is discussing a rape with Claire, a 26-year-old woman who has begun to talk about her experience for the first time as a part of therapy for depression. Claire says: "I am afraid all the time. When I see someone who looks like the rapist, my heart starts pounding. It is all I can do to keep from running the other way. I avoid everything that reminds me of the rape, but I still have these pictures in my head of the horrible event. I can't concentrate at work and I feel tired all the time. I can't sleep without medication. I am afraid to go to sleep because I often have nightmares of the rape. I feel totally out of control."

Reflection and Critical Thinking

- In addition to depression, what other disorders might Claire have or be at risk for?
- What responses from the nurse would be most therapeutic at this point?
- What things can the nurse do to help Claire function better in the short term?

Psychopharmacologic Interventions

Treatment with antidepressants (especially selective serotonin reuptake inhibitors) and antianxiety medications helps reduce symptoms of PTSD, depression, and anxiety. As a result, survivors can function normally and manage their worst symptoms. Antidepressants, notably the tricyclic antidepressants, commonly are used to induce and promote sleep.

Survivors with persistent obsessive thoughts or images of the trauma or with psychotic symptoms may benefit from "atypical" antipsychotics such as risperidone, olanzapine, and quetiapine.

Psychological Interventions

Although biochemical intervention is useful in symptom reduction, it does not address the issues of how to feel safe again or what to do about feelings of loss, anger, shame, guilt, and helplessness. It also does not address the numerous other areas of life affected by the sexual trauma. Trauma therapy frequently uses behavioral and cognitive approaches, individual and group treatment, as well as conjoint or family therapy as necessary.

Adjunctive techniques include biofeedback, relaxation training, assertiveness, hypnosis, bodywork (eg, dance, massage, yoga, self-defense training), meditation, guided imagery, journaling, grounding, and specialized groups for survivors. A controversial method for processing the traumatic memories of PTSD, called *eye movement desensitization and reprocessing* (Shapiro, 2005; van der Kolk et al., 2007), is being used extensively for treatment of trauma survivors. This method is thought to help reduce the debilitating symptoms of PTSD in sexual trauma survivors.

Checkpoint Questions

12. Which type of rape is least common?

13. What are the two phases of the rape trauma syndrome?

14. What two classes of medications are used to help a rape trauma survivor reduce the symptoms of PTSD, depression, and anxiety?

APPLYING THE NURSING PROCESS

Survivors of Rape Trauma

▲ ASSESSMENT

Assessment begins with the first contact with survivors of rape or sexual assault, whether by telephone or in person. Nurses convey attitudes of caring and support. Regardless of the circumstances, nurses suspend judgments to render care professionally. Moreover, nurses may compound the trauma if their attitude is not caring and supportive.

Not every nurse can work with survivors of rape. Even nurses who specialize in such care may encounter people with whom they cannot work effectively or therapeutically. Knowing how to recognize when personal feelings are likely to interfere with optimal care is part of the nurse's professional responsibility. Nurses must be emotionally available to all clients to empathize with their experience and at the same time view the information dispassionately. The ability to do so is directly proportional to the nurse's ability to acknowledge personal feelings (Case Vignette 33.3).

Instructions to those who call for information after a rape stress the importance of coming to the ED as is, without "cleaning up" in any way and especially without showering or bathing. Nurses tell survivors to bring a clean change of clothes with them for after the examination because they will need to leave their clothing at the hospital as evidence. If a survivor is not wearing the clothes in which the rape occurred, then he or she should bring them. If possible, a supportive person should accompany the survivor to the ED. Some survivors are reluctant to report the rape to the police. In such cases, nurses respect these wishes; however, they encourage clients to seek examination and treatment for potential pregnancy, sexually transmitted infections, AIDS, and impaired emotional and psychological well-being.

Once clients arrive at an ED, biopsychosocial assessment and documentation begin. In many communities, sexual assault nurse examiners conduct the physical examination. These registered nurses have special training in gathering evidence for use by the legal system in the arrest and prosecution of the perpetrator of rape. Nurses encourage survivors to allow such evidence gathering, even if a particular client is unsure whether

Case Vignette 33.3

One day, toward the end of a busy shift, a rape trauma survivor who was raped when she accepted a ride from a stranger comes into the emergency department. Nurse Monica is assigned to the survivor. She notices that the young woman is about her age and is attending nursing school. Monica finds herself stating to another nurse, "I can't understand why these women are so stupid. They deserve to be raped." The other nurse is surprised by Monica's comment and says so. He suggests that Monica is not in a "good place" to deal with this rape trauma survivor and that they switch clients to relieve Monica of working with the survivor. Later, this nurse sits down and talks with Monica about her feelings. Monica discovers that she overidentified with the survivor, who reminded her of herself and her willingness to hitch rides in younger days. Had Monica not received this timely intervention from her coworker, she may have communicated some of her judgmental attitude to the survivor. This action would not have been therapeutic for the survivor.

Reflection and Critical Thinking

- Discuss why nurses must be alert to their feelings about a client.
- Compare and contrast an overreaction and an underreaction to the client who has survived rape.
- Explain how Monica's feelings could have interfered with her ability to be therapeutic to, or even have harmed, the rape survivor.

---

to report the rape to the police. Nurses can turn over collected evidence to police in case a survivor decides to make a report.

ED nurses play a critical role. They often are the first professionals to talk with survivors and frequently remain throughout their stay in the hospital. These nurses express concern for survivors and are emotionally available to listen and provide support. Whether clients are emotional or stoic, nurses express concern. The primary goal is to establish a trusting relationship.

An accepting and caring attitude is critical for survivors to begin to trust nurses. Most clients feel tainted by the experience; they often feel "dirty" or somehow "bad" or guilty. They are especially sensitive to rejection or blame, partly because they already may have begun to blame themselves, but also because society frequently blames victims of rape. Many fear that no one will believe them. Sometimes just being present is the most therapeutic thing nurses can do to help clients feel safe and comfortable. Empowerment also is important, and nurses

may communicate this by respecting the survivor's right to self-determination. Nurses inform clients of everything being done or that will be done and respect their choices, even when nurses personally disagree with them.

During initial data gathering, nurses ask about any previous trauma, for example, physical or sexual abuse in childhood; previous unwanted sexual incidents; previous psychiatric treatment; other traumatic events, such as natural disasters, serious car accidents, or house fires. This information is especially useful in planning for care after discharge. Part of the nurse's assessment includes looking for any physical trauma that requires immediate attention. Although most rape victims do not have life-threatening injuries, some do. Nurses attend to these injuries with concern for the preservation of evidence of the crime.

▲ NURSING DIAGNOSIS, OUTCOME IDENTIFICATION, AND PLANNING

The most common diagnosis is **Rape Trauma Syndrome** (NANDA, 2007). Planning for treatment includes formulating goals and designing interventions for acute needs. It also necessitates considering longer-term needs as clients work to integrate and resolve their traumatic experience. See Case in Point 33.1 for a study of nursing care and outcomes for a client recovering from rape.

> **Think About It 33.1**
> Review Case in Point 33.1. Analyze the information provided and describe the signs and symptoms indicating that Alicia is in the acute phase of disorganization.

▲ IMPLEMENTATION

Immediate nursing care involves providing medical attention and gathering evidence for possible use in legal proceedings. Nurses provide rationales for each procedure (eg, medical and legal reasons for a pelvic examination). Nurses also plan when and with whom clients will leave the hospital and help notify significant others (eg, parents, spouse, or partner). They plan for survivors to speak with a crisis counselor either in the hospital or shortly after discharge. Client-Centered Education 33.1 contains key points for nurses to address with both victims and their families. To address long-term reorganization issues, nurses encourage clients to seek therapy or counseling services.

▲ EVALUATION

The general desired outcome is for clients to work through the feelings associated with rape and recover from the experience.

Case in Point 33.1

Alicia's Story

Alicia is a 20-year-old college student. She has been dating Jacob for 3 years, but recently they decided to see other people. Alicia began dating Tom, a young man whom she had met through her church. Four weeks earlier, Tom raped Alicia on their second date. She did not report the incident. Jacob has encouraged Alicia to seek counseling. During the initial session, Alicia, sobbing, relates the following:

"I had too much to drink; at first, I couldn't believe it was happening, I had let him kiss me, but he just kept going. I told him to stop, but he wouldn't. He ripped my clothes off and forced me to have sex with him several times. He told me if I told anyone, they would never believe me because everyone liked him and no one liked me. I never should have gone out with him. Now I'm so afraid; I cry all the time. I don't want to go to school; I can't think straight. And I will not go back to church. Every night I have nightmares, or I feel him holding me down . . . I never should have gone out with him. Even Jacob is sick of this; he says he doesn't know what to do and can't handle how I've changed."

Key Assessment Findings

- **Victim of rape 4 weeks earlier**
- **Reports of self-blame and guilt**
- **Statements of being afraid**
- **Increased startle response**
- **Recurring nightmares of event**
- **Inability to concentrate**

Nursing Diagnosis: Rape Trauma Syndrome related to experience of date rape 4 weeks prior as evidenced by feelings of guilt, self-blame, hyperalertness, fear, recurrent nightmares, and flashbacks

NOC: Abuse Recovery: The client will begin to demonstrate measures to integrate the trauma of rape into her personal history and take steps toward resolution.

NIC: Rape–Trauma Treatment
- Provide for a support person to stay with the client; demonstrate an accepting and caring attitude. *Support is key to assisting her to cope with the trauma and feel safe. Acceptance and concern are necessary to establish trust and to help the client express her feelings.*
- Implement crisis intervention counseling; assist the client to use techniques to reduce anxiety and fear. *Rape trauma is a crisis event. Crisis intervention counseling promotes positive coping and helps the client regain functioning. Techniques to reduce anxiety and fear help calm the autonomic nervous system, which causes many unpleasant physical symptoms and is overly sensitive during emotional trauma.*
- Use cognitive–behavioral therapy (CBT) strategies to address fears. Have the client talk through and gradually re-expose herself to the assault. Teach the cognitive technique of challenging automatic thoughts to help manage and defeat guilt and fear. *CBT has demonstrated effectiveness in short-term reduction of fear-related symptoms. Helping the client to remember and visualize the rape can aid in gradually reducing her anxiety and distress. Helping her recognize how automatic thoughts contribute to guilt, fear, and anxiety and to use more positive self-talk will empower the client and decrease her assumptions of self-blame and guilt.*
- Refer the client to a rape advocacy program; involve her in a rape survivors' support group. *Such participation can help her to understand that she is not to blame for the trauma. The ability to share experiences with others who have had similar events will be*

a source of support and compassion for the client who will need a place to express her feelings safely.
- Include a supportive partner in counseling sessions, if the client agrees. Help him work through his feelings of isolation, confusion, anger, powerlessness, and frustration. *The willingness of the client's partner to participate is crucial for the client to positively cope with the trauma. Partners of rape survivors often experience distress and frustration. The partner can be a greater resource for the client if his feelings are addressed.*

NIC: Crisis Intervention
- Reinforce anxiety reduction techniques; assist in redirecting the client's focus. *Increased anxiety interferes with the client's ability to focus and cope.*
- Assist in identifying past/present coping skills and their effectiveness. Assist in identifying personal strengths and abilities that the client can use to resolve the crisis. *Determining a baseline helps the nurse suggest skills that would be appropriate for use in this situation. Identifying and then using personal strengths and abilities to resolve a crisis promote empowerment. Use of positive coping skills and strengths and abilities aids in crisis resolution and fosters growth.*
- Assist client to develop new coping and problem-solving skills. *Development of new strategies enhances the client's ability to deal with stress; drawing on her strengths promotes feelings of control.*

NIC: Coping Enhancement
- Encourage the client to discuss feelings of guilt. *To help her adopt a more realistic appraisal, help her to identify evidence for and against these feelings.*
- Assist the client to develop an objective appraisal of the event. Discuss consequences of not dealing with guilt and shame. *Her emotional response is common but irrational and self-defeating. Asking her to examine rationally this emotional response will reveal no basis in reality for her self-blame.*

Case in Point 33.1 (continued)

Alicia's Story

- Encourage the client to talk about the event. Encourage verbalization of feelings, perceptions, and fears. Provide an atmosphere of acceptance; use a calm, reassuring approach. *All forms of avoidance behaviors are common and an attempt to reduce stress. However, fear levels will remain high until the client confronts the fear often enough for it to dissipate. Talking about the event is a form of exposure therapy.*

> 11/4/13: The client demonstrates a beginning level of acceptance of the trauma. She demonstrates moderate to substantial self-esteem and confidence. She expresses details and feelings about the trauma. She reports use of behaviors to reduce stress, increased involvement in pretrauma interests, and maintenance of role performance, social relationships, physical functioning, and control over life.

EPILOGUE

Alicia has been in treatment for nearly 5 months since the rape. She comes to the health care facility for follow-up. When the nurse asks how things are going, Alicia states, "I'm going to the support group, and that's really helped me a lot. I feel comfortable talking there. I'm not so afraid and jumpy anymore. I still have nightmares occasionally, but they are not as bad as they were. And I realize now that it wasn't my fault." Alicia also reports that she has resumed classes and is beginning to go out with her friends from time to time. "Jacob has been wonderful through all of this. He has been so supportive and helpful. I know it was hard for him, too, but he's been a really good friend."

Client-Centered Education 33.1

Coping with Rape Trauma Syndrome

Teaching Points

Family members, friends, and significant others frequently are at a loss about what to say or do to assist survivors of sexual trauma. Often, significant others exhibit strong feelings of anger and aggression toward the perpetrator. Although significant others generally have such feelings because they care for the survivor, these feelings are not helpful to the survivor who feels guilty about the rape. Nurses should allow significant others to express their feelings away from the survivor and then redirect them to discuss what the survivor needs from them now and in the future. Having some written information (a pamphlet or brochure) about rape trauma syndrome will be useful to survivors and those closest to them; written information should discuss what to expect, how to be helpful to a survivor, and what activities are beneficial to the survivor. Verbal discussion of the written information also helps because it allows survivors and their families to ask questions and relate their other concerns. Written information also is critical, however, because the participants frequently are in such a state of anxiety and concern that they do not remember what was said. Having a written guide to refer to as needed jogs the memory about what to do.

Instructions about rape trauma syndrome should include the following:

- Normal reactions to a traumatic event: cognitive, emotional, physical, and behavioral
- Negative coping strategies to avoid: use of drugs or alcohol, withdrawal
- Helpful ways to cope after the traumatic event, especially talking about the event with an experienced counselor
- Name of contact person to speak to about the rape

The information should include future medical and counseling appointments as well as guidance on symptom management (eg, exercise, relaxation, nutrition, sleep, resuming normal activities). In addition, the survivor should receive written information regarding whom to call for further information on legal issues related to the rape (eg, case number and name and number of the police investigator). Any medications needed by the survivor should be dispensed at the hospital if possible because the survivor already is overwhelmed with information and tasks related to coping with the event.

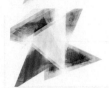

Reviewing and Applying Your Knowledge

Chapter Summary

• Community violence is an umbrella term for numerous forms of aggression that people inflict on one another. It includes phenomena such as youth violence, IPV, child maltreatment, elder abuse, and rape and sexual assault.

• One way to understand community violence is to consider not just traits of the perpetrator but also factors within the family, community, and culture that place people at risk for becoming a victim or perpetrator of violence.

• The tremendous increase in the incidence of youth violence has been explained by individual traits as well as family, school, community, and neighborhood influences.

• IPV affects many women, yet health professionals often fail to screen adequately for it.

• Maltreatment affects every aspect of the child, including his or her social, behavioral, emotional, intellectual, and physical development.

• Older adults are increasingly victims of abuse (ie, physical, sexual, psychological, or neglect) at the hands of their caregivers.

• Rape and sexual assault are acts of violence in the form of sexual behaviors forcefully perpetrated on others, violating their person and shattering their sense of safety and predictability.

• Rape trauma syndrome details the sequence of psychological events that rape victims may experience after an attack.

• The nursing care of the rape victim involves attending to both physical and psychological needs and requires particular sensitivity to the victim's reaction.

• To intervene with the rape victim effectively, nurses must attend to and control their own reaction to the event.

Study Questions

1. An 11-year-old student goes to the school nurse with a bloody nose after a fight with a peer. The fight ensued when the peer brushed against the client in the hall and knocked his books out of his hands. The client accosted the student, shoved him, and challenged him to a fight. What type of risk factor for continued youth violence does the client have?

    a. Peer risk factor

    b. Family risk factor

    c. Individual risk factor

    d. Neighborhood risk factor

2. The school nurse is concerned about the number of injuries she sees that have resulted from fighting. Which of the following interventions will likely have the greatest effect on youth violence in the school?

    a. A social problem-solving program

    b. Family therapy for students who have been involved in fighting

    c. Referral of students involved in fighting to the school counselor

    d. Distribution of handouts about youth violence to all students

3. A 5-year-old child is brought to the ED with a broken wrist. The mother states the child fell off a swing. The nurse notes multiple healing bruises on the child's back, which the mother states occurred when the child fell down the steps 5 days earlier. Based on these data, which action should the nurse take?

    a. Continue assessing the child for possible neurologic reasons for frequent falls.

    b. Report the family to the child protection agency for suspected physical abuse.

    c. Accept the mother's explanation and arrange for a cast to be applied to the arm.

    d. Inform the physician that she suspects child abuse.

4. A 78-year-old man with a history of atrial fibrillation and type 2 diabetes is brought to the ED by his 50-year-old son, who cares for him at home. On assessment, the nurse notes that the client is dehydrated, unkempt, and has a stage 3 pressure ulcer on his coccyx. He is weak but otherwise neurologically intact. The nurse asks if the client is being well cared for at home, to which the client replies, "He does the best he can, I guess." Which of the following interpretations of the findings and the client's statement is the most likely explanation for the client's condition?

    a. The client's age and weakness

    b. Physical abuse

    c. Physical neglect

    d. The client's underlying physical condition

5. A nurse in the ED is assessing a 42-year-old client who was brutally raped and beaten 3 hours earlier by her estranged boyfriend. The client has several facial fractures and multiple lacerations. She states, "He has done this before." Throughout the assessment, the client does not appear upset and is cooperating in a matter-of-fact manner with the examination. The nurse attributes the client's affect to which of the following explanations?

   a. The client is handling the assault well from an emotional standpoint.

   b. The client's reaction is abnormal and suggests an underlying psychological problem.

   c. The client is concerned more about her physical injuries at this time.

   d. The client's affect is a normal reaction and may represent an effort to regain control.

Critical Thinking Questions

1. When you read of a violent incident in the newspaper, do you usually feel removed from the event? Has that sense of distance changed since reading this chapter?

2. Do only particular types of people have the potential to become violent? Consider your own risk for becoming a victim or perpetrator of violence, as well as protective factors.

3. Of all the types of violence in this chapter (youth, IPV, child maltreatment, elder abuse, and rape), which seems completely implausible to you? Which do you believe could never happen to you or a member of your family?

4. Assess your community, schools, and neighborhood for risk factors of youth violence.

5. Of all sections of this chapter, which topic personally touched you or generated a great deal of feeling? Why?

References

American College of Emergency Physicians. (2007). *ACEP policy statement: Domestic family violence.* Retrieved from http://www.acep.org/content.aspx?id=29184

American College of Physicians. (1998). Firearm injury protection. *Annals of Internal Medicine, 128,* 236–241.

Anderson, M., Kaufman, J., Simon, T. R., Barrios, L., Paulozzi, L., Ryan, G., et al. (2001). School-associated violent deaths in the United States, 1994–1999. *Journal of the American Medical Association, 286,* 2695–2702.

Berg, A. O. (2004). Screening for family and intimate partner violence: Recommendation statement. *Annals of Family Medicine, 2,* 156–160.

Broidy, L. M., Nagin, D. S., Tremblay, R. E., Bates, J. E., Brame, B., Dodge, K., et al. (2003). Developmental trajectories of childhood disruptive behavior and adolescent delinquency: A six-site, cross-national study. *Developmental Psychology, 39,* 222–245.

Brook, D. W., Brook, J. S., Rosen, Z., Dela Rosa, M., Montoya, I., & Whiteman, M. (2003). Early risk factors for violence in Colombian adolescents. *American Journal of Psychiatry, 160,* 1470–1478.

Brown, E. J. (2003). Child physical abuse: Risk for psychopathology and efficacy of interventions. *Current Psychiatry Reports, 5*(2), 87–94.

Buckner, J. C., Mezzacappa, E., & Beardslee, W. R. (2003). Characteristics of resilient youth living in poverty: The role of self-regulatory processes. *Development and Psychopathology, 15,* 139–162.

Burgess, A. W., & Holmstrom, L. L. (1974). Rape trauma syndrome. *American Journal of Psychiatry, 131,* 981–999.

Campbell, S. B., Shaw, D. S., & Gilliom, M. (2000). Early externalizing behavior problems: Toddlers and preschoolers at risk for later maladjustment. *Development and Psychopathology, 12,* 467–488.

Cantu, M., Coppola M., & Lindner A. J. (2003). Evaluation and management of the sexually assaulted woman. *Emergency Medical Clinics of North America, 21*(3), 737–750.

Center for Mental Health Services (CMHS). (2001). *The CMHS approach to enhancing youth resilience and preventing youth violence in schools and communities.* Washington, DC: Substance Abuse and Mental Health Services Administration.

Centers for Disease Control and Prevention (CDC). (2002). Youth risk behavior surveillance—United States 2001. *Morbidity and Mortality Weekly Report, 51*(SS-04), 1–64.

Centers for Disease Control and Prevention (CDC). (2006a). *Costs of intimate partner violence against women in the United States.* Retrieved from http://www.cdc.gov/violenceprevention/pdf/IPV-Factsheet.pdf

Centers for Disease Control and Prevention (CDC). (2006b). Homicides and suicides—national violent death reporting system, United States, 2003–2004. *Morbidity and Mortality Weekly Report, 55*(26), 721–724.

Centers for Disease Control and Prevention (CDC). (2007a). *Injuries among older adults.* Retrieved from http://www.cdc.gov/homeandrecreationalsafety/falls/adultfalls.html

Centers for Disease Control and Prevention (CDC). (2007b). *Youth violence fact sheet.* Retrieved from http://www.cdc.gov/Violence Prevention/pdf/yv-factsheet-a.pdf

Child Welfare Information Gateway. (2006). *Child maltreatment 2004: Summary of key findings.* Retrieved from: http://www.childwelfare.gov/pubs/factsheets/canstats.cfm

Citrome, L. L. (2007). *Aggression.* Retrieved from http://emedicine.medscape.com/article/288689-overview

Cole, P. M., Teti, L. O., & Zahn-Waxler, C. (2003). Mutual emotion regulation and the stability of conduct problems between preschool and early school age. *Development and Psychopathology, 15,* 1–18.

Commission for the Prevention of Youth Violence. (2000). *Youth and violence: Medicine, nursing and public health. Connecting the dots to prevent violence.* Washington, DC: American Medical Association.

Cooper, W., Lutenbacker, M., & Faccia, K. (2000). Components of effective youth violence prevention programs for 7- to 14-year-olds. *Archives of Pediatric and Adolescent Medicine, 154,* 1134–1139.

Costello, E. J., Compton, S. N., Keeler, G., & Angold, A. (2003). Relationships between poverty and psychopathology: A natural experiment. *Journal of the American Medical Association, 290,* 2023–2029.

Dahlberg, L. L., & Potter, L. B. (2001). Youth violence: Developmental pathways and prevention challenges. *American Journal of Preventive Medicine, 20*(Suppl. 1), 3–14.

De Bellis, M. D., & Thomas, L. A. (2003). Biologic findings of post-traumatic stress disorder and child maltreatment. *Current Psychiatry Reports, 5*(2), 108–117.

Dodge, K. A. (2001). The science of youth violence prevention: Progressing from developmental epidemiology to efficacy to effectiveness to public policy. *American Journal of Preventive Medicine, 20*(Suppl. 1), 63–70.

Falsetti, S. A. (2007). Screening and responding to family and intimate partner violence in the primary care setting. *Primary Care, 34*(3), 641–657.

Fantuzzo, J. W., Borouch, R., Beriama, A., Atkins, M., & Marcus, S. (1997). Domestic violence and children: Prevalence and risk in five major U.S. cities. *Journal of the American Academy of Child and Adolescent Psychiatry, 36,* 116–122.

Ferris, L. E. (2004). Intimate partner violence. *British Medical Journal, 328,* 595–596.

Frick, P. J., Cornell, A. H., Bodin, S. D., Dane, H. E., Barry, C. T., & Loney, B. R. (2003). Callous-unemotional traits and developmental pathways to severe conduct problems. *Developmental Psychopathology, 39,* 2246–2260.

Fulmer, T., & Cahill, V. M. (1984). Assessing elder abuse: A study. *Journal of Gerontological Nursing, 10*(12), 16–20.

Fulmer T., Street, S., & Carr, K. (1984). Abuse of the elderly: Screening and detection. *Journal of Emergency Nursing, 10*(3), 131–140.

Gauthier, Y. (2003). Infant mental health as we enter the third millennium: Can we prevent aggression? *Infant Mental Health Journal, 24,* 296–308.

Gentile, D. A., & Stone, W. (2005). Violent video game effects on children and adolescents. A review of the literature. *Minerva Pediatrica, 57*(6), 337–358.

Gross, D., & Grady, J. (2002). Group based parent training for preventing mental health disorders in children. *Issues in Mental Health Nursing, 23,* 367–383.

Guerra, N. G., Huesmann, L. R., & Spindler, A. (2003). Community violence exposure, social cognition, and aggression among urban elementary school children. *Child Development, 74,* 1561–1576.

Gunter, J. (2007). Intimate partner violence. *Obstetric and Gynecological Clinics of North America, 34*(3), 367–368.

Hahn, R., Fuqua-Whitley, D., Wethington, H., Lowy, J., Liberman, A., Crosby, A., et al. (2007). The effectiveness of universal school-based programs for the prevention of violent and aggressive behavior: A report on recommendations of the Task Force on Community Preventive Services. *MMWR: Recommendations and Reports, 56*(RR-7), 1–12.

Halliday-Boykins, C. A., & Graham, S. (2001). At both ends of the gun: Testing the relationship between community violence exposure and youth violent behavior. *Journal of Abnormal Child Psychology, 29,* 383–402.

Hinderliter, D., Doughty, A., Delaney, K. R., Pitula, C., & Campbell, J. (2003). The effect of intimate partner violence education on nurse practitioner's feelings of competence and ability to screen patients. *American Journal of Nursing Education, 42,* 449–454.

Holmes, S. E., Slaughter, J. R., & Kashani, J. (2001). Risk factors in childhood that lead to the development of conduct disorder and antisocial personality disorder. *Child Psychiatry and Human Development, 31,* 183–193.

Huesmann, L. R. (2007). The impact of electronic media violence: Scientific theory and research. *Journal of Adolescent Health, 41* (6 Suppl 1), S6–S13.

Huesmann, L. R., Moise-Titus, J., Podolski, C. L., & Eron, L. D. (2003). Longitudinal relations between children's exposure to TV violence and their aggressive and violent behavior in young adulthood: 1977–1992. *Developmental Psychology, 39,* 201–221.

Jaycox, L. H., Stein, B. D., Kataoka, S. H., Wong, M., Fink, A., Escudero, P., & Zarogoza, C. (2002). Violence exposure, post-traumatic stress disorder and depressive symptoms among recent immigrant school children. *Journal of the American Academy of Child and Adolescent Psychiatry, 41,* 1104–1110.

The Joint Commission. (2012). *Comprehensive accreditation manual for hospitals.* Oak Brook, IL: Author.

Kelly, P. J. (2007). Integrating intimate partner violence prevention into daily practice. *Journal of Psychosocial Nursing and Mental Health Services, 45*(4), 8–9.

Krug, E. G., Dahlberg, L. L., Mercy, J. A., Zwi, A. B., & Lozano, R. (2002). *World report on violence and health.* Geneva, Switzerland: World Health Organization.

Leeb, R. T., Barker, L. E., & Strine, T. W. (2007). The effect of childhood physical and sexual abuse on adolescent weapon carrying. *Journal of Adolescent Health, 40*(6), 551–558.

McFarlane, J., Groff, J., O'Brien, J., & Watson, K. (2003). Behaviors of children who are exposed and not exposed to intimate partner violence: An analysis of 330 black, white and Hispanic children. *Pediatrics, 112,* 202–207.

Miller, C. A. (2009). *Nursing for wellness in older adults* (5th ed.). Philadelphia, PA: Lippincott Williams & Wilkins.

Mohr, W. K., Lutz, M. J., Fantuzzo, J. W., & Perry, M. A. (2000). Children exposed to family violence: A review of empirical research from a developmental–ecological perspective. *Trauma, Violence, and Abuse, 1,* 264–283.

Muris, P., Merckelbach, H., & Walczak, S. (2002). Aggression and threat perception abnormalities in children with learning difficulties and behavior problems. *Child Psychiatry and Human Development, 33,* 147–163.

NANDA International. (2007). *Nursing diagnoses: Definitions and classification (2007–2008).* Philadelphia, PA: Author.

National Institute of Justice, Bureau of Justice Statistics. (2002). The sexual victimization of college women. Retrieved from http://www.ojp.usdoj.gov/bjs

Olds, D. L., Robinson, J., O'Brien, R., Luckey, D. W., Pettitt, L. M., Henderson, C. R., et al. (2002). Home visiting by paraprofessionals and by nurses: A randomized controlled trial. *Pediatrics, 110,* 486–496.

Punukollu, M. (2002). Domestic violence: Screening made practical. *Journal of Family Practice, 52,* 537–543.

Reynolds, M. W., Wallace, J., Hill, T., Weist, M. D., & Nabors, L. A. (2001). The relationship between gender, depression, and self-esteem in children who have witnessed domestic violence. *Child Abuse and Neglect, 25,* 1201–1206.

Schore, A. N. (2001). The effects of early relational trauma on right brain development, affect regulation and infant mental health. *Infant Mental Health Journal, 22,* 201–269.

Scott, K. L., Wolfe, D. A., & Wekerle, C. (2003). Maltreatment and trauma: Tracking the connections in adolescence. *Child and Adolescent Psychiatric Clinics of North America, 12*(2), 211–230.

Self-Brown, S. R., LeBlanc, M., Kelley, M. L., Hanson, R., Laslie, K., & Wingate, A. (2006). Effects of community violence exposure and parental mental health on the internalizing problems of urban adolescents. *Violence and Victims, 21*(2), 183–198.

Shapiro, F. (2005). *EMDR solutions: Pathways to healing.* New York, NY: W. W. Norton.

Sourander, A., Jensen, P., Davies, M., Niemela, S., Elonheimo, H., Ristkari, T., et al. (2007). Who is at greatest risk of adverse long-term outcomes? The Finnish From a Boy to a Man Study. *Journal of the American Academy of Child and Adolescent Psychiatry, 46*(9), 1148–1161.

Springer, K. W., Sheridan, J., Kuo, D., & Carnes, M. (2003). The long-term health outcomes of childhood abuse: An overview and a call to action. *Journal of General Internal Medicine, 18*(10), 864–870.

Tenney-Soeiro, R., & Wilson, C. (2004). An update on child abuse and neglect. *Current Opinion in Pediatrics, 16*(2), 233–237.

Thornton, T. N., Craft, C. A., Dahlberg, L. L., Lynch, B. S., & Baer, K. (2000). *Best practices of youth violence prevention: A sourcebook for community action.* Atlanta, GA: CDC, National Center for Injury Prevention and Control.

Tolan, P. H., Gorman-Smith, D., & Henry, D. B. (2003). The developmental ecology of urban males' youth violence. *Developmental Psychology, 39,* 274–291.

Toth, S. L., & Cicchetti, D. (2010). The historical origins and developmental pathways of the discipline of developmental psychopathology. *Israel Journal of Psychiatry and Related Sciences, 47*(2), 5–14.

Tremblay, R. E., Nagin, D. S., Séguin, J. R., Zoccolillo, M., Zelazo, P. D., Boivin, M., et al. (2004). Physical aggression during early childhood: Trajectories and predictors. *Pediatrics, 114*(1), e43–e50.

U.S. Department of Justice. (2005). *Criminal victimization in the United States: Statistical tables index.* Retrieved from http://bjs .ojp.usdoj.gov/content/pub/pdf/cvus05.pdf

U.S. Department of Justice. (2007a). *Firearms and crime statistics.* Retrieved from http://bjs.ojp.usdoj.gov/content/guns.cfm

U.S. Department of Justice. (2007b). *Homicide trends in the US.* Retrieved from http://bjs.ojp.usdoj.gov/content/homicide/homtrnd. cfm

U.S. Public Health Service. (2003). Family violence as a public health issue. Retrieved from http://www.surgeongeneral.gov/news/ speeches/violence08062003.htm

Valentino, K., Cicchetti, D., Rogosch, F. A., & Toth, S. L. (2011). Mother–child play and maltreatment: A longitudinal analysis of emerging social behavior from infancy to toddlerhood. *Developmental Psychology, 47,* 1280–1294.

van der Kolk, B. A., Spinazzola, J., Blaustein, M. E., Hopper, J. W., Hopper, E. K., Korn, D. L., et al. (2007). A randomized clinical trial of eye movement desensitization and reprocessing (EMDR), fluoxetine, and pill placebo in the treatment of posttraumatic stress disorder: Treatment effects and long-term maintenance. *Journal of Clinical Psychiatry, 68*(1), 37–46.

Wilson, B. J., Smith, S. L., Potter, W. J., Kunkel, D., Linz, D., Colvin, C. M., et al. (2002). Violence in children's television programming: Assessing the risks. *Journal of Communication, 52,* 5–35.

Web Resources

Center for the Prevention of Sexual and Domestic Violence: http:// www.cpsdv.org

Child Abuse Prevention Network: http://http://child-abuse.com

National Center on Elder Abuse and the Clearinghouse on Abuse and Neglect of the Elderly (CANE): http://www.elderabusecenter.org

National Committee for the Prevention of Elder Abuse: http://www .preventelderabuse.org

National Domestic Violence Hotline: http://www.ndhv.org

Stop Family Violence: http://www.stopfamilyviolence.org

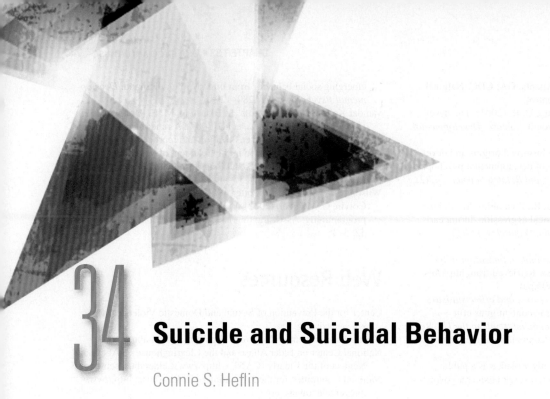

34

Suicide and Suicidal Behavior

Connie S. Heflin

KEY TERMS

ambivalence
death by suicide
hopelessness
suicidal behavior
suicidal ideation
suicidal intent
suicidal plan
suicide

LEARNING OBJECTIVES

On completion of this chapter, you should be able to accomplish the following:

- Explain the magnitude of suicide.
- Define suicide, suicidal behavior, and other key terms related to self-directed violence.
- Identify groups at risk for death by suicide.
- List the warning signs of suicide.
- Explain factors contributing to suicidal risk, including the relationship to culture and ethnicity, age, and gender.
- Discuss components and process of a comprehensive nursing assessment for people at risk for suicide.
- Develop nursing interventions for care of people at risk for suicide.
- Outline approaches to caring for survivors of suicide.

Suicide is a word that engenders various emotions: fear, pain, suffering, sadness, guilt, and anger, to mention a few. According to the Centers for Disease Control and Prevention (CDC), suicide is self-directed violent behavior that "deliberately results in injury or the potential for injury to oneself" (Crosby et al., 2011).

Suicide is a major public health concern, both in the United States and around the world. It is a word that every parent, child, friend, and health professional dreads. Although certain factors may increase risk for suicide, suicide knows no bounds of person, age, class, race, or gender.

This chapter presents an overview of suicide and suicidal behavior. It identifies warning signs, as well as risk and protective factors. The chapter outlines the content and process of a comprehensive nursing assessment of a client at risk for suicide. It also reviews general guidelines for caring for suicidal clients. The reader is urged to review this chapter in conjunction with discussions presented in Chapter 27 for a full understanding of depression and interventions to prevent suicide.

SUICIDE

Some definitions are important to understanding the context of suicide. This chapter considers a range of actions associated with suicide as **suicidal behaviors**. It uses the term **suicide** or **death by suicide** to describe the act of killing oneself. The chapter avoids terms such as completed suicide, failed suicide, or successful suicide.

Suicidal ideation is defined as thoughts of engaging in suicidal behavior. The term **suicidal intent** means that at the time of injury or death, the individual had thoughts of killing himself or herself, or wished to die. **Suicidal plan** refers to the organization of a time frame and method for killing oneself (Crosby et al., 2011).

Incidence and Prevalence

Globally, approximately 1 million people per year die by suicide, or one death every 40 seconds. Depression and alcohol use disorders are major risk factors for suicide in North America and Europe. In Asian countries, impulsivity is a contributing factor (World Health Organization [WHO], 2011a).

In the United States, more than 34,000 people each year die by suicide, or one death every 15 minutes. It is the 11th leading cause of death for all ages. Males take their own lives at nearly four times the rate of females and represent the majority of all U.S. suicides. This outcome may be because men generally tend to choose more violent methods. Two thirds of male suicide victims die by firearm. The most common cause of death by suicide in women is overdose or poisoning. However, women attempt suicide about two to three times as often as men (CDC, 2010).

As noted, suicide occurs across all ages of the lifespan. Young people (aged 15 to 24) are more likely to use firearms, suffocation, and poisoning than other methods of suicide.

Children (aged 10 to 14) are increasingly using suffocation as a means to end their lives (National Institute of Mental Health [NIMH], 2010). Suicide is a major concern in the latter years of life. White males over age 85 are at the greatest risk of all age-gender-race groups (American Association of Suicidology [AAS], 2009). This is a significant fact for nursing, because many of the people using nurses' services are elderly. A study of global elderly suicide rates by Shah (2011) showed the lowest rates to be in the Caribbean and Arabic/Islamic countries, with the highest rates in Europe and some Asian countries.

Sociocultural factors are also important when reporting statistics on suicide. In the United States, American Indian/Alaska Native suicide rates are high compared with the general population (CDC, 2010). Among Hispanics, the suicide rate is lower than that of non-Hispanics for all age groups. This may be due in part to social support by the family and a strong religious belief that suicide is a "sin" (Suicide Prevention Resource Center, n.d.). The rate of suicide for African Americans (all ages) is well below that of the Caucasian group. However, the rate has shown a slight increase since 2003. The suicide rate among African American females is the lowest of all racial/gender groups (AAS, 2010a, 2010b).

Suicide Prevention Efforts

The effects of suicide on families, the health care industry, and society at large are immeasurable. For every suicide that occurs, there are at least six survivors (AAS, 2010d).

One example of a global effort to stop suicide is the establishment of a World Suicide Prevention Day, held annually on September 10. The WHO designed it to promote worldwide strategies for education and prevention of suicide. Many countries around the world have established national suicide prevention strategies. Examples include Australia, Canada, England, Finland, France, Ireland, New Zealand, Norway, Scotland, Slovenia, Sweden, and the United States (WHO, 2011b).

> **Checkpoint Questions**
> 1. What method do males who die by suicide use most often?
> 2. Which group of people are at the highest risk of suicide and also comprise a large part of nurses' client base?

Etiology

People who die by suicide cannot explain their actions. Many theories have been proposed to explain suicide, but at best they are only guesses. Some people leave suicide notes before committing their acts, but these are not common. Fewer than one in five people who die by suicide leave a written note (Silverman et al., 2007).

"It is not possible to distinguish between patients with depression who will make a suicide attempt and those who will not" (Silverman et al., 2007, p. 1). This point is important because all clients with depression, except for those with the mildest symptoms, are potentially at risk for suicide.

Genetic Factors

Risk for suicide increases when there is a family history of suicide (Muzina, 2007). Risk of suicide is two to eight times higher in first-degree (parents, siblings, or children) relatives of people who died by suicide than in the general population. However, the question remains whether this link is specific to suicide factors or whether it is related to familial psychiatric disorders such as mood disorders, notably depression. Additional studies are clearly needed to delineate these factors.

It has been proposed that people who die by suicide may have an individual predisposition to it, as evidenced by certain personality traits. A recent study examined personality traits in adolescents as related to their suicidality. It was found that impulsive traits contributed to suicide attempts and self-injurious behaviors. Adolescents who displayed callous, unemotional traits (such as those seen in antisocial disorder) seemed protected from suicide (Javdani et al., 2011). Some examples of potential contributing factors may include sexual and physical abuse in childhood and recent life events. Aggressive personality traits also have been shown to correlate with suicidal behaviors (see Chap. 32).

Neurotransmitter changes are thought to occur during suicide attempts and completions. Lower levels of serotonin, which is also associated with depression, have been found in the brains of people with a history of suicide attempts (NIMH, 2011).

Psychological Factors

Mood disorders, particularly major depression, are predominant in most suicide deaths (see Chap. 27). In fact, the risk of suicide in people with major depression is 20 times greater than that of the general population. Almost two thirds of people who die by suicide are depressed at the time of their death (AAS, 2010c). Other mental disorders associated with suicide risk are personality disorders (borderline, antisocial, histrionic, and narcissistic), anxiety disorders (panic and obsessive–compulsive), somatoform disorders, and eating disorders (anorexia nervosa and bulimia). Although mental illness plays a significant role in death by suicide, more than 95% of people with mental illness do not die by suicide.

People who have a dependence on alcohol or drugs in addition to being depressed are at greater risk for suicide due to impaired judgment. A history of previous suicide attempts increases a client's risk substantially. It is noted to be the single most significant predictor of death by suicide. There is no clear evidence to date that the prescription of antidepressants for the treatment of depression increases suicidality in children, adolescents, or adults.

Dr. Thomas Joiner, an internationally recognized suicide expert and author of *Why People Die by Suicide,* has formed a research-based theory on the reasons people commit suicide. He has posited that the desire for death "is comprised of two psychological states. One is a perception of being a burden to others, having let everyone down, and the other is a feeling of not belonging, not feeling connected to a family or a relationship. Alone, neither of these states is enough to instill the desire for death, but together they produce a desire that can be deadly when combined with the ability to enact self-injury" (Florida State University, n.d.).

While theories attempt to explain suicidal behavior, they are less than adequate in explaining the diversity of experiences that characterize the range of suicidal behaviors and associated outcomes (see Case Vignette 34.1).

Physical Factors

Chronic physical illnesses contribute to higher suicide risk in some individuals. A study by Scott and colleagues (2010) investigated individuals with chronic physical conditions and their association with first onset of suicidal behavior. It was found that people with chronic conditions such as hypertension, heart attack/stroke, chronic headache or other chronic pain, and respiratory problems were associated with suicidal behavior. Those with epilepsy most strongly correlated with

Case Vignette 34.1

One of my dearest friends died by suicide. I have experienced the emotions described in this chapter. Months later, while the shock is not with me every moment, at times I still experience an overwhelming sadness and pain that can move me to tears and regret. It is a physical pain in my heart that hits with a crushing sensation. I know in my head that my friend made an intentional choice to end her life, but my heart still feels broken and torn. People who are bereaved feel like they are in a wilderness of grief. This grief in some ways is different than other kinds of grief because of the nature of the death.

Nurses may have an opportunity and privilege to walk alongside family members or friends of those who have been bereaved by suicide. It is important to acknowledge the pain and sorrow and to listen with care and compassion, to try and give survivors the opportunity to share their stories of love and loss. Alan Wolfelt, a psychologist and grief counselor in Colorado, identifies 10 touchstones that when embraced, offer hope of healing. He describes grief as a vast wilderness that has unfamiliar and brutal surroundings. His advice to those who are grieving is "you must journey through this wilderness…. You must become acquainted with its terrain and learn to follow the sometimes hard-to-find path that leads to healing" (Wolfelt, 2007, cover).

Reflection and Critical Thinking

- What special challenges might nurses, other health care providers, and people who belong to the helping professions face when dealing with personal experiences of suicide?
- What things could those whose loved ones have attempted or committed suicide do to move through their grief and protect their own psychological well-being?

suicidal outcomes. It is interesting to note that the individuals experiencing these physical conditions early in life had the strongest likelihood of suicidality. Another individual warranting the attention of nurses is the "suicidal mother" who experiences postpartum depression. Research has demonstrated that suicidal ideation is a frequent complication of pregnancy in both developed and developing countries (Gentile, 2011).

Other Factors

Environmental factors may be associated with suicidal behaviors. Loss of job with a resultant loss of status, relationships, and social contacts can be contributing factors. Natural disasters that have been experienced worldwide have created a multitude of mental health problems and possible suicidal behaviors. Veterans returning from war with post-traumatic stress disorder (PTSD) are also a high-risk group. Other difficult losses, such as the death of loved ones, divorce, financial problems, or other major stresses, may drive people to despair if coping mechanisms to handle them are inadequate.

Checkpoint Questions

3. What does a family history of suicide mean for a first-degree relative?

4. What is the single greatest risk factor for suicidality?

Protective Factors

Although numerous factors can increase risk for suicidal behavior, protective factors can help to prevent death by suicide. Improving social support, strengthening coping skills, and decreasing stigma associated with seeking help for mental health problems contribute to enhancing resilience and decreasing risk. The Suicide Prevention Resource Center (2001) notes the following definitive protective factors:

- Effective clinical care for mental, physical, and substance abuse disorders
- Easy access to various clinical interventions and support for help-seeking
- Close familial/friend relationships, which foster better coping with stress
- Restricted access to highly lethal means of suicide
- Strong connections to family and community support
- Support through ongoing medical and mental health care relationships
- Skills in problem solving, conflict resolution, and nonviolent handling of disputes
- Cultural and religious beliefs that discourage suicide and support self-preservation

Understanding both risk and protective factors can play an important role in nursing assessment and intervention for people at risk for suicide.

APPLYING THE NURSING PROCESS

Suicidal Clients

Nurses are frequently a first point of contact for clients who may be either overtly or covertly expressing suicidal ideation, suicidal behaviors, or both. Clients who may be considering taking their own life may be encountered across diverse practice settings: home care, community and public health agencies, inpatient and outpatient facilities, long-term care, and acute hospitals. Nurses are often first-line responders in the process for assessing risk and mobilizing the resources to intervene in a suicidal crisis.

Most people considering suicide are frequently ambivalent about their decision (Survivors of Suicide, n.d.). **Ambivalence** suggests that while they are sincere in their desire to die, at the same time, they wish that they could find another way to deal with their situation. Professional interventions are geared to work with these feelings of ambivalence and use them as a basis for instilling hope and preventing self-harm.

▲ ASSESSMENT

Determining suicide risk begins with understanding common warning signs of suicide. Most experts agree that suicide rarely occurs without warning. Warning signs, whether overt or covert, are generally present. See BOX 34.1.

None of the warning signs in BOX 34.1 alone are predictive of risk. A key to understanding a client's specific risk is to understand behaviors in terms of the person's normal context. Is a person's behaviors unusual? Has his or her behavior changed? See BOX 34.2.

Nursing assessment begins with a consideration of the therapeutic relationship and focuses on establishing a therapeutic alliance with clients at risk. Nurses should carry out assessment with a caring and compassionate approach in an attempt to understand the experience that the suicidal person is having. Such an approach provides the foundation for holistic assessment and intervention. Assessing clients at risk should involve understanding the person within his or her social and family context. Nurses should listen openly and nonjudgmentally. It is important to not act shocked or to negate the client's experiences or feelings (eg, "You can't feel that way. You have so much to live for!")

Nurses start with open-ended questions that invite clients to convey what is concerning them most at this particular time. Sensitivity and empathy allow nurses to gather information, engage clients, and develop the therapeutic relationship.

Understanding a client's current stressors helps nurses to determine what is happening at this particular time and how that person perceives those stressors. What symptoms is this person experiencing right now? Examples of questions for specific key areas are listed in Assessment Tool 34.1.

BOX 34.1 Warning Signs of Suicide

Emotional/Psychological Signs

- Feelings of hopelessness and helplessness
- Frequent mood changes
- Feelings of being a burden to others
- Anxiety and agitation
- Fatigue and tiredness
- Sadness
- Depression
- Inability to find enjoyment in anything
- Feelings of guilt
- Feelings of worthlessness
- Feelings of failure
- Feelings of isolation

Behavioral Signs

- Making a will
- Putting one's affairs in order
- Giving away prized possessions

- Making suicide threats
- Talking of wanting to kill oneself
- Talking about death, dying, or suicide
- Planning for death (stockpiling pills, seeking access to firearms)
- Previous suicide attempts
- Loss of interest in usual activities (sports, work, hobbies)
- Decreased interest in school (drop in grades and decreased achievement)
- Skipping school
- Running away from home
- Acting recklessly or engaging in risky behaviors seemingly without thinking (such as careless use of firearms, driving)
- Sexual promiscuity
- Withdrawal from friends and family
- Increased use of substances (alcohol or drugs)
- Change in sleep habits (difficulty sleeping or sleeping a great deal of the time)
- Change in eating habits (eating more or less with resultant weight changes)

Prior Suicidal Behavior

As previously mentioned, a key significant predictor of suicide risk is prior suicide attempts. Anyone who has had previous suicidal behavior or suicide attempts is at higher risk. Therefore, it is important to review the client's history of suicidality. Potential questions include the following:

- Have you ever had thoughts of harming yourself?
- When was that?
- What were you thinking and feeling at that time?
- Did you ever act on any thoughts of harming yourself?
- Tell me about those times.

BOX 34.2 Is Path Warm?

Several suicide prevention organizations such as the National Suicide Prevention Lifeline (http://www.suicidepreventionlifeline.org) use a mnemonic developed by the American Association of Suicidology to help remember the warning signs of suicide:

I	Ideation	(threatened or communicated)
S	Substance abuse	(excessive or increased)
P	Purposelessness	(feels no reason for living)
A	Anxiety	(agitation/insomnia)
T	Trapped	(feels there is no way out)
H	Hopelessness	(feels there is no hope, nothing to look forward to)
W	Withdrawal	(withdraws from family, friends, society)
A	Anger	(uncontrolled, rage, seeking revenge)
R	Recklessness	(risky behavior, without thinking)
M	Mood change	(severe and dramatic)

Current Suicide Plan

When clients have a suicide plan, risk for suicide is obviously increased because they are actively thinking about killing themselves. It is important to determine what methods clients plan to use. Asking directly is the best approach. Nurses should develop a style of asking that they are comfortable with, while not engaging in avoidance or hesitancy. Potential questions include the following:

- Are you thinking about killing yourself right now?
- Are you feeling so badly that you have thought of taking your own life?
- Have things been so bad that you feel you can't go on?
- What have you thought about doing?
- Have you thought about a specific time or place?
- Do you have access to a firearm, pills, knife? (Nurses ask this to learn whether the person has access to the means described.)

Lethality Assessment

A lethality assessment is conducted as part of a risk assessment. Once it is determined that someone is thinking of suicide, a lethality assessment is necessary. It is an attempt to predict how likely a person is to die by suicide. While there is no sure way to predict this, a few factors can assist nurses in helping to plan appropriate and informed interventions. The more lethal the method that the person is thinking about, the higher at risk he or she is. See Table 34.1.

Murray and Hauenstein (2008) note that while some people have a carefully laid-out plan to end their lives, others act on their suicidal ideas impulsively. Such clients tend to be adolescents or people with personality disorders, substance use disorders, or both. Frequently these clients may have lower intent of death, but they may be unable to control the outcome.

▲ **ASSESSMENT TOOL 34.1** ▲
Questions to Review Stressors for Suicidal Clients

Eating

* How is your appetite? What changes have you noticed and when? Have you had any weight gain or weight loss recently? Over what time period?

Sleeping

* How is your sleeping? What changes have you noticed? Do you have difficulty sleeping? Are you sleeping more or less than you usually do?

Mood

* Tell me what your mood has been like recently. What changes have you noticed? When was the last time that you felt really good or happy about something? What do you look forward to?

Health

* How is your physical health? Have you had any recent illnesses or physical health concerns?

Activities

* Tell me about a usual day for you. Do you spend your time at work, school, or home?
* What do you do for fun and enjoyment?

Coping

* How do you generally cope with problems and worries in your life?
* What are you doing to cope now?
* Do you ever take a drink to help you feel better? How often?
* Do you ever take medications or drugs to help you feel better? What are these and how often do you take them?

Current Resources

As noted earlier, the resources available to people can be a protective factor against suicidal behavior. If clients have friends, family resources, and people they feel they can confide in, risk may be decreased somewhat. Knowing about the available resources clients have also provides some options in terms of treatment. Questions nurses might ask are as follows:

* What are your living circumstances? Do you live alone or with someone? (If someone is living alone and socially isolated, he or she may be at increased risk.)
* Do you have people in your life who are supportive of you?
* Who do you have that you feel you can talk to and can understand you?

TABLE 34.1 Lethality of Suicide Attempts by Method

Less Lethal Methods	More Lethal Methods
Overdose of nonprescription drugs (except for acetaminophen and aspirin)	Firearms
	Hanging
	Overdose of antidepressants
Wrist slashing	Overdose of barbiturates and sleeping pills
	Overdose of aspirin and Tylenol
	Jumping
	Carbon monoxide poisoning

Checkpoint Questions

5. What is more important than determining any single risk factor for suicide in a client?
6. What is the best way for nurses to ask clients about suicidal thoughts?
7. What are some especially lethal methods of suicide?

▲ **NURSING DIAGNOSIS**

The most obvious diagnosis for clients is **Risk for Suicide** (NANDA, 2008). Other potential diagnoses include, but are not limited to, **Powerlessness, Hopelessness, Chronic Low Self-Esteem,** and **Ineffective Coping.**

▲ **OUTCOME IDENTIFICATION AND PLANNING**

The most important priority is maintaining the client's safety, as well as safety for others. Chapter 27 presents care planning and implementation for clients with depression who are at risk for self-harm. Possible outcomes for clients, integrating labels from the *Nursing Outcomes Classification* (*NOC*), may include the following (University of Iowa College of Nursing, n.d. b).

* **Suicide Self-Restraint**
* **Social Interaction Skills**
* **Depression Self-Control**
* **Distorted Thought Self-Control**
* **Will to Live**

▲ **IMPLEMENTATION**

Understanding a client's risk factors provides the foundation for intervening appropriately. Throughout assessment, nurses have had an opportunity to develop an awareness of the client at risk. Essentially, clients thinking of suicide are in need of help.

Common *Nursing Interventions Classification* (*NIC*) labels for suicidal clients include, but are not limited to, **Behavior Management: Self-Harm, Hope, Inspiration, Mood Management, Spiritual Support,** and **Suicide Prevention** (University of Iowa College of Nursing, n.d. a).

Immediate interventions involve removing the means of suicide to reduce the risk of it happening. If the person is hospitalized, methods may include ensuring pills or medications are not available to clients or that they are not taking any measures to accumulate needed drugs. If in a community or home care setting, nurses may enlist the help of family or friends to remove the means and to provide immediate support. M VIE viewing GUIDES

Nurses must communicate firmness in their intention to help. Acute suicide situations are psychiatric emergencies. Clients must not be left alone. Safety is the number one priority. It is also important to be clear about the limits of confidentiality in such situations. Nurses should not enter agreements to conceal the suicidal thoughts and behaviors of clients.

If a person is acutely suicidal, inpatient care is often the initial mode of treatment. Inpatient treatment is frequently short term, focused on crisis intervention, and followed up with outpatient approaches when the immediate danger has subsided.

Understanding the meaning of a client's suicidal thoughts and behavior is a good beginning point to planning ongoing care. Is the behavior a cry for help? Is it related to depression, substance abuse, social or family stressors, or all of these?

Although many health professionals advocate the use of no-harm contracts (NHC), these have not proven to lessen the suicide risk or to prevent death by suicide (Lewis, 2007). While little evidence supports the use of NHCs, many clinicians continue to use them. Clinicians may want to focus on safety plans that can provide guidance to people in crises and avoid using NHCs.

Think About It 34.1

The nurse is working with Joshua, a 47-year-old man with a history of three suicide attempts during the past 10 years. Joshua has recurrent episodes of depression. His family continues to try to support him through his illness, but they seem resigned to the fact that one day, Joshua will kill himself. What priorities should health care providers focus on in this situation? How can they intervene most effectively for Joshua and his loved ones?

General Overall Guidelines

An initial goal is to keep the person safe. Measures to optimize safety are as follows:

- Take any threat of suicide (ideation or attempt) seriously.
- If you have a concern that someone is thinking of suicide, ask directly. Asking the question will **not** give that person the idea. In fact, it may free him or her to discuss something perceived as "unmentionable" (Therapeutic Communication 34.1).

- Recognize the unique developmental circumstances and challenges of the client (adolescent, adult, older adult).
- When possible, remove methods of suicide from the person. In cases in which doing so is not possible (eg, jumping), remove the person from the means.
- Attempt to understand the person's suffering (stressors) that has led to this point.
- Be willing to discuss suicide openly without judgment. Accept the person without agreeing with the behavior.
- Encourage treatment of mental disorders. Mood disorders are common in people who die by suicide. Appropriate pharmacotherapy and treatment for these illnesses may go a long way in preventing death by suicide.
- Encourage treatment of substance abuse disorders. Often alcoholism or drug abuse co-occur with mood disorders, putting people at increased risk for suicide. Waern (2010) states that a review of studies from a number of Western settings demonstrates increased risk of suicide in elderly persons who have alcohol disorders, especially those with comorbid depression.
- Encourage adherence to medication regimens. Substantial evidence shows increased risk of suicide in clients (particularly those with bipolar disorder) who have discontinued their medication (Gonzalez-Pinto et al., 2006).
- Consult with other health care team members.
- Be aware that people who show improved mood may still be a significant suicide risk. (Often, they are more at risk as they improve because they have more energy to implement a plan).

Additional Guidelines for Hospitalized Clients

If a suicidal client is hospitalized, some additional guidelines may be useful:

- Decide with the rest of the health care team what level of suicide precaution is necessary; regularly monitor and update precautions as needed.
- Orient the client to the unit. Explain the significance of suicide precautions (including removing potentially harmful items such as pills, sharp objects, ropes, and belts).
- Develop care approaches with the person at risk, engaging his or her support as part of the planning.
- Consult with the client about his or her support people and who he or she would like to have contact with.
- Recognize that the client is probably experiencing guilt, shame, and emotional turmoil. Try to understand the experience through the client's perspective.
- Recognize issues of transference and countertransference (see Chaps. 3 and 13).
- Try to make sure the client is in a room close to the nurses' station.
- Look for opportunities to assist the person in finding or regaining hope. There are many examples of people who have clung to hope when their lives were filled with sorrow and darkness. One person explained her experience saying she had fallen into a deep depression and was full of darkness and sorrow. She described how she could not see any way out of

Therapeutic Communication 34.1

The Suicidal Client

Danny is an 18-year-old college freshman and amateur photographer. He had been seeing a school counselor because he was having trouble adjusting to college. The counselor became alarmed when Danny offered to give her his camera and photography equipment. She arranged for Danny to visit a psychiatrist. The psychiatrist determined that Danny had major depression and was at risk for suicide, although Danny denied having suicidal thoughts. He is being admitted to the adult open psychiatric unit. The nurse is conducting the admission interview.

INEFFECTIVE DIALOGUE

NURSE: Your counselor became upset when you wanted to give her your camera. Why were you giving it away?

DANNY: I don't need it anymore.

NURSE: Oh really? Why?

DANNY: *(Pauses a few seconds)* I'm not that interested in taking pictures.

NURSE: Yes, depressed people often lose interest in their usual activities. Do you have any other interests?

DANNY: No, not really. I spent most of my free time taking photos. *(Pauses)* Maybe someone will like looking at them someday.

NURSE: Don't worry, Danny, you'll start feeling better soon and then you can get back to your hobbies.

DANNY: *(With no expression whatsoever)* I'll never feel better as long as I'm here.

NURSE: You won't be here in the hospital too long. It may be hard to see it now, but once your medication takes effect, your mood will improve again and you'll go back home.

DANNY: *(Looks at the nurse for several seconds and replies somewhat sarcastically)* Okay, whatever you say.

EFFECTIVE DIALOGUE

NURSE: I know you wanted to give your camera to your counselor, Danny. Have you been thinking about killing yourself?

DANNY: The psychiatrist asked me that, too. Why do you think that?

NURSE: People who have decided to kill themselves often give away prized possessions first. I wondered if you've been thinking about dying.

DANNY: *(Stares out the window)* You call this a life … that's a joke.

NURSE: Does your life seem not worth living to you?

DANNY: *(Quietly)* Life is horrible. There's so much injustice in the world. What is the point of suffering? How about all the people who don't have food or live in countries where there are wars? I'm surprised more people aren't jumping out windows. Anyway, everyone would be better off without me to worry about.

NURSE: *(Repeats her first question gently)* Danny, are you thinking of killing yourself?

DANNY: Well, it's not crazy. It might be the sanest thing I can do.

NURSE: Do you have a plan for how you'd do it?

DANNY: I'd jump off a bridge. Just one small step is all it would take.

NURSE: Do you hear voices telling you to do this? Do you think about it often or once in a while?

DANNY: I don't hear voices, but I do think about it a lot. It's the only way out.

NURSE: Would anything stop you from suicide? What future hopes do you have?

DANNY: Well, I guess as long as I'm in here, I won't kill myself. This building isn't tall enough anyway. I'd probably just break my legs. *(Smiles wanly, looks to see the nurse's reaction)* If I have a future, which I'm not saying I do, I'd like to be a photographer. I'd take pictures of all the suffering people to let the world know to do something.

The nurse continues the interview. Danny is put on suicide precautions.

Reflection and Critical Thinking

- What clues to Danny's state of mind did the nurse miss in the first scenario? Did anything he said suggest ambivalence about dying?
- What comments by the nurse in the first scenario blocked communication?
- Why were the communication methods in the second scenario more effective than those in the first scenario?

the darkness. She explained how her mother gave her hope and helped her "fight for her life."

- Know that hope is strengthened in relationships. Hope is developed through trust in the interpersonal relationship as the nurse works with the client.
- As discharge planning occurs, work with the client to ensure that appropriate resources and follow-up are available upon discharge. Lack of these can very quickly increase the person's risk once again.
- Help the person at risk and the family understand the circumstances that led to the suicidal behavior. Establish a plan to address suicidal ideation should it occur in the future.

▲ EVALUATION

Nurses have a unique opportunity to walk with clients through many experiences: joy and sorrow, pain and relief, discovery and despair, hope and hopelessness. In the case of clients who are suicidal, nurses have the privilege of accompanying them through darkness and despair and helping them to discover or regain hope.

▲

SUICIDE AS A PUBLIC HEALTH PROBLEM

The focus to this point has been on the individual client. Suicide prevention also needs a broader approach. It must be treated as a public health problem with a focus on the community level where education is key.

Many people and organizations advocate for a national, public health approach to suicide prevention, intervention, and bereavement support (LivingWorks, 2007; Silverman et al., 2007). LivingWorks, a Canadian-based organization, has provided international leadership in education and training for suicide prevention. The group's work focuses on creating suicide-safer communities that preserve, protect, and promote life (LivingWorks, 2010). The staff at LivingWorks maintain that many intervention skills are known and can be learned. They advocate for a multilayered approach to education for communities that focus on teaching skills and raising awareness. Researchers at the Canadian Association for Suicide Prevention outline four broad strategies for inclusion in a public health approach to suicide prevention in their blueprint for a national suicide prevention strategy. See Box 34.3.

THOSE LEFT BEHIND

The cost of suicide goes far beyond years of life lost. Before concluding this chapter, there is one other important area to highlight—the people who are bereaved by suicide. As noted earlier in this chapter, it is believed that for every death by suicide, at least six other people are affected. In most cases, many more than six people are affected. Words seem inadequate to describe the overwhelming pain and devastation the people bereaved by suicide experience. Those left behind are left asking questions such as "Why? What did I do wrong? If only I had listened; what if I had phoned her?" The questions

---

BOX 34.3 Blueprint for a National Suicide Prevention Strategy

Awareness and Understanding

- Goal 1: Promote awareness in every part of the country that suicide is a national problem and is preventable.
- Goal 2: Develop broad-based support for suicide prevention and intervention (government, private and public stakeholders, professional and voluntary organizations).
- Goal 3: Develop and implement a strategy to reduce stigma, to be associated with all suicide prevention, intervention, and bereavement strategies.
- Goal 4: Increase media knowledge regarding suicide.

Prevention and Intervention

- Goal 1: Develop, implement, and sustain community-based suicide prevention programs, respecting diversity and culture at local, regional, and state levels.
- Goal 2: Reduce the availability and lethality of suicide methods.
- Goal 3: Increase training for recognition of risk factors, warning signs, and at-risk behaviors and provision of effective intervention, targeting key gatekeepers, volunteers, and professionals.
- Goal 4: Develop and promote effective clinical and professional practice (effective strategies, standards of care) to support clients, families, and communities.

- Goal 5: Improve access and integration with strong linkages between the continuum of care components/services/families.
- Goal 6: Prioritize intervention and service delivery for high-risk groups while respecting local and state uniqueness.
- Goal 7: Increase crisis intervention and support.
- Goal 8: Increase services and support to those bereaved by suicide.

Knowledge Development and Transfer

- Goal 1: Improve and expand surveillance systems.
- Goal 2: Promote and support the development of effective evaluation tools.
- Goal 3: Promote and develop suicide-related research.
- Goal 4: Increase opportunities for reporting.

Funding and Support

- Goal 1: Increase funding and support for all activities connected with a national suicide prevention strategy.
- Goal 2: Ensure access to appropriate and adequate health, wellness, and recovery services for all citizens.

Source: LivingWorks [2010]. Retrieved from http://www.livingworks.net/page/Experience%20Livingworks.

and frequent blaming seem endless. Sometimes the pain is so crushing, the person finds it difficult to breathe. He or she struggles to believe it has happened at the same time as wanting to relive those last days and weeks prior to the death by suicide in an effort to change the outcome.

Nurses have important roles to play in helping survivors of suicide. The loss of a loved one by suicide is not the same as the loss of a loved one to a physical health problem or even an accidental death. Suicide is stigmatized in society, and the survivors do not experience the same outpouring of support as others who experience a loss. In fact, suicide survivors don't "get over" the loss but instead are forever changed by it. They suffer a range of difficult emotions and may, themselves, develop depression, suicidality, or if they witnessed the suicide or found the body, PTSD (see Chap. 23). Some of the emotional responses suicide survivors may experience include:

- Feelings of unreality, shock, disbelief, and emotional numbness
- Grief, sadness, and despair
- Confusion over not knowing why the loved one chose suicide
- Anger toward the mental health practitioner, another family member, or a friend for failing to prevent the suicide

- Self-anger and guilt for failing to prevent the suicide
- Feelings of anger toward and betrayal by the loved one who committed suicide
- Social stigmatization and isolation

Nurses can offer support and guidance to survivors to help them come to terms with this agonizing loss by discussing emotions. They can explain that the emotions usually do subside with time, but there is no set time frame for the process. Nurses should let survivors know that painful feelings may recur, particularly during a special holiday or on the anniversary of the suicide.

In addition to helping the family member or friend work through the feelings of loss, grief, and anger, nurses suggest that they seek professional mental health counseling for a time after the suicide. Suicide survivors have a real risk for development of depression or PTSD, which can be prevented or appropriately treated with counseling or psychotherapy. In addition, nurses can help family members find a support group for suicide survivors and encourage them to talk openly with other relatives and friends of the deceased. It is important for survivors not to withdraw from others but to maintain social support systems.

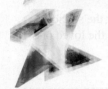

Reviewing and Applying Your Knowledge

Chapter Summary

- No one explanation can account for the tragic experience of death by suicide.

- Family history poses risks of suicide for clients. Other major risk factors include psychopathology and history of previous attempts.

- Psychiatric disorders that have risk for suicide as a major component of illness include depressive disorders, bipolar illness, schizophrenia, and substance abuse.

- Nurses commonly assess a client's risks, ideations, intent, plan, and lethality of the plan.

- Interventions against suicide include establishing a safe environment, implementation of suicide precautions, assistance in meeting basic human needs, medication management, and provision of client and family education.

- Suicide is a public health problem requiring interventions at all levels of health care and society.

- Survivors of suicide have long-term psychological consequences and are a grieving population that nurses and other health care providers should address.

Study Questions

1. Which of the following assessment findings would lead the nurse to suspect that a client is at a high risk for suicide? Select all that apply.

    a. Several available support persons

    b. Continual abuse of alcohol

    c. Hopelessness accompanied by withdrawal

    d. Marked hostility

    e. History of multiple previous attempts

2. A nurse is teaching a client group about depression and suicide. Which of the following behavioral clues would the nurse identify as suggestive of suicide?

    a. Going to see a psychiatrist

    b. Verbalizing feelings of hopelessness about problems

    c. Engaging in weekend drinking episodes

    d. Joking about stress

3. Which of the following statements about suicidal intent is most accurate?

    a. Following a suicidal gesture, all clients will be grateful to be alive.

    b. Clients expressing suicidal intent rarely follow through with the action.

    c. Degree of suicidal intent may change.

    d. Questions about the specific details of a suicide plan are not therapeutic.

Critical Thinking Questions

1. What feelings would you expect families in which a person has committed suicide to feel? How can nurses best help such families who come to their attention?

2. What interventions and measures would be the highest priorities for health care personnel who have not been able to prevent suicide in a client?

References

American Association of Suicidology [AAS]. (2009). *Elderly suicide fact sheet.* Retrieved from http://www.suicidology.org/c/document_library/get_file?folderId=232&name=DLFE-242.pdf

American Association of Suicidology [AAS]. (2010a). *African American suicide fact sheet.* Retrieved from http://www.suicidology.org/c/document_library/get_file?folderId=232&name=DLFE-241.pdfm

American Association of Suicidology [AAS]. (2010b). *Hispanic suicide fact sheet.* Retrieved from http://www.suicidology.org/c/document_library/get_file?folderId=232&name=DLFE-243.pdf

American Association of Suicidology [AAS]. (2010c). *Some facts about suicide and depression.* Retrieved from http://www.suicidology.org/c/document_library/get_file?folderId=232&name=DLFE-157.pdf

American Association of Suicidology [AAS]. (2010d). *Survivors of suicide fact sheet.* Retrieved from http://www.suicidology.org/c/document_library/get_file?folderId=232&name=DLFE-160.pdf

Centers for Disease Control and Prevention [CDC]. (2010). *Suicide: Facts at a glance.* Retrieved from http://www.cdc.gov/violenceprevention/pdf/Suicide_DataSheet-a.pdf

Crosby, A. E., Ortega, L., & Melanson, C. (2011). *Self-directed violence surveillance: Uniform definitions and recommended data elements.* Atlanta, GA: Centers for Disease Control and Prevention. Retrieved from http://www.cdc.gov/violenceprevention/pdf/Self-Directed-Violence-a.pdf

Florida State University (n.d.). *Thomas Joiner: Bright-Burton professor of psychology.* Retrieved from http://www.fsu.edu/profiles/joiner/

Gentile, S. (2011). Suicidal mothers. *Journal of Injury and Violence Research, 3*(2), 90–98.

Gonzalez-Pinto, A., Mosquera, F., Alonso, M., López, P., Ramirez, F., Vieta, E., & Baldessarini, R. J. (2006). Suicidal risk in bipolar I disorder patients and adherence to long-term lithium treatment. *Bipolar Disorders, 8*(5p2), 618–624.

Javdani, S., Sadeh, N., & Verona, E. (2011). Suicidality as a function of impulsivity, callous-unemotional traits, and depressive symptoms in youth. *Journal of Abnormal Psychology, 120*(2), 400–413.

Lewis, L. M. (2007). No-harm contracts: A review of what we know. *Suicide and Life Threatening Behavior, 37*(1), 50–57.

LivingWorks (2010). *Experience LivingWorks.* Retrieved from http://www.livingworks.net/page/Experience%20Livingworks

Murray, B. L., & Hauenstein, E. J. (2008). Self harm and suicidal behaviour: Children, adolescents, and adults. In W. Austin, & M. A. Boyd (Eds.), *Psychiatric nursing for Canadian practice* (pp. 898–922). Philadelphia, PA: Lippincott Williams & Wilkins.

Muzina, D. J. (2007). Suicide intervention: How to recognize the risk, focus on patient safety. *Current Psychiatry Online, 6*(9).

NANDA International. (2008). *NANDA International nursing diagnoses: Definitions and classification, 2009–2011.* Philadelphia, PA: Wiley-Blackwell.

National Institute of Mental Health [NIMH]. (2010). *Suicide in the U.S.: Statistics and prevention.* Retrieved from http://www.nimh.nih.gov/health/publications/suicide-in-the-us-statistics-and-prevention/index.shtml#risk

National Institute of Mental Health [NIMH]. (2011). *Suicide in America: Frequently asked questions.* Retrieved from http://www.nimh.nih.gov/health/publications/suicide-in-america/suicide-in-america-frequently-asked-questions.shtml

Scott, K. M., Chiu, W. T., Kessler, R. C., Sampson, N. A., Angermeyer, M., Beautrais, A., ... Nock, M. K. (2010). Chronic physical conditions and their association with first onset of suicidal behavior in the world mental health surveys. *Psychosomatic Medicine, 72*(2), 712–719.

Shah, A. (2011). Elderly suicide rates: A replication of cross-national comparisons and association with sex and elderly age bands using five-year suicide data. *Journal of Injury and Violence Research, 3*(2), 80–84.

Silverman, M., Berman, A., Sandaal, N., O'Carroll, P., & Joiner, T. (2007). Rebuilding the Tower of Babel: A revised nomenclature for the study of suicide and suicidal behaviors. Part I: Background,

rationale, and methodology. *Suicide & Life-Threatening Behavior, 37,* 248–263.

Suicide Prevention Resource Center. (n.d.). *Suicide among Hispanic Americans.* Retrieved from http://www.sprc.org/library/hispanic.am.facts.pdf

Suicide Prevention Resource Center. (2001). *Risk and protective factors for suicide.* Retrieved from http://www.sprc.org/library/srisk.pdf

Survivors of Suicide (n.d.). *Understanding suicide: Common elements.* Retrieved from http://www.survivorsofsuicide.com/understanding.shtml

University of Iowa College of Nursing (n.d. a). *Nursing interventions classification (NIC).* Retrieved from http://www.nursing.uiowa.edu/excellence/nursing_knowledge/clinical_effectiveness/niclabels.htm

University of Iowa College of Nursing (n.d. b). *Nursing outcomes classification (NOC).* Retrieved from http://www.nursing.uiowa.edu/excellence/nursing_knowledge/clinical_effectiveness/noclabels.htm

Waern, M. (2010). Alcohol and suicidal behavior in the elderly. *Internet and psychiatry.* Retrieved from http://www.internetandpsychiatry.com/joomla/suicidal-behavior-in-alcohol-and-drug-abuse-and-dependence/594-alcoholism-and-suicidal-behavior-in-the-elderly.html

Wolfelt, A. (2007). *The wilderness of grief: Finding your way.* Fort Collins, CO: Companion Press.

World Health Organization [WHO]. (2011a). *Mental health: Suicide prevention.* Retrieved from http://www.who.int/mental_health/prevention/suicide/suicideprevent/en/index.html

World Health Organization [WHO]. (2011b). *World suicide prevention day.* Retrieved from http://www.who.int/mediacentre/events/annual/world_suicide_prevention_day/en/index.html

Web Resources

American Association of Suicidology: http://www.suicidology.org

American Foundation for Suicide Prevention: http://www.afsp.org

National Institute of Mental Health: http://www.nimh.nih.gov

Suicide Prevention Advocacy Network USA, Inc.: http://www.spanusa.org

Survivors of Suicide: http://www.survivorsofsuicide.com

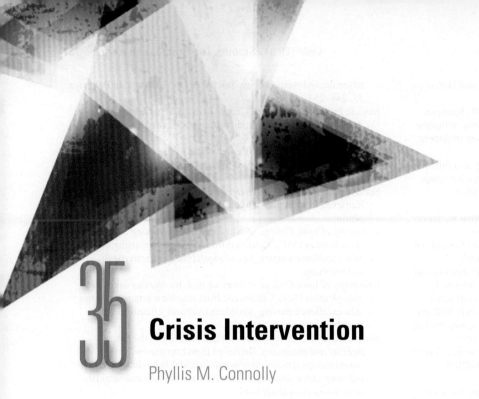

35

Crisis Intervention

Phyllis M. Connolly

KEY TERMS

adventitious crisis
crisis
crisis intervention
critical incidents
maturational or developmental crisis
resilience
situational crisis

LEARNING OBJECTIVES

On completion of this chapter, you should be able to accomplish the following:

- Discuss the phases of a crisis.
- Differentiate maturational, situational, and adventitious crises.
- Discuss the goals and methods of crisis intervention.
- Describe the relationship between evidence-based practice and crisis intervention.
- Discuss the need for critical incident stress debriefing for nurses experiencing violence.
- Apply the nursing process to a client, family, or community in crisis.

Crisis means a turning point. In written Chinese, two symbols communicate crisis: "danger" and "opportunity." *Crisis* and *stress* commonly are used interchangeably; however, they are not synonyms. Everyone experiences stressful events: a new job, diagnosis of a terminal illness, loss of a job, the death of a loved one, or loss of a friend. As long as a person can cope and is not overwhelmed, the event is not a crisis. Conversely, any event that causes enough stress can precipitate a crisis, depending on the person's perceptions, coping skills, and available support.

During a crisis, a person may not know what to do. Usual methods of problem solving are ineffective or unavailable. As anxiety and pain increase, the person may become willing to try new ways to handle the difficulties. In this willingness lies the opportunity for growth. Mental health is thought to result predominantly from a life history of successful crisis resolution and resilience (Erikson, 1963; Humphreys, 2001; Rew et al., 2001; Roberts & Yeager, 2009).

Intervention during crisis has been found to reduce the incidence and severity of mental disorders (Joy et al., 2006; Shepperd et al., 2009). There is little argument over the demand and increased need for cost-effective and well-organized crisis services (Dieterich et al., 2010). This chapter discusses the role of nurses in crisis intervention for clients. It discusses theories of crisis and techniques to address it, as well as practical ways that community-based care providers implement crisis intervention. The chapter includes a section that applies the nursing process to the care of clients in crisis. The content is congruent with *Crisis Intervention* (Registered Nurses Association of Ontario [RNAO], 2006) and the *Psychiatric–Mental Health Nursing: Scope and Standards of Practice* (American Nurses Association [ANA], American Psychiatric Nurses Association [APNA], & International Society of Psychiatric–Mental Health Nurses [ISPN], 2007).

CRISIS

One traditional definition of crisis is a threat to homeostasis (Caplan, 1964). During crisis, the magnitude of the problem and the immediate resources available to deal with it are imbalanced, with resultant confusion and disorganization (Figure 35.1). No person can tolerate such an imbalance for long. The active crisis state usually is short, approximately 4 to 6 weeks. Quick, appropriate intervention is crucial to help people return to optimal functioning (RNAO, 2006; Roberts & Yeager, 2009).

According to crisis theory, people strive to maintain constant emotional equilibrium (Aguilera, 1998; Roberts & Ottens, 2005). If they confront an overwhelming threat and cannot cope, crisis ensues. Crisis response is normal, not pathologic. Its outcome varies and sometimes can lead to problems. Following the high anxiety that accompanies crisis, people can (1) adapt and return to the previous state of mental heath, (2) develop more constructive coping skills, or (3) decompensate to a lower level of functioning.

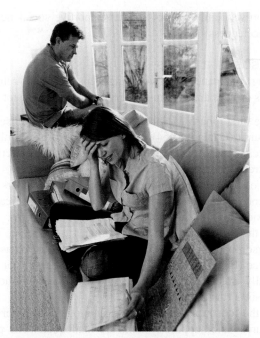

FIGURE 35.1 In a crisis state, stressors outweigh a person's or group's ability to respond and cope. Stressors that precipitate crisis vary; crisis can emerge from an accumulation of everyday problems, tensions, and challenges.

Factors that influence the outcome of a crisis include the following (RNAO, 2006; Roberts & Yeager, 2009):

- Previous problem-solving experience
- Perception or view of the problem
- Amount of help or hindrance from significant others
- Number and types of past crises
- Time since the last crisis
- Membership in a vulnerable population
- Sense of mastery
- Resilience

Risk factors that predict adverse outcomes in natural and human-caused disasters include the following (Aguilera, 1998; RNAO, 2006; Roberts & Yeager, 2009):

- Female sex
- Minority ethnicity
- Lower socioeconomic status
- Problematic predisaster functioning and personality

Studies have found **resilience** (National Center for Posttraumatic Stress Disorder [NCPTSD], 2011) to be a protective factor that contributes to success in coping with significant stresses. Resilience changes over time, and protective factors both within the person and from the external environment can enhance it (Rew et al., 2001). Resilient people have high self-esteem, self-efficacy, a repertoire of problem-solving skills, a sense of connectedness, and satisfying interpersonal relationships (Edward, 2005; Roberts & Yeager, 2009). Associated protective factors include social competence, problem-solving skills, autonomy, sense of purpose, educational aspirations, supportive family factors, and a supportive social network (connectedness).

Phases of a Crisis

During a traumatic or overwhelming event, people move through phases or steps that determine the level of the crisis state:

1. The first phase is increased anxiety in response to trauma (Caplan, 1964). A person tries to use familiar mechanisms to cope. If such mechanisms are effective, there is no crisis.
2. If coping mechanisms are ineffective, a person enters the second phase of crisis, which is marked by further increased anxiety from the failure of usual coping mechanisms.
3. In the third phase, anxiety continues to escalate. The person usually feels compelled to reach out for assistance (Figure 35.2). Those who are emotionally or socially isolated before the trauma usually experience a crisis at this point.
4. In the fourth phase, the active state of crisis, inner resources and support systems are inadequate. The precipitating event is not resolved, and stress and anxiety mount intolerably. The person has a short attention span, ruminates, and looks inward for possible reasons for the trauma and how he or she might have changed or avoided it. Anguish, apprehension, and distress accompany this rumination. Behavior becomes increasingly impulsive and unproductive. Relationships with others usually suffer. The person becomes less aware of the environment and begins to view others in terms of their ability to help solve the problem (RNAO, 2006). The high anxiety level may make people feel like they are "losing their mind" or "going crazy." Although anxiety greatly affects perceptive ability, the crisis state is not the same as psychosis. People in crisis often need others

to explain the difference and to give reassurance that when they feel less anxious, they will be able to think clearly again.

Types of Crises

There are three types of crises: maturational (developmental), situational, and adventitious. The following paragraphs define and explore features of each type.

Maturational Crisis

A **maturational (developmental) crisis** results from normal life events that cause stress. Erikson (1963) identified specific developmental periods when anxiety or stress normally increases and can precipitate a maturational crisis. Common examples in children include mastering control of body functions, starting school, and experiencing puberty. Events for adults that might precipitate maturational crises include getting married, becoming a parent or grandparent, and retiring (Figure 35.3).

Any transitional period in normal growth and development may precipitate a maturational crisis. The inability to master the tasks of one stage is thought to prevent growth and development in subsequent stages, which may compound stress and anxiety and lead to crisis.

Why are these times a crisis for some and not for others? One explanation is that some people cannot make the role transitions necessary to integrate the demands and expectations of the new level. For instance, the birth of a child requires parents to make numerous role changes and lifestyle accommodations. Some people adapt to the new situation more quickly and with greater ease than do others. In addition, factors outside of individual personality may influence response to new parenthood. A couple who has a strong and balanced partnership with adequate financial resources and

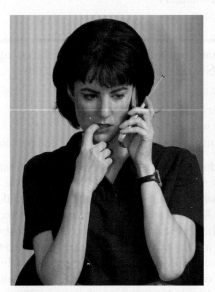
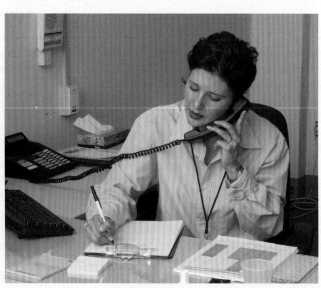

FIGURE 35.2 As anxiety mounts through the phases of a crisis, people usually eventually feel the need to reach out to others for assistance. They may turn to friends or loved ones, or they may consult health care providers or telephone/electronic mental health services.

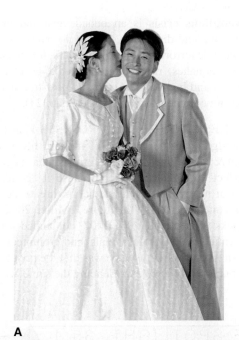

A

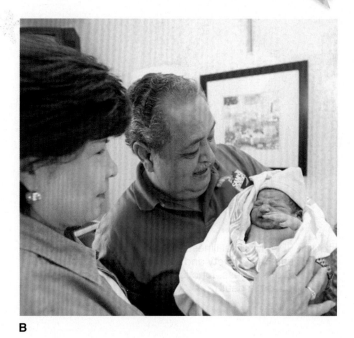

B

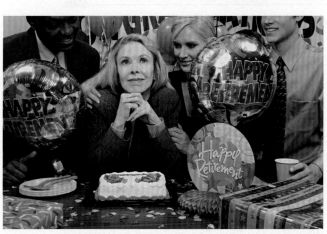

C

FIGURE 35.3 Even happy occasions such as (**A**) getting married, (**B**) becoming a grandparent, or (**C**) retiring may be precipitating factors for a maturational/developmental crisis, depending on the person's response to the resultant role transitions, his or her support systems, and the amount of preparation he or she has had to face the new paradigm.

reliable outside support may have an easier time adjusting than do parents with marital discord, financial stress, and no relatives or friends to help them (Collins, 2006).

In each stage of development, a person needs nurturance and resources from others to work through the risks of that phase and to obtain the necessary skills for the next phase (Erikson, 1963). Because maturational crises are predictable and gradual, preparing for them and preventing a crisis are possible. Examples of anticipatory guidance in crisis prevention include premarital counseling, prenatal parenting classes, and retirement planning.

Situational Crisis

A **situational crisis** develops as a response to a sudden and unavoidable traumatic event that dramatically alters a person's identity and roles. Stressful events that threaten physical, emotional, or social integrity are likely to precipitate crisis (Aguilera, 1998; Roberts & Ottens, 2005).

A situational crisis usually follows the loss of an established support. It disrupts the usual ways of presenting the self, and subsequently threatens self-image. Death of a spouse, divorce, job or academic failure, birth of a child with a disability, or diagnosis with a chronic or terminal illness affects self-perception and can lead to so much stress and anxiety that a crisis develops (Aguilera, 1998) (Figure 35.4). The most common response to loss or deprivation is depression.

The difficulty of dealing with a situational crisis is compounded when the person also is struggling with a maturational crisis. For example, an adolescent struggling through puberty whose parents are divorcing is experiencing maturational and situational crises. A person with serious mental illness may experience a crisis if there is a change in a significant health care provider or change in Social Security benefits.

For the results of the effectiveness of crisis intervention in the community for people with serious mental illness, see Evidence-Based Practice Spotlight 35.1.

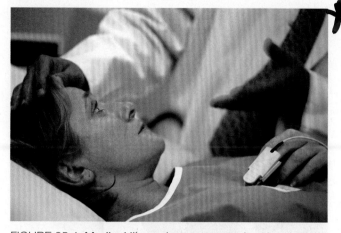

FIGURE 35.4 Medical illness is a common situational crisis. Many clients feel anxiety and depression when facing the possibility of sickness, functional loss, compromise to lifestyle, or possible death.

Adventitious Crisis

An **adventitious crisis** is an outside external event that causes trauma and disruption, usually to many people. Examples include terrorism, natural disasters, hurricanes, fires, floods, earthquakes, riots, unusual media events, kidnappings, wars, and bombings. Acute and post-traumatic stress reactions are common outcomes (see Chap. 23).

CRISIS RESPONSES TO TERRORISM. Fear of terrorism is a significant component of modern life worldwide (Milligan & McGuinness, 2009). Terrorism has been labeled the "perfect" traumatic stressor because it "combines the elements of malevolent intent, actual or threatened extreme harm, and unending fear of the future" (Miller, 2002, p. 284). The attacks of September 11, 2001, demanded a response from mental health professionals and volunteer disaster teams. An unusual circumstance was that the people helping others concurrently were experiencing the same crisis. They

---

▲ EVIDENCE-BASED PRACTICE SPOTLIGHT 35.1 ▲

Crisis Intervention for People With Severe Mental Illnesses Living in the Community

Overview of Effective Treatment: Fewer psychiatric hospitals and limited bed spaces in acute care facilities have led to a dramatic increase of people with severe mental illnesses living in the community. Many severe psychiatric illnesses are episodic, so that with treatment and adherence to a medical regimen, affected clients may have long periods of stability (Joy et al., 2006). Nevertheless, relapses occur in this vulnerable population and may not have an easily identifiable precipitating event.

Early studies of crisis intervention models developed in response to deinstitutionalization have shown cost effectiveness, a 50% reduction in hospitalizations, and less stigma related to institutionalization (Joy et al., 2006). The objective of the study by Joy et al. (2006) was to review the effects of the crisis intervention model compared with "standard care" for people with serious mental illness living in the community. They used the Cochrane Schizophrenia Group's register of trials from 2006 to update the 1998 and 2003 searches. They included all randomized controlled trials of crisis intervention models versus standard care (p. 3). The study included all people diagnosed with schizophrenia or other serious mental illnesses experiencing a psychosocial crisis and excluded all those with drug-induced psychosis or in a depressive crisis. The researchers examined five outcomes: (1) service utilization; (2) satisfaction with treatment; (3) clinical outcomes, such as death/suicide, improvement, compliance with medication, antipsychotic medication, and relapses; (4) social outcomes; and (5) cost of treatment. Results indicated that 45% of clients were unable to avoid hospital

treatment, although crisis intervention may help prevent repeat admissions. In addition, crisis intervention reduced family burden, and clients and family were more satisfied with care. Clients in crisis who received home care were more likely to remain in care for at least 1 year (p. 12). Home care was more cost effective than hospital care. The study findings were inconclusive for staff satisfaction, compliance with medications, general functioning, mental state, and number of relapses. The study raised more questions than answers regarding studies beyond the typical crisis stages, as well as the need for high-quality hospital care.

What Has Not Been Shown Effective: Repeated hospitalizations for acute phases or relapses of psychotic episodes and discharge back to the community are not effective.

Implications for Practice: Crisis intervention for people with serious mental illnesses living in the community reduces family burden. It is satisfactory for clients and cost effective. Nurses should assume an active role as team members of community crisis teams. Furthermore, they should educate clients and families about the trajectory of serious mental illnesses and prepare them to recognize the need for periodic crisis intervention. Helping clients and families to view periodic crises as just part of the illness with a plan for interventions during those times may help reduce stigma related to the experiences of relapses while encouraging clients to accept home care.

Reference

Joy, C. B., Adams, E. E., & Rice, K. (2006). Crisis intervention for people with severe mental illnesses. *Cochrane Database of Systematic Reviews, 2006*(4). doi:10.1002/14651858/CD001087.pub3.

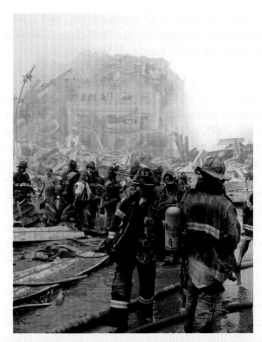

FIGURE 35.5 Terrorism is a unique type of adventitious crisis with holistic ramifications. Its wide-ranging consequences include physical harm, shattered psychological security, emotional instability, spiritual distress, and social upheaval. Many of those who responded to help during the attacks of September 11, 2001, also experienced a crisis state, with ongoing effects on their psychological health. (Photo courtesy of the American Red Cross.)

needed not only to rise to the challenge of assisting people but also to deal with their own reactions (Figure 35.5). Many volunteered, yet few actually were trained in the necessary skills for crisis work. The number of untrained volunteers made it clear that schools of nursing must prepare future nurses with disaster education (Kennedy, 2001; RNAO, 2006). Practicing nurses are encouraged to obtain training through the American Red Cross Disaster Assistance Team (http://www2.redcross.org/services/disaster).

Nurses responded immediately through hospitals and organizations such as the American Red Cross. By September 12, 2001, more than 1,000 nurses had donated blood. In addition, many national nursing organizations, including the ANA, the Visiting Nurses Association of America, the APNA, and the Nurse Practitioner Association, offered services. Saint Vincent's Medical Center and New York's Bellevue Hospital, the hospitals closest to the World Trade Center, immediately sent nurses; physicians from other New York City hospitals quickly arrived to help. The response was similar from the Virginia Hospital Center in Arlington, close to the Pentagon. Emergency response teams provided trained volunteers. The USNS *Comfort* sailed into New York harbor to assist in the care of exhausted workers. Again, nurses were the first people to assess rescue workers to determine if they needed more than sleep and a shower. If they needed further evaluation, nurses called the Special Psychiatric Rapid Intervention Team (SPRINT) (Kennedy, 2001).

Acts such as terrorism and mass shootings in schools or offices raise the need to evaluate early psychological interventions. The U.S. Departments of Defense, Justice, and Health and Human Services (National Institute of Mental Health [NIMH]), and Veterans Affairs and the American Red Cross met from October 30 to November 1, 2001, outside Washington, D.C., to examine the evidence of current practice, identify effective interventions, and determine future research areas. The complete report is *Mental Health and Mass Violence: Evidence-Based Early Psychological Intervention for Victims/Survivors of Mass Violence* (NIMH, 2002). Their consensus about effective interventions includes the following components:

- Early mental health assessment based on a hierarchy of needs
- Triage
- Orientation of survivors to immediate local services
- Communication with family, friends, and community
- Other forms of psychological first aid (NCPTSD, 2011)

Appendices A and B of the NIMH (2002) report contain specific guidelines for delivering interventions, including the roles of general helpers and specifically those of mental health professionals. Furthermore, the web site of the NCPTSD contains information for self-care for professionals and mental health care workers (see the Web Resources section at the end of the chapter).

A recent study of 1,112 employed adults who received worksite crisis intervention from mental health professionals for one to three brief sessions had positive outcomes for as long as 2 years. Outcomes included reduced alcohol dependence, binge drinking, depression, severity of post-traumatic stress syndrome (PTSD), and anxiety (Boscarino et al., 2006). People with mental illness may be more affected as a result of a disaster when their stability is disturbed, exacerbating their psychiatric symptoms (Milligan & McGuinness, 2009).

One important outcome of September 11 was the creation of guidelines for mental health professionals from the NCPTSD. Based on the NIMH (2002) report, they emphasize a natural recovery mechanism that focuses on resilience, rather than psychopathology. Their educational material states that symptoms decrease gradually and that those helping people in crisis should encourage them to use natural support systems at their own pace. Professionals working with those in immediate crisis should listen actively and supportively but not probe for details and emotional responses. They should allow clients to say what feels comfortable without pushing for more, and validate the normal natural recovery.

CRITICAL INCIDENT STRESS DEBRIEFING. Within this context, a brief discussion of critical incident stress debriefing (CISD) may help clarify its approach, use in some types of crisis intervention, and recent research. Mitchell (1983) reported on CISD in a description of a program for emergency services personnel at risk for cumulative critical incident stress. **Critical incidents** are sudden and unexpected situations that disrupt values and beliefs and challenge basic assumptions of how the world operates. People have strong emotional reactions to critical incidents and perceive them as life threatening. Some examples include witnessing a violent act, sudden infant death, violence in the workplace, mass shootings, and physical or psychological threats or losses, natural disasters, and unusual media events. Responses to the stress may occur in the following areas: cognitive, physical, emotional, and behavioral. Cognitive problems may include poor concentration, confusion, and memory lapses. Physical effects may include fatigue, gastrointestinal problems, insomnia, muscle tension, and heightened autonomic activity. Depression, anxiety, guilt, anger, and denial are possible emotional effects (Caine & Ter-Bagdasarian, 2003). Aggressiveness, substance abuse, social withdrawal, and listlessness are behavioral symptoms that might follow a critical incident.

Like crisis intervention (discussed later), CISD focuses on the present, is generally completed in one session, and requires an active nursing role (Ragaisis, 1994). Nurses can apply CISD to individuals, groups, and families. It usually takes place within 24 to 72 hours of the incident. Integrating the nursing process with CISD consists of seven phases: introductory, fact, thought, reaction, symptom, teaching, and re-entry. The first five phases are part of assessment, the teaching and re-entry phases are intervention, and evaluation takes place at the end (Ragaisis, 1994). Essential elements include establishing safety, enhancing calm, building self, reconnecting to social networks, and instilling hope (Pender & Prichard, 2009).

Best practice guidelines from the Association for Specialists in Group Work (Pender & Prichard, 2009) provide structure for planning, performing, and processing tasks for effective practice of critical incident stress debriefing. In fact, this is a similar approach to that put forth in the *Nursing Best Practice Guidelines Revised Supplement* (RNAO, 2006), by Roberts and Yeager (2009), and by this textbook. Current findings of the effectiveness of psychological debriefing have been mixed, especially when such debriefing has involved a single session only (Pender & Prichard, 2009). No evidence has shown that single-session crisis intervention prevents PTSD (Bledson, 2003; Rose et al., 2006). Some studies (Parkinson, 2001; Slomski, 2003) point out that CISD may not significantly decrease PTSD, which may be related to a lack of uniform research criteria. Thus, CISD may be misrepresented and misunderstood, and its outcome measurements may not truly reflect its effectiveness. An acute stress response may lead to PTSD for those genetically predisposed to it (see Chap. 23).

Clearly, when conducted by qualified mental health professionals using a traditional crisis intervention approach and building on the client's strengths and natural support systems, CISD still may be offered for traumatic events (Boscarino et al., 2006; Pender & Prichard, 2009; Roberts & Yeager, 2009). Some organizations use critical incident stress management programs that include precrisis preparation such as stress management education, crisis mitigation

training for individuals and organizations, and information on defusing and reevaluation for further services (Caine & Ter-Bagdasarian, 2003; Pender & Prichard, 2009).

SELF-CARE FOR PROVIDERS RESPONDING TO ADVENTITIOUS CRISES. According to Santandrea (2001), mental health professionals who assisted those who had witnessed the 2001 attacks at the World Trade Center needed support because they, too, were responding to stress and fear. They reported that the intensity of counseling sessions rose 3 weeks after the attacks. The need to work as a team became more important during the rescue work. Results of one study of 712 psychologists (Eidelson et al., 2003) indicated a need for training in trauma work because many felt unprepared for the challenge. Thirty-nine percent reported that their view of what constituted an irrational fear had changed, and 72% reported being slightly more fearful since the attacks. Many revealed that they felt increased positive feelings about their work, which counterbalanced the negative emotions.

Kinzel and Nanson (2000) discuss the issue of compassion fatigue that volunteers operating telephone crisis lines experience and strategies of education and psychological debriefing to combat it. Both the stages and methods of using group and individual debriefing are detailed based on the literature. The methods are most similar to graduate programs that use "supervision" to train future mental health workers. Zahourek (2003) emphasizes the role of nurses with trauma survivors as they assess for potential problems and make recommendations and referrals. She also reinforces the need for nurses to meet their own needs as they care for people during disasters. There is additional helpful information for victims at the NCPTSD (2011) website. Edward's (2005) phenomenological study findings recommend that organizations need to promote resilience in clinicians, which may reduce burnout and promote retention.

Gates and colleagues (2011) found that emergency department nurses (*N* = 224) experienced a high incidence of physical assaults from both clients and visitors, and 94% experienced at least one PTSD symptom. They also discovered a relationship between stress symptoms and a reduction in work productivity and quality of client care. These results suggest a need for CISD for emergency department nurses. A qualitative study of 35 nurses working in a number of areas in a hospital in Western Australia who had experienced workplace violence revealed that the nurses used cognitive adaptation to cope with the incident. They used the strategies of searching for meaning, gaining mastery, and self-enhancement (Chapman et al., 2010). The researchers recommended that critical incident debriefing be implemented to facilitate cognitive adaptation for future incidents.

CRISIS PREVENTION

Health care professionals can help clients and families prepare for possible maturational and situational crises (Aguilera, 1998; Roberts & Yeager, 2009). Although not all teens have difficulty during adolescence, many do. Providers can prepare families and assist them to deal with the conflicts and challenges common to this developmental stage with parenting classes, support groups, and school programs. Childbirth classes are another example of crisis prevention by helping prepare parents for both the physical aspects of birth and the demands of their new role (Figure 35.6). People considering divorce can seek counseling to ease their own and children's responses. Recognizing symptoms of relapse and seeking early interventions often prevent a crisis for those with chronic physical and mental illness (Dieterich et al., 2010; Joy et al., 2006). Encouraging people to establish balance in their lives and manage stress is an effective approach to crisis prevention.

Eating a healthy diet, exercising, playing and having fun, and meeting spiritual needs are means to maximize wellness and prevent crisis. Visualization, meditation, massage, acupressure, progressive relaxation, and water exercise may help (see Chap. 17). Added possibilities for people susceptible to stress include therapeutic touch, biofeedback, acupuncture, and hypnosis. Clients may benefit from formal courses in assertiveness training, stress management, or tai

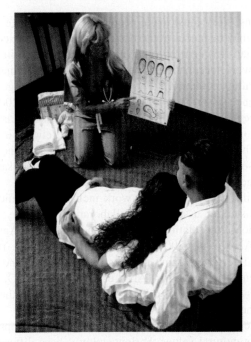

FIGURE 35.6 By participating in prenatal and childbirth classes, pregnant women and their partners may be able to prevent maturational crises associated with assuming parental roles and responsibilities

chi. Others may read self-help books or listen to self-help tapes (Aguilera, 1998). Groups such as the National Alliance on Mental Illness (NAMI) provide support, information, advice, and strategies for preventing and dealing with crises for family members and caregivers (see Chaps. 1 and 15).

Teaching or coaching clients may be a primary prevention strategy. Psychoeducational classes for consumers, families, and care providers can help them learn symptoms of relapse, triggers to symptoms, and how to develop a crisis plan (ANA et al., 2007; RNAO, 2006).

Crisis prevention is an ongoing role for staff members on any psychiatric unit. As the push for cost-effective care and restraint-free environments continues, clients are more acutely ill and have shorter stays in inpatient units (ANA et al., 2007). Their behaviors are more likely to increase risk for injury. Most facilities require staff to be trained; many use the intervention techniques of the National Crisis Prevention Institute.

CRISIS INTERVENTION AND STABILIZATION

Maladaptive crisis resolution increases the probability of unsuccessful responses to future crises (Aguilera, 1998; Roberts & Yeager, 2009). During a crisis, people usually are open to receiving professional help and learning new ways of problem solving. As a result, attitudes and behaviors are likely to change quickly (Aguilera, 1998; RNAO, 2006; Roberts & Yeager, 2009).

Crisis intervention focuses on the problem or stressor that precipitated the crisis, rather than on personality traits (Aguilera, 1998; RNAO, 2006; Roberts & Yeager, 2009). It views people in crisis as normal and capable of problem solving and growth with assistance from others (Aguilera, 1998; RNAO, 2006; Roberts & Yeager, 2009). The goal is to assist people in distress to resolve the immediate problem and regain emotional equilibrium. Problem solving should lead to enhanced coping to deal with future stressful events.

The role of the intervener is to actively participate in helping clients solve the current problem (Aguilera, 1998; RNAO, 2006; Roberts & Yeager, 2009). The crisis state is not an illness; the intervener does not take over and make decisions unless a person is suicidal or homicidal (Aguilera, 1998; ANA et al., 2007; RNAO, 2006; Roberts & Yeager, 2009). The underlying philosophy of crisis intervention is that, with varying degrees of assistance, people can help themselves. To maximize growth, clients must be actively involved in resolving the problem. Crisis intervention is a partnership.

Interveners help with the following (ANA et al., 2007; RNAO, 2006; Roberts & Yeager, 2009):

- Analyze the stressful event.
- Express feelings without probing.
- Explore ways to deal with stress and anxiety.
- Problem solve and identify actions and strategies.
- Seek support from family, friends, and community resource groups.

• Avert possible future crises through anticipatory guidance.
• Evaluate the postcrisis status.

Interveners validate the feelings of clients (which will vary) and reinforce strengths, protective factors, and resilience (RNAO, 2006; Roberts & Yeager, 2009).

Crisis Intervention Versus Traditional Therapies

Crisis intervention assists clients to resolve immediate problems that they perceive as overwhelming. Sometimes, the crisis stirs up unresolved past issues. Interveners do not explore or confront those. However, they may encourage clients to do so after the crisis resolves and usually with another therapist (Aguilera, 1998; RNAO, 2006; Roberts & Yeager, 2009).

Crisis intervention emphasizes healthy, not unhealthy, aspects of the personality. There is no diagnosis of mental illness; however, interveners would review that data during the assessment stage. Interveners evaluate clients in terms of coping skills, strengths, potential, and problem-solving ability. The focus is the client's social structures, rather than personality (Aguilera, 1998; RNAO, 2006; Roberts & Yeager, 2009). Interveners assume that clients will make appropriate decisions when given necessary information and support. Crisis intervention requires a more direct, but not directive, approach than that of traditional therapies (Aguilera, 1998; RNAO, 2006; Roberts & Yeager, 2009).

Crisis Intervention Across Contexts

The need for crisis prevention, intervention, and stabilization arises across all contexts: emergency departments, acute care settings, community and public health settings, schools, work settings, homes, jails, psychiatric inpatient units and day programs, primary care settings, nursing homes, and clinics. In colleges, crisis work is an increasing priority. Students have complex and severe problems such as depression, anxiety, suicidal ideation, sexual assault, and personality disorders (Benton et al., 2003). In addition, developmental problems, difficulties with academic skills, and situational problems have increased (Benton et al., 2003). See Case Vignette 35.1.

Health care professionals should carry out crisis intervention in the least restrictive environment possible (ANA et al., 2007; RNAO, 2006; Roberts & Yeager, 2009). Nurses need to be prepared and competent to perform such work (ANA et al., 2007; RNAO, 2006).

Characteristics and Skills of the Crisis Intervener

To intervene effectively, providers must be able to perform several broad therapeutic communication techniques that demonstrate calmness, caring, and empathy (RNAO, 2006). Because people in crisis tend to be confused, interveners must be able to identify facts and think clearly to plan

Case Vignette 35.1

Tanya, a 19-year-old college student living in the freshmen dormitory, has become increasingly concerned about feeling overwhelmed. She is having difficulty concentrating, cannot sleep, and deals with problems poorly. This is the second month of the semester, and a teacher recently returned her assignment as "not meeting expected academic standards." Tanya is beginning to doubt herself and her abilities to cope with college studies and life. She cannot prioritize assignments and frequently feels confused about course assignments and due dates.

Tanya graduated in the top 10% of her high school class and always was on the honor roll. Although she looked forward to going away to college, this is her first time away from her close family. None of her classmates were accepted to her college, and she has been so busy with her academic assignments that she has formed no close relationships on campus. Her roommate is not friendly.

After phoning her mother, Tanya feels some relief. Her mother suggests that Tanya ask about counseling services on campus. Tanya does so and receives an emergency appointment at the student services counseling center.

Reflection and Critical Thinking

• What might be some potential problems for Tanya if she does not seek help?
• Do you think Tanya's experience is common for people in her circumstances? What can be done to help students adjust?

solutions. They must make people in crisis feel safe. Interveners may be nurses at the basic or advanced practice level (see Chap. 13) or from other mental health disciplines (eg, social work, occupational therapy, psychology, counseling, therapeutic recreation). They must possess courage, self-confidence, assertiveness, and resilience (Edward, 2005).

The pain involved in a crisis is never pleasant. Listening to personal tragedies is difficult; however, clients in crisis need others to commit to working with them until the situation resolves. This may include tolerating anguish, sadness, and anger (RNAO, 2006; Roberts & Ottens, 2005).

Skills needed for crisis work include communication, active listening, assessment, collaboration, advocacy, documentation, consultation, teaching, and coaching (Aguilera, 1998; ANA et al., 2007; RNAO, 2006; Roberts & Yeager, 2009). Interveners must quickly establish trust and build therapeutic relationships (ANA et al., 2007; RNAO, 2006; Roberts & Yeager, 2009). The outcome is related to the quality of the established therapeutic relationship.

Interveners also must be nonjudgmental and appreciate different cultural values. Various cultures have different established patterns of response to death, illness, divorce, and pregnancy (Aguilera, 1998; ANA et al., 2007; de Chesnay, 2005). Interveners never impose their own value systems on clients. Crisis intervention, with its focus on immediate problem solving, direct approach, avoidance of psychiatric diagnoses, and time limitation, as well as emphasis on healthy personal strengths, may be more acceptable to people from some ethnic groups and cultures than do others (see Chap. 6).

> ### Checkpoint Questions
> **5.** What is the goal of crisis intervention?
> **6.** What aspects of the personality are the focus of crisis intervention?
> **7.** What skills are needed for crisis work?

Team Approach

Short-term inpatient psychiatric treatment facilities, as well as many emergency mental health services, use a crisis team approach. The team may consist of a psychiatrist, psychiatric–mental health nurse, psychologist, social worker, psychiatric aide, minister, and students in the mental health field (RNAO, 2006; Roberts & Yeager, 2009). In an inpatient facility, one clinician is primarily responsible for the management of a client; however, the system requires continuity of care because so many people are involved with the client (ANA et al., 2007; RNAO, 2006). The crisis team meets daily to discuss the client's progress and make decisions about care. A case manager or primary therapist outlines goals for the client; other team members implement the plan and decide on time of discharge and method and frequency of follow-up. These time lines also

may be subject to specific protocols from third-party payers, including managed care contracts. As with any crisis intervention mode, the team keeps the goals clearly in mind (Challenging Behaviors 35.1). As soon as clients reach their goals, they are discharged, even if it is the same day as admission. Some facilities develop crisis response teams with special training to improve the crisis management of assaultive and out-of-control clients (Loucks et al., 2010).

Crisis Groups

The goal of a crisis group is the same as that of individual crisis intervention. A crisis group helps members regain or improve their functioning and ability to problem solve.

Some clients find a crisis group more beneficial than one-to-one therapy, particularly those who have difficulty with interpersonal relationships. Crisis groups also benefit those with few support systems or difficulty accepting information from psychiatric professionals. Members may feel less isolated (Aguilera, 1998; Yalom & Leszcz, 2005). By observing others express their feelings, members realize that all people have similar feelings and problems. Often, reticent clients can express opinions more easily after observing others do so. Participants offer one another suggestions for coping and solving problems, which helps bolster members' self-esteem.

Crisis groups also have some disadvantages. Keeping each client's specific crisis in focus in a group setting is difficult. Members may suggest a destructive or maladaptive form of coping. These problems underscore the need for

Challenging Behaviors 35.1

The Client Who Pits Staff Members Against One Another

Situation: You are returning from lunch to the Crisis Intervention office. A coworker is counseling a client who has been identified as having an increased risk for violence. The client is not supposed to be brought into the office for counseling. The crisis plan clearly states for the client to be counseled in the emergency department (ED), where staff members are sufficient and the environment is safe. The client has visited many times at the Crisis Center and has a pattern of manipulating staff. He is a long-time client of the local mental health clinic. In addition, you saw the client earlier in the day in the ED, provided resources, and reinforced the mental health clinic plan.

Your Potential Feelings: Fear, anger

What Is Going On? Some coworkers may think that they can "handle" high-risk clients, disagree with others' assessment of the client, or have not fully read the client's chart. This coworker is disregarding safety issues and placing self, client, and colleagues at risk. Undoing earlier work encourages patterns of manipulation. It also leads colleagues to feel disregarded and slighted.

Strategy: Use your stress response and assertive communication techniques. Use the three **Rs: Relax**—take a deep breath; **Reflect**—use self-talk, "I can manage my response"; and **Respond**—if appropriate, you may ask to speak to the coworker outside the office, using assertive communication. State that the client needs to be moved to a safe location for further counseling. You may need to use the "broken record" technique, a form of repetitive communication in which you continue to say what you need. After the client leaves, you must discuss the issue and your feelings with the coworker.

Nurse Action/Communication: This situation presents major client and staff safety issues as well as inconsistencies in communication. It has the potential to increase worker conflicts and the risk for safety problems. The next time the client arrives at the Crisis Center, he or she must be managed in another environment, which adds to confusion and inconsistency in limit setting. The ability for crisis workers to work as a team is critical to the safety of the staff as well as the client. The situation may call for further evaluation and interventions with the supervisor of the unit to resolve tension between staff and to reinforce protocols that protect the working environment.

a trained and experienced crisis group leader (Roberts & Yeager, 2009). Crisis groups usually are scheduled for 90 to 120 minutes once a week for 6 to 8 weeks; 8 to 10 members is considered the ideal size. Some groups are homogeneous, with all members having a similar problem. For example, successful groups have been formed for people experiencing divorce, Alzheimer's disease, incest, cancer, and AIDS. Peer groups organized by lay people, rather than professionals, may be effective and supportive. Among the best known are Alcoholics Anonymous, self-help groups, and the family support groups of NAMI. In a heterogeneous group, all members are in crisis but have different problems. The group may be open, in which new members come in, work through their problems, and leave. This provides members with an opportunity to deal with feelings about intrusion and separation. A closed group does not accept new members after it is formed and continues for a specified time.

Families in Crisis

Seldom does a person live in total isolation. Usually, a crisis occurs within a family and affects all those in close contact with the client. Parents commonly struggle with midlife crises at the same time their adolescents are struggling to establish a separate identity (Aguilera, 1998; Erikson, 1963; Roberts & Yeager, 2009). People in crisis are either helped or hindered by their social networks: friends, family, doctors, teachers, employers, and everyone else with whom they interact routinely. Issues of crisis can be viewed within a social framework; the crisis is unresolved until severed social relationships are reestablished (Aguilera, 1998; ANA et al., 2007; RNAO, 2006; Roberts & Yeager, 2009).

While working with families in crisis, the intervener determines who is exhibiting crisis symptoms. Next, he or she attempts to identify what clients need to ensure safety and security for the entire family. In collaboration with the family, the intervener identifies strategies to reduce the most severe symptoms. He or she also assesses the family's resources and additional social resources. The intervener teaches about crisis and its resolution (Figure 35.7). Often, family members need respite during a crisis.

The intervener helps bring together a client in crisis and all members of his or her social system for a meeting. During the meeting, all those involved analyze the problem and its effect on each participant. All those involved have an opportunity to voice comments or concerns. They discuss available resources and possible solutions. Before ending, the participants should have developed a definite plan of action, including exactly who is to do what and when. The intervener sets up a follow-up meeting and helps the family decide the time, place, participants, and purpose. The social system approach is effective in dealing with many faceted family crisis situations (RNAO, 2006; Roberts & Yeager, 2009).

Telephone Counseling

With growing demands for health care services to be more responsive and cost effective, telephone counseling is

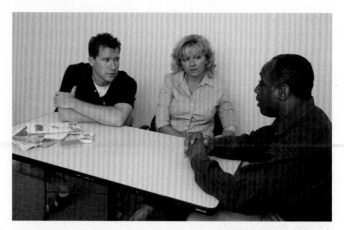

FIGURE 35.7 When intervening with families in crisis, the professional works to identify what is necessary to ensure the family's safety and security, pinpoint immediate strategies to reduce the most severe symptoms, assess the family's resources and additional external resources, and teach the family more about crisis and its resolution.

increasing (ANA et al., 2007). Medical advice "hotlines" operate all over the United States with more than 1 million calls per month (Figure 35.8). Estimates are that 12% to 18% of U.S. primary medical care is conducted over the telephone. Reese and colleagues (2002) found that telephone counseling was helpful and satisfying to recipients. In fact, they rated the counseling relationship and level of interpersonal influence as similar to that in face-to-face counseling.

During suicide crisis calls, the crisis worker keeps the caller talking to allow time for the call to be traced, to contact relatives or police if necessary, and to develop a relationship with the caller. Telephone advice lines also have been incorporated into emergency departments with specially trained staff to answer calls (ANA et al., 2007). Although less common, rural areas have used video conferencing for crisis intervention, with equipment installed in clients' homes, at remote service centers, or both (Hebda & Czar, 2009). The obvious benefit of video conferencing is that interveners can see clients and assess nonverbal behaviors.

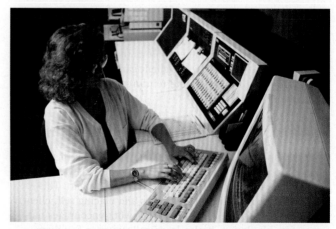

FIGURE 35.8 This woman is operating a switchboard at a telephone counseling hotline. Such resources are available across the United States and handle more than 1 million calls per month.

APPLYING THE NURSING PROCESS

Clients in Crisis

▲ ASSESSMENT

Assessment of the person in crisis is the most important, and often most difficult, step of crisis intervention. First, nurses determine whether the psychiatric symptoms are related to a physical problem (ANA et al., 2007; RNAO, 2006; Roberts & Yeager, 2009). One person in five with a brain disorder has a medical problem causing or exacerbating his or her psychiatric condition (see Chap. 39) (Chwastiak et al., 2006). A thorough health history and physical examination should help to identify any medical causes for the crisis response (Figure 35.9).

Nurses should examine the health history for use of substances that might cause psychiatric symptoms, including caffeine, nicotine, street drugs, and alcohol (RNAO, 2006; Roberts & Yeager, 2009). They also review current intake of any prescribed or over-the-counter medications, vitamins, supplements, or even herbal teas. Substance-related side effects, interactions, and reactions frequently explain symptoms (RNAO, 2006).

Tears or anger do not mean automatically that a person is overwhelmed (Aguilera, 1998). If clients are experiencing great anxiety, having difficulty thinking clearly, or failing to identify solutions, and if medical or substance-induced causes have been ruled out, then encouraging clients to discuss events that immediately preceded the distress is helpful (RNAO, 2006; Roberts & Yeager, 2009). This verbalization frequently calms clients and helps nurses to establish rapport with them.

During crisis intervention, nurses focus on the immediate problem. However, with improved access to data management systems, medical history and past treatment are readily available for review (Hebda & Czar, 2009). Usually, when people in

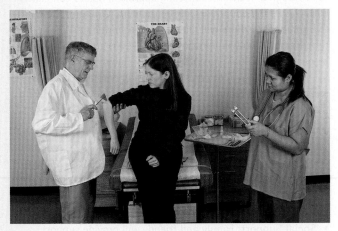

FIGURE 35.9 Health care providers should conduct a thorough health history and physical examination to ensure that clients are not experiencing a physical or medical problem that is generating a crisis response.

crisis seek help, the precipitating event is within the previous 14 days, sometimes within the last 24 hours (Aguilera, 1998; RNAO, 2006; Roberts & Yeager, 2009).

Evaluating Feelings

Feelings may be so overwhelming that clients have difficulty describing them. Some clients have little experience in identifying or discussing feelings. Nurses encourage clients to describe their feelings and accept them without judgment, thereby helping clients accept feelings as well. Nurses are careful to avoid probing, based on recent evidence and the controversy surrounding past practices (Parkinson, 2001; RNAO, 2006; Rose et al., 2006). They naturally may feel discomfort when others are expressing pain. The human inclination is to stop people from crying or talking about horrible or upsetting events. By avoiding the distressing topic, clients may seem to be in less pain. Nevertheless, expressing feelings and experiencing pain and frustration are beneficial to people in crisis. Therefore, nurses must learn to tolerate these feelings of discomfort as part of crisis intervention training (RNAO, 2006).

Usually, nurses are anxious about "saying the wrong thing" or feeling inadequate to deal with the situation. Examples of therapeutic communication are found in Nursing Spotlight 35.1 (RNAO, 2006). Nurses must understand both cognitively and emotionally that ultimately clients make their own decisions. In fact, it is not expedient or realistic to expect nurses to have all the answers. For clients to grow and develop intrinsic resilience, the work of problem solving must come from them (RNAO, 2006).

Determining Perception of the Event

Nurses first determine clients' perception of the stressful event (ANA et al., 2007; RNAO, 2006; Roberts & Yeager, 2009). How threatened is the client? Is the client realistic or distorting the meaning of the event?

Assessing Support Systems

After determining perception of the event, nurses focus on who is available to support clients. Questions that can help identify support systems include the following:

- "Whom do you trust?"
- "Who is your best friend?"
- "Are you particularly close with any member of your family?"

Children in crisis usually cope better if they are with their parents.

Nurses inquire about religious beliefs and spirituality (see Chap. 7). For many religious families, God is a source of comfort and strength. Religious affiliation and spirituality may be an excellent source of support (ANA et al., 2007; RNAO, 2006; Roberts & Yeager, 2009).

It is best to have several supportive people involved with a client. Because a crisis lasts briefly and nurses are involved only temporarily, clients need others from their natural support systems on whom to rely for continued support (RNAO, 2006; Roberts & Yeager, 2009).

Assessing Coping Skills

To assess coping skills, nurses ask what clients do when a problem is difficult to resolve or how clients deal with anxiety

NURSING SPOTLIGHT 35.1

Ten Tips for Crisis Prevention

1. **Be empathic.** Try not to be judgmental of your client's feelings. They are real, even if not based on reality, and you need to attend to them.

2. **Clarify messages.** Listen to what is really being said. Ask reflective questions and use both silence and restatement.

3. **Respect personal space.** Stand at least 1½ to 3 ft from the acting-out person. Encroaching on personal space tends to arouse an individual and escalate the situation.

4. **Be aware of body position.** Standing eye to eye and toe to toe with the client sends a challenge message. Standing one leg length away, at an angle off to the side, is less likely to incite an individual.

5. **Permit verbal expression when possible.** Allow the individual to release as much energy as possible by venting verbally. If this cannot be allowed, state directives and reasonable limits during lulls in the venting process.

6. **Set and enforce reasonable limits.** If the individual becomes belligerent, defensive, or disruptive, state limits and directives clearly and concisely.

7. **Avoid overreacting.** Remain calm, rational, and professional. How you, the staff person, respond directly affects the individual.

8. **Use physical techniques as a last resort.** Use the least restrictive method of intervention possible. Using physical techniques on an individual who is only acting out verbally can escalate the situation.

9. **Ignore challenge questions.** When the client challenges your authority, such as your position, training, or policy, redirect the individual's attention to the issue at hand. Answering these questions often fuels a power struggle.

10. **Keep your nonverbal cues nonthreatening.** Be aware of your body language, movement, and tone of voice. The more an individual loses control, the less he listens to your actual words. More attention is given to your nonverbal cues.

or depression (Aguilera, 1998; ANA et al., 2007; RNAO, 2006; Roberts & Yeager, 2009). Nurses encourage clients to describe specific coping methods and then determine whether they are adaptive or maladaptive. For example, clients may use alcohol or street drugs—maladaptive coping mechanisms. Is the client still working? Is he or she still attending school and fulfilling other roles, such as spouse and parent? How are significant others affected? Are they also upset? They may need crisis counseling as well (RNAO, 2006).

Determining Potential for Self-Harm

Nurses ask clients in crisis if they are having thoughts of hurting themselves. Most clients do not volunteer this information but, when asked, readily discuss suicidal thoughts (Aguilera, 1998; ANA et al., 2007; RNAO, 2006; Roberts & Yeager, 2009). In fact,

many people who commit suicide have seen a health care provider shortly before their death (Repper, 1999). Therefore, when clients arrive in any health care setting—emergency departments, primary care centers, hotlines—nurses should ask about suicidal ideation (Repper, 1999; Roberts & Yeager, 2009). Clients who have attempted suicide before or have decided how, when, and where to kill themselves need protection (Roberts & Yeager, 2009). They should not be left alone. Problem solving focused on immediate difficulties and identified actions frequently helps build the client's coping capacity and feelings of hope (Bilsker & Forster, 2003; RNAO, 2006).

▲ NURSING DIAGNOSIS

A crisis or precrisis state is neither a psychiatric illness nor a disabling, prolonged condition. While gathering data from clients and family members, nurses begin to formulate appropriate descriptions of the client's responses in terms of nursing diagnoses (ANA et al., 2007). Responses commonly evident in crisis intervention include the following (NANDA, 2007):

- Ineffective Coping
- Anxiety
- Disturbed Thought Processes
- Situational Low Self-Esteem
- Social Isolation
- Impaired Social Interaction

▲ OUTCOME IDENTIFICATION AND PLANNING

A crisis plan is necessary no matter how much time is available. After collecting data, nurses obtain the client's specific statement of the problem. Active involvement from clients in planning solutions helps ensure the plan's success (ANA et al., 2007; RNAO, 2006; Roberts & Yeager, 2009).

Nurses convey that clients will be able to solve the crisis and cope with life again (Figure 35.10). A basic principle is not to do things for clients that they can do for themselves. The more distraught and confused a client is, the more directive nurses must be. Together, the nurse, client, and available support people define goals and a time frame for crisis resolution.

Outlining the problem and available resources can be useful. Through a decision counseling approach, nurses can clarify with clients the boundaries of the problem. What are the tentative solutions? Where will clients try the solutions? What is the time frame? Who will do what? Follow-up is critical and should be part of the initial plan (RNAO, 2006; Roberts & Yeager, 2009).

The overall goal of crisis intervention is to help clients reestablish equilibrium. Supporting goals include the following (Aguilera, 1998; RNAO, 2006; Roberts & Yeager, 2009):

- **Participation in Healthcare Decisions:** The client will establish a working relationship with the nurse.
- **Concentration:** The client will identify the specific problem.
- **Distorted Thought Control:** The client will have a less distorted perception of the event.
- **Anxiety Self-Control:** The client's anxiety will decrease.
- **Social Support:** Family and friends will provide support.
- **Coping:** The client will use healthy coping mechanisms.

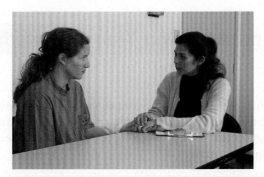

FIGURE 35.10 A primary nursing intervention during crisis is to reassure clients that the problems can be dealt with and that the situation is temporary.

Although it may be difficult, it is essential for nurses to accept that the goals of crisis intervention are different from those of other treatment strategies. In crisis intervention, the goal is not to deal comprehensively with various problems or to orchestrate major changes in a client's life (Aguilera, 1998; RNAO, 2006; Roberts & Yeager, 2009). Crisis intervention assists people to solve immediate problems that overwhelm the capacity for coping. Once clients have regained emotional equilibrium and can manage again, the work of crisis intervention has been accomplished.

▲ IMPLEMENTATION

The *Nursing Interventions Classification* (*NIC*) uses the label **Crisis Intervention** to represent "short-term counseling to help the client cope with a crisis and resume a state of functioning comparable to or better than the pre-crisis state" (Bulechek et al., 2008). Related interventions include, but are not limited to, **calming technique, coping enhancement, counseling, environmental management, rape-trauma treatment,** and **security enhancement.**

Realizing the Potential for Growth

Nurturing, caring, listening, and being willing to help are powerful and saving forces for clients in crisis. Clients facing overwhelming stressors have the potential to improve coping skills. Whether they realize this possibility for growth depends partly on the effectiveness of crisis intervention. Positive resolution of crisis results in growth and development.

> **Think About It 35.1**
> Recall Tanya from Case Vignette 35.1. What type of crisis is she experiencing?

Nurse and client reexamine any feelings that might interfere with adaptive coping. Extremely negative feelings may be especially difficult for clients to face. Helping clients change their thoughts regarding the crisis assists with adjusting negative feelings (RNAO, 2006).

Learning to Ask for Help

In a crisis, it is natural to withdraw and feel isolated. Therefore, nurses help clients communicate directly with significant others.

Clients who highly value independence may need particular assistance to recognize interdependence as healthy. Often, nurses must teach such clients how to ask for help. They can demonstrate this skill through role-playing.

Using Adaptive Coping

Nurses also help clients develop healthier coping skills (ANA et al., 2007; RNAO, 2006). Strategies include openly expressing feelings, recognizing that changing thoughts will change feelings, using positive self-talk, engaging in progressive relaxation, exercising, and using various sleep hygiene techniques to aid relaxation.

Focusing on Problem Resolution

Nurses keep clients focused on the problem and specific goals leading to its resolution. High anxiety may make it difficult for clients to concentrate on one issue. Therefore, they may need direction to avoid fragmentation. After clients have tried some alternative solutions, nurses help them to evaluate their effectiveness and decide whether additional plans are needed (ANA et al., 2007; RNAO, 2006; Roberts & Yeager, 2009). Nurses reinforce a client's abilities by reviewing the crisis event, coping skills, and newly acquired methods of problem solving or coping. Research studies have shown that cognitive–behavioral problem solving reduces the risk of suicidal behavior (Bilsker & Forster, 2003).

Using Information Technology

Internet resources may help reduce anxiety by providing quick access to needed information. For example, receiving a terminal medical diagnosis may trigger a crisis response. Providing clients with current information about options, research, outcomes, and resources for treatment is one way to reduce anxiety and, ultimately, a crisis response (Clarke et al., 2007; RNAO, 2006). Furthermore, clients themselves may access the Internet and need assistance in evaluating findings. Available modalities include e-mail, chat rooms, blogs, web sites, non-Internet video connections, Internet video connections, and Internet audio connections (ANA et al., 2007; Hebda & Czar, 2009).

▲ EVALUATION

In the evaluation process, the nurse and client together evaluate whether the crisis has been resolved (ANA et al., 2007; RNAO, 2006). Has the client regained equilibrium and usual level of functioning? The nurse must recognize when the client is ready for discharge. Before dissolving the partnership, the nurse and client engage in anticipatory planning to maximize the client's ability to avoid future crises (Aguilera, 1998; ANA et al., 2007; RNAO, 2006; Roberts & Yeager, 2009). Clients may need more information about community services or resources. After working through the crisis response, some clients are motivated to seek additional mental health services to resolve earlier issues or prior trauma; therefore, nurses may make referrals (Aguilera, 1998; ANA et al., 2007; RNAO, 2006; Roberts & Yeager, 2009).

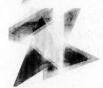

Reviewing and Applying Your Knowledge

Chapter Summary

• Crisis intervention differs from traditional psychotherapy primarily because it focuses on the here and now and immediate problem solving.

• A crisis occurs when a client cannot solve a problem that he or she perceives as overwhelming, when usual coping mechanisms fail to solve the problem, when perception of the event is distorted, or when others do not supply necessary support.

• The client in crisis has the potential to develop more adaptive coping and healthier functioning capabilities after the crisis experience.

• A crisis may be maturational, situational, or adventitious.

• Nurses often are the first health care professionals in contact with the client in crisis; therefore, they are uniquely positioned to intervene in crisis.

• The outcome of the crisis is related to the quality of the established therapeutic relationship.

• Nurses frequently experience incidents of workplace violence.

Study Questions

1. When assessing a client in the first phase of a crisis, which of the following would the nurse most likely observe?

   a. Increased levels of anxiety

   b. Effective problem solving

   c. Reaching out for help

   d. Short attention span

2. Which of the following would be an adventitious crisis? Select all that apply.

   a. Retirement

   b. Loss of a job

   c. Hurricane

   d. Birth of a child with a disability

   e. Bombing of a government building

   f. Diagnosis of a terminal illness

3. Which of the following would be the best indicator of a positive outcome for a client in crisis with the nursing diagnosis of ineffective coping related to an unexpected traumatic event?

   a. The client's report of fewer feelings of anxiety

   b. The client's use of agreed-on coping (problem-solving) strategies

   c. The client's ability to realistically interpret the crisis event

   d. The client's recognition of personal capabilities

4. When intervening in a crisis, the nurse would do which of the following? Select all that apply.

   a. Analyze the stressful event for the client.

   b. Express strong feelings while probing the client directly.

   c. Explore with the client ways to deal with stress and anxiety.

   d. Help the client problem solve and identify actions and strategies.

   e. Limit support from family and friends.

5. When intervening with families in crisis, which of the following would be the initial step?

   a. Ensure safety for all members.

   b. Identify the family member in crisis.

   c. Develop strategies for symptom reduction.

   d. Assess family resources.

6. Which of the following reflect the impact on nurses from workplace violence? Select all that apply.

   a. Disruption in client care

   b. Physical injury

   c. Absenteeism

   d. Job dissatisfaction

   e. Loss of sleep

Critical Thinking Questions

1. What aspects of crisis intervention might be useful in forensic settings?

2. What aspects of crisis intervention might homeless clients need?

3. What aspects of crisis intervention might be most appropriate for postpartum women?

4. How can cognitive adaptation facilitate nurses' recovery from experiencing workplace violence?

References

Aguilera, D. C. (1998). *Crisis intervention: Theory and methodology* (8th ed.). St. Louis, MO: Mosby-Year Book.

American Nurses Association (ANA), American Psychiatric Nurses Association (APNA), & International Society of Psychiatric–Mental Health Nurses (ISPN). (2007). *Psychiatric–mental health nursing: Scope and standards of practice.* Silver Spring, MD: American Nurses Publishing.

Benton, S. A., Robertson, J. M., Tseng, W., Newton, F. B., & Benton, S. L. (2003). Changes in counseling center clients' problems across 13 years. *Professional Psychology: Research and Practice, 34*(1), 66–72.

Bilsker, D., & Forster, P. (2003). Problem-solving intervention for suicidal crises in the psychiatric emergency service. *Crisis: The Journal of Crisis Intervention and Suicide Prevention, 24*(3), 134–136.

Bledson, B. E. (2003). Critical incident stress management (CISM): Benefit or risk for emergency services? *Prehospital Emergency Care, 7*(2), 272–279.

Boscarino, J. A., Adams, R. E., Foa, E. B., & Landrigan, P. J. (2006). A propensity score analysis of brief worksite crisis interventions after the World Trade Center disaster: Implications for intervention and research. *Medical Care, 44*(5), 454–462.

Bulechek, G. M., Butcher, H. K., & McCloskey Dochterman, J. (2008). *Nursing interventions classification (NIC)* (5th ed.). St. Louis, MO: Mosby.

Caine, R. M. N., & Ter-Bagdasarian, L. (2003). Early identification and management of critical incident stress. *Critical Care Nurse, 23*(1), 59–65.

Caplan, G. (1964). *Principles of preventive psychiatry.* New York, NY: Basic Books.

Chapman, R., Styles, I., Perry, L., & Combs, S. (2010). Nurses' experience of adjusting to workplace violence: A theory of adaptation. *International Journal of Mental Health Nursing, 19,* 186–194. doi:10.111/j.1447–0349.2009.00663.x

Chwastiak, L. A., Rosenheck, R. A., McEvoy, J. P., Keefe, R. S., Swartz, M. S., & Lieberman, J. A. (2006). Interrelationships of psychiatric symptom severity, medical comorbidity, and functioning in schizophrenia. *Psychiatric Services, 57*(8), 1102–1109.

Clarke, K., Rooksby, J., & Rouncefield, M. (2007). "You've got to take them seriously": Meeting information needs in mental health care. *Health Informatics Journal, 13*(1), 37–45.

Collins, R. (2006). What is the purpose of debriefing women in the postnatal period? *Evidence Based Midwifery, 4*(1), 4–9.

de Chesnay, M. (Ed.). (2005). *Caring for the vulnerable: Perspectives in nursing theory, practice, and research.* Sudbury, MA: Jones & Bartlett.

Dieterich, M., Irving, C. B., Park, B., & Marshall, M. (2010). Intensive case management for severe mental illness. *Cochrane Database of Systematic Reviews, 2010*(10). doi:120/1002/14651858. CD007906. pub2

Edward, K. (2005). The phenomenon of resilience in crisis care mental health clinicians. *International Journal of Mental Health Nursing, 14,* 142–148.

Eidelson, R. J., D'Alessio, G. R., & Eidelson, J. I. (2003). The impact of September 11 on psychologists. *Professional Psychology: Research and Practice, 34*(2), 144–150.

Erikson, E. (1963). *Childhood and society* (2nd ed.). New York, NY: W. W. Norton.

Gates, D. M., Gillespie, G. L., & Succop, P. (2011). Violence against nurses and its impact on stress and productivity. *Journal of Nursing Economics, 29*(2), 59–66.

Hebda, T. & Czar, P. (2009). *Handbook of informatics for nurses and healthcare professionals* (4th ed.). Upper Saddle River, NJ: Pearson/Prentice Hall.

Humphreys, J. C. (2001). Turnings and adaptations in resilient daughters of battered women. *Journal of Nursing Scholarship, 33*(3), 245–251.

Joy, C. B., Adams, E. E., & Rice, K. (2006). Crisis intervention for people with severe mental illnesses. *Cochrane Database of Systematic Reviews, 2006*(4). doi:10.1002/14651858/CD001087 .pub3

Kennedy, S. M. (2001). Disaster education and training are sorely needed. *American Journal of Nursing, 101*(11), 18.

Kinzel, A., & Nanson, J. (2000). Education and debriefing: Strategies for preventing crises in crisis-line volunteers. *Crisis: The Journal of Crisis Intervention and Suicide Prevention, 21*(3), 126–134.

Loucks, J., Rutledge, D. N., Hatch, B., & Morrison, V. (2010). Rapid response team for behavioral emergencies. *Journal of the American Psychiatric Nurses Association, 16*(2), 93–100.

Miller, L. (2002). Psychological interventions for terroristic trauma: Symptoms, syndromes, and treatment strategies. *Psychotherapy: Theory, Research, Practice, Training, 39*(4), 283–296.

Milligan, G., & McGuiness, T. M. (2009). *Mental health needs in a post disaster environment.* Retrieved May 26, 2012, from http://www.healio.com/~/media/Journals/JPN/2009/9_September/10_3928_02793695_20090731_01/10_3928_02793695_20090731_01.ashx.ber/10_3928_02793695_20090731_01/10_3928_02793695_20090731_01.ashx.

Mitchell, J. T. (1983). When disaster strikes: The critical incident stress debriefing process. *Journal of Emergency Medical Services, 8,* 36–39.

NANDA International. (2007). *Nursing diagnoses: Definitions and classification (2007–2008).* Philadelphia, PA: Author.

National Center for Posttraumatic Stress Disorder (NCPTSD). (2011). *Psychological first aid: Field operations guide.* Retrieved from http://www.ptsd.va.gov/professional/manuals/psych-first-aid.asp

National Institute of Mental Health (NIMH). (2002). *Mental health and mass violence: Evidence-based early psychological intervention for victims/survivors of mass violence. A workshop to reach consensus on best practices* (NIH Publication No. 02–5138). Washington, DC: U.S. Government Printing Office.

Parkinson, F. (2001). Debriefing and research. *CPR, 1*(3), 177–180.

Pender, D. A., & Prichard, K. K. (2009). ASGW best practice guidelines as a research tool: A comprehensive examination of the critical incident stress debriefing. *Journal for Specialists in Group Work, 34*(2), 175–192.

Ragaisis, K. M. (1994). Critical incident stress debriefing: A family nursing intervention. *Archives of Psychiatric Nursing, 8*(1), 38–43.

Reese, R. J., Conoley, C. W., & Brossart, D. F. (2002). Effectiveness of telephone counseling: A field-based investigation. *Journal of Counseling Psychology, 49*(2), 233–242.

Registered Nurses Association of Ontario (RNAO). (2006). *Crisis intervention.* Toronto, Ontario, Canada: Registered Nurses Association.

Repper, J. (1999). A review of the literature on the prevention of suicide through intervention in accident and emergency departments. *Journal of Clinical Nursing, 8*(1), 3–12.

Rew, L., Taylor-Seehafer, M., Thomas, N. Y., & Yockey, R. D. (2001). Correlates of resilience in homeless adolescents. *Journal of Nursing Scholarship, 33*(1), 33–40.

Robbins, I. (1999). The psychological impact of working in emergencies and the role of debriefing. *Journal of Clinical Nursing, 8*(3), 263–268.

Roberts (2005).

Roberts, A., & Ottens, A. (2005). The seven-stage crisis intervention model: A road map to goal attainment, problem solving and crisis resolution. *Brief Treatment and Crisis Intervention, 5*(4), 329–339.

Roberts, A., & Yeager, K. (2009). *Pocket guide to crisis intervention.* New York, NY: Oxford University Press.

Rose, S., Bisson, J., Churchill, R., & Wessely, S. (2006). Psychological debriefing for preventing post traumatic stress disorder. *Cochrane Database of Systematic Reviews, 2006*(4). doi:10.1002/14651858/CD001087.pub3

Santandrea, L. (2001). Salve. *American Journal of Nursing, 101*(11), 95.

Shepperd, S., Doll, H., Gowers, S., James, A., Fazel, M., Fitzpatrick, R., & Pollock, J. (2009). Alternatives to inpatient mental health care for children and young people. *Cochrane Database of Systematic Reviews, 2009*(2). doi:10.1002/14651858.CD006410.pub2

Slomski, G. (2003). Experts question value of psychological debriefing: The technique may do more harm than good to crisis survivors. *American Journal of Nursing, 103*(8), 64E.

Yalom, I., & Leszcz, M. (2005). *The theory and practice of group psychotherapy* (5th ed.). New York, NY: Basic Books.

Zahourek, R. (2003). Nurses have crucial role in debriefing: "Experts question value of psychological debriefing" falls short. *American Journal of Nursing, 103*(8), 64G.

Web Resources

American Psychiatric Nurses Association: http://www.apna.org

American Red Cross Disaster Services: http://www2.redcross.org/services/disaster

Centers for Disease Control and Prevention: Violence Prevention: http://www.cdc.gov/ViolencePrevention/suicide

Center for Mental Health Services (SAMHSA): http://www.samhsa.gov/index.aspx

Depression and Bipolar Support Alliance: http://www.ndmda.org

International Critical Incident Stress Foundation Articles: http://www.icisf.org

National Alliance for the Mentally Ill: http://www.nami.org

National Center for PTSD Guidelines for Mental Health Professionals' for Post Traumatic Stress Disorder, National Institute of Mental Health Public Information: http://www.nimh.nih.gov/publicat/index.cfm

Registered Nurses Association of Ontario Best Practice Guidelines: Crisis Intervention: http://www.rnao.org/Storage/15/930_BPG_Crisis_Rev06.pdf

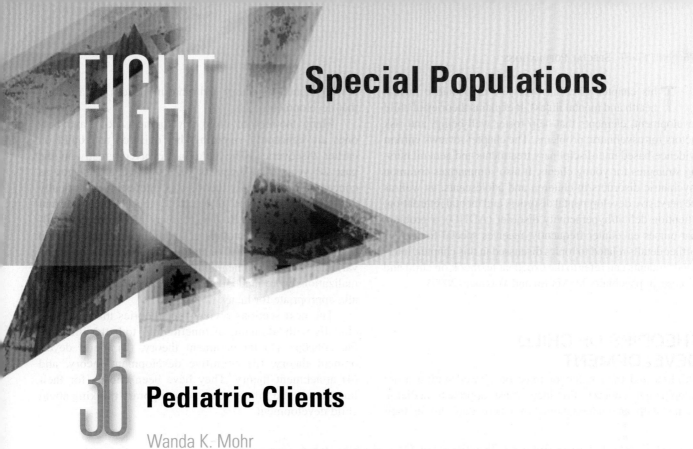

EIGHT

Special Populations

36

Pediatric Clients

Wanda K. Mohr

LEARNING OBJECTIVES

On completion of this chapter, you should be able to accomplish the following:

- Explain current theories related to child development.
- Outline factors that contribute to mental health in children and adolescents.
- Discuss the effects of childhood mental illness.
- Identify factors that contribute to psychiatric disorders in children and adolescents.
- Describe general interventions available for children or adolescents with psychiatric disorders.
- Discuss the role of the psychiatric–mental health nurse working with children and teens.
- Apply the nursing process to the care of children and adolescents with ADHD.
- Identify the most common childhood psychiatric and pervasive developmental disorders.
- Describe mental retardation and its criteria.
- Discuss the importance of self-care for nurses working with pediatric clients facing psychosocial challenges.

This chapter gives an overview of pediatric mental health and mental illness. It explains theories of child development, elements that help foster well-being, and risk factors for psychiatric problems. The chapter reviews current evidence-based interdisciplinary treatments and general nursing strategies for young clients. It also summarizes common psychiatric disorders in children and adolescents, as well as the pervasive developmental disorders and mental retardation. Attention deficit/hyperactivity disorder (ADHD), a problem that nurses encounter frequently, receives special focus. For further details related to topics discussed in this chapter, interested students can refer to the excellent textbook on child and adolescent psychiatry by Martin and Volkmar (2007).

THEORIES OF CHILD DEVELOPMENT

Children and their behavior must be viewed within a developmental context. Providers must approach pediatric clients with an understanding of where they are in their developmental trajectory and what influences are affecting that development.

Many theories of child development exist, and new ones are constantly emerging that question and build on earlier discoveries. The field has evolved greatly in the past 20 years. The linearity of developmental stages as conceptualized by past theorists is interesting historically (Table 36.1). However, global stages are no longer current thinking in the field. Rather, scholars recognize that children have different domains of functioning, which develop optimally, suboptimally, or not at all, depending on many variables and environmental factors. Moreover, past conceptualizations were inadequate because they were not culturally appropriate for many.

The next sections review four theories that deal specifically with "domains of functioning" to better illustrate the concept: (1) temperament theory, (2) moral development theory, (3) cognitive development theory, and (4) attachment theory. They have been chosen for their importance and influence on contemporary thinking about child development.

TABLE 36.1 **Overview of Traditional Developmental Theories**

Theory	Summary	Era	Proponents
Maturationist	Development is a biologic automatic process with predictable, sequential stages over time.	Very early to mid-20th century	Sigmund Freud Erik Erikson
Environmentalist	The child's environment shapes learning and behavior; in fact, human behavior, development, and learning are thought of as reactions to the environment.	Early to mid-20th century	John Watson B. F. Skinner Albert Bandura
Constructivist	Learning and development happen when children interact with their environments. Young children are active participants in the learning process and initiate most of the activities required for learning and development.	Later 20th century	Jean Piaget Maria Montessori Lev Vygotsky
Information processing	Children are active, sense-making beings who modify their own thinking in response to environmental demands. Thought processes are similar for people of all ages. The same thought processes in adults are found in children but to a lesser degree. Development is continuous.	Mid-20th century	George A. Miller
Ethology	Adaptation, survival, and the value of behavior in ensuring survival are prominent. This field has its origins in zoology and has become more influential in child development research in recent years. Observations of ethology scholars have led to the important concept of the *critical period*, which refers to a limited time span during which a child is prepared biologically to acquire certain adaptive behaviors but needs the support of appropriate environmental stimuli to do so.	Mid- to late 20th century	Konrad Lorenz Donald Dewsbury
Ecological systems theory	The child develops within complex environmental systems. Environment is a series of nested structures that includes, but extends beyond, home, school, and neighborhood.	Late 20th century	Uri Bronfenbrenner

Temperament Theory

Temperament represents the *how*, or style of behavior, as opposed to the *why*, or its motivation. Most researchers agree that humans are born with certain temperaments. Some scholars have put forth temperamental typologies. One such typology describes temperament as easy, difficult, or slow to warm up (Box 36.1).

Nurse researcher Sandee McClowry (2002) studied 883 children 4 to 12 years old and found that high-maintenance, cautious, and slow-to-warm-up children were deemed as having challenging temperaments. Industrious and social/eager to try were mirror images of those profiles and labeled easy. Some children fit both challenging and easy profiles. Challenging temperament profiles were disproportionately represented in boys, Hispanic children, and those from lower socioeconomic families. Girls were overrepresented in the group that included both types of easy temperaments. Social/eager-to-try children were more often from higher, rather than lower, socioeconomic status families.

Awareness of child temperament can help parents develop adaptive ways of coping with their children, regardless of temperament (Fox et al., 2001). According to McClowry (2002) temperament continues to influence children's development during their school-age years. She found that, just as with their parents, school-age children interact with teachers and peers in situations that contribute toward goodness or poorness of fit between the child and the other person.

Moral Development Theory

Lawrence Kohlberg, an American psychologist born in 1927, focused on moral development and proposed a stage theory of moral thinking (1984). He defined *moral reasoning* as judgments about right and wrong. His studies are based on the use of moral dilemmas or hypothetical situations in which people must make a difficult decision. Kohlberg noted that development of moral reasoning seemed related to age, but he also noted that many people did not reach the highest levels of moral reasoning.

Kohlberg's stages are as follows:

- **Level 1—Pre conventional:** People make judgments based solely on their own needs.

  - *Stage I: Punishment-obedience orientation.* People obey rules to avoid punishment. They determine good or bad actions based on physical consequences.
  - *Stage II: Personal reward orientation.* Personal needs determine right or wrong, along the lines of "you scratch my back, I'll scratch yours."
- **Level 2—Conventional:** People consider society's expectations and laws when making moral decisions.
  - *Stage III: Good boy–nice girl orientation.* "Good" means "nice." People determine behaviors based on what pleases and is approved by others. (Some feminist scholars criticize Kohlberg's theory as being biased against women.)
  - *Stage IV: Law-and-order orientation.* Authority must be respected and social order maintained. When deciding punishment for wrongdoing, laws are absolute.
- **Level 3—Postconventional:** People base judgments on abstract personal principles not necessarily defined by society's laws.
  - *Stage V: Social contract orientation.* People determine "good" by a socially agreed-on standard of individual rights. The U.S. Constitution is an example. People operating in this moral stage believe that different societies have different views of what is right and wrong.
  - *Stage VI: Universal ethical principle orientation:* What is right and good are matters of individual conscience and involve abstract concepts of justice, human dignity, and equality. People believe that there are universal points of view on which all societies should agree. Examples of famous people who reached this stage are Mahatma Gandhi and Nelson Mandela.

Cognitive Development Theory

The pioneer of cognitive development theory, Jean Piaget, was born in Switzerland in 1896 and became one of the 20th century's most influential thinkers, particularly among educators. Much of preschool and primary school education remains based on Piaget's concepts.

As a biologist, Piaget was interested in how organisms adapt to their environment. He called this environmental adaptation *intelligence*. The two major components of Piaget's theory are (1) the process of coming to know and (2) the stages people move through as they gradually acquire this ability to know. Table 36.2 presents an overview of Piaget's progression of cognitive development (1936).

Attachment Theory

John Bowlby, a British developmental psychologist, is credited with *attachment theory*. **Attachment** is the strong emotional bond that develops between infant and caregiver, providing babies with emotional security. By the second half of the first year, infants have become bonded to familiar people who have responded to their needs for physical care and stimulation. Bowlby (1969), who first applied this

---

> **BOX 36.1** Temperaments
>
> **Easy temperament:** Fairly regular feeding schedule and sleep–wake cycles; quickly adaptable to change and a predominantly positive mood of mild or moderate intensity.
>
> **Difficult temperament:** The opposite of easy; biologic irregularity, withdrawal tendencies to the new, slow adaptability to change, frequent negative emotional expressions of high intensity.
>
> **Slow to warm up:** Withdrawal tendencies to the new, slow adaptability to change, frequent negative emotional expressions of low intensity. These children often are labeled "shy."

TABLE 36.2 **Piaget's Theory of Cognitive Development**

Stage	Explanation
Sensorimotor (infancy) 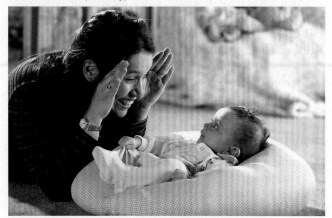	People demonstrate intelligence through motor activity without using symbols. Knowledge of the world is limited (but developing) because it is based on physical interactions and experiences. Children acquire *object permanence* (the ability to recognize that things still exist even if they are not directly visible) at approximately 7 months (memory). Physical development (mobility) allows them to gain new intellectual abilities. They have attained some symbolic (language) abilities at the end of this stage.
Preoperational (toddler and early childhood) 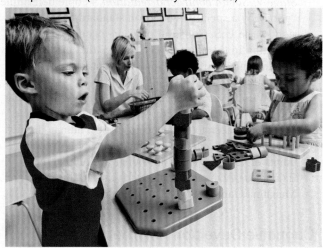	Children show intelligence through the use of symbols. Language use matures, and memory and imagination are developed, but thinking is nonlogical and non-reversible. Egocentric self-centered/self-referential thinking predominates during this period. Play is frequently parallel (side-by-side), rather than cooperative.
Concrete operational (elementary and early adolescence) 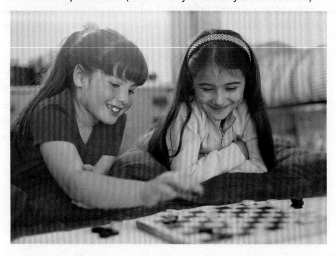	People demonstrate intelligence through logical and systematic manipulation of symbols related to concrete objects. Operational thinking develops (mental actions that are reversible). Egocentric thought diminishes. Group activity and cooperative play and projects emerge.

TABLE 36.2 **Piaget's Theory of Cognitive Development** (continued)

Stage	Explanation
Formal operational (adolescence and adulthood) 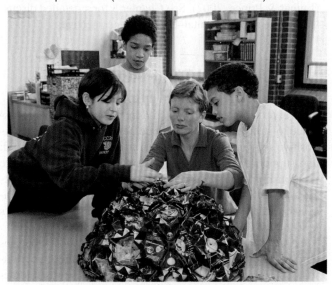	In this stage, people use symbols related to abstract concepts logically. Early in the period, there is a return to egocentric thought. Only 35% of high school graduates in industrialized countries reach this stage; many people do not think formally during adulthood.

idea to the infant–caregiver bond, was inspired by Lorenz's (1952) studies of imprinting in baby geese. Bowlby believed that human babies, like the young of most animal species, are equipped with built-in behaviors that help keep parents nearby, increasing the chances that they will protect infants from danger. Contact with parents also ensures that infants will be fed, but Bowlby emphasized that feeding is not the basis of attachment.

The infant's relationship to the parent begins as a set of innate signals that call the adult to the baby's side (Bowlby, 1980, 1988). Over time, true affection develops, which is supported by new cognitive and emotional capacities and a history of consistent, sensitive, responsive parental care. From this experience, children form an enduring bond with their caregivers and rely on this attachment as a base of security across time and distance. The inner representation of the parent–child bond becomes an important part of personality. It serves as an internal working model, or set of expectations about the availability of attachment figures, the likelihood of receiving support from them during times of stress, and ongoing interactions. This image becomes the basis for all future close relationships throughout a person's life (Figure 36.1).

Contemporary Views of Child Development

Scholars have entered a new era in understanding and appreciating the co-activity of nature and nurture in development (Shonkoff & Phillips, 2000). Beginning at conception, hereditary potential unfolds in concert with the environment. This dynamic interplay continues throughout life. The specialty of *behavioral genetics* has become increasingly influential in child psychiatry. However, in terms of physical traits, behaviors, or disorders, genes are just part of the

story. Various genetic and environmental factors contribute to the development of any trait. Having a genetic predisposition does not necessarily mean that a particular trait will emerge. Certain genetic factors can enhance or repress others. The proteins encoded by genes can be modified in ways that affect their ability to perform normal cellular functions.

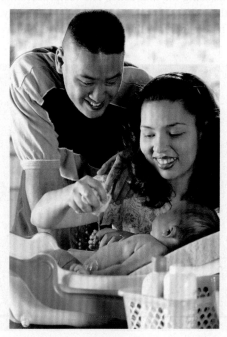

FIGURE 36.1 A child's image of his or her primary attachment figures serves as an internal working model that becomes the basis for all future close relationships throughout life.

Nature and nurture are partners in how developing people interact with the surrounding environment. Development is thought to depend on both stability and flexibility. Researchers focus attention not only on genetics, but also on how early events influence later experience. Early childhood is frequently an area of focus, not because the period serves as an unchangeable, deterministic map for adult well-being, but because early learning establishes capabilities, orientations to the world, and expectations about how things and people will behave.

Early learning also influences how people select and process new experiences throughout life. Infants who have learned that they can engage parents in play and make objects do what they want acquire a fundamental belief in their ability to affect their environment. Toddlers who have learned that people they depend on for comfort will help them in times of distress are more likely to approach others with empathy and trust than are toddlers whose worries and fears have been dismissed or belittled. Children who have routinely been read to are more likely to enter school with a keen interest in books and learning (Figure 36.2). Those who have missed these experiences may have a hard time recapturing them later. In short, getting off to a good start in life increases the odds of greater adult competence (Shonkoff & Phillips, 2000).

The National Academy of Sciences has recommended a developmental–ecological theoretical framework for research and practice with children (Cicchetti & Toth, 2009). This perspective is useful for conceptualizing the influences of risk and protective factors on children's development. It simultaneously addresses individual and environmental characteristics, emphasizing the interactive and reciprocal influences of children themselves, family, culture, and community. This integrative model includes the broader contexts of development and functioning and is informed by each person's genetic and neurophysiologic ontogenic variables. It posits that contextual characteristics and events may enhance or impede development and contribute to adaptation or psychopathology (Luthar & Prince, 2007). See Chapter 3 for a detailed discussion of the developmental–ecological perspective.

MENTAL HEALTH: PROTECTIVE INFLUENCES FOR RESILIENCE

Several protective factors in children can increase their resistance to stress. Examples include personality traits, such as positive self-image; family cohesion and absence of discord; and support from significant others. In addition, a positive relationship with at least one parent has been shown to exert a protective effect. Children with positive parental relationships have greater resistance to the effects of stressors (Cicchetti & Toth, 2009; Shonkoff & Phillips, 2000).

Developmental, ecological, and social systems theories emphasize the family's primary influence on child functioning. The family and other systems can be seen as interdependent spheres of influence. Current research and theory indicate that children learn much social behavior from their families of origin, suggesting that early family experiences play a key role in the development of social competence. Experiences in the primary social context of the parent–child relationship largely influence young children's abilities to prosper in any environment (Maccoby, 2000). Parenting styles also relate to the quality of children's social-emotional functioning, such as in developing peer relations and transitioning into the school context.

Family social support plays a strong role in promoting positive outcomes for both parents and children and in mitigating environmental and situational stressors (Kelly, 2000). For parents, strong external social supports strengthen positive social networks and feelings of connectedness, foster emotional well-being and coping, provide healthy outlets for stress and frustration, and increase access to community resources (Cicchetti & Toth, 2009). These positive effects enable parents to enhance their skills and, in turn, promote their children's social-emotional well-being. Specific child outcomes associated with strong family support include secure attachment with caregivers, positive parent–child interactions, healthy peer relationships, and healthy behavior patterns (Cicchetti & Toth, 2009). Thus, research suggests that child well-being and future competence are nested in a strong support network of parents and families. Healthy, well-supported families give rise to healthy, well-supported children.

OVERVIEW OF PEDIATRIC MENTAL ILLNESS

Youth is not a time of joy for all people. Many children and adolescents live in less-than-nurturing homes, face traumatic events, suffer maltreatment, become dependent on

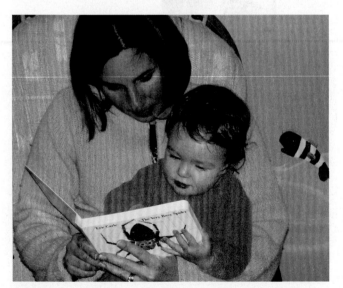

FIGURE 36.2 **Reading to children routinely can foster a lifelong love of books, learning, and knowledge. Early experiences that optimize cognitive and intellectual function increase the odds of successful adult competence.**

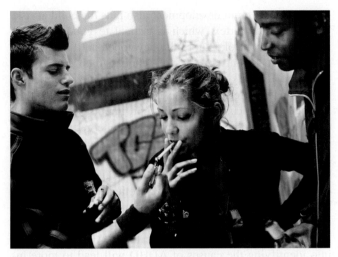

FIGURE 36.3 Psychiatric challenges such as substance abuse, depression, and conduct disorders affect many children and adolescents. Left untreated, such problems may have long-term negative consequence.

substances, fear that no one loves or will care for them, think of ways to hurt themselves, and develop illnesses such as mood and anxiety disorders (Figure 36.3).

Pediatric mental illness has staggering effects. Untreated psychiatric problems in childhood often result in long-term mental disorders in adulthood. For example, children with untreated depression frequently have dysthymia as adults, and children with conduct disorder may face serious ongoing problems into adulthood. The less obvious results—conflict, shame, guilt, lowered self-esteem, blame, unmet needs of siblings, thwarted development, and diminished productivity—are equally debilitating. Families, communities, child welfare programs, special education, juvenile justice, and health care systems bear the significant direct and indirect costs of mental illness in the young.

In December 1999, the first Surgeon General's report on the nation's mental health (see Chap. 1) also addressed pediatric mental illness and treatment (U.S. Department of Health and Human Services [USDHHS], 1999). It emphasized that psychiatric problems occur in children from all socioeconomic backgrounds. It also stressed that children and teens have unique developmental needs, which providers must assess in terms of each client's familial, social, and cultural backgrounds. The report also made the following points:

- Those who work with children must be familiar with what is and is not developmentally "normal."
- Services must be culturally appropriate and accessible.
- Preventive programs, including parent education and early childhood intervention, can improve children's social and emotional development and reduce risks for psychiatric disorders.
- Many interventions, both pharmacologic and psychosocial, could significantly help children and adolescents with depression, ADHD, and disruptive disorders.

Infrastructure and Availability of Care to Pediatric Populations

Report of the Surgeon General's Conference on Children's Mental Health: A National Action Agenda (USDHHS, 2001) called the state of children's mental health in the United States a "public health crisis." Approximately 5% to 10% of children and adolescents have illnesses severe enough to cause some impairment (National Institute of Mental Health [NIMH], 2006). Sadly, only 20% of those needing treatment actually receive it. The human and economic costs of pediatric psychiatric disorders are enormous.

Complicating the overall picture of access is the fact that only 5% to7% of youth are treated by mental health specialists each year (Substance Abuse and Mental Health Administration [SAMHA], 2003). The majority of mental health problems are first seen, and often only treated, in primary care settings by clinicians who are pressured to see more patients in less time. Moreover, an increasing number of problems (15% to 30%) are being identified by primary care providers who may have relatively little training or experience with psychiatric disorders in children and adolescents and who have added disincentives, such as decreased reimbursement, for identifying a mental health versus a somatic health problem (USDHHS, 2001). Also, rates of recognition (48% to 57%) are still low and connections to mental health specialists are inadequate among primary care providers (Institute of Medicine [IOM], 2001).

Moreover, children's mental health services are fragmented and spread across many different systems, including schools, child care centers, primary health care facilities, community mental health centers, the juvenile justice system, and the child welfare system. Historically, efforts to coordinate services for both families and children have been hampered because these services are administered by separate agencies and are not structured to facilitate coordination (SAMHA, 2003).

According to the IOM (2001), the workforce treating mental and/or substance use conditions is not uniformly and sufficiently equipped to provide access to and the quality of services needed by families. There are great variations in the types of clinicians licensed to diagnose and treat mental illnesses, and substantial differences in their training, knowledge, and skills. The present workforce is lacking in cultural diversity and understanding, and geographic distribution and numbers show a glut in some areas and a dearth in others.

In contrast to general health care, in which the diagnosis and treatment of medical conditions are typically provided by physicians, individuals licensed to diagnose and treat problems and illnesses include a wide range of practitioners: psychologists, psychiatrists, primary care and specialist physicians, social workers, psychiatric nurses, marriage and family therapists, addiction therapists, and a wide variety of counselors (eg, psychosocial rehabilitation, school, addiction, and pastoral counselors), many of whom are licensed to provide mental health services. In part this concern prompted discussion at the Surgeon General's Conference on Children's Mental Health (USDHHS, 2001) about inappropriate diagnosis, either over- or underdiagnosis, of children's mental health problems and about the availability of evidence-based (ie, scientifically proven) treatments and services for children and their families.

Thus, there is broad consensus and evidence that the nation lacks a unified infrastructure to help children with mental health problems. Many of those children who fail to be identified as having mental health problems and do not receive services end up in the legal system. Children and families suffer because of missed opportunities for early identification and prevention, fragmented treatment services, and low priorities for resources.

Cultural Barriers to Mental Health Care for Children

A child's ethnicity affects access to care and the likelihood of having mental health problems left untreated. The plight of minority and immigrant children and youth has been repeatedly documented, with numerous sources reporting that they face significant barriers to effective mental health care. They are the most likely to go without needed care (SAMHA, 2003). Documented barriers include population factors (socioeconomic disparities, stigma, poor health education, lack of documentation), provider dynamics (deficits in cross-cultural knowledge and skills and attitudinal sensitivity), and systemic factors (location and organization of services, lack of culturally competent services, etc.). Minority youth often reside in neighborhoods where services are unavailable, or they lack the public or private insurance necessary to obtain mental health services.

Risk Factors and Etiology

No single cause can explain child and adolescent psychopathology. Risk factors that may increase susceptibility include family history of mental illness; immature development of the brain; brain abnormality; family problems and dysfunction; poverty; mentally ill or substance-abusing parents; teen parents; abuse; discrimination based on race, creed, or color; chronic parental conflict or divorced parents; and chronic illness or disability (Cicchetti & Toth, 2009; Rutter, 2009). In recent years, researchers have realized that developmentally influential environments need to include possible prenatal as well as postnatal effects and also need to include physical environments as well as psychosocial environments. The effects of high levels of alcohol exposure in the first trimester of pregnancy constitute the best known example of prenatal effects, and the potential effect of cannabis on the emergence of psychosis in some children is an example of a postnatal effect (Arseneault et al., 2004; Rutter, 2009).

Biologic Influences

Biologic factors, such as a family history of a certain disorder, increase a child's likelihood of developing that disorder. For example, if one or both parents have depression, the child's risk for mood disorders is increased.

Immature brain development also puts the child at risk. The prefrontal cortex, which is critical to good judgment and impulse control, is not fully developed until at least age 20 years. In recent episodes of school violence, perpetrators were 15 years or younger; they are examples of people with immature prefrontal cortexes. Experts contend that they were not biologically ready to inhibit impulses, such as the desire to harm others when angry (Weinberger, 2001). Recent techniques have advanced the understanding of brain anatomy and physiology in mental illness. For example, neuroimaging and genetic studies of ADHD suggest that characteristic deficits result from genetically or environmentally influenced abnormalities in dopamine in the prefrontal circuitry. Problems in the basal ganglia, cerebellum, and parietal cortex have also been implicated in ADHD. Research into identifying the causes of ADHD will lead to more individualized, biologically targeted interventions and treatments (Casey et al., 2007). Similar studies are under way for other mental disorders as well (see Chap. 2).

Finally, temperament, which is thought to be at least partly determined genetically, plays a role in whether a child is at risk for maladjustment. An infant with a difficult temperament may be at risk for future maladjustment. However, it is important to remember that responses from caregivers and others can modify risks (Figure 36.4). Likewise, negative responses to infants with a difficult temperament may increase the risk for maladjustment.

Familial and Societal Influences

Some people think that parents do things "to" a child that affect development, as though parent–child transactions were one-way streets. In reality, they are two-way, reciprocal

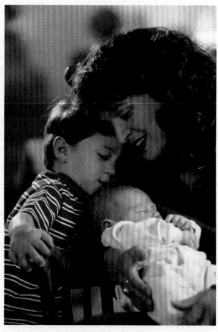

FIGURE 36.4 Positive and loving responses from family can help modify risks that may exist when children are born with challenging temperaments.

relationships. Children largely acquire the coordination of affect, cognition, and behavior, which they need to relate successfully to others, within the socialization context of the parent–child relationship (Cicchetti & Toth, 2009; Shonkoff & Phillips, 2000). Families do not operate in a vacuum—the behavior of each relative affects the others, and each person is influenced by other contexts to which he or she is exposed. Therefore, many situations affect family dynamics, and those dynamics may change from more to less adaptive, depending on specific contexts. For example, a family may function adaptively during the death of a grandparent, but maladaptively during parental unemployment.

Because children function within a family that helps to buffer the effects of social change, they are less susceptible to sociocultural influences than are adults. However, with growth and maturity, children have increasing contact with the larger society. Stable, nurturing forces at home help protect children from outside harm. Children without such stable, nurturing forces are at risk for maladjustment (see Chap. 3).

Parental fears, anxiety, depression, and aggression, as well as parents' love, nurturance, and concern, shape the youth's developing sense of self and the world. Parenting is an extension of self. What parents believe about their world is often reflected in their children's skills or deficits.

Parents also help to maintain two important family boundaries: generational and gender. *Generational boundaries* divide the family into parents who nurture, lead, and direct and children who are nurtured, follow, and learn. *Gender boundaries* divide the family into female and male members and promote gender awareness and identification.

Stressors

Exposure to stressors, especially many of them over time, can have damaging effects on development. However, small amounts of manageable stress can help "inoculate" the child to the effects of stress and can serve as a motivator. Children with buffers and protective factors, such as high intelligence, stable family, and comfortable socioeconomic status, demonstrate greater adaptability under stress. Children with fewer protective factors and more risk factors, such as poverty and exposure to domestic violence, tend to be less adaptable.

DIVORCE. Divorce involves a series of changes, transitions, and adjustments and subsequently affects children and adolescents in many ways. During divorce, children deal simultaneously with normal developmental challenges and the added problems that accompany separation. The father's or mother's absence, parental conflict, financial difficulties, multiple changes (eg, geographical moves, poverty, remarriage), level of parent adjustment, and short-term crisis are all factors that contribute to the stress of divorce for children and teens.

Preschool children are likely to regress after one parent's departure from the home, with the regression being in those domains of functioning most recently acquired. Children 5 to 8 years old grieve openly for the departed parent, while older children may develop fierce anger toward one or both parents (Wallerstein & Corbin, 2002).

Studies have shown that the effects of divorce are more detrimental than child development specialists once thought. Twenty-five years of longitudinal study (Wallerstein et al., 2000) revealed that ongoing as well as delayed effects surface during midadolescence to adulthood, when children of divorced parents begin to form their own romantic relationships. In addition to the adverse effect of sustained stress, children of divorce have decreased well-being and maladjustment across several domains of functioning. Conflict between parents leads to anger and anxiety in children because they want to be loyal to and please both parents (Figure 36.5). This feeling of being "caught in the middle" leads to depression, anxiety, and deviant behavior. Children exposed to ongoing demonstrations of hostility demonstrate higher levels of aggressive behavior. The less post-divorce conflict between parents, the greater is the children's well-being.

After divorce, many women and children become impoverished, with accompanying poor health care and nutrition, unsafe housing, and inferior schools. Children may display inadequate social skills, decreased academic performance, or drug and alcohol use. Children who are young at the time of divorce seem to experience greater emotional and social effects. Research also identifies gender-specific effects of divorce; girls tend to engage in precocious sexual activity and have difficulty establishing lasting adult heterosexual relationships, whereas boys demonstrate an unstable sense of masculinity (Marquardt, 2006).

Divorce is a current societal reality. To reduce its negative effects, parents should avoid hostile interactions with each other, reduce stressors in their children's lives, participate in

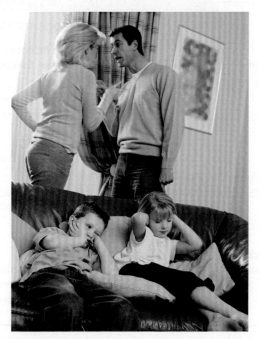

FIGURE 36.5 **Children who witness parental conflict experience confusion, depression, and anxiety. Ongoing demonstrations of discord and hostility can damage children's well-being and contribute to psychological dysfunction.**

divorce mediation to decrease conflict, and seek support for their children within schools and peer support groups. Referrals for therapy may be needed (Wallerstein & Corbin, 2002).

CHILD ABUSE. Each year, approximately 1 million children are reported to Child Protective Services (CPS) as being abused or neglected (see Chap. 33). Many more cases are unreported. Approximately 14 of every 1,000 children are mistreated in some way. Estimates of cases of sexual abuse are 25% of girls and 10% to 12% of boys. Exact figures are unknown (Centers for Disease Control and Prevention, 2007).

Abuse has long been associated with psychopathology and maladjustment. Abused children learn that the world is unsafe and not to trust others. Sequelae include anxiety, depression, interpersonal difficulties, anger management problems, disruptive conduct, dissociative symptoms, somatization, sleep and eating disorders, chemical dependency, and sexual acting out and dysfunction. Sexually abused children are at risk for symptoms of post-traumatic stress disorder, dissociative disorders, and depression. Maltreated children often are slow to trust and resistant to interventions; therapy may take many years.

Checkpoint Questions

1. What are two important family boundaries?
2. How do preschool children respond to the departure of one parent from the home with divorce?

Evidence-Based Interventions

Increasing recognition of the complexities of psychopathology has moved the field beyond a disease model and simple social explanations. Mounting knowledge of genetic, neurophysiologic, and environmental variables and their effects on behavior have provided new understanding of adaptation and maladaptation. For example, advances in the understanding of gender identity and behavior have led to a reexamination of the differences between how boys and girls think. Such discoveries, as well as an increased emphasis on the need for evidence-based practice (see Chap. 4), have led professionals to focus on optimal treatments with the best substantiated outcomes.

Although the knowledge base for child and developmental psychopathology has grown exponentially in the past decade, it has been, and continues to be, compromised by atheoretical, unsystematic, and somewhat fragmented research findings. Change comes slowly to the practice arena. Nurses may find interventions not based on current science being applied in facilities where they work. This is unfortunate for families and their children with mental illness.

Because the field of childhood psychopathology changes daily, nurses are ethically obligated to keep up with the research in the field. Evidence-Based Practice Spotlight 36.1 presents an overview of common psychiatric disorders in pediatric clients and the current levels of evidence supporting interventions for them with commentary.

EVIDENCE-BASED PRACTICE SPOTLIGHT 36.1

Interventions for Child and Adolescent Disorders

Problem	Level of Support	Positive Effects—Consistent Evidence	Inconsistent Evidence—Unproven	Comments
ADHD	Evidence-based treatments	*Psychosocial* Parent management, cognitive–behavioral therapy (CBT) *Pharmacologic* Methylphenidate (MPH)	Dietary replacement, exclusion; various vitamin, mineral, or herbal regimens; biofeedback; perceptual stimulation	It is not necessary to select one treatment at the expense of the other.
Adjustment disorders	Promising treatments	*Psychosocial* CBT, stress management, family therapy, group therapy		Medication is seldom used as monotherapy because the child needs assistance to cope with the stressor behind the maladaptive behavior.
Anorexia nervosa	Evidence-based treatments	*Psychosocial* Nutritional rehabilitation, family psychotherapy, inpatient behavioral programs *Pharmacologic* Selective serotonin reuptake inhibitors (SSRIs)	Individual psychotherapy, group therapy, 12-step programs, somatic treatments	Many clients display a limited response to treatment and require long-term monitoring and intervention.

EVIDENCE-BASED PRACTICE SPOTLIGHT 36.1   Interventions for Child and Adolescent Disorders (continued)

Problem	Level of Support	Positive Effects—Consistent Evidence	Inconsistent Evidence—Unproven	Comments
Anxiety disorders	Evidence-based treatments	*Psychosocial* CBT, modeling, CBT and family component, CBT and group component, systematic desensitization *Pharmacologic* SSRIs	Herbal supplements, which may impede diagnosis	Phobias may be treated through systematic desensitization. Parenting strategies and CBT are also effective. Medication should not be used as the sole intervention.
Binge eating disorder	None			Goals and strategies are similar to those for bulimia, except clients with binge eating disorder have difficulties associated with being overweight rather than malnourished.
Bipolar disorders	Evidence-based treatments	*Psychosocial* None *Pharmacologic* Lithium	Electroconvulsive therapy (ECT; no research with children)	Some evidence supports use of lithium in the acute phase; there is no current evidence for or against ECT.
Bulimia nervosa	Evidence-based treatments	*Psychosocial* CBT, combined treatments, group therapy *Pharmacologic* SSRIs	Bupropion, monoamine oxidase inhibitors (MAOIs)	Interventions include treatment of co-occurring disorders, establishment of regular, non-binge meals, and improvement of attitudes related to the disorder.
Fire setting	Promising treatments	*Psychosocial* CBT, fire safety education		No treatment is not beneficial because children usually do not outgrow this behavior.
Major depressive disorder and dysthymia	Evidence-based treatments	*Psychosocial* CBT, family systemic therapy, interpersonal therapy, combined treatments, group therapy *Pharmacologic* SSRIs	Dietary supplements such as omega-3, St. John's wort, SAM-e, which may have harmful side effects	Most studies fail to accommodate developmental differences in children, lack a culturally sensitive perspective, and pay little attention to cultural relevance of materials used.
Mental retardation	Evidence-based treatments	*Psychosocial* Individual therapy, family therapy, social skills training, cognitive therapy		Treatment is tailored for co-occurring disorders and is based on two guiding principles: normalization and community-based care.
Oppositional-defiant and conduct disorders	Evidence-based treatments	*Psychosocial* Parent training based on living with children, video-tape modeling, multisystem therapy, anger coping therapy, assertiveness training, delinquency prevention program, rational emotive therapy *Pharmacologic* Stimulants, mood stabilizers	Boot camps, psychiatric hospitalization, medication trials, brief courses of CBT	Interventions are usually performed in school or at home. Various modalities are used for these disorders as well as the comorbidities. Medications are prescribed only in conjunction with psychosocial interventions, such as parent training.

(continues on page 786)

EVIDENCE-BASED PRACTICE SPOTLIGHT 36.1   Interventions for Child and Adolescent Disorders (continued)

Problem	Level of Support	Positive Effects— Consistent Evidence	Inconsistent Evidence—Unproven	Comments
Pervasive developmental disorders (autism, Asperger's syndrome)	Promising treatments	*Behavior interventions* Educational and communication focused interventions, treatment and education of autistic and related communication-handicapped children (TEACCH) approach, natural language methods, picture exchange communication system, behavior intervention *Pharmacologic* Antipsychotics, psychostimulants		Approaches to treatment are of two types: 1. Focus on specific symptoms or learning needs. 2. Focus on reversing the level of impairment.
Schizophrenia	Evidence-based treatments	*Psychosocial* Psychoeducational therapy for the child and family, family intervention programs *Pharmacologic* Antipsychotics		Well-conducted psychopharmacology trials in children are few. Atypical medications are superior to neuroleptic drugs. Side effects are concerning. Best practice guidelines are based on extrapolation from adult studies or consensus of child clinicians.
Self-injury	Promising treatments	*Psychosocial* CBT, behavior modification, addictions model *Pharmacologic* SSRIs		Research continues on psychosocial interventions and medications. Hospitalization is used as last resort.
Sex offending	Promising treatments	Multisystemic therapy; residential sex offender treatment		Promising programs often combine an intensive, multimodal approach with early intervention. Comprehensive CBT programs focus on taking responsibility for sexual behavior, developing victim empathy, and building skills to prevent future offending. Approaches to treatment of juvenile sex offenders varies.
Substance abuse	Evidence-based treatments	*Psychosocial* CBT, group therapy, behavior therapies, skills development, family therapy, multisystemic therapy, individual psychotherapy, medical detoxification		Use of medication should be a last resort in the dually diagnosed population, because of the potential for misuse and overdose.

EVIDENCE-BASED PRACTICE SPOTLIGHT 36.1   Interventions for Child and Adolescent Disorders (continued)

Problem	Level of Support	Positive Effects—Consistent Evidence	Inconsistent Evidence—Unproven	Comments
Suicide prevention	Evidence-based treatments	*Psychosocial* Training of emergency professionals for follow-up and treatment *Pharmacologic* Lithium, clozapine, SSRIs (comorbid disorders)	Tricyclic antidepressants, medications that may increase disinhibition or impulsivity	All medications prescribed to the suicidal child must be carefully monitored by a third party, with any behavior change side effects reported immediately. Education about the benefits of follow-up treatment to reduce recurrent suicide attempts should be emphasized.
Tourette syndrome	Evidence-based treatments	*Psychosocial* Habit covariance, habit reversal *Pharmacologic* Neuroleptics	Plasma exchange or intravenous immunoglobulin	When tics interfere with functioning, other disorders are also present, or both, medication may be helpful.

Prevention and Early Identification

Primary prevention refers to any activity undertaken before a child or adolescent is diagnosed with a disorder. It would be wonderful if knowledge alone prevented problems; however, increased knowledge does not necessarily lead to behavior change (eg, education about weight and nutrition does not prevent eating disorders). Activities to enhance self-efficacy and a positive outlook on life, however, can foster protective factors. For example, the USDHHS website "Girl Power!" (http://www.girlpower.gov) was designed to help girls form healthy attitudes about their bodies. This site includes assessment of risk factors, programs to educate parents about the effects of their attitudes and comments about appearance, body image classes, exercise programs for obese children and teens, and esteem-building programs.

Another example of primary prevention is preschool programs (Figure 36.6). Research has documented relationships among children's social and emotional competencies, early learning behaviors, language use, cognitive abilities, and behavioral difficulties, and their ability to navigate present and future school environments successfully. Achievement in school is a significant protective factor for children; poor school outcomes are associated with maladjustment. Effective preschool programming is accordingly geared toward promoting developmental competencies. Head Start, the largest federally funded program committed to school readiness for children living in poverty, has served more than 15 million children since its inception in 1965. A review of 36 studies of Head Start found that children who completed the program had lower rates of enrollment in special education and higher rates of high school graduation. Head Start and other early childhood programs produce other less readily apparent benefits, such as better peer relations, less truancy, and lower rates of antisocial behavior (National Head Start Association, 2007).

Early identification and treatment are key to reducing the harm resulting from psychiatric disorders. Nurses play integral roles in detecting early symptoms, such as depression, and referring children and families to appropriate services. Screening for and preventing psychiatric disorders need to start with infants. Studies have shown that a fussy and demanding temperament in infancy predicts future maladjustment. However, when demanding infants and

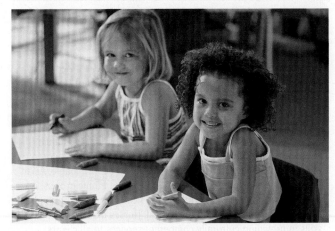

FIGURE 36.6 Preschool programs can serve as protective elements for children, helping to prevent future problems and promote social and emotional competence, learning, language and cognitive skills, and adaptation.

their parents are provided in-home family counseling that focuses on improving parent–child interaction, children are less likely to exhibit problems as adolescents (Shonkoff & Phillips, 2000). In addition, early intervention with at-risk children and teens can prevent more serious emotional turmoil later in life. For example, bereavement services through group sharing with peers can help ameliorate later adjustment difficulties for children whose parents have died.

Psychosocial Modalities

Several different forms of intervention are available for children and families. Types vary based on the specific disorder and the child himself or herself. Whichever therapy is used, providers must consider the child's and family's culture (Cultural Spotlight 36.1; see Chap. 6).

INDIVIDUAL THERAPY. Individual therapy for pediatric clients usually is cognitively or behaviorally oriented because these types of therapy have the greatest empirical support for efficacy. Individual therapy is something of a misnomer in that successful therapeutic interventions with any pediatric population, with the exception of older adolescents, will not be successful without parental involvement and support. Behavioral and cognitive therapies are based on the concept that psychiatric disorders represent learned behavior (see Chap. 3). Practitioners apply learning principles to help children modify their behavior and engage parents in helping new skills and behaviors to be reinforced and maintained at home.

Behavioral techniques include token economies, time-out (from positive reinforcement), and rewards for and reinforcements of desired behaviors. Parents and teachers also learn and use these techniques. Participation in a written behavioral contract is a common approach with adolescents to facilitate their adherence to treatment plans.

Cultural *Spotlight* 36.1

Considerations for Mental Health Services

Lack of culturally competent services is a barrier to children and adolescents receiving needed mental health services. Minority children are less likely to seek and receive needed treatment than are nonminority children. They also usually drop out of treatment earlier, enter treatment later in their illness, and are misdiagnosed more often (Bush, 2000).

Different cultural groups have different mental health needs. Native Americans are at highest risk for depression, substance abuse, anxiety, violence, and suicide. Services should be tailored to the needs of each distinct culture, which can be formidable. Asian Americans alone comprise at least 31 different ethnic groups. As diversity increases, demand for mental health services for children and adolescents becomes more critical. Nurses must refine their skills in providing culturally competent services to all clients (Bush, 2000).

Problem-solving skills training (PSST) is a cognitive therapy that has as its goal the development of interpersonal cognitive problem-solving skills. Like all cognitive therapies, it focuses on the thought processes in various situations and encourages clients to make a step-by-step analysis rather than jumping to a conclusion. Clients are taught to make self-statements that attend to all aspects of the situation rather than overemphasizing one facet. Therapists model prosocial behaviors for the client. With younger clients, games and stories may be part of the therapeutic tool kit. Older children appear to benefit more than younger children because of their greater cognitive development. Although cognitive processes change during treatment, evidence has not conclusively demonstrated them to be causative factors in treatment outcome (Kendall, 2006).

BRIEF PSYCHOTHERAPY. Brief psychotherapy addresses a central issue in a specified time. The provider and client do not discuss extraneous issues. The provider openly explores the central problem with the child and family.

PLAY THERAPY. Play is the child's work and natural medium for expression. *Play therapy* offers children an opportunity to express fears, anxieties, frustrations, and aggression. "Play therapy" is a misnomer; the play is the actual vehicle for the therapy to take place. The assumption is that children express and work out conflicts and problems through play. The symbolic interpretation of play behaviors as representational images is a psychoanalytic concept (see Chap. 3). In 1905, Freud suggested that the play of little children represents conscious and unconscious wishes and fears. Psychoanalytic therapists assume that children's behaviors can reveal troubling unconscious factors otherwise not available to either child or observer. Play therapy has been used as a treatment of choice since the early 1900s.

However, there is no support for the supposition that play therapy can be used to establish the truth of past events. Moreover, despite its ubiquity, empirical evidence to verify the effectiveness of play therapy is not available. Numerous play therapy books are on the market (Landreth et al., 2005; Schaefer & Kaduson, 2006). However, treatment effects for play therapy are conspicuously absent for specific behavioral disorders. In addition, play therapy does not improve the interpersonal adjustment of children who participate in it. Most "research" on play therapy consists of case reports, and even trials comparing play therapy with other forms do not account for the effects of the intense attention that the child undergoing it receives. Undoubtedly, it will not be possible to do Level I studies on play therapy because proponents describe this intervention as a creative and dynamic process (Schaefer & Kaduson, 2006). Therefore, it cannot be standardized to meet the rigorous criteria of an experimental design (see Chap. 4).

Although research to support claims of effectiveness is lacking, play therapy can be a useful tool for well-trained professionals to facilitate other interventions or to establish rapport during assessments (Karekla & Perdikogianni, 2006). With inexperienced practitioners, play therapy and its interpretation can have damaging consequences. Some children, such as those with autism spectrum disorders (who have interpersonal difficulties resulting from impaired communication, social interaction, and play skills), may benefit from play therapy as a way to establish human contact and engage in reciprocal interactions (Prendeville et al., 2006).

FAMILY THERAPY. The basic premise of family therapy is that the behavior of one member affects everyone else in the family. No behavior of one relative can be understood without appreciating the behavior of other relatives. Practitioners direct interventions at the behavior patterns of the entire family, not just at the identified client.

Family therapy promotes cohesion and addresses members' concerns, conflicts, and dynamics. The idea is that treating a child or adolescent successfully necessitates modifying how the home environment reinforces his or her behavior. See Chapter 15 for more discussion.

TRAUMA-INFORMED CARE. The majority of adults and children in psychiatric treatment settings have trauma histories (Lipschitz et al., 1999). Children are more vulnerable than adults to trauma. A "traumatic event" may encompass many experiences and may have many sources. These include neglect, physical abuse, psychological abuse, sexual abuse, the witnessing of domestic abuse and other violence, community violence, school violence, traumatic loss, medical trauma, natural disasters, war, terrorism, and refugee trauma (National Child Traumatic Stress Network, 2005).

Several factors mediate the outcome that children may experience after a traumatic event. These are the type, severity, duration, and chronicity of trauma, the child's age, prior or existing vulnerability or risk factors (ie, chronic illness, borderline IQ), and the response of primary caregivers. Traumatic events have the potential to affect every aspect of the child's development and functioning, including brain development, neurochemical pathways, psychosocial adaptation, and preferential responses to subsequent stress and other life experiences (Perry, 2004; Van der Kolk, 2003). Early identification, intervention, and support, and at times formal mental health treatment, may be indicated for children subjected to maltreatment and other trauma that disrupts their functioning and threatens their development. Early intervention is needed to interrupt trauma that is ongoing and to ensure the physical and emotional safety of the exposed child. Most scholars in this area strongly endorse screening all children who come into contact with mental health services for a history of trauma.

These children are difficult to treat, and they can try the patience of those who work with them unless staff members understand that the behaviors and mind-set that these children exhibit are part of the constellation of a trauma response. Traumatized children approach the world as a dangerous place, and their continual state of arousal may greatly interfere with efforts to soothe and de-escalate them, because children who are upset may no longer be able to *hear* and *process*. Too often staff members label these children as oppositional and "disruptive on purpose" or as "trying to put one over" on staff and as "manipulative." Rather than being malicious and "manipulative," such behaviors and responses may have been highly adaptive reactions to perceived danger in the past. In addition, they may reflect physical consequences of trauma exposure, and changes in cognitive beliefs triggered by such experiences. Table 36.3 lists some behaviors and cognitions that are typical of this population.

TABLE 36.3 Behaviors and Cognitions Associated With Traumatized Children

Behaviors	Cognitions, Beliefs, Mind-Set
Guarded, defensive, angry.	"The world is threatening and bewildering."
Difficult to redirect.	"The world is punitive, judgmental, humiliating, and blaming."
Dismisses support or attempts at engagement.	
Evidences intense reactivity to events.	"Control is external, not internal." Therefore, "I don't have control over my life."
Emotional outbursts appear to occur in response to seemingly unimportant events.	"People are unpredictable. Very few are to be trusted."
Outbursts are often inappropriate, offensive, and accompanied by physical aggression.	"When challenged, I must defend myself—my honor, and my self-respect. Above all else, I must defend my honor—at any price."
Has difficulty in recovering from outburst.	"If I admit a mistake, things will be worse than if I don't."
Holds on to perceived grievances or grudges.	
Unable to take personal responsibility and appears to lack insight and remorse.	
Oppositional and disruptive.	
Oversexualized behavior or loose personal boundaries.	
Seems to make the same mistakes over and over, and does not appear to learn from experience.	

Adapted from Garbarino, 1999; Hodas, 2006.

It is important for both parents and professionals to understand some of the variables that influence a child's response to traumatic exposure. Punitive and shaming interventions, rigid rules, and structure that is authoritarian are far too often characteristics of inpatient, residential, and juvenile justice milieus. Such approaches typically exacerbate behaviors of concern and alienate children from helpers and help. Such milieus are in contradistinction to respectful adult redirection and the maintaining of accountability (Mohr et al., 2009; Mohr & Pumariega, 2004). Yet such programming remains a common way of organizing therapeutic milieus; staff members resist giving up such programming despite the fact that alternate models exist and have been implemented successfully.

The provision of "trauma-informed care" is one such model that is emerging to address trauma in the lives of children, as well as adults. Trauma-informed care refers to the use of principles that include recognizing trauma and intervening early with appropriately designed interventions tailored to each individual child. As a practice and set of interventions, trauma-informed care involves professional relationships and interventions that take into account the individual's trauma history. There is no nursing care plan template for trauma-informed care. This model involves understanding the connection between presenting symptoms and behaviors and the individual's past trauma history. It involves providing services and interventions that do no harm, as opposed to such techniques as seclusion, restraints, counteraggression from staff, rigid rules, and humiliation. Characterized by individualized understanding and individualized approaches to each child, trauma-informed care promotes healing and growth by addressing the fundamental needs of persons subjected to significant trauma.

Until recently, there were few studies on trauma-informed interventions, but in the past decade, evidence-based practices incorporating this approach have been developed. For example, parent–child psychotherapy with young children exposed to violence has shown positive outcomes (Lieberman, 2005). Cohen and colleagues (2004a, 2004b) have described the use of trauma-focused cognitive–behavioral therapy (CBT) for treating childhood traumatic grief and the sequelae of sexual abuse. Others methods have offered positive data as well, such as cognitive–behavioral intervention for trauma in schools (Stein et al., 2003) and the trauma systems therapy approach (Saxe et al., 2005). A comprehensive discussion of these studies is beyond the scope of this chapter; the student is encouraged to access more information on other evidence-based treatments for childhood trauma at the website of the National Child Traumatic Stress Network (http://www.NCTSNet.org).

PARENT MANAGEMENT TRAINING AND MULTI-SYSTEMIC THERAPY. As expanded on in the later section on conduct disorder, parent management training (PMT) refers to procedures that teach parents to alter children's behavior in the home. Training reflects the idea that

problematic behavior develops inadvertently and is sustained by maladaptive parent–child interactions. Altering those interactions will reduce the problem behaviors. The goal is to replace coercive behavior with prosocial behavior in parent–child interchanges. PMT has been studied extensively and is a most promising treatment with solid supporting data. Despite the reasonably good empirical outcomes for PMT, however, it does have limitations. Some families do not learn social learning principles, some families will not implement these principles, and some families do not have the support or skills to follow through on the required "homework," which includes behavioral observation and recording and attending therapy sessions.

Multisystemic therapy (MST) is a superset of PMT that includes other factors. MST presumes that the problematic behavior is embedded within multiple systems (including the immediate family) and that these systems must be changed in order to modify behavior. MST includes contingency management, problem-solving skills therapy, and marital therapy. Treatment emphasizes problem assessment and planned intervention. MST is effective when properly implemented, and it has strong supportive evidence from multiple randomized controlled clinical trials (Type I studies) with very seriously disturbed youth. MST is more effective than hospitalization or institutionalization (Anderson et al., 2003; Henggeler et al., 1998, 1999). Limitations of MST include the fact that it is a very demanding and labor-intensive therapy for both clients and therapists. To be successful, MST must provide high-quality services across multiple areas (child, family, schools, and community).

GROUP THERAPY. Group interventions are especially helpful for adolescents because teens are more likely to accept feedback and suggestions from peers than from adults (Figure 36.7). Group therapy is less threatening than

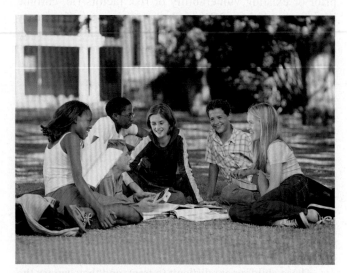

FIGURE 36.7 The peer group is of primary importance to adolescents. Thus, strategies, programs, and interventions that are group oriented can be especially successful with teens.

individual therapy and allows adolescents to identify with others who have similar problems. It provides opportunities to learn to identify and dismiss defeating cognitions and practice new behaviors. It is also cost-effective and often employed with little regard for client mix.

People with little training often lead group therapy. Questions exist about whether group therapy is appropriate for children with conduct disorder, with some scholars contending that this modality might provide an inadvertent outlet for peer reinforcement of antisocial behavior (Dishion et al., 1999). More recent literature suggests social cognitive group treatment may be efficacious in reducing aggressive behaviors associated with conduct disorder (vanManen et al., 2004). Results should be viewed with caution, however, because this study was conducted under ideal conditions with experienced group leaders. In addition, it took place in the Netherlands, a country with far greater governmental commitment to and policy support for youth well-being than the United States.

MILIEU THERAPY. Milieu therapy creates a therapeutic living environment through setting, structure, and relationships. In a therapeutic milieu, every interaction becomes an opportunity for therapeutic intervention with the child or teen. Providers model open, clear communication and supportive and respectful behavior, to give an example of cohesive adults dealing with others in healthy ways. Through the experiences of waking, dressing, eating, doing schoolwork, playing, interacting, and going to bed, children or teens can learn how to manage activities, deal with feelings, and get along with others. Inpatient milieu settings must offer safety, security, clear and reasonable limits, behavioral consequences, age-appropriate activities, and 24-hour availability from mature, caring adults. Unfortunately, because of very short lengths of stay in which children are only stabilized in inpatient settings, the notion of milieu as a healing force is becoming a thing of the past.

Milieu is an idea more prevalent in residential treatment; however, it can be less healing and more hurtful in some instances. An important contribution to the residential treatment literature is *Help at Any Cost: How the Troubled-Teen Industry Cons Parents and Hurts Kids* (Szalavitz, 2006). It is the first book to investigate and expose the troubled-teen industry that has arisen, in part, because of the lack of governmental attention paid to the mental health of children and adolescents. The rise of managed care and for-profit psychiatric hospital scandals have created a gap in the provision of pediatric mental health services at a time when the mental health field is making extraordinary progress. This gap has resulted in the growth of settings that offer distressed parents placement for their children with emotional disturbances. Many programs that purport to "treat" troubled children justify long lengths of residential stays and call their approach, in addition to milieu therapy, behavior modification schools, attitude adjustment schools, emotional growth schools, wilderness therapy programs,

attachment therapy institutes, and boot camps. Many residential facilities prey on desperate parents and cause great harm to families (Friedman et al., 2006). Scholars at the University of South Florida have formed a group that assists families with ways to evaluate residential facilities. See Client-Centered Education 36.1.

Pharmacologic Therapy

Pharmacologic therapy is an important part of any treatment program. However, medication alone does not solve all the child's or teen's problems. Combined with therapies such as family education, parent guidance, and special education, medication improves the likelihood that symptoms will decrease and functioning will improve (Green, 2007).

In 2004 the U.S. Food and Drug Administration (FDA) issued a black box warning about the use of antidepressants in children in response to reports that these drugs may increase suicidal thoughts (Schatzberg & Nemeroff, 2006). Pharmaceutical companies and the psychiatric community dispute this assertion. Nevertheless, all psychotropic medications must be administered cautiously to pediatric clients because of potentially idiosyncratic reactions (see Chap. 16).

Interdisciplinary Coordination

Many health professionals care for children and teens with psychiatric disorders. Examples include child and adolescent psychiatrists, social workers, nurse psychotherapists, testing psychologists, direct care providers, recreational therapists, psychiatric nurses, and occupational therapists (see Chap. 12). Although some areas overlap, each discipline contributes a unique service. For example, reviewing psychological testing results helps nurses develop a comprehensive picture of the client's diagnosis and condition.

TREATMENT SETTINGS AND CONTINUUM OF CARE. Treatment occurs in many different settings, from the most restrictive levels for seriously disturbed youths to outpatient resources for children with mild disabilities. Services within levels include prevention, early intervention, crisis stabilization, inpatient hospitalization, in-home crisis, residential treatment, partial hospitalization, day treatment, therapeutic foster care, case management, family support services, outpatient counseling, and medication management. Discharge planning, a collaborative process involving the client, family, and mental health team, begins with admission to any type of service.

WRAP-AROUND SERVICES AND SYSTEMS OF CARE. Since the early 1990s, several initiatives to improve coordination among the agencies that provide services for children with emotional and behavioral disabilities and their families have been implemented. In the past, these were called "wrap-around services." Current structures of service provision replacing the old models are called systems of care. The term **systems of care** refers to a comprehensive

Client–Centered Education 36.1

Warnings for Families Considering a Child's Residential Placement

Experts recommend that families beware of residential programs that:

1. Are not state licensed/accredited for *all* (1) educational, (2) mental health, *and* (3) residential aspects
2. Claim to be able to assess and make recommendations by Internet or phone and then urge parents to "act now" to prevent serious harm
3. Recommend or support private "escort" or "transport" services to take children to the program
4. Do not respect the family's wisdom and expertise. For example, they do not allow family visitation and meetings with staff before admission; tell parents to expect that children will lie to them while in the program; encourage parents not to believe reports of abuse; and discourage parental participation and feedback from children.
5. Restrict youth and family rights in terms of private contact with one another, child dress code, typical age-appropriate behavior, parental rights, and hotlines for youth and families to call at any time if they feel that their rights are being violated or they are being mistreated
6. Use harsh and excessive discipline: seclusion, restraint, corporal punishment, fear tactics, humiliation, peer-on-peer discipline, forced labor, sleep deprivation, or sedation by medication

7. Provide substandard therapeutic intervention. For example, they do not have individualized programs or offer therapies or supports recognized as most effective for the main problem, or they involve children with varying problems or do not have full-time licensed mental health professionals on staff.
8. Provide substandard education (eg, unlicensed teachers, high student:teacher ratios)
9. Admit youths with psychiatric diagnoses, but do not provide appropriate medical treatment
10. Require parents to sign contracts with unreasonable terms
11. Have been reported, investigated, or cited by at least one source for:
    • Unsanitary or unsafe living conditions
    • Nutritionally compromised diets
    • Exposing youth to extreme environmental conditions or physical overexertion
    • Lack of supervision by staff (low staff:youth ratio)
    • Medical neglect
    • Physical or sexual abuse of youths by program staff or by other program youths
    • Violation of youth/family rights

Adapted from University of South Florida. (2005). *A parent's checklist.* Retrieved from: http://astart.fmhi
.usf.edu/AStartDocs/factsheet.pdf.

---

spectrum of mental health and other necessary services organized into a coordinated network that changes with the needs of children and families. Integral to the systems-of-care concept is the belief that parents are full partners in the therapy and care of their children and are included in decisions about needed services (Anderson et al., 2003). Services may come from public or private mental health care, education, and juvenile justice (see Chap. 20).

COMMUNITY-RELATED FOCI. Estimates are that up to 20% of youths in juvenile justice facilities have serious mental illness and need immediate treatment (National Center for Mental Health and Juvenile Justice, 2006). School-based services, such as assessments of the child's emotional and academic status and educational modifications, are critical when a pediatric client has mental illness. In addition, many teens with psychiatric disorders, who are at risk for dropping out of school, require career services. These children and adolescents require coordination with mental health personnel and intensive and comprehensive case management.

SPECIAL EDUCATION. Children or adolescents with mental illness have the same developmental strivings as all youths: they want to succeed in school and take pride in their accomplishments. A dilemma for many schools is

how to manage disruptive behaviors while teaching academics. The goals of special education for youths with mental illness are to decrease disturbing behaviors, increase the rate of learning to enable children to remediate and progress, and reintegrate children into regular classes as soon as possible.

An essential classroom technique for those with psychiatric challenges is to maintain a high degree of structure. Clear expectations and defined limits diminish anxiety. Another valuable approach is to maximize group cohesion and peer influence in class. Because youths with mental illness typically have experienced little success with school, they may find it difficult to approach class work positively. The teacher's task is to help such children become motivated about learning (Figure 36.8). Coordination and collaboration among school and other care systems is critical.

General Nursing Care for Pediatric Clients With Psychiatric Disorders

Generally, all nursing care begins with assessment. Certain interventions apply in a wide variety of circumstances. The following sections focus on essentials of psychiatric–mental health nursing assessment for children and interventions that address common needs or clinical situations.

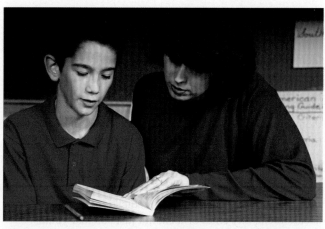

FIGURE 36.8 When working with children who have psychological, developmental, or emotional challenges, teachers must be creative in finding ways to motivate these students to learn and to succeed.

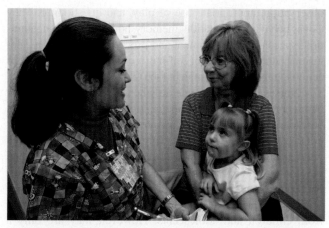

FIGURE 36.9 Nurses should include assessment of the family as part of the psychiatric evaluation of the child to ensure that expectations and perceptions are realistic and that adults have appropriate knowledge of their child's growth and development parameters.

Assessment

Assessment sets the tone for the entire nursing interaction. Nurses begin by welcoming clients and family and clarify that everyone is involved in treatment, not just the identified child or teen. Parents often worry that they "did something" to cause their child's problem. Nurses allow time to answer family members' questions, support their desire to be good parents, alleviate fears and guilt, and provide accurate information and teaching. Explaining that multiple factors contribute to mental disorders is helpful. Information from several informants, such as teachers and grandparents, gives a fuller picture of the issues.

FAMILY FUNCTIONING. *Family assessment*, usually performed before assessment of the client, reinforces the concept that everyone is involved in and expected to work on the identified problem. Nurses ask open-ended questions such as "How are things for this family?" This form of questioning allows the family members to respond with whatever information they wish to share; it gives nurses and other providers some insight into relatives' perceptions of the problem.

Nurses also assess family relationships, concern for one another, roles, empathy, decision making, and degree of autonomy or enmeshment. They elicit how family members view the child and whether their perceptions are unrealistic or grounded in knowledge of growth and development (Figure 36.9). For example, some parents erroneously think that an infant cries on purpose to "get back at the parent" or that a 7-year-old boy should be "the little man of the family."

CURRENT PROBLEM. Initial data include the nature, severity, and length of the *current problem* and any significant concomitant events. Nurses always ask, "How upsetting is this problem to the child and family?" and "Does anything make this problem better or worse?" It is essential to obtain parents' descriptions of the child's behavior at home,

to evaluate the child's response to discipline, and to learn whether the child is violent or defiant, cares about the rights of others, or has severe behavior problems (eg, cruelty to animals, fire-setting).

HISTORY. Nurses investigate and document responses in the following areas:

* *Previous treatment:* Type, length, and outcomes; testing results and diagnoses
* *Family history:* Any medical and mental health problem or symptoms in immediate and extended family members
* *Developmental history:* Prenatal history (maternal health or illness, substance use, or physical abuse), neonatal history (birth complications), and developmental milestones (sitting, walking, talking, self-care)
* *Social history:* Names, ages, and relationships of people with whom the child lives; relationships with parents, siblings, other relatives, and peers; activities or hobbies; legal charges against the child
* *Abuse history:* Exposure to physical, sexual, or emotional abuse, whether CPS was notified, and any treatment; exposure to family or community violence
* *Chemical history:* Use of substances by the child or adolescent, as well as by parents and other caretakers
* *Medical history:* History of seizures, head injuries, acute illnesses, other injuries and accidents, surgeries, loss of consciousness, asthma and other chronic illnesses, and vision and hearing deficits; current *medications*, their effects and side effects, and the names and effects of prior medications; *allergies*—drug, food, and seasonal
* *School history:* Current grade, regular or special education, any learning difficulties, and any behavior problems in school

MENTAL STATUS EXAMINATION. Nurses conduct the mental status examination of a child or adolescent through observation, appropriate use of play, and questioning. They assess behavior, orientation, memory, attention and concentration, speech, thought content and process, hallucinations, delusions, suicidal ideation, self-harm or homicidal thinking or actions, judgment, and insight (see Chap. 10) (Falsafi, 2001).

Nurses ask what clients do when they are angry, sad, or happy and try to elicit their perception of their behavior. It is best to ask children or teens privately about any drug or alcohol use and abuse experiences (Figure 36.10). Often children will respond, "I hit," "I kick," "I cry," or "I go to my room and play video games," which are indications of their coping skills. Nurses note any neurologic signs for further exploration.

Drawings are helpful tools for gathering information from children and adolescents. However, they are only a communication *tool*, and nurses must take care not to over-interpret what a child has drawn. In addition, children tell their stories through games and toys, especially when they have limited vocabularies to communicate their feelings.

PHYSICAL EXAMINATION. A complete physical examination should be done to rule out any nonpsychiatric condition that may be responsible for the client's problem or contributing to compromised mental health.

Interventions

Nursing interventions for pediatric clients with mental disorders vary for individual diagnoses, symptomatology, care settings, resources, and needs. The next several paragraphs highlight nursing roles and responsibilities that are consistently and generally applicable to all children/teens with psychiatric problems and their families.

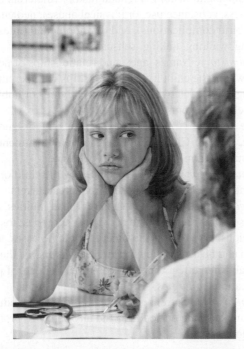

FIGURE 36.10 Nurses should conduct a private interview with the child or teen to discuss sensitive issues such as drug or alcohol use and abuse.

PROVIDING MEDICATION EDUCATION. Few psychotropic medications have FDA approval for use in children (Green, 2007). However, clinicians prescribe several of them "off label" because experience has proven them effective in treating mental illnesses in this age group.

Nurses should explain in simple terms the chemical basis for treating a disorder. Parents, other caregivers, and clients themselves (if mature enough to understand) need information about the medication, its purpose and intended effects, how to administer it, side effects, and what to do if dangerous effects develop. Nurses should also discuss the importance of keeping the medication in a safe and secure place to which only adults have access. These medications should never be accessible to any child or teen, not just suicidal youths.

Encouragement of honesty and openness about medication adherence is important. Clients may refuse to take their medicine or may throw it away for several reasons. In addition, some children believe that medications are punishment for bad behavior. Sometimes children agree to a time-limited trial of medication. At other times, parents may decide not to adhere to a prescribing schedule out of fear, misinformation, or a belief system incompatible with pharmacotherapy for children. Therefore, teaching about psychotropic medications for children, adolescents, and parents is an important nursing action to promote accuracy and adherence with prescribed dosing schedules.

It is also important to teach about drug–drug and herb–drug interactions. Some families think that because they can buy St. John's wort and other products over the counter, such agents must be "safe." However, these products can have dangerous interactions with prescribed medications (see Chap. 16).

MEETING FAMILIES' NEEDS. Families need support, continuity of care, and information about their child's diagnosis and treatment, as well as how to help. Parents may have other concerns, such as future planning for the child's care, feeling helpless about their child's condition, wanting to become an advocate for the child, respite, involvement in the school, financial support, and meeting the needs of siblings and themselves (Elder, 2001).

Evidence has shown that, despite efforts at education, nurses and other mental health care providers are not doing a stellar job at instructing families. One study found that parents of children with pervasive developmental delay thought that their child's behavior was the result of his or her wanting "attention" or "to test people." They did not understand their child's frustration at being unable to communicate wants and needs (Elder, 2001).

Children and their families need accurate information about their disorder and its treatment. Education should focus on correcting inaccurate beliefs and teaching ways to promote development and manage problems (Elder, 2001). Nurses should teach parents that children with biologically based risk factors for disorders such as ADHD are likely to be more vulnerable to negative self-perceptions as they develop and require extra support (Krueger & Kendall, 2001).

Teens and their families need to know that more biologic, psychological, and social role changes occur in adolescence than in any other life stage except infancy. Parents can help by being responsive to teens' needs for increasing responsibility and decision-making power while maintaining family cohesiveness.

PROMOTING THE RIGHTS OF CHILDREN IN TREATMENT SETTINGS. In 1999, the Association of Child and Adolescent Psychiatric Nurses (ACAPN), a division of the International Society of Psychiatric Nurses (ISPN), published a position paper on the rights of children in treatment settings (Nursing Spotlight 36.1).

The ISPN has also issued a position paper on the use of restraint and seclusion within treatment settings for all age groups; the paper espouses the rights of clients to be free of mechanical and chemical restraints (see Chap. 32). The first responsibility of nursing staff is prevention of use of restraint. The second step toward reducing aggression, similar to working with adults, is verbal intervention. If that fails, an alternative to seclusion and restraint for children may be what is euphemistically termed therapeutic holding. *Therapeutic holding* involves holding a client in a supported position for a brief period until he or she regains control to manage aggressive and self-injurious behavior (Berrios & Jacobowitz, 1998). A benefit of the technique is that parents can learn it to manage their child's behavior at home. However, it must be noted that therapeutic holding has also been associated with injury and death in children when used improperly. Indeed The Joint Commission (1998) did a root cause analysis

---

> ◢◣ **NURSING SPOTLIGHT 36.1** ◢◣
>
> ### Rights of Pediatric Clients in Health Care Settings
>
> Children have the following rights:
>
> - To be treated with dignity and not to be abused or mistreated in any way
> - To receive treatment in the least restrictive setting
> - To be free of physical restraints unless every other method to provide safety for the child and others has been tried and failed; if use of restraints or seclusion is necessary, children should never be left alone during that restriction of their freedom
> - To be treated in a developmentally appropriate way
> - To receive an individualized treatment plan that includes aftercare or follow-up measures
> - To have access to an advocacy group
> - To expect confidentiality and access to their records (ACAPN, 1999)
>
> Association of Child and Adolescent Psychiatric Nurses (ACAPN), division of the International Society of Psychiatric Nurses (ISPN). (1999). *A position on the rights of children in treatment settings.* Retrieved from http://www.ispn-psych.org/docs/children.pdf.

---

of restraint deaths on 21 clients reported under their sentinel event criteria. Of those clients, 30% died as a result of a "therapeutic hold." Therefore, parents require proper training before using this technique (Mohr & Anderson, 2001).

AVOIDING SECLUSION AND RESTRAINT. Although formerly seen as acceptable ways to deal with crises and keep clients and staff safe, seclusion and restraint are no longer interventions that nurses commonly use or encounter in inpatient settings. Restraint provides immediate containment of disruptive behavior, but limits client freedom. In addition, children view restraints as aversive and traumatic (Mohr et al., 1998). The use of restraints can also be dangerous to both staff members and clients, resulting in injury and death (Mohr et al., 2003). In particular, the metabolic syndrome resulting from some psychotropic medications can cause abdominal adiposity that makes prone restraint very dangerous. Such children are at particular risk for asphyxia from interference with the bellows action of the lungs. Death can come to such children within minutes (Siebert & Thogmartin, 2000).

Because of the misuse of restraints and subsequent related deaths, regulatory agencies since 2002 have tightly monitored the use of restraints. They have also curtailed the circumstances under which restraints are employed. Unfortunately they are still misused and children continue to die from their misuse (Nunno et al., 2006).

From the client's viewpoint, seclusion is a negative and overused intervention. Clients have described their experience in seclusion as feeling neglected, fearful, isolated, out of control, vulnerable, bad, and punished. No evidence has shown that seclusion or restraint leads to positive behavior change. Other interventions, such as instituting time-out, avoiding power struggles, talking with staff, listening to music, writing, or drawing may help children and teens de-escalate and calm down more effectively (Martinez et al., 1999).

PROVIDING ADVOCACY. The child is not a miniature adult, but a developing person in a family system. A child's concerns are those of any individual in an emotional and often confusing world. Children have legal rights and physical and emotional needs. In recent decades, the courts have expanded the rights of children and affirmed that they have many of the constitutional rights of adults (see Chap. 5).

> **Checkpoint Questions**
>
> 3. What are three protective factors in children that can increase their resistance to stress?
> 4. What two types of therapy are often used with individual therapy?
> 5. What are three goals of special education for youths with mental illness?
> 6. What is an alternative to seclusion and restraint for a child with aggression when verbal intervention fails?

COMMON PSYCHIATRIC DISORDERS OF CHILDREN AND ADOLESCENTS

Many psychiatric illnesses affect children and adolescents. Some of these disorders primarily are identified during infancy, childhood, or adolescence. Others are diagnosed across the lifespan, but manifestations, treatments, or both for children and adolescents may differ from those for adults. The disorders discussed in this section include the most common types from each category affecting children and teens.

DISRUPTIVE BEHAVIOR DISORDERS

Three disruptive behavior disorders commonly are seen in children and adolescents. They are ADHD, oppositional-defiant disorder (ODD), and conduct disorder.

Attention Deficit/Hyperactivity Disorder

Attention deficit/hyperactivity disorder (ADHD) is characterized by inattention, impulsivity, and hyperactivity. It is diagnosed through comprehensive clinical evaluation, as well as parents' and teachers' ratings of inattention, hyperactivity, and impulsivity. Approximately 5% to 12% of the population has ADHD, which runs in families (NIMH, 2006). If a child has ADHD, the chance of a sibling having ADHD is 30%; if a parent has ADHD, the risk for a child may be as high as 25% to 50% (Harmon, 2000).

Etiology

The complex etiology most likely involves genetic and environmental factors. Studies have found strong genetic influences and familial transmission (Spetie & Arnold, 2007). Magnetic resonance imaging studies have identified differences in brain function in clients with ADHD.

Signs and Symptoms/Diagnostic Criteria

Primary symptoms of ADHD are inattention and hyperactivity or impulsivity (*DSM-IV-TR* Box 36.1).

Common manifestations in children and adolescents include forgetting to do or to turn in homework; failing to hear or follow directions; daydreaming during school and at times when attention is required; talking excessively and inappropriately; constantly moving and climbing; not remaining seated during class or meals; taking extraordinary risks; and losing objects, particularly those needed for schoolwork, such as books, pencils, and paper. These symptoms eventually lead to poor performance or failure in school. Adolescents tend to have more inattentive and impulsive symptoms than hyperactivity and, therefore, may be ignored, underdiagnosed, and undertreated. Children

with ADHD also grow up with stigma and negative feedback from others about their behavior. As a result, they may view themselves as stupid, frustrated, "messing up," helpless, and worthless (Krueger & Kendall, 2001).

Most children with ADHD do not "grow out of it." The disorder continues into adulthood for at least 50% of diagnosed youth and causes impairment in 11% of them (NIMH, 2006). Teens and adults who seem to no longer have the same level of problems they had when younger most likely learned various compensatory and coping skills to help them increase focus and maintain attention during tasks.

Adults with ADHD may have a history of poor performance at work and school, inattention, distractibility, restlessness, procrastination, disorganization, impulsive behavior, and driving problems. They have a higher-than-average risk for drug and alcohol abuse and accompanying legal problems (Feinberg, 2000; NIMH, 2006).

Comorbidities

Comorbid psychiatric conditions often accompany ADHD, especially when untreated, in both children and adults. These include ODD, conduct disorder, depressive disorders, early-onset substance abuse disorders, and learning disorders (Kessler et al., 2005).

Interdisciplinary Goals and Treatment

The two treatment modalities endorsed by the American Academy of Child and Adolescent Psychiatry (1997) and the American Academy of Pediatrics (2001) are behavioral treatment and FDA-approved sympathomimetic agents (stimulants and atomoxetine). Behavioral treatments are based on learning theory (see Chap. 3). Parent management training and problem-solving skills training have also been found useful for ADHD (see Evidence-Based Practice Spotlight 36.1) (Spetie & Arnold, 2007). Medication in conjunction with other treatments is more effective than medication alone. The goals are to improve self-regulation and social functioning.

Behavioral Treatment and Other Psychosocial Interventions

Nonpharmacologic interventions include behavior therapy, education for client and family, organizational coaching, and supports at school and home. Behavior therapy refers to a wide range of interventions designed to diminish disruptive and encourage desirable behaviors. It is based on the idea that people repeat rewarded behaviors and abandon actions that generate negative consequences (see Chap. 3). Any behavior typically associated with ADHD, such as not completing tasks, interrupting, or using aggression, can be the target of behavioral therapy.

One school system uses specially trained, paraprofessional classroom aides who design and implement a behavioral program for struggling students. Adolescents may benefit from behavior management and cognitive therapy

Case in Point 36.1 (continued)

Michael's Story

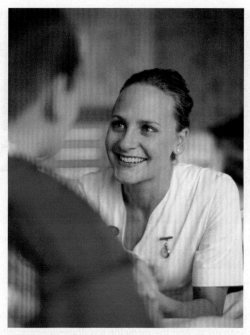

FIGURE E. The nurse works with Michael to discuss communication, body language, and social skills that help encourage friendships and positive responses from others.

- Discuss with the client how aggression affects others. Review how body language and facial expressions are clues to feelings (Figure E). Encourage respect for the rights of others and honesty in presenting oneself to others. Help him increase his awareness of strengths and limitations in communicating. *Increasing the client's sensitivity to others and teaching him how to interpret nonverbal communication provide tools for more effective interactions with his peers.*

NIC: Therapeutic Play
- Provide a quiet environment free from interruptions. *Such an atmosphere allows the child to focus on the task at hand.*
- Provide sufficient time for effective play; structure play session to facilitate the desired outcome. *Sufficient time is necessary to prevent overwhelming the child. Effective play enhances positive feelings of self-esteem.*
- Promote activities that require the child to use energy productively and focus on skills and accomplishments (Figure F). *Finding and focusing on a child's strengths promote a sense of self-pride.*
- Encourage the child to share feelings, knowledge, and perceptions. Validate and communicate acceptance of feelings he expresses during play. *Play helps the child communicate his perception of the world and gain mastery of his environment.*
- Facilitate interactions with other children as appropriate; provide positive reinforcement for effective interactions (Figure G). *Such interactions help the child become more aware of behaviors and their effects on others. Positive reinforcement promotes a more positive self-image.*

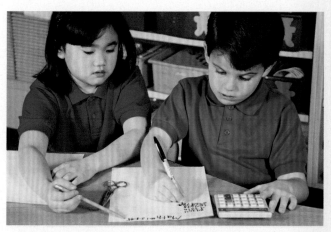

FIGURE F. The teacher sets up cooperative mathematics projects for Michael because it is a subject for which he shows aptitude and enjoys. Being able to work successfully in this subject area strengthens Michael's self-esteem, sense of accomplishment, and social competence.

- Develop a reward system based on a daily report from the client's teacher. For example, the client can earn tokens for each day he comes home with a good report on behavior with classmates. He can later trade the tokens for time on the computer or some other preferred activity (Figure H). *Establishing a reward system will reinforce positive behaviors.*

> 1/12/14: The client demonstrates appropriate social skills in his interactions with others. He demonstrates consideration of and sensitivity to others; use of compromise; ability to share and wait turns; improved daily reports of in-school behavior; decreased aggression; and satisfaction and enjoyment with play.
>
> Lily Zinoviev, RN, MSN

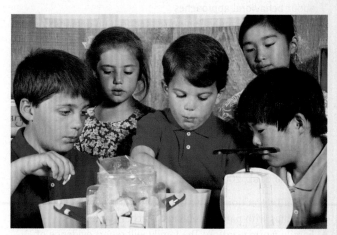

FIGURE G. Michael's treatment regimen allows him to participate more effectively in group projects and classroom activities.

(continues on page 802)

Case in Point 36.1 (continued)

Michael's Story

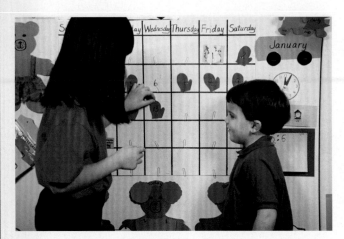

FIGURE H. Michael enjoys reviewing his behavior calendar and seeing his progress.

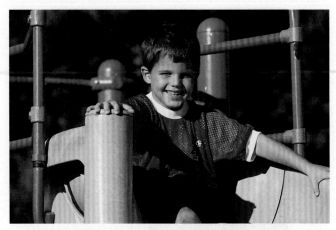

FIGURE I. After 3 months taking his medicine and adhering to his overall management plan, Michael is a happier and healthier boy.

EPILOGUE

It has been 3 months since Michael was first diagnosed with ADHD. His parents report that they have been implementing the behavioral strategies consistently and with good results. His father states, "His teacher has been great. And the medicine has done wonders. What a difference! His school performance has improved and he has being getting along so well with classmates." Michael continues to take methylphenidate three times a day with no evidence of side effects (Figure I).

▲ NURSING DIAGNOSIS

Diagnoses focus on the psychosocial, developmental, and academic side effects of living with ADHD, as well as on family issues that often arise. Appropriate diagnoses include the following (NANDA, 2007):

- Impaired Social Interaction related to behaviors associated with ADHD
- Ineffective Family Therapeutic Regimen Management related to high demands on family and insufficient knowledge about behavioral approaches
- Compromised Family Coping related to high demands on family and insufficient knowledge
- Risk for Delayed Development related to the effects of ADHD
- Chronic Low Self-Esteem related to the social dynamics of having ADHD

▲ OUTCOME IDENTIFICATION AND PLANNING

Goals vary with the client's specific circumstances. Some identified desired outcomes, organized according to the *Nursing Outcomes Classification (NOC)*, might include the following (Moorhead et al., 2008):

- Social Interaction Skills: The client will report improved relationships with parents, siblings, teachers, and peers.
- Family Normalization: The family will report evidence of increased independence by the child in age-appropriate self-care and other responsibilities.

- Family Coping: The family will report improved ability to cope with the child's illness and improved understanding of treatment strategies.
- Hyperactivity Level: The family will express decreased disruptive behaviors and improved academic performance on the part of the child.
- Self-Esteem: The client will verbalize an improved opinion of himself or herself.

▲ IMPLEMENTATION

Nurses use many types of interventions to assist clients with ADHD and their families. Common *Nursing Interventions Classification (NIC)* labels related to management of ADHD may include, but are not limited to, **Behavior Management: Overactivity/Inattention; Behavior Modification: Social Skills; Coping Enhancement; Developmental Enhancement: Child, Family; Involvement Promotion; Self-Esteem Enhancement;** and **Sibling Support** (Bulechek et al., 2008).

Teaching Social Skills

Various groups successfully advocated for the inclusion of children with mild and moderate disabilities in general classrooms. Such inclusion has benefits and risks for children with ADHD. Positively, they get to experience the same educational environment as their peers. Negatively, they may be subjected to social pressures and possibly ridicule from those same peers.

Teaching children with ADHD social skills and strategies is integral to their ability to maintain friendships. Childhood social skills include waiting for a turn, maintaining a conversation, sharing toys, asking for help, responding to teasing, playing cooperatively, handling frustration without aggression, apologizing, and showing concern for others (Figure 36.11). Many children with ADHD do not attend well to verbal and nonverbal communication (ie, they do not "read" facial expressions or interpret tone of voice and language subtleties). Although most children intuitively acquire these skills early (albeit to varying degrees), children with ADHD need specific instruction and ample opportunities to practice them.

Nurses can coach parents in helping children develop social skills or facilitate interactions with peers. In turn, such efforts will help clients become more aware of their behaviors and resulting effects on others. Social skills instruction should focus on one area at a time. For example, the parents (or group facilitator) may choose hitting as a behavior or apologizing as a skill. Children can role-play or act out a scenario involving the target behavior. A discussion should follow in which adults ask the child what happened, why he or she thinks it happened, how he or she felt, and what else might have been said or done. The role-playing can be videotaped and shown to the child to facilitate insight into the social situation. As the child progresses in one area, parents can then shift the focus to others.

Additional strategies include developing a reward system (discussed next) or creating a script for anticipated social situations, such as being wrongly accused of bad behavior, losing lunch money, or accidentally hurting someone. Practice and feedback from parents, teachers, siblings, and peers are fundamental to the success of teaching social skills.

Educating the Family

Nurses must educate parents and children about how ADHD affects learning, development, behavior, self-esteem, social skills, and family function. They must also teach the family how to develop and implement behavioral strategies and manage medications. Thorough understanding of the problem on the part of the family is essential before discussing treatment options. Nurses enhance the success of treatment when they address cultural values during education.

When assisting families with behavioral strategies, nurses must emphasize to parents the importance of focusing on only one or two behaviors at a time. They can teach a common technique that relies on positive reinforcement: earning "points" or "tokens" for good behaviors. Children can trade in a specific number of points for a reward, such as playing a computer game (Figure 36.12). Each family needs to develop its own system; however, rewards should not cost money, entail food, or manipulate parental time. Generally, the rewards should be everyday activities that children enjoy—bike riding, playing outdoors, watching television—and will miss if withheld. Nurses should inform parents to:

- Provide specific instruction about the desired behavior. They should not use a blanket statement such as "Obey me." Rather, they should give specific direction such as "Stay seated during dinner."
- Use short-term rewards. For example, a reward later in the day for good behavior now is more tangible than an incentive on the weekend for good behavior on Tuesday.
- Praise the child; give frequent reminders about the desired behavior and provide feedback.
- Let the child help choose the rewards. Parents should expect to change rewards when the child becomes bored with that incentive.
- Allow for early successes. As behavior improves, the measure for earning the reward can be increased gradually.
- Be consistent! Inconsistency will undermine the program and the child's trust.

Whereas parents use positive reinforcement to encourage desirable behavior, they can use negative consequences to reduce misbehavior. Again, consistency is key. If undesired behaviors lead to negative consequences only sometimes,

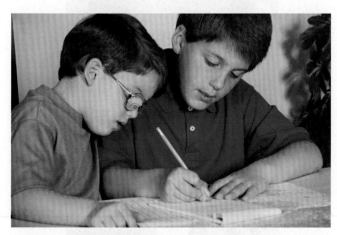

FIGURE 36.11 Children with ADHD often struggle with social skills as a result of their illness. Nurses, parents, and others involved in care can reinforce the need for these children to wait for turns in play, share, cooperate, apologize for mistakes, and show concern for others.

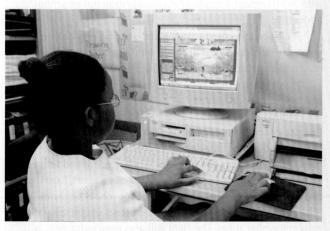

FIGURE 36.12 This child with ADHD follows a behavioral technique of trading in "points" that she has accumulated each day for appropriate actions and responses to be used on playing computer games.

children will continue them. Parents can use typical disciplinary consequences, such as forfeiting a planned activity, initiating time-out, or taking away television or computer time. Additionally, they can forfeit points a child has earned toward a reward for good behavior. As with the plan for earning rewards, parents should be specific about which negative behavior they are targeting, clearly define the consequences, and give frequent feedback and reminders.

Some children with ADHD may become defiant and angry when confronted with negative consequences; they may also simply refuse to perform the desired behavior. It is important to encourage parents not to relent. If they do so, children will learn that opposition and defiance achieve desired outcomes, thus reinforcing the original behavior *and* opposition and defiance.

Helping Families Cope

All types of chronic illness place emotional, physical, financial, and spiritual stress on families. Relatives of children with ADHD may experience disrupted routines and the strain of caregiving. Clients may victimize siblings, who may feel unprotected because parents are too emotionally overwhelmed to handle the situation appropriately. Chronic sorrow, worry, and sense of loss at being unable to enjoy a "normal" family life are also reported (Kendall, 1999).

Nurses can teach family coping skills, such as suggesting that parents make special time for themselves and for other children and encouraging everyone to verbalize feelings. All family members can learn relaxation techniques (see Chap. 17). Siblings may benefit from assertiveness skills or other appropriate social techniques for improving interactions with children who have ADHD.

Managing Developmental and Academic Issues

ADHD may be diagnosed after a child enters a structured educational program (ie, preschool, elementary school). The classroom environment usually requires children to sit still, patiently take turns, pay attention, and stay on task. Children with ADHD have difficulty doing these things, drawing attention to their disorder and compromising learning. As a result, many students with ADHD repeat a grade or eventually drop out of school altogether.

Poor academic performance and ongoing negative assessments thwart feelings of accomplishment and independence, resulting in pervasive feelings of low self-worth and failure. Classroom intervention is critical to children's social, academic, and developmental success.

Strategies to suggest to parents to help their children in the classroom include requesting that the child sit in an area with limited distractions (closer to the teacher), have a designated place to move around freely when needed, and follow a system of rules and rewards for desirable behaviors. Keeping a picture on the desk with specific rules for school behavior (eg, raising a hand and being called on before speaking) will help the child remember them. The child will also need extra help with directions. Reviewing directions, listing the materials that will be needed, and breaking down tasks into smaller components

helps disorganized, inattentive children focus on and complete schoolwork.

Improving Self-Esteem

Some but not all children can use help to improve their self-esteem. For example, children with conduct disorders often manifest high self-esteem (see Chap. 4). However, children whom peers perceive as being delayed in some areas or "different" frequently endure emotional attacks that can damage their self-esteem. Children with ADHD are frequently the targets of negative assessments ("Can't you pay attention?" "He loses everything!" "She's disrupting the entire class."). They internalize opinions from others and form similar opinions of themselves, leading to negative self-assessments and poor self-esteem. Additionally, all the problems discussed previously—disruptive behavior, lack of social skills, poor academic performance—exacerbate feelings of inferiority.

Implementing a behavioral program that helps children gain self-control and skills, use energy productively, and garner praise and rewards will help them mold a more positive self-image. Determining strengths, perhaps in sports or creative arts, and focusing on skills and accomplishments in that arena provide other sources of self-pride (Figure 36.13).

▲ EVALUATION

The family needs to understand that achieving the goals of treatment takes time and that therapeutic approaches will need to continue throughout childhood and adolescence. Indeed, clients with ADHD will continue to use strategies for overcoming their disorder into adulthood. Nevertheless, parents and teachers should see incremental improvement as long as they

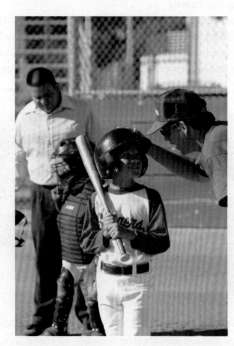

FIGURE 36.13 Success in sports, arts, or other areas can boost the self-esteem and confidence of children who struggle academically because of ADHD.

implement behavioral strategies consistently. Indicators that the plan of care is effective include the following:

- The client can maintain friendships.
- Family functioning improves according to family report.
- The client's academic performance improves.
- The client can better manage responsibilities.
- The client experiences improved views of himself or herself.

Oppositional-Defiant Disorder

Oppositional-defiant disorder (ODD) is marked by negativistic, defiant behaviors such as stubbornness, resistance to directions, and unwillingness to negotiate with adults or peers (*DSM-IV-TR* Box 36.2).

Clients with ODD persistently test limits, usually by ignoring rules, arguing, or failing to accept responsibility for behavior. They direct hostility at adults or peers through verbal aggression or deliberately annoying actions. They do not see themselves as defiant, but justify their behavior as a response to unreasonable demands. Symptoms may be present at home, but not seen at school.

ODD is one of the more common disorders seen in adolescents, although children have also it. Prevalence rates range from 6% to 10% (Tynan, 2006b). ODD is more common in boys before puberty, but equally prevalent in both sexes after puberty; symptoms are generally more confrontational and persistent in boys (Tynan, 2006b). Comorbidities include ADHD, depression, or learning problems. The etiology of ODD is unknown; however, there is a complex relationship between ODD and conduct disorder, for which risk factors are discussed below.

School-age children with ODD are likely to exhibit mood lability, low frustration tolerance, swearing, precocious substance abuse, and interpersonal conflicts. Parents and affected clients often bring out the worst in one another.

Youth with ODD are at risk for conduct disorder. Although teens are typically oppositional, those with ODD show more severe behaviors with more serious consequences and impairments in home, school, and social functioning.

Behavior modification techniques are effective in changing behaviors and violations of safety (eg, curfew violations, failure to report whereabouts). Family therapy can improve communication between parents and children. Medication is used to treat comorbidities such as ADHD and depression. The nurse's role in caring for the child with ODD does not differ substantially from his or her interventions in children with ADHD (see earlier discussion).

Conduct Disorder

Adolescents with *conduct disorder* are often unmanageable at home and disruptive in the community. They have little empathy or concern for others. They may be callous and lack appropriate feelings of guilt, although they may express remorse superficially to avoid punishment. They often blame others for their actions. Risk-taking behaviors such as drinking, smoking, using illegal substances, experimenting with sex, and participating in crime are typical. Cruelty to animals or people, destruction of property, theft, and serious violation of rules are diagnostic criteria (*DSM-IV-TR* Box 36.3).

Onset is usually late childhood or early adolescence. Conduct disorder in adolescents is seen frequently in mental

---

DSM-IV-TR BOX 36.2

Oppositional-Defiant Disorder

A. A pattern of negativistic, hostile, and defiant behavior lasting at least 6 months, during which four (or more) of the following are present:
  1. often loses temper
  2. often argues with adults
  3. often actively defies or refuses to comply with adults' requests or rules
  4. often deliberately annoys people
  5. often blames others for his or her mistakes or misbehavior
  6. is often touchy or easily annoyed by others
  7. is often angry and resentful
  8. is often spiteful or vindictive

Note: *Consider a criterion met only if the behavior occurs more frequently than is typically observed in individuals of comparable age and developmental level.*

B. The disturbance in behavior causes clinically significant impairment in social, academic, or occupational functioning.

C. The behaviors do not occur exclusively during the course of a Psychotic or Mood Disorder.

D. Criteria are not met for Conduct Disorder, and, if the individual is age 18 years or older, criteria are not met for Antisocial Personality Disorder.

DSM-IV-TR BOX 36.3

Conduct Disorder

A. A repetitive and persistent pattern of behavior in which the basic rights of others or major age-appropriate societal norms or rules are violated, as manifested by the presence of three (or more) of the following criteria in the past 12 months, with at least one criterion present in the past 6 months:

Aggression to people and animals
1. often bullies, threatens, or intimidates others
2. often initiates physical fights
3. has used a weapon that can cause serious physical harm to others (e.g., a bat, brick, broken bottle, knife, gun)
4. has been physically cruel to people
5. has been physically cruel to animals
6. has stolen while confronting a victim (e.g., mugging, purse snatching, extortion, armed robbery)
7. has forced someone into sexual activity

Destruction of property
8. has deliberately engaged in fire setting with the intention of causing serious damage
9. has deliberately destroyed others' property (other than by fire setting)

Deceitfulness or theft
10. has broken into someone else's house, building, or car
11. often lies to obtain goods or favors or to avoid obligations (i.e., "cons" others)
12. has stolen items of nontrivial value without confronting a victim (e.g., shoplifting, but without breaking and entering; forgery)

Serious violations of rules
13. often stays out at night despite parental prohibitions, beginning before age 13 years
14. has run away from home overnight at least twice while living in parental or parental surrogate home (or once without returning for a lengthy period)
15. is often truant from school, beginning before age 13 years

B. The disturbance in behavior causes clinically significant impairment in social, academic, or occupational functioning.

C. If the individual is age 18 years or older, criteria are not met for Antisocial Personality Disorder.

Reprinted with permission from *the Diagnostic and Statistical Manual of Mental Disorders, Fourth Edition, Text Revision* (Copyright © 2000). American Psychiatric Association.

health treatment centers. Prevalence rates range from 2% to 9% (Tynan, 2006a). A youth with conduct disorder may have comorbid ADHD, ODD, learning disorders, depression, anxiety disorders, or substance abuse. Risk factors for conduct disorder include physical and sexual abuse, inconsistent parenting with harsh discipline, lack of supervision, early institutional living or out-of-home placement, association with a delinquent peer group, and parental substance abuse.

Conduct disorder is exceedingly difficult with a very guarded prognosis. Behavioral techniques may reduce some symptoms; however, their application requires great consistency. Aggression and impulsivity can be treated with several medications, including the atypical antipsychotics, lithium, and other mood stabilizers such as valproic acid (see Chap. 16). Parent management training (PMT) has shown the greatest promise in treating conduct disorder (Frick & Dickens, 2006; Woolfenden et al., 2006). See Evidence-Based Practice Spotlight 36.2, which contains further information about PMT and additional references.

The nurse's role in caring for children with conduct disorder does not differ substantially from intervention for children with ADHD (see earlier discussion).

ADJUSTMENT DISORDERS

An **adjustment disorder** is marked by clinically or behaviorally significant symptoms within 3 months of the onset of an identifiable stressor. Stress temporarily overwhelms the client's capacity to solve problems, resulting in impaired functioning.

The course of an adjustment disorder may be acute or chronic. It may accompany depression, anxiety, or conduct disturbances.

Clients with adjustment disorder may have difficulty at school or with peers or family members. Risk of suicidal actions is increased. The response to the stressor is greater than normally expected. This maladaptive reaction may occur when a child becomes ill, is hospitalized, or faces surgery (Figure 36.14). Signs may include regressed, fearful, or acting-out behavior. After leaving the hospital, the child may cling to a parent, cry, have nightmares, eat poorly, and need a diaper even though he or she is toilet trained.

Treatment requires understanding, support, and encouragement to move beyond the event as the youth works through feelings associated with the stressor. The nurse teaches and reinforces adaptive coping skills. Signs of depression or anxiety are managed with appropriate medications.

ANXIETY DISORDERS

Children and adolescents with anxiety disorders often have symptoms of fear, anxiety, physical complaints, and sleep disturbances, including nightmares and night terrors. In all age groups, sleep problems are associated with mental illness.

Obsessive-Compulsive Disorder

Obsessive-compulsive disorder (OCD) is characterized by recurrent intrusive thoughts (*obsessions*) and repetitive behaviors that the client recognizes as senseless but feels must

Parent Management Training and Conduct Disorder

Effective treatments: Parent management training (PMT) refers to procedures in which parents are trained to alter their child's behavior in the home. Parents meet with a therapist or trainer who teaches them to use specific procedures to alter interactions with their child, to promote prosocial behavior, and to decrease deviant behavior. Outcome studies support several conclusions. PMT has led to marked improvements in child behavior on parent and teacher reports of deviance and in direct observation of behavior at home and at school. PMT is effective and highly cost-effective when provided in small parent groups in neighborhoods where the families reside.

What has not been shown to be effective: Variations of psychodynamic therapy, relationship-based treatment, and play therapy have been shown less effective than PMT or other evidence-based approaches. Current research

suggests that placing deviant youths together can impede therapeutic change, have deleterious effects, and sustain deviance through the process of bonding with other problematic peers. Level-point systems, although widely used, have also not been studied as a way of structuring programs for youth.

Implications for practice: Insofar as PMT has been studied and found efficacious, the nurse should strive to encourage parents to be closely involved in treatment planning and provide them with educational materials describing such programs. Nurses have also an affirmative obligation to bring to the attention of program directors and other professionals, as well as to parents, what the research shows, as well as the lack of research about practices that may be in common use in treatment settings, and advocate for more evidence-based approaches.

References

Dishion, T. J., McCord, J., & Poulin, F. (1999). When interventions harm: Peer groups and problem behavior. *American Psychologist, 54,* 755–764.

Irvine, A. B., Biglan, A., Smolkowski, K., Metzler, C. W., & Ary, D. V. (1999). The effectiveness of a parenting skills program for parents of middle school students in small communities. *Journal of Consulting and Clinical Psychology, 68,* 811–825.

Kazdin, A. E. (2004). Evidence-based treatments: Challenges and priorities for practice and research. *Child & Adolescent Psychiatric Clinics of North America, 13*(4), 923–940.

Mohr, W. K., & Pumariega, A. (2004). Level systems: In-patient programming whose time has passed. *Journal of Child and Adolescent Psychiatric Nursing, 17*(3), 113–125.

Reid, M. J., Webster-Stratton, C., & Baydar, N. (2004). Halting the development of conduct problems in Head Start children: The effects of parent training. *Journal of Clinical Child & Adolescent Psychology, 33*(2), 279–291.

Weiss, B., Cantron, T., Harris, V., & Phung, T. M. (1999). The effectiveness of traditional child therapy. *Journal of Consulting and Clinical Psychology, 67,* 82–94.

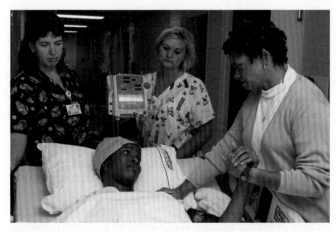

FIGURE 36.14 A child or teen may develop an adjustment disorder in response to illness or hospitalization.

be performed (*compulsions*). Obsessions and compulsions consume hours of the day and cause great distress. OCD occurs in families; if a parent has OCD, the child has an increased likelihood of having OCD as well.

Treatment of pediatric OCD involves behavioral and psychopharmacologic intervention. Behavioral techniques include *exposure* (deliberately confronting the client with stimuli that trigger obsessions and provoke the urge to

perform rituals) and *response prevention* (either instructing the client to delay the ritual or blocking the child from performing it). These two techniques allow the child to experience the rise and fall of anxiety. Some effective medications for OCD are clomipramine, fluoxetine, and sertraline. Clomipramine and sertraline are the only FDA-approved medications for OCD, with clomipramine showing greater efficacy than any selective serotonin reuptake inhibitor (SSRI) (Schatzberg & Nemeroff, 2006). Students are warned that the FDA has issued a black box warning regarding the use of antidepressants in children (see Chaps. 16 and 23).

Separation Anxiety Disorder

A child or adolescent with **separation anxiety disorder** experiences severe anxiety to the point of panic when apart from a parent or attachment figure. When threatened with parental separation, the child may fear accidents or injuries befalling the parent, cling to or shadow the parent, have nightmares, or refuse to attend school or spend the night away from home. During actual separation, he or she may complain of headaches and stomachaches, suffer severe homesickness, and vomit. These children often have sleep disturbances (eg, inability to fall asleep apart from the parent). Teens usually complain of physical ailments and refuse

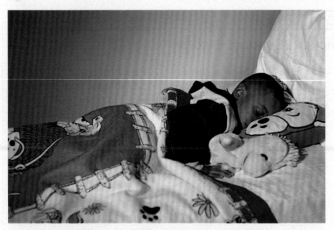

FIGURE 36.15 Parents should strive to provide soothing nighttime rituals and reassurance to help children who struggle with separation anxiety. Taking a security object to bed may be one method of easing stress associated with being apart from family during sleep. (Copyright © B. Proud.)

to attend school. Separation anxiety tends to abate as the young person moves into adolescence.

Clients with separation anxiety usually experience good response (ie, anxiety decreases) to SSRIs. Behavioral therapy includes imagery, self-talk, and cognitive techniques. Nursing interventions include reassuring the child and teaching the parents helpful responses to the child's fears and calming bedtime activities (Figure 36.15).

Phobias

Phobias are morbid, irrational, and persistent fears. They are so common in childhood that mild, passing fears are considered part of normal development.

A child may express the anxiety of a specific phobia by crying, clinging, or having tantrums. Frequently, children fear animals, storms, or traveling in certain vehicles. They may ask repeated questions about illness or death, kidnappers, or criminals. For example, the child with a dog phobia is preoccupied with the thought of possibly meeting a dog, feels constantly anxious about it, and may not want to leave the house over fear of seeing a dog. Phobias can be incapacitating.

Treatment of specific phobias includes pharmacotherapy with SSRIs (see Chap. 16); preparation of children for traumatic experiences; behavioral training such as relaxation, desensitization, and modeling; and psychotherapy for youth who have experienced traumatic events (eg, an attack by a dog; see Chap. 23).

Social Anxiety Disorder (Social Phobia)

Children and adolescents with *social anxiety disorder* avoid contact with unfamiliar people and performing or speaking in front of others. This behavior interferes with typical functioning, such as with peers or at school. Clients appear socially withdrawn, embarrassed, shy, self-conscious, and anxious if asked to interact with strangers. Avoidance and anxious anticipation cause marked distress in new or forced social situations.

Treating social anxiety disorder requires both pharmacologic and psychosocial interventions. SSRIs, particularly paroxetine (Paxil), have anxiety-reducing properties (see Chap. 16). In addition, clients need support in learning and using social skills through role-playing and other forms of practice and through reading and discussing books about children who have overcome their social reticence. Providers and family members should encourage children to take calculated risks and reinforce their progress.

Generalized Anxiety Disorder

Children with *generalized anxiety disorder (GAD)* have excessive or unrealistic fears; they worry about past and future events, the weather, their own school performance or health, the family's finances, and the welfare of others. For example, a child with GAD might say, "I'm worried about whether my father is going to get another kidney stone and whether we're going to have another tornado. I don't like it when there are clouds in the sky because there could be a storm." Physical symptoms of anxiety such as stomachache, headache, nausea, shortness of breath, and dizziness often accompany GAD.

The anxiolytic buspirone (BuSpar) or the SSRI paroxetine (Paxil) helps reduce anxiety and promotes well-being. In addition, reassuring clients of their safety and that of loved ones, teaching relaxation techniques, and helping them relax standards to realistic levels of performance are appropriate nursing interventions.

Post-Traumatic Stress Disorder

Post-traumatic stress disorder (PTSD) can result in children who are exposed to the pervasive trauma of inner-city life, suffer abuse, witness community or family violence, or watch the wounding or death of a close family member. Whether a child or adolescent develops PTSD in response to trauma depends on several factors, including environmental risk and protective factors and individual vulnerabilities and strengths (Silva et al., 2000) (see Chap. 3).

Interventions for PTSD include psychotherapy with a skilled therapist and medications to treat symptoms. Effective treatment for PTSD should address stages of grief, risk and protective factors, and self-care techniques and should include pharmacotherapy (O'Donnell et al., 2007). Clients with severe PTSD may need an antipsychotic medication for auditory hallucinations, an antidepressant for depressive symptoms and thoughts of self-harm, or both types of drugs.

Checkpoint Questions

9. What are four diagnostic criteria used to determine conduct disorder?
10. What two behavioral techniques are used to treat OCD in children?

MOOD DISORDERS

Mood disorders, including unipolar depression and bipolar disorder, occur in all age groups (see Chaps. 27 and 28). The most prominent signs and symptoms are specific to the age and developmental level of the affected client (Case Vignette 36.1).

Some signs and symptoms of mood disorders in children and adolescents are similar to the normal mood swings that all people have at different developmental stages. Therefore, families and health care providers may fail to recognize mood disorders in pediatric clients. Mood disorders in young people often co-occur with other problems, such as anxiety, disruptive behavior, or substance use disorders, and with physical illnesses, such as diabetes.

Several factors contribute to the failure to recognize depressive disorders in youth. The way that young people express symptoms is a function of their developmental stage. Adolescence is a time of emotional turmoil, mood swings, and rebelliousness. Substance abuse may also contribute to a missed diagnosis. Another problem is that children and adolescents sometimes have difficulty expressing their internal feelings and emotions. Sometimes, the only way they can do

so is by acting out and behaving inappropriately. However, parents, teachers, and other adults may misinterpret such clues as disobedience or insolence.

Early diagnosis and treatment of mood disorders are essential for continued healthy development. Identifying and treating mood disorders early reduce their duration, severity, and resulting functional impairment.

Depression

Many adults do not take childhood depression seriously. However, childhood depression is real and takes a serious toll on U.S. youth. According to Costello et al. (2003), 1% to 2% of prepubertal children and 3% to 8% of adolescents are depressed at any point in time; moreover, 50% of all adults with depression report that their illness began before age 20 years. Adolescents disclose their depression more readily through self-reports than to their parents (Pullen et al., 2000). As with adult depression, depression in children involves some combination of genetic vulnerability and psychosocial or environmental factors.

Dysthymia, a mild form of depression, lasts 1 year or more in a child or teen. Because the symptoms are less debilitating than with major depression, nurses in school and clinic settings may see youth with dysthymia who are at risk for major depression (Bhatia & Bhatia, 2007; Klein et al., 2000). When dysthymia and major depression occur together, it is called **double depression**.

Signs and Symptoms

Depression affects all areas of physical, emotional, and cognitive development. The duration and intensity of symptoms differentiate depression from sadness. Depressive behavior differs significantly from the child's usual behavior and interferes with his or her family, schoolwork, and friends (Box 36.2).

Depression in children and adolescents is easily confused with other childhood disorders, such as ADHD. Because children often cannot tell adults what they are feeling, they communicate by acting out. Prepubertal children with depression often exhibit irritability and separation anxiety; adolescents may be negative, antisocial, defiant, socially withdrawn, and failing at school.

Signs of depression in children and adolescents are as follows:

- Depressed or irritable mood, low frustration level, overreaction to simple requests, loss of joy, and moodiness
- Psychomotor agitation or retardation; the child may talk slowly and pause before responding
- Changes in appetite and sleep; the child may eat everything or very little, not sleep restfully, have trouble falling or staying asleep, or awaken very early
- Physical complaints such as headache, stomachache, fatigue, and loss of energy
- Depressive themes expressed in play, dreams, or verbalizations; examples include feeling worthless or guilty, minimizing strengths and maximizing failures, and blaming self over family problems

Case Vignette 36.1

Eight-year-old Sarah and her parents come to the child outpatient clinic after she wrote a note to her father about how badly she feels when she bites herself. Sarah has bruised her arms and legs with the biting that started 3 months ago. She has several fears, including the dark, being alone, and getting sick and dying. Her parents say she is irritable, cries excessively, and "gets upset over any little thing."

Sarah's appetite has decreased, and her sleeping is restless—she often awakens early in a "cranky mood." Her maternal grandmother died 1 year ago, and Sarah continues to talk about how much she misses her. She is demanding, has temper tantrums, and throws things. She yells at her parents and 6-year-old sister. She "forgets things" and is inattentive and impulsive but not hyperactive.

The psychiatric nurse practitioner evaluates Sarah. Her diagnoses are Major Depressive Disorder, single episode, moderate; ADHD, inattentive type; Anxiety Disorder, NOS; and rule out ODD.

Reflection and Critical Thinking

- In order of priority, what are the mental health needs of Sarah and her family?
- Identify the appropriate level of treatment for Sarah. Justify your answer.
- Create a teaching plan for Sarah and her parents; include learning outcomes, teaching content, and strategies.
- How would you respond to Sarah's mother when she says, "Why is she depressed?" and "I don't want her to become addicted to any medicine"?

BOX 36.2 What Does a Child Have to Be Depressed About?

Only decades ago, the general view held that children could not suffer depression. After all, what do they have to be depressed about? Children do not have to hold down a job to pay for food and shelter. All they must do is attend school and play. We idealize the period of childhood as a time of joy and learning.

Even today parents may ask, "What could he or she possibly have to be depressed about?" Depression does not only occur after a sad or traumatic event. Depression (like other mental disorders) "runs in families," just as heart disease and diabetes are familial disorders.

Children of any age can experience depression. However, the expression of mood disorders, depression, and bipolar disorder in children does not mirror the symptoms seen in adults. Whereas adults with depression are sad, children are usually irritable or angry. They may have rages. Adolescents may show disruptive behavior and end up in trouble at both home and school.

When parents have mood disorders such as depression, it is particularly crucial that their children be screened for a mood disorder. Early detection and treatment are essential to promote children's and adolescents' recovery from depression and return to wellness. Every October, National Depression Screening Day offers anyone the opportunity to take part in a screening.

- Social withdrawal
- Intense anger or rage
- **Anhedonia**—loss of pleasure in hobbies or activities of interest
- Acting-out behaviors: substance abuse, truancy, dropping out of school, running away, antisocial behaviors, self-injury, or sexual promiscuity
- Decreased ability to think, concentrate, or make decisions, often manifested in poor academic performance
- Thoughts of and verbalizations about death or wishing one had never been born; teens may express their thoughts through music, films, or writing with morbid themes
- Stressors, such as a breakup with a boyfriend or girlfriend, which may trigger suicidal thoughts (Kuchta, 2001)

Think About It 36.1

Review Case Vignette 36.1. After analyzing the scenario, describe the manifestations Sarah exhibits that would apply to the diagnosis of major depression.

Comorbidities

Half of children and adolescents with depression have another psychiatric illness, such as GAD, OCD, ADHD, or conduct disorder. In addition, they may abuse drugs or alcohol (see Chap. 30).

Prevention

Early identification and treatment are essential to prevent depression, especially long-term depression in adulthood. Facilitating a strong sense of self, trust, and resiliency; providing a stable home life; practicing open and honest communication; teaching how to deal with disappointment and frustration; and providing activities that build on the youth's abilities and talents may diminish the incidence of depression.

Interdisciplinary Goals and Treatment

The recovery rate from a single episode of pediatric major depression is relatively high; 70% to 80% of affected clients are treated effectively. However, depression has a high rate of recurrence; 40% of children with one depressive episode will experience another within 2 years (Bhatia & Bhatia, 2007). Therefore, the goal is no longer to help children or teens respond to treatment; instead, it is for them to become well. In addition, youths with dysthymic disorder are at risk for major depression (Klein et al., 2000). Anyone with depression needs close monitoring; ongoing treatment is needed to prevent recurrences.

CBT or play therapy for younger children, parent and family consultation, and medication constitute the necessary interventions for these clients. Neither therapy alone nor medication alone has been found as effective as combination treatment.

Cognitive–Behavioral Therapy and Family Consultation

CBT can decrease errors in thinking and improve developmental skills. Techniques include using self-talk to promote coping in certain situations, active participation in planning activities, and self-monitoring by writing about moods or feelings in a journal (Figure 36.16).

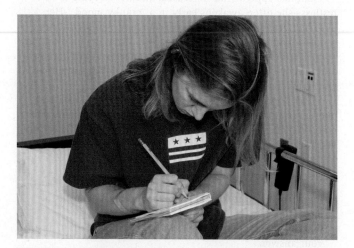

FIGURE 36.16 Some young clients with depression and other mood disorders benefit from writing about their moods or feelings in a journal. Over time, they can evaluate whether reactions or emotions show any type of pattern and what sorts of coping mechanisms were most effective in addressing their problems.

Family consultation helps relatives understand mood disorders, support the client, and develop more effective parenting skills. Through consultation, parents learn strategies to develop and maintain effective family communication. Especially important is the need to listen to and communicate openly and respectfully with adolescents. Parents also learn to identify risk factors that will worsen depression, such as alcohol and nicotine use.

Pharmacologic Therapy

The most commonly used antidepressants for children and adolescents are the SSRIs. Side effects, especially nausea, headache, and stomachache, are minimal, especially when the starting dose is low and gradually increased to a therapeutic level. Although the client and family may see improvement in 1 to 2 weeks, it may take 12 weeks to assess the full response to the medication. Antidepressants are given for 6 to 24 months to treat depression fully and decrease its likelihood of recurrence.

TCAs are older drugs with greater side effects, including potentially life-threatening dysrhythmias. Because of their potential lethality in an overdose, TCAs are rarely given to pediatric clients. Imipramine (Tofranil) and amitriptyline (Elavil) are useful to treat both enuresis in very small doses and ADHD symptoms (especially for those with concomitant anxiety) in children with depression.

For clients who also experience aggression, severe agitation, or delusions and hallucinations, antipsychotic medications, particularly the atypical antipsychotics, are used. Drugs from this class most likely to be given to children or teens are risperidone (Risperdal), quetiapine (Seroquel), and olanzapine (Zyprexa). They cause some sedation, especially initially. Of these three, quetiapine causes the least weight gain. Little research on the use of aripiprazole (Abilify) in children is available because of its relatively recent introduction. Traditional antipsychotic medications are used less frequently in children because of increased risk of tardive dyskinesia (see Chaps. 16 and 29). Note that all atypical antipsychotics, with the possible exception of aripiprazole, have been associated with metabolic syndrome (see Chap. 16).

Nurses must stay abreast of the latest research on the efficacy, utility, and risk of psychotropic medications with children. Compared with the research base and longitudinal study of antidepressants with adults, knowledge about psychopharmacologic effects on children and adolescents is relatively scant. Several medications have been pulled from state formularies because of concerns over liver toxicity and risk of suicide.

Bipolar Disorder

When the book *The Bipolar Child* by Demitri and Janice Papolos was published in 1999 (revised 2002), many parents of children with unusual patterns of disturbing behavior described a revelation in their lives. These authors have proposed a definition of juvenile-onset *bipolar disorder*, marked by rapid, wide swings of emotion; arousal; excitability; and movement (see Chap. 28). Bipolar disorder has a strong familial component. Its etiology involves some combination of genetic vulnerability and environmental factors. Consensus on key diagnostic issues for juvenile bipolar disorder remains unclear (Axelson et al., 2006).

Studies indicate that 70% to 100% of children and adolescents with bipolar disorder will eventually recover from their first episode; however, of those who recover, up to 80% will experience one or more recurrences in a period of 2 to 5 years. The condition is characterized by fluctuations, recovery, and recurrences. It can cause enormous psychosocial impairment and have a negative impact on families.

Signs and Symptoms

Bipolar disorder is a mood disorder, and the primary symptoms are mood related. Severely irritable, dysphoric, and agitated children who have "affective (or emotional) storms" or rages (ie, prolonged, aggressive temper outbursts), are prone to violence, show poor school performance, have sleep disturbances, and experience rapid mood swings that may occur hourly or every 2 hours may have bipolar disorder. Children do not show the classic manic picture of elated mood seen in adults with bipolar disorder. Sometimes, identifying episodes of cycling (ie, switching from one mood to another) is difficult because symptoms seem to be chronic (Birmaher et al., 2006). Children may also exhibit delusions, hypersexuality, pressured speech, or flight of ideas. Adolescents may have hallucinations, delusions, labile mood, or idiosyncratic thinking (Birmaher et al., 2006). Although teens may have symptoms that resemble those in adults, determining the cycling of moods remains difficult. The incidence of substance abuse is high in teens with bipolar disorder.

Symptoms of bipolar disorder overlap with those of ADHD, but children with bipolar disorder always have a mood disturbance. Childhood-onset bipolar disorder may have comorbidity with ADHD, ODD, or conduct disorder, or the bipolar disorder may have features of ADHD, ODD, or conduct disorder.

Interdisciplinary Goals and Treatment

Pediatric clients with bipolar disorder and their families need several types of treatment, such as education, family therapy, special education or school modifications, support groups, individual or play therapy, and mood-stabilizing medication (Mohr, 2001). The goals are to alleviate symptoms and improve day-to-day functioning.

Importance of Early Identification and Treatment

Studies suggest that clients with prior episodes of bipolar disorder may have a poorer response to lithium and that past history in terms of episodes and mood instability affects treatment response (Birmaher et al., 2007). Scientists believe that the cause of these disparities is spontaneous neuronal sensitization as the illness and its cycles progress. If bipolar disorder remains unrecognized and unchecked in children, future episodes may occur independently of any stimulus, and with greater frequency (Papolos & Papolos,

2002). Therefore, early identification of bipolar disorder in children is urgent.

Strong evidence also suggests that medications such as TCAs and stimulants may induce sensitization (see Chap. 16). As stated previously, bipolar disorder appears to be comorbid with ADHD. Both stimulants and antidepressants are used to manage ADHD; both may be implicated in the precipitation of mania in genetically vulnerable children (Birmaher et al., 2007; Papolos & Papolos, 2002). Altshuler and colleagues (1995) found that 35% of clients with bipolar disorder had a manic episode rated as likely to have been induced by antidepressants. Moreover, an acceleration of cycling was associated with antidepressant treatment in 26% of subjects, and a younger age at first treatment was a predictor of vulnerability to antidepressant-induced cycle acceleration. Therefore, because of the confusion regarding the diagnosis of juvenile-onset bipolar disorder, it is essential for clients to undergo a detailed, thorough, longitudinal history before medications are prescribed. Rushing to judgment can have unintended consequences; drugs completely appropriate for ADHD may worsen the course and prognosis of bipolar disorder.

Pharmacologic Therapy

Mood-stabilizing medications, including lithium, divalproex (Depakote), and carbamazepine (Tegretol), have calming and antiaggressive effects and help to prevent depressive and manic symptoms. Lithium, which affects serotonin, norepinephrine, and dopamine systems, is particularly effective in clients whose behavior is manic or elated. During mania, lithium diminishes the action of dopamine; during depression, it enhances the action of serotonin. Moreover, lithium has strong suicide-preventive properties and generally is recommended as a first-line treatment for bipolar disorder. The anticonvulsant mood stabilizers divalproex and carbamazepine are more effective in treating rapid cycling and angry or depressed states. Other medications for mood stabilization and augmentation are discussed in Chapters 16 and 28. Children with bipolar disorder who also have psychosis may be given an antipsychotic medication, most likely an atypical antipsychotic (Green, 2007).

Although the medications discussed previously are used frequently in adults with bipolar disorder (see Chaps. 16 and 28), some concerns are specific to children and adolescents. For example, children and teens often spend more time outside playing and engaging in sports. Parents need to be careful that their children do not become dehydrated while taking lithium, which could elevate their lithium levels. Many schools allow children and teens taking lithium to keep a water bottle with them in class for hydration. Other side effects of lithium are nausea, polyuria with resulting enuresis, and polydipsia.

AUTISM SPECTRUM DISORDERS

Autism spectrum disorders (ASD), also called *pervasive developmental disorders*, have three core features: (1) impairments in socialization, (2) impairments in communication,

and (3) restricted repertoire of behavior. They are found in approximately 1 of 300 to 500 children up to 3 years old.

Signs and Symptoms/Diagnostic Criteria

DSM-IV-TR Box 36.4 outlines diagnostic criteria for two major types of autism-spectrum disorders. These are autism and Asperger's syndrome.

Autism

Autism, a genetic disorder of neuronal organization, occurs more frequently in boys than girls. Chromosomal abnormalities are present in 5% to 6% of affected children. Children with autism develop language slowly or not at all. They may use words without attaching meaning to them or communicate with only gestures or noises. They spend time alone and show little interest in making friends. Probably 50% of children with ASD exhibit some degree of intellectual deficiency (mental retardation). IQ scores are strongly correlated with adaptive outcomes. A few persons with ASD exhibit truly remarkable, isolated activities (eg, memory for dates, mathematical skills, musical talents), but most do not. Cognitive defects become noticeable in infancy (Volkmar et al., 2007). However, their most distinctive feature is their seeming isolation from the world around them. This detachment and aloofness help distinguish people with autism from those who are solely mentally retarded. Children with autism are less responsive to social cues (eg, smiles, eye contact). They often have some sensory impairment, including sensitivity in sight, taste, hearing, touch, or smell (Volkmar et al., 2007).

Children with autism do not play spontaneously or imaginatively. They do not imitate others' actions or participate in pretend games. They may act aggressively and throw tantrums for no obvious reason. In addition, they may *perseverate* (show an obsessive interest in some item or activity and engage in ritualistic behavior). They often adhere to routines and do not tolerate change well. These characteristics are evident before 3 years of age.

Asperger's Syndrome

Asperger's syndrome, also occurring more frequently in boys, is characterized by major difficulties with social interaction and restricted, unusual interests and behaviors. Although there is no significant delay in language, people with Asperger's syndrome use monotone speech and rigid vocabulary. They cannot understand jokes and are taken advantage of easily. Despite not grasping nonverbal communication cues and an inability to show empathy, they want to meet people and make friends. Mental retardation usually does not accompany Asperger's syndrome, although occasional cases of concomitant mild mental retardation have been noted (Volkmar et al., 2007).

People with Asperger's syndrome are obsessed with facts about circumscribed and odd topics. For example, they may be tremendously interested in, and talk incessantly about, subjects of little appeal to others (eg, deep-fat fryers, state counties, video game characters). They are often perfectionists and hate to fail.

DSM-IV-TR BOX 36.4

Autism Spectrum Disorders

Autistic Disorder

A. A total of six (or more) items from (1), (2), and (3), with at least two from (1), and one each from (2) and (3):

1. qualitative impairment in social interaction, as manifested by at least two of the following:
   a. marked impairment in the use of multiple nonverbal behaviors such as eye-to-eye gaze, facial expression, body postures, and gestures to regulate social interaction
   b. failure to develop peer relationships appropriate to developmental level
   c. a lack of spontaneous seeking to share enjoyment, interests, or achievements with other people (eg, by a lack of showing, bringing, or pointing out objects of interest)
   d. lack of social or emotional reciprocity

2. qualitative impairments in communication as manifested by at least one of the following:
   a. delay in, or total lack of, the development of spoken language (not accompanied by an attempt to compensate through alternative modes of communication such as gesture or mime)
   b. in individuals with adequate speech, marked impairment in the ability to initiate or sustain a conversation with others
   c. stereotyped and repetitive use of language or idiosyncratic language
   d. lack of varied, spontaneous make-believe play or social imitative play appropriate to developmental level

3. restricted repetitive and stereotyped patterns of behavior, interests, and activities, as manifested by at least one of the following:
   a. encompassing preoccupation with one or more stereotyped and restricted patterns of interest that is abnormal either in intensity or focus
   b. apparently inflexible adherence to specific, nonfunctional routines or rituals
   c. stereotyped and repetitive motor mannerisms (eg, hand or finger flapping or twisting, or complex whole-body movements)
   d. persistent preoccupation with parts of objects

B. Delays or abnormal functioning in at least one of the following areas, with onset prior to age 3 years: (1) social interaction, (2) language as used in social communication, or (3) symbolic or imaginative play.

C. The disturbance is not better accounted for by Rett's Disorder or Childhood Disintegrative Disorder.

Asperger's Disorder

A. Qualitative impairment in social interaction, as manifested by at least two of the following:

1. marked impairment in the use of multiple nonverbal behaviors such as eye-to-eye gaze, facial expression, body postures, and gestures to regulate social interaction
2. failure to develop peer relationships appropriate to developmental level
3. a lack of spontaneous seeking to share enjoyment, interests, or achievements with other people (eg, by a lack of showing, bringing, or pointing out objects of interest to other people)
4. a lack of social or emotional reciprocity

B. Restricted repetitive and stereotyped patterns of behavior, interests, and activities, as manifested by at least one of the following:

1. encompassing preoccupation with one or more stereotyped and restricted patterns of interest that is abnormal either in intensity or focus
2. apparently inflexible adherence to specific, nonfunctional routines or rituals
3. stereotyped and repetitive motor mannerisms (eg, hand or finger flapping or twisting, or complex whole-body movements)
4. persistent preoccupation with parts of objects

C. The disturbance causes clinically significant impairment in social, occupational, or other important areas of functioning.

D. There is no clinically significant general delay in language (eg, single words used by age 2 years, communicative phrases used by age 3 years).

E. There is no clinically significant delay in cognitive development or in the development of age-appropriate self-help skills, adaptive behavior (other than in social interaction), and curiosity about the environment in childhood.

F. Criteria are not met for another specific Pervasive Developmental Disorder or Schizophrenia.

Due to the close overlap of certain symptoms of Asperger's syndrome with those of autism, there is strong indication from the American Psychiatric Association that Asperger's syndrome will be subsumed under the overall category of Autism Spectrum Disorders in the new edition of the *DSM*.

Interdisciplinary Goals and Treatment

Early detection improves outcomes. An easy screening tool for 18-month-olds is the Checklist for Autism in Toddlers (CHAT), used to evaluate the ability to pretend, enjoyment in peekaboo games, attempts to engage parents, and eye contact (visit http://www.aheadwithautism.com/chat_screening.html).

Treatment for clients with autism spectrum disorders centers on behavioral interventions, particularly CBT, special education, social skills training in groups, language therapies, occupational therapy, and sometimes pharmacotherapy. Behavior modification techniques include those used to enhance and reduce certain behaviors. For example, social skills training:

- Uses role-playing, coaching, and social stories to help clients play like same-age peers
- Teaches flexibility in how to engage in an activity and recognize cues and actions for specific social situations
- Teaches ways to reduce stress, anxiety, and inattention

Medication may help manage symptoms of hyperactivity, irritability, aggression, self-injury, ritualism, and obsessive-compulsive behavior. Common drug classes for these problems include neuroleptics, anticonvulsants, and mood stabilizers.

Needs change with the child's development. Speech and language therapy and parental assistance are critical for very young children. Older children or adolescents may need CBT and medication to deal with obsessive-compulsive symptoms. Prognosis is more positive when language development and social interaction are less impaired. Researchers hope that, someday, it may be possible to treat autism with neuronal growth factors.

Children with autism spectrum disorders need a structured environment and social-emotional training. The goal may be to learn to imitate social behavior that other children learn intuitively. In addition, special education placement in public school settings with measurable goals and objectives for the child is necessary. Public Law 94-142, the Education for All Handicapped Children Act of 1975, requires that all children between ages 3 and 21 years with diagnosed ASDs receive free, appropriate education. A newer law ensures service provision from birth, although such services may be given by an agency outside the school system.

Parents need accurate information, training in becoming advocates, respite programs, and inclusion in individualized, collaborative treatment planning to understand and help their children. Future needs of children with autism spectrum disorders might involve vocational training and placement, use of sheltered workshops, supported employment, and community-based programs such as group home or supervised apartment living.

Checkpoint Questions

11. What is the most commonly used class of antidepressants for children and adolescents?
12. Although the symptoms of bipolar disorder overlap with ADHD, what is always present for children with bipolar disorder?
13. What three core features are present with pervasive developmental disorders?

EATING DISORDERS

Eating disorders develop in adolescents and sometimes children. Prevalence estimates for teens is 0.5% for anorexia and 0.5% to 5.8% for bulimia. Many girls have some symptoms of eating disorders, but do not meet all criteria for the illness

(White, 2000). These long-term, complex disorders affect both physical and psychological well-being. They are explored in depth in Chapter 26.

SUBSTANCE ABUSE

Adolescents primarily are polysubstance abusers. They most widely use tobacco, alcohol, and marijuana. Nicotine and alcohol are termed "gateway" drugs because they may "open the gates" to further and heavier drug use. Choice of drugs among youths often is related to fashions, such as "club drugs," which refer to dangerous, even lethal, substances that young people use at all-night parties (raves or trances), dance clubs, and bars. Examples of club drugs are 3,4-methylenedioxymethamphetamine (MDMA or Ecstasy), gamma hydroxybutyric acid (GHB), flunitrazepam (Rohypnol), ketamine, methamphetamine, and lysergic acid diethylamide (LSD). See Chapter 30 for more information.

Substance abuse is associated with other problems such as criminality and sexual promiscuity. It provides teens with a maladaptive escape from frustration, disappointment, boredom, and emptiness. Teens who abuse drugs and alcohol are at increased risk for health problems, depression, suicidal ideation, and conduct disorder (Box 36.3).

In addition, they are more likely to drive while intoxicated, putting them at great risk for motor vehicle accidents. Adolescent substance abuse is related to premature involvement in sex, increased incidence of sexually transmitted infections, and teen pregnancy. Prevalence of substance use disorders among adolescents is 32% and higher among teens with mental illness. Mood disorders, anxiety disorders, and disruptive behavior disorders are comorbid conditions.

Prevention of Drug and Alcohol Abuse

Protective factors against substance use include positive relationships with parents, satisfaction of basic needs, religious involvement, and activities that instill values

---

BOX 36.3	Signs and Symptoms of Substance Abuse in Adolescents

All of the following can be signs that an adolescent is using substances:

- Poor academic performance, failure, or truancy
- Withdrawal from family and friends
- Change in or loss of friends
- Physical complaints
- Aggression or risk-taking behavior
- Depression and suicidal thoughts or actions
- Continuous use of the substance, even though it interferes with the adolescent's ability to perform at school, home, or work and causes interpersonal or social problems
- Use of the substance in situations in which it is dangerous, for example, when driving a car, which may lead to legal problems (eg, driving while intoxicated [DWI])

(Mainous et al., 2001). High-risk youth whose parents are substance abusers must be identified and given prevention education and support. The goals should be to foster self-worth, assist with impulse control, and enhance coping through behavioral and cognitive measures.

Interdisciplinary Goals and Treatment

The first step in treating adolescent substance abuse is awareness and recognition of the problem, especially considering that parents, teachers, and communities frequently deny or underestimate it. It is critical that nurses ask direct questions of the client and family about the child's substance use; embarrassment or fear should not be excuses for not inquiring (Therapeutic Communication 36.1).

Nurses and other mental health professionals must aim to redirect the substance-abusing family toward health and strength.

Interventions should address the reasons teens give for using substances, including avoiding peer pressure, getting "high," cheering up, alleviating boredom, having more

energy (cocaine or stimulant users), and escaping from problems. Adolescents may also express feelings of unmet needs as important factors in their substance abuse (Mainous et al., 2001). Substance abuse and its treatment are presented fully in Chapter 30.

TIC DISORDERS

A **tic** is a sudden repetitive movement, gesture, or utterance. Tics are brief and may occur in bouts. They tend to increase with stress and lessen during absorbing activities. Tics can be motor or vocal, simple or complex.

Tourette syndrome, the most severe tic disorder, is characterized by multiple motor tics and one or more vocal tics many times throughout the day for 1 year or more. The disorder impairs functioning at home, in school, and with peers. Obsessions, compulsions, hyperactivity, disinhibited speech or behavior, and impulsivity may be associated features. Children may also have depression and school and behavioral problems.

Therapeutic Communications 36.1

Discussing Peer Pressure and Substance Use With Adolescents

Luis, 14 years old, has come for a regular physical examination. The nurse is interviewing him before the physical assessment.

INEFFECTIVE DIALOGUE	EFFECTIVE DIALOGUE
NURSE: How are things going for you at school?	NURSE: How are things going for you at school?
CLIENT: *(Shrugs)* Okay.	CLIENT: *(Shrugs)* Okay.
NURSE: Have you been facing any peer pressure lately?	NURSE: Many teenagers face issues involving peer pressure, especially related to drugs and alcohol. *(Pauses)* Have you used any of these substances recently?
CLIENT: *(Looks confused)* No.	
NURSE: A lot of kids your age start using drugs. I'm giving you a bunch of pamphlets about the dangers of drinking and doing drugs. Please read them. If you have questions, let me know.	CLIENT: *(Looks down at the floor)* A few weeks ago, my friend tried to get me to drink beer with him. I took a sip, but I didn't like it. I don't want to do it again.
CLIENT: *(Seems to stifle a laugh)* Okay.	NURSE: Were there reasons why you didn't say no?
	CLIENT: I didn't want to seem like a nerd or have him laugh at me.
	NURSE: It's difficult to say no. We all want to be part of the crowd. Let's talk more about how to handle these situations and why drugs and alcohol can be dangerous. I also have pamphlets that you can read on your own. What questions do you have?

Reflection and Critical Thinking

* Why do you think the first nurse failed to learn the information that the client divulged to the second nurse?
* How did the second nurse achieve rapport with the client? Cite specific ways in which the nurse made the client feel comfortable and encouraged him to share information.
* What assumptions about teenagers do nurses need to try to avoid? How can such assumptions block communication?

Tic disorders may be treated with supportive counseling, school modifications, parent guidance, and individual therapy. Pharmacotherapy with haloperidol, pimozide, clonidine, clomipramine, desipramine, fluoxetine, and sertraline helps diminish tics. Anticipatory guidance can help clients and their families learn that tics improve and worsen in response to many variables and stressors.

TRICHOTILLOMANIA

Clients with **trichotillomania** have an irresistible urge to pull out their hair. They feel tension before and relief or pleasure during and after pulling. They may then examine, chew on, or eat the hair. The hair loss is noticeable (Figure 36.17). Trichotillomania is a chronic impulse-control condition that impairs social and academic life. Typically, people with trichotillomania try to deny or hide their behavior, pulling hair privately. The result is social withdrawal because clients fear that they may have a strong urge to pull hair while with others. Feelings of shame and humiliation, poor self-image, and problems with mood, anxiety, or addictions are common associations (Enos & Plante, 2001).

At least 2.5 million people in the United States have trichotillomania. It affects boys and girls with equal frequency. The average age of onset is 12 to 13 years, although many younger children have the problem. Clients most commonly pull out scalp hair, then eyelashes, eyebrows, and pubic hair. Some clients pull hair in certain circumstances, such as while watching television, reading or studying, or lying in bed waiting to fall asleep. Causes for the disorder seem to be biologic (links have been seen between trichotillomania and Tourette syndrome) and behavioral (eg, hair pulling reduces tension and becomes a habit).

Treatment includes both behavior therapy and pharmacotherapy with clomipramine, fluvoxamine, fluoxetine, or another SSRI. *Habit reversal therapy* is used to increase awareness of the hair pulling. In addition, teaching alternative coping activities (eg, relaxing, pulling weeds) and maintaining motivation through social support may be effective (Enos & Plante, 2001).

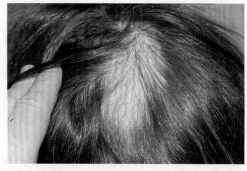

FIGURE 36.17 The hair loss of the compulsive behavior of trichotillomania is noticeable and can cause clients struggling with the problem further embarrassment and anxiety.

SUICIDE

Another major concern among youths, particularly adolescents, is suicide. Although pediatric clients with depression are generally recognized as a group at risk for suicide, they are not alone. Young people with bipolar disorders, substance use disorders, and homosexual orientation are also at risk for self-harm. Those younger than 25 years (35% of the population) account for approximately 15% of all U.S. suicides. Suicide is the second leading cause of death among college students, third among those 15 to 24 years, and sixth among children younger than 15 years. As many as 10% of children may attempt suicide during high school. However, between 1990 and 2003, the rate in this age group decreased by 35% (Shain, 2007).

Signs

Although no specific tests are capable of identifying a suicidal person, specific risk factors exist. Nurses and other clinicians should use care when interpreting risk factors, however, because risk factors are common, whereas suicide is infrequent, and the absence of most risk factors does not make a child safe from suicide.

Fixed risk factors include family history of suicide or suicide attempts, male gender, parental mental health problems, gay or bisexual orientation, a history of physical or sexual abuse, and a previous suicide attempt. Social and environmental risk factors include the presence of firearms in the home, impaired parent–child relationship, living outside of the home (homeless or in a corrections facility or group home), difficulties in school, neither working nor attending school, social isolation, and presence of stressful life events such as legal or romantic difficulties or an argument with a parent. Personal mental health problems that predispose to suicide include depression, bipolar disorder, substance abuse or dependence, psychosis, PTSD, panic attacks, and a history of aggression, impulsivity, or severe anger. More than 90% of adolescent suicide victims met criteria for a psychiatric disorder before their death. Immediate risk factors include agitation, intoxication, and a recent stressful life event (Shain, 2007).

Parents, teachers, and other adults may miss warning signs of suicidal thoughts or behavior, which include the following:

- Statements such as "I won't be around for you to yell at" or "You won't have to worry about me much longer"
- Lack of emotional responsiveness
- Social withdrawal

- Inability to enjoy previously enjoyed activities
- Drug or alcohol abuse
- Threat-making and giving away possessions
- Sudden cheerfulness after being depressed

Prevention

There is a nationwide call for increased awareness of, focus on, and interventions targeted at decreasing suicide rates, particularly for adolescents (Center for Mental Health Services, 2001). Early screening and prompt intervention can help lower the incidence of youth suicide. The American Foundation for Suicide Prevention aims to teach that suicide results from undiagnosed or untreated mental illness.

Interdisciplinary Goals and Treatment

Safety concerns are the priority for suicidal children and teens. Nurses must take all threats of self-harm seriously. They must help parents establish a safety plan that (1) provides for a safe and unrestrictive environment, (2) offers alternatives to self-harm, and (3) enables families to quickly get children in crisis to hospital emergency departments. If a child refuses to participate in a contract to refrain from self-harm, parents must take the child to health care providers for an appropriate level of care assessment (Kuchta, 2001).

To assess suicide risk, nurses talk openly with clients and family about specific factors. These include presence of a suicide plan and such a plan's lethality, availability of lethal weapons such as guns, history of substance abuse, prior suicide attempts, exposure to suicidal people who could inspire imitative behavior, and level of depression and hopelessness. Children and adolescents, like adults, require close observation and monitoring when recovering from depression because they may have regained enough energy to act on suicidal thoughts or plans.

A safety contract contains a written promise not to hurt oneself or another intentionally or accidentally for a specific period, as well as a list of actions or coping skills to prevent suicidal behavior. Young people may benefit from being taught how to differentiate and rank the intensity of feelings.

CHILDREN WITH MEDICAL ILLNESS OR DISABILITY

Medical illness in a child is a stressor in the life of a family system. Whether the problem is congenital, acute, or chronic, it interrupts the developmental process and disrupts the lives of all family members. Children may regress to earlier forms of behavior (eg, throwing tantrums, refusing to use the toilet, demanding a bottle). Visits to health care settings alter daily routines. Hospital stays can affect parents' sleeping arrangements and family responsibilities. Siblings experience disruptions as they become secondary to ill children and are cared for by neighbors or relatives. Hospital bills, medication costs, and time away from work result in

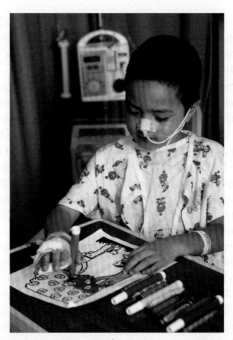

FIGURE 36.18 Health care facilities and providers can be enormously influential in shepherding children and families during their experiences with illness and hospitalization. Providing normal age-appropriate activities and outlets can mitigate the disruptive and traumatic effects that the challenges of sickness can pose.

financial strains. As one child assumes the client role, other relatives shift in their roles and functions. Changes to daily living, routines, and roles require adaptation by all family members.

How families perceive these stresses influence how they cope. Benefits can occur when children and families view illness as a stressful event that can result in positive adaptation and that can increase self-confidence and mastery. By providing support and assistance in mastering stress, nurses mediate adaptive responses (Figure 36.18).

MENTAL RETARDATION

Mental retardation refers to substantial limitations in functioning and is characterized by significantly subaverage intellectual functioning. *DSM-IV-TR* diagnostic criteria for mental retardation include the following (American Psychiatric Association, 2000):

- An intelligence quotient (IQ) of approximately 70 or below
- Concurrent deficits or impairments in present adaptive functioning in at least two of the following areas: communication, self-care, home living, social/interpersonal skills
- Onset before 18 years

Retardation affects 2% to 3% of the general population, although some experts argue that only approximately 1% should receive the diagnosis. Most affected clients fall in the mild range of retardation (IQ = 55 to 70); smaller numbers are moderately (IQ = 40 to 54), severely (IQ = 25 to 39), and profoundly (IQ = 0 to 24) retarded. Retardation affects more boys than girls and can coexist with psychological disorders and physical disabilities.

Knowledge of the normal developmental sequence has proved useful in early behavioral interventions with children with mental retardation. Studies of programs serving retarded children younger than 5 years have shown that particular types of cognitive and social stimulation can increase levels of functioning. Ever-expanding abilities to screen for and diagnose retardation in infancy, along with the early identification of at-risk children, make it increasingly possible for interventions to reach more retarded children at early ages.

Research on older retarded children has shown that motivational factors play the major role in determining how productive and independent they ultimately become (Figure 36.19). As they face increased failures compared with normal children, however, children with mental retardation may develop traits that work against independence. They often become overly wary of adults and do not expect to succeed at challenging tasks. At the same time, retarded children are more likely to become dependent on adult approval and to accept adult (as opposed to their own) solutions to difficult problems. The net effect is frequent performance below the level of intellectual ability on various experimental and real-life tasks.

Checkpoint Questions

16. What intervention is crucial for a child with suicidal thoughts?

17. Based on the *DSM-IV-TR*, what level of intellectual functioning and IQ denotes mental retardation?

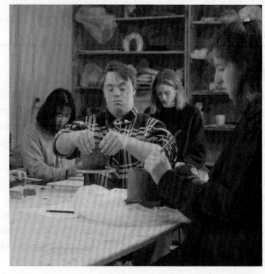

FIGURE 36.19 Early intervention and ongoing management can benefit clients with mental retardation as they mature. This teenager with Down syndrome participates in a "mainstream" pottery class at his high school. (Richard Hutchings/Photo Researchers, Inc.)

NURSES' SELF-CARE

Working with pediatric clients who have psychiatric challenges and their families can be emotionally draining (Figure 36.20). The idea of children having such problems is upsetting for some and frightening to others. Nurses are no different from other people. Their own backgrounds and upbringing range from optimal to destructive. They carry many messages from their youth and may see themselves in the children whom they encounter.

Nurses may find the care of children who are ill or disabled difficult. There are times of helplessness: physical pain continues, disability cannot be reversed, disease cannot be arrested, or death approaches. Anger is a natural response. How nurses manage such anger is important.

To care for themselves, nurses need to recognize and discuss their job-related stressors. They should acknowledge and deal with issues that remind them of their own childhood and adolescence. Equally important, they need to attend to their own physical and mental health. Proper nutrition, rest and sleep, exercise, health care, maturity, and balance in personal and professional lives maximize the energy available to work therapeutically with youth and their families. Furthermore, in clinical settings, nurses must consider whether their expectations are realistic and what they can actually accomplish.

The concept of hardiness may play an important role in preventing burnout. Nurses can assess and determine ways to increase their own hardiness. To establish a sense of control and minimize the effects of uncertainty, they need adequate education and continued mentoring. Orientation programs that facilitate mentoring are advantageous. The importance of relationships between novice and more experienced nurses cannot be overemphasized. They build personal hardiness by nurturing competent practice. Verbal and nonverbal support from mentors can reduce uncertainty and increase sense of mastery.

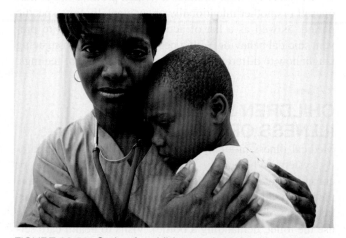

FIGURE 36.20 Caring for children and teens with mental disorders, illness, and developmental challenges can be draining and emotionally challenging for nurses. Many nurses take comfort in their ability to serve as a source of comfort and support for children, and find their positive influence on others to offset the difficulties inherent in such caregiving.

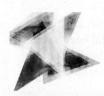

Reviewing and Applying Your Knowledge

Chapter Summary

- The effects of child and adolescent mental illness include the increased likelihood of the disorder continuing into later life, feelings of guilt and blame, unmet needs of siblings and other family members, marital stress and conflict, diminished productivity of lives, and direct and indirect costs.

- Factors placing the child or adolescent at risk for development of mental health disorders include biologic ones, such as a family history of a mental illness, immature development of the brain, or a brain abnormality; psychological ones, including family problems and dysfunction; and stressors, including poverty, parents with mental illness or substance abuse problems, teen parents, abuse, discrimination because of race, creed, or color, chronic parental conflict or divorced parents, and chronic illness or disability.

- Early intervention with children and adolescents at risk can prevent more serious mental disturbance later in life. Child and adolescent mental illness is treated by biologic interventions such as psychotropic medication, psychosocial interventions, therapeutic approaches designed for each client, school modifications, and community-based services.

- The role of the nurse in child and adolescent mental health care is essential. The nurse performs a thorough assessment, including an assessment of family functioning and current problems, a history, and a mental status examination. The nurse also provides medication education, meets the needs of the families, and promotes the rights of children in treatment settings, which includes avoiding seclusion and restraints and providing advocacy.

- Children and adolescents are affected by many psychiatric illnesses, including ones that are usually first diagnosed during infancy, childhood, or adolescence and ones that, although common in adults, have different manifestations and require different treatment in children and adolescents. The most common from each category include ADHD, conduct disorder, ODD, adjustment disorder, OCD, phobias, social anxiety disorder, GAD, separation anxiety disorder, PTSD, depression, bipolar disorder, autism spectrum disorders, eating disorders, substance abuse, tic disorders, and trichotillomania.

- Nursing care of the child with ADHD focuses on the family as a whole and involves educating family members about treatment and behavioral strategies, helping the family cope, managing developmental and academic issues, teaching social skills, and improving self-image.

Study Questions

1. A 6-year-old girl was hospitalized for a bowel obstruction. When visiting the child at home after discharge, the nurse assessed the following: flat affect, reports of nightmares, and new onset of bed-wetting. The nurse suspects which of the following?

   a. Conduct disorder

   b. Adjustment disorder

   c. Dysthymia

   d. Generalized anxiety disorder

2. The parents of a child newly diagnosed with ADHD relate that their son cannot focus on school activities for more than a minute or two at a time. Which of the following responses by the nurse would be most appropriate regarding the child's planned treatment?

   a. "We can develop a system of negative consequences for inattentive behavior that will help your son focus on schoolwork."

   b. "A system of rewards will be the most helpful intervention for improving his ability to focus."

   c. "Medication therapy can be most helpful in improving your son's ability to focus on activities."

   d. "We will begin social skills training to help improve his behavior at school."

3. The nurse is planning a discussion group for parents of children and adolescents with depression. Which of the following would the nurse include as the major reason for this condition being underdiagnosed in this age group?

   a. Teenagers and children often deliberately cover up their true feelings.

   b. Transient depression is a normal part of growing up.

   c. Teenagers and children may be unable verbally to express their feelings and act out instead.

   d. Health care providers do not believe childhood depression is real.

4. Substance abuse is a significant problem among adolescents, one that puts them at risk for other mental health disorders, negative life events, and injury. When assessing the adolescent client for signs and symptoms of substance abuse, the nurse should consider which of the following as a possible indicator of a substance problem?

a. Change in or loss of friends

b. Family history of substance abuse

c. Sleep disturbances and rapid mood swings

d. Avoidance of contact with unfamiliar people

Critical Thinking Questions

1. Reread Case in Point 36.1. Develop a rewards-based program for school performance for Michael.

2. Based on all the information in this chapter, identify what you think is the most pressing mental health issue confronting children and adolescents. Identify ways in which the social environment contributes both positively and negatively to this issue.

3. Discuss how families from various cultural backgrounds approach mental health issues in children and adolescents. Compare and contrast the suicide and depression rates in the United States with those of other countries. Suggest reasons these rates may differ.

References

Altshuler, L. L., Post, R. M., Leverich, G. S., Mikalauskas, K., Rosoff, A., & Ackerman, L. (1995). Antidepressant-induced mania and cycle acceleration: A controversy revisited. *American Journal of Psychiatry, 152*(8), 1130–1138.

American Academy of Child and Adolescent Psychiatry. (1997). Practice parameters for the assessment and treatment of children, adolescents and adults with ADHD. *Journal of the American Academy of Child and Adolescent Psychiatry, 36*(10S), S855–S1218.

American Academy of Pediatrics. (2001). Clinical practice guideline: Treatment of the school age child with ADHD. *Pediatrics, 108,* 1033–1044.

American Psychiatric Association. (2000). *Diagnostic and statistical manual of mental disorders* (4th ed., text rev.). Washington, DC: Author.

Anderson, J. A., Wright, E. R., Kooreman, H. E., Mohr, W. K., & Russell, L. A. (2003). The Dawn Project: A model for responding to the needs of children with emotional and behavioral challenges and their families. *Community Mental Health Journal, 39*(1), 63–74.

Arseneault, L., Cannon, M., Witton, J., & Murray, R. (2004). Causal association between cannabis and psychosis: Examination of the evidence. *British Journal of Psychiatry, 184,* 110–117.

Association of Child and Adolescent Psychiatric Nurses (ACAPN). (1999). *On the rights of children in treatment settings: Position paper.* Philadelphia, PA: Author.

Axelson, D., Birmaher, B., & Strober, M. (2006). Phenomenology of children and adolescents with bipolar spectrum disorders. *Archives of General Psychiatry, 63,* 1139–1148.

Berrios, C. D., & Jacobowitz, W. H. (1998). Therapeutic holding: Outcomes of a pilot study. *Journal of Psychosocial Nursing, 36*(8), 14–18.

Bhatia, S. K., & Bhatia, S. C. (2007). Childhood and adolescent depression. *American Family Physician, 75*(1), 73–80.

Birmaher, B., Axelson, D., & Pavuluri, M. (2007). Bipolar disorder. In A. Martin & F. R. Volkmar (Eds.), *Lewis's child and adolescent psychiatry: A comprehensive textbook* (4th ed., pp. 513–528). Philadelphia, PA: Lippincott Williams & Wilkins.

Birmaher, B., Axelson, D., Strober, M., Gill, M. K., Valeri, S., Chiappetta L., et al. (2006). Clinical course of children and adolescents with bipolar spectrum disorders. *Archives of General Psychiatry, 63,* 175–183.

Bowlby, J. (1969). *Attachment and loss. Vol. 1. Attachment.* New York, NY: Basic Books.

Bowlby, J. (1980). *Attachment and loss. Vol. 3. Loss.* New York, NY: Basic Books.

Bowlby, J. (1988). *A secure base: Parent–child attachment and healthy human development.* New York, NY: Basic Books.

Bulechek, G. M., Butcher, H. K., & McCloskey Dochterman, J. (2008). *Nursing interventions classification (NIC)* (5th ed.). St. Louis, MO: Mosby.

Bush, C. T. (2000). Cultural competence: Implications of the Surgeon General's Report on Mental Health. *Journal of Child and Adolescent Psychiatric Nursing, 13*(4), 177–178.

Casey, B. J., Nigg, J. T., & Durston, S. (2007). New potential leads in the biology and treatment of attention deficit-hyperactivity disorder. *Current Opinion in Neurology, 20*(2), 119–124.

Center for Mental Health Services. (2001). National strategy for suicide prevention (NSSP). Retrieved from http://www.mentalhealth.org

Centers for Disease Control and Prevention. (2007). Child maltreatment: Fact sheet. Retrieved from http://www.cdc.gov/ncipc/factsheets/cmfacts.htm

Cicchetti, D., & Toth, S. L. (2009). The past achievements and future promises of developmental psychopathology: The coming of age of a discipline. *Journal of Child Psychology & Psychiatry, 50*(1–2), 16–25.

Cohen, J., Deblinger, E., Mannarino, A., & Steer, R. (2004a). A multisite, randomized controlled trial for children with sexual abuse-related PTSD symptoms. *Journal of the American Academy of Child and Adolescent Psychiatry, 43*(4), 393–402.

Cohen J., Mannarino, A., & Knudsen, K. (2004b). Treating childhood traumatic grief: A pilot study. *Journal of the American Academy of Child and Adolescent Psychiatry, 43*(10), 1225–1233.

Costello, E. J., Mustillo, S., Erkanli, A., Keeler, G., & Angold, A. (2003). Prevalence and development of psychiatric disorders in childhood and adolescence. *Archives of General Psychiatry, 60,* 765–794.

Dishion, T., McCord, J., & Poulin, F. (1999). When interventions harm: Peer groups and problem behavior. *American Psychologist, 54,* 755–764.

Elder, J. H. (2001). A follow-up study of beliefs held by parents of children with pervasive developmental delay. *Journal of Child and Adolescent Psychiatric Nursing, 14*(2), 55–60.

Enos, S., & Plante, T. (2001). Trichotillomania: An overview and guide to understanding. *Journal of Psychosocial Nursing, 39*(5), 10–18.

Falsafi, N. (2001). Pediatric psychiatric emergencies. *Journal of Child and Adolescent Psychiatric Nursing, 14*(2), 81–88.

Feinberg, A. G. (2000, March/April). Diagnosis and treatment of AD/HD in adults. *Attention*, pp. 20–22.

Fox, N. A., Henderson, H. A., & Marshall, P. J. (2001).The biology of temperament: An integrative approach. In C. A. Nelson & M. Luciana (Eds.), *The handbook of developmental cognitive neuroscience* (pp. 631–645). Cambridge, MA: MIT Press.

Frick, P. J., & Dickens, C. (2006). Current perspectives on conduct disorder. *Current Psychiatry Reports, 8*(1), 59–72.

Friedman, R. M., Pinto, A., Behar, L., Bush, N., Chirolla, A., Epstein, M., et al. (2006). Unlicensed residential programs: The next challenge in protecting youth. *American Journal of Orthopsychiatry, 76*(3), 295–303.

Garbarino, J. (1999). *Lost boys: Why our sons turn violent and how we can save them*. New York. NY: Free Press.

Green, W. H. (2007). *Child and adolescent clinical psychopharmacology*. Philadelphia, PA: Lippincott.

Harmon, P. L. (2000, March/April). One-on-one with Russell Barkley. *Attention*, pp. 12–14.

Henggeler, S. W., Rowland, M. D., Randall, J., Ward, S. L., Edwards, J., Zealberg, J. J., et al. (1999). Home-based multisystemic therapy as an alternative to hospitalization of youths in psychiatric crisis: Clinical outcomes. *Journal of the American Academy of Child and Adolescent Psychiatry, 38*, 1331–1339.

Henggeler, S. W., Schoenwald, S. K., Borduin, C. M., Rowland, M. D., & Cunningham, P. B. (1998). *Multisystemic treatment of antisocial behavior in children and adolescents*. New York, NY: Guilford Press.

Hodas, G. R. (2006, February). Responding to childhood trauma: The promise and practice of trauma informed care. Retrieved from http://www.nasmhpd.org/general_files/publications/ntac_pubs/Responding%20to%20Childhood%20Trauma%20-%20Hodas.pdf

Institute of Medicine, Committee on Quality of Health Care in America (2001). *Crossing the quality chasm: A new health system for the 21st century*. Washington, DC: National Academies Press.

The Joint Commission. (1998). *Preventing restraint death*. Washington, DC: Author.

Karekla, M., & Perdikogianni, M. (2006). Treating children through play. *PsychCritiques, 51*(26), Electronic Collection: 2006-06323-001.

Kelly, J. G. (2000). Wellness as an ecological enterprise. In D. Ciccetti, J. Rappaport, I. Sandler, & R. P. Weissberg (Eds.), *The promotion of wellness in children and adolescents* (pp. 29–58). Washington, DC: CWLA Press.

Kendall, J. (1999, Spring). Sibling accounts of ADHD. *Family Process, 38*, 117–136.

Kendall, P. C. (2006). *Child and adolescent therapy: Cognitive–behavioral therapy*. New York, NY: Guilford Press

Kessler, R. C., Chiu, W. T., & Demler, O., Merikangas, K. R., & Walters, E. E. (2005). Prevalence severity and comorbidity of 12-month DSM-IV disorders in the National Comorbidity Survey Replication. *Archives of General Psychiatry, 62*, 617–627.

Klein, D. N., Schwartz, J. E., Rose, S., et al. (2000). Five-year course and outcome of dysthymic disorder: A prospective, naturalistic follow-up study. *American Journal of Psychiatry, 157*(6), 931–939.

Kohlberg, L. (1984). *The psychology of moral development: The nature and validity of moral stages*. San Francisco, CA: Harper and Row.

Krueger, M., & Kendall, J. (2001). Descriptions of self: An exploratory study of adolescents with ADHD. *Journal of Child and Adolescent Psychiatric Nursing, 14*(2), 61–72.

Kuchta, M. (2001, Spring/Summer). Depression in pre-teen and adolescent children. *Nursing in Pediatrics*, pp. 4–7.

Landreth, G. L., Sweeney, D. S., Ray, D. C., Homeyer, L. E., & Glover, G. J. (2005). *Play therapy interventions with children's problems: Case studies with DSM IV-TR diagnoses* (2nd ed.). Northvale, NJ: Jason Aronson.

Lieberman, A. (2005). Child–parent psychotherapy with young children exposed to violence. Presentation at Institute 2 (Treating Traumatized Children, Adolescents, and Families), American Academy of Child and Adolescent Psychiatry, October 19, 2005. Retrieved from http://www.kindertraumainstitut.de/download.php?name=aktuelles_24.pdf

Lipschitz, D. S., Winegar, R. K., Hartnick, E., Foote, B., & Southwick, S. M. (1999). Posttraumatic stress disorder in hospitalized adolescents: Psychiatric comorbidity and clinical correlates. *Journal of the American Academy of Child and Adolescent Psychiatry, 38*, 385–392.

Lorenz, K. Z. (1952). *King Solomon's ring*. New York, NY: Crowell.

Luthar, S. S., & Prince, R. P. (2007). Developmental psychopathology. In A. Martin & F. R. Volkmar (Eds.), *Lewis's child and adolescent psychiatry: A comprehensive textbook* (4th ed.). Philadelphia, PA: Lippincott Williams & Wilkins.

Maccoby, E. E. (2000). Parenting and its effects on children: On reading and misreading behavior genetics. *Annual Review of Psychology, 51*, 1–27.

Mainous, R. O., Mainous, A. G., Martin, C. A., Oler, M. J., & Haney, A. S. (2001). The importance of fulfilling unmet needs of rural and urban adolescents with substance abuse. *Journal of Child and Adolescent Psychiatric Nursing, 14*(1), 32–40.

Marquardt, E. (2006). *Between two worlds: The inner lives of children of divorce*. Bethel, CT: Crown Publishing.

Martin, A., & Volkmar, F. R. (Eds.). (2007). *Lewis's child and adolescent psychiatry: A comprehensive textbook* (4th ed.). Philadelphia, PA: Lippincott Williams & Wilkins.

Martinez, R. J., Grimm, M., & Adamson, M. (1999). From the other side of the door: Patient views of seclusion. *Journal of Psychosocial Nursing, 37*(3), 13–22.

McClowry, S. G. (2002). The temperament profiles of school-age children. *Journal of Pediatric Nursing, 17*(1), 3–10.

Mohr, W. K. (2001). Bipolar disorder in children. *Journal of Psychosocial Nursing, 39*(3), 12–23.

Mohr, W. K., & Anderson, J. A. (2001). Faulty assumptions associated with the use of restraints with children. *Journal of Child and Adolescent Psychiatric Nursing, 14*(3), 141–151.

Mohr, W. K., Mahon, M. M., & Noone, M. J. (1998). A restraint on restraints: The need to reconsider the use of restrictive interventions. *Archives of Psychiatric Nursing, 12*(2), 95–106.

Mohr, W. K., Olson, J. N., Martin, A., Pumariega, A. J., & Branca, N. (2009). Beyond point and level systems: Moving toward child-centered programming. *American Journal of Orthopsychiatry, 79*(1), 8–18.

Mohr, W. K., Petti, T. A., & Mohr, B. D. (2003). Adverse effects associated with the use of physical restraints. *Canadian Journal of Psychiatry, 48*, 330–337.

Mohr, W. K., & Pumariega, A. J. (2004). Level systems: Inpatient programming whose time has passed. *Journal of Child and Adolescent Psychiatric Nursing, 17*(3), 113–125.

Moorhead, S., Johnson, M., Maas, M. L., & Swanson, E. (2008). *Nursing outcomes classification (NOC)* (4th ed.). St. Louis, MO: Mosby.

NANDA International. (2007). *Nursing diagnoses: Definitions and classification (2007–2008)*. Philadelphia, PA: Author.

National Center for Mental Health and Juvenile Justice. (2006). *Blueprint for change: A comprehensive model for the identification and treatment of youth with mental health needs in contact with the juvenile justice system*. Retrieved from http://www.ncmhjj.com/Blueprint/cornerstones/Identification_background.shtml

National Head Start Association. (2007). *Benefits of Head Start and Early Head Start programs*. Retrieved from http://www

.nhsa.org/files/static_page_files/399E0881-1D09-3519-AD-56452FC44941C3/BenefitsofHSandEHS.pdf

National Institute of Mental Health (NIMH). (2006). *Attention deficit hyperactivity disorder*. Retrieved from http://www.nimh.nih.gov/publicat/adhd.cfm

Nunno, M. A., Holden, M., & Tollar, A. (2006). Learning from tragedy: A survey of child and adolescent restraint fatalities. *Child Abuse and Neglect, 30*, 1333–1342.

O'Donnell, D. A., Joshi, P. T., & Lewin, S. M. (2007). Innovations: Child & adolescent psychiatry: Training in developmental responses to trauma for child service providers. *Psychiatric Services, 58*(1), 12–14.

Papolos, D., & Papolos, J. (2002). *The bipolar child*. New York, NY: Broadway Books.

Perry, B. (2004). Understanding traumatized and maltreated children: The core concepts—Living and working with traumatized children. The Child Trauma Academy. Retrieved from http://www.ChildTrauma.org

Piaget, J. (1936). *Origins of intelligence in the child*. London, United Kingdom: Routledge & Kegan Paul.

Pliszka, S. R., Browne, R. G., Olvera, R. L., & Wynne, S. K. (2000a). A double-blind, placebo-controlled study of Adderall and methylphenidate in the treatment of attention-deficit/hyperactivity disorder. *Journal of the American Academy of Child and Adolescent Psychiatry, 39*(5), 619–626.

Pliszka, S. R., Greenhill, L. L., Crismon, M. L., Sedillo, A., Carlson, C., Conners, K., et al. (2000b). The Texas Children's Medication Algorithm Project: Report of the Texas Consensus Conference Panel on medication treatment of childhood attention-deficit hyperactivity disorder. Part I. *Journal of the American Academy of Child and Adolescent Psychiatry, 39*(7), 908–919.

Prendeville, J. A., Prelock, P. A., & Unwin, G. (2006). Peer play interventions to support the social competence of children with autism spectrum disorders. *Seminars in Speech & Language, 27*(1), 2–46.

Pullen, L. M., Modrcin-McCarthy, M. A., & Graf, E. V. (2000). Adolescent depression: Important facts that matter. *Journal of Child and Adolescent Psychiatric Nursing, 13*(2), 69–75.

Rutter, M. (2009). Understanding and testing risk mechanisms for mental disorders. *Journal of Child Psychology and Psychiatry, 50*(1–2), 44–52.

Saxe, G., Ellis, H., Fogler, J., et al. (2005). Comprehensive care for traumatized children: An open trial examines treatment using trauma systems therapy. *Psychiatric Annals, 35*, 443–448.

Schaefer, C. E., & Kaduson, H. G. (2006). *Contemporary play therapy: Theory, research, and practice*. New York, NY: Guilford Press.

Schatzberg, A. F., & Nemeroff, C. B. (2006). *Essentials of clinical pharmacology*. Washington, DC: American Psychiatric Press.

Shain, B. N. (2007). Suicide and suicide attempts in adolescents. *Pediatrics, 120*(3), 669–676.

Shonkoff, J. P., & Phillips, D. A. (2000). *From neurons to neighborhoods: The science of early childhood development*. Washington, DC: National Academy Press.

Siebert, C. F., Jr., & Thogmartin, J. R. (2000). Restraint-related fatalities in mental health facilities: Report of two cases. *American Journal of Forensic Medicine and Pathology, 21*(3), 210–212.

Silva, R. R., Alpert, M., Munoz, D. M., Singh, S., Matzner, F., & Dummit, S. (2000). Stress and vulnerability to posttraumatic stress disorder in children and adolescents. *American Journal of Psychiatry, 157*(8), 1229–1236.

Spetie, L. & Arnold, E. L. (2007). Attention deficit hyperactivity disorder. In A. Martin & F. R. Volkmar (Eds.), *Lewis's child and adolescent psychiatry: A comprehensive textbook* (4th ed., pp. 430–449). Philadelphia, PA: Lippincott Williams & Wilkins.

Stein, B., Jaycox, L., Kataoka, S., Wong, M., Tu, W., Elliot, M., et al. (2003). A mental health intervention for schoolchildren exposed to violence: A randomized controlled trial. *Journal of the American Medical Association, 290* (5), 603–611.

Substance Abuse and Mental Health Administration (SAMHA). (2003). *Achieving the promise, transforming mental health care in America*. Washington, DC: President's New Freedom Commission on Mental Health.

Szalavitz, M. (2006). *Help at any cost: How the troubled-teen industry cons parents and hurts kids*. New York, NY: Riverside Books.

Tynan, W. D. (2006a). *Conduct disorder*. Retrieved from http://www.emedicine.com/ped/topic2793.htm

Tynan, W. D. (2006b). *Oppositional defiant disorder*. Retrieved from http://www.emedicine.com/ped/topic2791.htm

U.S. Department of Health and Human Services (USDHHS). (1999). *Mental health: A report of the surgeon general*. Rockville, MD: U.S. Department of Health and Human Services, Substance Abuse and Mental Health Services Administration, Center for Mental Health Services, National Institutes of Health, National Institute of Mental Health.

U.S. Department of Health and Human Services (USDHHS). (2001). *Report of the Surgeon General's Conference on Children's Mental Health: A national action agenda*. Rockville, MD: U.S. Department of Health and Human Services, Substance Abuse and Mental Health Services Administration, Center for Mental Health Services, National Institutes of Health, National Institute of Mental Health. Retrieved from http://www.surgeongeneral.gov/cmh/childreport.htm

Van der Kolk, B. (2003, April). The neurobiology of childhood trauma and abuse. *Child and Adolescent Psychiatric Clinics of North America, 12*(2), 293–317.

vanManen, T. G., Prins, T. J. M., & Emmelkamp, P. M. G. (2004). Reducing aggressive behavior in boys with a social cognitive group treatment: Results of a randomized, controlled trial. *Journal of the American Academy of Child and Adolescent Psychiatry, 43*(12), 1478–1487.

Volkmar, F. R., Lord, C., Klin, A., & Cook, E. (2007). Autism and the pervasive developmental disorders. In M. Lewis (Ed.), *Child and adolescent psychiatry: A comprehensive textbook* (pp. 384–400). Philadelphia, PA: Lippincott Williams & Wilkins.

Wallerstein, J. S., & Corbin, S. B. (2002). The child and the vicissitudes of divorce. In M. Lewis (Ed.), *Child and adolescent psychiatry: A comprehensive textbook* (pp. 1276–1285). Philadelphia, PA: Lippincott Williams & Wilkins.

Wallerstein, J. S., Lewis, J., & Blakeslee, S. (2000). *The unexpected legacy of divorce: Report of a 25-year landmark study*. New York, NY: Hyperion.

Weinberger, D. R. (2001, March 10). A brain too young for good judgment. *New York Times*. Retrieved from http://www.nytimes.com/2001/03/10/opinion/a-brain-too-young-for-good-judgment.html

White, J. H. (2000). The prevention of eating disorders: A review of the research on risk factors with implications for practice. *Journal of Child and Adolescent Psychiatric Nursing, 13*(2), 76–88.

Woolfenden, S. R., Williams, K., & Peat, J. (2006). Family and parenting interventions in children and adolescents with conduct disorder and delinquency aged 10–17. *Cochrane Database of Systematic Reviews, 2006*.

Web Resources

Academy for Eating Disorders: http://www.aedweb.org

American Academy of Child and Adolescent Psychiatry: http://www.aacap.org

American Association of Intellectual and Developmental Disabilities: http://www.aaidd.org

American Autism Society: http://www.autism-society.org

American Foundation for Suicide Prevention: http://www.afsp.org

Association of Child and Adolescent Psychiatric Nurses: http://www.ispn-psych.org/html/acapn.html

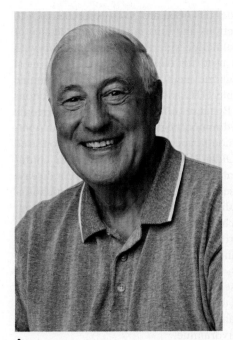

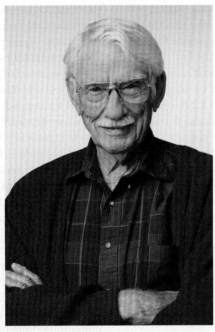

A   **B**

FIGURE 37.2 The age range for people belonging to the older adult age group can span 40 years or more. Differences in ability, physiologic status, and interests can vary greatly for people in their 60s (**A**) versus those in their 80s (**B**).

weight loss. Vascular dementia and delirium may appear with psychiatric symptoms of delusions, agitation, and mood and behavior changes (see Chap. 31). Similarly, chronic medical conditions are associated with psychiatric illness, particularly depression, which can increase both morbidity and mortality (Sadock & Sadock, 2007). Depression can accompany such conditions as stroke, cancer, arthritis, myocardial infarction, and chronic obstructive pulmonary disease (COPD). Medications used to treat chronic diseases, such as beta blockers for hypertension and steroids for COPD and

arthritis, can also contribute to depression because of their effects on the CNS (see Chap. 39).

Medications

Older adults use 33% of all prescription and 40% of all OTC medications in the United States. They are twice as likely as younger people to have adverse drug reactions (Roose et al., 2004). Age-related changes in the central nervous, gastrointestinal, and renal systems are most responsible for the variations in drug reactions in older compared with younger clients.

Pharmacokinetics refers to how the body absorbs, distributes, metabolizes, and excretes medications (see Chap. 16). With aging, fat and protein distribution and renal function change significantly. Decreased gastrointestinal acid secretion and peristalsis may impair absorption. Decreased lean body mass and increased fat alter distribution, which results in longer storage of lipid-soluble drugs. Nearly all drugs that affect the CNS must be lipid soluble to cross the blood–brain barrier. Deceased hepatic function can affect metabolism. Most significantly, blood flow though the renal system decreases by almost 50%, impairing drug excretion. Resulting compromises in urine concentration can lead to medication toxicity.

Pharmacodynamics refers to actions of medications on the person (see Chap. 16). Absorption, actions, and possible side effects can be very different even when the same drug in the same dose is given to two people of the same age and sex with the same condition. Factors such as activity level and medical conditions can influence pharmacodynamics. Knowing where a drug is metabolized is important because when medications are not metabolized

---

BOX 37.1   Ten Tips for Healthy Aging

1. Eat a balanced diet.
2. Exercise regularly.
3. Get regular checkups.
4. Do not smoke. It is never too late to quit.
5. Practice safety habits at home to prevent falls and fractures. Add grab bars, bath mats, and rails in the bathroom as needed. Always wear your seat belt when traveling by car.
6. Maintain contacts with family and friends, and stay active through work, recreation, and community.
7. Avoid overexposure to the sun and the cold.
8. If you drink, do so in moderation. When you drink, let someone else drive.
9. Keep personal and financial records to simplify budgeting and investing. Plan long-term housing and financial needs.
10. Keep a positive attitude toward life. Do things that make you happy.

Adapted from the National Institute on Aging, National Institutes of Health. (2007). Rockville, MD: Author.

as intended, drugs can accumulate and cause toxicity or overdose. For instance, the liver metabolizes acetaminophen. Thus, this drug might not be the best choice for people with liver disorders.

One of the most significant age-related changes is decreased CNS functional reserve. Disease or drug effects in any part of the body may present with CNS changes. Any drug affecting the CNS puts older adults at risk. To be effective, a medication must bind with appropriate receptor sites. Chapter 16 addresses psychopharmacology in detail; however, nurses must understand this action and the CNS effects in specific reference to older adults. The neurotransmitter acetylcholine (ACh) serves as an illustration. ACh is the bioamine thought most involved in cognition; problems related to ACh can lead to delirium and other cognitive disorders. ACh is a necessary component of cognition; without it, confusion and memory impairment occur. As the brain ages, and especially in clients with Alzheimer's disease (see Chap. 31), the functioning of neurons decreases significantly. See also Understanding Biologic Foundations 37.1.

Too many prescribed medications can also interfere with ACh, because many drugs have anticholinergic effects (Sadock & Sadock, 2007). Because the need to preserve ACh in the synaptic junction is so important, nurses should be aware of drugs that interfere with this process. Anticholinergics often are given before surgery to decrease oral secretions and thus minimize the chance of aspiration. Anticholinergic side effects are common with many medications used for depression. One of the most common anticholinergic medications is diphenhydramine (Benadryl), available OTC and used for allergy reactions and as a sleep aid. Because of its side effects, many people who use diphenhydramine begin to feel dizzy and lightheaded, get a dry mouth, and sometimes become confused and disoriented. Older adults who already have confusion and disorientation secondary to Alzheimer's disease will be compromised significantly if they take anticholinergic drugs. In addition to decreased cognition and confusion, other anticholinergic effects such as dry mouth, dizziness, and blurred vision can predispose older clients to falls. Giving anticholinergics routinely to any older adult is dangerous, even if the older adult does not have Alzheimer's disease. Nurses should be aware of the effects of anticholinergics to prevent adverse reactions and should teach older adults and family members to avoid OTC drugs containing diphenhydramine.

The term that describes the use of many drugs simultaneously in the same client is **polypharmacy** (see Chap. 16). Because the number of physical problems tends to increase with age, many clients have several different medical conditions that require treatment. They may receive medications

UNDERSTANDING BIOLOGIC FOUNDATIONS 37.1

Acetylcholine and Aging

The presynaptic neuron releases ACh, which travels to specific receptors on the postsynaptic neuron. In the *synapse* between the neurons, the enzyme acetylcholinesterase (AChE) is released and rapidly breaks down ACh before it can bind to the receptor sites on the postsynaptic neuron. Sufficient levels of ACh must circulate among neurons for optimal functioning. Drugs that inhibit AChE and allow ACh to bind with receptor sites on the postsynaptic neuron are called AChE inhibitors. They are the cornerstone of current treatment for Alzheimer's disease (Sunderland et al., 2004).

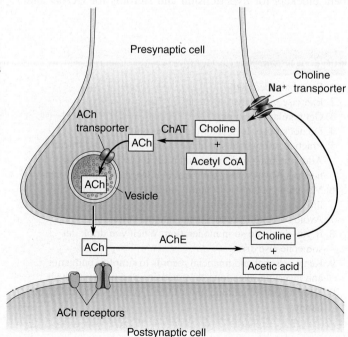

from both their regular health care providers and several specialists. Problems arise when no single physician oversees all the medications for compatibility and client adherence. When a client adds OTC medications, medical repercussions can be severe. As routine parts of their assessment, nurses should consistently assess clients' medication use, including prescriptions, OTC medications, and herbal supplements.

> **Checkpoint Questions**
> 1. What are three normal age-related changes in the renal system of an older adult?
> 2. How does pharmacokinetics differ in older adults?

Psychosocial Issues and Influences of Aging

Conflicting theories have been proposed to explain psychological adaptation to aging. Those who posit the *disengagement theory* believe that healthy aging involves a voluntary "stepping back" from earlier life activities. Proponents of the *activity theory* suggest that psychological health in old age depends on staying active and involved. A third choice, the *continuity theory,* is a bridge connecting these views. It suggests that healthy adaptation is based on each person's preferences for involvement or solitary pursuits (Grossman, 2006).

Tasks of old age include conserving strength and resources as necessary and adapting to age-related changes and losses. The ability to adapt and thrive is contingent on physical health, personality, early life experiences, and societal support, such as adequate finances, shelter, medical care, social roles, and recreation.

Flood (2005) suggests that an older person's ability to adapt predicts successful aging. Her theory focuses on spiritual and existential domains, in addition to the traditional biopsychosocial perspective. Drawing on Reed's (2009) work on theories of self-transcendence, Tornstam's (2005) work on gerotranscendence, and Roy's (1997) adaptation model, she outlines how integrating coping, adaptation, and spirituality provides a foundation for older persons to experience gerotranscendence, which in turn leads to "more meaning and purpose in life and greater life satisfaction—indicators of successful aging" (p. 38). Lander McCarthy (2011) illustrates how Flood's model can be applied to older adults living in a low-income retirement community.

Retirement

One of the first adjustments that older adults face is retirement. Many people base their sense of identity on the position they hold in the workforce. Those with a common employment experience frequently develop friendships and social relationships. Occupational identity largely is responsible for a person's social position and accompanying social roles.

Upon leaving an occupation, some retirees have difficulty adjusting to aspects of the transition, such as reduced income and perhaps lowered prestige. Retirement may force spouses or life partners to reestablish and renegotiate family or household roles. Each partner, whether working outside the home or not, had a daily routine that provided a sense of identity and accomplishment. Retirement requires significant adjustments for both partners. Preparing for retirement is a preventive intervention that helps clients plan for transitions and maximizes the potential for health and well-being (Client-Centered Education 37.1).

Although most people eventually retire, increasing numbers of people are choosing to work full time or part time after 65 years for financial reasons, personal rewards, or both. As they become a bigger segment of the overall population, society will need to find additional ways to continue using the skills older adults have to offer.

Client–Centered Education 37.1

Preretirement Planning

When working with older adult clients, helping them to prepare for retirement transitions can be an important nursing intervention. The following guidelines are important teaching points:

- Establish and practice good health habits, such as following a nutritious diet and regular exercise program and avoiding alcohol, drug, and tobacco use.
- Develop interests unrelated to work, such as leisure activities, hobbies, and participation in civic, religious, and other group activities.

- Develop roles outside the employment area. Use experiences to assist others. Develop the role of a community or volunteer helper.
- Recognize the realities versus the fantasies of retirement. Establish goals and routines to provide stability for the future.
- Establish financial security. Develop a budget that is realistic yet provides for desired activities.
- If married or in a long-term partnership, begin to establish renegotiated roles. Plan to share household activities and responsibilities. Provide for separate and joint activities.

Relocation

Giving up their homes and moving into assisted living or long-term care facilities is a transition for some older people. Many clients view moving to such facilities as a sign of relinquishing freedom and assuming a dependent role. They may have difficulty coping and suffer from related depression.

Older people facing an unscheduled, possibly permanent move need all possible resources to cope with stress. Relocation is difficult at any age, but may be especially difficult for older adults experiencing several other changes. People who see themselves as hardy, that is, committed, in control, and challenged, are less likely to experience depression after moving to a nursing home (Murrell et al., 2003). Psychiatric–mental health nurses can influence the day-to-day care of older clients positively and assist them with their transition to new residences by acting as teachers, advocates, facilitators, and role models. Involving the client's family before, during, and after transition to long-term care can help both the older adult and his or her family make a successful transition (Figure 37.3).

Bereavement

Older adults often confront several concurrent losses, including the deaths of significant others. Older women outnumber older men, as the mortality rate for women has declined rapidly during the past 40 years. The difference in mortality rate between genders may be partly related to the adjustment of men and women to the loss of a spouse or significant other, although recent data on this issue are inconclusive. What

seems clear is that lack of social support for both men and women tends to affect health and may lead to increased mortality. Noting the need for social support during this difficult time, a study by Wilcox and colleagues (2003) found that older women were more resilient and better able to reestablish social connections after the loss of a spouse than were men.

Deaths of spouses, partners, siblings, and friends may lead older people to become more aware of their own declining function and mortality. Before they can help older people deal with death and bereavement, nurses must acknowledge their own feelings about death. Contemplating mortality and working through the grief process assists clients to find meaning in their remaining lives. Nurses also need to assess cultural values, personal characteristics, health beliefs, health practices, and social support systems to help each client achieve optimal functioning and quality of life. See Case Vignette 37.1.

Case Vignette 37.1

Barbara, a 74-year-old widowed and retired teacher, lives in a home she and her husband shared. Her husband Don died 4 months ago after a battle with lung cancer. During the last few months of his life, Barbara primarily cared for her husband at home, with assistance from hospice. Barbara is generally in good health; she takes Fosamax and calcium supplements for osteoporosis and an occasional ibuprofen when she experiences osteoarthritic pain.

Initially, after Don's death, Barbara managed her grief and dealt with all the arrangements and financial matters, with help from friends and her daughters. After staying with Barbara for 2 weeks after Don's death, her daughters returned to their families in distant states.

In the past 2 weeks, Barbara has begun to have difficulty sleeping and has lost her appetite, resulting in a 10-lb weight loss. Her osteoarthritis has been more painful, and she has increased use of ibuprofen without much relief. In addition, she has begun to experience some midsternal pain. A friend remarks on Barbara's weight loss and tired appearance and convinces her to see her family physician. A complete physical examination reveals a normal electrocardiogram and no new or obvious cause for difficulty sleeping and weight loss. The physician wants Barbara to have a colonoscopy and a mammography, screening tests she neglected while caring for Don. He also refers her to the geriatric nurse practitioner in his office for further evaluation and a plan of care.

Reflection and Critical Thinking

- What are some possible reasons for Barbara's symptoms?
- What types of interventions should the nurse consider implementing?
- Based on your knowledge learned in this and other chapters, which psychiatric disorders might be risks for Barbara?

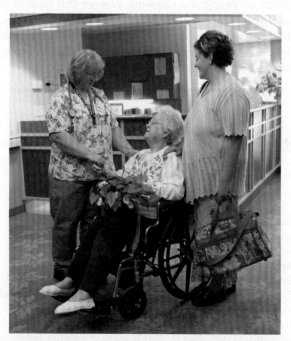

FIGURE 37.3 When an older adult moves to a residential facility, involving his or her family in the process can facilitate a more positive and pleasant transition for everyone.

Responses to Life Transitions

Older adults facing the loss of loved ones, multiple health problems, and decreasing abilities for self-care require support and hope. Sources of hope may include religious symbols, relationships, and activities. Well-designed environments can be encouraging; clinicians should work with older clients to choose or plan any new environments as much as possible. Self-efficacy is associated positively with mental wellness (Murrell et al., 2003). By participating in decisions related to relocation, older clients retain a sense of control over an event that can seem chaotic and jarring. Methods of assisting people to maintain control include planning for social, spiritual, and physical care needs. Providing spiritual care for clients requires developing an understanding of where they are on their spiritual journey and assisting them to adapt to losses and find meaning in late-life struggles (Lavretsky, 2010) (see Chap. 7).

Sociopolitical Issues and Influences
Ageism, Myths, and Prejudices

Sometimes health care providers, family members, and older people themselves incorrectly believe that depression, confusion, memory loss, and other mental or emotional problems are part of normal aging. These attitudes prevent many from seeking treatment, and unfortunately, some providers with these attitudes avoid aggressive diagnosis and management. For example, depression, the most common disorder in older adults, is *not* normal and can be diagnosed and treated.

Many older people are reluctant to seek assistance, particularly for mental or emotional disorders, because they grew up at a time when people hid mental problems. The need for self-determination and independence often impedes their willingness to seek care. They may endure problems in an attempt to preserve independence. Those with cognitive disturbances may not be motivated or aware of the need for care.

Often health care professionals tend to focus on physical problems when treating older adults, rather than considering mental health issues. Identifying and treating psychiatric disorders in the older population are especially challenging for nurses. Failure to distinguish disease-related psychiatric symptoms from manifestations of normal aging may blur their understanding of healthy mental functioning. Health professionals cannot treat the mental health problems of older adults adequately if they assume a client's behavior is part of normal aging. For example, a health care professional may find it difficult to determine if a client is experiencing dementia or depression. The distinction is important because—unlike dementia—depression can be treated successfully. On the other hand, dementia and depression may be misdiagnosed as physical problems because mental and physical illnesses in older people often occur simultaneously, and older adults are more likely to report physical symptoms. Depression and dementia may co-occur and be difficult to distinguish from each other. For example, an older adult with severe depression may present with cognitive impairment. Each condition tends to mimic

or exacerbate the symptoms of the other. To identify and differentiate for various causes of cognitive impairment, care providers should conduct detailed assessments of all clients with a diagnosis of dementia.

Fragmentation of Health Care

Until recently, society largely neglected the care of older adults with mental health problems. Epidemiologic studies since the 1950s have documented a 15% to 25% prevalence rate of serious mental disorders in clients 65 years or older. Current estimates are that approximately 25% of older adults in the community, 30% of those in hospitals, and nearly 50% of those in nursing homes have symptoms of mental illness (Bartels et al., 2005). Yet, most people with mental health issues never receive treatment as a result of systemic barriers to care.

Because of evolving changes in the U.S. health care delivery system, essential mental health services sometimes are difficult for clients to locate and finance. Mental health services are underfunded, and the system is fragmented across a wide array of health, mental health, aging, social services, long-term care, and private and public entities. No specific mental health authority for older adults exists. Finding appropriate services can be frustrating and confusing. Narrow criteria for entrance into community mental health, home health, and other treatment programs frequently present further challenges. Nursing homes are generally funded poorly and are inadequate to care for the number of residents with a mental illness. Insurance does not cover or restricts access to mental health services. Managed care policies with a focus on prevention sometimes seem to overlook that mental health disorders are leading risk factors for premature institutionalization and can turn a minor medical problem into a life-threatening and costly condition. Most older adults receive health care from a primary care provider. Reports indicate that primary care providers fail to detect 50% to 70% of psychiatric conditions. Even when such problems are recognized, treatment may be inadequate (Charney et al., 2003).

> **Checkpoint Questions**
> 3. What is one of the first adjustments that many older adults face?
> 4. Research has identified which factor as most protective for older adults experiencing significant loss?

OLDER ADULTS WITH PSYCHIATRIC DISORDERS

Many mental health disorders occur across the lifespan. As clients age, some disorders become more prevalent, and the resulting prognoses are more serious. Targeting reversible or at least controllable disorders is essential for prompt action and positive outcomes. Table 37.1 lists some conditions most prevalent in older adults, with usual onset, identifying symptoms, assessment techniques, treatment options, and

TABLE 37.1 Common Psychiatric Conditions in Older Adults

Disorder	Onset	Symptoms	Assessment and Treatment	Prognosis
Delirium	Rapid (from hours to days)	Fluctuating loss of concentration, confusion, disorientation, disturbed sleep, impaired memory and cognition, incoherent speech, good insight when lucid	Score on Mini-Mental Status Examination improves as condition improves. Treatment should address underlying medical condition as indicated.	Reversible
Dementia, Alzheimer's type	Gradual (from months to years)	Confusion, disorientation, labile affect, impaired memory and cognition, disorganized speech and behavior, delusions, poor insight and judgment	Score on Mini-Mental Status Examination decreases over time. Treatment aims at controlling psychosis.	Irreversible: mental condition deteriorates, as does physical condition eventually.
Vascular dementia	Rapid—immediately after vascular incident (eg, cerebrovascular accident and transient ischemic attack)	Confusion, disorientation, labile affect, impaired memory and cognition, delusions, poor insight and judgment	Score on Mini-Mental Status Examination decreases over time. Treatment aims at controlling psychosis. Condition remains the same over time, unless there is an additional vascular incident.	Irreversible: initial improvement is possible with therapeutic intervention, but condition tends to stabilize and becomes irreversible after 3 to 6 months.
Delusional disorder	Fluctuates: can be gradual or rapid	Possible visual or auditory hallucinations, often paranoia, difficulty distinguishing between reality and delusions	Thorough physical examination is necessary to rule out medical conditions (usually infections). Treatment aims at eliminating the delusions through medication and reality orientation.	Reversible
Depression	Usually gradual, unless there is a sudden personal loss	Sleep disturbance, appetite changes, decreased pleasure in usual activities, feelings of sadness, worthlessness, and guilt	Use of a depression scale is essential, as is assessment of suicidal ideation and lethality. Treatment may include antidepressants, psychotherapy, and various somatic therapies.	Improvement occurs with medication and psychotherapy; somatic therapies may also be needed. Without treatment, deterioration to the point of suicide is a risk.
Anxiety disorders	Usually rapid	Feelings ranging from apprehension, to dread, to panic	Treatments include psychotherapy, anti-anxiety agents, and biofeedback.	Improvement occurs with treatment, but can recur with increased stressors.
Late-onset schizophrenia	Usually develops over 6 months; usually first noted in client's early 20s	Delusions, hallucinations, flat affect, disorganized speech and behaviors	Mini-Mental Status Examination is necessary. Treatment includes antipsychotic medication and psychotherapy aimed at adherence to medication regimen.	Remission is possible with adherence to treatment plan.

TABLE 37.1 **Common Psychiatric Conditions in Older Adults** (continued)

Disorder	Onset	Symptoms	Assessment and Treatment	Prognosis
Substance abuse (drugs, alcohol, caffeine, tobacco)	May be rapid or gradual	Inability to hold a job or meet obligations, substance use in dangerous situations (driving, caring for children, operating machinery), legal problems related to substance use	Thorough psychosocial assessment, history, and physical examination are needed to rule out emergency and other secondary medical conditions. Treatment includes detoxification, psychotherapy, and medication management.	Remissions are possible with treatment; however, relapses are common. There can be long-term medical consequences of any substance abuse. Suicidal and homicidal ideation is not uncommon during initial treatment.
Elder abuse	May be rapid or gradual	Unexplained bruising, malnutrition, social isolation, and withdrawal	A detailed history and physical examination are necessary, as is a psychosocial assessment. Treatment can include removal of client from residence and appropriate medical and legal interventions.	With quick, appropriate interventions, prognosis is positive. There may be long-term consequences of injuries and malnutrition.

prognosis. Because most of these disorders are discussed in other parts of this book, they are covered here briefly in terms of presentation in older adults. Depression, the second leading primary care condition after hypertension for all ages and very prevalent in older adults, is considered more extensively.

Although many of these conditions are discussed elsewhere, nurses must understand that presentation in older adults often differs from that in the general population. The seriousness of the illness and treatment modalities may differ as well.

Sleep Disorders

Sleep disorders (see Chap. 22) are notable in older adults because becoming older is the most important factor associated with difficulty sleeping (Sadock & Sadock, 2007). Sleep disorders result from several complex interacting factors, including medical conditions, medications, lack of or disruption in daily routines, and changes in sleep–wake cycles thought to be age related. Certainly, as with any other mental illness, older adults are at increased risk for adverse reactions secondary to sleep disorders.

Anxiety Disorders

Most anxiety disorders (see Chap. 23) begin early in life, although some appear after 60 years. More than 15% of those older than 60 years have an anxiety disorder (Kessler et al., 2005). Anxiety disorders may be more incapacitating in older adults because of concurrent medical problems. With many Vietnam veterans entering the older adult category, rates of post-traumatic stress disorder are likely to increase in this population.

Somatoform Disorders

Eighty percent of people older than 65 years have at least one chronic disease and present with somatic concerns (Sadock & Sadock, 2007). Some of them believe that receiving help for a physical concern is more acceptable than receiving care for mental illness (see Chap. 24). The interplay of psychiatric and physical illness in older adults makes detection of each difficult. Health care providers may focus on the physical and miss psychological components.

Mood Disorders

Although many older people maintain highly functional lives, others have deficits associated with age-related sensory losses, failing physical health, difficulty performing activities of daily living, and social deprivation or isolation. Life changes related to work roles and retirement often result in reduced social contacts and support. Other losses may be associated with the death of a spouse, other family members, or friends. At some time, virtually all adults experience a tragic or unexpected loss or a serious setback with accompanying profound grief or distress. Given adequate support and adaptation, most resume their lifestyles after the death of a loved one despite their sadness. For others, reduced social networks and contacts that accompany such life events can influence mood and contribute to serious depression (Figure 37.4). Specific physiologic stressors and medical conditions may also trigger depression in older adults because the aging brain is more vulnerable (Alexopoulos, 2005).

Major Depression

Major depressive disorder differs both in intensity and duration from normal sadness or grief. Depression is one disorder that can cause serious emotional pain and suffering in late life, but it is potentially one of the most treatable (Blazer, 2009). Serious and persistent symptoms include sleep and appetite changes, loss of interest in activities previously enjoyed, sad mood, physical complaints, anxiety, and inability to concentrate resulting in memory loss (see Chap. 27). In older adults, physical and mental conditions are intertwined closely. A physical illness may first present with psychiatric symptoms; depression may be expressed through physical concerns. Although not all older people with depressive symptoms may meet diagnostic criteria for major depression, even chronic and persistent relatively low levels of depression may disrupt relationships and functions.

The National Institute of Mental Health (NIMH) (2007) reported depression as the second leading primary care condition after hypertension in all ages. Two million Americans 65 years or older have a diagnosable depressive illness; an estimated 5 million have subsyndromal depression, which increases the risk for major depression. Depression affects 11.9% of adults older than 65 years. Rates in older adults in hospitals and nursing homes are even higher. Statistics are deceptive because of the "cohort effect." Current depression is not well detected or reported in older adults, and rates will rise as subsequent generations enter old age with the increased incidence of depression they had as a younger cohort (NIMH, 2007).

Available medications and psychological treatment can help 80% of those with depression, yet many clients do not seek help. Those with depression are more likely to visit a physician for some other reason. The mental health condition may remain undetected and untreated because of atypical presentations; misguided expectations that depression is normal as one grows older; complexities of interrelated physical illness, symptoms, and treatments; stigma; and attribution of symptoms of depression to physical illness (Frederick et al., 2007).

Depression is costly in terms of dollars, suffering, and death. It increases functional decline and morbidity, especially in those with other chronic conditions. High health care use for depression-related conditions results in an estimated expenditure of $43 billion annually. Perhaps the greatest cost is the loss of human life and its effects on family, whether through the exacerbation of physical illness or suicide resulting from undetected and untreated depression. Ragan and Kane (2010) offer a motivational client-oriented interviewing strategy for mental health nurses to employ with older persons who are experiencing depression. The nurse, using a warm, empathic style in a directive way that employs reflective listening, focuses on identifying discrepancies and establishes a collaborative relationship that fosters hope.

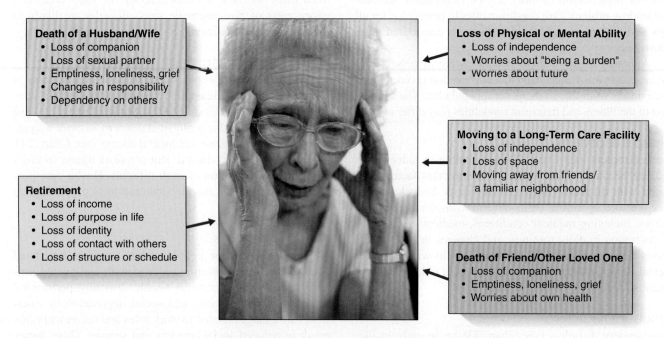

Death of a Husband/Wife
• Loss of companion
• Loss of sexual partner
• Emptiness, loneliness, grief
• Changes in responsibility
• Dependency on others

Loss of Physical or Mental Ability
• Loss of independence
• Worries about "being a burden"
• Worries about future

Moving to a Long-Term Care Facility
• Loss of independence
• Loss of space
• Moving away from friends/
  a familiar neighborhood

Retirement
• Loss of income
• Loss of purpose in life
• Loss of identity
• Loss of contact with others
• Loss of structure or schedule

Death of Friend/Other Loved One
• Loss of companion
• Emptiness, loneliness, grief
• Worries about own health

FIGURE 37.4 **Aging presents many challenges. Accompanying stresses can put older adults at risk for clinical depression and other mental illnesses.**

Suicide

In 2004, suicide was the 11th leading cause of death for all Americans (CDC, 2007). Although suicide prevention strategies often focus on the young, older adults have the highest rate of U.S. suicide. Currently older people account for less than 13% of the national population, but the ratios of attempts to completed suicides are 150 to 1 in the young but 4 to 1 in older adults. Older people use methods that are more likely to be lethal, have a greater motivation to die, have poorer recuperative powers, are more socially isolated, and have more chronic conditions and disability.

One suicide occurs among older adults every 97 minutes (American Association of Suicidology [AAS], 2010). The risk of suicide accrues with age and is gender related. White men older than 65 years account for 8% of all suicides, with a rate of 31 per 100,000 deaths. The highest rate of suicide is in white men 85 years or older. This population has 45.42 suicide deaths per 100,000, or 2.5 times the current rate for men of all ages (AAS, 2010). These estimates may be conservative because passive or accidental suicides are not reported. Most people who kill themselves have depression or another diagnosable mental illness or substance abuse disorder. Other risk factors include prior suicide attempts, stressful life events, having been widowed or divorced, and access to lethal methods. In fact, firearms accounted for 72% of all suicide deaths in those older than 65 years (AAS, 2010).

Suicide is tragic and often preventable. Every suicide intimately affects at least six other people (McIntosh, 2006). The CDC (2007) reports that 20% of older people who committed suicide had visited a physician within 24 hours of their act, 41% within 1 week, and 75% within 1 month. Because suicide is a significant public health problem, it is important for nurses and others to understand prevalence within age groups, behavior patterns, and prevention strategies (see Chap. 34).

Nursing and Health Care Responses

Because depression and suicide are so prevalent in older adults, how do health care providers miss the signs? Identifying and treating mental disorders in the older population are especially challenging. Failure to distinguish disease-related psychiatric symptoms from manifestations of normal aging may result in undue suffering and even death. Depression is missed because of individual, provider, and system barriers to detection. Older adults may associate mental health issues with stigma or the fear of becoming dependent on others and might not report emotional distress. Somatic concerns are more acceptable and indeed part of depression. Difficulty with sleep or weight loss may result from several other conditions. Atypical presentations in older adults are common, particularly depression without significant mood change, making detection difficult. Providers may focus only on physical problems and attribute behavioral or emotional symptoms to old age. Further barriers to the detection and treatment of mental illness include lack of provider time, inadequate funding for mental health programs, and insufficient training of long-term care staff.

Thought Disorders

Schizophrenia, a severe and persistent mental illness with onset in early adulthood, is not usually associated with older adults. In fact, prevalence was thought to decline with aging as a result of early mortality, decreased symptom severity, and recovery. However, prevalence in late life is underestimated severely because of problems with epidemiologic studies, which did not sample those living in institutions, assisted-living facilities, and transient housing. People with schizophrenia live into their 60s and 70s, although their mortality rates continue to be higher than those of the general population.

Late-onset schizophrenia (after 45 years) is more prevalent in women than in men and characterized by paranoid delusions. It has varying degrees of impairment, but the psychopathology decreases with age (Sadock & Sadock, 2007).

Delusional disorders usually occur between 40 and 55 years of age, but may develop at any time. Both persecutory and somatic delusions may develop after physical or psychological stress (eg, loss of a spouse). *Paraphrenia* is a late-onset delusional disorder (after age 65) characterized by persecutory delusions. Some believe that paraphrenia is late-onset schizophrenia because the incidence is higher in those with a family history of schizophrenia. Delusions can accompany any psychotic illness, delirium, or dementia. However, a delusional disorder is diagnosed by excluding other causes (Sadock & Sadock, 2007).

Substance Use Disorders

Discerning the incidence of alcohol abuse in older adults is difficult. Substance use disorders have increased during the past 10 years and are predicted to continue to rise for all gender and racial/ethnic groups in the coming decade (Wu & Blazer, 2011). Estimates even at the high end are probably conservative because of the covert nature of the problem. Substance abuse is underdiagnosed and undertreated because of associated stigma, ageism, failure to recognize symptoms, different presentations in older adults, underreporting, and minimizing of symptoms. Older adults with alcohol impairment do not come to the attention of those who might insist on treatment. They may no longer drive and are more likely to be socially isolated (Figure 37.5).

Nurses should further investigate for substance abuse in clients who present with alcohol-related physical problems, such as delirium, fractures, or gastrointestinal distress. Unexplained changes in behavior and functional decline are further clues.

Polypharmacy and misuse of medications are prevalent and additional forms of substance abuse. The use of medications to control symptoms of anxiety, promote sleep, or quell pain can extend beyond safe limits. Often, medication overuse first presents with psychiatric symptoms. As noted previously, many medications used to treat physical and mental

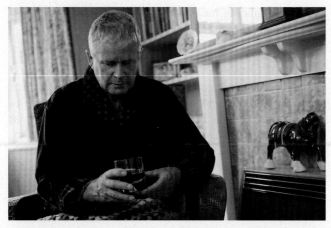

FIGURE 37.5 Older clients with substance use disorders are at risk for social isolation, depression, numerous health problems, and suicide. The incidence of alcoholism and other addictions in this population tends to be underreported and undertreated.

conditions in older adults can cause depression and delirium, along with falls, fractures, and the cascade of functional and physical decline associated with immobility. Underuse of appropriate medications because of financial, cognitive, or psychiatric constraints creates further mental health distress.

Cognitive Disorders

Chapter 31 discusses delirium and dementia. Remember that delirium, dementia, and depression are not mutually exclusive: the same person can have all three at any given time. Depression may present with symptoms suggestive of cognitive impairment and must be differentiated from both delirium and dementia. Fifty percent of those with Alzheimer's disease also have depression at some time during their illness, particularly in the early stages (Sadock & Sadock, 2007).

> ### Checkpoint Questions
> 5. What term is used to refer to a late-onset delusional disorder characterized by persecutory delusions?
> 6. What is the single most important factor associated with the development of difficulty sleeping?

COMMUNICATING EFFECTIVELY WITH OLDER ADULTS

To detect and treat mental health problems and improve outcomes for older adults, nurses must first be able to communicate sensitively. Effective communication is one of the most important nursing techniques (see Chap. 11) because it is the foundation of the therapeutic nurse–client relationship. Effective communication is essential for providing comprehensive and holistic nursing care and for engaging clients in health-related endeavors. A relationship based on good communication may make the difference in whether clients

understand and trust health care providers enough to take a new medication or try a new intervention.

Although principles of therapeutic communication are applicable across the lifespan, older adults require some special adaptations because of age-related changes (Box 37.2). Physical factors, such as decreased vision or hearing, may interfere with communication. Age-related changes in hearing require nurses to use a lower-pitched voice and eliminate background noise. Speaking in a somewhat louder voice may be necessary if hearing loss is clear. However, nurses must not assume that all older people have difficulty hearing and speak to them unnaturally loudly, which can be irritating. Nurses should assess for hearing and visual deficits early and then implement various helpful techniques based on findings.

Although memory impairment is not a normal part of aging, older adults do have a slower reaction time and need a bit longer to retrieve information. Clients with depression may present with speech latency and psychomotor retardation or may not have the energy to communicate. Allowing

---

BOX 37.2   Useful Communication Skills With Older Adults

Metacommunication and Body Language

- Use nonverbal language indicating undivided attention.
- Use direct eye contact. Sit or stand at the same level as the client.
- Evaluate acceptability of touch. Personal distance and response to touch vary.
- Identify yourself by name.
- Call the client by his or her preferred name. Use the client's first name *only* if he or she prefers you to do so.

Sensory Changes

- Keep yourself in the client's view so that he or she can see your face. Talking at his or her side or behind the client may cause some difficulty with communication or confusion.
- Be sure the client is wearing his or her glasses or hearing aids.
- Use a calm, clear, slightly slower, lower-pitched voice. Do not speak loudly.
- Eliminate background noise (eg, television, other conversation). Provide the client with a hearing amplification device if needed.
- Be sure there is adequate nonglare light.
- Provide large-type reading and teaching materials.

Cognitive Changes

- Ask one question at a time. Use open-ended questions to elicit information when possible.
- Allow time and wait for responses. It may take a little longer than you expect.
- Do not interrupt the person; doing so discourages responses.
- Listen attentively and actively.

Compiled from lecture notes based on Arnold, E. & Ryan, J. W. (2007). Communicating with older adults. In E. Arnold & K. U. Boggs (Eds.), *Interpersonal relationships: Professional communication skills for nurses* (5th ed., pp. 417–431). St. Louis, MO: W. B. Saunders.

more time and short interactions can facilitate communication. Strategies for communicating with clients who have cognitive impairment are addressed in Chapter 31.

Nurses and other health care professionals must take care to use respectful terms when talking with or about older people, regardless of diagnosis, symptoms, or both. They must avoid the degrading terminology associated with ageism in all cases. Many of these terms can decrease feelings of self-esteem, thus contributing to depression in older people. Examples of inappropriate terms and more sensitive substitutes are listed in Table 37.2.

CARE OF OLDER ADULTS

Care of older adults with mental health issues can be challenging but rewarding. Assessment and intervention modified to a client's special needs are most effective. Atypical presentations of illness are common in older adults, and physical and psychiatric illnesses are interwoven. Clinicians must rule out all physical possibilities before diagnosing a psychiatric illness (see Table 37.1).

Comprehensive assessment and intervention require a multidisciplinary approach because each member of the health care team brings valuable expertise. Clinicians consider family members to be part of the team because they bring practical expertise and knowledge. Assessment is not complete without family input, particularly if a client has cognitive problems. Assessment through evaluation of care should be multidimensional. Expression of illness varies greatly, so knowing how the illness affects daily functioning is critical. Because of the comprehensive nature of geriatric assessment, individual differences in energy, and special communication needs noted previously, more time might be needed to gather information. Allowing more time for intervention is also important.

Comprehensive Geriatric Mental Health Assessment

Assessment includes not only a detailed history and physical examination, but also a mental status examination, functional assessment, and review of psychosocial factors, including guardianship and power-of-attorney issues (see Chap. 31). Documentation includes certified copies of all legal papers, as well as advance directives and living wills. If the nurse finds a client to be cognitively impaired and lacking capacity to make health care decisions, the family (or the treating institution if no family is available) must take legal action immediately to ensure appropriate and timely treatment (see Chap. 5).

Recognizing the physical changes of aging is important because these factors play an important role in assessment and treatment. Many factors can cause such changes, including heredity, environment, and chronic medical conditions. Changes and concurrent medical processes often overlap. A gradual hearing deficit combined with tinnitus can result in not only additional hearing problems but also problems with equilibrium, increasing the risk of falling. Visual problems

such as cataracts can cause impairments that increase the dangers associated with self-medication. When previously mentioned concerns are combined with medical issues (eg, diabetes, arthritis, malnutrition), psychosocial concerns (eg, moving, loss of spouse, increased dependence on others), and cognitive changes (eg, Alzheimer's disease), a comprehensive assessment clearly is imperative.

One of the most important aspects of a comprehensive assessment is to determine what medications clients may be using, including OTC drugs and herbal supplements. Because many clients have several different medical conditions requiring treatment, many medications often are prescribed. Problems begin when no single physician or practitioner oversees all medications for compatibility and client adherence. When the client adds OTC drugs and alternative herbal supplements, medical repercussions can occur. See Case Vignette 37.2.

Think About It 37.1

Consider Graham in Case Vignette 37.2. Review the list of medications he is taking and determine the reason for each drug. Propose possible explanations for how the medications may have contributed to his current change in cognition.

Case Vignette 37.2

Graham, 77 years old, experiences an episode of decreased level of consciousness and syncope. After calling emergency services, his frantic wife gathers all his medications, which she takes with her in the ambulance as she accompanies her husband to the emergency department. On arrival, the triage nurse empties the sack of medications and discovers the following:

- Lasix (furosemide), Trental (pentoxifylline), Clinoril (sulindac) (prescribed by Dr. Abruzzi)
- NPH insulin (prescribed by Dr. Elihu)
- Zoloft (sertraline), Aricept (donepezil) (prescribed by Dr. Perkins)
- Depakote (divalproex sodium) (prescribed by Dr. Neville)
- Nexium (esomeprazole) (prescribed by Dr. Goldberg)
- Aspirin, one-a-day vitamins, Tylenol PM, milk of magnesia, ginkgo biloba

The nurse approaches the wife and asks what medications Graham had taken before fainting. The wife looks bewildered and states that she is unsure because her husband took his own medications. The wife reports that the client has taken vitamins daily for more than 40 years. She also states that for the past several days, he had been complaining of poor sleep and had been taking aspirin several times a day and Tylenol PM at night. He had also complained of stomach problems and had taken at least one full bottle of milk of magnesia during the past day. She noted that the donepezil was just prescribed and that he had been taking ginkgo biloba for memory problems.

▲

TABLE 37.2 Age-Sensitive Terminology

Do Not Use	Substitute
Adult day care (similar to child care)	Adult day services (may include needed health care)
Adult diaper (implies being a baby)	Pants, pads, briefs, trade name (product)
Afflicted	Affected by
Aged	Older people
Bed bound (not tied to the bed)	In bed much of the time
Bed sore	Pressure ulcer (area)
Bib	Clothes protector
Cerebral palsied	People with cerebral palsy
Childish, childlike	None (never use)
Convalescent home	Nursing facility (home)
Crazy	Mentally ill (often with a physical cause)
Crippled	Disabled
Deaf and dumb	Hearing and speech impaired
Elderly (implies people ages 50–110 all alike)	Older people
First name or familial title (granny)	Only if the family, friend, or by request
Formula (relates to babies)	Nutritional supplement
Frail, fragile (What does this mean?)	Disabled, or description of specific problem
Golden agers	None (never use)
Greedy geezers (odd character)	None (never use)
Handicapped	Persons with disabilities
Homebound, shut-in (not tied to the house)	Rarely leaves home
Honey, deary, sweetie, grandpa, grandma	Mr., Ms.
Incompetent	Incapacitated (legal term)
Little old lady (man)	Older woman (man)
Older generation	Older people
Oldsters	Older people
Old-timer's disease (implying Alzheimer's)	None (never use)
Poor	Low income
Rest home	Nursing facility (home) or assisted living facility
Role reversal	Role reversal (dependent parent becomes child) does not occur; a mature adult-to-adult relationship
Senile	None (never use)
Senior	Older adult
Senior moment (implies forgetfulness)	Never use (all ages forget at times)
Sitter (used for babies)	Companion
Suffers (from a disease)	Has a disease
Symptoms or problems due to age	Diagnose symptoms and treat
Victim (of a disease)	None (never use)
Wheelchair bound (not tied to the wheelchair)	Wheelchair user, person who uses a wheelchair
Young man (lady)—when obviously older	None (never use)

Nurses should be aware of several words and terms not to use when talking with or about or writing about older people or those with disabilities. Many of the *terms are disrespectful and demeaning*. Others have unclear meanings open to various interpretations.

Note: Some words have been contributed by REACH Resource Center on Independent Living, in Fort Worth, Texas.

Adapted from Hogstel, M. O. (1998). *Community resources for older adults: A guide for case managers.* St. Louis, MO: Mosby. Used with permission.

Intervention and Treatment

Intervention occurs across all health care settings. Both inpatient and outpatient treatment options for mental health disorders almost always involve pharmacotherapy and psychotherapy. Some adjunct somatic therapies also apply. Problems arise when clients cannot administer or receive prescribed treatments because of physical and cognitive barriers. Examples range from an inability to swallow secondary to a stroke to a client's refusal to swallow a pill because of a delusion that the pill is poison. To stay within the legal and ethical parameters of good care, nurses must anticipate and resolve possible barriers before they inhibit needed interventions.

General Medication Management

Nurses are in a position to help resolve polypharmacy issues and prevent problems. The first step is to implement the *all* system. Nurses request that *all* clients bring in *all* medications (including OTC and herbal supplements) they are taking at *all* visits. Health conditions can change often (eg, seasonal allergies, trauma from a fall), and clients use many OTC medications to relieve temporary problems. Doing so can have effects on overall health. An example is a client with diabetes who takes an OTC medication for nausea and vomiting after eating spicy food. The nurse would be concerned about the client's blood glucose level and suggest that during this period, the client use a sliding scale to determine an appropriate insulin dosage. Another situation is a client taking aspirin and ginkgo biloba, both of which have anticoagulant effects.

Once nurses have noted all the medications, the next step is to list them, times and routes of administration, and names and phone numbers of each physician who ordered them. They would also list OTC medications. Obviously, documenting this information in the chart is important. It is possibly more important for clients (and family) also to have a copy of this list. If Graham in Case Vignette 37.2 had had such a list, the triage nurse could have notified his physicians about the medication information more quickly. Another important item to add to this medication card is a list of medical conditions. In an emergency this information could be vital.

All medications have side effects and adverse reactions. Because of polypharmacy in older adults, checking drug compatibility is vital. Even when a medication is not contraindicated secondary to drug interactions or known allergies, awareness of potential problems is essential. Teaching clients about their medications is a serious responsibility. In addition to a medication list, a medication administration sheet might be helpful. This plan not only serves as a reminder about what clients should take and when, but its check-off format enables supervision of medication adherence. Clients should bring this form, along with current medications, to all health care and hospital visits.

Psychotropic Medication Management

Since the late 1990s, researchers have conducted many studies regarding psychotropic medications and older adults. Findings have resulted in new drugs for cognitive disorders (used most commonly in this population) and many dosage alterations for long-established treatments. Selective serotonin reuptake inhibitors (SSRIs) have greatly advanced the treatment of depression in older adults because these drugs have a decreased risk of anticholinergic effects. Integration of research findings into care have improved the length and quality of life dramatically. Nurses need to learn about changing treatments and advocate for the highest level of care for older clients.

Although newer medications for depression and psychosis are generally thought to be safer and to have fewer side effects than earlier drugs, they still have serious adverse effects. Neuroleptic malignant syndrome (NMS), a potentially fatal reaction to antipsychotic medications, is characterized by intense body rigidity and a sudden high temperature with no other explanation (eg, urinary tract infection). Although rare, NMS is usually not recognized immediately in older adults. An antipsychotic drug could be a new prescription or something that a client has taken for days, weeks, months, or years. It is crucial to stop the antipsychotic drug and transport the client to the hospital immediately for supportive therapy. A delay in hospitalization usually results in death.

Routes of medication administration have expanded dramatically during the past several years. Oral medications are available in tablet, capsule, chewable, and liquid forms. Many drugs are also available as injections, intravenous solutions, suppositories, drops, sprays, aerosols, ointments, creams, and patches. Which method is best? The answer depends on the specific medication ordered, routes of administration available, the client's physical and cognitive abilities, side effects, caregiver abilities, and cost.

Many older adults residing in institutions have feeding tubes. Nurses must carefully consider whether such tubes are also to be the chosen delivery route for drugs. Not all oral medications (such as timed-release capsules) may be administered through a feeding tube. Also, the distal end of the tube may be in the stomach, duodenum, or jejunum, which would affect absorption. Because of physical impairments (such as hepatic or renal insufficiency), clients might require alternate dosing schedules to avoid toxicity. An important approach is the collaborative care model, a cost-effective means of addressing psychotropic medication management, as well as other care approaches for older persons with mental health issues (Ahn et al., 2011).

Electroconvulsive Therapy

Although not widely used, electroconvulsive therapy (ECT) remains an intervention for intractable or drug-resistant depression and some other psychiatric conditions (see Chap. 18). Advances since the 1980s have made ECT safe and effective for older adults who cannot tolerate the side effects of antidepressants. Although ECT's precise mechanism of action remains unclear, positron emission tomography scans done during ECT show increased use of oxygen and glucose in the brain (Sadock & Sadock, 2007). Sometimes a client's condition improves dramatically with just two or three treatments. The nurse's role is to educate and prepare the client using therapeutic communication to discuss concerns. Nurses also assist in preoperative and postoperative care because ECT is done under general anesthesia.

Psychosocial Interventions

Psychosocial interventions strive to support both clients and families. Antai-Otong (2003) and Ragan and Kane (2010) note the importance of a therapeutic, empathetic environment and cite research supporting the importance of frequent follow-up contacts with a caring professional in the treatment and management of depression and prevention of suicide. Many nurses serve as milieu managers and have a pivotal role in creating such an environment. Enhancing protective factors that strengthen a client's social support and coping skills is another nursing role. Interpersonal or cognitive–behavioral approaches are effective for older adults with depression. Adjunctive therapies such as recreation and occupational therapy can stimulate participation, creativity, cognition, and self-esteem and decrease isolation. Wiggs and colleagues (2011) found that maintaining relationships with family, friends, and colleagues is important in helping people find meaning in life and look toward the future with anticipation. Group therapy can also diminish loneliness and increase a sense of belonging and support. All these modalities can enhance protective factors and promote mental health. Jones (2011) advocates for person-centered care that focuses on the older adult's quality of life.

Because of evolving changes in the U.S. health care delivery system, essential mental health services sometimes are difficult for clients to locate and finance. Few mental illnesses are treated in hospital settings for several reasons. Some people prefer to and can stay at home and receive outpatient treatment in a physician's office or clinic, especially if they have available supportive family members and friends (Figure 37.6). Some home health agencies have psychiatric–mental health nurses on staff to provide limited services to clients in their homes (see Chap. 20). Some hospitals and community clinics provide partial hospitalization on a day basis, which Medicare covers. Geriatric psychiatrists, geriatric nurses, and social workers provide diagnoses, medication management, various forms of counseling and therapy, nutrition, and activities. However, decreasing coverage for such services by Medicare and Medicare health maintenance organizations has led to decreased availability. Nursing facilities (homes) in some areas have become more aware of the mental health needs of their residents and are employing, as either part-time staff members or consultants, geriatric psychiatrists, gerontological clinical psychologists, and geropsychiatric or mental health nurses.

Role of Nurses

Care of older adults has become highly sophisticated. The number of nurses who focus on the care of older adults has grown enormously. The American Nurses Credentialing Center certifies several hundred nurses every year in gerontological nursing. There is national certification in psychiatric and mental health nursing and three types of gerontological nursing, but none in geropsychiatric nursing. The specialty has advanced rapidly and will continue to grow as the challenges of and demand for specialized nursing of older adults become more apparent.

One expanded role for geropsychiatric nurses is to provide education, support, and consultation to staff members in long-term care facilities. Some facilities have used a combined consultation and training program to meet their clients' needs. Approximately 40% to 70% of all nursing home residents have a chronic mental condition, yet nursing home staff members frequently are unprepared to deal with mental illness. Because they have less education and experience in caring for clients who exhibit difficult behaviors, nurses may become withdrawn, terminate their employment, or even physically or psychologically abuse their clients. Current facts and knowledge about mental health conditions in a specific population, experience in caring for these clients, and a support group for staff in the health care setting can help. If no such support group is available, nurses could initiate and plan such an activity. Other technical and support staff members should also be encouraged to participate in these support groups. Selecting and using personal strategies, such as family visits, activities with friends, and exercise that can reduce stress, help people cope when working conditions become difficult. Although such programs cannot completely replace direct professional intervention, they may help nursing home staff effectively manage behavioral problems (Wiggs et al., 2011).

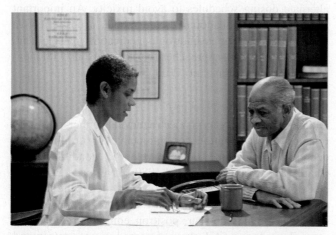

FIGURE 37.6 **Many older adults with long-term psychiatric challenges live at home and receive care for their illnesses from primary care practitioners.**

Checkpoint Questions

7. What is the advantage of using SSRIs in older adults?

8. What factors need to be considered when deciding on the best route for medication administration?

PROMOTING MENTAL HEALTH AND WELLNESS IN OLDER ADULTS

In addition to caring for clients with diagnosed mental health problems, nurses in all settings who have contact with older people must teach and promote activities that will help these clients maintain mental health and wellness. Psychological well-being depends greatly on and is interrelated with physical integrity. Areas of concern for older adults include nutrition, activity, and relationships. Older people who eat poorly, are inactive, and have minimal contact with family members or friends are more likely to become lonely and depressed, experience more physical and mental problems, and possibly become suicidal. Positive psychological states have been associated with both protective factors (less disease) and promotion factors (more vitality) (Murrell et al., 2003; Ragan & Kane, 2010). The following sections discuss these areas in more detail. See also Client-Centered Education 37.2.

Health promotion education programs for older adults have demonstrated effectiveness in improving both knowledge and behavior (Newman et al., 2010). Those who are better educated, have a more positive outlook, and are younger tend to engage in health promotion activities (Murrell et al., 2003). Nevertheless, programs can be effective across all settings and groups. As with many programs, ongoing follow-up and monitoring of health status help to improve outcomes (Newman et al., 2010). McAuley and colleagues (2003) found that social support and coaching made the difference in predicting who would continue to engage in health-promoting behaviors. "There is an emerging evidence base that supports the efficacy of mental wellness interventions for older adults and adults with a disability" (Hirst et al., 2011, p. 18). This most extensive evidence is found in support of psychological and pharmacologic interventions as well as interventions for dementia. A strength-based approach refers to a way of working with and intervening with individuals, families and groups that is grounded in the following principles (adapted from Hirst et al., 2011, p. 5):

- Individuals have existing competencies and resources.
- Individuals have the capacity to learn new skills and to problem solve.
- Individuals can draw on their own resources in identifying and addressing their concerns.
- Individuals can participate in the process of healing and wellness.

The Substance Abuse and Mental Health Services Administration (2011) has developed an excellent online toolkit that is available for mental health professionals for use in promoting mental health and preventing suicide.

By promoting mental health and wellness and detecting and intervening in mental illness, nurses can make a significant difference in the lives of older adults, in terms of their quality of life and their ability to find or renew a sense of purpose and meaning for living (Evidence-Based Practice Spotlight 37.1).

Nutrition and Fluids

Good nutrition and fluids are essential to physical health. Decreasing calories, fats, salt, and sugar and increasing complex carbohydrates, fresh vegetables, fruits, and calcium-rich foods are basic suggestions. Eating four to five small meals a day is better than eating two or three large meals. Moderation is key. Clients must obtain essential vitamins and minerals from foods. Because of various factors related to aging, including decreased absorption of some substances, older people probably should take at least one basic multivitamin and mineral supplement.

Some older people are increasing their use of alternative medicines, including large doses of some vitamins. Nurses should caution all clients that excessive doses could be dangerous, and some herbs and other health food products could react with prescription medications and cause dangerous adverse effects.

Client–Centered Education 37.2

Suggestions About Mental Wellness

Nurses should teach clients as follows:

- Keep active, both mentally and physically. Reduce stress.
- Take as few medicines as possible, but do not stop taking any medication without discussing it with the physician. Discuss the possible need for a vitamin, mineral, and calcium supplement with the physician.
- Ask the physician for a written explanation of the benefits and risks of specific medicines, treatments, and surgery.
- Prepare for all physician's office visits by writing down questions and concerns a few days before the visit and do not leave until questions have been answered.

- Keep a written record of the dates of physician visits.
- Select physicians and hospitals that have the special services, staff, and equipment to provide quality care to older people, noting that a quality to look for in a physician and nurse is the ability to listen well.
- Be *assertive* in seeking quality health care.
- Report poor care to the appropriate person or agency.
- Take responsibility for your own health.
- Do not sign anything that you do not completely understand.

EVIDENCE-BASED PRACTICE SPOTLIGHT 37.1

Interventions to Increase Health Promotion Activities in Older Adults

Overview of Effective Treatment: Risk factors associated with depression in older adults include disability, new medical illness, poor health status, prior depression, poor perceived health status, and bereavement. Three modifiable lifestyle behaviors are associated with the development of chronic diseases: smoking, diet, and physical inactivity. People with chronic diseases are at increased risk to become less active, gain weight, and take more OTC and prescribed medications. Adverse drug events are common in older people and increase with the number of medications prescribed. People with chronic illness and those using multiple medications are also at higher risk for falls. A multidisciplinary, multimodal assessment and intervention approach using screening tools to detect emerging problems along with education and encouragement of healthy behaviors has been demonstrated as most effective in decreasing chronic disease-associated morbidity in older adults. Serious medication occurrences are preventable through careful prescribing, avoiding new prescriptions, incorporating computerized medication lists, and reviewing all medications

at each contact with health care providers. When nurses are involved in obtaining current medication lists, reviewing adverse effects, and improving the client's knowledge through medication education, adverse drug effects decline. The use of motivational interviewing has been demonstrated as effective for enabling health behavior change.

What Has Not Been Shown Effective: Visits to a health care provider that focus only on the disease rather than on counseling regarding lifestyle modifications are less effective.

Implications for Practice: Health care providers should integrate screening of older adults and counseling them about health behaviors into every contact to lower rates of related morbidity and mortality. Every visit should include review of medications and behavior, lifestyle changes, and losses. Motivational interviewing approaches help facilitate the provider–client relationship and enable clients to receive coaching through efforts to change behavior.

References

Chang, J. T., Morton, S. C., Rubenstein, L. Z., Mojica, W. A., Maglione, M., Suttorp, M. J., et al. (2004). Interventions for the prevention of falls in older adults: Systematic review and meta-analysis of randomized clinical trials. *BMJ (Clinical Research Ed.), 328,* 680.

Cole, M. G., & Dendukuri, N. (2003). Risk factors for depression among elderly community subjects: A systematic review and meta-analysis. *American Journal of Psychiatry, 160*(6), 1147–1156.

Cung, B., & Dickman, R. L. (2007). Minimizing adverse drug events in older patients. *American Family Physician, 76*(12), 1837–1844.

Levensky, E. R., Forcehimes, A., O'Donohue, W. T., & Beitz, K. (2007). Motivational interviewing: An evidence-based approach to counseling helps patients follow treatment recommendations. *American Journal of Nursing, 107*(10), 50–58.

McGuire, L. C, Strine, T. W., Oloro, C. A., Ahluwalia, I. B., & Ford, E. S. (2007). Healthy lifestyle behaviors among older U.S. adults with and without disabilities (Behavioral Risk Factor Surveillance System, 2003). *Prevention of Chronic Disease.* Retrieved from http://www.ced.gov/pcd/issues/2007/jan/06.

Taylor, A. H., Cable, N. T., Faulkner, G., Hillsdon, M., Narici, M., & Van Der Bij, A. K. (2004). Physical activity and older adults: A review of health benefits and the effectiveness of interventions. *Journal of Sports Science, 22*(8), 703–725.

Mental and Physical Activities

Physical activity remains an important aspect of healthy aging throughout the lifespan (Figure 37.7). Simple walking is probably best. Nurses may wish to suggest to most clients (unless contraindicated because of other physical factors) that they exercise at least 30 minutes a day, three times a week. Keeping active mentally is also important. More older people are working after retirement, participating in volunteer organizations and community activities, and being actively involved in church and political groups. A basic recommendation related to muscles and bones as well as mental functioning is to stay active. Sensory stimulation and creative activities along with avoidance of stress and adequate sleep and nutrition may help clients maintain and enhance brain function (Vance et al., 2011).

Support Systems

The third major criterion for healthy aging is a good support system, which means that older people need family members, friends, neighbors, and church or other organizations to provide support and assistance. Clients may benefit from a daily telephone call from people who care about them or

assistance with transportation for shopping. Family caregivers may also need education about aging and mental health issues as well as participation in a support group.

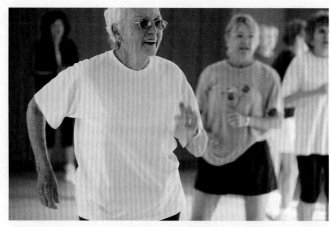

FIGURE 37.7 Nurses and other health care providers should encourage ongoing exercise and physical activity in older adults to promote holistic wellness for clients.

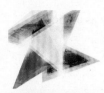

Reviewing and Applying Your Knowledge

Chapter Summary

- The age 65 years has arbitrarily become the point at which people are considered old.

- To be more precise about the relationship between age and needs, the National Institute on Aging has defined chronologic categories of young old (65 to 74 years), middle old (75 to 84 years), old old (85 to 94 years), and elite old (95 years and older).

- As more people live longer, there will be a greater diversity of physical and mental health needs for society to recognize.

- Tasks of aging include conserving strength and resources as necessary and adapting to accompanying changes and losses.

- Changes and issues that most older adults confront include retirement, relocation, and bereavement.

- Effective communication with older adults is one of the most important nursing interventions. Nurses need to use specific techniques for those with a hearing, visual, or cognitive deficit or who display aggressive tendencies related to a health condition. They must also avoid using any degrading terminology.

- Approximately 25% of older adults in the community and more than 50% of those in nursing homes have symptoms of mental illness. Identifying and treating mental disorders in the older population are challenging because health care providers may confuse signs of normal aging with problems in mental functioning or may misdiagnose physical problems as mental illness.

- Geriatric psychiatrists, geriatric nurses, and social workers can provide diagnoses, medication management, various forms of counseling and therapy, nutrition, and activities for older adults. However, Medicare and Medicare health maintenance organizations have decreased coverage for such services in recent years.

- Nurses must understand that the presentation of several psychiatric disorders can differ in older adults from findings in the general population. Comprehensive assessment is vital.

- When administering and monitoring psychopharmacotherapy to older adults, nurses must handle issues involving adjustments in method of administration, polypharmacy, age-related differences in pharmacokinetics and pharmacodynamics, and the increased possibility of adverse and side effects.

- Areas of mental health promotion for nurses to address when working with older adults include maintaining adequate nutrition and fluids, engaging in mental and physical activities, ensuring adequate support systems, and fostering hope.

Study Questions

1. Which of the following statements from a married older man who is to retire in 2 weeks would alert the nurse to possible future problems?

    a. "She's going to do some volunteer work while I help out with household chores."

    b. "We're going to travel all year long to all sorts of foreign and exotic places."

    c. "I'm finally going to learn how to play golf like I've wanted all these years."

    d. "I have a good pension, but we're planning a budget so we don't overspend."

2. An 80-year-old woman who wears a hearing aid in her left ear is being admitted to an extended care facility. When obtaining the client's history, which of the following would be most appropriate for the nurse to do?

    a. Keep the television on to provide stimulation during the interview.

    b. Hug the client as part of the introduction and greeting.

    c. Speak calmly but loudly, directing the voice to the client's left ear.

    d. Ask one question at a time, allowing the client ample time to answer.

3. Which of the following older adults would the nurse assess as being at greatest risk for mental health problems?

    a. A 72-year-old man with severe degenerative joint disease who is recently widowed and lives alone

    b. A 67-year-old man who lives with his daughter and volunteers twice a week at a community center

    c. A 70-year-old woman who lives with her 72-year-old husband in an assisted-living community

    d. A 68-year-old woman with a history of osteoporosis who lives with her 74-year-old spouse and works part time

(continues on page 844)

4. The nurse is completing an assessment of an 84-year-old client with Alzheimer's disease. Which of the following statements by the client's son would alert the nurse to a potential problem?

 a. "He has a night-light in his bedroom, and there's one in the hallway on the way to the bathroom."

 b. "We make sure that somebody is in the house with him at all times, day or night."

 c. "He's been having trouble sleeping over the past week or so, so we're giving him Benadryl."

 d. "I've been giving him a liquid nutritional supplement because he's such a poor eater."

5. A recently widowed 73-year-old woman with a history of hypertension and diabetes has just moved to an assisted-living facility. During a follow-up nursing assessment, the client states, "I can't eat. I can't sleep. I get up so early in the morning. I don't know how much longer I can live like this." Further assessment reveals that she has not been taking her antihypertensive medications. Which

of the following would the nurse identify as a priority need for this client?

 a. Lack of medication compliance

 b. Difficulty sleeping

 c. Inadequate nutrition

 d. Feelings of loss

Critical Thinking Questions

1. What factors may cause a society to neglect mental health problems in older adults?

2. What factors interfere with accurate mental status assessments of older adult clients?

3. How can nurses become more interested in and committed to the field of geropsychiatric nursing?

4. What is meant by a strengths-based approach and what are some ways that nurses can incorporate this into their practice?

References

Administration on Aging (AOA), U.S. Department of Health and Human Services. (2010). *A profile of older Americans: 2010.* Washington, DC: Author.

Ahn, S., Tai-Seale, M., Huber, C., Smith, M. L., & Ory, M. G. (2011). Psychotropic medication discussions in older adults' primary care office visits: So much to do, so little time. *Aging & Mental Health, 15*(5), 618–629.

Alexopoulos, G. S. (2005). Depression in the elderly. *Lancet, 365,* 1961–1970.

American Association of Geriatric Psychiatry (2008). *Geriatrics and mental health—The facts.* Retrieved from http://www.aagponline .org/prof/facts_mh.asp.

American Association of Suicidology (AAS). (2010). *Elderly suicide fact sheet.* Washington, DC: Author.

Antai-Otong, D. (2003). Suicide: Life span considerations. *Nursing Clinics of North America, 28,* 137–150.

Anton, B., Vitetta, L., Cortino, F., & Sali, A. (2005). Can we delay aging? The biology and science of aging. *Annuals of New York Academy of Science, 1057,* 525–535.

Bartels, S. J., Blow, F. C., Brockmann, L. M., & Van Citters, A. D. (2005). *Substance abuse and mental health amongv older Americans: The state of knowledge and future directions.* Rockville, MD: WESTAT. Retrieved from: http://www.samsha.gov/OlderAdultsTAC/

Blazer, D. (2009). Depression in late life: Review and commentary. *Journal of Lifelong Learning in Psychiatry, VII*(I), 118–136.

Centers for Disease Control and Prevention (CDC). (2007). *Suicide: Facts at a glance.* Retrieved from http://www.cdc.gov/injury

Centers for Disease Control (CDC) and Prevention and National Association of Chronic Disease Directors. (2008). *The state of mental health and aging in America issue brief 1: What do the data tell us?* Atlanta, GA: National Association of Chronic Disease Directors.

Charney, D. S., Reynolds, C. F., Lewis, L., Lebowitz, B. D., Sunderland, T., Alexopoulos, G. S., ... Young, R. C. (2003). Depression and Bipolar Support Alliance consensus statement on the unmet needs in diagnosis and treatment of mood disorders in late life. *Archives of General Psychology, 60,* 664–672.

Federal Interagency Forum on Aging-Related Statistics. (2006). *Older Americans update 2006: Key indicators of well-being.* Washington, DC: U.S. Government Printing Office.

Flood, M. (2005). A mid-range nursing theory of successful aging. *Journal of Theory Construction and Testing, 9*(2), 35–39.

Frederick, J. T., Steinman, L. E., Prohaska, T., Satariano, W. A., Bruce, M., Bryant, L., ... Snowden, M. (2007). Community-based treatment of late life depression: An expert panel-informed literature review [Review]. *American Journal of Preventive Medicine, 33*(3), 222–249.

Grossman, S. (2006). *Medical surgical nursing.* Albany, NY: Thomson Gale.

Hirst, S. P., Lane, A. M., & LeNavenec, C. (2011). Strengths-based approaches for mental wellness in seniors and adults with disabilities. Alberta, Canada: Alberta Health Services–Addiction and Mental Health.

Jones, C. (2011). Person-centered care: The heart of cultural change. *Journal of Gerontological Nursing, 37*(6), 18–23.

Kessler, R. C., Berglund, P., Demler, O., Jin, R., Merikangas, K. R., & Walters, E. E. (2005). Lifetime prevalence and age of onset distributions of *DSM-IV* disorders in the National Comorbidity Survey Replication. *Archives of General Psychiatry, 63,* 593–602.

Lander McCarthy, V. (2011). A new look at successful aging: Exploring a mid-range nursing theory among older adults in a low-income retirement community. *Journal of Theory Construction and Testing, 15*(1), 17–23.

Lavretsky, H. (2010). Spirituality and aging. *Aging Health, 6*(6), 749–769.

McAuley, E., Jerome, G. J., Elavsky, S., Marquez, D. X., & Ramsey, S. N. (2003). Predicting long-term maintenance of physical activity in older adults. *Preventative Medicine, 37*(2), 110–118.

McIntosh, J. L. (2006). *Suicide: 2004. Official final data.* Washington, DC: American Society of Suicidology.

Murrell, S. A., Salsman N. L., & Meeks, S. (2003). Educational attainment, positive psychological mediators, and resources for health and vitality in older adults. *Journal of Aging and Health, 15*(4), 591–615.

National Institute of Mental Health (NIMH). (2007). *Older adults: Depression and suicide facts.* Retrieved from http://www.nimh .nih.gov/publications/older-adults-depression-and-suicide-facts

Newman, A. B., Bayles, C. M., Milas, C. N., McTigue, K., Williams, K., Robare, J. F., ... Kuller, L. H. (2010). The 10 keys to healthy aging: Findings from an innovative prevention program in the community. *Journal of Aging and Health, 22*(5), 547–566.

Ragan, M., & Kane, C. F. (2010). Meaningful lives: Elders in treatment for depression. *Archives of Psychiatric Nursing, 24*(6), 408–417. doi:10.1016/j.apnu.2010.04.002

Reed, P. G. (2009). Demystifying self-transcendence for mental health nursing practice and research. *Archives of Psychiatric Nursing, 23*(5), 397–400. doi:10.1016/j.apnu.2009.06.006

Roose, S. P., Pollock, B. G., & Devanand, D. P. (2004). Treatment during late life. In A. F. Schatzberg & C. B. Nemeroff (Eds.), *Textbook of psychopharmacology* (3rd ed.). Washington, DC: American Psychiatric Publishing.

Roy, C. (1997). Future of the Roy model: Challenge to redefine adaptation. *Nursing Science Quarterly, 10,* 42–48.

Sadock, B. J., & Sadock, V. A. (2007). Geriatric psychiatry. In B. J. Sadock & V. A. Sadock (Eds.), *Kaplan and Sadock's synopsis of psychiatry* (9th ed., pp. 1318–1337). Philadelphia, PA: Lippincott Williams & Wilkins.

Sloane, P. D. (2007). Clinical implications of normal aging. In R. J. Ham, P. D. Sloane, G. A. Warshaw, M. A. Bernard, & E. Flaherty (Eds.), *Primary care geriatrics. A case-based approach* (5th ed.). St. Louis, MO: Mosby.

Substance Abuse and Mental Health Services Administration. (2011). *Promoting emotional health and preventing suicide: A toolkit for senior living communities (SPARK kit).* Retrieved from http://store.samhsa.gov/product/SMA10-4515?WT.ac=EB_20110505_ SMA10-4515

Sunderland, T., Mirza, N., & Linker, G. (2004). Cognitive enhancers. In A. F. Schatzberg & C. B. Nemeroff (Eds.), *Textbook of psychopharmacology* (3rd ed., pp. 639–650). Washington, DC: American Psychiatric Publishing.

Tornstam, L. (2005). *Gerotranscendence: A developmental theory.* New York, NY: Springer.

U.S. Department of Health and Human Services (USDHHS). (1999). *Mental health: A report of the Surgeon General.* Rockville, MD: U.S. Department of Health and Human Services, Substance Abuse and Mental Health Services Administration, Center for Mental Health Services, National Institutes of Health, National Institute of Mental Health.

Vance, D. E., Eagerton, G., Harnish, B., McKie, P., & Fazeli, P. L. (2011). Cognitive prescriptions: A nursing approach to increasing cognitive reserve. *Journal of Gerontological Nursing, 37*(4), 22–29.

Wilcox, S., Evenson, K. R., Aragake, A., Wassertheil-Smoller, S., Mouton, C. P., & Loevinger, B. L. (2003). The effects of widowhood on physical and mental health, health behaviors, and health outcomes: The Women's Health Initiative. *Health Psychology, 22*(5), 513–522.

Wiggs, C. M., Young, A., Mastel-Smith, B., & Mancuso, P. (2011). Rediscovering: The lived experience of women journeying toward aging. *Journal of Gerontological Nursing, 73*(1), 20–27.

Wu, L., & Blazer, D. G. (2011). Illicit and nonmedical drug use among older adults: A review. *Journal of Aging and Health, 23*(3), 481–504.

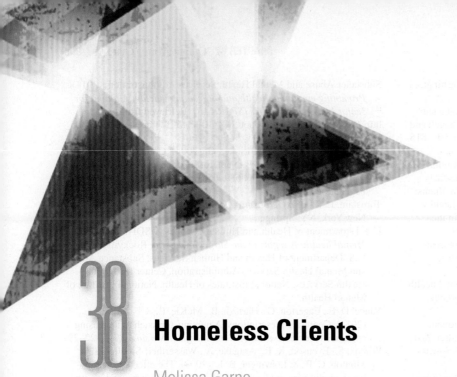

38

Homeless Clients

Melissa Garno

KEY TERMS

affordable housing
homelessness
period prevalence count
point-in-time count

LEARNING OBJECTIVES

On completion of this chapter, you should be able to accomplish the following:

- Identify current trends in the homeless population.
- Discuss factors that contribute to homelessness in people with mental illness.
- Discuss barriers that prevent homeless people with mental illness from receiving care and measures to promote access.
- Describe specific health care concerns of homeless people with mental illness.
- Apply the nursing process to the care of homeless clients with mental illness.

The McKinney-Vento Act of 1987 defines **homelessness** as lacking a regular and adequate nighttime residence. Consequently, homeless people spend nighttime hours in a shelter, institution, or nonresidential location under temporary conditions. Using this definition, over 3 million people in the United States annually are homeless, with 1.5 million being children and one third being families (National Law Center on Homelessness and Poverty, 2010). For most affected people, homelessness is a short-term situation. However, for some, including many people with concomitant mental illness, homelessness is a long, difficult, and frequently chronic state. Approximately 16% of the total homeless population suffers from chronic mental illness (National Coalition for the Homeless [NCH], 2009h).

Nurses can play significant roles in the lives of people experiencing homelessness, regardless of whether the situation is a one-time aberration or a chronic, recurring problem. Opportunities to help range from assisting families displaced by a fire or natural disaster to obtain needed resources to facilitating the long and slow engagement process that people with untreated psychiatric disorders and living on the streets require. Nurses in all settings and working in all specialties will, at some point, need to address homelessness with clients.

DEMOGRAPHICS

The main contributors to the growth in the number of homeless people in recent years are a shortage of affordable housing, an increase in foreclosures, eroding work opportunities and lagging incomes, and a decline in public services and government assistance (NCH, 2009h; National Law Center on Homelessness and Poverty, 2010). In 2009, there was a 32% increase in foreclosures from the previous year, displacing nearly 40% of families who are renters (National Low Income Housing Coalition, 2011). In 2009 the official unemployment rate was 9.4%, reflecting a loss of 6 million jobs since the start of the 2008 recession (NCH, 2009h). With rising unemployment and a 47% increase in housing rental rates in the past decade (National Low Income Housing Coalition, 2011), the trend toward increased homelessness continues. Recent policy may be having a positive impact. The *Annual Homeless Assessment Report to Congress* based on 2010 data shows a 1% increase in overall homelessness from 2009 to 2010 (National Alliance to End Homelessness, 2011).

Factors contributing to homelessness may be different for individuals than for families. In 2008, the top three causes for family homelessness were lack of affordable housing, poverty, and unemployment. For single individuals the most prevalent causes were substance abuse, lack of affordable housing, and mental illness (U.S. Conference of Mayors, 2008).

Studies of the number of homeless people use operational definitions that vary according to state or federal agency, resulting in methodological problems. Some researchers continue to use convenience samples of persons in shelters or who are on the streets, leading to gross underestimates of homelessness. One way to estimate numbers of homeless people is to calculate results on a given day or week; this process is called a **point-in-time count.** Another method is to count homeless people over a more extended period, which is called a **period prevalence count** (NCH, 2009d). The magnitude of homelessness is likely to be most accurate when a study includes not only people in shelters, but also those displaced by domestic violence, families living together in single-family dwellings, street youth, incarcerated people, and the "invisible" homeless in camps, under bridges, and in rural areas.

Most homeless people are unaccompanied adults in central parts of cities, although they also exist in suburbs and rural areas. Approximately 39% are Caucasians, 42% are African American, 13% are Hispanic, 4% are Native American, and 2% are Asian (NCH, 2009d). Of the adult homeless population, approximately 51% are single men, and 17% are single women (U.S. Conference of Mayors, 2008). Families with children are the fastest growing homeless subpopulation. Children younger than 18 years make up approximately 39% of the homeless population, with 42% of these children younger than 5 years. Unaccompanied youth comprise approximately 5% of the homeless population (NCH, 2009g).

Homeless children commonly experience developmental delays, depression, anxiety, and learning difficulties (Figure 38.1) (NCH, 2009c). Their homelessness may be a source of shame. However, they may also demonstrate resiliency to their multiple stressors. Because of the lack of policies and programs that target prevention, homelessness is becoming intergenerational, with more children growing up in a climate of poverty.

The homeless population encompasses a diverse array of people. Some have disabilities or chronic illnesses, with benefits that do not provide permanent housing. Some have fixed incomes and simply cannot afford to rent or buy

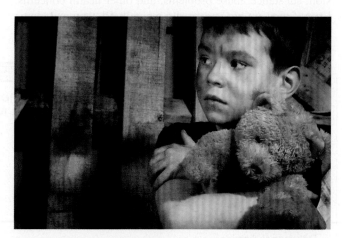

FIGURE 38.1 The most rapidly growing segment of the homeless population consists of families with children. Children and adolescents make up almost 40% of people living without a home.

housing. Veterans may be homeless following estrangement from support systems, whereas youth may have wound up on the streets after rejection from families. Other segments of the homeless population include documented and undocumented immigrants, those incarcerated in the criminal justice system, and unemployed and underemployed (work, but do not make enough to afford permanent housing) people.

HOMELESSNESS AND MENTAL ILLNESS

People with serious mental illness account for a significant percentage of the homeless population, at an estimated 26% (NCH, 2009h). In a survey of 23 American cities, 26% of homeless people suffered from serious mental illness, in comparison with an estimated 6% of the overall population (U.S. Conference of Mayors, 2008). Clients with serious mental illness have great difficulty escaping homelessness. Compared with those who are mentally healthy, people with psychiatric problems often are homeless for longer periods, have less contact with family, encounter more barriers to obtaining employment, display poorer physical health, and have more encounters with the legal system (NCH, 2009b).

Schizophrenia is one of the most common chronic mental illnesses affecting homeless people (see Chap. 29). This disorder is most distressing to people who lack support and are too ill to negotiate the bureaucratic mental health system. Mood and substance use disorders also have higher prevalence rates in homeless people than in the general population. See *DSM-IV-TR* Box 38.1 for frequently observed psychiatric diagnoses among the homeless mentally ill (American Psychiatric Association, 2000).

Even when clients are homeless, but not experiencing a psychiatric disorder, they are at risk for problems. Homelessness adversely affects mental health. People who become homeless because of economic stressors, unemployment, domestic violence, or eviction are prone to anxiety, depression, substance abuse problems, and other health concerns. Even if they are not necessarily mentally ill, they may come to the attention of nurses and other health care personnel. For example, staff may associate behavioral characteristics in a person staying at a shelter with stress reactions, impaired intellectual functioning, or maladaptive behaviors.

Checkpoint Questions

1. Which subpopulation of homeless people is the fastest growing?

2. What problems do homeless children commonly experience?

3. What psychiatric diagnosis most commonly affects the homeless population?

Contributing Factors

Homelessness in people with mental illness has many different causes. A unique set of circumstances has contributed to the difficult outcome of homelessness for each person. Nevertheless, common societal factors have helped to foster conditions that have led to increased homelessness. Examples include a deficient mental health care system, the disabling functional deficits of mental illness, substance abuse, the effects of poverty, inadequate housing, and mobility.

Deficient Mental Health Care System

The current mental health care system has shifted from an institutional to a community orientation. Resulting gaps in care have contributed to increased rates of homelessness. The system has not adequately addressed the comorbidity of mental illness and substance abuse. Housing options have been reduced, clients frequently have not received benefits to which they are entitled, and many have lost contact with families and social supports (National Resource Center on Homelessness and Mental Illness, 2010). All these issues have helped to increase the risks for people with mental illness to become homeless.

Because of problems that resulted after the deinstitutionalization of people with psychiatric problems during the

---

DSM-IV-TR BOX 38.1

Common Diagnoses in Homeless People with Mental Illness

- Alcohol dependence
- Alcohol-related disorder
- Amphetamine abuse
- Antisocial personality disorder
- Bipolar I disorder
- Bipolar II disorder
- Borderline personality disorder
- Delusional disorder
- Hallucinogen-related disorder
- Major depressive disorder

- Nicotine dependence
- Obsessive-compulsive disorder
- Opioid dependence
- Personality disorder NOS
- Polysubstance dependence
- Post-traumatic stress disorder
- Psychotic disorder NOS
- Schizoaffective disorder
- Schizophrenia (paranoid, disorganized, undifferentiated, residual)

past 30 to 35 years, a new generation of people with severe mental illness has spent only brief times in hospitals. The implementation of managed care has resulted in more frequent denial of services and premature discharges. Many of these people have never received the care or treatment they require for their conditions to be truly stabilized. They also face a national shortage of affordable housing (NCH, 2009e). As a result, these noninstitutionalized, often younger people with mental illness are increasingly joining the ranks of the homeless. The course of their condition usually demonstrates a common pattern. They are referred to treatment in the community, yet often do not follow through. In many cases, their condition worsens, perhaps leading to a brief hospitalization. Frequently, hospitals discharge such clients without their symptoms being fully stabilized. These people return to a stressful environment without needed structure and support. Some of them complicate their mental illness by using drugs or alcohol to self-medicate their psychiatric symptoms. Others perceive taking psychotropic drugs as an acknowledgment that their lives are no longer "normal" and thus fail to adhere to their treatment regimens. Thus, a vicious cycle continues.

Creative and innovative measures to fill gaps in the mental health system and decrease the risk of homelessness are necessary. Each community must decide what is best and most realistic according to its resources. Examples of interventions that may prevent and decrease homelessness include intensive case management, a continuum of housing supports, respite and crisis stabilization facilities, and a wider range of subsidized housing.

Functional Abilities and Deficits

Characteristics of severe mental illness often are exaggerated in clients who also are homeless. Distorted perceptions, lack of situational supports, and poor symptom control may cause them to be unable to handle the crisis of homelessness. Some of the most challenging problems include difficulties with basic activities of daily living (eg, personal hygiene, cooking, housekeeping). Other significant deficits include difficulty relating to others, lack of self-confidence and self-esteem, dependency needs, difficulty with self-direction, and limited motor capacity from side effects of medications.

Substance Abuse

Substance abuse is much more common among homeless people than the general population whether it is the cause of homelessness through financial and functional losses or the result of homelessness as an attempt to cope (NCH, 2009g). Many people with mental illness misguidedly attempt to self-medicate psychiatric symptoms with mood-altering drugs or alcohol (Figure 38.2). Common psychosocial characteristics of homeless people with dual diagnoses include denial of illness, psychiatric symptoms, housing instability, lack of family support, involvement with the criminal justice system, and increased risk for suicide. Given that rates of substance abuse among the homeless range from 35%

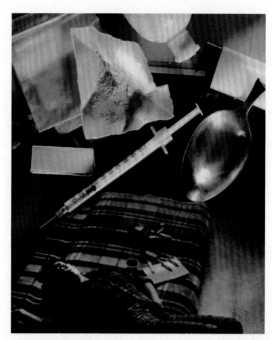

FIGURE 38.2 Substance abuse complicates the problems and treatment of many homeless people, including many of those also struggling with mental illness. In fact, many clients with psychiatric problems turn to drugs and alcohol as a way to deal with their psychiatric symptoms.

to 65%, their drinking and drug abuse patterns are highly visible. Substance abuse depletes available resources and may alienate family members who could provide support. It may also have led to a state of unemployment or underemployment. Criminal offenses related to substance use are often grounds for eviction (Phinney et al., 2007). Those experiencing both mental illness and substance abuse are more likely to have higher rates of medical illness, specifically hypertension, epilepsy, organic brain disorders, diabetes, and hepatitis (Dickey et al., 2002).

Crack cocaine has changed the economic status of many, including homeless people who are mentally ill. Such people may spend their limited funds on this highly potent and rapidly addictive drug, instead of on housing or food. New drugs appear on the street each year; others reemerge, such as LSD (see Chap. 30). Marketing of such drugs often targets vulnerable populations. The street use of heroin and methamphetamines has created a higher incidence of crime, death by overdose, and unpredictability in criminal behavior.

Poverty

The gap between rich and poor continues to widen in the United States. For many people, the margin between poverty and homelessness is narrow. The most seriously affected groups are people of color, children, and older adults (Figure 38.3). High unemployment rates, cuts in funding for public assistance, inadequate insurance for debilitating illnesses including psychiatric disorders, and increased domestic violence all contribute to a cycle of poverty that promotes

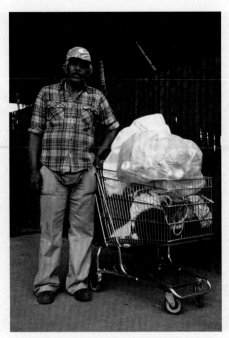

FIGURE 38.3 People of color are overrepresented in both the poor and homeless populations. Unemployment, inadequate insurance, and lack of family and social supports all contribute to a debilitating cycle of poverty.

despair, poor self-esteem, and feelings of alienation. Homelessness is one of the most visible consequences. Employed Americans are not immune; many are only one missed paycheck away from homelessness as has been seen during the recent recession.

Inadequate Housing
In general, people with low incomes are paying proportionately more for housing. According to the definition of **affordable housing**, a worker should spend approximately 30% of his or her income on housing. However, based on the nationwide average of housing in cities, a worker earning minimum wage would have to work 102 hours each week to afford a two-bedroom apartment (National Low Income Housing Coalition, 2011). At the same time, housing assistance programs have become limited, rents have increased, and waiting lists for public housing have become longer.

In recent years, the focus of attempts to address the problem of homelessness have shifted away from creating emergency shelters to developing more permanent housing options (*Federal report takes snapshot*, 2007). A significant problem for clients with mental illness has been the reduced availability of single-room occupancy housing. This decline has rendered homeless many people with addictions, mental illness, or both (NCH, 2009r). In many areas, those receiving entitlements through Social Security pay a certain percentage of their income for subsidized housing. Some require assistance with management of their monthly income to ensure their rent is paid and basic needs are met. The reality for

people with mental illness in such situations is that the incidence of eviction is high and support for maintaining housing is lacking. People with mental illness, particularly those who have been homeless for a long time, experience difficulty establishing residential stability. They may be evicted because of psychiatric symptoms; for example, a person living in a multi-unit apartment may respond verbally to auditory hallucinations in the middle of the night, disrupting other tenants. Often, community-based nurses need to advocate for clients in the process of eviction prevention. To accommodate the diverse functioning levels of people with mental illness, a wide array of community housing and support is needed.

High Mobility
Restlessness affects many homeless people with mental illness. Their homelessness may be episodic, meaning that they move in and out of residential and outpatient treatment facilities. Their mobility may be seasonal. For example, a person may move from city to city because of impaired thought processes, "voices" that give directions, diminished judgment, or simply frustration with symptoms. Young adults who are mentally ill struggle with the desire to obtain independence from their families and may find autonomy in being homeless (Figure 38.4). Nevertheless, they face lack of treatment, use of street drugs, and inability to cope with mental illness. Homeless people with mental illness who are frequently mobile may become disconnected from disability entitlements, complicating their ability to obtain housing, food, and health care.

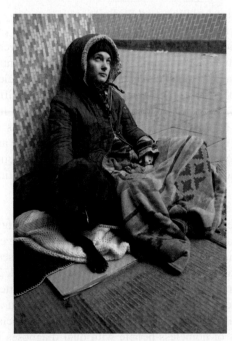

FIGURE 38.4 Many young adults may wind up living on the streets following difficulties with their families of origin. This situation can be particularly problematic for those with psychiatric illness, laying the foundation for long-term, chronic homelessness.

Critical Issues Affecting the Homeless Population with Mental Illness

Homeless people incur losses far greater than that of a house; they also lose the psychological senses of "belonging" and "home." Additional losses may include family ties, friends, work, health, and community support. When newly homeless, people with mental illness find themselves in a culture filled with fears. They may face a mental health system that is difficult to negotiate and multiple barriers to improving their plights. Clients who cannot turn this process around are at risk for chronic homelessness. When attempting to cope with the multiple losses of homelessness, clients are likely to disaffiliate from the larger society and identify with the homeless culture. In this sense, they use acculturation to survive. Early intervention is crucial.

A Changing Mental Health System

In the 1960s and 1970s, deinstitutionalization began as a positive process in support of the civil rights of clients with psychiatric disorders. The negative effects of deinstitutionalization came not from its intentions, but rather from minimal and unprepared community support, fragmented services, and few housing alternatives in the community. Deinstitutionalization has become more of an ongoing process of social change. The current homeless population with mental illness includes not only clients who have been deinstitutionalized, but also those who no longer meet criteria for hospitalization because of changes in commitment laws. These laws vary in each state, but shared issues include the right to receive treatment, the right to refuse treatment, and the right to be treated in the least restrictive environment (see Chap. 5). The troublesome question arises as to whether the least restrictive setting is also the most therapeutic. Involuntary commitment occurs if a client is judged to be a danger to self or others.

Often, those with financial resources do not experience the negative effects of deinstitutionalization as harshly as do those without such resources. Most people receiving mental health care do so in a managed care environment that limits coverage. In the current system, a client is likely to receive limited hospitalization and to experience incomplete remission of symptoms. At times, a client may receive follow-up care under an outpatient commitment or trial visit; this process can be difficult when a client is homeless.

Barriers to Care

One of the first steps in promoting access to care for homeless people with mental illness is to identify barriers to care (Box 38.1). This is especially significant because homeless people are three to six times more likely to become ill, and three to four times more likely to die than housed people (National Health Care for the Homeless Council, 2008). In 2007, an estimated 15% of the population did not have health insurance. That number rises to nearly 70% in the homeless population (DeNavas-Walt et al., 2008). Data analyzed in the 2003 National Health Care for the Homeless User survey revealed that individuals who had been unemployed in

BOX 38.1   Barriers to Health Care for the Homeless Population

- Lack of knowledge about where to get treated
- Lack of access to transportation
- Lack of identification
- Embarrassment
- Nervousness about filling out the forms and answering questions properly
- Self-consciousness about appearance and hygiene when living on the streets
- Cost

From Whitbeck, L. B. (2009). *Mental Health and Emerging Adulthood Among Homeless Young People.* New York, NY: Psychology Press, Taylor & Francis Group.

the past year were more likely than those who had not been unemployed to be uninsured and to have unmet health care needs. The most common unmet health care needs included an inability to obtain needed medical or surgical care, prescription medications, mental health care, eyeglasses, and dental care (Baggett et al., 2010).

Some community mental health programs may exclude homeless people with mental illness because they cannot meet admission criteria or they lack an address. Fragmented services with limited coordination of care do not address the complex co-occurrence of physical illness, mental illness, and substance abuse that characterizes many homeless people (Baggett et al., 2010). People with mental illness routinely experience inconsistent treatment approaches, frequent medication changes, overmedication, and poor coordination of care, which leaves them feeling justifiably distrustful of the system.

Clinician bias toward clients may present a barrier. One study identified homelessness and low social class as the two most common bases for discriminatory treatment (Wen et al., 2007). In these instances, homeless clients may feel dehumanized or disempowered. Other studies exploring homeless persons' perceptions of their health care revealed mixed perceptions of health care services, specifically a perceived mismatch between expectations and provision, disputes with health care providers, dissatisfaction with the degree to which they have choice in their care, and suspicions about the intentions of health professionals (Bhui et al., 2006; Jenkins & Parylo, 2011). The process of withdrawal by nurses from the therapeutic relationship may cause an internal psychological barrier to care. When professional expectations do not balance with practice realities, nurses may withdraw psychologically from clients. The effects of poverty and alienation may promote threatening and abusive behavior from these clients, compounding their alienation from care providers. Nurses should be cautious regarding frustration that may develop and not allow this to interfere with the treatment plan.

The traditional health care delivery system usually does not reach the homeless population. Services that can

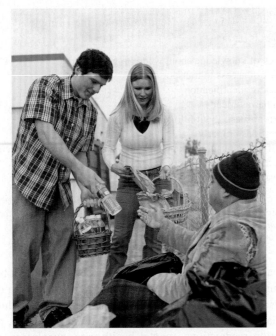

FIGURE 38.5 Street outreach teams work to deliver supplies and assistance to homeless people.

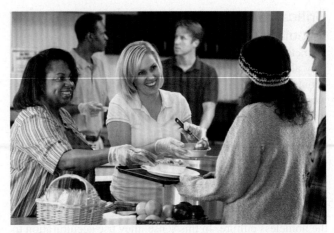

FIGURE 38.6 Volunteers, including nurses, serve at many homeless shelters to provide assistance to those in need.

improve access include shelter-based clinics, clinical day programs, freestanding clinics specific to the needs of homeless people, respite care services, mobile outreach units, and street outreach teams (Nuttbrock et al., 2003) (Figure 38.5). As of 2012 there was only one federally funded program, Health Care for the Homeless (HCH), that provided primary health care, substance abuse services, emergency care, outreach, and assistance to homeless persons in qualifying for housing (NCH, 2009b). In providing these services, nurses frequently work on multidisciplinary teams.

The Shelter System

Many urban settings have given shelters the impossible task of replacing mental institutions. Shelters are a necessary stopgap, not the solution, to homelessness. They vary in capacity and services. Some provide cots or beds; others offer only floor space. Some provide meals, reading materials, laundry facilities, a mailing address, and clothing. Others offer support services for recovery from substance abuse, spiritual guidance, and psychiatric and medical services.

Shelters commonly are staffed by paid personnel, as well as volunteers, both professional and nonprofessional (Figure 38.6). Staff must balance provision for all residents against the special needs of some. There may be differences in mission or philosophy. Staff members may need instruction about symptoms of mental illness, communicable diseases, communication skills, conflict resolution, and substance abuse. Nurses who work to instruct shelter staff should understand that specific institution's structure and dynamics when devising a training program. Such teaching opportunities are valuable ways for nurses to provide health education and build alliances.

Health Concerns

Homeless people have increased rates of trauma, foot problems, sexual health problems, dental disease, emphysema and asthma, gastrointestinal reflux disease, dermatologic conditions, and cardiac disease (Atherton et al., 2004; Brush & Powers, 2001; Poulton et al., 2006). These conditions lower life expectancy significantly. Other conditions, such as tuberculosis, HIV/AIDS, diabetes, hypertension, substance use disorders, and mental disorders, are extremely difficult to manage successfully in the homeless population. Health problems specific to urban homeless people are related to exposure, high population density, poor ventilation, and dependent positioning of the lower extremities. The risk of all illnesses increases in a shelter environment (Case Vignette 38.1).

In addition, homeless people are at increased risk of acute trauma resulting from muggings, beatings, and hate crimes. Documented hate crimes against the homeless in 2010 involved dosing individuals with gasoline and setting them aflame, rape in exchange for shelter, spray painting and stomping on sleeping individuals, and repeated incidence of gang initiations involving stabbings and beatings (NCH, 2010a).

Tuberculosis (TB) is one disease increasing globally because of increases in HIV infection, poverty, poor nutrition, and crowded conditions (Davies, 2003). U.S. cases of TB are rising in the homeless even though they are declining in the general population. Homeless people with TB are most likely to be men 25 to 44 years of age. The co-occurrence of TB with homelessness, positive HIV status, and substance abuse is significant. Homeless people with TB are far more likely to have the disease diagnosed while they are residing in a correctional facility than are people with TB who have homes. Because the association between homelessness and lack of adherence to treatment for TB is significant, homeless people with TB have higher rates of hospitalization and longer hospital stays (Moss et al., 2004). Most county health departments require and provide TB testing through Mantoux skin testing or chest x-rays. Nurses are instrumental in either provision of or referral for this testing. A client's ability to stay in a shelter may depend on having tested negative for TB.

Case Vignette 38.1

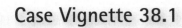

Police have asked a mental health outreach team to help a woman about whom they have received multiple calls. Community members have noticed the woman sleeping on a bench outside the supermarket. When team members arrive, they notice that the woman has a cart stuffed with belongings and a soiled sleeping bag. She has sores on her legs. The woman refuses to speak, although she accepts clean socks. The team persuades her to accompany them to a homeless shelter, where she receives soup, blankets, and clothes.

At the shelter, the woman reveals that her name is Louise. She reports that she recently spent time in a hospital where she "was poisoned with medication." She adds that she has been poisoned several other times in other cities. She believes that the poison caused her leg ulcers. She states that she left the hospital because "the police chief bugged the sewer system."

Louise says she has an adult son in another state but hasn't spoken to him in years. She adds that she was getting a check from the Social Security Administration until 2 months ago when she left the city where she was hospitalized. She has lost her identification card and refuses a test for tuberculosis.

Reflection and Critical Thinking

- What were your initial thoughts reading this scenario?
- Prioritize this client's immediate needs. What issues might a nurse wish to defer when working with this client?
- What services might be particularly helpful for Louise?

▲

Acute clinical situations that may require nursing attention include infestation by lice, scabies, or insects (Figure 38.7A) and thermoregulatory problems such as heat stroke or frostbite. Underlying every acute and chronic illness is the poor nutritional state of most homeless people compounded by minimal resources for treatment, which frequently results in severe dental disease (Seirawan et al., 2010).

Special challenges exist in the management of diabetes in an environment where dietary factors are mostly outside the person's control. Seizure disorders may result in bodily injuries from falls.

Trauma is a significant problem for urban homeless people. Sexual assaults, stabbings, fractures, and contusions secondary to assaults are common (Figure 38.7B). Because of their anonymity, homeless people often are victims of crimes. Some health-compromising behaviors are simply part of being homeless; the longer people are homeless, the more likely they are to engage in such behaviors. Examples include drug and alcohol use, sleeping outdoors, aggression, and risky sexual practices. They are more prevalent in homeless who already perceive their health to be poor. Exposure to violence, either as witness or victim, increases health-compromising and violent behaviors (Taylor et al., 2008) and significantly leads to more mental health problems (Kim et al., 2010).

Another significant health concern is the increased risk of exposure to disease of younger homeless people with mental illness. Because of certain aspects of their illnesses, such as sexual promiscuity, poor impulse control, or hypersexuality associated with mania, they may participate in unprotected sexual practices. Substance abuse may involve sharing needles for IV drug use, thus increasing exposure to infectious agents such as hepatitis and HIV.

Criminal Justice System

Many people detained in jails and prisons have a chronic mental illness (see Chap. 21). Crimes leading to incarceration may result from psychiatric symptoms, such as command hallucinations or diminished capacity to make clear judgments. Other crimes simply may arise from being homeless. For example, stealing or prostitution may be an attempt to maintain daily needs; sleeping in an abandoned building may lead to charges of criminal trespassing. If mental illness is associated with drug and alcohol use, the likelihood of arrest increases.

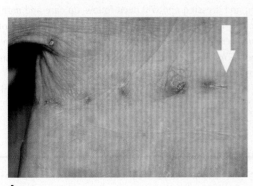
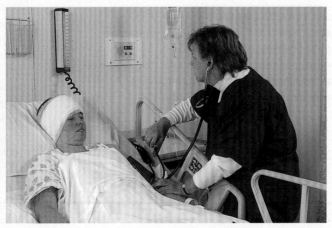

A   **B**

FIGURE 38.7 Homeless people are at risk for a host of health problems related to their harsh living conditions. Examples include (**A**) infestations and (**B**) trauma as a result of violence.

As a result of the recent recession and subprime housing crisis, 2009 saw a 32% increase in housing foreclosures from 2008. As of 2009, 6 million jobs had been lost. Forty-nine percent of people facing foreclosure report that medical problems played a role in losing their homes (NCH, 2009e). Legislation has been enacted to assist the growing segment of the population that is homeless due to foreclosures. This includes the American Recovery and Reinvestment Act of 2009, which created a $1.5 billion Homelessness Prevention and Rapid Re-Housing Program (HPRP) to help cover housing expenses for people who are either homeless or at risk of becoming homeless, and the Protecting Tenants at Foreclosure Act (H.R. 1247), which protects the renters' rights of those who are occupying housing units undergoing foreclosure (NCH, 2010b).

The housing and homelessness crisis has worsened. In 2008, 19 of 25 cities reported an average 12% increase in homeless populations (U.S. Conference of Mayors, 2008). This rise in the number of homeless has led cities and states to increase their measures against criminalization. Such measures have added another barrier to homeless people with mental illness who are trying to sustain life on the streets. Many cities have made it illegal to sleep, eat, sit, or beg in public spaces. Some cities are placing restrictions on providers serving food to poor and homeless people in public spaces (NCH, 2009f). The criminalization of services represents a growing trend of cracking down on homeless clients and families. Nurses must develop an understanding of the complexities contributing to the cause and perpetuation of homelessness and advocate for services to empower the homeless poor or those with mental illness.

The growing number of homeless people with mental illness in the criminal justice system underscores the need for prevention, outreach, mental health services within jails, and planning for treatment after release. Because homeless clients with mental illness are more often victims than perpetrators of crimes, mental health providers must also support and advocate for clients in the criminal justice system when appropriate to their treatment.

Checkpoint Questions

4. What common factors contribute to homelessness in people with mental illness?
5. How does a homeless client use acculturation to survive?
6. What measure provides a necessary stopgap to homelessness?

APPLYING THE NURSING PROCESS

Homelessness

▲ ASSESSMENT

Nurses consider how daily living conditions are affecting homeless clients, regardless of current mental state. Box 38.2 lists common stressors that may influence mental health in homeless clients.

BOX 38.2 Stressors of Homelessness That Influence Mental Health

- The effect of constant vigilance for safety, resulting in lack of sound sleep, fearfulness, suspicion, and insecurity
- Social isolation, being shunned by others, or feelings of "invisibility"
- Use of drugs or alcohol in a futile attempt to create comfort or a sense of community
- Poor diet, which may contribute to biochemical imbalances and mood changes
- Susceptibility to physical illness
- Constant uncertainty and disruptions
- Lack of medical, psychiatric, or other needed assistance
- Pervasive sense of hopelessness and uncertainty

From Haus, A. (1988). *Working with homeless people.* New York, NY: Columbia University Press.

Assessment of clients living in a shelter presents special challenges for nurses because of the lack of privacy, noise level, and clients' fear of being stigmatized. Clients may not want to be identified with a psychiatric care provider and may agree to meet with nurses only under pressure from shelter staff. Nurses must consider and appreciate the effects that undergoing assessment might have on clients.

While conducting a thorough mental status examination can be difficult, nurses proceed within the limits of a client's cooperation. They assess for neurologic problems, including a careful history for head trauma or other organic damage. If possible, they contact the client's family or health care agencies for collateral information. Other screening may be indicated; for example, most shelters require TB screening before admittance. Assessment may involve sensitive questioning, particularly with clients who have psychiatric disorders. See Box 38.3.

Think About It 38.1

A homeless client with a history of paranoid schizophrenia arrives at the emergency department by ambulance after being struck by a motor vehicle. He is disheveled and unshaven and has a strong body odor. The client has sustained a minor concussion and multiple bruises and cuts. Lacerations on his left leg require suturing and dressing and will need follow-up care and monitoring. The client rouses and begins screaming, "I'm getting out of here. I know you're part of the conspiracy to get me to tell you my secret formula." As the client screams and flails, two prescriptions for antipsychotic drugs fall from his jacket.

Propose possible ways to promote effective communication with this client, applying the information in Box 38.3.

▲ NURSING DIAGNOSIS

Nurses formulate nursing diagnoses cautiously. They first become familiar with the norms and necessities of street life because some unusual behaviors may be adaptive mechanisms in these circumstances. For example, clients may wear excessive

Communication Suggestions With Homeless Clients Who Have a Mental Illness

- Be aware of your own feelings, fears, and even your breathing.
- Create physical space so that both you and the client can leave the room if either of you decide to do so; it creates a safety zone.
- Involve significant others in communication if it facilitates a client's sense of security; don't involve others until you have asked the client's permission to do so.
- Discuss basic needs—it may be the best starting place for communication.
- Promote the client's sense of control and choice within the current environment; it may simply involve giving the client a choice of placement for his or her bedroll or whether you should give an injection in the left or right side.
- Be mindful and respectful of confidentiality issues.
- Be sensitive to possible feelings of not wanting to be identified with a psychiatric nurse or program.
- Be concrete in your interactions, avoiding metaphors, until you understand the client's cognitive functioning.
- For clients experiencing psychotic symptoms, let them know that you are not afraid of them and that your presence is not intrusive or demanding.
- For clients responding to internal stimuli, it may be helpful to ask if you could have their attention for a little while.
- For clients with delusions, let them experience that you have some sensitivity and understanding of the situation (or desire understanding); attempt to connect with the symbolism of the delusion.
- For clients with paranoia, it may be helpful to sit side by side rather than in front of them; it is possible to identify with the feeling more than the content of the paranoia and let clients know you understand that feeling.
- For clients who are suicidal, be direct in your concern and your questions in assessing for suicidality.
- Be aware of clients' varying insights into their illness.
- It may be helpful to summarize with clients, expressing your observations of their situation, then assessing with them if your observations are congruent with theirs.

clothing to prevent theft or to keep others from disturbing them, not because they have schizophrenia or other psychiatric challenges. Likewise, they may consciously exhibit bizarre behaviors to keep others away. Nursing diagnosis addresses clients in relation to their illness, family, and community.

Possible nursing diagnoses for homeless clients with mental illness include the following (NANDA, 2008):

- Interrupted Family Processes related to recent displacement
- Social Isolation related to new onset of homelessness
- Ineffective Coping related to family disruption
- Powerlessness related to lack of personal control over environment
- Chronic Low Self-Esteem related to onset of psychotic illness
- Social Isolation related to mistrust of others and lack of social support system

- Risk for Infection related to congested environment and poorly ventilated shelter setting
- Risk for Injury related to inability to maintain personal boundaries

▲ OUTCOME IDENTIFICATION AND PLANNING

In planning any treatment program, nurses recognize the realities of available local resources, client perception of needs, the conditions under which clients must function, and the nature of and symptoms related to mental illness. Another important consideration is that over time, the shelter lifestyle may have become the most important organizing factor in a client's life, providing needed structure and support. Preparing for a new life typically produces anxiety and may cause exacerbation of symptoms or new problems to emerge. Despite reality-based and reasonable goals, nurses may have to function without a tangible treatment outcome.

Possible goals for clients with mental illness who are homeless may include the following (Moorhead et al., 2008):

- **Personal Safety Behavior:** The client will satisfy physical needs and remain safe.
- **Knowledge: Disease Process:** The client will understand the symptoms of his or her mental illness.
- **Client Satisfaction: Psychological Care:** The client will build a therapeutic alliance with providers.
- **Social Support:** The client will identify and use supports and assistance from others.

Outcome criteria should be reasonable and attainable. For example, an outcome criterion for a homeless client with paranoid schizophrenia might be that paranoid thoughts are controlled long enough for the client to spend a complete night in a shelter. Other examples include that the client will demonstrate increased appropriate independent functioning, increased contact with case management services, or increased use of clinic services. Nurses must be willing to evaluate outcomes in terms of small and client-focused successes. They should not necessarily designate the end of homelessness as an outcome criterion or view the client's episodic homelessness as a failure. Clients with mental illness may move in and out of homelessness as part of a lengthy adjustment process to residential stability.

▲ IMPLEMENTATION

Nurses use many types of interventions to assist homeless clients, with or without mental illness (Evidence-Based Practice Spotlight 38.1). Specific interventions will be as varied as clients themselves. Common *Nursing Interventions Classification (NIC)* labels include, but are not limited to, **Abuse Protection Support, Case Management, Communicable Disease Management, Community Health Development, Crisis Intervention, Emotional Support, Financial Resource Assistance, Medication Management, Relocation Stress Reduction, Substance Use Treatment: Alcohol Withdrawal,** and **Substance Use Treatment: Drug Withdrawal** (Bulechek et al., 2008).

▲ EVIDENCE-BASED PRACTICE SPOTLIGHT 38.1 ▲

Meeting the Needs of Homeless People

Overview of Effective Treatment: Evidence-based guidelines state that nurses should perform a holistic assessment of homeless clients. The history should include current living conditions, prior homelessness, acute/chronic illness, current medications, prior health providers, mental illness/cognitive deficits, developmental/behavioral problems, alcohol/nicotine/other drug use, health insurance/prescription drug coverage, sexual history, history and current risk of abuse, legal/violence history, regular/strenuous activities, work history, literacy, nutrition/hydration, cultural heritage/affiliations/supports, and client strengths such as coping skills, abilities, and resourcefulness. The physical exam should include a dental assessment, along with tuberculosis testing and screening for asthma, sexually transmitted infections, and interpersonal violence. Care should address basic needs, be available after hours, and should be communicated in simple language. Medication management should address simplicity of regimen, onsite dispensing, storage of/access to medications, client

financial assistance, potential for misuse, side effects, and need for preauthorization. Special recognition should be given to associated problems and complications, such as having no place to heal, fragmented care, masked symptoms/misdiagnosis, developmental discrepancies, functional impairments, dual diagnoses, and loss of child custody. Service delivery design should include multiple points of service, integrated and interdisciplinary services, a flexible service system, assured access to mainstream health system, and access to convalescent care/supported housing.

Implications for Practice: Nurses should make several practice adaptations when providing care to the homeless. They should verify contact information with each visit. Communication with and visits to health care providers should be more frequent. Allow unscheduled visits, assist with transportation, and enhance collaboration with case managers to facilitate adherence and follow-up care.

Reference

Bonin, E., Brehove, T., Carlson, T., Downing, M., Hoeft, J., Kalinowski, A., et al. (2010). Adapting your practice: General recommendations for the care of homeless patients. Nashville (TN): Health Care for the Homeless Clinicians' Network, National Health Care for the Homeless Council, Inc. Retrieved from http://www.guidelines.gov/content.aspx?id=16325&search=homeless

Forming a Therapeutic Alliance

Homeless clients with mental illness may distrust anyone who represents the mental health system. Thus, nurses initiate the helping relationship in a nonthreatening manner, giving clients as much control as possible. They avoid wanting to "fix" the client's problems. Rather, nurses need to display behaviors that convey acceptance of clients as people worthy of dignity and respect. Nurses advocate for their clients while knowing their own limits. They avoid making

quick referrals before building trust with clients (Challenging Behaviors 38.1).

Nurses may need to postpone interventions (or even discussions of them) for the most disturbing symptoms to avoid creating a negative therapeutic experience for clients. Discussing medical conditions before psychiatric problems may help build trust with clients and improve the therapeutic relationship. An alliance can develop as clients experience a consistent and nonjudgmental attitude from nurses.

Challenging Behaviors 38.1

The Client Lost in the System

Situation: During a practicum at a homeless soup kitchen, you have been assigned to work with a man who presents there almost every day. The client avoids others and frequently talks to himself. Your assessment reveals that he cannot independently meet his basic needs and is at health risk because of foot sores. You believe strongly that he should be hospitalized. He is unwilling to be evaluated more closely and refuses hospitalization. You call the mobile crisis team. They tell you they cannot mandate a hospitalization at this time.

Your Potential Feelings: Discounted, frustrated, angry

Strategy: Ask for clarification from the clinicians on the mobile team regarding what criteria are required before the client can be hospitalized. Try to separate your feelings from clinical opinions regarding the client's best interests.

Nurse Action/Communication: Continue to build an alliance with the client. Monitor closely and document his abilities to care for himself. You might say to the client "I was concerned about how you were doing, so I asked these people to talk with you. I was hoping that over time we would be able to talk more about how you are doing and things you might need. If it's okay, I'd like to just sit here with you for awhile."

Managing Medications

Homeless clients with mental illness have special medication management needs. Many psychotropic drugs have sedating or otherwise unwanted side effects that place clients in danger in relation to life on the streets. Because homeless people must stay consistently vigilant for safety reasons, they cannot afford drowsiness. Issues of access and storage of medications pose another problem. Carrying medications increases the risk of assault or theft because most medications have street value. Nurses must also caution clients against combining medications with alcohol and drugs.

Nurses provide specific instructions to clients taking certain medications. For instance, they instruct clients taking lithium to maintain adequate fluid intake, which may be difficult, depending on the availability of water. Clients taking certain antipsychotic medications must know the importance of skin protection to prevent sunburn, which may be difficult in warm climates. Nurses involve clients in medication management. Clients alone must determine when they have access to their medication, how they can carry the medication safely, and specific daily risk factors (Understanding Psychopharmacology Box 38.1).

Teaching Clients

Homeless clients need information to promote health and to use pertinent health care resources. Client education may include topics such as personal hygiene, recognizing and treating infestation, thermoregulatory disorders, TB screening, respiratory problems, sexually transmitted infections, signs of domestic violence, emergency services, and substance abuse issues. Nurses also educate clients about the nature of mental illness; symptoms to expect; side effects, risks, and benefits of prescribed medications; and ways to negotiate the complexities of the mental health system.

Providing Case Management

Case management is the key intervention that connects clients with the community. Nurse case managers coordinate services to ensure that clients receive the structure and support needed to achieve and maintain optimal functioning. Case management encompasses health teaching, crisis intervention, symptom monitoring, assistance with federal or local entitlements, assistance with transportation, teaching about money management, and consumer advocacy. For some homeless clients, case management relationships extend for years, long after they have a home. In a managed care environment, transfer of case management may be difficult because of waiting lists, increased caseloads, and fears that clients will become lost in the system. For clients who already have experienced multiple episodes of decompensation, the anxiety produced by such a change can be challenging.

Becoming Politically Involved

Regardless of practice setting, nursing responsibilities involve interventions in the lives of homeless clients with mental illness. Hospital nurses will see homeless clients; nursing administrators will set policies for caring for homeless clients; nursing educators will devise curricula regarding homeless issues. Nurses should be knowledgeable about governmental influences on health care and willing to testify from their knowledge and experience. They must influence policies regarding health care, employment, housing, and the effects of poverty on the health status of all citizens. Nurses can stay informed on such policies by using informational resources such as the websites of many national advocacy agencies for homeless people with mental illness.

▲ EVALUATION

Reviewing the effects of the nursing care plan is an integral part of the nursing process. Without evaluation, there is no learning or improvement. To measure effects, nurses define behavioral criteria. For example, measures might include how often a client accomplished target activities, how much time he or she spent on them, the degree of insight he or she gained, or the number of symptoms relieved. In addition, nurses must reevaluate care plans in terms of new problems that may have arisen or to clarify nursing diagnoses.

In qualitatively evaluating services, the nurse performs an overall review of the program's characteristics. Such evaluative criteria address the quality of the continuum of care provided and measure a program's ability to be comprehensive, individualized, flexible, and meaningful to the client.

UNDERSTANDING PSYCHOPHARMACOLOGY 38.1

Medication Management Suggestions for the Homeless Person

- When possible, simplify the dosage and times of administration.
- Assist in locating a secure place to keep medications (refrigeration if needed).
- Assist client to locate screening clinics to evaluate ongoing therapeutic effectiveness of medications.
- Provide a telephone call service for shelters or agency providers to answer their questions and concerns about medications.

- Show clients how to carry medications on their person (if necessary) so that they don't make noise. (Rattling noises may identify homeless people as "targets" for drug theft.)
- Provide written and verbal education to the client and providers on medication, side effects, and measures to control side effects.
- Assist clients in obtaining adequate fluids, dietary needs, and sun protection; the nurse frequently needs to be creative in mobilizing volunteer services.

Reviewing and Applying Your Knowledge

Chapter Summary

- The homeless population is heterogeneous and encompasses the young, older adults, families with children, unemployed, victims of domestic violence, street youth, veterans, those released from jails, immigrants, and people with mental illness.

- Homelessness is a result of personal crises, economic crises, lack of community and family support, symptoms of chronic illness, and pervasive effects of poverty.

- Homeless people with mental illness are at increased risk for both acute and chronic illnesses. Their access to health care may be limited by attitudes of care providers, symptoms of mental illness, and the complexities of a bureaucratic mental health system.

- Shelters and programs for the homeless are crucial, but they do not offer the solution to the deeper structural problems of poverty, inadequate housing, and prejudice toward people with mental illness.

- The process of returning from homelessness to the community is a complex and anxiety-producing experience for anyone with a chronic mental illness who has been on the street for any length of time.

- The role of the nurse is crucial in identifying and removing barriers to care, providing fair and thorough assessments, and providing quality care to those who are so alienated in the margins of society that they are incapable of using the traditional mental health system.

Study Questions

1. The nurse leader is teaching a group about factors contributing to the significant increase in the number of people with mental illness living outside the hospital. Which of the following stated by the group as a factor indicates a need for additional teaching?

   a. The introduction of major tranquilizers

   b. The reduction of low-income housing

   c. An increase in U.S. immigration

   d. The civil rights movement

2. When describing characteristics of the homeless population that differ from the general population, which of the following areas would the instructor include? Select all that apply.

   a. Higher incidence of schizophrenia

   b. Greater likelihood of having an addictive disorder

   c. Higher incidence of major affective disorders

   d. Increased access to a variety of health care services

   e. Higher incidence of tuberculosis

3. When evaluating service access for the homeless population, which of the following would the nurse identify as the most likely barrier preventing a homeless person with a mental illness from seeking services?

   a. Type of symptoms the person experiences

   b. Family history of disease

   c. Clinic eligibility criteria

   d. Length of time of homelessness

4. Which of the following factors would the nurse identify as contributing to the increased risk for homelessness in people with mental illness?

   a. Increased options for available housing

   b. Gaps in care related to community treatment

   c. Movement toward greater access to institutionalization

   d. Isolated incidences of comorbidities

5. Which action would be most appropriate for a therapist who is communicating with a homeless client with a mental illness in a shelter setting?

   a. Identifying self as a mental health nurse

   b. Using short, concrete sentences without metaphors

   c. Discussing the symptoms perceived that the client may be experiencing

   d. Being gently indirect in expressing concerns regarding suicidal thoughts

Critical Thinking Questions

1. If you were to lose your income and residence today, immediately becoming homeless, what three belongings would you take with you to a shelter? Remember that you must carry these items with you and be accountable for them 24 hours a day.

2. What types of changes or circumstances would be necessary to motivate federal, state, and local governments to make the concerns of homeless people a higher priority? What would motivate health care providers?

References

American Psychiatric Association. (2000). *Diagnostic and statistical manual of mental disorders* (4th ed., text rev.). Washington, DC: Author.

Atherton, L., Stepney, J., Hamilton, J., & Smart, B. (2004). Care for the homeless: A nurse-run PMS. *Practice Nursing, 15*(3), 114–117.

Baggett, T. P., O'Connell, J. J., Singer, D. E., & Rigotti, N. A. (2010). The unmet health care needs of homeless adults: A national study. *American Journal of Public Health, 100,* 1326–1333.

Bhui, K., Shanahan, L., & Harding, G. (2006). Homelessness and mental illness: A literature review and a qualitative study of perceptions of the adequacy of care. *International Journal of Social Psychiatry, 52,* 152–165. doi:10.1177/0020764006062096

Brush, B., & Powers, E. (2001). Health and service utilization patterns among homeless men in transition: Exploring the need for on-site, shelter-based nursing care. *Scholarly Inquiry of Nursing Practice, 15,* 143–154.

Bulechek, G. M., Butcher, H. K., & McCloskey Dochterman, J. (2008). *Nursing interventions classification (NIC)* (5th ed.). St. Louis, MO: Mosby.

Davies, P. (2003). The worldwide increase in tuberculosis. *Annals of Medicine, 35*(4), 235–243.

DeNavas-Walt, C., Proctor, B. D., & Smith, J. (2008, August). *Income, poverty, and health insurance coverage in the United States: 2007* (pp. 60–233). United States Census Bureau. Retrieved from http://www.census.gov

Dickey, B., Normand, S. L., Weiss, R. D., Drake, R. E., & Azeni, H. (2002). Medical morbidity, mental illness, and substance use disorders. *Psychiatric Services, 53*(7), 861–867.

Federal report takes snapshot of country's homeless population. (2007). *Nation's Health,* Retrieved from Health Source: Nursing/Academic Edition database.

Jenkins, M., & Parylo, C. (2011). Evaluation of health services by homeless families in Leicester. *Community Practitioner, 84*(1), 21–24.

Kim, M. M., Ford, J. D., Howard, D. L., & Bradford, D. W. (2010). Assessing trauma, substance abuse, and mental health in a sample of homeless men. *Health and Social Work, 35*(1), 39–48.

Moorhead, S., Johnson, M., Maas, M. L., & Swanson, E. (2008). *Nursing outcomes classification (NOC)* (4th ed.). St. Louis, MO: Mosby.

Moss, A. R., Hahn, J. A., Perry, S., Charlebois, D., Clark, R. A., & Bangsburg, D. R. (2004). Adherence to highly active antiretroviral therapy in the homeless population in San Francisco: A prospective study. *Clinical Infectious Diseases, 39,* 1190–1198.

NANDA International. (2008). *NANDA International nursing diagnoses: Definitions and classification, 2009–2011.* Philadelphia, PA: Wiley-Blackwell.

National Alliance to End Homelessness. (2011). *No increase in homelessness despite recession.* Retrieved from http://www.endhomelessness.org/content/article/detail/4011

National Coalition for the Homeless [NCH]. (2009a). *Foreclosure to homelessness: The forgotten victims of the subprime crisis.* Retrieved from http://www.nationalhomeless.org/factsheets/foreclosure.html

National Coalition for the Homeless [NCH]. (2009b). *Health care and homelessness.* Retrieved from http://www.nationalhomeless.org/factsheets/health.html

National Coalition for the Homeless [NCH]. (2009c). *Homeless families with children.* Retrieved from http://www.nationalhomeless.org/factsheets/families.html

National Coalition for the Homeless [NCH]. (2009d). *How many people experience homelessness?* Retrieved from http://www.nationalhomeless.org/factsheets/How_Many.html

National Coalition for the Homeless [NCH]. (2009e). *Mental illness and homelessness.* Retrieved from http://www.nationalhomeless.org/factsheets/Mental_Illness.html

National Coalition for the Homeless [NCH]. (2009f). *Substance abuse and homelessness.* Retrieved from http://www.nationalhomeless.org/factsheets/addiction.html

National Coalition for the Homeless [NCH]. (2009g). *Who is homeless?* Retrieved from http://www.nationalhomeless.org/factsheets/who.html

National Coalition for the Homeless [NCH]. (2009h). *Why are people homeless?* Retrieved from http://www.nationalhomeless.org/factsheets/why.html

National Coalition for the Homeless [NCH]. (2010a). *Hate crimes against the homeless: America's growing tide of violence.* Retrieved from http://www.nationalhomeless.org/publications/hatecrimes/hatecrimes2009.pdf

National Coalition for the Homeless [NCH]. (2010b). *NCH public policy recommendations: Foreclosure and homelessness prevention.* Retrieved from http://www.nationalhomeless.org/factsheets/PPR/2010/5%20-%20Foreclosure%206-10-10.pdf

National Health Care for the Homeless Council (2008). *The basics of homelessness.* Retrieved from http://www.nhchc.org

National Law Center on Homelessness and Poverty. (2010). *Homelessness and poverty in America.* Retrieved from http://www.nlchp.org/hapia.cfm

National Low Income Housing Coalition. (2011). *Out of reach.* Retrieved from http://www.nlihc.org/oor/oor2011

National Resource Center on Homelessness and Mental Illness. (2010). *Mental health: Co-occurring disorders.* Retrieved from http://www.nrchmi.samhsa.gov/Channel/Co-Occurring-Disorders-457.aspx

Nuttbrock, L., Rosenblum, A., Magura, S., & McQuiston, H. (2003). Broadening perspectives on mobile medical outreach to homeless people. *Journal of Health Care for the Poor and Underserved, 14*(1), 5–16.

Phinney, R., Danziger, S., Pollack, H. A., & Seefeldt, K. (2007). Housing instability among current and former welfare recipients. *American Journal of Public Health, 97*(5), 832–837.

Poulton, B., McKenna, H., Keeney, S., Hasson, F., & Sinclair, M. (2006). The role of the public health nurse in meeting the primary health care needs of single homeless people: A case study report. *Primary Health Care Research and Development, 7,* 135–146.

Seirawan, M., Elizondo, L., & Mulligan, R. (2010). The oral health conditions of the homeless in downtown Los Angeles. *Journal of the California Dental Association, 38,* 681–688.

Taylor, C. A., Boris, N. W., Heller, S. S., Clum, G. A., Rice, J. C., & Zeanah, C. H. (2008). Cumulative experiences of violence among high risk urban youth. *Journal of Interpersonal Violence, 23,* 1618–1635.

U.S. Conference of Mayors. (2008). *A status report on hunger and homelessness in America's cities: A 25-city survey.* Retrieved from http://www.usmayors.org/pressreleases/documents/hungerhomelessnessreport_121208.pdf

Wen, C. K., Hudak, P. L., & Hwang, S. W. (2007). Homeless people's perceptions of welcomeness and unwelcomeness in health care encounters. *Journal of General Internal Medicine, 22*(7), 101–117.

Web Resources

National Alliance to End Homelessness: htttp://www.endhomelessness.org

National Coalition for the Homeless: htttp://www.nationalhomeless.org

National Data Resource Center on Homelessness and Mental Illness: htttp://www.nrchmi.samhsa.gov

National Law Center on Homelessness and Poverty: htttp://www.nlchp.org

U.S. Department of Veterans Affairs Homeless Assistance Information: htttp://www.va.gov/homeless

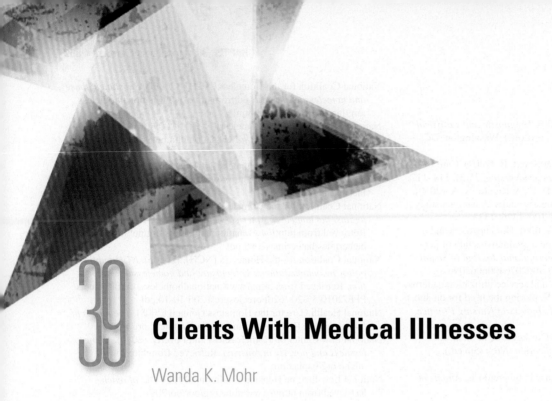

39

Clients With Medical Illnesses

Wanda K. Mohr

KEY TERMS

adjustment disorder
medical mimics
mental disorder due to a general
medical condition

LEARNING OBJECTIVES

On completion of this chapter, you should be able to accomplish the following:

• Identify the effects of medical illness on mental health.
• Explain the term "medical mimics," as well as the nurse's role relative to them.
• Discuss nursing implications for clients with adjustment disorders.
• Explain how a client's reaction to a medical condition might contribute to a psychiatric disorder.
• Identify common medical conditions that can have accompanying psychiatric complications or symptoms.
• Describe general nursing implications for clients experiencing psychiatric disorders that are intertwined with other nonpsychiatric illnesses.

Many nursing programs divide their curricula into specialties, offering individualized courses in medical–surgical care, maternal–child health, gerontology, and so forth. They also frequently teach psychiatric nursing as a separate specialty, with its own classes, texts, and clinical rotations. Such segmentation may mistakenly give students a dualistic (composed of two separate entities) impression related to the mind and body—that is, that mental health and physical health are different, and never shall they meet. Some nursing students are apprehensive about psychiatric–mental health and try to put the course quickly behind them. Others erroneously believe it is "less important" and divorced from the rest of their learning. However, unlike some specialties, mental health infuses *all* aspects of client care. Every child, pregnant woman, adult, and older adult, whether receiving primary, secondary, or tertiary care in a clinic, nursing home, hospital, or community-oriented setting, has mental health needs (Figure 39.1).

Many clients with nonpsychiatric illnesses and medical conditions develop emotional reactions to their altered health. Nurses should be sensitive to and aware of this

possibility. All nurses in all clinical specialties encounter two common diagnoses found in the *Diagnostic and Statistical Manual,* 4th edition, text revision (*DSM-IV-TR*) not often emphasized in psychiatric nursing textbooks (American Psychiatric Association [APA], 2000). These are "**mental disorder due to a general medical condition**" and "psychological factor affecting medical condition." Studies have shown that many health challenges (eg, diabetes, asthma, paralysis) have diverse psychiatric manifestations. Likewise, people may find a new diagnosis or unexpected illness to be stressful and fundamentally life changing. When they experience emotional distress and difficulty adjusting to the new reality, they may also qualify as having a psychiatric diagnosis.

This chapter is designed to help all nurses understand the problems and conditions that can arise when medical illness is, in some way, intimately linked with psychiatric manifestations. It discusses how nurses can assess and implement care for clients who experience (1) psychiatric symptoms caused by a medical condition, (2) emotional upheaval as a consequence of an adjustment disorder, or

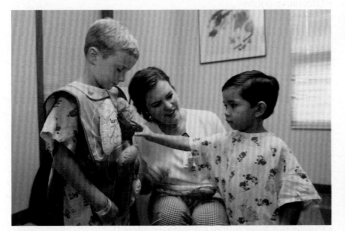

A

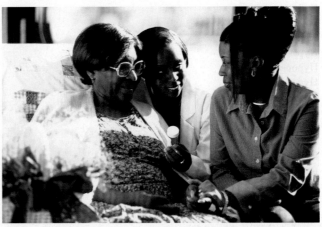

B

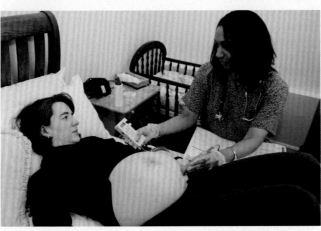

C

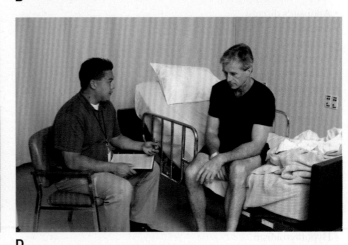

D

FIGURE 39.1 Clients of all ages and backgrounds have mental health needs. This is true whether they are receiving medical, obstetric, psychiatric, or pediatric care, and also whether they are in an institutional, hospital, community, or residential setting.

(3) mental distress concomitantly with a physical illness. The content is organized according to these diagnostic categories, with pertinent examples and associated nursing care for each.

MENTAL DISORDER DUE TO A GENERAL MEDICAL CONDITION

According to the *DSM-IV-TR*, this classification represents underlying medical conditions that directly cause psychiatric symptoms. Such disorders sometimes are called **medical mimics** of mental disorders. The causal relationship between the medical disorder and psychiatric symptoms is the most critical concept with this classification. In other words, evidence must support that the medical condition actually is the etiology of the mental problems. Thus, the psychiatric symptoms are not a reaction to being ill or to receiving a medical diagnosis, which might be true with an adjustment disorder (discussed later).

Medical mimics can have diverse psychiatric manifestations. Because of space constraints, the following paragraphs explore seizure disorder in detail as an example of this category. A comprehensive list of common medical mimics is found in Box 39.1.

BOX 39.1 Common Medical Disorders Associated With Psychiatric Symptoms

Associated With Psychotic Symptoms

- Addison's disease
- Cerebrovascular diseases
- Central nervous system (CNS) infections, including HIV
- CNS neoplasms
- CNS trauma
- Cushing's disease
- Epilepsy
- Folic acid deficiency
- Huntington's disease
- Hyperthyroidism
- Hypoparathyroidism
- Hypothyroidism
- Liver failure
- Migraine
- Multiple sclerosis
- Pancreatitis
- Porphyria
- Renal failure
- Vitamin B deficiencies
- Wilson's disease

Associated With Mood Disorders

- Addison's disease
- Anemia
- Asthma
- Chronic infections
- Cerebrovascular accident
- CNS tumors
- Cushing's disease
- Dementia
- Diabetes mellitus
- Fibromyalgia/chronic fatigue syndrome
- HIV infection
- Huntington's disease
- Hyperparathyroidism
- Hyperthyroidism
- Hypoparathyroidism
- Hypothyroidism
- Liver failure
- Malignancies, especially abdominal

- Mononucleosis
- Multiple sclerosis
- Parkinson's disease
- Sleep apnea
- Syphilis
- Systemic lupus erythematosus (SLE)
- Traumatic brain injury
- Ulcerative colitis
- Uremia
- Vitamin B_{12} deficiency
- Wilson's disease

Associated With Anxiety Disorders

- Acute infection
- Anemia
- Carcinoid syndrome
- Cardiac arrhythmia
- Cardiovascular disease
- Cerebrovascular disease
- chronic obstructive pulmonary disease (COPD)
- CNS infection
- CNS neoplasms
- Congestive heart failure (pulmonary edema)
- Cushing's disease
- Encephalitis
- Epilepsy
- Hyperthyroidism
- Hyperventilation
- Hypoglycemia
- Hypothyroidism
- Hypoxia, any cause
- Migraine
- Pheochromocytoma
- Pneumonia
- Porphyria
- Pulmonary embolism
- Rheumatoid arthritis
- SLE
- Traumatic brain injury
- Vestibular dysfunction
- Vitamin B_{12} deficiency
- Wilson's disease

General Features

The following features generally suggest a medical origin for psychiatric symptoms:

- Known underlying medical condition
- Atypical presentation of a specific psychiatric diagnosis
- No personal or family history of psychiatric illness
- No history or indication of substance abuse
- Medication use
- Sudden onset of mental symptoms
- Abnormal vital signs
- Waxing and waning of mental status

The *DSM-IV-TR* further categorizes mental disorders due to a general medical condition in three primary ways (*DSM-IV-TR* Box 39.1):

1. Diagnoses that fall within the *DSM-IV-TR* classification of cognitive disorders (see Chap. 31)
2. Diagnoses that do not fit within cognitive disorders or other specific psychiatric disorders
3. Diagnoses organized within another specific type of *DSM-IV-TR* disorder

An example of the third category is "psychotic disorder caused by a general medical condition." This diagnosis is appropriate when a person's medical history, physical examination, or laboratory test results suggest that one or more medical problems have led to psychoses (eg, hallucinations, delusions). Hallucinations linked to medical illness tend to involve phenomena less commonly found in primary psychotic disorders (eg, schizophrenia). Examples of such phenomena include olfactory and tactile elements, as well as vivid visual hallucinations. However, the hallucinations can be of any sensory type and can range from simple to complex. Delusions may also be present, with paranoia being the most common type (Mayou et al., 2001; Morrison, 2006).

Example: Seizure Disorder (Epilepsy)

According to the National Institutes of Health (NIH) (2007), more than 2 million people in the United States (approximately 1% of the overall population) have been diagnosed with epilepsy or have experienced an unprovoked seizure. Of those, 30% to 50% may manifest psychiatric symptoms during their illness (NIH, 2007). Researchers have identified more than 30 different types of seizures; however, epileptic seizures can be categorized as generalized or partial.

Generalized seizures involve both hemispheres of the cerebrum, simultaneously with classic symptoms of loss of consciousness, tonic-clonic limb movements, tongue biting, and incontinence. Delirium that resolves gradually over a few minutes to many hours characterizes the postictal state.

Partial seizures have focal signs and symptoms resulting from electrical discharge in a limited site in one brain hemisphere. Simple partial seizures have no accompanying impairment of consciousness and usually stem from primary motor, sensory, or visual cortical regions. Complex partial seizures are associated with impaired consciousness and usually originate from a focal point in the temporal lobe. Such seizures may have psychiatric manifestations, including memory dysfunction, affective auras, perceptual changes

---

DSM-IV-TR BOX 39.1

Mental Disorders Due to a Medical Condition

Diagnostic Criteria

- There is evidence from the history, physical examination, or laboratory findings that the disturbance is the direct physiologic consequence of a general medical condition.
- The disturbance is not better accounted for by another mental disorder.
- The disturbance does not occur exclusively during the course of a delirium.

Categories

- Diagnoses organized within cognitive disorders
  - Delirium due to a general medical condition
  - Dementia due to a general medical condition
  - Amnestic disorder due to a general medical condition
- Diagnoses that do not fit a category for a specific type of disorder
  - Catatonic disorder due to a general medical condition
- Personality change due to a general medical condition
- Mental disorder not otherwise specified due to a general medical condition
- Substance-induced disorders are also organized under the specific type of disorder (ie, psychosis, mood, anxiety or sleep disorder) in *DSM-IV-TR* with the exception of intoxication, abuse, and dependence
- Diagnoses organized under the specific type of disorder in the *DSM-IV-TR*
  - Psychotic disorder due to a general medical condition
  - Mood disorder due to a general medical condition
  - Anxiety due to a general medical condition
  - Sexual dysfunction due to a general medical condition
  - Sleep disorder due to a general medical condition

Reprinted with permission from the *Diagnostic and Statistical Manual of Mental Disorders, Fourth Edition, Text Revision* (Copyright © 2000). American Psychiatric Association.

(eg, hallucinations), and depersonalization. With temporal lobe epilepsy, the most common psychiatric abnormality is personality change. Hyper-religiosity, hypergraphia, and hyposexuality are other associated manifestations of this form, as is psychosis (Kaufman, 2006).

Fear and anxiety are the most common ictal affective states (NIH, 2007). Estimates are that 4% to 27% of clients with complex partial epilepsy may have psychoses such as paranoid ideation, thought disorder, and hallucinations. Symptoms of mood disorders occur most often with foci in the temporal lobe. Recent statistics indicate that 30% of clients with epilepsy have a history of suicide attempts, with more women than men completing suicide. This underscores the importance of diagnosing depression in these clients.

Treatment

It is axiomatic that proper diagnosis of a psychiatric illness necessitates investigation of all appropriate medical causes or explanations of the symptoms. When a medical problem is the cause of mental problems, treatment of the medical condition dramatically improves psychiatric health. However, while medical treatment is being planned and initiated, symptoms of anxiety, psychosis, or mood disturbance should be handled no differently than for any client with these manifestations. Of course, individualized management depends on various factors, including pharmacodynamics and metabolic issues (see Chap. 16).

Nursing Implications

Failure to identify underlying medical causes for psychiatric problems is potentially dangerous because serious and frequently reversible conditions can be overlooked. The nurse's role relative to medical mimics is to be aware of the classification itself and to understand that common psychiatric symptoms often arise from medical illnesses. Nurses should perform accurate and thorough health histories and physical examinations of all clients to gather data that can help pinpoint the specific etiology of problems. They should also be alert to abnormal laboratory test results and report such findings to physicians or advanced practice nurses immediately.

Checkpoint Questions

1. What is meant by the term "medical mimics?"
2. Which type of delusion occurs most commonly in a psychotic disorder caused by a general medical condition?

ADJUSTMENT DISORDERS

Adjustment disorder (AD) is an appropriate psychiatric diagnosis when an identifiable stressor leads to impaired relationships or functional occupational or social limitations. It is also appropriate when a person's symptoms seem excessive and disproportionate to the amount of stress he or she has experienced. A physical disorder in oneself or a family member can be a stressor leading to adjustment disorder. The qualifier "excessive" leaves significant room for the clinician's subjective judgment and interpretation (Katzman & Tomori, 2004).

The diagnosis of AD accounts for as many as 10% of consultations in general hospitals, even though researchers have criticized this construct for lack of scientific foundation (Despland et al., 1995; Katzman & Tomori, 2004). Some clinicians think that the development of psychiatric symptoms in response to difficult events is a normal part of being human. AD is one of the few *DSM-IV-TR* categories that links a stressful event to the development of symptoms.

General Features

Diagnostic criteria for AD are listed in *DSM-IV-TR* Box 39.2. The *DSM-IV-TR* further identifies six types of ADs:

- *AD with depressed mood:* Symptoms are that of a minor case of depression.
- *AD with anxious mood:* Symptoms of anxiety dominate the clinical picture.
- *AD with mixed anxiety and depressed mood:* Symptoms are a combination of depression and anxiety.
- *AD with disturbance of conduct:* Symptoms are demonstrated in behaviors that break societal norms or violate the rights of others.
- *AD with mixed disturbance of emotions and conduct:* Symptoms include combined affective and behavioral

DSM-IV-TR BOX 39.2

Adjustment Disorder

A. The development of emotional or behavioral symptoms in response to an identifiable stressor(s) occurring within 3 months of the onset of the stressor(s).
B. These symptoms or behaviors are clinically significant as evidenced by either of the following:
 1. Marked distress that is in excess of what would be expected from exposure to the stressor

2. Significant impairment in social or occupational (academic) functioning
C. The stress-related disturbance does not meet the criteria for another specific Axis I disorder and is not merely an exacerbation of a preexisting Axis I or Axis II disorder.
D. The symptoms do not represent Bereavement.
E. Once the stressor (or its consequences) has terminated, the symptoms do not persist for more than an additional 6 months.

Reprinted with permission from the *Diagnostic and Statistical Manual of Mental Disorders, Fourth Edition, Text Revision* (Copyright © 2000). American Psychiatric Association.

characteristics of AD with mixed emotional features and AD with disturbance of conduct.

• *AD NOS:* This residual diagnosis is used when a maladaptive reaction that is not classified under other ADs occurs in response to stress (APA, 2000).

Other subtypes include *acute AD,* which lasts for less than 6 months, and *chronic AD,* which lasts for 6 months or more.

Reactions to Physical Illness

The far-reaching effects of illness extend beyond the sick person to touch all those with whom he or she comes in contact. Medical illness can affect social and family relations, vocational and recreational activities, and general well-being. The very definition of AD is that of a psychological response to an identifiable stressor. Devastating and chronic illnesses constitute such stressors and automatically tend to trigger significant emotions. Many physical illnesses produce reactions that involve affective or other symptoms; some of them induce people to engage in substance abuse or other maladaptive coping strategies. Reactions to physical illness vary and how a person specifically responds depends on several factors, as outlined in Box 39.2 (Gledhill et al., 2000; Katzman & Tomori, 2004).

Treatment

Because ADs often present with subthreshold symptoms (ie, symptoms are distressing, but not severe enough to merit a psychiatric diagnosis such as major depression), they have no single treatment or intervention approach. Moreover, little information on this topic is available in the research literature (Strain, 2007). Effective treatments for other stress-related disorders may be constructive for clients with AD, provided that such interventions are geared toward the alleviation of psychiatric symptoms in conjunction with the physical illness. Specific examples might include individual supportive therapies, group therapies, and involvement in support groups. Medications and other somatic therapies are usually unnecessary, except in the instance of a client's subjective levels of distress (ie, the person feels uncomfortable enough emotionally to warrant medication).

Nursing Implications

When nurses care for clients with medical diagnoses, they should be cognizant of potential idiosyncratic reactions to them. They should also reassure clients and family members

---

BOX 39.2 Factors That Influence Reactions to Illness

• Nature of the condition—acuteness or chronicity, alterations to lifestyle, potential of associated death
• Pre-illness personality of the client
• Meaning of the illness to the client
• Other life circumstances
• Degree of social support in the client's environment

---

that an AD is a common, natural, and usually time-limited reaction to a new diagnosis (or situation). Nurses can be instrumental in teaching families that an AD may occur when a medical condition temporarily challenges their relative's capacity for coping. They can also encourage the client (and family) to identify relatives, friends, and spiritual advisors to provide support during acute periods of psychological discomfort.

Foundations have established a plethora of support groups for many medical disorders. Clients and families can obtain information about them simply by entering the name of the condition (eg, cancer) into an Internet search engine such as Google. Likewise, nurses can advise clients and families of the integrity of the "dot.gov" sites, where they can access current empirically supported research reported through various federal agencies on various conditions.

Checkpoint Questions

3. What are five factors that can affect a person's reaction to physical illness?
4. How do the symptoms of AD differ from those of an Axis I disorder?

MENTAL DISORDER NOT OTHERWISE SPECIFIED DUE TO A GENERAL MEDICAL CONDITION

This category is used when symptoms *appear* to be associated with a general medical condition; however, they do not qualify for the full criteria of an Axis I disorder (see Chap. 1). Thus, although a designation of "almost Axis I" is not a true categorization of these conditions, it may be useful to think of them this way.

Just because a condition is not in the *DSM-IV-TR,* it does not mean that the condition does not exist. The *DSM-IV-TR* categories are not written in stone, but change over time (Morrison, 2006). Major psychiatric texts tend to give little attention to the emotional reactions of clients to physical disorders. Nevertheless, the topic is important because emotional reactions can contribute to morbidity, recovery, and mortality (Bane et al., 2006). In fact, emotional responses to medical conditions and associated behaviors have far-reaching implications for all nurses, regardless of specialty. Specifically, this classification represents those instances in which clients face medical conditions and develop symptoms similar to a major Axis I disorder other than an AD. (The exception is the supraordinate designation of cognitive disorders due to a general medical condition; see Chap. 31.)

Evaluation of specific *DSM-IV-TR* criteria can be challenging when clients are dealing with an "almost Axis I" problem. For example, the diagnostic criteria for major depression (see Chap. 27) state that "symptoms are not due to the direct physiologic effects of a substance or a general medical condition" (APA, 2000). Yet, major depression

(Axis I) can coexist with a medical condition such as diabetes (Axis III). Moreover, the diabetes may have preceded the depression. Likewise, some researchers have posited a relationship between a psychological condition and its effect on a medical condition. For example, a client with borderline personality disorder may have a different experience with cardiovascular illness than is typical because of his or her preexisting psychiatric illness. The *DSM-IV-TR* calls this category "psychological factor affecting medical condition." However, readers are cautioned that many authors have questioned the reliability and validity of this loosely constructed diagnosis. This classification is understudied and not well described or delineated in the psychiatric literature, although the medical literature contains discussions of such phenomena (National Institute of Mental Health [NIMH], 2005).

The immune, neurologic, and psychological systems have many interacting and overlapping functions. Examples include communication pathways from the brain to the immune system, particularly the hypothalamic-pituitary-adrenal (HPA) axis and the autonomic nervous system. These pathways help mediate the influence of stress and emotions on a person's immunity and resistance to disease (Figure 39.2). Clients with physical illnesses may have a depressed mood, anxiety, anorexia, weight loss, altered sleep patterns, fatigue, motor retardation, reduced interest in the environment, and impaired cognition as a result of the influence of the interactions among immune systems and neurologic systems.

Clients with medical conditions often have to change their aspirations, expectations, lifestyle, and employment. Many grieve about their predicament before accepting it and adapting accordingly. Others develop psychiatric disorders, most commonly depression or anxiety. A prospective study of general medical admissions found that 13% of men and 17% of women had an affective disorder (Mayou et al., 2001). The proportion of clients with chronic conditions such as

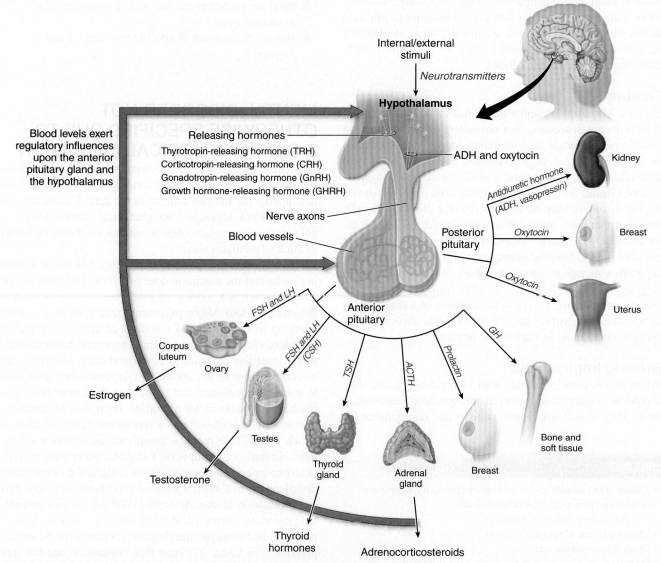

FIGURE 39.2 The HPA axis is one of the body's pathways that mitigates the effects that stress and emotions can have on immunity and disease resistance.

diabetes or rheumatoid arthritis who have an affective disorder is 20% to 40% (Dunn et al., 2006; Egede, 2006). Among clients admitted to the hospital for acute care and among clients with cancer, rates of affective disorders can exceed 30% (Stover, 2003). These numbers are significantly higher than the prevalence of depression in the community, which is approximately 4% to 8% (NIMH, 2005). However, because depression is often unrecognized and undertreated in sick people, most studies probably underestimate its prevalence (Drucker, 2004).

Clinicians find it difficult to separate depression in people with medical illnesses from the medical conditions themselves. Symptoms such as disturbed sleep, impaired appetite, and lack of energy may already exist because of the medical problem. Moreover, treatments may affect mood. For example, steroids used for acute exacerbations of Crohn's disease may have psychological side effects. The disease itself can influence psychological state, such as when a person has hypoxia from chronic obstructive pulmonary disease (COPD).

The functional limitations that a disease imposes may result in "understandable" distress. Some physicians and nurses, as well as clients and family members, may find it difficult to conceptualize such distress as a psychiatric disorder. A further complication is that the differences among AD, major depression, anxiety, and acute stress disorder are often not clear.

Great attention to ways to achieve correct diagnoses and the complexities of such determinations are beyond the scope of this chapter. The focus of the subsequent sections is the examination of examples of common medical illnesses and related literature findings about emotional reactions to such predicaments.

Cardiovascular Illness

Critically ill clients with life-threatening myocardial infarctions may present with altered emotions, cognition, and behaviors requiring prompt attention, not only from the medical team, but also from consulting psychiatric clinicians. Acute cardiac changes can severely compromise normal coping strategies (Davidson et al., 2006). Furthermore, the trauma of being attended to amid the controlled chaos of an emergency department and the highly technological environment of the coronary care unit (CCU) is foreign and frightening to most people (Figure 39.3).

Client Reactions

The uncertainty that accompanies being suddenly physically ill is probably what makes clients who have experienced dramatic cardiovascular problems feel most vulnerable and in danger, regardless of how attentive, empathic, and reassuring CCU personnel are. Health care providers must remember that admission to the CCU followed a major crisis in heart function. Cardiac arrest, cardiogenic shock, or severe heart failure may have complicated an initial myocardial infarction (MI).

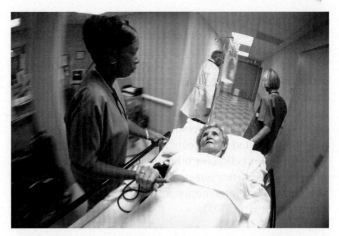

FIGURE 39.3 The stress of emergency care related to a cardiovascular problem can compound a client's trauma and capacity for responding psychologically, emotionally, and spiritually to it.

Psychological problems that accompany cardiac difficulties may result from the following factors:

- The effect of the medical illness or its treatment on the central nervous system (eg, secondary to diminished cardiac output)
- The client's subjective response to how the cardiac illness will impair his or her future (ie, a client may feel that any worthwhile life is over)
- The client's worry and preoccupation about physical symptoms, which may worsen the clinical state (eg, failure to cooperate in rehabilitative efforts)
- Interactions with family or life circumstances (eg, stresses already present prior to the MI may be magnified)
- Fear of another episode

Admission to the CCU following a life-threatening medical event may lead to acute anxiety and fear in clients. Although these emotions may not qualify as an anxiety disorder (see Chap. 23), they may be uncomfortable and disconcerting to clients and their loved ones. Initially, fear of death is most acute. The complexity of human personality is revealed in the CCU setting by the numerous manifestations of anxiety that clients and relatives can display. Examples include outbursts of anger and impatience, threats to leave the hospital against medical advice, paranoia, frequent calls for the nurse, and silent withdrawal.

Once fear of death subsides, concerns about the illness and its treatments may become the focus. Subjective preoccupation may lead to more sustained depression or anxiety. Depression commonly occurs alongside of cardiovascular disease. Depressive symptoms often go unrecognized in pursuit of medical stability (eg, control of hypertension and cholesterol levels). Nevertheless, persistent depression or anxiety may impede recovery and influence adherence to rehabilitation regimens. In fact, the magnitude of the effects of depression on morbidity and mortality in cardiovascular disease is on a par with the effects of factors the contributing variables that are commonly recognized as medical risk factors (Shapiro, 2005).

Symptoms of anxiety are also frequent in clients with heart disease, during acute coronary events and arrhythmias. Anxiety and anxiety disorders can also adversely affect outcomes in cardiovascular diseases. Anxiety's adverse effects on outcome in coronary artery disease may be mediated by effects on heart rate variability, QT interval prolongation, or other abnormalities in autonomic nervous system responses (Levenson, 2008). Thus, early recognition and intervention are crucial (Bane et al., 2006; Rumsfeld & Ho, 2005).

Treatment and Nursing Implications

During the acute phase of cardiovascular illness, nurses can provide quiet reassurance and as much support to families and clients as possible. Although Health Insurance Portability and Accountability Act (HIPAA) legislation may limit how much information health care providers can share, it is well accepted that uncertainty increases anxiety. HIPAA was not enacted to be an obstruction to communication, but a way to protect clients. However, HIPAA rules sometimes impede communication between staff and family members and limit important interventions, such as family education. Nurses can help alleviate distress by having clients sign HIPAA waiver of confidentiality forms when they are in stable condition. In this way, nurses are enabled to appropriately communicate with and educate families, who can afford substantial relief and support to clients.

Evidence-based findings of an association between depression and cardiovascular morbidity and mortality have grown and been more consistent during the past decade. Davidson et al. (2006) concluded that because cardiovascular disease and depression are the two most prevalent causes of death and disability worldwide, it is important for more research efforts to develop effective interventions unique to these comorbidities. The group opined that a "one-size-fits-all" intervention that focuses only on depression without considering its context is likely to be an ill fit for these clients. Although further studies are pending, health care providers should be cognizant that these disorders often occur together, recognize the coexistence when it happens, and intervene with modalities known to "work" for depression. Reducing isolation, evaluating social support structures, and making referrals to support groups and for cognitive therapy are some suggested strategies, with interventions tailored to the specific needs of clients (Arthur, 2006).

Pulmonary Illness

Dyspnea, the major symptom associated with acute exacerbations of COPD, is a subjective experience. Extensive research has been done on the pathophysiology and affective components of dyspnea; however, the precise physical mechanism of breathlessness remains elusive (Bailey, 2004).

Client Reactions

Chronic or acute dyspnea must be not only exceedingly anxiety evoking, but also agonizing for people experiencing it. Panic about breathing can worsen dyspnea. Anxiety and depression frequently complicate chronic airflow obstruction and probably other forms of advanced lung disease. Anxiety, a common and sometimes disabling symptom among clients with respiratory disease, seems to be most prevalent in clinical samples of clients. This should surprise no one with any imagination who can put himself or herself in the place of a person who cannot breathe.

Anxiety in clients with expiratory airflow obstruction can result in a breathing pattern that precipitates physiologic changes that produce dyspnea (West, 2007). As respiratory rates rise (a common manifestation of anxiety), clients with expiratory airflow obstruction have insufficient time to exhale. This leads to hyperinflation with an increased work of breathing and a sense of greater effort being required to breathe.

Research suggests that pulmonary disease constitutes a risk factor for panic related to repeated experiences with dyspnea and life-threatening exacerbations of pulmonary dysfunction, repeated episodes of hypercapnia or hyperventilation, use of anxiolytic medications, and stress of coping with chronic disease. Panic in clients with pulmonary disorders may also contribute to significant morbidity, including phobic avoidance of activity, overly aggressive treatment with anxiolytic medications, and more prolonged and frequent hospitalizations (Smoller et al., 1999; West, 2007).

Despite the development of many new therapeutic options, anxiety, panic, and depressive conditions remain underrecognized and undertreated in this client population (Frownfelter, 2005; Wingate & Hansen-Flaschen, 1997). Underdiagnosis may partly result from the challenge of distinguishing between the somatic manifestations of psychiatric disease and the physical symptoms of severe respiratory dysfunction. A complication is that clients with anxiety disorders frequently report dyspnea, chest pain, palpitations, and a tingling or prickling sensation in the extremities (paresthesias). Clients experiencing an acute anxiety disorder may also experience hyperventilation and hypocapnia. Recognition that the differential diagnosis of dyspnea and anxiety includes both pulmonary and psychiatric conditions can be crucial to appropriate medical management and to minimizing iatrogenic harm and suffering (West, 2007).

Treatment and Nursing Implications

Above all, nurses should carefully assess and evaluate whether clients have dyspnea secondary to anxiety or anxiety from dyspnea and hypoxia. This matter is not to be taken lightly because clients with COPD have been known to suffer unnecessarily and to be severely compromised by sedation when their agitation was erroneously assumed to be anxiety and not recognized as the effects of impaired respiratory functioning. In some cases, clients have died.

If a client has a diagnosis of COPD, asthma, or any other respiratory illness, *the nurse's first assumption should*

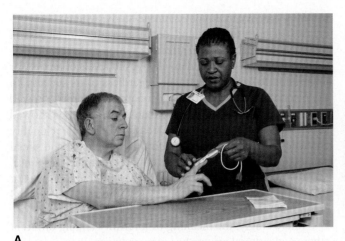 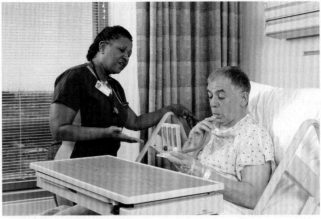

A   **B**

FIGURE 39.4 Clients with hypoxia, regardless of the source, require quick evaluation. Examples of common measures include (**A**) pulse oximetry and (**B**) incentive spirometry.

be that the client is hypoxic and that manifestations of anxiety or agitation are the result of hypoxia. This assumption should hold until proven otherwise.

In these instances, quick evaluation with spirometry, a pulse oximeter, drawing of blood gases, and other measures to reverse the hypoxia are in order (Figure 39.4). When the client's oxygen levels and blood pH have been restored, the level of agitation also will subside. While instituting these measures, it is appropriate for the nurse to quietly reassure the client that he or she is receiving treatment that will act very soon. Telling the client to "Calm down and take deep breaths" is a waste of time and counterproductive. Such exhortations serve only to agitate clients. Clients who could calm down and breathe most assuredly would do so without a nurse's or other clinician's direction.

Breathing retraining techniques, commonly used in pulmonary rehabilitation programs, are designed to break the cycle of rapid breathing, hyperinflation, more distress, and even faster, shallower breaths (Smoller et al., 1999). To the extent that nurses and other clinicians can provide clients with strategies for dealing with their symptoms and attendant fears, clients may establish a sense of control over their bodies that may preempt anxiety and hyperventilation. Exercise training that repeatedly exposes clients to breathing discomfort may also "desensitize" them to the fear associated with dyspneic sensations. Such training should be undertaken only by a pulmonary specialist and psychologist under safe, monitored conditions.

Think About It 38.1

A 23-year-old man comes to the emergency department reporting dyspnea and palpitations. He is tachycardic and tachypneic. He also reports tingling in his fingers. He is visibly anxious, apprehensive, and irritable. "I feel like I want to jump out of my skin." The client has a history of asthma. What should the nurse do?

Reproductive Challenges

The fertility rate is a measure of the number of live births to women of childbearing age. A woman's fertility drops sharply after she is 30 years old. Despite this, increasing numbers of women are postponing pregnancy until after 30 years. Many reasons have contributed to this outcome, including economic factors and women's choices to pursue higher education and career objectives before starting families (Kohler & Rodgers, 2003). This shift in many European countries and the United States has resulted in an increasing concentration of childbearing to a relatively narrow interval during the late stage of the reproductive span (Kohler & Ortega, 2002). The lower fertility rates and relative affluence of women older than 30 years have also spawned new techniques to assist them in their desire to have biological children. Examples include hormonal stimulation, intracytoplasmic sperm injection (ICSI), gamete intrafallopian transfer (GIFT), and in vitro fertilization (IVF).

Client Reactions

Surprisingly little research has been done in the past 10 years on emotional reactions to infertility. Most existing studies have been conducted outside the United States, although more have been conducted in the past 5 years, and a major journal (*Human Reproduction*) has published numerous studies in this area. The relationship between psychological factors and infertility is a particularly difficult area for study because it involves potential psychological factors in both members of the couple, the interactions between the two, as well as their effects on sexual behavior and fertility (Cwikel et al., 2004).

Most psychological distress seen in infertile couples is a result of infertility and not a cause of it (Levenson, 2008). When couples are dealing with infertility, feelings of grief and loss are common as they accept that they cannot conceive naturally. Different emotional coping styles between men and women may add to an already stressful situation

(Alesi, 2005). The effects of infertility on couples' psychological well-being are significant and can be deeply distressing. For almost 10 years, researchers have noted that health problems, loss of self-esteem, feelings akin to mourning, sexual distress, depression, guilt, anxiety, frustration, emotional distress, and marital problems are associated with infertility (Domar et al., 1999; Guerra et al., 1998; Lapane et al., 1995). Several studies have demonstrated that anxiety has a detrimental effect on fertility and that reduced anxiety increases pregnancy rates. Other research has failed to support a relationship between anxiety and infertility. Lapane et al. (1995) indicated that depression could play an important role in the pathogenesis of infertility.

Emotional tensions such as anxiety, interpersonal problems, suppressed anger, frustration, feelings of inferiority, depression, feelings of rejection, and unconscious guilt can sometimes accompany infertility (Figure 39.5). The overall percentage of couples dealing with psychological problems related to infertility ranges from 25% to 60%, with one study finding that 74.6% of clients reported changes in their mood (Dhaliwal et al., 2004).

In sum, ample evidence supports that lower stress levels mean better female and male natural fertility, although no conclusive experimental evidence shows that lower stress levels result in better fertility treatment outcome. Accumulating evidence points to the need to tailor medical fertility treatment, bearing in mind both chronic and acute stress levels, and to treat for their reduction before commencing the actual fertility treatment (Campagne, 2006). Psychological difficulties of infertile clients are complex. Several factors influence such problems, such as gender differences, cause and length of infertility, and history of coping.

In addition to the emotional factors related to infertility itself and the effects of those factors on fertility, women and their partners may also have psychological reactions to failed fertility treatments. In one study, women show increases in both anxiety and depression after unsuccessful treatment and decreases in affective symptoms after successful treatment. Men showed no changes in levels of anxiety or depression following treatment, regardless of its success. In the 6 months after unsuccessful treatment, women showed no recovery. At follow-up, more than 20% of women showed subclinical forms of anxiety, depression, or both. Personality characteristics, meaning of the fertility problems, and social support determined the course of the emotional response. Most women adjusted well to unsuccessful treatment, but at follow-up, a considerable proportion still showed substantial emotional problems (Verhaak et al., 2005).

Interestingly, the meaning of infertility among different ethnic and cultural groups has garnered virtually no research in the United States. A Medline search of the literature from 1996 to 2010 combining the terms "infertility" and "culture" (and ethnicity) yielded 12 articles dealing with the phenomenon in Malawi, India, Greece, Bangladesh, Israel, South Africa, and Egypt. Only one article (Nasseri, 2000) speaks to cross-cultural differences among ethnic groups in the United States. Clearly, more research needs to be done in the United States comparing how different ethnic groups experience and cope with infertility.

Treatment and Nursing Implications

Nurses and other health care professionals should be sensitive to the emotional experiences of couples receiving a diagnosis of infertility or during infertility treatment. They can help identify factors that contribute to stress or that may be targets for intervention. Group and couples therapy, as well as individual cognitive–behavioral psychotherapy, have been shown to decrease clients' anxiety and depression (deLiz & Straus, 2005). Some couples continue to provide support to one another or to others after a formal group has disbanded. Nurses should encourage such social support and informal group interactions. In addition, nurses can refer couples to free support and educational groups online. Some helpful organizations are included in the Web Resources list at the end of this chapter.

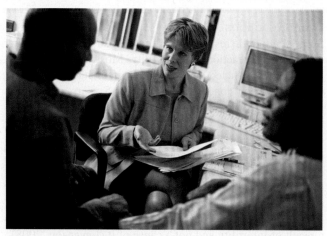

FIGURE 39.5 When working with clients who have faced fertility challenges, health care providers must strive to help clients through the emotional roller coaster that many of them face, in addition to trying to assist them in their quest to have children.

> **Checkpoint Questions**
> **5.** Why do clinicians find it difficult to separate depression in people with medical illnesses from the medical conditions themselves?
> **6.** What are two common feelings associated with couples dealing with infertility?

Neoplastic Diseases (Cancer)

At one time, receiving a diagnosis of cancer was synonymous with receiving a confirmation of impending death. Although this is no longer the case, attitudes change slowly. Being diagnosed with cancer often is a devastating emotional experience; however, an individual's psychological response to cancer is influenced by specific aspects of the cancer. It may change over the course of the illness and depends on medical, psychological, and social factors, previous coping style, social support, and religious and cultural backgrounds, as well as aspects of the disease itself (eg, site, stage, clinical course, cancer treatment, and complications).

Client Reactions

The physical suffering associated with cancer and cancer treatment causes significant distress. Although some clients with advanced cancer do not consider themselves to be suffering, research conducted by Wilson et al. (2007) showed that almost half (49.2%) of all clients do. That suffering is multidimensional, related most strongly to physical symptoms, but with psychological, existential, and social-relational elements. Adverse effects of chemotherapy on quality of life are well documented. People with cancer who are undergoing chemotherapy experience several symptoms (eg, nausea, vomiting, fatigue, sleep disturbance) and physical limitations (eg, task performance and activity restrictions) accompanied by declines in physical and mental well-being (Wilson et al., 2006). Distress in clients with cancer can significantly affect quality of life and response to treatment. In fact, Holland and Bultz (2007) of the National Comprehensive Cancer Network suggest that distress should be considered the sixth vital sign for health care providers to evaluate in people with cancer.

Overall, studies of distress in people with cancer yield similar findings, with rates of clinically significant symptoms, such as depression and anxiety, being as high as 42%. In a study of more than 3,000 outpatients in Scotland, almost 25% of those receiving treatment for colorectal, breast, cervical, genitourinary, skin, and mixed forms of cancer reported significant emotional distress as measured by the Hamilton Inventories (Hamilton Depression and Hamilton Anxiety Inventory). Women had more significant scores of distress than did men, particularly those who were younger than age 65 years. Reduced activity status predicted increased distress, as did cancer in an active phase versus cancer in remission. No difference in distress scores emerged relative to the specific type of cancer (Strong et al., 2007). Results from an interesting qualitative study of suffering in cancer showed that distress was part of the experience of clients with cancer and that often such suffering remained unalleviated (Daneault et al., 2006). The study's researchers speculated that the impersonal and rushed nature of a bureaucratic health care environment directly influenced how much suffering clients reported.

Treatment and Nursing Implications

The research literature supports that nurses can do much to alleviate the distress of clients with cancer. Clients report that very simple interventions, such as providing humanizing touches, chatting about life events, asking about family,

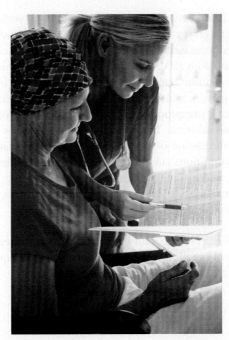

FIGURE 39.6 Basic nursing interventions (such as individualized and thorough teaching) can help clients with cancer to better cope with their illness.

and individualizing care, would help them to cope better with their diagnosis and situation (Daneault et al., 2006) (Figure 39.6). Nurses can provide stress reduction exercises, such as instruction in paced abdominal breathing, progressive muscle relaxation with guided imagery, and the use of coping self-statements. In addition, they can encourage clients to practice such techniques before the start of chemotherapy and to use them after each round of treatment. Mock and colleagues (2001) reported that clients who spent more time per week exercising experienced less decline in physical functioning. Nurses can encourage such exercise and help clients to tailor it to their own needs and within their own limitations. In addition, nurses can encourage clients with cancer and their families to avail themselves of the many support and education groups available to them (see Web Resources).

Finally, nurses should address the needs of caregivers. Although an in-depth discussion of this issue is beyond the scope of this chapter, caregiver burden and the distress of an impending death can cause significant pain. Nurses should recognize this and provide the same levels of support and empathy to caregivers as they do to clients with cancer.

NURSING STRATEGIES FOR PSYCHOSOCIAL CARE IN MEDICAL ILLNESS

The preceding discussions review medical mimics of psychiatric disorders, adjustment disorders, and the coexistence of medical disorders with psychological symptoms. Because of space limitations, many specific conditions within these general categories have not been explored. For example, much has been written about the emotional consequences of infection with HIV, multiple sclerosis, rheumatoid arthritis, other autoimmune diseases, and other various illnesses. Chronic pain is another condition with intense emotional distress and inappropriate coping that nurses should recognize and address. The space limitations of this chapter preclude discussion of psychiatric sequelae associated with medical conditions such as substance abuse, anorexia, loss of libido, and insomnia. Regardless of the specific medical problem experienced by a client, several important conclusions can be drawn:

• A client is a holistic entity. What affects one system or domain of functioning often has important consequences on others.

• The emotional dimensions of medical conditions often may be overlooked in medical–surgical or primary care settings.
• Diagnosing depression or other mental alterations in people with medical illness may be challenging, but accurate identification and treatment are essential.
• Nurses and other clinicians may be well equipped for the biomedical aspects of care but not always for the challenges of understanding the psychological, social, and cultural dimensions of illness and health.
• Nurses can play an important part in helping clients maintain healthy coping skills.
• Nurses should reflect on the emotional dimensions of their work, including whether they truly are applying a psychosocial-spiritual model of assessment and intervention to clients with a disorder that falls on Axis III of the *DSM-IV-TR* (see Chap. 1).

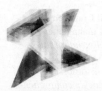

Reviewing and Applying Your Knowledge

Chapter Summary

- Two common diagnoses from the *DSM-IV-TR* may occur in all clinical specialties: *mental disorder due to a general medical condition* and *psychological factor affecting medical condition*. When people with medical illnesses experience emotional distress and difficulty adjusting to a new reality, they may receive the psychiatric diagnosis of an adjustment disorder.

- Disorders that present with psychiatric symptoms directly resulting from an underlying medical condition are sometimes called medical mimics of mental disorders. The medical illness is the actual cause of the psychiatric symptoms.

- Adjustment disorder is a diagnosis used when an identifiable stressor leads to impaired relationships or functional limitations in a client's work or social life, or when symptoms seem excessive or disproportionate to the amount of stress. The symptoms are distressing, but are not severe enough to merit a separate *DSM-IV-TR* Axis I diagnosis.

- Mental disorder not otherwise specified due to a general medical condition is used when symptoms seem to be associated with a general medical condition and do not qualify for the full criteria of an Axis I disorder. Examples may include depression with diabetes, depression and myocardial infarction, and anxiety or panic and chronic obstructive pulmonary disease.

- Clinicians need to view the client holistically and consider the emotional dimensions of the medical condition for the client.

Study Questions

1. When describing adjustment disorders to the class, the nursing instructor identifies which of the following as crucial to this diagnosis?

   a. An identifiable stressor

   b. Evidence of a mood change

   c. Fear of separation

   d. Violation of another's rights

2. A client is diagnosed with a psychotic disorder caused by a general medical condition. Which of the following would the nurse most likely expect to assess?

   a. Mental status changes

   b. Anxiety

   c. Depression

   d. Paranoid delusions

3. A client has temporal lobe epilepsy. Which of the following would be least likely?

   a. Hyper-religiosity

   b. Dementia

   c. Hypergraphia

   d. Psychosis

4. Which of the following would be least appropriate to include when developing the plan of care for a client with an adjustment disorder and his family?

   a. Reassuring them that this is often a natural reaction to a new situation

   b. Offering suggestions to the client and family about possible support groups

   c. Telling them that it may take quite a long time for this condition to resolve

   d. Informing them that their coping ability is being challenged by the client's condition

5. After reviewing information about emotional reactions and infertility, which of the following would the nurse identify as most accurate?

   a. Evidence supports that lower stress levels seem to improve natural fertility.

   b. Psychological problems facing infertile clients typically relate to one area.

   c. Men and women react similarly to fertility treatment successes and failures.

   d. Much research has been done to evaluate the meaning of infertility among cultural groups.

Critical Thinking Questions

1. A client is exhibiting signs and symptoms of depression. He also has a history of epilepsy. Describe how the nurse would proceed in attempting to determine if the client's depression is separate from or related to the epilepsy.

2. Compare and contrast the following: mental disorder due to a general medical condition and mental disorder not otherwise specified due to a general medical condition. How do they differ from adjustment disorder?

References

Alesi, R. (2005). Infertility and its treatment—An emotional roller coaster. *Australian Family Physician, 34*(3), 135–138.

American Psychiatric Association (APA). (2000). *Diagnostic and statistical manual of mental disorders* (4th ed., text rev.). Washington, DC: Author.

Arthur, H. M. (2006). Depression, isolation, social support and cardiovascular disease in older adults. *Journal of Cardiovascular Nursing, 21*(55), 52–57.

Bailey, P. H. (2004). The dyspnea-anxiety-dyspnea cycle—COPD patients' stories of breathlessness: "It's scary when you can't breathe." *Qualitative Health Research, 14*(6), 760–778.

Bane, C., Hughes, C. M., & McElnay, J. C. (2006). The impact of depressive symptoms and psychosocial factors on medication adherence in cardiovascular disease. *Patient Education and Counseling, 60,* 187–193.

Campagne, M. (2006). Should fertilization treatment start with reducing stress? *Human Reproduction, 21*(7), 1651–1658.

Cwikel, J., Gidron, Y., & Sheiner, E. (2004). Psychological interactions with infertility among women. *European Journal of Obstetrics, Gynecology, and Reproductive Biology, 117,* 126–131.

Daneault, S., Lussier, V., Mongeau, S., Hudon, E., Paille, P., Dion, D., et al. (2006). Primum non nocere: Could the health care system contribute to suffering? In-depth study from the perspective of terminally ill cancer patients. *Canadian Family Physician, 52,* 1574–1575.

Davidson, K. W., Kupfer, D. J., Bigger, J. T., Califf, R. M., Carney, R. M., Coyne, J. C., et al. (2006). Assessment and treatment of depression in patients with cardiovascular disease: National Heart, Lung, and Blood Institute Working Group Report. *Psychosomatic Medicine, 68,* 645–650.

deLiz, T. M., & Straus, B. (2005). Differential efficacy of group and individual/couple psychotherapy with infertile patients. *Human Reproduction, 20*(5), 1324–1332.

Despland, J. N., Monod, L., & Ferrero, F. (1995). Clinical relevance of adjustment disorder in *DSM III-R* and *DSM IV. Comprehensive Psychiatry, 36,* 454.

Dhaliwal, L. K., Gupta, K. R., Gopalan, S., & Kulhara, P. (2004). Psychological aspects of infertility due to various causes—Prospective study. *International Journal of Fertility and Women's Medicine, 49*(1), 44–48.

Domar, A. D., Zuttermeister, P. C., & Friedman, R. (1999). Distress and conception in infertile women. *Journal of the American Medical Women's Association, 54,* 196–198.

Drucker, M. A. (2004). Other cognitive disorders and mental disorders due to a general medical condition. In B. J. Sadock, & V. A. Sadock, *Kaplan & Sadock's comprehensive textbook of psychiatry* (8th ed., pp. 1107–1136). Philadelphia, PA: Lippincott Williams & Wilkins.

Dunn, S. L., Corser, W., Stommel, M., & Holmes-Rovner, M. (2006). Hopelessness and depression in the early recovery period after hospitalization for acute coronary syndrome. *Journal of Cardiopulmonary Rehabilitation, 26*(3), 152–159.

Egede, L. E. (2006). Disease-focused or integrated treatment: diabetes and depression. *Medical Clinics of North America, 90*(4), 627–646.

Frownfelter, D. (2005). *Cardiovascular and pulmonary physical therapy: Evidence and practice.* St. Louis: Mosby.

Gledhill, J., Rangel, L., & Garralda, E. (2000). Surviving chronic physical illness: Psychosocial outcome in adult life. *Archives of Diseases in Childhood, 83*(2), 104–110.

Guerra, D., Liobra, A., Veiga, A., & Barri, P. N. (1998). Psychiatric morbidity in couples attending a fertility service. *Human Reproduction, 13,* 1733–1736.

Holland, J. C., & Bultz, B. D. (2007). The National Comprehensive Cancer Network (NCCN) guideline for distress management: A case for making distress the sixth vital sign. *Journal of the National Comprehensive Cancer Network, 5*(1), 3–7.

Katzman, J. W., & Tomori, O. (2004). Adjustment disorders. In B. J. Sadock, & V. A. Sadock, *Kaplan & Sadock's comprehensive textbook of psychiatry* (8th ed., pp. 2055–2062). Philadelphia, PA: Lippincott Williams & Wilkins.

Kaufman, D. M. (2006). *Clinical neurology for psychiatrists.* St. Louis, MO: Elsevier.

Kohler, H. P., & Ortega, J. A. (2002). Tempo-adjusted period parity progression measures, fertility postponement and completed cohort fertility. *Demographic Research, 6*(6), 91–144.

Kohler, H. P., & Rodgers, J. L. (2003). Education, fertility and heritability: Explaining a paradox. In K. W. Wachter, & R. A. Bulatao (Eds.), *Offspring: Human fertility behavior in biodemographic perspective* (pp. 46–90). Washington, DC: National Academies Press.

Lapane, L. K., Zierler, S., Lasatar, T. M., Stein, M., Barbout, M. M., & Hume, A. L. (1995). Is a history of depressive symptoms associated with an increased risk of infertility in women? *Psychosomatic Medicine, 57,* 509–513.

Levenson, J. L. (2008). Psychological factors affecting physical condition. In A. Tasman, J. Kay, J. A. Lieberman, M. B. First, & M. Maj (Eds.), *Psychiatry* (3rd ed., Vol. 2, pp. 1754–1772). West Sussex, UK: John Wiley & Sons.

Mayou, R., Hawton, K., & Feldman, E. (2001). Psychiatric problems among medical admissions. *International Journal of Psychiatry and Medicine, 21,* 71–84.

Mock, V., Pickett, M., Ropka, M. E., Lin, E. M., Stewart, K. J., Rhodes, V. A., et al. (2001). Fatigue and quality of life outcomes of exercise during cancer treatment. *Cancer Practice, 9,* 119–127.

Morrison, J. (2006). *Diagnosis made easier: Principles and techniques for mental health clinicians.* New York, NY: Guilford Press.

Nasseri, M. (2000). Cultural similarities in psychological reactions to infertility. *Psychological Reports, 86*(2), 375–378.

National Institute of Mental Health (NIMH). (2005). *Biological rhythms in psychiatry and medicine.* Washington, DC: Author.

National Institutes of Health (NIH). (2007). *NINDS epilepsy information page.* Retrieved from http://www.ninds.nih.gov/disorders/epilepsy/epilepsy.htm

Rumsfeld, J. S., & Ho, M. (2005). Depression and cardiovascular disease: A call for recognition. *Circulation, 1111,* 250–253.

Shapiro, P. (2005). Heart disease. In J. J. Levenson (Ed.), *American Psychiatric Publishing textbook of psychosomatic medicine* (pp. 423–444). Washington, DC: American Psychiatric Publishing Press.

Smoller, J. W., Simon, N. M., Pollack, M. H., Kradin, R., & Stern T. (1999). Anxiety in patients with pulmonary disease: Comorbidity and treatment. *Seminars in Clinical Neuropsychiatry, 4*(2), 84–97.

Stover, E. (2003). Depression and comorbid medical illness: The National Institute of Mental Health perspective. *Biological Psychiatry, 54*(3), 184–186.

Strain, J. J. (2007). Adjustment disorders. In G. O. Gabbard (Ed.), *Treatments of psychiatric disorders* (4th ed., pp. 1656–1665). Washington, DC: American Psychiatric Association Press.

Strong, V., Waters, R., Hibberd, C., Rush, R., Cargills, A., Storey, D., et al. (2007). Emotional distress in cancer patients: The Edinburgh Cancer Symptom Study. *British Journal of Cancer, 96,* 868–874.

Verhaak, C. M., Smeenk, J. M. J., van Minnen, A., Kremer, J. A. M., & Kraaimaat, F. W. (2005). A longitudinal prospective study on emotional adjustment before, during and after consecutive fertility treatment cycles. *Human Reproduction, 20*(8), 2253–2260.

West, J. B. (2007). *Pulmonary pathophysiology: The essentials.* Philadelphia, PA: Lippincott Williams & Wilkins.

Wilson, K. G., Chochinov, H. M., McPherson, C. J., LeMay, K., Allard, P., Chary, S., et al. (2007). Suffering with advanced cancer. *Journal of Clinical Oncology, 25*(13), 1691–1696.

Wilson, R. W., Taliaferro, L. A., & Jacobsen, P. B. (2006). Pilot study of a self administered stress management and exercise intervention during chemotherapy for cancer. *Supportive Care in Cancer, 14,* 928–935.

Wingate, B. J., & Hansen-Flaschen, J. (1997). Anxiety and depression in advanced lung disease. *Clinics in Chest Medicine, 18*(3), 495–505.

Web Resources

Fertility
American Academy of Family Physicians: http://www.familydoctor.org
American College of Obstetricians and Gynecologists: http://www.acog.org
American Fertility Association: http://www.theafa.org
American Society for Reproductive Medicine (ASRM): http://www.asrm.org

American Urological Association: http://www.urologyhealth.org
IVillage: http://parenting.ivillage.com
RESOLVE: http://www.resolve.org

Cancer Education and Support
Ameripros: http://www.ameripros.org
Bloch Cancer Foundation: http://www.blochcancer.org
CureSearch: http://www.nccf.org
NABCO: National Network of Breast Cancer Organizations. Education and support: http://www.nabco.org
National Cancer Institute: http://www.cancer.gov
National Cervical Cancer Coalition: http://www.ncc-online.org
ONCOCHAT: http://www.oncochat.org

Pulmonary Diseases
American Lung Association: http://www.lungusa.org

Cardiovascular Diseases
Adult Congenital Heart Association: http://www.achaheart.org
American Heart Association: http://www.americanheart.org
Congenital Heart Information Network: http://tchin.org/support__groups/index
Mended Hearts Inc.: http://www.mendedhearts.org

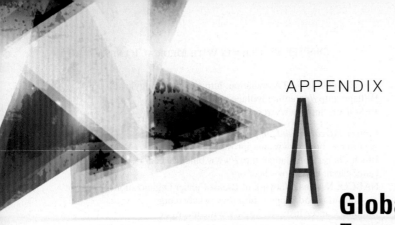

Global Assessment of Functioning (GAF) Scale

Consider psychological, social, and occupational functioning on a hypothetical continuum of mental health–mental illness. Do not include impairment in functioning due to physical (or environmental) limitations. *Note:* Use intermediate codes when appropriate (e.g., 45, 68, 72).

Code	
100 | 91	**Superior functioning in a wide range of activities, life's problems never seem to get out of hand, is sought out by others because of his or her many positive qualities. No symptoms.**
90 | 81	**Absent or minimal symptoms** (e.g., mild anxiety before an exam), **good functioning in all areas, interested and involved in a wide range of activities, socially effective, generally satisfied with life, no more than everyday problems or concerns** (e.g., an occasional argument with family members).
80 | 71	**If symptoms are present, they are transient and expected reactions to psychosocial stressors** (e.g., difficulty concentrating after family argument); **no more than slight impairment in social, occupational, or school functioning** (e.g., temporarily falling behind in schoolwork).
70 | 61	**Some mild symptoms** (e.g., depressed mood and mild insomnia) **OR some difficulty in social, occupational, or school functioning** (e.g., occasional truancy, or theft within the household), **but generally functioning pretty well, has some meaningful interpersonal relationships.**
60 | 51	**Moderate symptoms** (e.g., flat affect and circumstantial speech, occasional panic attacks) **OR moderate difficulty in social, occupational, or school functioning** (e.g., few friends, conflicts with peers or co-workers).
50 | 41	**Serious symptoms** (e.g., suicidal ideation, severe obsessional rituals, frequent shoplifting) **OR any serious impairment in social, occupational, or school functioning** (e.g., no friends, unable to keep a job).
40 | 31	**Some impairment in reality testing or communication** (e.g., speech is at times illogical, obscure, or irrelevant) **OR major impairment in several areas, such as work or school, family relations, judgment, thinking, or mood** (e.g., depressed man avoids friends, neglects family, and is unable to work; child frequently beats up younger children, is defiant at home, and is failing at school).
30 | 21	**Behavior is considerably influenced by delusions or hallucinations OR serious impairment in communication or judgment** (e.g., sometimes incoherent, acts grossly inappropriately, suicidal preoccupation) **OR inability to function in almost all areas** (e.g., stays in bed all day; no job, home, or friends).
20 | 11	**Some danger of hurting self or others** (e.g., suicide attempts without clear expectation of death; frequently violent; manic excitement) **OR occasionally fails to maintain minimal personal hygiene** (e.g., smears feces) **OR gross impairment in communication** (e.g., largely incoherent or mute).
10 | 1	**Persistent danger of severely hurting self or others** (e.g., recurrent violence) **OR persistent inability to maintain minimal personal hygiene OR serious suicidal act with clear expectation of death.**
0	Inadequate information.

From American Psychiatric Association. (2000). *Diagnostic and statistical manual of mental disorders* (4th ed., text rev.). Washington, DC: Author.

The rating of overall psychological functioning on a scale of 0 to 100 was operationalized by Luborsky (1962) in the Health-Sickness Rating Scale. Spitzer and colleagues developed a revision of the Health-Sickness Rating Scale called the Global Assessment Scale (GAS) (Endicott et al., 1976). A modified version of the GAS was included in the *Diagnostic and statistical manual of mental disorders,* third edition, revised (American Psychiatric Association, 1987) as the Global Assessment of Functioning Scale.

This rating scale highlights important areas in the assessment of functioning. Because many of the judgments are subjective, experienced clinicians use this tool as a guide when planning care, and also draw on their knowledge of their clients.

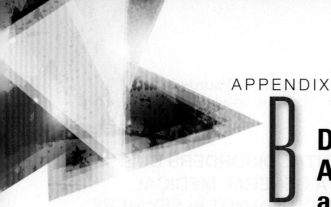

DSM-IV-TR Classification: Axes I and II Categories and Codes

DISORDERS USUALLY FIRST DIAGNOSED IN INFANCY, CHILDHOOD, OR ADOLESCENCE

Mental Retardation
Note: These are coded on Axis II.

317	Mild Mental Retardation
318.0	Moderate Mental Retardation
318.1	Severe Mental Retardation
318.2	Profound Mental Retardation
319	Mental Retardation, Severity Unspecified

Learning Disorders

315.00	Reading Disorders
315.10	Mathematics Disorders
315.2	Disorder of Written Expression
315.9	Learning Disorder NOS

Motor Skills Disorder

315.4	Developmental Coordination Disorder

Communication Disorders

315.31	Expressive Language Disorder
315.32	Mixed Receptive-Expressive Language Disorder
315.39	Phonological Disorder
307.0	Stuttering
307.9	Communication Disorder NOS

Pervasive Developmental Disorders

299.00	Autistic Disorder
299.80	Rett's Disorder
299.10	Childhood Disintegrative Disorder
299.80	Asperger's Disorder
299.80	Pervasive Developmental Disorder NOS

Attention-Deficit and Disruptive Behavior Disorders

314.xx	Attention-Deficit/Hyperactivity Disorder
.01	Combined Type
.00	Predominantly Inattentive Type
.01	Predominantly Hyperactive-Impulsive Type
314.9	Attention-Deficit/Hyperactivity Disorder NOS
312.8	Conduct Disorder
	Specify type: Childhood-Onset/ Adolescent-Onset
313.81	Oppositional Defiant Disorder
312.9	Disruptive Behavior Disorder NOS

Feeding and Eating Disorders of Infancy or Early Childhood

307.52	Pica
307.53	Rumination Disorder
307.59	Feeding Disorder of Infancy or Early Childhood

Tic Disorders

307.23	Tourette's Disorder
307.22	Chronic Motor or Vocal Tic Disorder
307.21	Transient Tic Disorder
	Specify if: Single Episode/Recurrent
307.20	Tic Disorder NOS

Elimination Disorders

—.-	Encopresis
787.6	With Constipation and Overflow Incontinence
307.7	Without Constipation and Overflow Incontinence
307.6	Enuresis (Not Due to a General Medical Condition)
	Specify type: Nocturnal Only/Diurnal Only/ Nocturnal and Diurnal

Other Disorders of Infancy, Childhood, or Adolescence

309.21	Separation and Anxiety Disorder
	Specify if: Early Onset
313.23	Selective Mutism

NOS = not otherwise specified.

An *x* appearing in a diagnostic code indicates that a specific code number is required.

An **ellipsis** (. . .) is used in the names of certain disorders to indicate that the name of a specific mental disorder or general medical condition should be inserted when recording the name (eg, 293 Delirium Due to Hypothyroidism).

*Indicate the General Medical Condition.

**Refer to Substance-Related Disorders for substance-specific codes.

***Indicate the Axis I or Axis II Disorder.

American Psychiatric Association. (2000). *Diagnostic and statistical manual of mental disorders.* (4th ed., text revision). Washington, DC: Author.

313.89	Reactive Attachment Disorder of Infancy or Early Childhood
	Specify type: Inhibited/Disinhibited
307.3	Stereotypic Movement Disorder
	Specify if: With Self-Injurious Behavior
313.9	Disorder of Infancy, Childhood, or Adolescence NOS

DELIRIUM, DEMENTIA, AND AMNESTIC AND OTHER COGNITIVE DISORDERS

Delirium

293.0	Delirium Due to . . .*
—.-	Substance Intoxication Delirium**
—.-	Substance Withdrawal Delirium**
—.-	Delirium Due to Multiple Etiologies (code each of the specific etiologies)
780.09	Delirium NOS

Dementia

294.xx	Dementia of the Alzheimer's Type, With Early Onset
.10	Without Behavioral Disturbance
.11	With Behavioral Disturbance
294.xx	Dementia of the Alzheimer's Type, With Late Onset
.10	Without Behavioral Disturbance
.11	With Behavioral Disturbance
290.xx	Vascular Dementia
.40	Uncomplicated
.41	With Delirium
.42	With Delusions
.43	With Depressed Mood
	Specify if: With Behavioral Disturbance
294.1x	Dementia Due to HIV Disease
294.1x	Dementia Due to Head Trauma
294.1x	Dementia Due to Parkinson's Disease
294.1x	Dementia Due to Huntington's Disease
294.10	Dementia Due to Pick's Disease
290.10	Dementia Due to Creutzfeldt-Jakob Disease
294.1	Dementia Due to . . . [Indicate the General Medical Condition not listed above]
—.-	Substance-Induced Persisting Dementia**
—.-	Dementia Due to Multiple Etiologies (code each of the specific etiologies)
294.8	Dementia NOS

Amnestic Disorders

294.0	Amnestic Disorder Due to . . .*
	Specify if: Transient/Chronic
—.-	Substance-Induced Persisting Amnestic Disorder**
294.8	Amnestic Disorder NOS

Other Cognitive Disorders

294.9	Cognitive Disorder NOS

MENTAL DISORDERS DUE TO A GENERAL MEDICAL CONDITION NOT ELSEWHERE CLASSIFIED

293.89	Catatonic Disorder Due to . . .*
310.0	Personality Change Due to . . .*
	Specify type: Labile/Disinhibited/ Aggressive/Apathetic/Paranoid/Other/ Combined/Unspecified
293.9	Mental Disorder NOS Due to . . .*

SUBSTANCE-RELATED DISORDERS

The following specifiers may be applied to Substance Dependence:
With Physiological Dependence/Without Physiological Dependence
Early Full Remission/Early Partial Remission
Sustained Full Remission/Sustained Partial Remission
On Agonist Therapy/In a Controlled Environment
The following specifiers apply to Substance-Induced Disorders as noted:
[I]With Onset During Intoxication
[W]With Onset During Withdrawal

Alcohol-Related Disorders

Alcohol Use Disorders

303.90	Alcohol Dependence
305.00	Alcohol Abuse

Alcohol-Induced Disorders

303.00	Alcohol Intoxications
291.8	Alcohol Withdrawal
	Specify if: With Perceptual Disturbances
291.0	Alcohol Intoxication Delirium
291.0	Alcohol Withdrawal Delirium
291.2	Alcohol-Induced Persisting Dementia
291.1	Alcohol-Induced Persisting Amnestic Disorder
291.x	Alcohol-Induced Psychotic Disorder
.5	With Delusions[I, W]
.3	With Hallucinations[I, W]
291.8	Alcohol-Induced Mood Disorder[I, W]
291.8	Alcohol-Induced Anxiety Disorder[I, W]
291.8	Alcohol-Induced Sexual Dysfunction[I]
291.	Alcohol-Induced Sleep Disorder[I, W]
291.9	Alcohol-Related Disorder NOS

Amphetamine (or Amphetamine-Like)-Related Disorders

Amphetamine Use Disorders
304.40   Amphetamine Dependence*
305.70   Amphetamine Abuse

Amphetamine-Induced Disorders
292.89   Amphetamine Intoxication
         Specify if: With Perceptual Disturbances
292.0   Amphetamine Withdrawal
292.81   Amphetamine Intoxication Delirium
292.xx   Amphetamine-Induced Psychotic Disorder
  .11   With Delusions[I]
  .12   With Hallucinations[I]
292.84   Amphetamine-Induced Mood Disorder[I, W]
292.89   Amphetamine-Induced Anxiety Disorder[I]
292.89   Amphetamine-Induced Sexual Dysfunction[I]
292.89   Amphetamine-Induced Sleep Disorder[I, W]
292.9   Amphetamine-Related Disorder NOS

Caffeine-Related Disorders

Caffeine-Induced Disorders
305.90   Caffeine Intoxication
292.89   Caffeine-Induced Anxiety Disorder[I]
292.89   Caffeine-Induced Sleep Disorder[I]
292.9   Caffeine-Related Disorder NOS

Cannabis-Related Disorders

Cannabis Use Disorders
304.40   Cannabis Dependence*
305.20   Cannabis Abuse

Cannabis-Induced Disorders
292.89   Cannabis Intoxication
         Specify if: With Perceptual Disturbances
292.81   Cannabis Intoxication Delirium
292.xx   Cannabis-Induced Psychotic Disorder
  .11   With Delusions[I]
  .12   With Hallucinations[I]
292.89   Cannabis-Induced Anxiety Disorder
292.9   Cannabis-Related Disorder NOS

Cocaine-Related Disorders

Cocaine Use Disorders
304.20   Cocaine Dependence*
305.60   Cocaine Abuse

Cocaine-Induced Disorders
292.89   Cocaine Intoxication
         Specify if: With Perceptual Disturbances

292.0   Cocaine Withdrawal
292.81   Cocaine Intoxication Delirium
292.xx   Cocaine-Induced Psychotic Disorder
  .11   With Delusions[I]
  .12   With Hallucinations[I]
292.84   Cocaine-Induced Mood Disorder[I, W]
292.89   Cocaine-Induced Anxiety Disorder[I, W]
292.89   Cocaine-Induced Sexual Dysfunction[I]
292.89   Cocaine-Induced Sleep Disorder[I, W]
292.9   Cocaine-Related Disorder NOS

Hallucinogen-Related Disorders

Hallucinogen-Use Disorders
304.50   Hallucinogen Dependence*
305.30   Hallucinogen Abuse

Hallucinogen-Induced Disorders
292.89   Hallucinogen Intoxication
292.89   Hallucinogen Persisting Perception Disorder (Flashbacks)
292.81   Hallucinogen Intoxication Delirium
292.xx   Hallucinogen-Induced Psychotic Disorder
  .11   With Delusions[I]
  .12   With Hallucinations[I]
292.84   Hallucinogen-Induced Mood Disorder[I]
292.89   Hallucinogen-Induced Anxiety Disorder[I]
292.9   Hallucinogen-Related Disorder NOS

Inhalant-Related Disorders

Inhalant Use Disorders
304.60   Inhalant Dependence*
305.90   Inhalant Abuse

Inhalant-Induced Disorders
292.89   Inhalant Intoxication
292.81   Inhalant Intoxication Delirium
292.82   Inhalant-Induced Persisting Dementia
292.xx   Inhalant-Induced Psychotic Disorder
  .11   With Delusions[I]
  .12   With Hallucinations[I]
292.84   Inhalant-Induced Mood Disorder[I]
292.89   Inhalant-Induced Anxiety Disorder[I]
292.9   Inhalant-Related Disorder NOS

Nicotine-Related Disorders

Nicotine Use Disorder
305.10   Nicotine Dependence*

Nicotine-Induced Disorder
292.0   Nicotine Withdrawal
292.9   Nicotine-Related Disorder NOS

Opioid-Related Disorders

Opioid Use Disorders
304.00   Opioid Dependence*
305.50   Opioid Abuse

Opioid-Induced Disorders
292.89   Opioid Intoxication
         Specify if: With Perceptual Disturbances
292.0   Opioid Withdrawal
292.81   Opioid Intoxication Delirium
292.xx   Opioid-Induced Psychotic Disorders
   .11   With Delusions[I]
   .12   With Hallucinations[I]
292.84   Opioid-Induced Mood Disorder[I]
292.89   Opioid-Induced Sexual Dysfunction[I]
292.89   Opioid-Induced Sleep Disorder[I, W]
292.9   Opioid-Related Disorder NOS

Phencyclidine (or Phencyclidine-Like)-Related Disorders

Phencyclidine Use Disorders
304.90   Phencyclidine Dependence*
305.90   Phencyclidine Abuse

Phencyclidine-Induced Disorders
292.89   Phencyclidine Intoxication
         Specify if: With Perceptual Disturbances
292.81   Phencyclidine Intoxication Delirium
292.xx   Phencyclidine-Induced Psychotic Disorders
   .11   With Delusions[I]
   .12   With Hallucinations[I]
292.84   Phencyclidine-Induced Mood Disorder[I]
292.89   Phencyclidine-Induced Anxiety Disorder[I]
292.9   Phencyclidine-Related Disorder NOS

Sedative-Hypnotic- or Anxiolytic-Related Disorders

Sedative-Hypnotic- or Anxiolytic Use Disorders
304.10   Sedative, Hypnotic, or Anxiolytic Dependence*
305.40   Sedative, Hypnotic, or Anxiolytic Abuse

Sedative, Hypnotic, or Anxiolytic-Induced Disorders
292.89   Sedative, Hypnotic, or Anxiolytic Intoxication
292.0   Sedative, Hypnotic, or Anxiolytic Withdrawal
         Specify if: With Perceptual Disturbances
292.81   Sedative, Hypnotic, or Anxiolytic Intoxication Delirium
292.81   Sedative, Hypnotic, or Anxiolytic Withdrawal Delirium
292.82   Sedative-, Hypnotic-, or Anxiolytic-Induced Persisting Delirium
292.83   Sedative-, Hypnotic-, or Anxiolytic-Induced Persisting Amnestic disorder

292.xx   Sedative-, Hypnotic-, or Anxiolytic-Induced Psychotic Disorder
   .11   With Delusions[I, W]
   .12   With Hallucinations[I, W]
292.84   Sedative-, Hypnotic-, or Anxiolytic-Induced Mood Disorder[I, W]
292.89   Sedative-, Hypnotic-, or Anxiolytic-Induced Anxiety Disorder[W]
292.89   Sedative-, Hypnotic-, or Anxiolytic-Induced Sexual Dysfunction[I]
292.89   Sedative-, Hypnotic-, or Anxiolytic-Induced Sleep Disorder[I, W]
292.9   Sedative-, Hypnotic-, or Anxiolytic-Induced Disorder NOS

Polysubstance-Related Disorder
304.80   Polysubstance Dependence*

Other (or Unknown) Substance-Related Disorders

Other (or Unknown) Substance Use Disorders
304.90   Other (or Unknown) Substance Dependence*
305.90   Other (or Unknown) Substance Abuse

Other (or Unknown) Substance-Induced Disorders
292.89   Other (or Unknown) Substance Intoxication
         Specify if: With Perceptual Disturbances
292.0   Other (or Unknown) Substance Withdrawal
         Specify if: With Perceptual Disturbances
292.81   Other (or Unknown) Substance-Induced Delirium
292.82   Other (or Unknown) Substance-Induced Persisting Dementia
292.83   Other (or Unknown) Substance-Induced Persisting Amnestic Disorder
292.xx   Other (or Unknown) Substance-Induced Psychotic Disorder
   .11   With Delusions[I, W]
   .12   With Hallucinations[I, W]
292.84   Other (or Unknown) Substance-Induced Mood Disorder[I, W]
292.89   Other (or Unknown) Substance-Induced Anxiety Disorder[I, W]
292.89   Other (or Unknown) Substance-Induced Sexual Dysfunction[I]
292.89   Other (or Unknown) Substance-Induced Sleep Disorder[I, W]
292.9   Other (or Unknown) Substance-Induced Disorder NOS

SCHIZOPHRENIA AND OTHER PSYCHOTIC DISORDERS
295.xx   Schizophrenia

The following Classification of Longitudinal Course applies to all subtypes of Schizophrenia:

Episodic With Interepisode Residual Symptoms
   (*Specify if:* With Prominent Negative Symptoms)/
Episodic With No Interepisode Residual Symptoms/
   Continuous
   (*Specify if:* With Prominent Negative Symptoms)
Single Episode in Partial Remission
   (*Specify if:* With Prominent Negative Symptoms)
Single Episode in Full Remission
Other or Unspecified Pattern
   .30   Paranoid Type
   .10   Disorganized Type
   .20   Catatonic Type
   .90   Undifferentiated Type
   .60   Residual Type
295.40   Schizophreniform Disorder
         Specify if: Without Good Prognostic
         Features/With Good Prognostic Features
295.70   Schizoaffective Disorder
         Specify if: Bipolar/Depressive
297.1   Delusional Disorder
         Specify if: Erotomanic/Grandiose/Jealous/
         Persecutory Somatic/Mixed/Unspecified
298.8   Brief Psychotic Disorder
         Specify if: With Marked Stressor(s)/Without
         Marked Stressor(s)/With Postpartum Onset
297.3   Shared Psychotic Disorder
293.xx   Psychotic Disorder Due to . . .*
   .81   With Delusions
   .82   With Hallucinations
—.-   Substance-Induced Psychotic Disorder
         (refer to Substance-Related Disorders for
         substance-specific codes)
         Specify if: With Onset During Intoxication/
         With Onset During Withdrawal
298.9   Psychotic Disorder NOS

MOOD DISORDERS

*Code current state of Major Depressive Disorder or Bipolar
I Disorder in fifth digit*
1 = Mild
2 = Moderate
3 = Severe Without Psychotic Features
4 = Severe With Psychotic Features
   Specify: Mood-Congruent Psychotic Features/
      Mood-Incongruent Psychotic Features
5 = In Partial Remission
6 = In Full Remission
0 = Unspecified

*The following specifiers apply (for current or most current
episode) to Mood Disorders as noted:*
[a]Severity/Psychotic/Remission Specifiers/[b]Chronic/[c]With
Catatonic Features/[d]With Melancholic Features/[e]With
Atypical Features/[f]With Postpartum Onset
The following specifiers apply to Mood Disorders as noted:
[g]With or Without Full Interepisode Recovery/[h]With
Seasonal Pattern/[i]With Rapid Cycling

Depressive Disorders
296.xx   Major Depressive Disorder,
   .2x   Single Episode[a,b,c,d,e,f]
   .3x   Recurrent[a,b,c,d,e,f,g,h]
300.4   Dysthymic Disorder
         Specify if: Early Onset/Late Onset
         Specify if: With Atypical Features
311   Depressive Disorder NOS

Bipolar Disorders
296.xx   Bipolar I Disorder,
   .0x   Single Manic Episode[a,c,f]
         Specify if: Mixed
   .40   Most Recent Episode Hypomanic[a,h,j]
   .4x   Most Recent Episode Manic[a,c,f,g,h,i]
   .6x   Most Recent Episode Mixed[a,c,f,g,h,i]
   .5x   Most Recent Episode Depressed[a,b,c,d,e,f,g,h,i]
   .7   Most Recent Episode Unspecified[g,h,i]
296.89   Bipolar II Disorder[a,b,c,d,e,f,g,h,i]
         Specify (current or most recent episode):
         Hypomanic/Depressed
301.13   Cyclothymic Disorder
296.80   Bipolar Disorder NOS
293.83   Mood Disorder Due to . . .*
         Specify type: With Depressive Features/
         With Major Depressive-Like Episode/
         With Manic Features/With Mixed Features
—.-   Substance-Induced Mood Disorder**
         Specify type: With Depressive Features/
         With Manic Features/With Mixed Features
         Specify if: With Onset During Intoxication/
         With Onset During Withdrawal
296.90   Mood Disorder NOS

ANXIETY DISORDERS
300.01   Panic Disorder Without Agoraphobia
300.21   Panic Disorder With Agoraphobia
300.22   Agoraphobia Without History of Panic Disorder
300.29   Specific Phobia
         Specify type: Animal Type/Natural Environ-
         ment Type/Blood-Injection-Injury Type/Situ-
         ational Type/Other Type
300.23   Social Phobia
         Specify if: Generalized
300.3   Obsessive-Compulsive Disorder
         Specify if: With Poor Insight
309.81   Posttraumatic Stress Disorder
         Specify if: Acute/Chronic
         Specify if: With Delayed Onset
308.3   Acute Stress Disorder
300.2   Generalized Anxiety Disorder
293.80   Anxiety Disorder Due to . . .*
         Specify if: With Generalized Anxiety/
         With Panic Attacks/With Obsessive
         Compulsive Symptoms . . .*

293.84   Substance-Induced Anxiety Disorder
         Specify if: With Generalized Anxiety/
         With Panic Attacks/With Obsessive-Compul-
         sive Symptoms/With Phobic Symptoms
         Specify if: With Onset During Intoxication/
         With Onset During Withdrawal
300.00   Anxiety Disorder NOS

SOMATOFORM DISORDERS

300.81   Somatization Disorder
300.82   Undifferentiated Somatoform Disorder
300.11   Conversion Disorder
         Specify type: With Motor Symptom or Deficit/
         With Sensory Symptom or Deficit/
         With Seizures or Convulsions/With Mixed
         Presentation
307.xx   Pain Disorder
   .80   Associated With Psychological Factors
   .89   Associated With Both Psychological Factors and a
        General Medical Condition
         Specify if: Acute/Chronic
300.7   Hypochondriasis
         Specify if: With Poor Insight
300.7   Body Dysmorphic Disorder
300.82   Somatoform Disorder NOS

FACTITIOUS DISORDERS

300.xx   Factitious Disorder
   .16   With Predominantly Psychological Signs and
        Symptoms
   .19   With Predominantly Physical Signs and
        Symptoms
   .19   With Combined Psychological and Physical Signs
        and Symptoms
300.19   Factitious Disorder NOS

DISSOCIATIVE DISORDERS

300.12   Dissociative Amnesia
300.13   Dissociative Fugue
300.14   Dissociative Identity Disorder
300.6   Depersonalized Disorder
300.15   Dissociative Disorder NOS

SEXUAL AND GENDER IDENTITY DISORDERS

Sexual Dysfunctions

The following specifiers apply to all primary Sexual Dysfunctions:
Lifelong Type/Acquired
Type Generalized Type/Situational Type
Due to Psychological Factors. Due to Combined Factors

Sexual Desire Disorders

302.71   Hypoactive Sexual Desire Disorder
302.79   Sexual Aversion Disorder

Sexual Arousal Disorders

302.72   Female Sexual Arousal Disorder
302.72   Male Erectile Disorder

Orgasmic Disorders

302.73   Female Orgasmic Disorder
302.74   Male Orgasmic Disorder
302.75   Premature Ejaculation

Sexual Pain Disorders

302.76   Dyspareunia (Not Due to General Medical Condition)
306.51   Vaginismus (Not Due to a General Medical Condition)

Sexual Dysfunction Due to a General Medical Condition

625.8   Female Hypoactive Sexual Desire Disorder Due to . . .*
608.89   Male Hypoactive Sexual Desire Disorder Due to . . .*
607.84   Male Erectile Disorder Due to . . .*
625.0   Female Dyspareunia Due to . . .*
608.89   Male Dyspareunia Due to . . .*
625.8   Other Female Sexual Dysfunction Due to . . .*
608.89   Other Male Sexual Dysfunction Due to . . .*
—.-   Substance-Induced Sexual Dysfunction**
         Specify if: With Impaired Desire/
         With Impaired Arousal/With Impaired
         Orgasm/With Sexual Pain
         Specify if: With Onset During Intoxication
302.70   Sexual Dysfunction NOS

Paraphilias

302.4   Exhibitionism
302.81   Fetishism
302.89   Frotteurism
302.2   Pedophilia
         Specify if: Sexually Attracted to Males/
         Sexually Attracted to Females/Sexually
         Attracted to Both
         Specify if: Limited to Incest
         Specify if: Exclusive Type/Nonexclusive type
302.83   Sexual Masochism
302.84   Sexual Sadism
302.3   Transvestic Fetishism
         Specify if: With Gender Dysphoria
302.82   Voyeurism
302.9   Paraphilia NOS

Gender Identity Disorders

302.xx   Gender Identity Disorder
   .6   in Children

.85   in Adolescents or Adults
     Specify if: Sexually Attracted to Males/
     Sexually Attracted to Females/Sexually
     Attracted to Both/Sexually Attracted to Neither

302.6   Gender Identity Disorder NOS
302.9   Sexual Disorder NOS

EATING DISORDERS

307.1   Anorexia Nervosa
     Specify type: Restricting, Binge-Eating/Purging
307.51   Bulimia Nervosa
     Specify type: Purging/Nonpurging
307.50   Eating Disorder NOS

SLEEP DISORDERS
Primary Sleep Disorders

Dyssomnias

307.42   Primary Insomnia
307.44   Primary Hypersomnia
     Specify if: Recurrent
347   Narcolepsy
380.59   Breathing-Related Sleep Disorder
307.45   Circadian Rhythm Sleep Disorder
     Specify type: Delayed Sleep Phase/
     Jet Lag/Shift Work/Unspecified
307.47   Dyssomnia NOS

Parasomnias

307.47   Nightmare Disorder
307.46   Sleep Terror Disorder
307.46   Sleepwalking Disorder
307.47   Parasomnia NOS

Sleep Disorders Related to Another Mental Disorder

307.42   Insomnia Related to . . .***
307.44   Hypersomnia Related to . . .***

Other Sleep Disorders

780.xx   Sleep Disorder Due to . . .*
  .52   Insomnia Type
  .54   Hyposomnia Type
  .59   Parasomnia Type
  .59   Mixed Type
—.-   Substance-Induced Sleep Disorder (refer to
    Substance-Related Disorders for substance-
    specific codes)
     Specify type: Insomnia/Hypersomnia/
     Parasomnia/Mixed
     Specify if: With Onset during Intoxication/
     With Onset During Withdrawal

IMPULSE-CONTROL DISORDERS NOT ELSEWHERE CLASSIFIED

312.34   Intermittent Explosive Disorder
312.32   Kleptomania
312.33   Pyromania
312.31   Pathological Gambling
312.39   Trichotillomania
312.30   Impulse-Control Disorder NOS

ADJUSTMENT DISORDERS

309.xx   Adjustment Disorder
  .0   With Depressed Mood
  .24   With Anxiety
  .28   With Mixed Anxiety and Depressed Mood
  .3   With Disturbance of Conduct
  .4   With Mixed Disturbance of Emotions
    and Conduct
  .9   Unspecified
     Specify if: Acute/Chronic

PERSONALITY DISORDERS

Note: These are coded on Axis II

301.0   Paranoid Personality Disorder
301.20   Schizoid Personality Disorder
301.22   Schizotypal Personality Disorder
301.7   Antisocial Personality Disorder
301.83   Borderline Personality Disorder
301.50   Histrionic Personality Disorder
301.81   Narcissistic Personality Disorder
301.82   Avoidant Personality Disorder
301.6   Dependent Personality Disorder
301.4   Obsessive-Compulsive Personality Disorder
301.9   Personality Disorder NOS

OTHER CONDITIONS THAT MAY BE A FOCUS OF CLINICAL ATTENTION
Psychological Factors Affecting Medical Condition

316 . . . [Specified Psychological Factor] Affecting . . .*
Choose name based on nature of factors:
Mental Disorder Affecting Medical Condition
Psychological Symptoms Affecting Medical Condition
Personality Traits or Coping Style Affecting Medical
   Condition
Maladaptive Health Behaviors Affecting Medical
   Condition
Stress-Related Physiological Response Affecting
   Medical Condition
Other or Unspecified Psychological Factors Affecting
   Medical Condition

Medication-Induced Movement Disorders

332.1   Neuroleptic-Induced Parkinsonism
333.92   Neuroleptic Malignant Syndrome
333.7   Neuroleptic-Induced Acute Dystonia
333.99   Neuroleptic-Induced Acute Akathisia
333.82   Neuroleptic-Induced Tardive Dyskinesia
333.1   Neuroleptic-Induced Postural Tumor
333.90   Neuroleptic-Induced Movement
          Disorder NOS

Other Medical-Induced Disorder

995.2   Adverse Effects of Medication NOS

Relational Problems

V61.9   Relational Problem Related to a Mental
          Disorder or General Medical Condition
V61.1   Partner Relational Problem
V61.20   Parent-Child Relational Problem
V61.8   Sibling Relational Problem
V62.81   Relational Problem NOS

Problems Related to Abuse or Neglect

(*Code 995.5 if focus of attention is on victim*)
V61.21   Physical Abuse of Child
V61.21   Sexual Abuse of Child
V61.21   Neglect of Child
V61.12   Physical Abuse of Adult

V61.1   Sexual Abuse of Adult
V62.83   Person Other Than Partner

Additional Conditions That May be Focus of Clinical Attention

V15.81   Noncompliance With Treatment
V65.2   Malingering
V71.01   Adult Antisocial Behavior
V71.02   Child or Adolescent Antisocial Behavior
V62.89   Borderline Intellectual Functioning
          Note: This is coded on Axis II.
780.9   Age-Related Cognitive Decline
V62.82   Bereavement
V62.3   Academic Problem
V62.2   Occupational Problem
313.82   Identity Problem
V62.89   Religious or Spiritual Problem
V62.4   Acculturation Problem
V62.89   Phase of Life Problem

ADDITIONAL CODES

300.9   Unspecified Mental Disorder (nonpsychotic)
V71.09   No Diagnosis or Condition on Axis I
799.9   Diagnosis or Condition Deferred on Axis I
V71.09   No Diagnosis on Axis II
799.9   Diagnosis Deferred on Axis II

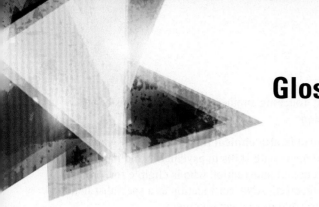

Glossary

A

Action potential The change in electrical potential on the surface of a nerve or muscle cell, often initiated by a change in cellular ionic balance.

Acute stress disorder An anxiety disorder in which symptoms of post-traumatic stress disorder appear within 4 weeks of exposure to the trauma and usually last less than 3 months.

Adaptation In the context of family therapy, the outcome of a family's successful adjustment to stress.

Adaptive plasticity An irreversible change in nervous tissue that usually affects the expression of a genotype into a phenotype.

Addiction A behavioral pattern of drug abuse characterized by overwhelming involvement with use of a drug (compulsive use) and securing its supply, and by a high tendency to relapse after discontinuation.

Adherence A client's willingness to receive recommended drug treatment as prescribed by a caregiver.

Adjustment disorder A psychiatric disorder marked by clinically or behaviorally significant symptoms that develop within 3 months after the onset of an identifiable stressor.

Adventitious crisis A crisis precipitated by an unexpected event (e.g., natural disasters, bombings, mass shootings).

Advocacy Formal or informal promotion of children's rights.

Affect An observable behavior that expresses feeling or emotional tone; it refers to more fluctuating changes in emotional "weather." It is of shorter duration, more variable, and more reactive than underlying mood, which is more pervasive and stable.

Affective flattening A reduced intensity of emotional expression and response.

Affinity A drug's tendency to be found at a given receptor site.

Aggregate group A group identified as having at least one commonality among its members.

Aggregate mental health The degree to which families and groups within a given environment contribute to,

enhance, or intensify interaction among individuals along the mental health-illness continuum.

Aggression Harsh physical or verbal responses that indicate rage and a potential for destructiveness.

Aggressiveness Behavior marked by belittling, threatening, moralizing, coercing, or communicating in a condescending way.

Agnosia An inability to recognize or identify familiar objects (e.g., the parts of a telephone).

Agonist A drug that initiates a therapeutic effect by binding to a receptor.

Agoraphobia A marked fear of being alone or in a public place from which escape would be difficult or help would be unavailable in the event of becoming disabled.

Alcohol (ethanol) A legal chemical substance (drug) that commonly leads to abuse and dependency.

Alogia A poverty of thinking that is inferred from observing the client's language and speech.

Alter Two or more identities or personality states.

Altruism The desire to contribute something valuable to society.

Ambivalence Having conflicting feelings about something.

Amenorrhea Absence of or abnormal cessation of menstruation.

Anger An emotional response to perceived frustration of desires or needs.

Anhedonia Loss of pleasure in hobbies or activities of interest; a characteristic of depression.

Anorexia nervosa A life-threatening eating disorder characterized by disturbed body image, emaciation, and intense fear of becoming obese.

Antagonist A drug that binds to receptors without causing any regulatory effect; its action is to block the binding of an endogenous agonist.

Anxiety A sense of psychological distress that may or may not have a focus; it is a state of apprehension that may represent a response to environmental stress or a physical disease state.

Anxiety disorder A group of conditions in which the affected person experiences persistent anxiety that he or she cannot dismiss and that interferes with his or her daily activities.

Apathy A sense of detachment and the belief that nothing a person does makes any difference, leading to a lack of concern about the problem or outcome.

Aphasia Difficulty with finding the appropriate words in conversation.

Applied behavior analysis A systematic way of examining and analyzing behaviors as they relate to the environment and basing appropriate interventions on this analysis.

Apraxia An inability to perform motor tasks despite intact motor function.

Aromatherapy The use of essential oils to treat symptoms for physiological and psychological benefits.

Arousal Physiological stimulation, such as touching, kissing, fondling, licking, or biting erogenous body parts, that causes changes in the genitals.

Assertiveness A technique by which a person communicates what he or she thinks, feels, or wants directly and respectfully.

Assessment Gathering, classifying, categorizing, analyzing, and documenting information about a client's health status.

Assimilation The prevailing expectation during most of the 20th century for immigrants and minority groups in the United States to become like the majority (white) culture.

Assumptions Assertions taken for granted or supposed that may be either explicit or hidden.

Attention-deficit disorder (ADD) A psychiatric disorder characterized by inattention without hyperactivity or impulsivity.

Attention-deficit hyperactivity disorder (ADHD) A psychiatric disorder characterized by inattention, impulsiveness, and hyperactivity.

Autism A genetic disorder of neuronal organization that requires early detection and treatment.

Autocratic leader A leader who exercises significant authority and control over group members; rarely, if ever, seeks or uses input from the group; and does not encourage participation or interaction from the group.

Autonomy The right to make decisions for oneself.

Avolition The inability to start, persist in, and carry through to its logical conclusion any goal-directed activity.

Axon A cylindrical neuron structure that relays information away from the cell body.

B

Battery Touching another person without his or her permission.

Behavioral health clinical nurse specialist A master's-prepared nurse with skills in psychiatric and mental health assessment and intervention who is eligible for, or has already received, ANA certification as a specialist in adult psychiatric and mental health nursing.

Behavioral statement A statement in a nursing plan of care in which the verb represents an observable behavior.

Beneficence The principle of doing good, not harm.

Bibliotherapy The use of literature to help clients gain insight into feelings and behavior and learn new ways to cope with difficult situations.

Binge eating Uncontrollable consumption of large amounts of food.

Binge eating disorder An eating disorder characterized by recurrent episodes of binge eating, with accompanying marked distress and impaired control over such behavior.

Bisexuality An equal or almost equal attraction to or preference for either sex as a sexual partner.

Blackout A phenomenon in which a person functions normally while drinking but later has no memory of what occurred during that period, with no accompanying loss of consciousness.

Blood alcohol level (BAL) Milligrams of alcohol per milliliter of blood.

Blood–brain barrier A protective system in the lining of blood vessels composed of endothelial cells with tight junctions, thus limiting access of blood constituents to the central nervous system.

Blunting A reduced intensity of emotional expression and response.

Body dysmorphic disorder A somatoform disorder in which the client is preoccupied with an imagined defect in his or her appearance (e.g., a facial flaw or spot) when no abnormality or disturbance actually exists.

Bulimia nervosa An eating disorder characterized by binge eating, followed by purging.

C

Caring A core value of nursing that consists of three primary behaviors: (1) giving of self, (2) meeting the client's needs in a timely manner, and (3) providing comfort measures for clients and family members.

Case-control study A study for which a researcher uses specific criteria to identify participants.

Case manager A person who coordinates the various services that address the individual needs (e.g., housing, health care, mental health treatment, social contacts, work-ups) of a mentally ill client.

Channel The route or method a communicator chooses to convey his or her message.

Circadian rhythm A rhythmic activity cycle lasting approximately 24 hours.

Clinical trials Tests that compare a treatment's or medication's effects against a placebo.

Club drugs A group of synthetic drugs used commonly in nightclubs and as recreational drugs.

Cognitions Beliefs and thoughts that color a person's construction of his or her world.

Cognitive mental disorders A group of disorders characterized by a disruption of or deficit in cognitive functioning.

Communication The process of conveying information through a complex variety of verbal and nonverbal behaviors.

Communicator A person who simultaneously sends and receives messages through words and nonverbal behaviors.

Community support system A network of caring and responsible people committed to assisting a vulnerable population to meet its needs and develop its potential without becoming unnecessarily isolated or excluded from the community.

Compulsions Ritualistic behaviors that a person feels compelled to perform either in accord with a specific set of rules or in a routine manner.

Concepts The building blocks of theories.

Concordance rate The rate at which a trait expressed in one twin is expressed in another.

Conditioning A basic form of learning by which a subject begins to associate a behavior with a previously unrelated stimulus. There are two kinds of conditioning: operant and respondent.

Confabulation A characteristic of cognitive disorders in which an affected individual fills in gaps in memory with fabricated or imagined data.

Confrontation The skill of pointing out, in a caring way, concern about another person's behavior or discrepancies between what the other person says and what he or she does.

Contemplation Mental exercises that involve calmly limiting thought and attention.

Conversion disorder A somatoform disorder in which the client has at least one symptom or deficit of sensory or voluntary motor function (e.g., paralysis) that cannot be explained by a neurological or general medical condition.

Countertransference The feelings and thoughts that a mental-health service provider has toward a client that may be related to the provider's own unconscious or repressed emotions, feelings, and experiences.

Crisis A turning point in a disease or another condition.

Crisis intervention Methods and techniques used to assist a person in distress to resolve the immediate problem and regain emotional equilibrium.

Critical incidents Sudden and unexpected situations that disrupt values and beliefs and challenge basic assumptions of how the world operates.

Critical periods Periods during which children should be most exposed to certain stimuli for optimum development to take place. These periods vary according to different domains of functioning.

Cultural competence The skills, both academic and interpersonal, that allow persons to understand and appreciate cultural differences and similarities within, between, and among groups.

Cultural congruence Verbal and nonverbal validation of a client's culture.

Culturally competent care Care provided in a manner acceptable to a client's cultural background, regardless of whether the health care professional who delivers the care is from the same ethnic or minority group as the client.

Culture The integration of human behavior (including thoughts, communications, actions, customs, beliefs, values, and institutions) of a racial, ethnic, religious, or social group.

Culture bound A term used to describe a person whose understanding of other cultures is limited because he or she refuses to go beyond the parameters of his or her personal culture.

Culture-bound syndromes Forms of mental illness found only in one particular culture, symbolizing that culture's unique expression of physical or mental distress.

Culture care theory A theory developed by Dr. Madeleine Leininger that emphasizes learning principles related to culture care, culturalogical assessments, the universality of culture care diversity, and the importance of fit between the client's health care values and services provided.

Cyclothymia A disorder resembling bipolar disorder, with less severe symptoms, characterized by repeated periods of nonpsychotic depression and hypomania for at least 2 years (1 year for children and adolescents).

D

Decoding The process by which one communicator discerns or interprets what another communicator is saying.

Defense mechanisms Unconscious measures that people use to defend their personal stability and protect against anxiety and threat resulting from conflicts between the id, ego, and superego.

Deinstitutionalization The massive discharge of clients from state hospitals that began in the 1950s, accelerated in the 1960s and 1970s, and continues today as psychiatric treatment continues to move from inpatient to outpatient settings.

Delirium A cognitive disorder caused by an acute disruption of brain homeostasis that is characterized by a rapid onset of cognitive dysfunction and disruption in consciousness; when the cause of that disruption is eliminated or subsides, the cognitive deficits usually resolve within a few days or sometimes weeks.

Delirium tremens (DTs) Most serious form of withdrawal from alcohol; occurs after cessation or reduction in prolonged heavy drinking; can be a medical emergency and needs immediate treatment.

Delusions Fixed, false beliefs about external reality that reasoning cannot correct; these include, but are not limited to the following types: grandiose (beliefs involving inflated self-worth, power, or knowledge); persecutory (belief that one is being attacked, harassed, cheated, or conspired against); and somatic (beliefs that give false attributions to the appearance or functioning of one's body).

Dementia A cognitive disorder resulting from primary brain pathology that is usually not amenable to treatment; prognosis depends on whether the cause can be identified and the condition reversed.

Democratic leader A leader who encourages group interaction and participation in group problem-solving and decision-making, values the input and feedback of each group member, seeks spontaneous and honest interaction among group members, creates an atmosphere that rewards members for their contributions, solicits the group's opinions, and tailors the group's work to their common goals.

Dendrites Branched processes that extend from and relay information to the cell body and receive signals from numerous neurons.

Depersonalization disorder A dissociative disorder characterized by a recurring or persistent feeling that one is detached from one's own thinking. Affected clients feel that they are outside their mind or body, much like an observer.

Depressive/Manic Depressive Association (DMDA) A national support and advocacy association with regional chapters for people with depressive and bipolar disorders and their families.

Desire Activation of areas in the brain that produce sexual appetite or drive.

Diagnostic and Statistical Manual of Mental Disorders **(DSM)** A criteria-based psychiatric diagnostic system that specifies the type, intensity, duration, and effect of the various behaviors and symptoms required for the diagnosis.

Dialectical therapy An approach for clients with borderline personality disorder in which the therapist attempts to assist them to overcome debilitating experiences with an "invalidating environment" by achieving goals of stabilization, behavioral control, emotional calmness, effectiveness, joy, and wholeness. The therapist uses acceptance, validation, and problem-solving to assist the client to synthesize inner contradictions and conflicts.

Discrimination (1) Differential treatment based on race, class, gender, or other variables rather than on individual merit. (2) The process by which a person learns to distinguish between and respond differently to similar stimuli.

Dissociation Altering one's usual level of self-awareness in an effort to escape an upsetting event or feeling.

Dissociative amnesia A dissociative disorder characterized by loss of memory that is not organic and involves an inability to recall events or facts too extensive to be labeled as mere forgetfulness.

Dissociative disorders A disruption in the usually integrated functions of consciousness, memory, identity, or perception, causing disturbance that may be sudden or gradual, transient or chronic.

Dissociative fugue A dissociative disorder that involves sudden travel away from home coupled with an inability to remember the past and confusion about identity or the adoption of a new identity.

Dissociative identity disorder A dissociative disorder in which the person acquires two or more identities or personality states (alters), who take control over the client's behavior.

Dissociative trance A dissociative state in which a person's awareness of his or her immediate surroundings narrows, and he or she exhibits stereotyped behaviors, such as immobilization, collapse, or loud, uncontrollable shrieking.

Double-blind approach A trial in which neither the clients nor the researchers know which treatment a subject receives.

Double depression A diagnosis given when dysthymia and major depression occur together.

Dual diagnosis A diagnosis of a coexisting substance abuse or dependency disorder and a major psychiatric disorder; the disorders are unrelated and meet the DSM-IV-TR diagnostic criteria for each specific disorder.

Dyads Relationships between two people.

Dyspareunia Genital pain associated with sexual intercourse in either a man or woman.

Dyssomnias Abnormalities in the amount, quality, or timing of sleep.

Dysthymia A mild form of depression that lasts 1 year or more in a child or adolescent.

E

Ecological model A perspective that holds that certain behaviors result from the interaction of individuals' traits with contextual factors arising from the family, community, and culture in which they reside.

Ecomap An illustration of a family's interaction with larger systems.

Efficacy The information encoded in a drug's chemical structure that causes the receptor to change accordingly when the drug is bound.

Elder abuse Mistreatment of older adults, which includes physical abuse, physical neglect, sexual abuse, psychological abuse or neglect, financial abuse, and violation of personal rights.

Electroconvulsive therapy (ECT) A therapy that involves the application of a small dose of electricity to one or both sides of the brain to induce a seizure.

Elite old A chronological category used to designate those 95 years of age or older.

Emergency admission Admission to a psychiatric hospital that occurs when a client acts in a way that indicates that he or she is mentally ill and, as a consequence of the particular illness, is likely to harm self or others. State statutes define the exact procedure for the initial evaluation and the possible length of detainment.

Emotional reasoning A cognitive distortion by which a person relies on his or her subjective emotions to determine reality.

Empathy Emotional knowing of another person.

Empiricism The philosophical view that all knowledge and ideas come from experience.

Enabler A social worker who improves social functioning by helping clients resolve their own issues.

Encoding The process by which a communicator puts into words or behaviors the ideas or feelings that he or she is trying to convey.

Environment In communication, the personal experiences and cultural background that a communicator brings to an interaction.

Ethical dilemma A situation in which there are conflicting moral claims or in which two ethical principles conflict.

Ethics Principles that serve as a code of conduct about right and wrong behavior to guide the actions of individuals.

Ethnocentrism The belief that one's own cultural practices and values are inherently correct or superior to those of others.

Evidence-based care Conscientious, explicit, and judicious use of current best evidence in making decisions about the care of a client.

Excitement Psychological stimulation during the desire phase such as sexual fantasies or romantic communication.

Expressive violence Interpersonal violence, usually between people known to one another and of similar age, ethnicity, and cultural background.

External noise Factors outside a communicator that create distractions.

Extrapyramidal side effects (EPS) The most common and distressing side effects associated with traditional antipsychotic medications; they include akathisia (severe restlessness), dystonia (muscle spasm or contraction), chronic motor problems such as tardive dyskinesia, and the pseudoparkinsonian symptoms of rigidity, mask-like facies, and stiff gait.

F

Family In the context of family therapy, any unit that defines itself as "family."

Family burden The effects of serious mental illness on the family (see iatrogenic burden, objective burden, and subjective burden).

Family consultation A professional service offered to families to reduce family burden; a type of secondary prevention, originally called supportive counseling.

Family education Educational programs of varying duration to increase family members' knowledge about mental illness, caregiving, and self-care, with the objective of improving the entire family's quality of life.

Family empowerment Supporting family members' sense of self-worth.

Family psychoeducation A lengthy educational program for families (including the client) that is team taught by professionals and includes, in addition to didactic content about mental illness, extensive training in behavioral skills intended to create a home environment conducive to reducing relapse and recidivism.

Family resilience The family's capacity to rebound from the effects of mental illness.

Family support services Opportunities for mutual support available without cost to families through groups organized by family organizations (e.g., NAMI, DMDA).

Family therapies Nursing interventions made with families that include health promotion and improvement of family functionality.

Family therapy A specialized type of psychiatric practice aimed at modifying family behavior.

Feedback The discernible response that a receiver makes to a sender's message when communicating.

Fetal alcohol syndrome A syndrome characterized by a group of congenital birth defects caused by the mother's drinking while pregnant.

Fidelity Faithfulness to duties, obligations, and promises.

First messengers Neurotransmitters that are responsible for transmitting impulses between nerve cells.

First-order change A change that does not affect family functioning.

Flexibility The ability to embrace change by modifying expectations, readjusting old operating norms and stereotypes, and trying new behavior

Foreplay Petting and fondling behaviors that cause arousal during the excitement phase.

Formal group A group with structure and authority, which usually emanates from above; interaction in the group is usually limited.

Free association A technique in which a client says the first thing that comes to his or her mind, without restrictions, in response to something the therapist says.

Friendly visiting Historical tradition in which members of the upper classes socialized with members of the lower classes to motivate them to change their conditions.

Functional behavioral assessment (FBA) In educational settings, a problem-solving process that focuses on identifying significant, pupil specific social, affective, cognitive, and environmental factors associated with specific behaviors.

G

Gang violence Violence associated with group membership and committed for retaliation or revenge (Labecki, 1994; Sigler, 1995).

Genogram An illustration of a family tree that shows genetic connections, family transitions, and health conditions.

Generalization The process by which a person learns to associate a conditioned response with similar stimuli.

Generalized anxiety disorder An anxiety disorder characterized by chronic and excessive worry and anxiety more days than not for at least 6 months and involving many aspects of the person's life; the worry and anxiety cause such discomfort as to interfere with daily life and relationships.

Genuineness A nursing value that involves being a real person and truly engaged in knowing the client in open, human exchanges.

Glial cells In the nervous system, non-neural cells that serve supporting and nutritive roles for neurons.

Group Three or more people with related goals.

Group norm The development, over time, of a pattern of interaction within a group to which certain behavioral expectations are attached.

H

Half-life The time required for normal biological processes to metabolize or eliminate half the quantity of a drug or other substance.

Hallucinations Sensory perception with a compelling sense of reality; types include auditory (involving the perception of sound); gustatory (involving the perception of taste); olfactory (involving the perception of odor); tactile (involving the perception of being touched or of something under the skin); visual (involving sight such as seeing images, people, flashes of light); and somatic (involving perception of a physical experience localized within the body).

Healing touch A method of energetic healing that incorporates the therapist's intention to heal, through either actual touch or non-touch re-patterning, energy fields around the person; also called *therapeutic touch.*

Heterosexuality An attraction to and preference for members of the opposite sex as sexual partners.

Hippotherapy In occupational therapy, use of the movement of a horse as a treatment for clients with movement dysfunction.

Home care Part of a comprehensive health and mental health care system that aims to provide an array of health-related services to clients and families in their places of residence.

Homosexuality An attraction to and preference for members of the same sex as sexual partners.

Horizontal violence Anger or negativity a nurse directs toward another nurse.

Hostility-related variables Emotions, attitudes, and behaviors that occur regularly and predictably in people prone to aggression and violence.

Hypervigilance A common symptom of somatoform disorders in which the client's heightened focus on the body and its sensations leads to chronic, prolonged misinterpretation and overreaction to physical signs.

Hypochondriasis A somatoform disorder characterized by a client's unwarranted fear or belief that he or she has a serious disease, without significant pathology.

Hypomania A subcategory of mania, slightly less severe and without the psychotic features or severely impaired functioning that would require hospitalization.

Hypothesis An assumptive statement about the relationship between two or more concepts (or variables).

Hysteria An historical term (preceding somatoform disorder) coined in the early 1900s by Sigmund Freud to describe a condition in which people could not use certain body parts despite having no physiological damage or dysfunction.

I

Iatrogenic burden Iatro, from Greek iatros (physician) and iasthai, to heal. Used here to mean family burden exacerbated by the mental health system or mental health professionals.

Impulsivity A symptom of an underlying disorder or a pervasive personality trait that causes a person to perform actions with little or no regard for the consequences.

Individualized Education Program (IEP) Legal document that outlines a student's educational, social, and behavioral goals and objects and provides a school-based plan to meet them.

Informal group A group that provides much of a person's education and contributes greatly to his or her cultural values; members do not depend on one another.

Informed consent Consent that a recipient of health care gives to treating providers that enables the recipient to understand a proposed treatment, including its administration, prognosis after treatment, side effects, risks, possible consequences of refusal, and other alternatives.

Instrumental violence Violent acts that are usually premeditated and motive driven (frequently economic gain), usually involving people unknown to one another.

Intimate partner violence Violence occurring between persons (same or opposite sex) who have a current or former relationship (i.e., dating, marital, or cohabiting). Violent acts include both physical and sexual violence as well as threats and psychological/emotional abuse.

Involuntary admission Admission to a psychiatric hospital that occurs when a person with mental illness who refuses psychiatric hospitalization or treatment poses a danger to self or others and cannot safely be cared for in a less restrictive setting.

Insomnia Perception of insufficient sleep or not feeling rested after a habitual sleep episode.

J

Junk science Faulty data collection and analysis used to further a special agenda.

L

La belle indifference In conversion disorder, a remarkable lack of affect or concern shown by a client despite a symptom that imposes significant physical disability (e.g., paralysis).

Laissez-faire leader A leader who allows group members to operate as they choose.

Learning A process that occurs when organisms take in and store information as a function of experience.

Licensure A nonvoluntary process through which a government agency regulates a profession.

Listening Focusing on all behaviors exhibited by a person who is communicating.

Loss of efficacy The loss of ability to achieve a drug's maximum benefit.

M

Malpractice A tort action that a consumer plaintiff brings against a defendant professional from whom the plaintiff believes that he or she has received injury during the course of the professional–consumer relationship; professional negligence.

Maltreatment Behavior toward another person that is outside the norms of conduct and involves a significant risk of causing physical or emotional harm; four categories are recognized: physical abuse, sexual abuse, neglect, and emotional maltreatment.

Manic episodes Periods of abnormally and persistently elevated, expansive, or irritable mood.

Mantras Sounds, short words, or phrases repeated in the mind.

Masturbation Self-stimulation of erogenous areas to the point of orgasm.

Maturational or developmental crisis A crisis precipitated by the normal stress of development.

Maturity The ability to integrate aspects of life into a whole and find balance in one's outlook and attitudes toward others.

Maximal efficacy The maximal effect a drug can produce.

Medication adherence The actual taking of medications as prescribed; also called medication compliance.

Meditation A state of consciousness and an experience of the mind in which one tries to achieve awareness without thought.

Memory Information that is stored as a result of learning.

Mental disorders Health conditions marked by alterations in thinking, mood, or behavior that cause distress, impair ability to function, or both.

Mental health The successful performance of mental function, resulting in productive activities, fulfilling relationships, and the ability to adapt to change and cope with adversity.

Mental health nursing The care of well and at-risk populations to prevent mental illness or provide immediate treatment for those with early signs of a psychiatric disorder.

Mental illness A clinically significant behavioral or psychological syndrome experienced by a person and marked by distress, disability, or the risk of suffering, disability, or loss of freedom.

Mental status examination A tool for assessing objective and observational data that yields information about the client's appearance, level of consciousness, motor status and behavior, affect and mood, attitude, intellectual functioning, speech, cognitive status (including attention and concentration), judgment, abstraction, content of thought, and insight.

Middle old A chronological category used to designate those 75 to 84 years of age.

Modeling The demonstration of desired behavior patterns to a learner.

Mood A pervasive, sustained emotional coloring of one's experience; a sustained emotional "climate."

Multidisciplinary teams Groups of professionals from diverse disciplines, who provide assessments for, establish and carry out interactions with, and engage in consultations about the progress of clients.

Multigenerational family A family consisting of at least three generations.

Multiple sleep latency testing (MSLT) A procedure that determines the extent of daytime sleepiness by evaluating how long it takes a client to fall asleep during a series of daytime naps.

Myths Complete inventions, often rooted in cultural beliefs and difficult to dispel.

N

NAMI, The Nation's Voice on Mental Illness Formerly known as the National Alliance for the Mentally Ill, a national advocacy organization with state and local affiliates dedicated to improving the lives of persons with serious mental illness and their families.

Narcolepsy A disorder of unknown etiology characterized by excessive daytime sleepiness and associated with cataplexy and other REM-sleep phenomena.

Naturopathy An umbrella term used in most Western countries to cover a range of therapies referred to as natural medicine; a way of life wherein the body innately knows how to maintain health and heal itself.

Negative reinforcement Removal of an aversive stimulus that results in an increase in behavior or response.

Neuroleptic malignant syndrome A serious and potentially fatal side effect that accompanies use of certain antipsychotic agents. Characteristics include severe muscular rigidity, altered consciousness, stupor, catatonia, hyperpyrexia, and labile pulse and blood pressure.

Neurons Nerve cells; the fundamental units of the nervous system.

Neuropeptides The newest class of neurotransmitters, which includes endorphins and enkaphalins, vasoactive intestinal peptide, cholecystokinin, and substance P.

Neuroplasticity The ability of nervous tissue to change in its structure and functioning.

Neurotransmitters Chemical substances that relay messages between presynaptic and postsynaptic cells and are synthesized, stored, and released by neurons.

Nocturnal polysomnography A test that employs continuous monitoring of at least one channel of electroencephalography (EEG) to monitor brain waves, an electrooculogram (EOG) to monitor eye movements, and chin electromyography (EMG). Depending on the purposes of the study, the examiner may obtain other physiologic measurements. By reviewing the results, sleep specialists can determine quantity and stages of sleep and evaluate for cardiorespiratory disorders.

Noise Any forces within communicators or in the environment that interfere with effective communication.

Nontherapeutic communication Interactions in which the nurse uses ineffective responses that result in clients feeling defensive, misunderstood, controlled, minimized, alienated, or discouraged from expressing their thoughts and feelings.

Nursing diagnosis A clinical judgment about individual, family, or community responses to actual or potential health problems or life processes it is the product of the analysis of data collected during the assessment step of the nursing process.

Nursing process A problem-solving method of five steps (assessment, nursing diagnosis, planning, intervention, and evaluation) that nurses systematically apply to the care of clients.

O

Objective burden The practical problems associated with caregiving (e.g., employment issues, financial drain).

Objective data Phenomena that a person other than the client observes to be present.

Obsessions Recurrent, intrusive, and persistent ideas, thoughts, images, or impulses.

Obsessive-compulsive disorder An anxiety disorder marked by recurrent obsessions or compulsions that are time-consuming (taking more than 1 hour per day) or cause significant impairment or distress.

Obstructive sleep apnea-hypopnea syndrome A syndrome associated with repetitive episodes of reduced airflow or cessation of airflow resulting from collapse of the upper airway.

Occupational therapists Professionals who provide treatment that helps people achieve independence in all facets of their lives.

Old old A chronological category used to designate those 85 to 94 years of age.

Operant conditioning A type of conditioning by which a subject responds to a stimulus to achieve something rewarding or to avoid something aversive.

Oppositional-defiant disorder (ODD) A psychiatric disorder marked by negativistic, defiant behaviors such as stubbornness, resistance to directions, and unwillingness to negotiate with adults or peers.

Orgasm The peak of sexual pleasure. In the female it consists of 3 to 15 strong rhythmic contractions of the orgasmic platform of the vagina. In the male, it consists of emission and ejaculation.

P

Panic attack A discrete period of intense apprehension or terror without any real accompanying danger, accompanied by at least 4 of 13 somatic or cognitive symptoms.

Panic disorder An anxiety disorder marked by recurrent, unexpected panic attacks that cause the affected person to persistently worry about recurrences or complications from the attacks or to undergo behavioral changes in response to the attacks for at least 1 month.

Paraphilias Sexual expressions for at least 6 months that are characterized by recurrent, intense sexual urges, fantasies, or behaviors that generally involve nonhuman objects or animals, suffering or humiliation of self or partner, or children or other nonconsenting persons.

Parasomnias Abnormal behavioral or physiological events associated with sleep.

Passive-aggressive communication Communication that uses indirect aggression through backstabbing, sabotaging, ignoring, or "forgetting" to do something.

Paternalism An ethical principle by which the intent is to do good; however, professional determine what is considered "good" and may override a client's wishes and self-determination.

Perception check A confrontational communication technique that uses a three-step formula to clarify another person's behavior. The three steps are to (1) describe the inconsistent or confusing behavior; (2) offer at least two possible interpretations of that behavior; and (3) ask for feedback.

Period prevalence count An attempt to count something over an extended period.

Periodic limb movement disorder A condition in which the legs move repetitively during the night.

Personality The totality of a person's unique biopsychosocial characteristics that consistently influences his or her inner experience and behavior across the lifespan.

Personality disorder A collection of personality traits that have become fixed and rigid to the point that they impair the affected client's functioning and cause distress; also can be considered a lifelong pattern of behavior that affects many areas of the client's life, causes problems, and is not produced by another disorder or illness.

Pharmacodynamics The study of biochemical and physiological effects of drugs and their mechanisms of action.

Pharmacokinetics Various factors that, grouped together, affect the concentration of a drug at the site of action. The factors are absorption, distribution, biotransformation, and excretion.

Phobia A persistent, irrational fear attached to an object or situation that objectively does not pose a significant danger.

Phototherapy Use of artificial light therapy to prevent and treat depression with a seasonal pattern.

Physiologic noise Physical factors within a communicator that detract from effective communication.

Placebos Inert substances given to determine the efficacy of a medication.

Point-in-time count An attempt to count a number of something at a given time.

Polypharmacy Use of two or more psychotropic drugs, two or more drugs of the same chemical class, or two more drugs with the same or similar pharmacologic actions to treat different conditions.

Positive reframing A communication technique in which the mental health care provider specifically states the behavior changes a client should make rather than criticizing the client's negative behavior.

Positive reinforcement The addition of something that increases the probability of a behavior or response.

Possession trance A dissociative state that involves acquiring a new identity attributed to the influence of a spirit, power, deity, or other person.

Post-traumatic stress disorder An anxiety disorder marked by the development of characteristic symptoms after exposure to a severe or extraordinary stressor (e.g., natural disasters, accidental or intentional human-made disasters), in which there is actual or threatened death, serious injury, or maiming to the self or others; occurs only in response to a traumatic life experience.

Potency The concentration of a drug in plasma.

Power The perceived ability to control appropriate reward, therefore lending influence.

Prayer A kind of communication or conversation with a power that a person recognizes as divine.

Prejudice Negative preconceived opinions about other people or groups based on hearsay, perception, or emotion.

Premature ejaculation A persistent or recurrent onset of orgasm and ejaculation with minimal sexual stimulation before, on, or shortly after penetration and before the person wishes it.

Primary gain The main benefit a person derives from the "sick role," which, in the case of somatoform disorders, is the blocking of psychological conflict from conscious awareness.

Primary group A group that has face-to-face contact, boundaries, norms, and explicit and implicit interdependent roles.

Primary prevention Health care interventions designed to prevent mental disorders or to reduce identified mental disorders and disabilities within a population.

Professional A person who applies a specific background of knowledge and skills.

Professional certification A voluntary process that grants recognition to people for having met certain qualifications.

Proof Concentration of ethyl alcohol in a beverage.

Pseudoscience Therapies or treatments employed without empirical or theoretical support.

Psychiatric home care Services in the home appropriate for different age groups, clients with acute psychoses, clients with serious and persistent mental illnesses, and clients with AIDS.

Psychiatric home care nursing Specialty service in which home health care nurses provide holistic psychiatric nursing care on a visiting basis.

Psychiatric nursing The care and rehabilitation of people with identifiable mental illnesses or disorders.

Psychiatric-mental health nursing The diagnosis and treatment of human responses to actual or potential mental health problems.

Psychiatrist Physician who specializes in the prevention, diagnosis, and treatment of mental illnesses and emotional problems.

Psychological noise Emotional and cognitive forces within a communicator that interfere with accurately expressing or understanding a message.

Psychology Science-based profession that studies how people think, act, react, and interact.

Psychoneuroimmunology An emerging field that focuses on the links between a person's emotions, the functioning of his or her immune system, and how both factors alter central nervous system functioning.

Psychopharmacology The study of the chemistry, disposition, actions, and clinical pharmacology of drugs used to treat psychiatric disorders.

Psychopharmacotherapeutics The study of the uses of drugs in the treatment of mental illness.

Psychosocial assessment The assessment of psychological, sociological, developmental, spiritual, and cultural data commonly derived from interviews with a client.

Psychosocial rehabilitation Model that focuses on client rehabilitation in a normal daily environment.

Psychosomatic medicine The clinical and scientific study of the connections between the mind and body.

Public health approach A method of addressing social problems that holds that multiple causes of the phenomena must be met with solutions that address each level of the problem.

Punishment Presentation of a negative or aversive stimulus or event that results in a decrease in a response or behavior.

Purging Attempting to eliminate the body of excess calories; examples of purging methods include self-induced vomiting, use of laxatives, and excessive exercise.

Q

Quack A person who pretends to have medical skill.

Quackery The use of methods not scientifically accepted or the practice of fraudulent medicine.

R

Rape A crime of forced or coerced sexual penetration (oral, anal, or vaginal) of a nonconsenting person.

Reactive plasticity A rapid, usually reversible, functional change in nervous tissue.

Reasonable person test A legal concept that refers to how a reasonable and prudent health care professional is expected to perform with regard to their professional role in a practice situation.

Registered dietitian Health care provider who works to improve the nutritional health of clients, households, and communities by addressing the causes of nutritional problems.

Receptor A component of the cell membrane with the capacity to bind to a specific neurotransmitter.

Refractoriness A state of desensitization in which a drug's effect diminishes with repeated or subsequent use of the same concentration.

Refractory mania Bipolar disorder with mania that is completely unresponsive or marginally responsive to drug therapy with conventional mood-stabilizing agents.

Reinforcement The process by which a stimulus, whether pleasant (positive) or aversive (negative), strengthens a new response by its repeated association with that response.

Reinforcer A stimulus that strengthens a new response (behavior) by its repeated association with that response.

Religion The outward practice of a spiritual system of beliefs, values, codes of conduct, and rituals.

Repressed Pushed out of consciousness.

Resilience An identified protective behavior that studies have found to contribute to success coping with significant stresses; components include high self-esteem, self-efficacy, a repertoire of problem-solving skills, and satisfying interpersonal relationships.

Respondeat superior A Latin term meaning that acts of employees are attributable to their employer, whom the court also will find responsible for damages to injured third parties.

Respondent conditioning The process by which a response and a stimulus become connected.

Restless legs syndrome Syndrome associated with disagreeable leg sensations, such as pain, cramping, and itching, which often interfere with the onset of sleep.

Restraint The use of a physical or mechanical device to involuntarily restrict the free movement of all or a portion of a person's body to control his or her physical activity.

Reuptake The process of the terminal of a presynaptic nerve cell taking back released neurotransmitter molecules for storage and subsequent release.

Ritual abuse A severe form of abuse in which a child is repeatedly physically and sexually abused in ceremonies by an organized group of perpetrators.

Rituals Ceremonies, rites, or acts such as prayer, singing hymns, fasting, or abstaining from food, water or sexual relations, and partaking of sacramental emblems.

S

Schema or core beliefs An accumulation of the person's learning and experience within the family, religion, ethnicity, gender, regional subgroups, and broader society.

Schizophrenia A heterogeneous disorder of the brain with features including thought disturbances and preoccupation with frightening inner experiences (e.g., delusions and hallucinations), affect disturbances (e.g., flat or inappropriate affect), and behavioral/social disturbances (e.g., unpredictable, bizarre behavior or social isolation).

Science The attempt to make sense of natural phenomena by creating a simple conceptual framework to account for observed facts.

Scientific method A self-correcting system that relies on the application of logic and empirical processes to test theories against observable data.

Seclusion The placement of a client alone in a hazard-free room that is often locked and in which others can maintain direct observation of him or her.

Second hit Environmental factors hypothesized to contribute to the expression and characteristics of a person's illness.

Second messengers Secondary chemicals produced by the binding of a neurotransmitter to a receptor coupled with a G protein.

Second-order change Change that affects an entire family.

Secondary data analysis Analysis of data that the analyst did not collect or collected for a different reason.

Secondary gain Additional benefits that a person derives from the "sick role"; examples include being released from expected responsibilities and receiving attention from others.

Secondary group A group that usually is larger and more impersonal than a primary groups; members do not have the relationship bonds or emotional ties of members of a primary group.

Secondary prevention (1) An intervention to prevent further damage after a traumatic event; in this context, interventions to prevent families subjected to the trauma of mental illness from experiencing further adverse consequences (e.g., caregiver burnout, disrupted interpersonal relationships, psychiatric and medical health problems). (2) Health care interventions designed to identify mental health problems early and reduce their duration and prevalence.

Sensory integration The brain's integration and interpretation of sensory stimulation from the environment.

Separation anxiety disorder A childhood psychiatric disorder in which a child experiences severe anxiety to the point of panic when separated from a parent or attachment figure.

Serious mental illness A term given to a psychiatric disorder that meets the criteria for duration (at least 1 year), disability (relatively severe functional impairment), and diagnosis (including schizophrenia, bipolar disorder, and major depression) (National Advisory Mental Health Council, 1993).

Service coordination Connecting the various systems, agencies, and people participating in a person's care through effective, ongoing communication.

Sexual assault Forced or coerced sexual acts performed on a nonconsenting person.

Sexual dysfunction Sexual expressions characterized by a disturbance in the processes that characterize the sexual response cycle or by pain associated with sexual intercourse.

Sexual intercourse (coitus) Penetration of the vagina by the penis.

Sexuality The experience of the sexual self.

Sham treatments Counterfeit treatments or forms of therapy administered to a control group in a research study.

Shaping A procedure employed in behavioral therapy when a person lacks a certain behavior in his or her inventory, so that reinforcement of that behavior might take place.

Sick role The role that all chronically ill clients assume that releases them from usual responsibilities; in somatoform disorders, clients unconsciously assume the sick role to meet their dependency needs.

Side effects Dysfunctions and discomforts that a client experiences directly as a result of taking a medication.

Situational crisis A crisis precipitated by a sudden traumatic event (e.g., job loss).

Sleep hygiene Strategies to manipulate environmental conditions and personal behaviors to support effective sleep.

Social broker/advocate A social worker who connects clients with resources and services and acts as an intermediary for them.

Social phobia An anxiety disorder characterized by a persistent, irrational fear of and compelling desire to avoid situations in which the person may be exposed to unfamiliar people or to the scrutiny of others; fear of behaving in a way that may prove humiliating or embarrassing.

Social worker A professional whose work requires knowledge of human development and behavior; of social, economic, and cultural institutions; and of how all these factors interact.

Somatization disorder A somatoform disorder characterized by many physical complaints over several years that cannot be explained by pathology or a general medical condition.

Somatoform disorders A group of psychiatric disorders in which clients complain of extreme physiologic discomfort or disability without any identifiable pathology on testing or examination.

Spirituality A person's experience of, or a belief in, a power apart from his or her own existence; an individual search for meaning.

Splitting Perceiving people and life experience in terms of "all good" or "all bad" categories.

Statutory rape Rape of a minor.

Stereotyping Believing that one member of a cultural group will display certain behaviors or hold certain attitudes (usually negative) simply because he or she is a member of that cultural group.

Stigmatization The attribution of negative characteristics or identity to one person or group, causing the person or group to feel rejected, alienated, and ostracized from society.

Strengths-based philosophy Recognition that all children, families, and environments possess assets that can be used to overcome challenges and meet needs.

Structural and functional analysis An assessment of the functional relationships between various purported motivational variables and the rate of occurrence of certain behaviors.

Subjective burden The emotional response the client and family have to mental illness and caregiving (e.g., grief, fear, guilt, anger). (Note: Some researchers define subjective burden differently, as perceived objective burden.)

Subjective data Data that the nurse gathers by interviewing the client.

Substance abuse Use of alcohol or other drugs repeatedly to the extent that functional problems occur; it does not include compulsive use or addiction.

Substance dependency Continued used of alcohol or other drugs despite negative consequences, such as significant functional problems in daily living.

Substituted consent Authorization that another person gives on behalf of a client who needs a procedure or treatment but cannot provide consent for it independently.

Sundowning A characteristic feature of dementia by which most behavior changes are more pronounced in the evenings after sunset.

Synapse The area involving the membrane of a presynaptic neuron (sender), the synaptic cleft, and the membrane of the postsynaptic neuron (receiver), across which a nerve impulse passes.

Synaptic cleft A gap between the cellular membranes of the terminal of the presynaptic neuron and dendritic processes of the postsynaptic neuron.

Systems of Care Comprehensive spectrums of mental health and other necessary services organized into coordinated networks so that providers can more appropriately address the various and changing needs of children and adolescents with serious emotional disturbances and their families.